Hydroxyzine	Meperidine	Metoclopramide	Midazolam	Morphine	Nalbuphine	Pentazo	Pentob	Perphe	Prochlo	Promaz	Prometh	Ranitidin	Scopolam	Secobarbi	Thiethylperazine
C	C	C	C	C	C	C	C	C	C	C	C	C	C	I	
C	C	C	C	C		C	I	C	C		C		C	I	C
C	C	C	C	C		C	I	C	C	C	C	C	C	I	
							I							I	
I	I	I		I	I	I	I	I	I	I	I		I	I	I
I	C	C	I	C		C	I	C	I	I	I	C	C	I	
C	C	C	C	C		C	I	C	C	C	C	C	C	I	
C	C	C		C	C	C	I	C	C	C	C		C	I	
C	C	C		C		C	I	C	C	C	C	C	C	I	
C	C			C		I	I		C	C	C	C	C	I	
	I			I		I					I				
	C	C		C	C	C	I		C	C	C	I	C	I	
C		C		I		C	I	C	C	C	C	C	C	I	
C	C			C		C		C	C	C	C	C	C	I	
C		C		C	C		I	I	I	C	C	I	C		C
C	I	C				C	I	C	C	C	C	C	C	I	
C							I		C		C	C	C	I	C
C	C	C		C			I	C	C	C	C	C	C	I	
I	I			I	I	I		I	I	I	I		C	I	
	C	C		C		C	I		C		C	C	C	I	I
C	C	C		C	C	C	I	C		C	C	C	C	I	
C	C	C		C		C	I		C		C		C	I	
C	C	C		C	C	C	I	C	C	C		C	C	I	
	C	C	I	C	C	C		C	C		C		C		C
C	C	C		C	C	C	C	C	C	C	C	C		I	
I	I	I		I	I	I	I	I	I	I	I		I		I
					C			I				C		I	

Parenteral compatibility occurs when two or more drugs are successfully mixed without liquefaction, deliquescence, or precipitation.

Drug Monographs New to This Edition

(See Appendix A, Selected New Drugs)

anagrelide
ardeparin
azelastine
bromfenac
cabergoline
cerivistatin
clopidogrel
delavirdine
dolasetron
follitropin alfa/follitropin beta
grepafloxacin
interferon alfacon-1
irbesartan
letrozole
mibefradil
nelfinavir
pramipexole
quetiapine
ropinirole
sildenafil
sodium hyaluronate
tamsulosin
tiagabine
tiludronate
tizanidine
toremifene
trandolapril

NEW! FREE INTERNET DRUG UPDATES!

Your purchase of this book entitles you to receive our NEW free online drug updates!

To help you keep pace with the constant changes in pharmacology, Mosby now provides periodic drug information updates on our Web site. By visiting us at

www.mosby.com

you'll be assured of receiving the most up-to-the-minute drug information, including*:

- New drug monographs
- Brief updates on other recently approved drugs
- Names and brief descriptions of new OTC drugs
- Drug alerts, including information about drugs taken off the market, significant new contraindications and dosage changes, and more
- Updated drug information, such as new uses and other information of interest to health care professionals
- Hyperlinks to additional useful drug information Web sites

Visit our Web site at **www.mosby.com** today to access this important information!

*Not every update will include each of these items. Information released by the FDA and other developments will determine the contents of each update.

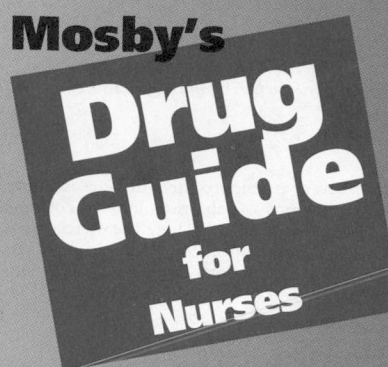

Third Edition

Linda Skidmore-Roth, R.N., M.S.N., N.P.
Skidmore-Roth Publishing, Inc.
Englewood, Colorado
Formerly, Nursing Faculty,
New Mexico State University,
Las Cruces, New Mexico;
El Paso Community College,
El Paso, Texas

Mosby's Pharmacology Patient Teaching Disk Version 2.0 by

Leda McKenry, Ph.D., R.N.
Associate Professor,
Director of Undergraduate Studies,
School of Nursing, University of Massachusetts,
Amherst, Massachusetts

with 30 *illustrations and* 1 *color insert*

Mosby

St. Louis Baltimore Boston Carlsbad
Chicago Minneapolis New York Philadelphia Portland
London Milan Sydney Tokyo Toronto

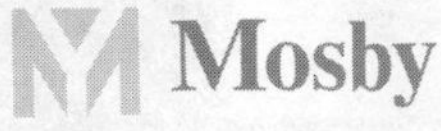

Dedicated to Publishing Excellence

A Times Mirror Company

Publisher: Nancy Coon
Editor: N. Darlene Como
Senior developmental editor: Dana L. Knighten
Project manager: Deborah L. Vogel
Designer: Bill Drone
Cover illustrator: Ken Joudrey
Manufacturing manager: Linda Ierardi

A NOTE TO THE READER

The author and publisher have made every attempt to check dosages and nursin content for accuracy. Because the science of pharmacology is continuall advancing, our knowledge base continues to expand. Therefore we recommenc that the reader always check product information for changes in dosage o administration before administering any medication. This is particularly impor tant with new or rarely used drugs.

Printed in the United States of America
Composition by Graphic World, Inc.
Printing/binding by R.R. Donnelley & Sons Company

Mosby, Inc.
11830 Westline Industrial Drive
St. Louis, Missouri 63146

Library of Congress Cataloging-in-Publication Data

Skidmore-Roth, Linda.
Mosby's drug guide for nurses / Linda Skidmore-Roth. — 3rd ed.
p. cm.
Includes bibliographical references and index.
ISBN 0-323-00308-7
1. Drugs—Handbooks, manuals, etc. 2. Nursing—Handbooks, manuals, etc. I. Title.
[DNLM: 1. Pharmaceutical Preparations—administration & dosage nurses' instruction handbooks. 2. Drug Therapy nurses' instruction handbooks. QV 39 S628mb 1999]
RM301.12.S56 1999
615′.1—dc21
DNLM/DLC
for Library of Congress

98-2377
CIP

98 99 00 01 02 / 9 8 7 6 5 4 3 2 1

Consultants

Bob Aucker, Pharm.D
Clinical Pharmacist, St. Joseph Hospital,
Atlanta, Georgia

Barbara A. Brunow, R.N., M.S.N.
Instructor, Providence Hospital,
School of Nursing,
Sandusky, Ohio

Connie L. Bush, R.N., M.S.
Associate Professor, Nursing,
Niagara County Community College,
Sanborn, New York

Shari L. Clarke, R.N.C.
Nursing Unit Coordinator,
Emory at Crawford Long Hospital,
Fayetteville, Georgia

Judy E. Davison, R.N., M.S., C.C.R.N.
Clinical Nurse Specialist,
University of California San Diego Medical Center,
San Diego, California

Jane Doyle, R.N., B.S.N., M.S., M.B.A.
Nursing Faculty,
Mount Wachusett Community College,
Gardner, Massachusetts

Laurel A. Eisenhauer, R.N., Ph.D.
Professor of Nursing,
Boston College School of Nursing,
Chestnut Hill, Massachusetts

Tim Engelhardt, B.Sc., Pharm.D.
Manager, Pharmacy Services,
Calgary District Hospital Group,
Calgary, Alberta

Linda A. Howe, R.N., M.S., M.A.E.
Director,
Roper Hospital School of Nursing,
Charleston, South Carolina

Theresa M. Hulub, R.N., M.S.Ed., M.S.N.
Professor of Nursing Education,
Niagara County Community College,
Sanborn, New York

Kimberly A. Hunter, Pharm.D.
Assistant Professor of Pharmacy Practice,
Washington State University College of Pharmacy;
Geriatric Clinical Pharmacist,
Sacred Heart Medical Center,
Spokane, Washington

Jon E. Lewis, B.A., Ph.D.
Senior Research Scientist and Director,
Respiratory Diseases,
Marion Merrell Dow Research Institute,
Cincinnati, Ohio

Edwina A. McConnell, R.N., Ph.D.
Independent Nurse Consultant,
Madison, Wisconsin

Janet R. Paul, B.S.N., M.S.N., R.N.
Assistant Professor of Nursing,
Hahnemann University,
Philadelphia, Pennsylvania

Rosemary A. Pine, R.N., M.S.N.
Assistant Professor of Nursing,
Department Chair, ADN Program,
Houston Baptist University,
Houston, Texas

Carolyn Smith Powell, A.D.N., B.S.N., M.S.N.
Assistant Professor of Nursing,
Abraham Baldwin College,
Tifton, Georgia

Mary Quintas, R.N.
Miles Community College,
Department of Nursing,
Miles City, Montana

Robert T. Reilly, Pharm.D.
Associate Director of Pharmacy, Clinical Services,
Thomason Hospital,
El Paso, Texas

Roberta Roynayne, R.N., B.Sc.N., M.Sc.
Assistant Professor,
University of Ottawa,
School of Nursing,
Ottawa, Ontario

Carol Ruscin, R.N., B.S.
Level I Faculty,
Baptist Medical System,
School of Nursing,
Little Rock, Arkansas

Lori Schoonover, Pharm.D.
Assistant Professor, Pharmacy,
Washington State University,
Spokane, Washington

Roberta J. Secrest, Ph.D., Pharm.D., R.Ph.
Associate Scientist,
Marion Merrell Dow Research Institute,
Cincinnati, Ohio

Denice Sheehan, R.N., M.S.N., O.C.N.
Nursing Supervisor,
Hospice of the Western Reserve,
Mentor, Ohio

John R. White, Jr., Pharm.D.
Assistant Professor,
Washington State University,
College of Pharmacy,
Spokane, Washington

Preface

Mosby's Drug Guide for Nurses, third edition, presents more than 4000 generic and trade name drugs—those most commonly administered by students—as well as more than 2900 drug fact updates. To keep our readers up-to-date, the new edition also contains 27 detailed new monographs for drugs recently approved by the FDA, in addition to the 49 monographs comprising the 1998 update to the *Drug Guide,* which have been integrated into Section II of the book. The new drug monographs, which are found in Appendix A, "Selected New Drugs," include sildenafil (Viagra), used to treat impotence; nelfinavir (Viracept), used to treat HIV/AIDS; irbesartan (Avapro), used for hypertension; delavirdine (Rescriptor), used for HIV-1 in combination with zidovudine or didanosine; and ropinirole (Requip), used to treat parkinsonism. In addition, new Appendix B, "Recent FDA Drug Approvals," provides generic/trade names and uses for 19 of the most recently approved drugs, about which complete information was not yet available at the time this book went to press.

The third edition of *Mosby's Drug Guide for Nurses* also includes several other useful new features. Appendix C, "Combination Products," provides a handy alphabetical listing of more than 500 combination products, their generic ingredients, and component dosages. Appendix D, "Rarely Used Drugs," provides abbreviated monographs for 10 infrequently used products. Also new to this edition are two special icons to identify information within monographs that is of special inportance to students. More than 100 "Nursing Alert" icons, ◆, highlight situations that potentially could put the patient at risk; and more than 60 "Do Not Crush" icons, ⊘, denote drugs that may not be administered in crushed form. An updated Windows disk is included inside the back cover, providing patient teaching guides for 25 of the most commonly prescribed drugs. For the first time, *Mosby's Drug Guide for Nurses* also includes free Internet updates on the Mosby Web site (www.mosby.com). The information found on this site will be updated periodically throughout the year to provide users with the very latest drug information.

Brief introductory chapters on drug calculations and drug therapy across the lifespan, as well as a four-color photo atlas of drug administration, provide invaluable reviews for practitioners and students. Key drugs are highlighted with a special icon, O-π, at the individual monograph and within the drug classifications section to call attention to important drugs. More than 60 drug classifications are provided.

Individual drug monographs also include IV content, featuring detailed coverage of both drug compatibilities and incompatibilities as well as site-specific information. The five-step nursing process format includes rationales. To aid application of the nursing process, therapeutic outcomes are prominently stated at the beginning of each monograph, and positive therapeutic outcomes are highlighted under the evaluation heading. Treatment of overdose is included after evaluation when appropriate.

Drug monographs are arranged in alphabetical order by generic name, and trade names are given for all medications commonly used in the United States and Canada. Drugs available only in Canada are identified by a maple leaf, ♣. The following information is provided whenever possible for safe and effective administration of each drug:

Pronunciations: Pronunciations are provided to help the nursing student master the more complex generic names.

Functional and chemical classifications: All known broad functional and chemical classifications are given. These classifications allow the nurse to see similarities and dissimilarities among drugs that are in the same functional class and different chemical classes.

Pregnancy category: FDA pregnancy categories A, B, C, D, or X are noted at the beginning of the monograph and under *precautions.* Appendix F provides a detailed explanation of each category.

Controlled substance schedule: Schedules are included for the United States (I, II, III, IV, V) and Canada (F, G, H). Appendix E provides a chart correlating the two systems with examples.

Action: Pharmacologic properties are described in detail. Action is discussed to the cellular level when known.

Therapeutic outcome: All possible results of medication use are detailed.

Uses: Provides drug application.

Investigational uses: Provides drug application for those uses a student may encounter in practice, although they are not FDA approved.

Dosage and route: May be given if known for uses not FDA approved but encountered in practice.

Available forms: All available forms — including tablets, capsules, extended-release, injectables (IV, IM, SC, ID, IC), solutions, creams, ointments, lotions, gels, shampoos, elixirs, suspensions, suppositories, sprays, aerosols, and lozenges — are provided.

Adverse effects: Grouped by body system, common side effects are in *italic type,* and life-threatening reactions are in **boldface type,** allowing the student to quickly identify common and life-threatening reactions. All adverse effects are reported for an incidence of 1% or greater.

Contraindications: Contraindications are instances in which a medication absolutely should not be given. When the FDA has assigned pregnancy safety category D or X, it appears here.

Precautions: Special precautionary steps are given here, including FDA pregnancy safety categories A, B, and C.

Pharmacokinetics: If known, onset, peak, and duration appear in an easily accessible chart format.

Pharmacodynamics: Absorption, distribution, elimination, and half-life are reported, when known, also in a handy chart format.

Interactions/incompatibilities: This section includes confirmed drug, food, and smoking interactions. The drugs are listed in alphabetical order, followed by the reaction(s) caused by that drug.

Lab test interferences: When known, lab test interferences are provided. Lab interference includes false negative and false positive results and increase or decrease interferences.

Nursing considerations: Highlighted nursing considerations are organized to foster use of the nursing process: Assessment; Nursing diagnoses; Implementation, including special instructions for administering drugs IM, IV, SC, PO, topically, and rectally; Patient/family education; and Evaluation, with positive therapeutic outcomes.

Treatment of overdose: Drugs and treatment for overdoses are provided for appropriate drugs.

Appendixes: The following appendixes are included to further enhance the usefulness of this reference: Selected New Drugs, Recent FDA Drug Approvals, Combination Products, Rarely Used Drugs, Controlled Substance Chart, FDA Pregnancy Categories, Nomogram for Calculation of Body Surface Area, Commonly Used Abbreviations, Bibliography, IV Drug/Solution Compatibility Chart, and Ophthalmic, Nasal, and Topical Products.

Disorders index: This book includes both a general index and a disorders index, both of which have been expanded in this edition. For easy application with integrated medical-surgical nursing courses, the disorders index lists major disorders and major drugs used in their management, followed by the page number for each drug listed. More than 40 new entries have been included.

Inside the covers: A syringe compatibility chart is printed inside the front cover for quick access, and installation instructions for the software disk appear inside the back cover.

Design: This book features a functional, user-friendly, two-color design that includes alphabetical tabs; icons for key drugs, therapeutic outcome, and lifespan content G P; the two new icons, "Nursing Alert" and "Do Not Crush"; colored monograph headings; and screened pages for the category drugs and index to facilitate information retrieval. The type and format of the book are spacious to enhance visual appeal and user-friendliness.

I am indebted to the nursing and pharmacology consultants who reviewed the manuscript, and I thank them for their thoughtful comments and encouragement. I would also like to thank Darlene Como and Dana Knighten, my editors, whose active encouragement and enthusiasm have made this book better than it might otherwise have been. In addition, I want to extend a special note of gratitude to Don Ladig, who has supported and encouraged my efforts since I began my relationship as an author with Mosby.

Linda Skidmore-Roth

Contents

Chapter 1

Drug Calculations Review

CALCULATION METHODS

Calculating dosages involves the following three steps:

1. Determine whether the drug dosage desired (what is written in the prescriber's order) is in the same measurement system as the drug dosage available. If they are not in the same measurement system, convert between the two systems.
2. Simplify by reducing to the lowest terms whenever possible.
3. Calculate the dosage quantity to be administered. This may be done by using fractions, ratios, or proportions.

Fraction method

When using fractions to compute drug dosages, write an equation consisting of two fractions. First set up a fraction showing the number of units to be given over *x*, the unknown number of tablets or milliliters. For example, if the physician's order states "ibuprofen 600 mg, "you would put $\frac{600 \text{ mg}}{x}$. On the other side of the equation, write a fraction showing the drug dosage as listed on the medication bottle over the number of tablets or milliliters. The ibuprofen bottle label states "200 mg per tablet," so the second fraction would be $\frac{200 \text{ mg}}{1}$. The fractions then read:

$$\frac{600 \text{ mg}}{x \text{ tab}} = \frac{200 \text{ mg}}{1 \text{ tab}}$$

You will note that the same units of measure are in both numerators and the same measures are in both denominators. Now, solve for *x:*

$$\frac{600 \text{ mg}}{x \text{ tab}} = \frac{200 \text{ mg}}{1 \text{ tab}}$$

$$\frac{600}{x} = \frac{200}{1}$$

$$200\,x = 600$$

$$x = 3 \text{ tablets}$$

Ratio method

In using the ratio method, first write the amount of the drug to be given and the quantity of the dosage *(x)* as a ratio. Using the example above this would be 600 mg : x tab. Next, complete the equation by forming a second ratio consisting of the number of units of the drug in the dosage form and the quantity of that dosage form, as taken from the bottle. Again, using the example above, the second ratio would be 200 mg : 1 tablet. Solving for x determines the dosage.

$$200 \text{ mg} : 1 \text{ tab} :: 600 \text{ mg} : x \text{ tab}$$

Multiply the means (inside); divide by the extremes (outside).

$$600 \times 1 = 600$$

$$200x \overline{)600} = 3$$

$$600$$

This, again, gives us three tablets.

Desired over available method

A third method for drug dosage calculation combines the conversion of ordered units into available units and the computation of drug dosage into one step. The equation for doing this is:

$$\frac{\text{DESIRED}}{\text{Units}} \times \frac{\text{Conversion}}{\text{Factor}} \times \frac{\text{Quantity (Caps, tabs, etc)}}{\text{Dosage AVAILABLE}} = \frac{x\text{(Quantity}}{\text{to give)}}$$

If a physician orders 10 grains of a drug and the drug is available only in 300 mg tablets, the dose may be easily calculated with this formula.

Substitute 10 gr (DESIRED) for the first element of the equation. Then use the conversion fraction $^{60\text{ mg}}/_{1\text{ gr}}$ as the second portion of the formula. The third element of the equation shows the quantity of dosage form (capsule or tablet) for the dosage AVAILABLE. One tablet contains 300 mg. The completed equation then is:

$$10 \text{ gr} \times \frac{60 \text{ mg}}{1 \text{gr}} \times \frac{1 \text{ tab}}{300 \text{ mg}} = x = 10 \times \frac{60}{1} \times \frac{1}{300} = \frac{600}{300} = 2 \text{ tablets}$$

Solving for x, the patient should receive two 300 mg tablets.

All three methods of drug calculation (fractions, ratios, or proportions) use the same information and much of the same format in solving problems. With minor variations, they do the same thing. Some methods will make more sense to you or be easier for you to follow. Throughout the calculation sections, use the method that makes the most sense to you. Return here for review if you have trouble.

CALCULATING DOSAGES

Oral medications

Although there are many forms of oral products, oral medications usually come in capsules, tablets, or liquids. Medications dispensed via the unit-dose system are packaged according to the dosage ordered.

When medication is ordered individually or through an open-stock system, the nurse usually calculates the proper drug dosage. These drug calculations are required when the drug available:

1. Is in a smaller dose than that ordered.
2. Is in a larger dose than that ordered.
3. Is in a different unit of measure than that ordered.

Capsules and tablets

Capsules cannot be broken or divided. This makes calculating the drug dosage more difficult. More than one capsule may be given to provide an accurate dosage; a part of one capsule cannot be given. Manufacturers provide capsules in different dosages to help in arriving at the proper dosage. If your calculations specify that you should give a fraction of a capsule, give an additional capsule if the fraction is ½ or more; do not give an additional capsule if the fraction is less than ½. (For example, if the calculation is 2¾, give three capsules; if it is 2¼, give two.)

Some tablets may be easily divided if they are "scored." Examples of unscored tablets include coated tablets and layered tablets. If a tablet is not scored, it should *not* be broken or cut apart.

The medication order usually states the dosage of grams, grains, or milligrams to give. The nurse understands the dosage DESIRED. The order also specifies how often the medication is to be given, such as twice a day (bid) or four times a day (qid). It may or may not specify for how many days it is to be given. If the order does not indicate a specific length of time (such as give for 5 days), the drug is given on a continuous basis, unless the institution has a policy limiting the length of time a drug may be given without reordering. Therefore the nurse may also need to calculate how much medication to order, depending on the length of time the patient will receive the medication. The nurse needs to know how much medication is NEEDED.

For example, the order reads: diazepam (Valium) 10 mg PO stat and 2 mg bid × 10 days. The medication DESIRED is diazepam 10 mg and diazepam 2 mg. The nurse must know the dosage AVAILABLE of the medication. A check with the pharmacy reveals that diazepam comes in 2 mg, 5 mg, and 10 mg tablets.

The nurse NEEDS one 10 mg diazepam tablet and enough 2 mg tablets for 10 days, or enough 2 mg tablets to fill the whole order (bid means twice a day). Thus the nurse needs to order:

One 10 mg tablet plus
One 2 mg tablet × 2 times a day × 10 days =
$1 \times 2 \times 10 = 20$ 2 mg tablets plus 1 10 mg tablet

or because five 2 mg tablets are the same as one 10 mg tablet, the nurse may order:

Five 2 mg tablets plus one 2 mg tablet ×
2 times a day × 10 days =
$5 + (1 \times 2 \times 10) = 25$ tablets

The formula to calculate the number of capsules or tablets to order is a basic proportion problem

$$\frac{\text{Dose}}{\text{DESIRED}} : \frac{\text{Dose}}{\text{AVAILABLE}} :: \begin{matrix}\text{Tablets or}\\ \text{capsules}\\ \text{per dose}\end{matrix} : \begin{matrix}\text{Drug form}\\ \text{(tablets or capsules)}\end{matrix} = \begin{matrix}\text{Numbers of tablets}\\ \text{or capsules per dose}\end{matrix}$$

For example, the order reads: sulfadiazine 1.0 gm q6h × 3 days. Sulfadiazine comes in 300 or 500 mg tablets.

DESIRED: 1.0 gm
AVAILABLE: 500 mg = 0.5 gm (converted from mg to gm)

$$\frac{1.0 \text{ gm}}{0.5 \text{ gm}} = 2 \text{ tablets}$$

Therefore give two 500 mg tablets every 6 hours for 3 days. Two tablets given four times a day for 3 days equals 24 tablets total. Simply:

$$\frac{\text{(Dose DESIRED)}}{\text{(Dose AVAILABLE)}} \times \begin{matrix}\text{Tablet}\\ \text{or capsule}\end{matrix} = \begin{matrix}\text{Number of tablets}\\ \text{or capsules per dose}\end{matrix}$$

To illustrate, let's try a few examples. Order: ASA gr *x* stat and prn for temperature elevation. ASA is labeled as 0.3 gm/tab.

$$\frac{\text{(Dose DESIRED)}}{\text{(Dose AVAILABLE)}} \; \frac{\text{gr } x}{0.3 \text{ gm}}$$

(gr 16 = 1 gm, so $\frac{\text{gr } x}{16} = 0.6$ gm)

$$\frac{D}{A} = \frac{0.6 \text{ mg}}{0.3 \text{ mg}} \times 1 = 2 \text{ tablets}$$

Order: methocarbamol 1.5 gm qd. The medication comes in 750 mg tablets.

$$\frac{\text{(Dose DESIRED)}}{\text{(Dose AVAILABLE)}}\ \frac{1.5\text{ gm}}{750\text{ mg}} \times 1 = ?$$

$$(1.5\text{ gm} = 1500\text{ mg})$$

$$\frac{D}{A} = \frac{1500\text{ mg}}{750\text{ mg}} \times 1 = 2\text{ tablets}$$

Liquids

The process and formulas used to calculate dosages of liquids are the same as those used to compute dosages of capsules or tablets. Only the unit of measure is different.

To review:

$$\frac{\text{(Dose DESIRED)}}{\text{(Dose AVAILABLE)}} \times \frac{\text{Drug form}}{\text{(minims, ml, drams)}} = \frac{\text{Amount of liquid}}{\text{per dose}}$$

Order: phenobarbital elixir 0.2 gm hs. The drug is available in 20 mg/5 ml.

$$\frac{\text{(Dose DESIRED)}}{\text{(Dose AVAILABLE)}}\ \frac{0.2\text{ gm}}{20\text{ mg/5 ml}} = \frac{200\text{ mg}}{20\text{ mg/5 ml}}$$

$$20\text{ mg} : 5\text{ ml} :: 200\text{ mg} : x\text{ ml} = 50\text{ ml/dose}$$

Parenteral medications

When medication is to be injected, it comes in the following three different forms:

1. A prefilled syringe labeled with a certain dosage in a certain volume (for example, meperidine [Demerol] 100 mg in 1 ml).
2. A single- or multiple-dose ampule labeled with a certain dosage in a certain volume (for example, epinephrine [Adrenalin] 1:1000 in 0.1 ml).
3. A vial with a powder or crystals that must be mixed or reconstituted with sterile water or normal saline solution. The drug may be measured in grains, grams, milligrams, or units. The amount of solution to be added varies and must be calculated according to the instructions with the vial. Medications given intradermally or subcutaneously generally involve very small amounts of solution, whereas IV preparations may involve 50 ml or more of solution.

Again, proportion is the standard method for calculating this dosage.

$$\text{Drug AVAILABLE} : \text{Dilution} :: \text{Drug DESIRED} : x$$

To illustrate, let's try a few examples.
Order: digoxin 0.2 mg IM. Drug is available as 0.5 mg/ml.

$$\frac{\text{(Dose DESIRED)}}{\text{(Dose AVAILABLE)}} \frac{0.2\text{mg}}{0.5\text{ mg}} \times 1\text{ ml} = \frac{2}{5} \times 1\text{ ml} = 0.4\text{ ml or 6 minims}$$

Order: KCl 24 mEq stat PO. Solution labeled potassium chloride contains 20 mEq/10 ml.

$$\frac{\text{(Dose DESIRED)}}{\text{(Dose AVAILABLE)}} \frac{24\text{ mEq}}{20\text{ mEq}} \times 10\text{ ml} = \frac{6}{5} = 12\text{ ml}$$

Order: Cedilanid-D 0.6 mg IM qd. Drug is available in 0.8 mg/4 ml ampules.

$$\frac{\text{(Dose DESIRED)}}{\text{(Dose AVAILABLE)}} \frac{0.6\text{ mg}}{0.8\text{ mg}} \times 4\text{ ml} = \frac{3}{4} \times 4\text{ ml} = 3\text{ ml (0.6 mg)}$$

Some medications come as powders or crystals, making them more stable. When the medication is ordered, liquid must be added to the drug to dissolve the medication in the solution (reconstitute the drug). The medication must then be given within a few hours or it will decay.

Some chemicals come in a single-dose vial. When the medication is ordered, usually 1 to 2 ml of liquid is added, the solution is gently shaken to dissolve it, and it is all drawn into a syringe and injected.

At other times, an ampule will contain several doses of the powdered medication. The instructions for adding the liquid (diluent) must be followed carefully. Some multiple-dose vials for steroids contain the diluent in the top part of the bottle, separated from the powder in the bottom part. Pushing on the top part forces the liquid into the bottom part, dissolving the medication. The instructions are usually found on the package, on the ampule label, or on the package insert in the box, and they must be followed exactly. If instructions are not included, it is common to dissolve the drug in enough diluent so that the dose ordered may be given in no more than 0.5 to 1 ml.

Once powders have been dissolved in liquid or reconstituted, the bottle must be carefully labeled so that further doses may be accurately given from it. It is very important to note the date/time the powder was dissolved, as well as the concentration of the reconstituted medication.

If instructions are not given for diluting the medication, the following modification of the familiar proportion formula may be used:

$$\text{Dose desired : 1 ml :: Total drug available : } x$$

The dose desired to the known amount of liquid is compared to the total amount of the drug to an unknown amount of liquid.

Multiply the means, divide by the extremes. (In this formula, the dose AVAILABLE is on the top, the dose DESIRED is on the bottom. Think clearly as you establish your problems. Keep the logic of the proportions clear. DESIRED doesn't always go over AVAILABLE!)

For example, order: cephalothin (Keflin) 500 mg q6h IM. It comes in a multiple-dose vial containing 3 gm of powder. Prepare it so that 500 mg equals 1 ml. Convert 3 gm to 3000 mg.

500 mg : 1 ml :: 3000 mg : x = 6 ml diluent to add to obtain 1 ml = 500 mg/ml

or

$$\frac{\text{(Dose AVAILABLE)}}{\text{(Dose DESIRED)}} \frac{3000 \text{ mg}}{500 \text{ mg}} \times 1 \text{ ml} = 6 \text{ ml to add}$$

Order: give 500,000 U penicillin IM. Dilute 1,000,000 U penicillin so that 500,000 U equals 1 ml.

1,000,000 U : x :: 500,000 U : 1 ml = 2 ml diluent

or

$$\frac{\text{(Dose AVAILABLE)}}{\text{(Dose DESIRED)}} \frac{1{,}000{,}000 \text{ U}}{500{,}000 \text{ U}} \times 1 \text{ ml} = 2 \text{ ml diluent added}$$

Order: Give cephalosporin 200 mg in 1 ml IM. The drug comes in 1 gm units of powder. What is the amount of diluent to add?

$$\frac{\text{(Dose AVAILABLE)}}{\text{(Dose DESIRED)}} \frac{1 \text{ gm}}{200 \text{ mg}} = \frac{1000 \text{ mg}}{200 \text{ mg}} \times 1 \text{ ml} = 5 \text{ ml diluent}$$

Hypodermic tablets

Some narcotics come as sterile tablets. A tablet is put into a syringe, 1 to 2 ml of diluent is drawn into the syringe, and the medication is dissolved by gently turning the syringe. Rather than breaking the tablet, the proper amount is calculated and any extra solution is discarded before the medication is injected. The usual dilution is 1 ml. The following standard formula is used:

Amount available : 1 ml :: Amount desired : x ml

For example, the order reads: give morphine gr ⅙. The available tablets are gr ¼.

$$\frac{\text{(Dose DESIRED)}}{\text{(Dose AVAILABLE)}}\ \frac{\text{gr } 1/6}{\text{gr } 1/4} \times 1 \text{ ml} = \frac{1}{6} \times \frac{4}{1} \times 1 \text{ ml}$$

$$= \frac{2}{3} \text{ ml or 11 minims}$$

Insulin

Great accuracy is important in preparing and administering insulin because the quantity given is very small and even minor variations in dosage may produce adverse symptoms in the patient.

Calculating and preparing insulin dosage is unique in three ways:

1. There are many kinds of insulin, but they all come in a standardized measure called a *unit.* Insulin is available in 10 ml vials and in two strengths (concentrations): U-100 (100 units per 1 ml solution) and U-500 (500 units per 1 ml solution). U-500 is five times stronger (more concentrated) than U-100, and rarely used.
2. Insulin should be drawn up in a special insulin syringe that is calibrated in units. If an insulin syringe is not available, a tuberculin syringe that is calibrated in minims may be used.
3. The insulin order, the insulin bottle, and the insulin as drawn up should always be rechecked by another nurse for maximum accuracy. Small errors can cause big problems.

Let's try some examples.

Order: 48 U Lente insulin U-100 (insulin zinc suspension) 1 hour before breakfast.

$$\frac{\text{(Dose DESIRED)}}{\text{(Dose AVAILABLE)}}\ \frac{48 \text{ U}}{100 \text{ U}} \times 1 = 48 \text{ U}$$

It is easy to see that if the insulin and the syringe are both U-100, all you have to do is draw up the number of units ordered.

When the order calls for two different types of insulin, both may be given at the same time in the same syringe. One will be short-acting (regular) insulin and the other will be an intermediate or longer-acting type (NPH or zinc suspension). Draw up the regular insulin first, then the longer acting. Give both in the same syringe.

For example, order: 20 U regular (Iletin) insulin U-100 and 30 U NPH (isophane insulin suspension) U-100 before breakfast. Using a U-100 syringe, draw up 20 U regular insulin; then draw up 30 U NPH insulin to equal 50 U in the syringe.

Sometimes U-100 syringes are not available and a tuberculin (TB) syringe must be used. The number of minims that will equal the units ordered must be calculated. The formula for determining insulin dosage when a TB syringe is used is as follows:

$$\frac{\text{(Insulin DESIRED)}}{\text{(Insulin AVAILABLE)}} \times 16 \text{ minims} = \begin{array}{c}\text{Number of minims}\\ \text{to administer}\end{array}$$

Order: 80 U of regular (Iletin) U-100 insulin, given in TB syringe.

$$\frac{\text{(Dose DESIRED)}}{\text{(Dose AVAILABLE)}} \frac{80\text{ U}}{100\text{ U}} \times 16 = \frac{64}{5} = 12.8 \text{ minims}$$

Intravenous infusions

Flow rates: Regulating the intravenous infusion rate is a common nursing task. The completeness of prescribers' orders for intravenous infusions varies widely. Some prescribers are more specific in their instructions than others. A complete order specifies the type of solution and the volume to be infused (usually 500 or 1000 ml), as well as the length of time that the medication should be given. Usually, the nurse calculates the flow rate, or how fast the infusion will be completed.

There are three mathematical procedures that the nurse must be familiar with regarding intravenous infusions:

1. Calculating the flow rate for IV fluid administration.
2. Making modifications in flow rates for infants.
3. Calculating total administration time for IV fluid.

To *calculate the flow rate for IV fluid administration,* two concepts must be understood—the flow rate and the drop factor. The rate at which IV fluids are given is the flow rate, and this is measured in drops per minute. The drop factor is the number of drops per milliliter of liquid and is determined by the size of the drops. The drop factor is different for different manufacturers of IV infusion equipment, and it must be checked by reading it on the infusion set itself. Regular infusion sets generally range between 10 and 15 drops per milliliter. Infusion sets have different drop factors for use with blood infusion sets (usually 10 to 12 drops per milliliter) because the drops are larger, whereas pediatric setups use very small drops called microdrops (often with 50 or 60 microdrops per milliliter).

Once the nurse has learned the drop factor for the equipment being used, the flow rate may be calculated by using the following formula:

$$\text{Drop factor} \times \text{Milliliters per minute} = \text{Flow rate (drops/minute)}$$

Order: IV infusion to run at a slow rate to keep vein open. The rate is to be at 2 ml/minute. The IV infusion set delivers 10 drops/ml. The goal is to determine the flow rate in drops/minute.

$$10 \text{ (drop factor)} \times 2 \text{ ml/min} = 20 \text{ drops/minute}$$

Order: 1000 ml NS to be administered in 5 hours. The drop factor is 15. Use:

$$\frac{\text{Total of fluid to give}}{\text{Total time (minutes)}} \times \text{Drop factor} = \text{Flow rate (drops/minute)}$$

$$\frac{1000\text{ ml}}{300\text{ min}} \times 15 = \frac{15{,}000\text{ ml}}{300\text{ min}} = 50\text{ drops/minute}$$

Flow rates for infants and children: Infants and small children are very sensitive to extra amounts or volumes of fluids. Smaller total amounts of IV fluids are often given, and the infusions are given in very small drops to avoid quickly overloading the infant's circulation. This is a built-in safety mechanism to prevent fluid overload resulting from accidental delivery of too much fluid.

The drop factor must be determined from the infusion setup. Usually 60 microdrops per ml is the drop factor for infants. For calculating the flow rates in infants, the same formula is used, but the microdrop drop factor is substituted for the adult drop factor.

$$\frac{\text{Total of fluid to give}}{\text{Total time (minutes)}} \times \text{Drop factor} = \text{Flow rate (drops/minute)}$$

For example, give 50 ml of D_6W IV in 4 hours. The drop factor is 60 microdrops/ml.

$$\frac{50\text{ ml}}{240\text{ min}} \times 60 = \frac{300}{24} = 12.5\text{ microdrops/minute}$$

Total infusion time

Sometimes prescribers order how fast they want infusions to run. To plan nursing care and to anticipate when new IV bottles may be needed, the nurse needs to calculate the total time the infusion will run.

Calculating the total administration time for IV fluid depends on calculating the total number of drops to be infused. Using this information, plus the drop factor, the total infusion time can be easily determined by using the following formula:

$$\frac{\text{Total drops to be infused}}{\text{Flow rate (drops/min)} \times 60} = \text{Total infusion time (hours or minutes)}$$

For example, if the prescriber orders 1000 ml 5% dextrose in water (D_5W) to be given at 50 drops per minute with a drop factor of 10 drops/ml:

1. *Determine the total number of drops ordered.* The total number of drops to be infused comes from the prescriber's order for the amount of fluid (such as 1000 ml) × the drop factor (read from the infusion setup).
2. *Determine the number of minutes that the IV is to flow.* The number of drops per minute (50) is multiplied by 60 to give the number of drops infused in 1 hour (3000). This figure is then divided into the total number of drops. This will give the number of minutes for the total infusion. For example:

$$1000 \text{ ml} \times 10 \text{ drops/ml} = 10{,}000 \text{ drops}$$

$$\frac{10{,}000 \text{ drops}}{3{,}000 \text{ drops/hr}} = 3.33 \text{ hr or 3 hours, 20 minutes}$$

Other factors influencing flow rates: There are many other factors that influence the flow rate of an infusion. The nurse has no control over many of them, such as the age, size, and condition of the patient, the size of the vein, the type of fluid, and the need for the fluid. Other factors, such as the size of the needle, the needle's position in the vein, the height of the IV pole, the condition of the filter, the air in the air vent, and movement of the patient, may be altered to assist in infusion of IV fluids. If the fluid does not infuse at the calculated rate, the IV should be carefully checked from the IV bottle to the site of the needle's insertion.

Chapter 2

Drug Therapy Across the Life Span

CHILD-BEARING CLIENTS

Any substance ingested or absorbed by a pregnant or nursing woman is likely to reach the fetus by way of maternal circulation or to be transferred to the breast-fed neonate by way of breast milk if the substance is in sufficient concentration and is well distributed. These drugs taken by the mother potentially can cause serious harm to the fetus or neonate. No drug is known to be *absolutely* safe for the developing embryo, but some oral medications that are inactivated in the mother's stomach or not absorbed by the maternal gastrointestinal tract are assumed to be relatively safe. However, many drugs and other substances have yet to be identified as harmful to the fetus.

Considerations for drug therapy in the child-bearing client center on the effects of drugs administered to the mother on the developing fetus or nursing infant. The child-bearing client takes, on average, four or more drugs (other than vitamins) during pregnancy, and the fetal effects of these drugs are unknown. Based on animal experiments, there are more than 600 substances with some degree of "teratogenicity," or ability to cause developmental abnormalities of offspring when taken by a parent. Only about 25 substances are known to cause human malformations.

Parents now ask health professionals more questions than in the past. Nurses are called on to supply accurate information, provide rationales, discuss the options available, and support parents' decisions. Prescribers and parents may have to make difficult choices between the benefits to the mother and the risks to the fetus or neonate. A judgment may need to be made between the risks to both if the mother's illness is not treated by a certain drug and the risks to the fetus if the drug is administered.

Drug transfer to the fetus

Pregnancy does not seem to have much effect on drug absorption from the gastrointestinal tract, but protein binding is decreased, freeing more drug for placental transfer. Biotransformation of drugs in the liver is probably delayed in pregnancy, but renal excretion may be more rapid because renal blood flow increases dramatically as a result of increased cardiac output and glomerular filtration rate.

At the placental interface, transfer of drugs and other substances is affected primarily by simple diffusion and partly by active transport.

Drugs That Cross the Placenta Rapidly*	
ampicillin	meperidine
barbiturates	penicillin G
cephalothin	phenytoin
diazepam	propranolol
ethanol	salicylates
kanamycin	streptomycin
lidocaine and other local anesthetics	sulfonamides
	tetracycline

*Especially if administered intravenously.

Transfer across the placenta depends on the chemical properties of the drug: its molecular weight, spatial configuration, protein-binding capabilities, pK_a (the point when half the amount of drug in the body is ionized and half is nonionized), and lipid solubility, as well as its distribution and concentration gradient. The potential for transfer is proportional to the period of time the drug remains in the maternal bloodstream. Transfer is greater during late gestation because of enhanced uteroplacental blood flow, increased placental surface at the interface, thinner membranes separating maternal blood flow and placental capillaries, and an increased proportion of free drug available to the circulation. Pathologic processes in the placenta, such as inflammation, degeneration, or partial separation, can increase blood flow and thus drug transfer. Not much is known about drug metabolism in the placenta itself, but it is thought to be a less active process. Certain drugs can alter placental enzyme activity necessary for degradation of substances and for energy-dependent transport mechanisms.

Many drugs are carried across the placenta within minutes (see box above). Thus the historical concept of the placenta as a completely protective barrier to circulating substances must be discarded. Most drugs that cross the placenta stabilize in the fetus at a level between 50% and 100% of the maternal level. Some (such as diazepam and local anesthetics) stabilize at levels even higher than the mother's blood levels. However, continued exposure of the fetus to a drug is more important than the rate of placental transport.

Within the fetus, drug effects may be more significant and prolonged than in the mother because of (1) probable lower enzyme concentrations and enzymatic reaction rates of drug metabolism and (2) slower excretion rates. Fetal excretion of drugs takes place via maternal resorption and by excretion by the fetal kidneys into amniotic fluid, which, under ordinary circumstances, the fetus often swallows.

On occasion, various fetal complications such as anemia and syphilis exposure have been actively treated by drugs in utero. The drug delivery routes chosen have been either the passive, transplacental approach or direct instillations into the amniotic fluid. These modes are still controversial.

It is, however, well documented that many unintended fetal drug doses via maternal circulation produce harmful fetal effects. The embryo or fetus runs the risk of developing the usual side or toxic effects, just as the mother does. Also, doses can be lethal or **teratogenic** (causing fetal organ defects), **mutagenic** (causing genetic mutation), or **carcinogenic** (causing or accelerating the development of cancer, sometimes much later).

Every embryo undergoes a series of precisely programmed steps from cell proliferation, differentiation, and migration to organogenesis. The critical periods for drug effects on the fetus are the first 2 weeks of rapid cell proliferation, when drug exposures can be lethal to the embryo, and the third through the tenth weeks of pregnancy, when the axial skeleton, muscles, limbs, and organs are developing most rapidly. Beyond the tenth week of pregnancy, the results are more likely to be physiologic or behavioral alterations and delays in growth.

Abuse of cocaine by pregnant women has resulted in reports of frequent miscarriages, fetal hypoxia, and low-birth-weight infants in the United States. In utero, cocaine exposure has induced fetal tremors, strokes, and an increase in stillbirth rates. Exposed infants are also at high risk for developing congenital heart disease, skull defects, and other congenital malformations. The newborn often has symptoms of increased irritability, increased respiratory and heart rates, diarrhea, irregular sleeping patterns, and poor appetite. It has been reported that behavioral patterns of infants born from cocaine-abusing mothers may also be affected—that is, they may have poor attention spans and a decrease in organizational skills.

Advice that all drugs be avoided during pregnancy and breast-feeding cannot always be followed. Some maternal conditions (hypertension, epilepsy, diabetes, and infection) put both mother and fetus in jeopardy if left untreated. Although literature and drug package inserts routinely warn that drugs have not been tested for use in pregnancy, during breast-feeding, or for infants, much empiric data and some research data are accumulating. The FDA now rates drugs as to their safety for use during pregnancy. (See Appendix F)

Certain categories of drugs are expressly contraindicated during pregnancy or are used only when the risk-benefit situation has been carefully considered and thoroughly discussed with the client. These are listed in the box on p. 15. Some drugs are considered relatively safe during pregnancy, depending on the situation. However, their use should be severely curtailed, being limited to only those pregnant women whose life or that of the fetus would be in jeopardy without drug treatment. One variable to be considered is the dose that reaches the embryo or fetus. This depends on the maternal dosage, the maternal volume of distribution, and the metabolic clearance rate of the

Drugs Contraindicated in Pregnant Women*	
aminopterin	oral contraceptives
sodium iodide (^{125}I, ^{131}I)	clomiphene
iodinated glycerol	measles vaccine
diethylstilbestrol (DES)	mumps vaccine
chlorotrianisene	rubella vaccine
dienestrol	smallpox vaccine
estradiol	vitamin A, high doses (25,000 units or more daily)
estrogens, conjugated	isotretinoin
estrone	menadione
ethinyl-estradiol	menadiol
mestranol	phencyclidine

*These are listed in category X on the FDA pregnancy scale.

mother. The fetal gestational age at time of exposure, duration of therapy planned, fetal and maternal genotypes, and any other drugs administered concurrently are also factors in prescribing decisions. Dosages, dosing intervals, and duration of treatment may be manipulated carefully to avoid harmful effects. Ethyl alcohol, especially at or near time of conception, is associated with the **fetal alcohol syndrome,** which produces both growth and mental retardation. Other very common substances such as aspirin, vitamin supplements, caffeine, and nicotine are suspected to cause adverse reactions in the fetus.

One difficulty with these and other substances is that effects on the embryo may occur before the woman is aware that she is pregnant. Women of child-bearing age who are not using contraceptives and who are sexually active should be prescribed for carefully and should be instructed to use over-the-counter medications cautiously. Education and prevention are considered the best therapy.

Medication administration in childbearing clients

Most nursing goals related to these topics should be aimed at ensuring that parents know that any foreign substance absorbed by the mother may have lifelong effects on the child. A balance must be maintained between protecting the child and dealing constructively with the family; creating unnecessary family concern is not appropriate. Essential to these aims is cooperating with the prescribing clinician, providing an environment for free exchange of information, and, if possible, forestalling parental feelings of guilt or fear associated with drug administration, whether planned or inadvertent. Convey that:

1. Potential harm to the child resulting directly from substances the mother is exposed to and potential danger to both mother and child if treatment is not begun must both be weighed. These

decisions must be made with the prescriber whenever exposure to an unfamiliar substance or drug is contemplated. Not everything is known at this time about effects on the child; and as more information becomes available, accepted guidelines may change.
2. Over-the-counter medications and common substances such as aspirin, high-dose or multiple vitamins, alcohol, caffeine, and nicotine may also have detrimental effects on the fetus.
3. Any prescription written by a professional who is not a specialist in the care of pregnancies or nursing mothers should be evaluated by an obstetrician or pediatrician. The prescription may need to be changed by the specialist to a safer drug or dosage.
4. If a questionable substance is absorbed by the mother, close health care supervision is essential. If real potential for fetal or infant injury results, the parents need ongoing support to endure the sometimes long wait for effects to be manifested. If birth defects or toxic effects are present or if invasive diagnostic tests or a therapeutic abortion is to be performed, objective psychologic intervention may help the parents endure this critical period.

PEDIATRIC CLIENTS

Neonates

Because newborns are small and immature, lacking many of the protective mechanisms that allow older children and adults to be relatively resistant to stressors of all kinds, they require special considerations. Their skin is thin and permeable, their stomachs lack acid, and their lungs lack much of the mucous barrier. Neonates regulate body temperature poorly and become dehydrated easily. Their liver and kidneys are immature and cannot manage foreign substances as well as those of older children and adults.

Breast-fed infants

Almost *all* forms of drugs in maternal circulation can be readily transferred to the colostrum and breast milk. Because drugs or their biotransformed products are handled by different pathways in the infant and the fetus, the impact of maternal medications on the infant probably differs (is probably less) from that on the fetus. This difference can serve as a guide in prescribing for the breast-feeding mother. Typical nontherapeutic outcomes in the breast-fed infant are signs of the drug's usual side or toxic effects. Adverse effects may occur, such as gray-brown stains of the later-erupting teeth as a result of tetracycline therapy more than 10 days in length or allergic sensitization to penicillin. Most drug products that reach the neonate via breast milk have undergone maternal biotransformation and are probably less than the original dose. However, immaturity of the neonate's liver and kidney systems limits its capacity for further metabolism and excretion.

Data about infants' capabilities for drug absorption, digestion, distribution, metabolism, and excretion are scant and conflicting. In general, the proved benefits of continuing breast-feeding must be weighed on an individual basis against the risks of maternal medication to the infant. Although the mammary glands are a relatively insignificant route for maternal drug excretion and the drug level in breast milk is usually less than the actual maternal dose, the infant's actual dose depends largely on the volume of milk consumed. Thus a single measurement of a drug in human milk will not accurately reflect the total dose the infant receives.

The concentration of the drug in maternal circulation depends on the relationship among several factors: dosing and route of administration, the drug's distribution, its protein binding, and maternal metabolism and excretion. The mammary alveolar epithelium presents to any potentially transferable substance a lipid barrier with water-filled pores. It is more permeable to drugs during the colostrum stage of milk production—during the first week of life. Drug factors that enhance drug excretion into milk are nonionization, low molecular weight, solubility in fat, and plasma binding versus milk-protein binding. Transfer of an active or passive form of a drug's metabolites into maternal plasma and then to milk depends mainly on passive diffusion. The absorptive processes of the infant's gastrointestinal tract and drug distribution are estimated to be similar to those in the adult, which means that lipid-soluble substances are well absorbed. The infant's age (thus the amount of drug-containing milk consumed) and the relative immaturity of the infant's important organs bear greatly on the outcome. If the drug is fat soluble, it may be more highly concentrated in breast milk at the end of feedings and at midday. Because the infant's total serum protein is lower in comparison to the adult's, more free drug is available to the circulation. Metabolic reactions in the infant's liver are slower than in the older child's; consequently, drug biotransformation may likewise be delayed. Other factors in the neonatal period may present risks: inadequate body temperature control, hypoxemia, or inadequate nutrition, for example. Drug excretion is delayed in the neonate because it is largely via the kidneys, where immature glomerular filtration rates and tubular functioning are maintained for several months. The extreme variability among drug effects and infants' capabilities makes it difficult to decide whether the mother should take a drug and whether or not she should breast-feed.

Human milk contains small, fixed amounts of many substances absorbed by the mother. Considerable evidence shows that certain other substances are incontrovertibly contraindicated unless necessary for survival and unless their effects are closely monitored. The usual recommendation is that breast-feeding be temporarily interrupted (usually for 24 to 72 hours) and the breasts pumped to remove drug-containing milk. Less often, it is advisable to stop breast-feeding.

Drugs Contraindicated During Breast-Feeding	
The American Academy of Pediatrics committee on drugs has suggested that the following drugs be avoided in the woman who is breast-feeding:	
bromocriptine	gold salts
cimetidine	methimazole
clemastine	methotrexate
cyclophosphamide	thiouracil
ergotamine	

Dosages and routes may also be changed. It is recommended that certain drugs be avoided while breast-feeding; see the box above.

Drug effects may be minimized by substituting formula for the midday breast-feeding, since that is the feeding highest in fat content and thus more likely to contain higher amounts of fat-soluble drug products. In addition, breast-feeding mothers who must be treated with medications can time their doses to be taken right *after* breast-feeding so as much time as possible elapses and the drug can reach a relatively low concentration before the next feeding.

With radioactive substances, therapy is of short duration; or if merely a diagnostic radioisotope test is to be done, breast-feeding must be interrupted until all radiation is absent from milk samples. Breast-feeding will probably be terminated when the drug is so potent that minute amounts may profoundly affect the infant, when the drug has high allergenic potential, when the mother exhibits evidence of decreased renal function (which augments drug excretion into breast milk), or when serious pathologic conditions require prolonged drug administration of high dosages.

Changes in the activity levels of the fetus or nursing infant signal dangerous effects resulting from drug administration; parents should be taught how to assess and report unusual fetal inactivity or infant apathy.

Alternatives to drug therapy. Both health professionals and clients place high value on pharmaceutical solutions to health concerns. However, many illnesses are self-limited or cause only minor discomforts that end or decrease without medication or with non-drug alternatives, such as relaxation techniques rather than tranquilizers. The effect of any medication should be weighed against the mother and child's physical and psychologic stress of abrupt weaning.

Other considerations might be to delay the mother's pharmacologic therapy until the infant is weaned on his or her own or to select another drug to meet the therapeutic goal without interfering with breast-feeding. The age and maturity of the child must be considered also; as the infant develops physiologically the drug's ability to cause harmful effects will diminish. The frequency of feedings should also be considered. An infant dependent on breast milk for total nutrition will receive higher doses of drugs than an infant breast-feeding only once or twice a day and taking other forms of nourishment.

Other pediatric clients

Drug administration to pediatric clients requires special knowledge and approaches. Physicians may prescribe the dosage of medication, but it is the nurse's responsibility to know the safe dosage range of any medication administered to children. A standard dosage of medication is nonexistent in pediatrics; medications are usually ordered according to the weight or body surface area of the child. Some pharmaceutical companies continue to supply medications in a standard adult dosage strength, and the nurse must be able to evaluate the correct dosage before administering the medication.

Weight as a basis. Following is a formula for calculating estimated safe dosages based on weight alone (Clark's rule). Because this is based on weight alone, it is a somewhat imprecise calculation for children.

$$\frac{\text{Average adult dose} \times \text{Weight of child in pounds}}{150} = \text{Estimated safe dose}$$

A nurse preparing calculated dosages of digitalis, insulin, barbiturates, and narcotics should have the calculations as well as the prepared medication dosage checked by another nurse or pharmacist before the drug is administered. Pediatric dosages are often minute, and a slight mistake in calculating the amount of medication to be administered results in greater proportional error.

Pediatric dose calculation based on weight alone implies that the pediatric client is a small adult, which is not true. Physiologic differences in the infant when compared to an adult may definitely affect the amount of drug needed to produce a therapeutic effect. For example, infants have a body composition that is approximately 75% water (adults have 50% to 60%) and less fat content than the adult. Therefore, water-soluble drugs are generally administered in larger doses to infants and children per body weight than to an adult.

Rules based on weight, such as Clark's rule, are generally taught and used by students in clinical areas to assess pediatric dosages. While useful as a guide, their accuracy for a number of drugs is questionable.

Body surface area as a basis. More than 100 years ago, Hufeland suggested that drug doses should be calculated on size or proportional amount of body surface area (BSA) to weight. Many physicians continue to use weight as the basis for calculating drug doses and body surface area for calculating fluid requirements. Most clinicians advocate using body surface area for determining drug dosage for adults as well as children. Physicians usually carry a simple slide rule or nomogram, such as the West nomogram (see Appendix G) to make rapid BSA conversions from weight and height. It is believed that the larger amount of total body water (TBW) in children, as well as the percentage of water in body weight and the part of that percentage formed by extracellular water, accounts for the fact that children tolerate or require larger doses of some drugs on a mg/m^2 basis.

For the 75% of drugs that have no established pediatric dosage, calculating the child's dosage as a fraction of the average adult dose using Clark's rule is really too imprecise for most applications, yet it may be used (mg per kg) where the dosage according to body surface area has not been established. The surface area rule is the most accurate. As a relationship between height and weight, it can provide a more precise guide to the maturity of the child's organs and metabolic rate of functioning for effective pharmacokinetics. The dosage should be tailored to the child according to the amount of medication per square meter of body surface area. The BSA rule for children's dosages:

$$\text{Child's approximate dose} = \frac{\dfrac{\text{Child's BSA in square meters (from nomogram)}}{} \times \text{Adult dose}}{1.73}$$

Medication administration in pediatric clients

Although these rules have been devised for relating adult doses to infants and children, it must be emphasized that *no rules or charts are adequate to guarantee safety of dosage at any age,* particularly in the neonate. No method takes into account all variables, particularly individual tolerance differences. Astute, accurate nursing observations of how individual children react to drugs can assist in choosing drugs and dosages.

The administration of medications to infants and children is both challenging and frustrating. Giving injections skillfully will enhance security and help gain a child's cooperation. A sound knowledge of growth and development also provides the nurse with information about how a child might be approached, whether reasoning will help or hinder the process, and whether assistance will be needed. The principles of safe administration of medication apply to all age groups, but children differ from adults, and the nurse has added responsibilities. (See box on p. 21.)

Ideally, a child will cooperate more readily with a nurse who has established a positive relationship. The child may also find it easier to

Pediatric Drug Administration

1. Parents are good sources of information about successful methods or vehicles of giving medications to their children.
2. Avoid using essential foods such as milk, cereal, or orange juice; the child may refuse to accept that food in the future.
3. Never underestimate children's reactions. They may not require that the taste of medication be disguised.
4. A sip of cold fruit juice, ice chips, a frozen fruit-bar, or a mint-flavored substance before and after the administration of an unpalatable medicine may effectively dull its taste.
5. Sugarless vehicles such as those sweetened by saccharin should be used to disguise the taste of medications given to diabetic children or those on a ketogenic diet.
6. Honey and syrup are ideal for suspending drugs that do not dissolve easily in water.
7. Since fruit syrups are usually acid, they should not be used for medicines that react in an acid medium (such as sodium bicarbonate, soluble barbiturates, and penicillin).
8. Elixirs have an alcohol base that, when undiluted, may cause the child either to refuse them or to cough and choke; they may also cause a drug-drug interaction. Small amounts of water added to elixirs of phenobarbital or chloral hydrate occasionally help.
9. Nursing time can be saved by recording the most successful method of administering medications and pertinent nursing orders on the child's care plan. This notation also saves the child frustration, fear, and anxiety.

accept the discomforts accompanying injections and some oral medications from the nurse who is associated with daily hygiene, feeding, holding, play, and happy times. In addition, the nurse will feel less guilty when the child associates the nurse with pleasure and comfort most of the time, and discomfort only when necessary to get well.

When a child is afraid or anxious, the natural response is to strike out at the frustration or avoid it. By accepting this behavior as a natural response, the nurse will be able to deal with it and be honest when a medication or procedure will be unpleasant or painful.

Truthful explanations to children are essential. Children have a right to some explanation of any procedure that concerns them. The timing and type of explanation should be geared to the child's ability to perceive and understand. For the child 2 years of age or younger very simple explanations such as "I have some medicine for you to drink" or

"I have an injection to give you, and it will hurt a little" are sufficient. Long explanations to children through 5 years of age do little more than prolong the anticipation and increase anxiety or fear. Telling 4-year-olds to stop kicking, hitting, or other avoidance behavior only conveys to them that they are not understood and they will receive little or no help with their feelings of frustration about being medicated. Providing the preschool-age child opportunities at play (for example, to give a doll an "injection" [empty syringe without a needle] or "drops") affords an important outlet and allows the child to work through the trauma of the experience.

Many children are courageous, or like to be considered so, and appealing to their courage is sometimes effective. Children 4 years old or over may choose to hold their own medicine cup, or drink unassisted, and to take pills from the container without any assistance from the nurse. Children of this age are motivated by social reinforcers, such as being praised for their cooperation, or "your job is to stay very still," which enhance their self-esteem and feelings of competence. Because of the sense of achievement that follows, they may want to save the medicine cups to show their parents.

Oral medications. Success in administering oral medications usually requires a kind yet firm approach with a positive attitude. No doubt that the child will take the medicine should be reflected in choice of words or tone of voice. The nurse might say, "Jimmy, it's time to take your yellow medicine" or "Do you want to take your pill now or with your Jell-O?" This indicates that Jimmy is expected to cooperate and to do it willingly. It also allows the child some control over the situation. An unwise approach that reveals doubt on the nurse's part might be: "I have your yellow pill, Jimmy. Will you take it for me, please?"

Nurses should try to be aware of how a medicine tastes so that they can answer such questions as, "Does it taste bad? Will it burn my mouth?" A helpful reply would be, "It tastes like cherry to me. Tell me what it tastes like to you." Often the child will accept the suggestion to taste and find out. However, if the medication is bad tasting, deceit or lying to the child is as futile and destructive as it is to an adult.

Disagreeable-tasting medications should be disguised if at all possible. Small amounts of honey, syrup, jam, fruit, and some fruit juices are suitable sweet vehicles for less palatable drugs. Some pills can be crushed and suspended in small amounts of these substances as long as the two are compatible. Infants and children swallow many liquid medications more readily if mixed with a sweet substance or diluted with a small amount of water. (If large amounts of water or other substances are used and the child refuses to take all of the mixture, estimating the amount of medication the child received is difficult.) Fortunately, many drugs are available in palatable syrups or suspension form well suited for administration to infants and children. Suspensions, however, should be thoroughly agitated to ensure that doses are not offered in unequal concentrations.

Caution must be exercised to prevent aspiration when giving oral medications to children. Medications must be given to infants slowly and in small amounts to avoid choking. Liquid medications may be administered by nipple, plastic medicine cup, plastic dropper, or a plastic syringe without the needle. Water should be swished through the inside of these *first* to prevent medication from sticking, thereby undermedicating. Glass cups, droppers, or syringes should be avoided because of the obvious danger of breakage in the child's mouth. A dropper or syringe is best suited for placing a liquid medication along one side of the infant's tongue. Older infants and toddlers seem to prefer to take their medications from a plastic medicine cup. If children are held or placed in a sitting position, they are less likely to aspirate the medication than if lying on their backs. When administering a medication with a dropper or syringe, the nurse may purse the infant's lips with one hand to keep the medicine from running out of the mouth. Droppers and syringes used for medication should be kept clean, they should be reserved for only one client's use, and they should be rinsed or washed before being returned to the medication bottle.

If the child refuses to cooperate even after explanations and encouragement, the nurse may have to ask whether the child will take the medication alone or will need the nurse to give it. Physical coercion is seldom necessary, but if used, it should be mild and used with dispatch and firmness, since aspiration is a danger. The nurse must not combine force with anger or resort to force when one nurse has been unable to administer the medication. Careful consideration should be given to such factors as: Why does the child resist? Does the child disapprove only of one nurse? Have past experiences with medications given at home or in the hospital frightened the child? Will forcing a medication cause a struggle that will negate the effects of a drug given for sedation? If mild restraint is necessary, the nurse should explain to the child that this form of treatment is necessary. The child will not cooperate if force is seen as a punishment for inability to cooperate; often the child loses confidence in all personnel.

Topical medications. Children have a large skin surface area in proportion to total body weight. Their skin, especially neonates', is particularly thin, permeable, and without much protective oil. Although adults absorb much more medication through intact skin than was previously believed, the child is at increased risk for systemic medication administration. The discovery that hexachlorophene can cause encephalopathy in newborns and that topically applied boric acid can cause systemic poisoning testifies to the hazard of applying drugs to children's skin, especially for prolonged contact or over broken skin areas. Plain soap and water may be preferred for abrasions or open lesions, replacing medicated dressings.

Subcutaneous injections. There are wide swings in the amounts of subcutaneous fat during the childhood years. Neonates have proportionately smaller amounts; these increase slightly to 23% by 1 year of age. From 1 to 5 years of age they drop to between 8% and 12%. Then the amounts of bodily fat climb to about 20% when the child reaches age 10. Lipid-soluble drugs have an affinity for fat tissue; less subcutaneous fat means that lower dosages of drugs such as diazepam and barbiturates are necessary to maintain blood levels. In addition, less subcutaneous tissue for injections may be available. An alternate route may need to be selected—oral, intramuscular, or intravenous.

Intramuscular injections. The principles and techniques of the administration of injections are similar to those for adults.

Most authorities believe that the risk of sciatic nerve injury is too great to warrant the use of the gluteal site of administration. The sciatic nerve is the largest nerve in the body; its normal pathway is the hollow midway between the ischial tuberosity and the greater trochanter, covered by the gluteus maximus muscle. This pathway, however, varies a great deal from individual to individual. In addition, the small size of the gluteal mass in the infant or neonate and the potential neurotoxicity of many drugs enhance the possibility of iatrogenic trauma secondary to IM injections. Trauma of this kind is the leading cause of sciatic neuropathy in infancy. A lesion at this height of the sciatic nerve is usually tragically associated with marked permanent disability.

The younger the child, the less muscle tissue may be available for IM injections anywhere on the body. If repeated injections are necessary, the available sites may become overused, inflamed, or dystrophic, requiring concerted efforts by the nurse to develop systematic plans for rotating sites and communicating them to the rest of the staff. The vastus lateralis muscle is the site of choice for IM injections in children under 3 (see Plate 8). The ventrogluteal site is preferred for the child over 3 years old who has been walking for a year or two (see Plate 9). The dorsogluteal muscles should not be used in the child under 6 years old if other IM sites are available. These muscles should not be used at all until the child has been walking for at least 1 year.

For injection into the left gluteals, the thumb is placed on the trochanter and the middle finger on the iliac crest. The index finger placed midway between the thumb and middle finger will indicate a safe injection area. Infants should receive no more than 0.5 ml in each injection site. Small children can tolerate a volume of up to 1 ml at each site. The deltoid muscle is likewise not used for children under 5 years of age because of its underdevelopment. Rather than the skin being held taut, as for adults, the muscle mass may instead be pinched up. The needle will thus avoid striking deeper-lying structures such as nerves, bones, or blood vessels. The IM injection is still made at a 90-degree angle to the top of the massed flesh. Preferred needle sizes for pediatric IM injections are 25- to 27-gauge and ½ to 1 inch in length. A 21- or 22-gauge needle may be preferred if a viscous medication such as procaine penicillin is to be given. In the interest of safety, the child should usually be restrained for an injection, and the injection should be given rapidly. Two or more persons should be available for children over 4 years of age despite promises that they will "hold still." An extra sterile needle may be carried in a pocket in case a needle becomes contaminated when a child moves unexpectedly. A child's attention may be distracted from the injection by asking the youngster to wiggle the toes. Because children enjoy trying out each other's beds, the identifying armband must be checked before giving each medication.

Rectal administration. When oral administration is difficult or contraindicated, the rectal route is often advised. Many children perceive use of the rectal route as an extreme invasion of their bodies or anticipate pain as a result. It may help to let them insert the suppository. Several drugs, such as sedatives, aspirin, and antiemetics, are available in suppository form. Suppositories made with a cocoa butter base will melt rapidly at normal body temperature, releasing the drug for absorption. After a suppository is inserted in an infant, the buttocks should be held or taped together for 5 to 10 minutes to relieve pressure on the anal sphincter and thereby help to ensure retention and absorption of the medication. Infants and children with diarrhea, however, may easily expel suppositories with explosive stools. Likewise, a suppository inserted into a child with a constipation problem or a rectum full of stool will be surrounded with stool and will have little chance for absorption of its contents.

Pharmacists and nurses often divide suppository doses by cutting them to obtain correct doses. This is a dangerous practice because all the medication might be contained in one area of the suppository. If divided doses must be administered, the pharmacist should be contacted for alternate product advice and guidance.

Nose drops, eardrops, and eyedrops. Aqueous preparations of nose drops are the only safe preparations to use, if it is deemed necessary to use them at all, because of the danger of aspiration. Many nose drop preparations contain vasoconstrictors, and prolonged or excessive use may be harmful. Infants are nose breathers, and nasal congestion will inhibit their sucking. For this reason, nose drops, if necessary, should be instilled 20 to 30 minutes before feedings. To instill *nose drops:*

1. Hold the infant in your arm, allowing the head to fall back over the edge of your arm, or place a small pillow under the shoulders and allow the head to fall back over the edge of the pillow.

2. Place your free arm so that the forearm is around the far side of the child's head, stabilizing the head between your forearm and your body. Use your hand to stabilize the arms and hands.
3. With your free hand you can then instill the prescribed drops with minimum struggle and maximum accuracy.

The instillation of *eardrops* requires a knowledge of anatomic structure because the shape of the auditory canal of a young child is different from that of an adult. Gentle massage of the area immediately anterior to the ear will facilitate the entry of the drops into the canal. Before the initial administration of a course of therapy with eardrops, the nurse should assess whether the child has excessive cerumen. If so, it may be necessary to consult with the physician about its removal with cerumen softeners and/or irrigation.

Eyedrop instillation is done in the same way with children as with adults except that the head may be stabilized by an assistant. Many eyedrops cause a burning sensation for a few seconds, so if both eyes are to be medicated it is wise to do the second instillation quickly before the client begins to blink and tear as a reaction to the burning sensation occurring in the first eye medicated. Mild pressure for 30 seconds over the inner canthus next to the nose will prevent premature drainage of the medication away from the eye.

Aqueous preparations of nose, ear, and eye drops may support the growth of bacteria and fungi. For this reason small volumes of such medications are ordered and should be used for only *one* individual (not shared by family members). The dropper (especially eye droppers) should not be permitted to become contaminated by touching anything but medication or rinsing water from the tap at any time. It should never be inverted so that medication or water runs into the rubber bulb to form a medium for microbiologic growth or to flavor the medication with a rubber taste. A dropper from one medication should usually not be used to measure and administer another type of medication because droppers are not standardized—all droppers are not manufactured to deliver drops of the same volume. Viscosity of drugs also varies, affecting the drop size.

Eyedrops and eardrops are more comfortably tolerated if they are warmed (if not contraindicated) before instillation. Warming can be achieved by running warm water over the side of the bottle without the label or immersing the bottle in some warm water in a medicine cup. Even carrying the bottle in a pocket for half an hour or so will take the chill off the drops.

Intravenous medications. The use of IV drug therapy is widespread on most pediatric services for several reasons. In children with vomiting and diarrhea, medications given by mouth may be vomited, losing precious time in drug management. These same children may have poor absorption of drugs and fluids as a result of dehydration or

Pediatric IV Drug Administration

1. IV drug therapy should be used only if other channels of drug administration are impracticable. Pediatric nurses skilled in giving medications to children via other routes may be able to influence prescribers' decisions regarding successful routes of drug administration.
2. For small infants a scalp vein or a superficial vein of the wrist, hand, foot, or arm may be most convenient and most easily stabilized. Scalp veins have no valves, and thus infusions may be in either direction. They are the most frequent sites for infant infusions. Older children may receive infusions through any accessible vein.
3. A too-rapid IV infusion or injection may cause "speed shock": rapid fall in blood pressure, respiratory irregularity, blood incoagulability, and even death. Preventive measures include: use of the minidropper (note that the milliliter per hour in the order translates to the drops per minute with this tubing), calibrated volume control chambers, infusion pumps.
4. Total parenteral nutrition (TPN) solutions are usually infused into the vena cava or innominate or subclavian veins approached via the external or internal jugular veins. Occasionally the inferior vena cava is entered via the femoral vein.
5. Once a drug is injected intravenously, the drug's action is relatively irreversible.
6. Drugs must be properly diluted. Too much emphasis cannot be placed on the caution: GIVE THE SMALLEST POSSIBLE DOSE AT THE SLOWEST POSSIBLE RATE.

peripheral vascular collapse, so that drugs administered via the IM route may be equally ineffective. For premature or physiologically distressed neonates, it may be preferable to give certain high-osmolality drugs by IV rather than give the syrup or elixir forms by the oral route. These infants are prone to necrotizing enterocolitis (NEC) and death when administered feedings or oral drugs that have an osmolality greater than that of body fluids. Although elixirs of theophylline, phenobarbital, calcium, digoxin, and dexamethasone all have osmolalities 10 times greater than body fluids and have been implicated in causing NEC, analysis shows that the contained additives actually raise the medication's osmolality. Related studies continue.

The pediatric nurse responsible for the administration of IV drugs may find the suggestions in the box above helpful. Most older children may be given fluids or drugs intravenously following the same principles and techniques used for adults. The younger and smaller the child, the greater the margin for error.

Neonates, infants, and children must be adequately restrained so as not to dislodge or pull out an infusion needle or catheter once it is in place. Helpful hints while caring for a client receiving IV therapy:

1. The needle or catheter should be fixed with plastic tape.
2. When a loop of tubing directly above the needle is secured to the tape, tension is relieved from the needle should it be pulled by sudden movement.
3. Because most children move about or are restless, it is necessary to support the limb with a padded arm board and immobilize the site of IV therapy. Support should extend to the joints above and below the site (with arm boards or IV boards).
4. If the infusion bottle is too high, the pressure in the vein will increase, causing fluid seepage into the surrounding tissues.

Other factors influencing drug dosages. Again, the dosage of most agents is related to the child's age, weight, and height. A child's bodily systems grow and develop at varying rates. This makes for unpredictable primary and secondary effects in pediatric medication administration. One example of secondary effects specific to children is discoloration of teeth and depression of enamel growth in the child under 8 years of age with administration of tetracycline liquid medications. (This adverse reaction is well-documented, but many prescriptions for this drug are still being written for this age group, according to the FDA.) Skeletal growth of children receiving long-term adrenocortical steroids is similarly impaired.

Individual variations are noted in children's response to digitalis, insulin, opiates, and oral enzyme products; dosages require careful titration. Paradoxical responses are noted with a few drugs; responses may be directly opposite that which could be expected in the adult. Excessive reactivity to atropine by infants may be related to immaturity of the central nervous system. In addition, many drugs that are safe and effective for adults have not been tested for use with children, nor have dosages been established, because of the complex medicolegal issues involved in experimentation on children.

GERIATRIC CLIENTS

Although individuals age 65 and over represent 12% of the total population in the United States today, they use approximately 35% of all health care goods and services, 25% to 30% of all prescribed drugs, and considerable quantities of OTC, self-treatment medications. Today the elderly comprise 1 of every 9 Americans, but within 50 years (by the year 2040) it has been projected that 1 of every 5 Americans will be 65 years or older (Lamy, 1988; Sloan, 1986).

At the turn of the century, only 1 person in 25 was over 65 years old. People died from parasitic and infectious diseases (pestilence and famine) then, while today the primary causes of death result from degenerative, chronic diseases. Three out of every four elderly deaths today are caused by heart disease, cancer, or stroke.

The elderly are usually affected by age-related, altered pharmacokinetics and pharmacodynamics and an increased incidence of chronic diseases, which generally result in an increase in physician's prescriptions or self-treatment with various medications and home remedies. The age of specialization has added to this problem in that multiple physicians usually prescribe a variety of medications often without discontinuing any previous drugs the client is taking. This practice, referred to as *polypharmacy,* too often has a disastrous outcome.

The practice of polypharmacy has resulted in an increased risk of inducing drug interactions, adverse reactions, and the need for, or prolonging of, hospitalization. Pray (1989) has reported that persons receiving two medications have a 5.6% potential for having a drug interaction, while clients that receive five or eight different medications have a 50% and 100% drug interaction risk, respectively. Dr. Robert Kane (1989) reported that "adverse drug reactions in the elderly in 1985 were responsible for 243,000 hospitalizations; 32,000 hip fractures; 160,000 mental impairments, and 2,000,000 addictions." While the magnitude of problems with polypharmacy is enormous, it is frequently overlooked as the causative factor. It is important that health care providers realize that the vast majority of undesirable drug effects resulting from polypharmacy are preventable.

Physiologic changes

As people age they undergo a variety of physiologic changes that increase their sensitivity to drugs and drug-induced disease. General loss in body weight of many elderly clients may require reevaluation of dosages used for them; the criterion for dosage should be shifted from age to weight. Some older clients weigh no more than the average large child, and some weigh a lot less; yet they are prescribed the larger "adult" doses. In another case, stimulants are generally less effective in elderly individuals, and large doses are often necessary. However, CNS depressants produce intensified effects in the elderly. Sedatives and hypnotics can produce paradoxical side effects of irritability, incontinence, confusion, and disorientation.

Pharmacokinetics are altered in the aging client because of reduced gastric acid and slowed gastric motility, resulting in unpredictable rates of dissolution and absorption of drugs. Changes in absorption may occur when acid production decreases, altering the absorption of weakly acidic drugs such as barbiturates. However, few studies of drug absorption have shown clinically significant changes occurring with advanced age.

Changes in body composition, such as increased proportion of body fat and decreased total body water, plasma volume, and extracellular fluid, have been noted in the elderly. The increased proportion of body fat increases the body's ability to store fat-soluble compounds such as phenothiazines and barbiturates, and thus increase the accumulation of those drugs. The reduced lean body mass affects drug distribution by decreasing the volume in which the drug circulates, thereby causing higher peak levels. The risk of toxicity with water-soluble drugs increases as total body water decreases. Decreased serum albumin for binding drugs leads to increased amounts of free drug in the circulation. Disorders common to the aging person such as congestive heart failure (CHF), which may impair liver function, influence biotransformation by decreasing the metabolism of drugs and increasing the risk of drug accumulation and toxicity. Renal function may be impaired because of loss of nephrons, decreased blood flow, and glomerular filtration rate. A reduction in renal function is also secondary to CHF. Decreased renal clearance may cause increased plasma drug concentrations and longer half-lives of drugs and active metabolites that the kidney usually excretes. Special precautions include careful monitoring of the elderly client for a safe drug regime.

Problem medications in the elderly

The potent medications available to treat the diseases or illnesses of the elderly often have a narrow index between drug effectiveness and toxicity.

Responsibility of health care providers. The primary responsibility of a health care provider is to reduce or eliminate the potentially adverse risk factors associated with various drug regimens. To do this:

1. Identify the client at special risk, such as the elderly person with potential altered pharmacokinetics, multiple illnesses, or liver or kidney impairment. Other factors that may affect selected medications include a history of alcoholism, smoking, or specific dietary habits.
2. Take a complete medication history, preferably in the client's home. Note all medications on hand, ordering physician(s), expiration dates, and their storage. A thorough history should include prescribed drugs, OTC medications, and home remedies (such as herbal or health food store purchases), if used.
3. If unfamiliar with a drug, look it up for its primary and secondary effects. Also check recommended dosage, side and adverse effects, and contraindications.
4. Check all medications for possible drug interactions by using a current reference guide or by consulting a pharmacist.
5. Discuss drug regimen with the primary physician (or encourage the client to do so) if problem areas are identified (for example, duplicate medications have been prescribed, possible drug interactions are present, or the client has had side effects that may be attributable to one or more of the medications).

6. Educate clients on their medications, safe storage, and proper method of disposing of discontinued medications.
7. Monitor therapy closely so that therapeutic response and development of side effects or adverse effects can be detected early in treatment.

Ideally the prescriber will individualize and simplify drug therapy for the client. Keeping medications to a minimum with the least frequent dosage administration necessary will help reduce the potential for drug interactions and also improve client compliance with the drug regimen.

Nursing management of medication administration for geriatric clients

In view of the effects just outlined and the multiplicity of drugs prescribed for elderly clients, their occasionally unreliable memories and senses, inadequate financial status, and propensity for adverse secondary effects, nurses must make every attempt to simplify the geriatric drug therapy plan. Suspect medications as the cause whenever you note a change in an elderly client's behavior, particularly restlessness, irritability, and confusion. These alterations of thought processes may be the earliest signs of drug toxicity. Encourage nursing assistants to report to a nurse any changes they notice in the client's behavior. Often what passes for senility is drug-induced lethargy or confusion.

In the administration of medications, the geriatric client may have special needs. The elderly frequently have dry mucous membranes, which impede swallowing, so offer water before and after oral medications if the client's condition permits. Position the elderly client so that gravity will assist the drug through the esophagus and minimize the possibility of aspiration. Because of diminished sensation, the client may be unaware that the tablet is stuck between the lip and gum, so examine the client's mouth to ensure that the medication has been swallowed. Geriatric clients may have slowed reflexes and reduced understanding of treatment. It helps to organize the dispensing of medication so that enough time is allowed for clients who require a great deal of attention, possibly by medicating them last, and yet so that all clients will receive their medication on time. A nurse has roughly an hour's range in which to distribute all the medications during one administration period.

Diminished taste sensation usually keeps unpalatable drugs from being much of a problem, but many older individuals may have difficulty swallowing, especially if they have sustained a cerebrovascular accident (stroke).

Selection of sites for injectable medications in elderly clients may present a challenge. Because muscle mass declines with age, suitable sites for intramuscular injection may be fewer than in younger individuals and will require more skill and effort in palpating to detect muscles of adequate body and size. Yet, decreased sensory perception, including that of pain, may make injections less painful.

Physical problems often interfere with the ability of the older client to comply with prescribed drug regimens. Some older clients may be unable to read labels or locate drugs because of failing eyesight; others, such as arthritic clients, may have difficulty opening bottles (particularly child-proof containers) or handling small pills, while the hard-of-hearing client may not hear all of the instructions. The logistics of obtaining drugs and the economic cost may be a deterrent to complying with therapy. Multiple drug therapy may simply be too complex for the client to manage without assistance. The nurse can simplify drug administration and scheduling as much as possible. Dosage schedules and calendars often help the forgetful client. Drug packaging that is easy to use and clearly labeled, as well as printed directions and drug information, help ensure compliance in the older client.

The elderly client's functional capabilities must be assessed to determine the educational requirements for safe and accurate self-administration of medications in the home. The nurse's creativity and skill are essential in devising teaching plans to enhance client compliance with the home medication regimen. Discuss OTC medications with clients and their family and friends and have them describe in detail how and when they take all medications.

Probably the most important part of the nursing process for aging clients is the nurse's ability to communicate patience, warmth, and understanding and to treat the elderly as persons with dignity and with the ability to reason, to feel, and to contribute.

abciximab (℞)

(ab-six'i-mab)

ReoPro

Func. class.: Platelet aggregation inhibitor

Pregnancy Category C

Action: Decreases platelet aggregation by binding to receptors on platelet surfaces (glycoproteins)

Therapeutic Outcome: Prevention of cardiac ischemia

Uses: Used with heparin and aspirin to prevent acute cardiac ischemia following percutaneous transluminal angioplasty (PTCA) in patients at high risk for reclosure of affected arteries

Dosage and routes

Adult: **IV** 250μg (0.25 mg)/kg bolus 10-60 min prior to PTCA, followed by 10μg/min CONT INF for 12 hr

Available forms: Inj 2 mg/ml

Adverse effects

CNS: Dizziness, abnormal thinking, hyperesthesia, confusion

CV: Hypotension, atrial fibrillation/flutter, bradycardia, vascular disorder, supraventricular tachycardia, weak pulse, AV block, peripheral edema

HEMA: Bleeding, *thrombocytopenia,* anemia, leukocytosis

RESP: Pleural effusion

Contraindications: Hypersensitivity to this drug or murine protein; GI, GU bleeding; CVA within 2 yr, bleeding disorders, intracranial neoplasm, intracranial arteriovenous malformations, intracranial aneurysm, platelet count <100,000 cells/mm^3, recent surgery, aneurysm, uncontrolled severe hypertension, vasculitis

Precautions: GI disease, pregnancy **C,** lactation, children, patients >65 yr or <75 kg

Pharmacokinetics

Absorption	Complete
Distribution	Unknown
Metabolism	Bound to platelet receptor sites for 10 days
Excretion	Unknown
Half-life	½ hr

Pharmacodynamics

Onset	1 min
Peak	2 hr
Duration	24-48 hr

Interactions

Individual drugs

Dipyridamole: ↑ bleeding

Heparin: ↑ bleeding

Drug classifications

NSAIDs: ↑ bleeding

Oral anticoagulants: ↑ bleeding

Thrombolytics: ↑ bleeding

NURSING CONSIDERATIONS

Assessment

- Assess for bleeding at all possible sites: (catheter, puncture sites, GI, GU, and retroperitoneal sites) during therapy; if bleeding occurs, stop the infusion; provide bed rest for 8 hr after infusion to prevent bleeding
- Assess hypersensitivity reactions: rash, pruritus, laryngeal edema, wheezing during treatment; if hypersensitivity reaction occurs, infusion should be stopped and appropriate action taken to treat the reaction; have epinephrine, antihistamines, corticosteroids in case of anaphylaxis

• Check distal pulses of affected legs frequently while femoral artery sheath is in place and for several hr after sheath is removed
• Monitor ECG and vital signs during treatment

Nursing diagnoses

✓ Tissue perfusion, altered (uses)
✓ Injury, risk for (adverse reactions)
✓ Knowledge deficit (teaching)

Implementation

• Visually inspect solution for opaque particles, do not use if these particles are present
IV • Give by direct **IV** after withdrawing the amount of drug needed using a sterile, nonpyrogenic low-protein-binding 0.2-0.22 μm filter into a syringe; give by bolus dose 10-60 min before the start of PTCA
• Give by continuous infusion after withdrawing 4.5 ml of drug through a sterile, nonpyrogenic low-protein-binding 0.2-0.22 μm filter into a syringe; inject into 250 ml of 0.9% NaCl or D_5 Wa; give at a rate of 17 ml/hr (10 μg/min) for 12 hr using an infusion pump and with an inline filter as above
• Discard any unused portion
• Discontinue heparin therapy at least 4 hr prior to removal of femoral artery sheath
• Provide pressure to the femoral artery using manual compression or a mechanical device for hemostasis; bed rest should be maintained for several hr after sheath removal
• Maintain affected limb in straight position and complete bed rest with HOB at 30° while the femoral artery sheath is in place

Patient/family education

• Advise reason for the medication and extent of treatment; hypersensitivity reaction including rash, bleeding, dyspnea
• Advise reason for bed rest, leg immobilization, and to avoid injury

Evaluation

Positive therapeutic outcome

• Prevention of cardiac ischemia after PTCA

acarbose (℞)

(a-kar'bose)

Precose

Func. class.: Oral hypoglycemic

Chem. class.: α-Glucosidase inhibitor

Pregnancy category B

Action: Delays the digestion of ingested carbohydrates, results in a smaller rise in blood glucose after meals; does not increase insulin production

➔ Therapeutic Outcome: Decreased blood glucose levels in diabetes mellitus

Uses: Stable adult-onset diabetes mellitus (type II) NIDDM

Dosage and routes

Initial dose

Adult: PO 25 mg tid with first bite of meal

Maintenance dose

Adult: PO may be increased to 50 mg tid; may increase to 100 mg tid if needed only in patients >60 kg, dosage adjustment at 4-9 wk intervals

Available forms: Tabs 50, 100 mg

A

Adverse effects

GI: Abdominal pain, diarrhea, flatulence

Contraindications: Hypersensitivity, diabetic ketoacidosis, cirrhosis, inflammatory bowel disease, colonic ulceration, partial intestinal obstruction, chronic intestinal disease

P **Precautions:** Pregnancy **B**, ↓renal disease, lactation, children, hepatic disease

Pharmacokinetics	
Absorption	Unknown
Distribution	Unknown
Metabolism	GI tract
Excretion	Kidneys as intact drug
Half-life	Elimination 2 hrs

Pharmacodynamics

Unknown

Interactions

Individual drugs

Insulin: ↑ hypoglycemia

Drug classifications

Digestive enzymes: ↓ effect of acarbose

Intestinal absorbents: ↓ effect of acarbose

Sulfonylureas: ↑ hypoglycemia

Lab test interferences

↑ AST

↓ Hct

NURSING CONSIDERATIONS

Assessment

- Assess for hypoglycemia, hyperglycemia; even though this drug does not cause hypoglycemia, if on a sulfonylurea or insulin, hypoglycemia may be additive

Nursing diagnoses

- ✓ Nutrition altered, more than body requirements (uses)
- ✓ Nutrition altered, less than body requirements (adverse reactions)
- ✓ Knowledge deficit (teaching)
- ✓ Noncompliance (teaching)

Implementation

- Give tid with first bite of each meal
- Provide storage in tight container in cool environment

Patient/family education

- Teach patient the symptoms of hypoglycemia, hyperglycemia and what to do about each
- Instruct that medication must be taken as prescribed; explain consequences of discontinuing the medication abruptly
- Tell patient to avoid OTC medications unless approved by prescriber
- Teach patient that diabetes is a life-long illness; drug will not cure condition
- Instruct patient to carry/wear Medic Alert ID as diabetic
- Teach patient that diet and exercise regimen must be followed

Evaluation

Positive therapeutic outcome

- Decreased signs, symptoms of diabetes mellitus (polyuria, polydipsia, polyphagia, clear sensorium, absence of dizziness, stable gait)

acebutolol (℞)

(a-se-byoo' toe-lole)

Monitan ✦, Rhotral ✦, Sectral

Func. class.: Antihypertensive

Chem. class.: Selective β_1-blocker; group II antidysrhythmic

Pregnancy category B

Action: Competitively blocks stimulation of β-adrenergic receptors within vascular smooth muscle; produces chronotropic, inotropic activity (decreases rate of SA node discharge, increases recovery time), slows conduction of AV node, decreases heart rate, which decreases O^2 consumption in myocardium; also decreases renin-aldosterone-angiotensin system at high doses, inhibits β_2-receptors in bronchial system (high doses)

Therapeutic Outcome: Decreased B/P, heart rate, AV conduction, control of dysrhythmias

Uses: Mild to moderate hypertension, sinus tachycardia, persistent atrial extrasystoles, tachydysrhythmias

Investigational uses: Prophylaxis of MI, treatment of angina pectoris, tremor, mitral valve prolapse, thyrotoxicosis, idiopathic hypertrophic subaortic stenosis

Dosage and routes

Hypertension

Adult: PO 100 mg qd or in 2 divided doses; may be increased to desired response; maintenance 200-1200 mg/qd in 2 divided doses

Ventricular dysrhythmia

Adult: PO 200 mg bid, may increase gradually; usual range 600-1200 mg daily; should be tapered over 2 wk before discontinuing

Available forms: Caps 200, 400 mg; tabs 200, 400 mg ✦

Adverse effects

CNS: ***Insomnia, fatigue, dizziness, mental changes,*** memory loss, hallucinations, depression, lethargy, drowsiness, strange dreams, catatonia

CV: Profound hypotension, bradycardia, CHF, cold extremities, postural hypotension, 2nd or 3rd degree heart block

EENT: Sore throat, dry burning eyes

ENDO: Increased hypoglycemic response to insulin

GI: Nausea, diarrhea, vomiting, ***mesenteric arterial thrombosis, ischemic colitis***

GU: Impotence, decreased libido, dysuria, nocturia

HEMA: Agranulocytosis, thrombocytopenia, purpura

INTEG: Rash, fever, alopecia, dry skin

MS: Joint pain, cramping

RESP: Bronchospasm, dyspnea, wheezing, cough

Contraindications: Hypersensitivity to β-blockers, cardiogenic shock, heart block (2nd or 3rd degree), sinus bradycardia, CHF, cardiac failure

Precautions: Major surgery, pregnancy **B,** lactation, diabetes mellitus, renal disease, thyroid disease, COPD, asthma, well-compensated heart failure, aortic or mitral valve, hepatic disease

Pharmacokinetics

Absorption	Well
Distribution	Crosses placenta, minimal CNS
Metabolism	Liver to diacetolol
Excretion	Kidneys, unchanged
Half-life	8-13 hr diacetolol, 3-4 hr acebutolol

Pharmacodynamics

	PO (ANTIHYPERTENSIVE)	PO (ANTIDYSRHYTHMIAS)
Onset	1-1½ hr	1 hr
Peak	2-4 hr	4-6 hr
Duration	12-24 hr	8-10 hr

Interactions

Individual drugs

Alcohol: ↑ hypotension (large amounts)
Hydralazine: ↑ hypotension, bradycardia
Indomethacin: ↓ antihypertensive effect
Insulin: ↑ hypoglycemia
Prazosin: ↑ hypotension, bradycardia
Thyroid: ↓ effectiveness
Verapamil: ↑ myocardial depression

Drug classifications

Antihypertensives: ↑ hypertension
Cardiac glycosides: ↑ bradycardia
Nitrates: ↑ hypotension
Theophyllines: ↓ bronchodilatation

Lab test interferences

Interference: Glucose/insulin tolerance tests
↑ Uric acid, ↑ potassium, ↑ triglyceride, ↑ lipoproteins

NURSING CONSIDERATIONS

Assessment

- Monitor B/P during beginning treatment, periodically thereafter; pulse q4h; note rate, rhythm, quality; apical/radial pulse before administration; notify prescriber of any significant changes (pulse <50 bpm)
- Check for baselines in renal, liver function tests before therapy begins
- Assess for edema in feet, legs daily, monitor I & O, daily weight; check for jugular vein distention, rales bilaterally, dyspnea (CHF)
- Monitor skin turgor, dryness of mucous membranes for hydration status, especially G elderly

Nursing diagnoses

- ✓ Cardiac output, decreased (side effects)
- ✓ Injury, risk for physical (side effects)
- ✓ Knowledge deficit (teaching)
- ✓ Noncompliance (teaching)

Implementation

- Given ac, hs; tablet may be crushed or swallowed whole; give with food to prevent GI upset; reduced dosage in renal dysfunction; check pulse before giving, hold dose and notify prescriber if pulse is <50 bpm
- Store protected from light, moisture; place in cool environment

Patient/family education

- ❗ Teach patient not to discontinue drug abruptly, taper over 2 wk; may cause precipitate angina if stopped abruptly
- Teach patient not to use OTC products containing α-adrenergic stimulants (such as nasal decongestants, cold preparations); to avoid alcohol, smoking; to limit sodium intake as prescribed
- Teach patient how to take pulse and B/P at home, advise when to notify prescriber
- Instruct patient to comply with weight control, dietary

adjustments, modified exercise program
• Tell patient to carry/wear Medic Alert ID to identify drug(s) that patient is taking, allergies; tell patient that drug controls symptoms but does not cure
• Caution patient to avoid hazardous activities if dizziness or drowsiness is present; that drug may cause sensitivity to cold
• Teach patient to report symptoms of CHF: difficult breathing, especially on exertion or when lying down, night cough, swelling of extremities or bradycardia, dizziness, confusion, depression, fever
• Teach patient to take drug as prescribed, not to double or skip doses; take any missed doses as soon as remembered if several hours until next dose

Evaluation

Positive therapeutic outcome
• Decreased B/P in hypertension (after 1-2 wk)
• Absence of dysrhythmias

Treatment of overdose: Lavage, **IV** atropine for bradycardia, **IV** theophylline for bronchospasm, digitalis, O_2, diuretic for cardiac failure, hemodialysis, **IV** glucose for hyperglycemia, **IV** diazepam (or phenytoin) for seizures

acetaminophen 🔑 (OTC)

(a-seat-a-mee'noe-fen)

Acetaminophen Uniserts, Anacin-3 Infant's Drops, Anacin-3 Maximum Strength, Apacet, Aspirin Free Pain Relief, Atasol ✤, Banesin, Campain ✤, Children's Feverall, Dapa Extra Strength, Datril Extra-Strength, Dolane, Dorcol Children's Fever and Pain Reducer, Genapap Extra Strength, Genapap Infant's Drops, Genebs Extra Strength, Halenol Children's, Junior Strength Feverall, Liquiprin Elixir, Liquiprin Infant Drops, Meda Cap, Myapap Drops, Oraphen PD, Panadol, Panadol Infant's Drops, Panex-500, Parten, Pedric, Phenaphen Caplets, Redutemp, Robigesic ✤, Rounax ✤, St. Joseph Aspirin-free Infant Drops, Tapanol Extra Strength, Tempra, Tempra Drops, Tylenol, Tylenol Caplets, Tylenol Extra Strength, Tylenol Infant's Drops

Func. class.: Nonnarcotic analgesic

Chem. class.: Nonsalicylate, paraaminophenol derivative

Pregnancy category B

Action: May block pain impulses peripherally that occur in response to inhibition of prostaglandin synthesis; does not possess antiinflammatory properties; antipyretic action results from inhibition of prostaglandins in the CNS (hypothalamic heat-regulating center)

Therapeutic Outcome: Decreased pain, fever

Uses: Mild to moderate pain or fever

Dosage and routes

P ***Adult and child >10 yr:*** PO 325-650 mg q4h prn, not to exceed 4 g/day; REC 325-650 mg q4h prn, not to exceed 4 g/day

P ***Child 0-3 mo:*** 40 mg/dose

P ***Child 4-11 mo:*** 80 mg/dose

P ***Child <1 yr:*** PO/REC 15-60 mg/dose q4-6h, not to exceed 65 mg/kg/day

P ***Child 1-2 yr:*** PO/REC 60 mg/dose

P ***Child 2-3 yr:*** PO/REC 120 mg/dose

P ***Child 3-4 yr:*** PO/REC 180 mg/dose

P ***Child 4-5 yr:*** PO/REC 240 mg/dose

P ***Child 5-10 yr:*** PO/REC 325 mg/dose

Available forms: Rec supp 120, 125, 325, 600, 650 mg; chewable tabs 80, 160 mg; caps 500 mg; elix 120, 160, 325 mg/5 ml; liq 120, 160 mg/5 ml, 500 mg/15 ml; sol 100 mg/1 ml, 120 mg/2.5 ml; tabs 160, 325, 500, 650 mg; granules 80 mg/pkg or cup

Adverse effects

CNS: Stimulation, drowsiness
GI: Nausea, vomiting, abdominal pain, ***hepatotoxicity***
HEMA: Leukopenia, neutropenia, hemolytic anemia (long-term use), thrombocytopenia, pancytopenia
INTEG: Rash, urticaria, ***angioedema***
SYST: Anaphylaxis
TOXICITY: Cyanosis, anemia, neutropenia, jaundice, pancytopenia, CNS stimulation, delirium followed by vascular collapse, convulsions, coma, death

Contraindications: Hypersensitivity; intolerance to tartrazine (yellow dye no. 5), alcohol, table sugar, saccharin

Precautions: Anemia, hepatic disease, renal disease, chronic alcoholism, pregnancy **B**, G elderly, lactation

Pharmacokinetics

Absorption	Well absorbed (PO), variable (rec)
Distribution	Widely distributed; crosses placenta in low concentrations
Metabolism	Liver 85%-95%; metabolites are toxic at high levels
Excretion	Kidneys—metabolites, breast milk
Half-life	3-4 hr

Pharmacodynamics

	PO	REC
Onset	½-1 hr	½-1 hr
Peak	1-3 hr	1-3 hr
Duration	3-4 hr	3-4 hr

Interactions

Individual drugs

Alcohol: ↑ hepatotoxicity
Caffeine: ↑ effects of acetaminophen
Cholestyramine: ↓ effects of acetaminophen
Colestipol: ↓ effects of acetaminophen

Lab test interferences

Interference: Chemstrip G, Dextrostix, Visidex II, 5-HIAA

NURSING CONSIDERATIONS

Assessment

- Monitor liver function

studies: AST (SGOT), ALT (SGPT), bilirubin, creatinine before therapy if long-term therapy is anticipated

- Monitor renal function studies: BUN, urine creatinine, occult blood; albumin indicates nephritis
- Monitor blood studies: CBC, pro-time if patient is on long-term therapy
- Check I&O ratio; decreasing output may indicate renal failure (long-term therapy)
- Assess for fever and pain: type of pain, location, intensity, duration, temperature, diaphoresis
- Assess mucosa, fingernail beds for cyanosis; inquire about dyspnea, vertigo, headache, weakness; symptoms indicate methemoglobinemia; notify prescriber immediately
- Assess for chronic poisoning: rapid, weak pulse, dyspnea, cold, clammy extremities; report immediately to prescriber
- Assess hepatotoxicity: dark urine, clay-colored stools, yellowing of skin and sclera; itching, abdominal pain, fever, diarrhea if patient is on long-term therapy
- Assess allergic reactions: rash, urticaria; if these occur, drug may have to be discontinued

Nursing diagnoses

✓ Pain (uses)
✓ Mobility, impaired physical mobility (uses)
✓ Injury, risk for (side effects)
✓ Knowledge deficit (teaching)

Implementation

- Administer to patient crushed or whole; chewable tabs may be chewed
- Give with food or milk to decrease gastric symptoms; give 30 min before or 2 hr after meals; absorption may be slowed

Patient/family education

- ❗ Teach patient not to exceed recommended dosage; acute poisoning with liver damage may result; acute toxicity includes symptoms of nausea, vomiting, and abdominal pain; prescriber should be notified immediately
- Tell patient to read label on other OTC drugs; many contain acetaminophen and may cause toxicity if taken concurrently
- Teach patient to recognize signs of chronic overdose: bleeding, bruising, malaise, fever, sore throat
- Inform patient that urine may become dark brown as a result of phenacetin (metabolite of acetaminophen)
- Tell patient to notify prescriber for pain or fever lasting over 3 days

Evaluation

Positive therapeutic outcome

- Decreased pain
- Decreased fever

Treatment of overdose:

Drug level q4h, gastric lavage, activated charcoal; administer oral acetylcysteine to prevent hepatic damage (see acetylcysteine monograph, p. 46)

acetazolamide (℞)
(a-set-a-zole′-a-mide)
Apo-Acetazolam ✱, Generic acetazolamide, AK-ZOL, Diamox, Diamox sequels, Hydrazol, Diamox Parenteral, Storzolamide
Func. class.: Diuretic carbonic anhydrase inhibitor; antiglaucoma agent, antiepileptic
Chem. class.: Sulfonamide derivative
Pregnancy category C

Action: Decreases the aqueous humor in the eye, which lowers intraocular pressure by the inhibition of carbonic anhydrase; also inhibits carbonic anhydrase activity in proximal renal tubules to decrease reabsorption of water, sodium, potassium, bicarbonate; decreases carbonic anhydrase in CNS, increasing seizure threshold; prevents uric acid or cysteine buildup in the renal system by the decrease in pH causing alkaline urine

➔ **Therapeutic Outcome:** Decreased intraocular pressure; control of seizures; prevention and treatment of acute mountain sickness; prevention of uric acid/cysteine renal stones; decreased edema in lung tissue and peripherally; decreased B/P

Uses: Open angle glaucoma, narrow angle glaucoma (preoperatively if surgery delayed), epilepsy (petit mal, grand mal, mixed), edema in CHF, drug-induced edema, acute mountain sickness

Investigational uses: Prevention of uric acid/cysteine renal stones

Dosage and routes

Closed angle glaucoma
Adult: PO/IM/**IV** 250 mg q4h or 250 mg bid, to be used for short-term therapy or 500 mg ES bid

Open angle glaucoma
Adult: PO/IM/**IV** 250 mg-1g/day in divided doses for amounts over 250 mg

Edema in CHF
Adult: IM/**IV** 250-375 mg/day in AM

P ***Child:*** IM/**IV** 5 mg/kg/day in AM

Seizures
Adult: PO/IM/**IV** 8-30 mg/kg/day, usual range 375-1000 mg/day in divided doses tid or qid, or 300-900 mg/m^2/day, not to exceed 1.5 g/day

Mountain sickness
Adult: PO 250 mg q8-12h

Renal stones
Adult: PO 250 mg hs

Available forms: Tabs 125, 250 mg; caps ext rel 500 mg; inj 500 mg

Adverse effects
CNS: Drowsiness, paresthesia, anxiety, depression, headache, dizziness, confusion, stimulation, fatigue, ***convulsions,*** sedation, nervousness
EENT: Myopia, tinnitus
ENDO: Hyperglycemia, hypokalemia, hypocalcemia, hypomagnesemia, hyponatremia, hyperchloremia
GI: Nausea, vomiting, anorexia, constipation, diarrhea, melena, weight loss, ***hepatic insufficiency,*** taste alterations
GU: Frequency, hypokalemia, polyuria, ***uremia,*** glucosuria,

hematuria, dysuria, crystalluria, renal calculi
HEMA: **Aplastic anemia, hemolytic anemia, leukopenia, agranulocytosis, thrombocytopenia, purpura, pancytopenia**
INTEG: Rash, pruritus, urticaria, fever, ***Stevens-Johnson syndrome,*** photosensitivity

Contraindications: Hypersensitivity to sulfonamides, severe renal disease, severe hepatic disease, electrolyte imbalances, (hyponatremia, hypokalemia), hyperchloremic acidosis, Addison's disease, long-term use in narrow angle glaucoma

Precautions: Hypercalcemia, pregnancy **C**

Pharmacokinetics

Absorption	GI tract–65% if fasting (75%) with food); IV—complete
Distribution	Crosses placenta; widely distributed
Metabolism	None
Excretion	Kidneys, unchanged (80% within 24 hr); breast milk
Half-life	2½-5½ hr

Pharmacodynamics

	PO	PO–EXT REL	IV
Onset	1½ hr	2 hr	2 min
Peak	1-4 hr	3-6 hr	15 min
Duration	6-12 hr	18-24 hr	4-5 hr

Interactions
Individual drugs
Amphotericin B: ↑ hypokalemia
Aspirin: ↑ excretion of aspirin
Lithium: ↑ excretion of lithium
Drug classifications
Amphetamines: ↑ action
Barbiturates: ↑ excretion
Diuretics: ↑ hypokalemia
Salicylates: ↑ toxicity
Lab test interferences
False positive: Urinary protein, 17-hydroxysteroids

NURSING CONSIDERATIONS
Assessment
- Assess patient for tinnitus, hearing loss, ear pain; periodic testing of hearing is needed when high doses of this drug are given by **IV** route
- Monitor manifestations of hypokalemia: *RENAL:* acidic urine, reduced urine osmolality, nocturia, polyuria, polydipsia; *CARDIAC:* hypotension, broad T wave, U wave, ectopy, tachycardia, weak pulse; *NEURO:* muscle weakness, altered LOC, drowsiness, apathy, lethargy, confusion, depression; *GI:* anorexia, nausea, cramps, constipation, distention, paralytic ileus; *RESP:* hypoventilation, respiratory muscle weakness
- Monitor for CNS, GI, cardiovascular, integumentary, neurologic manifestations of hypocalcemia: *CNS:* personality changes, anxiety, disturbances, depression, psychosis, nausea, vomiting; *GI:* constipation, abdominal pain from muscle spasm; *CV:* decreased contractility, decreased cardiac output, hypotension, lengthened ST segment, prolonged QT interval; *INTEG:* scaling eczema, alopecia, hyperpigmentation; *NEURO:* tetany, muscle twitching, cramping, grimacing, seizure, altered deep tendon reflexes, spasm
- Monitor for manifestations of hypomagnesemia: *CNS:* agitation; *NEURO:* muscle twitching, paresthesias, hyperactive reflexes, positive Babinski's reflex, dysphagia, nystag-

mus, seizures, tetany; *GI:* nausea, vomiting, diarrhea, anorexia, abdominal distention; *CARDIAC:* ectopy, tachycardia, broad, flat, or inverted T waves, depressed ST segment, prolonged QT, decreased cardiac output, hypotension

• Monitor for manifestations of hyponatremia: *CV:* increased B/P, cold, clammy skin, hypovolemia, or hypervolemia, vomiting, diarrhea, abdominal cramps; *NEURO:* lethargy, increased intracranial pressure, confusion, headache, seizures, coma, fatigue, tremors, hyperreflexia

• Monitor for manifestations of hyperchloremia: *NEURO:* weakness, lethargy, coma; *RESP:* deep, rapid breathing

• Assess fluid volume status: I&O ratio and record, count or weigh diapers as appropriate, distended neck veins, crackles in lung, color, quality and sp gr of urine, skin turgor, adequacy of pulses, moist mucous membranes, bilateral lung sounds, peripheral pitting edema; dehydration symptoms of decreasing output, thirst, hypotension, dry mouth, and mucous membranes should be reported

• Monitor electrolytes: potassium, sodium, calcium, magnesium; also include BUN, blood pH, ABGs, uric acid, CBC, blood sugar

• Assess B/P before and during therapy with patient lying, standing, and sitting as appropriate; orthostatic hypotension can occur rapidly

• Monitor blood, urine glucose in diabetic patients; glucose levels may be increased

• Assess for eye pain, change in vision when using drug for intraocular pressure

• Assess neurologic status when using drug for seizures

• Assess for decreased symptoms of acute mountain sickness: headache, nausea, vomiting, dizziness, fatigue, drowsiness, shortness of breath, insomnia

Nursing diagnoses

- ✓ Sensory-perceptual alterations: visual (uses)
- ✓ Fluid volume deficit (side effects)
- ✓ Fluid volume excess (uses)
- ✓ Knowledge deficit (teaching)

Implementation

• Give in AM to avoid interference with sleep

• Administer fluids 2-3 L/day to prevent renal calculi, unless contraindicated

• Potassium replacement if potassium level is <3.0

PO route

• Give with food, if nausea occurs, crush tabs and mix with sweet substance to counteract bitter taste; ES caps may be opened and sprinkled on food

• Do not crush or chew caps

IV route

• Do not use solution that is yellow or has a precipitate or crystals

IV*:* Dilute 500 mg of drug/5 ml or more sterile water for inj: use within 24 hr

Direct* IV:* Give over 1 min or more

Intermittent infusion: May be added to NS, D_5W, $D_{10}W$, 0.45% NaCl; give over 4-8 hr

Additive compatibility:
Cimetidine

Additive incompatibilities:
Multivitamins

Patient/family education

- Teach patient to take the medication early in the day to prevent nocturia
- Instruct patient to take with food or milk if GI symptoms of nausea and anorexia occur
- Teach patient to maintain a record of weight on a weekly basis and notify prescriber of weight loss of >5 lb
- Caution patient that this drug causes a loss of potassium, so food rich in potassium should be added to the diet; refer to a dietician for assistance in planning
- Advise patient to wear protective clothing and sunscreen in the sun to prevent photosensitivity
- Teach patient not to use alcohol or any OTC medications without prescriber's approval; serious drug reactions may occur
- Emphasize the need to contact prescriber immediately if muscle cramps, weakness, nausea, dizziness, or numbness occurs
- Teach patient to take own B/P and pulse and record
- Teach patient to continue taking medication even if feeling better; this drug controls symptoms but does not cure the condition
- Teach patient to see ophthalmologist periodically; glaucoma is a slow process

Evaluation

Positive therapeutic outcome

- Decreased intraocular pressure
- Decreased edema
- Decreased seizures
- Prevention of mountain sickness
- Prevention of uric acid/cysteine stones

Treatment of overdose: Lavage if taken orally, monitor electrolytes, administer dextrose in saline, monitor hydration, CV, renal status

acetohexamide (℞)

(a-set-oh-hex'a-mide)

acetohexamide, Dimelor ✱, Dymelor

Func. class.: Antidiabetic, oral

Chem. class.: Sulfonylurea (1st generation)

Pregnancy category C

Action: Causes functioning β-cells in pancreas to release insulin, leading to drop in blood glucose levels; may improve binding between insulin and insulin receptors or increase number of insulin receptors with prolonged administration; may also reduce basal hepatic glucose secretion; not effective if patient lacks functioning β-cells

➔ Therapeutic Outcome: Decreased blood glucose levels in diabetes mellitus

Uses: Stable adult-onset diabetes mellitus (type II), NIDDM

Dosage and routes

Adult: PO 250 mg-1.5 g/day; usually given before breakfast, unless large dose is required, then dose is divided in two

Available forms: Tabs 250, 500 mg scored

Adverse effects

CNS: Headache, weakness, tinnitus, fatigue, dizziness, vertigo

ENDO: ***Hypoglycemia,*** hyponatremia
GI: Nausea, vomiting, diarrhea, ***hepatotoxicity, jaundice,*** heartburn
HEMA: ***Leukopenia, thrombocytopenia, agranulocytosis, aplastic anemia, hemolytic anemia,*** increased AST (SGOT), ALT (SGPT), alkaline phosphatase
INTEG: Rash, allergic reactions, pruritus, urticaria, eczema, photosensitivity, erythema

Contraindications: Hypersensitivity to sulfonylureas, juvenile or brittle diabetes, renal failure

Precautions: Pregnancy C, G elderly, cardiac disease, renal disease, hepatic disease, thyroid disease, severe hypoglycemic reactions

Pharmacokinetics

Absorption	Well absorbed
Distribution	Bile
Metabolism	Liver to metabolites
Excretion	Kidneys
Half-life	Parent drug 1.3 hr, metabolites 6 hr

Pharmacodynamics

Onset	10-30 min
Peak	½-2 hr
Duration	3-4 hr

Interactions
Individual drugs
Cimetidine: ↑ hypoglycemia
Chloramphenicol: ↑ hypoglycemia
Diazoxide: ↓ effect of both drugs
Guanethidine: ↑ hypoglycemia
Insulin: ↑ hypoglycemia
Methyldopa: ↑ hypoglycemia
Phenytoin: ↓ action of acetohexamide
Rifampin: ↓ action of acetohexamide
Drug classifications
Anticoagulants, oral: ↑ hypoglycemia
Corticosteroids: ↓ action of acetohexamide
Diuretics, thiazide: ↓ action of acetohexamide
Estrogens: ↓ action of acetohexamide
MAOI: ↑ hypoglycemia
NSAIDs: ↑ hypoglycemia
Oral contraceptives: ↓ action of acetohexamide
Phenothiazines: ↓ action of acetohexamide
Salicylates: ↑ hypoglycemia
Sulfonamides: ↑ hypoglycemia

NURSING CONSIDERATIONS
Assessment
- Assess for hypoglycemic/hyperglycemic reactions that can occur soon after meals; hypoglycemic reactions: sweating, weakness, dizziness, anxiety, tremors, hunger
- Monitor glucose levels often; may need insulin therapy during severe stress surgery
- Monitor CBC (baseline, q3mo) during treatment; check liver function tests (AST [SGOT], LDH) periodically and renal studies (BUN, creatinine) during treatment

Nursing diagnoses
- ✓ Nutrition, altered: More than body requirements (uses)
- ✓ Nutrition altered: Less than body requirements (adverse reactions)
- ✓ Injury, risk for physical (adverse reactions)
- ✓ Knowledge deficit (teaching)
- ✓ Noncompliance (teaching)

Implementation

- Conversion from other oral hypoglycemic agents or insulin dosage of <40 U/day, change may be made without gradual dosage change; patients taking insulin of >40 U/day convert gradually by receiving oral hypoglycemic and 50% of previous insulin dosage for 3-5 days; monitor serum or urine glucose and ketones 3 times/day during conversion

PO route

- Give drug 30 min before breakfast; if large dose is required, may be divided into two; give with meals to decrease GI upset and provide best absorption
- Give tabs crushed and mixed with meal or fluids for patients with difficulty swallowing
- Store in tight container in cool environment

Patient/family education

- Teach patient to check for symptoms of cholestatic jaundice: dark urine, pruritus, yellow sclera; if these occur, notify prescriber
- Teach patient to use capillary blood glucose test or Chemstrip 3 times a day
- Teach patient symptoms of hypoglycemia and hyperglycemia and what to do about each
- Tell patient that drug use must be continued daily; explain consequence of discontinuing drug use abruptly
- Teach patient to take drug in AM to prevent hypoglycemic reactions at night
- Tell patient to avoid OTC medications unless prescribed
- Teach patient that diabetes is lifelong illness; that this drug is not a cure
- Tell patient that all food included in diet plan must be eaten to prevent hypoglycemia
- Tell patient to carry Medic Alert ID for emergency purposes and to carry a glucagon emergency kit

Evaluation

Positive therapeutic outcome

- Decrease in polyuria, polydipsia, polyphagia; clear sensorium, absence of dizziness, stable gait, blood glucose, WNL

Treatment of overdose:

Glucose 25 g **IV**, via dextrose 50% sol, 50 ml or 1 mg glucagon

acetylcysteine 🔑 (℞)

(a-se-teel-sis'tay-een)

Airbron ✦, Mucomyst, Mucosal

Func. class.: Mucolytic; antidote—acetaminophen

Chem. class.: Amino acid L-cysteine

Pregnancy category B

Action: Decreases viscosity of secretions in respiratory tract by breaking disulfide links of mucoproteins; increases hepatic glutathione, which is necessary to inactivate toxic metabolites in acetaminophen overdose

➔ Therapeutic Outcome: Decreased hepatotoxicity from acetaminophen overdose (PO); decreased viscosity of mucus in respiratory disorders (inh)

Uses: Acetaminophen toxicity; bronchitis; pneumonia; cystic fibrosis; emphysema; atelectasis; tuberculosis; complications of thoracic surgery and cardiovascular surgery; diagnosis in bronchial lab tests

Dosage and routes

Mucolytic

P ***Adult and child:*** INH 2-20 ml (10% sol) q1-4h prn, or 1-10 ml (20% sol)

Acetaminophen toxicity

P ***Adult and child:*** PO 140 mg/kg, then 70 mg/kg q4h × 17 doses to total 1330 mg/kg

Available forms: Sol 10%, 20%

Adverse effects

CNS: Dizziness, drowsiness, headache, fever, chills

CV: Hypotension

EENT: Rhinorrhea, tooth damage

GI: Nausea, stomatitis, constipation, vomiting, anorexia, ***hepatotoxicity***

INTEG: Urticaria, rash, fever, clamminess

RESP: ***Bronchospasm,*** burning, ***hemoptysis,*** chest tightness

Contraindications: Hypersensitivity, increased intracranial pressure, status asthmaticus

Precautions: Hypothyroidism, Addison's disease, CNS depression, brain tumor, asthma, hepatic disease, renal disease, COPD, psychosis, alcoholism, convulsive disorders, lactation, pregnancy **B**

Pharmacokinetics

Absorption	Extensive (PO), locally (INH)
Distribution	Unknown
Metabolism	Liver
Excretion	Kidneys
Half-life	Unknown

Pharmacodynamics

	PO	INH
Onset	Unknown	1 min
Peak	Unknown	Unknown
Duration	up to 4 hr	5-10 min

Interactions

Individual drugs

Activated charcoal: ↓ absorption of acetylcysteine

Iron, copper, rubber: Do not use with acetylcysteine

NURSING CONSIDERATIONS

Assessment

Mucolytic use

- Assess cough: type, frequency, character, including sputum
- Assess characteristics, rate, rhythm of respirations, increased dyspnea, sputum; discontinue if bronchospasm occurs; ABGs for increased CO_2 retention in asthma patients
- Monitor VS, cardiac status including checking for dysrhythmias, increased rate, palpitations

Antidotal use

- Assess liver function tests, acetaminophen levels, protime, glucose, electrolytes; inform prescriber if dose is vomited or vomiting is persistent; provide adequate hydration; decrease dosage in hepatic encephalopathy
- Assess for nausea, vomiting, rash; notify prescriber if these occur

Nursing diagnoses

✓ Injury, risk for physical (uses) (antidote)

✓ Impaired gas exchange (uses) (mucolytic)

✓ Airway clearance ineffective (uses) (mucolytic)

✓ Poisoning, risk for (uses) (antidote)
✓ Knowledge deficit (teaching)

Implementation

- Give decreased dosage to elderly patients; their metabolism may be slowed; give gum, hard candy, frequent rinsing of mouth for dryness of oral cavity
- Use only if suction machine is available

PO route: *Antidotal use*

- Lavage, then give within 24 hr; give with cola or soft drink to disguise taste; can be given with H_2O through tubes; use within 1 hr

INH route: *Mucolytic use*

- Use ac ½-1 hr for better absorption, to decrease nausea; only after patient clears airway by deep breathing, coughing
- Give by syringe 2-3 doses of 1-2 ml of 20% or 2-4 ml of 10% sol; 20% sol diluted with NS or water for injection; may give 10% sol undiluted
- Store in refrigerator: use within 96 hr of opening
- Provide assistance with inhaled dose: bronchodilator if bronchospasm occurs; wash face and rinse mouth after use to remove sticky feeling
- Use mechanical suction if cough insufficient to remove excess bronchial secretions

Patient/family education

Mucolytic use

- Tell patient to avoid driving or other hazardous activities until patient is stabilized on this medication; avoid alcohol, other CNS depressants; will enhance sedating properties of this drug
- Teach patient that unpleasant odor will decrease after repeated use; that discoloration of solution after bottle is opened does not impair its effectiveness; avoid smoking, smoke-filled rooms, perfume, dust, environmental pollutants, cleaners

Evaluation

Positive therapeutic outcome

- Absence of purulent secretions when coughing (mucolytic use)
- Clear lung sounds bilaterally (mucolytic use)
- Absence of hepatic damage (acetaminophen toxicity)
- Decreasing blood toxicology (acetaminophen toxicity)

acrivastine/pseudoephedrine (℞)

Semprex-D

Func. class.: Antihistamine

Chem. class.: H_1-histamine antagonist

Pregnancy category B

Action: Acts on blood vessels, GI, respiratory system by competing with histamine for H_1-receptor site; decreases allergic response by blocking pharmacologic effects of histamine; less sedation rate than with other histamines; causes increased heart rate, vasodilation, increased secretions

Therapeutic Outcome: Absence of allergy symptoms and rhinitis

Uses: Rhinitis, allergy symptoms, chronic idiopathic urticaria

Dosage and routes

Adult and child >12 yr: PO 8 mg q4-6h

Available forms: Caps 8 mg/60 mg

Adverse effects
CNS: Headache, dizziness, nervousness, insomnia
GI: Nausea, dry mouth
GU: Dysmenorrhea
RESP: Cough, pharyngitis

Contraindications: Hypersensitivity to this drug or triprolidine, severe hypertension, cardiac disease

Precautions: Pregnancy **B,** G elderly, children, respiratory P disease, hypertension, diabetes mellitus, ischemic heart disease, increased intraocular pressure, prostate hypertrophy

Pharmacokinetics

Absorption	Well absorbed rapidly
Distribution	Not known
Metabolism	Liver
Excretion	Kidneys, feces
Half-life	1½ hr

Pharmacodynamics

Onset	Unknown
Peak	1-1½ hr
Duration	12 hr

Interactions
Individual drugs
Alcohol: ↑ CNS depression
Drug classifications
β-agonists: Hypertensive crisis
MAOI: Hypertensive crisis
Narcotics: ↑ CNS depression
Sedative/hypnotics: ↑ CNS depression
Lab test interferences
False negative: Skin allergy tests (discontinue antihistamine 3 days before testing)

NURSING CONSIDERATIONS
Assessment
- Assess respiratory status: rate, rhythm, increase in bronchial secretions, wheezing, chest tightness; provide fluids to 2L/day to decrease secretion thickness

Nursing diagnoses
✓ Airway clearance, ineffective (uses)
✓ Knowledge deficit (teaching)

Implementation
- Give with food or fluid for GI symptoms
- ⊘ Do not crush, chew caps
- Store in tight, light-resistant container

Patient/family education
- Teach all aspects of drug usage; to avoid driving or other hazardous activity if drowsiness occurs; to avoid alcohol or other CNS depressants that may potentiate effect
- Caution patient not to exceed recommended dose
- Advise patient hard candy, gum, frequent rinsing of mouth may be used for dryness

Evaluation
Positive therapeutic response
- Absence of running or congested nose, rashes

Treatment of overdose: Administer ipecac syrup or lavage, diazepam, vasopressors, barbiturates (short-acting)

activated charcoal (OTC)

Acta-char, Acta-Char Liquid-A, Actidose-Aqua, Aqueous Charcodote ✤, Charac-50 ✤, Charcoaide, Charcocaps, Charcodote, Charcotabs, Digestalin, Insta-Char, Insta-Char Aqueous Suspension, Liqu-Char, Super-Char, Super-Char Aqueous

Func. class.:
Antiflatulent/antidote

Pregnancy category C

Action: Binds poisons, toxins, irritants; increases adsorption in GI tract; inactivates toxins and binds until excreted

➔ **Therapeutic Outcome:** Prevention of toxicity and death resulting from absorption of drugs

Uses: Flatulence, poisoning, dyspepsia, distention, deodorant in wounds, diarrhea

Dosage and routes

Poisoning

P ***Adult and child:*** PO 5-10 × weight of substance ingested; minimum dosage 30 g/250 ml of water; may give 20-40g q6h for 1-2 days in severe poisoning

Flatulence/dyspepsia

Adult: PO 520-975 mg pc up to 4.16 g/day

Available forms: Powder 15, 30, 40, 120, 125, 240 g/container; oral susp 12.5 g/60 ml, 15 g/72 ml, 15 g/120 ml, 25 g/120 ml, 30 g/120 ml, 50 g/240 ml; ✤ 15 g/120 ml, 25 g/125 ml, 50 g/225 ml, 50 g/250 ml

Adverse effects

GI: Nausea, black stools, vomiting, constipation, diarrhea

Contraindications: Hypersensitivity to this drug, unconsciousness, semiconsciousness, poisoning of cyanide, mineral acids, alkalies

Precautions: Pregnancy **C**

Pharmacokinetics	
Absorption	None
Distribution	None
Metabolism	None
Excretion	Feces (unchanged)
Half-life	Unknown

Pharmacodynamics	
Onset	1 min
Peak	Unknown
Duration	4-12 hr

Interactions

Individual drugs

Ipecac: ↓ effectiveness of both drugs

Drug classifications

Laxatives: ↓ effectiveness of both drugs

Food

Dairy products: ↓ effect of activated charcoal

NURSING CONSIDERATIONS

Assessment

- Assess neurologic status including LOC, pupil reactivity, cough reflex, gag reflex, and swallowing ability before administration; do not give if neurologic status is impaired; aspiration may occur unless a protected airway is present
- Assess toxin, poison ingested, time of ingestion, and amount
- Monitor respiration, pulse, B/P to determine charcoal effectiveness if taken for barbiturate/narcotic poisoning

A

Nursing diagnoses
- ✓ Injury, risk for (uses)
- ✓ Poisoning, risk for (uses)
- ✓ Knowledge deficit (teaching)

Implementation
- Give after inducing vomiting unless vomiting contraindicated (i.e., cyanide or alkalies); mix with 8 oz water or fruit juice to form thick syrup; do not use dairy products to mix charcoal; repeat dose if vomiting occurs soon after dose
- Space at least 2 hr before or after other drugs, or absorption will be decreased; use a laxative to promote elimination; constipation occurs often
- Give alone; do not administer with ipecac; give through a nasogastric tube; if patient unable to swallow, dilute to a less thick sol; keep container tightly closed to prevent absorption of gases

Patient/family education
- Tell patient stools will be black
- Teach patient about overdose/poison prevention and about keeping poison control chart available

Evaluation
Positive therapeutic outcome
- Alert, PERL (poisoning)
- Absence of distention
- Absence of odor in wounds

acyclovir (℞)
(ay-sye'kloe-ver)
Zovirax
Func. class.: Antiviral
Chem. class.: Acylic purine nucleoside analog
Pregnancy category C

Action: Interferes with DNA synthesis by conversion to acyclovir triphosphate, causing decreased viral replication, time of lesional healing

Therapeutic Outcome: Decreased amount and time of healing of lesions

Uses: Mucocutaneous herpes simplex virus, herpes genitalis (HSV-1, HSV-2), herpes zoster; simple mucocutaneous herpes simplex in immunocompromised clients with initial herpes genitalis; herpes simplex encephalitis, cytomegalovirus, HSV after transplant

Dosage and routes
Herpes simplex
P ***Adult and child >12 yr:*** **IV** inf 5 mg/kg over 1 hr q8h × 5 days

P ***Child <12 yr:*** **IV** inf 250 mg/m^2 over 1 hr q8h × 5 days

Genital herpes
Adult: PO 200 mg q4h 5 times a day while awake × 5 days to 6 mo depending on whether initial, recurrent, or chronic

P ***Adult and child:*** TOP apply to all lesions q3h while awake, 6 times a days × 1 wk

Herpes simplex encephalitis
P ***Child >6 mo:*** **IV** 500 mg/m^2 q8h × 10 days

Herpes zoster
Adult: PO 800 mg q4h while

awake × 7-10 days; **IV** 5 mg/kg q8h

Children with immunosuppression

P ***Child >2 yr:*** 20 mg/kg qid × 5 days

Available forms: Caps 200 mg; inj **IV** 500 mg; top ointment 5% (50 mg/g); tabs, susp

Adverse effects

CNS: Tremors, confusion, lethargy, hallucinations, ***convulsions, dizziness, headache,*** encephalopathic changes

EENT: Gingival hyperplasia

GI: Nausea, vomiting, diarrhea, increased ALT (SGPT), AST (SGOT), abdominal pain, glossitis, colitis

GU: Oliguria, proteinuria, hematuria, vaginitis, moniliasis, ***glomerulonephritis, acute renal failure,*** changes in menses, polydipsia

INTEG: Rash, urticaria, pruritus, pain or phlebitis at **IV** site, unusual sweating, alopecia, stinging, burning, vulvitis

MS: Joint pain, leg pain, muscle cramps

Contraindications: Hypersensitivity

Precautions: Lactation, hepatic disease, renal disease, electrolyte imbalance, dehydration, pregnancy **C**

Pharmacokinetics

Absorption	Minimal (PO)
Distribution	Widely distributed, crosses placenta, CSF concentration 50% plasma
Metabolism	Liver, minimal
Excretion	Kidneys, 95% unchanged
Half-life	2.0-3.5 hr, increased in renal disease

Pharmacodynamics

	PO	IV	TOP
Onset	Unknown	Rapid	Unknown
Peak	1½-2½	Infusion's end	Unknown

Interactions

Individual drugs

Amphotericin B: ↑ neurotoxicity, nephrotoxicity

Interferon: ↑ neurotoxicity, nephrotoxicity

Methotrexate: ↑ neurotoxicity

Probenecid: ↑ neurotoxicity, nephrotoxicity

Drug classification

Aminoglycosides: ↑ neurotoxicity, nephrotoxicity

NURSING CONSIDERATIONS

Assessment

- Monitor for signs of infection, type of lesions, area of body covered, purulent drainage
- Check I&O ratio; report hematuria, oliguria, fatigue, weakness; may indicate nephrotoxicity; check for protein in urine during treatment
- Monitor any patient with compromised renal system, since drug is excreted slowly in poor renal system function; toxicity may occur rapidly
- Monitor liver studies: AST (SGOT), ALT (SGPT)
- Monitor blood studies: WBC, RBC, Hct, Hgb, bleeding time; blood dyscrasias may occur; drug should be discontinued
- Monitor renal studies: urinalysis, protein, BUN, creatinine, CrCl; increased BUN, creatinine indicates renal failure
- Obtain C&S before drug therapy; drug may be taken as soon as culture is taken; repeat

C&S after treatment; determine the presence of other sexually transmitted diseases
• Monitor bowel pattern before, during treatment; if severe abdominal pain with bleeding occurs, drug should be discontinued
• Assess allergies before treatment, reaction of each medication; place allergies on chart in bright red letters; allergic reaction: burning, stinging, swelling, redness, rash, vulvitis, pruritus

Nursing diagnoses

✓ Infection, risk for (uses)
✓ Knowledge deficit (teaching)

Implementation

PO route

• Give with food to lessen GI symptoms
• Store at room temperature in dry place

Topical route

• Use finger cot or rubber glove to prevent further infection
• Enough medication to cover lesions completely
• After cleansing with soap and water before each application, dry well

IV **IV route**

• Provide increased fluids to 3 L/day to decrease crystalluria when given **IV**
• Give by int inf after reconstituting with 10 ml sterile water for injection/500 mg of drug (50 mg/ml); shake; dilute in 0.9% NaCl, LR, D_5W, D_5/0.25% NaCl, D_5/0.45% NaCl, D_5/0.9% NaCl (7 mg/ml); give over at least 1 hr (constant rate) by infusion pump to prevent nephrotoxicity; do not reconstitute with sol containing benzyl alcohol or parabens; check infusion site for redness, pain, induration; rotate sites
• Lower dosage in acute or chronic renal failure
• Store at room temperature for up to 12 hr after reconstitution; if refrigerated, sol may show a precipitate that clears at room temperature

Y-*site compatibilities:*
Allopurinol, amikacin, ampicillin, cefamandole, cefazolin, cefonicid, cefoperazone, ceforanide, cefotaxime, cefoxitin, ceftazidime, ceftizoxime, ceftriaxone, cefuroxime, cephapirin, chloramphenicol, cimetidine, clindamycin, co-trimoxazole, dexamethasone sodium phosphate, dimenhydrinate, diphenhydramine, doxycycline, erythromycin lactobionate, filgrastim, fluconazole, gallium, gentamicin, heparin, hydrocortisone sodium succinate, hydromorphone, imipenem/cilastatin, lorazepam, magnesium sulfate, melphalan, meperidine, methylprednisolone sodium succinate, metoclopramide, metronidazole, morphine, multivitamin infusion, nafcillin, oxacillin, paclitaxel, penicillin G potassium, pentobarbital, perphenazine, piperacillin, potassium chloride, ranitidine, sodium bicarbonate, tacrolimus, teniposide, tetracycline, theophylline, thiotepa, ticarcillin, tobramycin, vancomycin, zidovudine

Y-*site incompatibilities:*
Dobutamine, dopamine, ondansetron, verapamil

Additive compatibilities:
Fluconazole

Additive incompatibilities:
Blood products, protein-

containing solutions, dobutamine, dopamine

Patient/family education

Topical route

- Tell patient not to use in eyes; for use when there is no evidence of infection; apply with glove to prevent further infection
- Instruct patient to avoid use of OTC creams, ointments, lotions unless directed by prescriber; may cause reinfection, delayed healing
- Teach patient to use asepsis (hand washing) before, after each application and avoid contact with eyes; to adhere strictly to prescribed regimen to maximize successful treatment outcome

PO route

- Teach patient that drug may be taken orally before infection occurs; that drug should be taken when itching or pain occurs, usually before eruptions; that partners need to be told that patient has herpes; they can become infected, so condoms must be worn to prevent reinfections; that drug does not cure infection, just controls symptoms and does not prevent infection to others
- Tell patient to report sore throat, fever, fatigue; may indicate superinfection; that drug must be taken in equal intervals around the clock to maintain blood levels for duration of therapy
- Tell patient to notify prescriber of side effects: bruising, bleeding, fatigue, malaise; may indicate blood dyscrasias
- Tell patient to seek dental care during treatment to prevent gingival hyperplasia
- Teach female patients with genital herpes to have regular Pap smears to prevent undetected cervical cancer
- Do not crush or chew caps

Evaluation

Positive therapeutic outcome

- Absence of itching, painful lesions
- Crusting and healed lesions

Treatment of overdose: Discontinue drug, hemodialysis, resuscitate if needed

adenosine (℞)

(ah-den'oh-seen)

Adenocard

Func. class.: Antidysrhythmic misc.

Chem. class.: Endogenous nucleoside

Pregnancy category C

Action: Slows conduction through AV node, can interrupt reentry pathways through AV node, and can restore normal sinus rhythm in patients with paroxysmal supraventricular tachycardia (PSVT)

Therapeutic Outcome: Normal sinus rhythm in patients diagnosed with PSVT

Uses: PSVT

Dosage and routes

Adult: **IV** bol 6 mg; if conversion to normal sinus rhythm does not occur within 1-2 min, give 12 mg by rapid **IV** bol; may repeat 12 mg dose again in 1-2 min

Available forms: Inj 3 mg/ml

Adverse effects

CNS: Lightheadedness, dizziness, arm tingling, numbness, apprehension, blurred vision, headache
CV: Chest pain, ***atrial tachydysrhythmias,*** sweating, palpitations, hypotension, *facial flushing*
GI: Nausea, metallic taste, throat tightness, groin pressure
RESP: *Dyspnea, chest pressure,* hyperventilation

Contraindications: Hypersensitivity, 2nd- or 3rd-degree heart block, AV block, sick sinus syndrome, atrial flutter, atrial fibrillation

Precautions: Pregnancy **C,** P lactation, children, asthma, G elderly

Pharmacokinetics

Absorption	Complete bioavailability
Distribution	Erythrocytes, cardiovascular endothelium
Metabolism	Liver, converted to inosine and adenosine monophosphate
Excretion	Kidneys
Half-life	10 sec

Pharmacodynamics

Onset	Rapid
Peak	Unknown
Duration	1-2 min

Interactions

Individual drugs

Caffeine: ↓ effects of adenosine
Carbamazepine: ↑ heart block
Dipyridamole: ↑ effects of adenosine
Theophylline: ↓ effects of adenosine

Smoking

↑ tachycardia

Lab test interferences

↑ Liver function tests

NURSING CONSIDERATIONS

Assessment

- Monitor I&O ratio, electrolytes (potassium, sodium, chloride)
- Assess cardiac status: pulse, respiration, ECG intervals (PR, QRS, QT); check for transient dysrhythmias (PVCs, PACs, sinus tachycardia, AV block); B/P continuously for fluctuations
- Assess respiratory status: rate, rhythm, lung fields for rales, watch for respiratory depression; lung fields, bilateral rales may occur in CHF patient; if increased respiration, increased pulse occurs, drug should be discontinued
- Assess CNS effects: dizziness, confusion, paresthesias; drug should be discontinued

Nursing diagnoses

- ✓ Cardiac output, decreased (uses)
- ✓ Impaired gas exchange (adverse reactions)
- ✓ Knowledge deficit (teaching)

Implementation

- Give **IV** bol undiluted; give 6 mg or less over 1 min; if using an **IV** line, use port near insertion site, flush with NS (50 ml); warm to room temperature before giving
- Store at room temperature; sol should be clear; discard unused drug

Patient/family education

- Tell patient to report facial flushing, dizziness, sweating, palpitations, chest pain
- Instruct patient to rise from sitting or standing slowly to prevent orthostatic hypotension

Evaluation

Positive therapeutic outcome

- Decreased B/P, dysrhythmias

albumin, human (℞)

(al-byoo'min)

Albuminar 5%, Albutein 5%, Buminate 5%, Plasbumin 5%, Albuminar 25%, Albutein 25%, Buminate 25%, Plasbumin-25%

Func. class.: Blood derivative—volume expander

Chem. class.: Placental human plasma

Pregnancy category C

Action: Exerts colloidal oncotic pressure, which expands volume of circulating blood by pulling fluid from extravascular to intravascular spaces, and maintains cardiac output

Therapeutic Outcome: Restoration of plasma volume by extravascular to intravascular fluid shift

Uses: Restores plasma volume in burns, hyperbilirubinemia, shock, hypoproteinemia, prevention of cerebral edema, cardiopulmonary bypass procedures, ARDS, hemorrhage; also replacement in nephrotic syndrome, hepatic failure

Dosage and routes

Burns

Adult: **IV** dose to maintain plasma albumin at 30-50 g/L, use 5% sol initially, then 25% sol after 24 hr

Shock

Adult: **IV** 500 ml of 5% sol q30 min, as needed

P ***Child:*** ¼-½ adult dose in nonemergencies

Hypoproteinemia

Adult: **IV** 1000-2000 ml of 5% sol qd, not to exceed 5-10 ml/min or 25-100 g of 25% sol qd, not to exceed 3 ml/min, titrated to patient response

Hyperbilirubinemia/erythroblastosis fetalis

P ***Infant:*** **IV** 1 g of 25% sol/kg before transfusion

Available forms: Inj 50, 250 mg/ml (5%, 25%)

Adverse effects

CNS: Fever, chills, flushing, headache

CV: ***Fluid overload,*** hypotension, erratic pulse, tachycardia

GI: Nausea, vomiting, increased salivation

INTEG: Rash, urticaria

RESP: Altered respirations, ***pulmonary edema***

Contraindications: Hypersensitivity, CHF, severe anemia, renal insufficiency

Precautions: Decreased salt intake, decreased cardiac reserve, lack of albumin deficiency, hepatic disease, renal disease, pregnancy **C**

Pharmacokinetics	
Absorption	Complete bioavailability
Distribution	Intravascular spaces
Metabolism	Liver
Excretion	Unknown
Half-life	Unknown

Pharmacodynamics	
Onset	15-30 min
Peak	Unknown
Duration	Unknown

Interactions: None

Lab test interferences

False ↑ Alkaline phosphatase

NURSING CONSIDERATIONS

Assessment

- Monitor blood studies: Hct, Hgb; if serum protein declines, dyspnea, hypoxemia can result; check for decreasing B/P, erratic pulse, respiration
- Monitor CVP: pulmonary wedge pressure will increase if overload occurs; I&O ratio: urinary output may decrease; CVP reading: distended neck veins indicate circulatory overload; shortness of breath, anxiety, insomnia, expiratory rales, frothy blood-tinged sputum, cough, cyanosis indicate pulmonary overload
- Assess for allergy: fever, rash, itching, chills, flushing, urticaria, nausea, vomiting, hypotension; requires discontinuation of infusion, use of new lot if therapy reinstituted

Nursing diagnoses

✓ Fluid volume deficit (uses)
✓ Injury, risk for physical (uses)
✓ Fluid volume excess (adverse reactions)
✓ Knowledge deficit (teaching)

Implementation

- Check type of albumin; some are stored at room temperature, some need to be refrigerated; use only amber-colored sol without precipitate, solution should be clear
- Give **IV** slowly to prevent fluid overload; 5% may be given undiluted; 25% may be given diluted (D_5W, 0.9% NaCl) or undiluted; give over 4 hr, use infusion pump
- Provide adequate hydration before, during administration; whole blood may need to be given to prevent anemia; monitor hydration during treatment

Solution compatibilities: 0.9% NaCl, D_5W, D_5/0.9% NaCl, D_5/0.45%, D_5/LR, LR

Y-site compatibilities: Diltiazem, lorazepam

Patient/family education

- Explain use, reason for albumin; provide information on what to report to prescriber (hypersensitivity, fluid overload)

Evaluation

Positive therapeutic outcome

- Increased B/P, decreased edema (shock, burns)
- Increased serum albumin levels
- Increased plasma protein (hypoproteinemia)

albuterol (Rx)

(al-byoo'ter-ole)

albuterol, Gen-Salbutamol ♣, Novo-salmol ♣, Proventil, Proventil HFA, Proventil Repetabs, Salbutamol ♣, Ventodisk ♣, Ventolin, Ventolin Rotacaps, Volmax

Func. class.: Bronchodilator

Chem. class.: Adrenergic β_2-agonist

Pregnancy category C

Action: Causes bronchodilatation by action on β_2 (pulmonary) receptors by increasing levels of cyclic adenosine monophosphate (cAMP), which relaxes smooth muscle; produces bronchodilatation; CNS, cardiac stimulation, increased diuresis, and increased gastric acid secretion; longer acting than isoproterenol

Therapeutic Outcome: Increased ability to breathe because of bronchodilatation

Uses: Prevention of exercise-induced asthma, bronchospasm

Investigational uses: Hyperkalemia in dialysis patients

Dosage and routes

To prevent exercise-induced asthma

Adult: INH 2 puffs 15 min before exercising, NEB/IPPB 5 mg tid-qid

Bronchospasm

Adult: INH 1-2 puffs q4-6h; PO 2-4 mg tid-qid, not to exceed 8 mg

Available forms: Aerosol 90, 100 μg/actuation; tabs 2, 4 mg; oral sol 2 mg/5 ml, ✤ ext rel 4, 8 mg; inh sol 0.83, 1, ✤ 5 mg/ml; inh caps (Rotacaps) 200 mg

Adverse effects

CNS: Tremors, anxiety, insomnia, headache, dizziness, stimulation, *restlessness,* hallucinations, flushing, irritability

CV: Palpitations, tachycardia, hypertension, angina, hypotension, dysrhythmias

EENT: Dry nose, irritation of nose and throat

GI: Heartburn, nausea, vomiting

MS: Muscle cramps

Contraindications: Hypersensitivity to sympathomimetics, tachydysrhythmias, severe cardiac disease

Precautions: Lactation, pregnancy **C,** cardiac disorders, hyperthyroidism, diabetes mellitus, hypertension, prostatic hypertrophy, narrow angle glaucoma, seizures, exercise-induced bronchospasm (aerosol) in children <12 years

Pharmacokinetics

Absorption	Well absorbed (PO)
Distribution	Unknown
Metabolism	Liver extensively, tissues
Excretion	Unknown, breast milk
Half-life	3-4 hr

Pharmacodynamics

	PO	PO–EXT REL	INH
Onset	½ hr	½ hr	5-15 min
Peak	2½ hr	2-3 hr	1-1½ hr
Duration	4-6 hr	12 hr	4-6 hr

Interactions

Drug classifications

β-Adrenergic blockers: Block therapeutic effect

Bronchodilators, aerosol: ↑ action of bronchodilator

MAOI: ↑ chance of hypertensive crisis

Sympathomimetics: ↑ adrenergic side effects

NURSING CONSIDERATIONS

Assessment

- Assess respiratory function: vital capacity, forced expiratory volume, ABGs, lung sounds, heart rate, rhythm (baseline and during therapy)
- Determine that patient has not received theophylline therapy before giving dose, to prevent additive effect; client's ability to self-medicate
- Monitor for evidence of allergic reactions; paradoxic bronchospasm; withhold dose; notify prescriber

Nursing diagnoses

✓ Airway clearance, ineffective (uses)
✓ Impaired gas exchange (uses)
✓ Knowledge deficit (teaching)

Implementation

PO route

• Give PO with meals to decrease gastric irritation; oral sol P for children (no alcohol, sugar)

Aerosol route

• Give after shaking; have patient exhale and place mouthpiece in mouth, inhale slowly, hold breath, remove inhaler, exhale slowly; allow at least 1 min between inhalations

• Store in light-resistant container; do not expose to temperatures over 86° F (30° C)

Patient/family education

• Tell patient not to use OTC medications before consulting prescriber; extra stimulation may occur; instruct patient to use this medication before other medications and allow at least 5 min between each to prevent overstimulation; to limit caffeine products such as chocolate, coffee, tea, and cola

• Teach patient to use inhaler; review package insert with patient; to avoid getting aerosol in eyes or blurring may result; to wash inhaler in warm water and dry qd; to rinse mouth after using; to avoid smoking, smoke-filled rooms, persons with respiratory infections

• Teach patient that if paradoxic bronchospasm occurs to stop drug immediately and notify prescriber

• Instruct patient on administration of dose, not to use more than prescribed; serious side effects may occur; if taking PO regularly and dose is missed, take when remembered; space other doses on new time schedule; do not double doses

Evaluation

Positive therapeutic outcome

• Absence of dyspnea and wheezing after 1 hr

• Improved airway exchange

• Improved ABGs

Treatment of overdose: Administer a β_1-adrenergic blocker

aldesleukin (interleukin-2, IL-2) (℞)

(al-dess-loo'kin)

Proleukin

Func. class.: Miscellaneous antineoplastics

Chem. class.: Interleukin-2, human recombinant, cytokine

Pregnancy category C

Action: Enhancement of lymphocyte mitogenesis and stimulation of IL-2–dependent cell lines; enhancement of lymphocyte cytotoxicity; induction of killer cell activity; induction of interferon-γ production; results in activation of cellular immunity and cytokines and inhibition of tumor growth

Therapeutic Outcome: Prevention of rapid growth of malignant cells

Uses: Metastatic renal cell carcinoma in adults, phase II for HIV in combination with zidovudine, melanoma

Investigational uses: Kaposi's sarcoma given with zidovudine, metastatic melanoma given with cyclophosphamide, non-Hodgkin's lymphoma given with lymphokine-activated killer cells, AIDS (phase I) given with zidovudine

Dosage and routes

Adult: **IV** inf 600,000 IU/kg (0.037 mg/kg) q8h over 15 min × 14 doses; off 9 days; repeat schedule for another 14 doses, for a maximum of 28 doses/course

Available forms: Powder for inj, lyophilized

Adverse effects

CNS: Mental status changes, dizziness, sensory dysfunction, syncope, motor dysfunction, fever, chills, headache

CV: Hypotension, sinus tachycardia, dysrhythmias, bradycardia, PVCs, PACs, myocardial ischemia, ***myocardial infarction, cardiac arrest,*** capillary leak syndrome

GI: Nausea, vomiting, diarrhea, stomatitis, anorexia, GI bleeding, dyspepsia, constipation, ***intestinal perforation/*** ileus, jaundice, ascites

GU: ***Oliguria/anuria, proteinuria, hematuria,*** dysuria, ***renal failure***

HEMA: Anemia, ***thrombocytopenia, leukopenia, coagulation disorders, leukocytosis, eosinophilia***

INTEG: Pruritus, erythema, rash, dry skin, ***exfoliative dermatitis,*** purpura, petechiae, urticaria

MS: Arthralgia, myalgia

RESP: Pulmonary congestion, dyspnea, ***pulmonary edema, respiratory failure,*** tachypnea, pleural effusion, wheezing

SYST: Infection

Contraindications: Hypersensitivity, abnormal thallium stress test or pulmonary function tests, organ allografts

Precautions: CNS metastases, bacterial infections, renal/hepatic, cardiac/pulmonary disease, pregnancy **C**, lactation, P children, anemia, thrombocytopenia

Pharmacokinetics

Absorption	Complete bioavailability
Distribution	Rapid extracellular, intravascular
Metabolism	Kidneys (convoluted tubules)
Excretion	Kidneys
Half-life	85 min

Pharmacodynamics

Unknown

Interactions

Individual drugs

Indomethacin: ↑ toxicity

Radiation: ↑ toxicity, bone marrow suppression

Drug classifications

Aminoglycosides: ↑ toxicity

Antihypertensives: ↑ hypotension

Antineoplastics: ↑ toxicity, bone marrow suppression

Corticosteroids: ↓ tumor effectiveness

Lab test interferences

↑ Bilirubin, ↑ BUN, ↑ serum creatinine, ↑ transaminase, ↑ alkaline phosphatase, ↑ hypomagnesemia, ↑ acidosis hypocalcemia, ↑ hypophosphatemia, ↑ hypokalemia, ↑ hyperuricemia, ↑ hypoalbuminemia, ↑ hypoproteinemia, ↑ hyponatremia, ↑ hyperkalemia, ↑ alkalosis

NURSING CONSIDERATIONS

Assessment

• Monitor CBC, differential, platelet count weekly; withhold drug if WBC is <4000/mm³ or platelet count is <75,000/mm³; notify prescriber of these results; transfusion of RBCs, platelets may be required

- Identify capillary leak syndrome (CLS), including a drop in mean arterial pressure (2-12 hr after initiating therapy); hypotension and hypoperfusion will occur; monitor ECG, CVP in cardiac patients
- Monitor renal function studies: BUN, serum uric acid, urine CrCl, electrolytes before, during therapy; I&O ratio; report fall in urine output to <30 ml/hr
- Monitor temperature q4h; fever may indicate beginning infection
- Check liver function tests before, during therapy: bilirubin, AST (SGOT), ALT (SGPT), alkaline phosphatase as needed or monthly
- Monitor ECG; watch for ST-T wave changes, low QRS and T, possible dysrhythmias (sinus tachycardia, PVCs)
- Monitor baselines in pulmonary function; document FEV >2 L or ≥75% before therapy; check daily VS, pulse oximetry, dyspnea, rales, ABGs
- Obtain stress thallium study before therapy; document normal ejection fraction, unimpaired wall motion
- Assess for bleeding: hematuria, guaiac, bruising or petechiae, mucosa, or orifices q8h
- Assess for GI symptoms: frequency of stools, cramping
- Assess for acidosis, signs of dehydration: rapid respirations, poor skin turgor, decreased urine output, dry skin, restlessness, weakness
- Assess for cardiac status: B/P, pulse, character, rhythm, rate, ABGs, ECG
- Assess for infection: sore throat; antibiotics may be prescribed prophylactically

Nursing diagnoses

- ☑ Injury, risk for (adverse reactions)
- ☑ Body image disturbance (adverse reactions)
- ☑ Infection, risk for (adverse reactions)
- ☑ Knowledge deficit (teaching)

Implementation

- Give by intermittent **IV** inf after diluting 22 million IU (1.3 mg)/1.2 ml sterile (1.1 mg/ml) H_2O for inj at side of vial and swirl, do not shake; dilute dose with 50 ml D_5W and give over 15 min; use plastic bag; do not use an in-line filter; give through Y-tube or 3-way stopcock
- Give prophylactic antibiotics because of ↑ risk of infection
- Give dopamine 1-5 kg/min before onset of hypotension; ↓ dose preserves kidney output
- Give hydrocortisone, dexamethasone, or sodium bicarbonate (1 mEq/1 ml) for extravasation, apply ice compresses
- Store in refrigerator any diluted drug; do not freeze; administer within 48 hr; bring to room temperature before infusing; discard unused portion

Y-site compatibilities:

Amikacin, IV fat emulsion, gentamicin, morphine, piperacillin, ticarcillin, tobramycin, TPN #145, amphotericin B, calcium gluconate, diphenhydramine, dopamine, fluconazole, foscarnet, heparin, magnesium sulfate, metoclopramide, ondansetron, KCI, ranitidine, trimethoprim/sulfamethizole

Patient/family education

- Teach patient to avoid use of products containing aspirin or

ibuprofen, razors, commercial mouthwash because bleeding may occur; to report symptoms of bleeding hematuria, tarry stools
- Tell patient to report signs of anemia: fatigue, headache, irritability, faintness, shortness of breath
- Tell patient to report any changes in breathing or coughing even several months after treatment
- Advise patient that contraception will be necessary during treatment; teratogenesis may occur
- Teach patient to report signs/symptoms of infection: fever, chills, sore throat; patient should avoid crowds or persons with known infections

Evaluation

Positive therapeutic outcome
- Decreased spread of malignancy

alendronate (℞)
(al-en'droe-nate)

Fosamax

Func. class.: Bone-resorption inhibitor

Chem. class.: Biphosphonate

Pregnancy category C

Action: Absorbs calcium phosphate crystal in bone and may directly block dissolution of hydroxyapatite crystals of bone; inhibits bone resorption, apparently without inhibiting bone formation and mineralization

➔ **Therapeutic Outcome:** Decreased symptoms of osteoporosis, Paget's disease

Uses: Osteoporosis in postmenopausal women, Paget's disease

Dosage and routes

Osteoporosis in postmenopausal women

G ***Adult and elderly:*** PO 10 mg qd

Paget's disease

G ***Adult and elderly:*** PO 40 mg qd × 6 mo

Available forms: Tabs 10, 40 mg

Adverse effects

META: Anemia, hypokalemia, hypomagnesemia, hypophosphatemia

GI: Abdominal pain, anorexia, constipation, nausea, vomiting

MS: Bone pain

CV: Hypertension

GU: UTI, fluid overload

Contraindications: Hypersensitivity to biphosphonates

P **Precautions:** Children, lactation, pregnancy **C,** renal disease

Pharmacokinetics

Absorption	Unknown
Distribution	Mainly to bones
Metabolism	Unknown
Excretion	Via kidneys
Half-life	Unknown

Pharmacodynamics

Unknown

NURSING CONSIDERATIONS

Assessment
- Monitor renal studies and Ca, P, Mg, K
- Assess for hypercalcemia: paresthesia, twitching, laryngospasm, Chvostek's, Trousseau's signs

Implementation
- Give PO for 6 mo to be effective in Paget's disease

• Store in cool environment out of direct sunlight

Evaluation

Positive therapeutic outcome

• Increased bone mass, absence of fractures

alfentanil (℞)

(al-fen'ta-nil)

Alfenta, Rapifen ✱

Func. class.: Narcotic analgesic

Chem. class.: Opiate, synthetic

Pregnancy category C

Controlled substance schedule II

Action: Inhibits ascending pain pathways in limbic system, thalamus, midbrain, hypothalamus by binding to opiate receptor sites; this alters pain perception and response

Therapeutic Outcome: Relief of pain (moderate, severe pain), anesthesia

Uses: In combination with other drugs in general anesthesia; as a primary anesthetic in general surgery usually used with barbiturates, oxygen, nitrous oxide, monitored anesthesia care (MAC)

Dosage and routes

Anesthesia <30 min

Combination

Adult: **IV** 8-50 μg/kg, may increase by 3-15 μg/kg

Anesthetic induction

Adult: **IV** 3-5 μg/kg, then 0.5-1.5 μg/kg/min; total dose is 8-40 μg/kg

Anesthesia 30-60 min

Induction

Adult: **IV** 20-50 μg/kg

Maintenance

Adult: **IV** 5-15 μg/kg; may give up to 75 μg/kg total dose

Continuous anesthesia >45 min

Induction

Adult: **IV** 50-75 μg/kg

Maintenance

Adult: **IV** 0.5-3.0 μg/kg/min; rate should be decreased by 30%-50% after 1 hr maintenance inf; may be increased to 4 μg/kg/min or bol doses of 7 μg/kg

Induction of anesthesia >45 min

Adult: **IV** 130-245 μg/kg, then 0.5-1.5 μg/kg/min or general anesthesia

MAC

Adult: **IV** duration ≤ ½ hr, 3-8 μg/kg; maintenance: 3-5 μg/kg at 5-20 min to 1 μg/kg/min; total dose 3-40 μg/kg

Available forms: Inj 500 μg/ml

Adverse effects

CNS: Drowsiness, dizziness, confusion, headache, sedation, euphoria, delirium, agitation, anxiety

CV: Palpitations, bradycardia, change in B/P, facial flushing, syncope, asystole

EENT: Tinnitus, blurred vision, miosis, diplopia

GI: Nausea, vomiting, anorexia, constipation, cramps, dry mouth

GU: Urinary retention, dysuria

INTEG: Rash, urticaria, bruising, flushing, diaphoresis, pruritus

MS: Rigidity

RESP: Respiratory depression, apnea

P **Contraindications:** Child <12 yr, hypersensitivity

Precautions: Pregnancy **C**, lactation, increased intracranial pressure, acute MI, severe heart disease, renal disease, hepatic disease, asthma, respiratory conditions, convulsive G disorders, elderly

Pharmacokinetics

Absorption	Complete
Distribution	Crosses placenta; 90% bound to plasma proteins
Metabolism	Liver, up to 100%
Excretion	Kidneys
Half-life	1-2 hr

Pharmacodynamics

Onset	Immediate
Peak	1-1½ min
Duration	30 min

Interactions

Individual drugs

Alcohol: ↑ respiratory depression, hypotension, ↑ sedation
Cimetidine: ↑ recovery time
Erythromycin: ↑ recovery time
Nalbuphine: ↓ analgesia
Pentazocine: ↓ analgesia

Drug classifications

Antihistamines: ↑ respiratory depression, hypotension
Benzodiazepines: ↑ hypotension
CNS depressants: ↑ respiratory depression, hypotension
MAOI: Do not use within 2 wk of alfentanil
Phenothiazines: ↑ respiratory depression, hypotension
Sedative/hypnotics: ↑ respiratory depression, hypotension

Lab test interferences

↑ Amylase, ↑ lipase

NURSING CONSIDERATIONS

Assessment

- Respiratory status: respiratory depression, character, rate, rhythm; notify prescriber if respirations are <12/min; CV status; bradycardia, syncope; monitor ECG continuously

Nursing diagnoses

✓ Pain (uses)
✓ Sensory perceptual alteration: visual, auditory (adverse reactions)
✓ Breathing pattern, ineffective (adverse reactions)
✓ Knowledge deficit (teaching) (preoperatively)

Implementation

General

- Administer pain medications for postoperative pain, since alfentanil effect is short; medication for severe pain may be required
- Benzodiazepines are given after surgery to reduce alfentanil dosage and reduce anesthesia recovery time
- Give direct **IV** over 1½-3 min; use tuberculin syringe for accurate dosing
- Give cont **IV** by diluting 20 ml of drug in 230 ml of diluent (0.9% NaCl, D_5W, LR) (40 μg/ml); discontinue infusion 15 min before surgery is completed
- Store in light-resistant area at room temperature

Syringe compatibilities: Atracurium

Y-site compatibilities: Etomidate

Patient/family education

- Tell patients to avoid CNS depressants (alcohol, sedative/hypnotics) for at least 24 hr after use of this drug
- Discuss with patient that dizziness, drowsiness, and

confusion are common; to avoid getting up without assistance

- Discuss in detail all aspects of the drug and the purpose of this drug and what to expect after anesthesia
- Tell patient to make position changes to lessen orthostatic hypotension

Evaluation

Positive therapeutic outcome

- Maintenance of anesthesia
- Absence of motor activity during surgery

Treatment of overdose: Narcan 0.2-0.8 **IV**, O_2, **IV** fluids, vasopressors; have resuscitation equipment available

allopurinol (℞)

(al-oh-pure'i-nole)

Generic allopurinol, Apo Allopurinol ♣, Lopurin, Purinol ♣, Zyloprim

Func. class.: Antigout drug

Chem. class.: Xanthine enzyme inhibitor

Pregnancy category C

Action: Inhibits the enzyme xanthine oxidase, reducing uric acid synthesis

➡ **Therapeutic Outcome:** Decreasing serum uric acid levels, decreasing joint pain

Uses: Chronic gout, hyperuricemia associated with malignancies, recurrent calcium oxalate calculi, Chaga's disease, cutaneous/visceral leishmaniasis

Dosage and routes

Gout/hyperuricemia

Adult: PO 200-600 mg qd depending on severity, not to exceed 800 mg/day

P ***Child 6-10 yr:*** 300 mg qd

P ***Child <6 yr:*** 150 mg qd

Impaired renal function

Adult: PO 200 mg qd when CrCl is 20-10 ml/min

Recurrent calculi

Adult: PO 200-300 mg qd

Uric acid nephropathy prevention

Adult: PO 600-800 mg qd × 2-3 days

Available forms: Tabs 100, 300 mg

Adverse effects

CNS: Headache, drowsiness, neuritis, paresthesia

EENT: Retinopathy, cataracts, epistaxis

GI: Nausea, vomiting, anorexia, malaise, metallic taste, cramps, peptic ulcer, diarrhea, stomatitis

HEMA: ***Agranulocytosis, thrombocytopenia, aplastic anemia, pancytopenia, leukopenia, bone marrow depression, eosinophilia***

INTEG: Fever, chills, dermatitis, pruritus, purpura, erythema, ecchymosis, alopecia

MISC: Myopathy, arthralgia, hepatomegaly, ***cholestatic jaundice, renal failure***

Contraindications: Hypersensitivity

Precautions: Pregnancy **C**, lactation, renal disease, hepatic P disease, children

Pharmacokinetics	
Absorption	80%
Distribution	Widely distributed
Metabolism	Liver to oxypurinol
Excretion	Kidneys
Half-life	2-3 hr, terminal 18-30 hr

Pharmacodynamics	
Onset	Unknown
Peak	2-4 hr
Duration	Unknown

Interactions

Individual drugs

Ampicillin: ↑ risk of rash
Azathioprine: ↑ bone marrow depression
Chlorpropamide: ↑ action of chlorpropamide
Cyclophosphamide: ↑ action of allopurinol
Mercaptopurine: ↑ bone marrow depression
Theophylline: ↑ action of chlorpropamide

Drug classifications

ACE inhibitors: ↑ action of ACE inhibitors
Aluminum salts: ↓ effects of allopurinol
Anticoagulants, oral: ↑ action of oral anticoagulants
Diuretics, thiazide: ↑ hypersensitivity

Lab test interferences

↑ AST (SGOT), ↑ ALT (SGPT), ↑ alkaline phosphatase
↓ Hct/Hgb, ↓ leukocytes, ↓ serum glucose

NURSING CONSIDERATIONS

Assessment

- Assess for pain including location, characteristics, onset/duration, frequency, quality, intensity or severity of pain, precipitating factors
- Monitor uric acid levels q2wk; normal uric acid levels are 6 mg/dl; check I&O ratio; increase fluids to 2-3 L/day to prevent stone formation, toxicity
- Monitor CBC, AST (SGOT), BUN, creatinine before starting treatment, monthly; check blood glucose in diabetic patients receiving oral antidiabetic agents
- Nutritional status: discourage organ meat, sardines, salmon, legumes, gravies (high-purine foods)

Nursing diagnoses

✓ Nutrition, more than body requirements (uses)
✓ Knowledge deficit (teaching)

Implementation

- Give with meals to prevent GI symptoms; crush and mix with food or fluids for patients with swallowing difficulties
- Give a few days before antineoplastic therapy if using for hyperuricemia associated with malignancy

Patient/family education

- Tell patient to increase fluid intake to 3-4 L/day; to avoid taking large doses of vitamin C; kidney stone formation may occur; to maintain a diet enhancing urine alkalinity (e.g., milk, other dairy products)
- Tell patient to report skin rash, stomatitis, malaise, fever, aching; drug should be discontinued
- Advise patient to avoid hazardous activities if drowsiness or dizziness occurs; response may take several days to determine
- Tell patient to avoid alcohol, caffeine; these substances increase uric acid levels and decrease allopurinol levels
- Teach patient to report side effects and adverse reactions to prescriber, including rash, itching, nausea, vomiting

Evaluation

Positive therapeutic outcome

- Decreased pain in joints
- Decreased stone formation in kidney

- Decreased uric acid level to 6 mg/dl

alpha$_1$-proteinase inhibitor, human (℞)

Prolastin

Func. class.: Enzyme inhibitor

Pregnancy category C

Action: Prevents elastase destruction on alveolar tissue

Therapeutic Outcome: Absence of signs/symptoms of alpha$_1$-antitrypsin deficiency

Uses: Replacement in patients with alpha$_1$-antitrypsin deficiency

Dosage and routes

Adult: **IV** 60 mg/kg q wk; may give at a rate of 0.08 ml/kg/min or more

Available forms: Inj 500 mg, 1000 mg vials

Adverse effects

HEMA: Leukocytosis, *viral transmission possible*

CNS: Dizziness, lightheadedness

MISC: Fever, delayed

Contraindications: Hypersensitivity to polyethylene glycol, emphysema associated with alpha$_1$-antitrypsin

Precautions: Irreversible destruction of lung tissue secondary to alpha$_1$-antitrypsin deficiency, pregnancy **C**, lactation, children

Pharmacokinetics

Absorption	Complete
Distribution	Epithelial fluids-lungs
Metabolism	Intravascular space
Excretion	Intravascular space
Half-life	4½-5½ days

Pharmacodynamics

Unknown

Interactions

Smoking: ↓ effects

NURSING CONSIDERATIONS

Assessment

- Assess respiratory status: rate, lung sounds, rhythm, prior to and weekly during treatment
- Assess for fluid overload: hypertension, dyspnea, rales/crackles, jugular vein distention
- Assess for fever, chills, dizziness, lightheadedness

Nursing diagnoses

- ✓ Gas exchange impaired (uses)
- ✓ Knowledge deficit (teaching)

Implementation

- Give by direct **IV** after bringing to room temperature, reconstitute with sterile water for inj to a concentration of 20 mg/ml; use instructions for vacuum transfer using filter needle, swirl to mix, do not shake; may be diluted in 0.9% NaCl; give at a rate 0.08 mg/kg/min or greater

Additive incompatibilities:

- Do not mix with other drugs or diluents

Patient/family education

- Teach purpose for medication and need for weekly treatment; tell patient to avoid smoking and report changes in breathing or sputum production
- Teach that fever may be delayed for up to 12 hr after inj and resolves by 24 hr
- Advise that periodic pulmonary function test may be required to determine progression of disease
- Advise not to smoke during treatment

Evaluation
Positive therapeutic outcome
- Prevention of destruction of lung tissue

alprazolam (℞)
(al-pray'zoe-lam)
Apo-Alpraz ✤, Novo-Alprazol ✤, Nu-Alpraz ✤, Xanax
Func. class.: Antianxiety/sedative/hypnotic
Chem. class.: Benzodiazepine

Pregnancy category D
Controlled substance schedule IV

Action: Depresses subcortical levels of CNS, including limbic system, reticular formation; potentiates GABA (γ-aminobutyric acid)

➔ Therapeutic Outcome: Decreased anxiety

Uses: Anxiety, panic disorders, anxiety with depressive symptoms

Investigational uses: Depression, social phobia, premenstrual syndrome

Dosage and routes
Anxiety disorder
Adult: PO 0.25-0.5 mg tid, not to exceed 4 mg/day in divided doses
G ***Elderly:*** PO 0.25 mg bid-tid
Panic disorder
Adult: PO 0.5 mg may ↑ g 3-4 days by 1 mg/day or less
Premenstrual syndrome
Adult: PO 0.25 mg tid
Social phobia
Adult: PO 2-8 mg/day

Available forms: Tabs 0.25, 0.5, 1, 2 mg

Adverse effects
CNS: Dizziness, drowsiness, confusion, headache, anxiety, tremors, stimulation, fatigue, depression, insomnia, hallucinations
CV: Orthostatic hypotension, ***ECG changes, tachycardia,*** hypotension
EENT: Blurred vision, tinnitus, mydriasis
GI: Constipation, dry mouth, nausea, vomiting, anorexia, diarrhea
INTEG: Rash, dermatitis, itching

Contraindications: Hypersensitivity to benzodiazepines, narrow angle glaucoma, P psychosis, pregnancy **D,** child <18 yr

G **Precautions:** Elderly, debilitated, hepatic disease, renal disease

Pharmacokinetics	
Absorption	Slow, complete
Distribution	Widely distributed; crosses placenta; crosses blood-brain barrier
Metabolism	Liver, to active metabolites
Excretion	Kidneys, breast milk
Half-life	12-15 hr

Pharmacodynamics	
Onset	1 hr
Peak	1-2 hr
Duration	4-6 hr, therapeutic response 2-3 days

Interactions
Individual drugs
Alcohol: ↑ CNS depression
Cimetidine: ↑ action of alprazolam
Disulfiram: ↑ action of alprazolam

Levodopa: ↑ action of alprazolam

Drug classifications

Anticonvulsants: ↑ CNS depression

Antidepressants: ↑ CNS depression

Antihistamines: ↑ CNS depression

Oral contraceptives: ↑ action of alprazolam

Sedative/hypnotics: ↑ CNS depression

Lab test interferences

↑ AST (SGOT)/ALT (SGPT), ↑ serum bilirubin

False ↑ 17-Hydroxycorticosteroids

↓ RAIU

NURSING CONSIDERATIONS

Assessment

- Assess mental status: mood, sensorium, anxiety, affect, sleeping pattern, drowsiness, **G** dizziness, especially elderly; physical dependency, withdrawal symptoms: anxiety, panic attacks, agitation, convulsions, headache, nausea, vomiting, muscle pain, weakness; suicidal tendencies; indications of increasing tolerance and abuse; withdrawl seizures may occur after rapid-decrease dose or abrupt discontinuation
- Monitor B/P (with patient lying, standing), pulse; if systolic B/P drops 20 mm Hg, hold drug, notify prescriber
- Monitor blood studies: CBC during long-term therapy; blood dycrasias have occurred rarely; decreased hematocrit, neutropenia may occur
- Monitor hepatic studies: AST (SGOT), ALT (SGPT), bilirubin, creatinine LDH, alkaline phosphatase
- Monitor I&O; indicate renal dysfunction

Nursing diagnoses

✓ Anxiety (uses)
✓ Depression (uses)
✓ Injury, risk for (adverse reactions)
✓ Knowledge deficit (teaching)

Implementation

- Give with food or milk for GI symptoms; tab may be crushed, if patient is unable to swallow medication whole, and mixed with foods or fluids
- Give sugarless gum, hard candy, frequent sips of water for dry mouth

Patient/family education

- Tell patient that drug may be taken with food or fluids, and tabs may be crushed or swallowed whole
- Tell patient not to use for everyday stress or longer than 3 mo unless directed by prescriber; not to take more than prescribed amount; may be habit forming; not to double doses or skip doses
- Tell patient to avoid OTC preparations unless approved by prescriber; alcohol and CNS depressants will increase CNS depression
- Tell patient to avoid driving, activities that require alertness, since drowsiness may occur; to avoid alcohol ingestion or other psychotropic medications; to rise slowly or **G** fainting may occur, especially elderly; that drowsiness may worsen at beginning of treatment
- Tell patient not to discontinue medication abruptly after long-term use; withdrawal symptoms include vomiting, cramping, tremors, seizures

Evaluation

Positive therapeutic outcome

- Decreased anxiety, restlessness, sleeplessness (short-term treatment only)

Treatment of overdose: Lavage, VS, supportive care

alprostadil (℞)

(al-pros'ta-dil)

Caverject, Edex, Muse, PGE_1 prostaglandin E_1, Prostin VR Pediatric, Prostin VR ✦

Func. class.: Hormone

Chem. class.: Prostaglandin E_1

Pregnancy category C

Action: Relaxes smooth muscles of ductus arteriosus; results in increased O_2 content perfusion throughout body; causes erection by dilation of cavernosal arteries and relaxation of trabecular muscle, leads to the trapping of blood

Therapeutic Outcome: Maintenance of patent ductus arteriosus with increased O_2 in neonates with congenital heart defects

Uses: To maintain patent ductus arteriosus (temporary treatment), erectile dysfunction

Dosage and routes

Patent ductus arteriosus

P ***Infants:*** **IV**/intraarterial inf 0.1 μg/kg/min, until desired response, then reduce to lowest effective amount; 0.4 μg/kg/min not likely to produce greater beneficial effects

Erectile dysfunction of vasculogenic or mixed etiology, psychogenic

Men: Intracavernosal 2.5 μg may increase by 2.5 μg, may then increase by 5-10 μg until adequate response occurs

Intraurethral

Men: Administer as needed to achieve erection

Available forms: Inj 500 μg/ml; lyopholized powder for inj 6.15, 11.9 μg/23.2 μg, 5, 10, 20, 40 μg/single dose vial; pellets 125, 250, 500, 1000 μg

Adverse effects

CNS: Fever, ***convulsions,*** lethargy, hypothermia, stiffness, hyperirritability, ***cerebral bleeding***

CV: ***Bradycardia, tachycardia, hypotension, CHF, ventricular fibrillation, shock,*** flushing, **cardiac arrest,** edema

GI: Diarrhea, regurgitation, hyperbilirubinemia

GU: Oliguria, hematuria, ***anuria***

HEMA: ***DIC, thrombocytopenia,*** anemia, ***bleeding***

Local (Caverject): Penile pain, prolonged erection, penile fibrosis, penile rash, edema, hematoma, ecchymosis

MISC: ***Sepsis,*** hypokalemia, ***peritonitis,*** hypoglycemia, hyperkalemia

RESP: ***Apnea, bradypnea, wheezing, respiratory depression***

Systemic (Caverject): Headache, dizziness, flu symptoms, sinusitis, nasal congestion, hypertension, back pain, prostatic disorder

Contraindications: Hypersensitivity, respiratory distress syndrome (RDS)

Precautions: Bleeding disorders, pregnancy **C**

Pharmacokinetics	
Absorption	Complete bioavailability (IV)
Distribution	Unknown
Metabolism	80% lungs, rapidly
Excretion	Kidneys to metabolites
Half-life	Up to 10 min

Pharmacodynamics	
Onset	1½-3 hr
Peak	Up to 11 hr
Duration	Infusion's end

Interactions: None

NURSING CONSIDERATIONS

Assessment

- Monitor ABGs, arterial pH, arterial pressure, continuous ECG; if arterial pressure decreases, reduce or stop drug; check for increased pH, B/P, urinary output, decreased ratio of PA to AP (restricted systemic blood flow)
- Assess neurologic status: level of consciousness, reflexes, muscle tone, response to stimuli during administration; if convulsions, stiffness, or hyperirritability occurs, drug should be discontinued; have P ventilator available; neonates <2 kg or infusion >48 hr means increased risk for CNS adverse reactions
- Assess respiratory and cardiac status: rate, rhythm, depth, and effort of respirations; check for bradypnea, tachypnea, apnea, wheezing, respiratory depression; monitor arterial B/P by use of umbilical artery catheter, auscultation, Doppler transducer; check for bradycardia, hypotension
- P Assess neonate with bleeding tendencies for DIS
- P Check neonate for flushing, which indicates a need to reposition the intraarterial catheter

Nursing diagnoses

- ✓ Tissue perfusion, altered (cardiopulmonary, cerebral) (uses)
- ✓ Injury, risk for physical (uses, adverse reactions)
- ✓ Impaired gas exchange (uses)
- ✓ Knowledge deficit (teaching)

Implementation

- Give only with emergency equipment available by trained clinicians
- Administer by cont inf, after diluting with 0.9% NaCl or D_5W inj to a concentration of 500 μg/ml; dilute further with 0.9% NaCl, D_5W; 500 μg of drug/250 ml = 2 μg/ml; 0.1 μg/kg/min; run at 0.05 ml/kg/min, (2 μg/ml); at 0.02 ml/kg/min (5 μg/ml) use inf pump and arterial pressure measurement during inf; do not use sol with benzyl alcohol; stable for 24 hr at room temperature
- Refrigerate drug; discard all mixed unused portion
- Do not mix with other drugs or sol

Patient/family education

- Teach family about diagnosis, prognosis, treatment; P inform parents of neonate's condition
- Teach method for self-injection (erectile disorder), amount to be used, disposal of needle

Evaluation

Positive therapeutic outcome

- Increased urine output (noncyanotic heart disease)
- Increased PO_2 (cyanotic heart disease)
- Absence of metabolic acidosis
- Erection (Caverject)

Treatment of overdose: Discontinue drug, provide supportive measures

alteplase (℞)

(al-ti-plaze')

Activase, Activase rt-PA ✦, tissue plasminogin activator, t-PA, TPA

Func. class.: Thrombolytic

Chem. class.: Tissue plasminogen activator (TPA)

Pregnancy category C

Action: Produces fibrin conversion of plasminogen to plasmin; able to bind to fibrin, convert plasminogen in thrombus to plasmin, which leads to local fibrinolysis, limited systemic proteolysis

➡ **Therapeutic Outcome:** Lysis of thrombi in MI, pulmonary emboli (life threatening)

Uses: Lysis of obstructing thrombi associated with acute MI; conditions requiring thrombolysis, (e.g., PE, DVT, unclotting arteriovenous shunts)

Investigational uses: Unstable angina

Dosage and routes

Adult: **IV** a total of 100 mg; 6-10 mg given **IV** bol over 1-2 min, 60 mg given over 1st hr, 20 mg given over 2nd hr, 20 mg given over 3rd hr; or 1.25 mg/kg given over 3 hr for smaller patients

Accelerated inf

Adult: **IV** bol 15mg; then 50 mg over ½ hr; 35 mg over 1 hr

Available forms: Powder for inj 50 mg (29 million IU/vial), 100 mg (58 million IU/vial)

Adverse effects

CV: ***Sinus bradycardia, ventricular tachycardia, accelerated idioventricular rhythm***

INTEG: Urticaria, rash

SYST: ***GI, GU, intracranial, retroperitoneal bleeding, surface bleeding***

Contraindications: Hypersensitivity, active internal bleeding, recent CVA, severe uncontrolled hypertension, intracranial/intraspinal surgery/trauma, aneurysm

Precautions: Pregnancy **C**, Ⓟ lactation, children

Pharmacokinetics

Absorption	Complete
Distribution	Unknown
Metabolism	>80% liver
Excretion	Kidneys
Half-life	30 min

Pharmacodynamics

Onset	Unknown
Peak	½-2 hr
Duration	Unknown

Interactions

Individual drugs

Aspirin: ↑ bleeding

Dipyridamole: ↑ bleeding

Heparin: ↑ bleeding

Plicamycin: ↑ bleeding

Valproic acid: ↑ bleeding

Drug classifications

Cephalosporins: ↑ bleeding

Anticoagulants, oral: ↑ bleeding

NSAIDs: ↑ bleeding

Lab test interferences

↑ PT, ↑ APTT, ↑ TT

NURSING CONSIDERATIONS

Assessment

• Monitor VS q15 min, B/P, pulse, respirations (including peripheral), neurologic signs, temp at least q4h; temp >104° F (40° C) indicates internal bleeding; monitor rhythm closely; ventricular dysrhythmias may occur with hyperfusion; monitor heart, breath sounds, neurologic status, and peripheral pulses

- Assess for bleeding during first hr of treatment: hematuria, hematemesis, bleeding from mucous membranes, epistaxis, ecchymosis, puncture sites; guaiac all body fluids and stools; obtain blood studies (Hct, platelets, PTT, PT, TT, APTT) before starting therapy; PT or APTT must be less than 2 times control before starting therapy; TT or PT q3-4h during treatment; draw CPK—MB drawn to identify drug effectiveness
- Assess allergy: fever, rash, itching, chills; mild reaction may be treated with antihistamines; report to prescriber
- Monitor ECG; on monitor, watch for segment changes, changes in rhythm: sinus bradycardia, ventricular tachycardia, accelerated idioventricular rhythm may occur due to reperfusion

Nursing diagnoses

- ✓ Pain (uses)
- ✓ Tissue perfusion, altered (uses)
- ✓ Injury, risk for (adverse reactions)

Implementation

- Give after reconstituting with provided diluent; add appropriate amount of sterile water for injection (no preservatives); 20-mg vial/20 ml or 50-mg vial/50 ml (1 mg/ml); mix by slow inversion or dilute with NaCl, D_5W to a concentration of 0.5 mg/ml further dilution; 1.5 to <0.5 mg/ml may result in precipitation of drug; use 18-gauge needle; flush line with NaCl after administration; use reconstituted **IV** sol within 8 hr, within 6 hr of coronary occlusion for best results
- Do not use 150 mg or more total dose; intracranial bleeding may occur
- Give heparin therapy after thrombolytic therapy is discontinued and when TT, ACT, and APTT less than 2 times control (about 3-4 hr)
- Avoid invasive procedures, inj, rec temp; apply pressure for 30 sec to minor bleeding sites; 30 min to sites of atrial puncture, followed by pressure dressing; inform prescriber if this does not attain hemostasis; apply pressure dressing
- Store powder at room temperature or refrigerate; protect from excessive light

Y-site incompatibilities:
Dobutamine, dopamine, heparin, nitroglycerin

Y-site compatibilities:
Lidocaine, metoprolol, propranolol

P ***Additive compatibilities:***
Lidocaine, morphine, nitroglycerin

Patient/family education

- Teach patient reason for alteplase, signs and symptoms of bleeding, allergic reactions, when to notify prescriber

Evaluation

Positive therapeutic outcome

- Lysis of pulmonary thrombi
- Adequate hemodynamic state
- Absence of congestive heart failure

altretamine (℞)

(al-tret'a-meen)

Hexalen, hexamethylmelamine

Func. class.: Misc. antineoplastic

Chem. class.: *S*-Triazine derivative (formerly known as hexamethylmelamine)

Pregnancy category D

Action: Products of metabolism form covalent bonds with tissue macromolecules including DNA, which may be responsible for cytotoxicity; activity is not cell cycle phase specific

➔ **Therapeutic Outcome:** Prevention of rapid growth of malignant cells

Uses: Palliative treatment of recurrent, persistent ovarian cancer following first-line treatment with cisplatin or alkylating agent–based combination

Dosage and routes

Adult: PO 260 mg/m^2 day for 14 or 21 days in a 28-day cycle; give in 4 divided doses pc and hs

Available forms: Caps 50, 100 ✦ mg

Adverse effects

CNS: Peripheral sensory neuropathy, fatigue, ***seizures,*** mood disorders, disorders of consciousness, ataxia, dizziness, vertigo

*GI: **Nausea, anorexia, vomiting,*** increased alkaline phosphatase, ***hepatic toxicity***

GU: Increased BUN, serum creatinine

*HEMA: **Leukopenia, thrombocytopenia, anemia***

INTEG: Rash, pruritus, alopecia

Contraindications: Hypersensitivity, severe bone marrow depression, severe neurologic toxicity

Precautions: Pregnancy **D**, P lactation, children

Pharmacokinetics

Absorption	Well
Distribution	Concentrated in liver, kidneys, small intestine
Metabolism	Liver (99%)
Excretion	Kidneys
Half-life	4½-10½ hrs

Pharmacodynamics

Onset	Unknown
Peak	½-3 hr
Duration	Unknown

Interactions

Individual drugs

Cimetidine: ↑ toxicity

Radiation: ↑ toxicity

Drug classifications

Antineoplastics: ↑ bone marrow depression

MAOI: ↑ orthostatic hypotension

NURSING CONSIDERATIONS

Assessment

- Monitor CBC, differential, platelet count weekly; withhold drug if WBC is <4000 or platelet count is <75,000; granulocytes <1000 mm^3, notify prescriber of results; nadir (leukopenia/ thrombocytopenia) occurs in 1 mo; resolves in 6 wk
- Monitor renal function studies: BUN, serum uric acid, urine CrCl before, during therapy; I&O ratio; report fall in urine output of 30 ml/hr; monitor for decreased hyperuricemia

- Monitor for cold, fever, sore throat (may indicate beginning infection)
- Assess for bleeding: hematuria, guaiac, bruising or petechiae, mucosa or orifices q8h; no rec temp; identify inflammation of mucosa, breaks in skin; use viscous lidocaine (Xylocaine) for oral pain
- Identify food preferences; list likes, dislikes
- Identify edema in feet, joint or stomach pain, shaking
- Assess neurologic status: paresthesia, numbness, tingling; pyridoxine may minimize neurologic reaction

Nursing diagnoses

- ✓ Injury, risk for (adverse reactions)
- ✓ Infection, risk for (adverse reactions)
- ✓ Knowledge deficit (teaching)

Implementation

- Give 1 hr before or 2 hr after meals to lessen nausea and vomiting or antacid before oral agent; give drug after evening meal, before bedtime; antiemetic 30-60 min before giving drug to prevent vomiting
- Antibiotics for prophylaxis of infection may be prescribed, since infection potential is high
- Store in tight container

Patient/family education

- Tell patient that contraceptive measures are recommended during therapy; teratogenic effects occur
- Teach patient to avoid use of products containing alcohol, aspirin, or ibuprofen, razors, hard bristle toothbrush, and commercial mouthwash because bleeding may occur; to report symptoms of bleeding (hematuria, tarry stools)
- Tell patient to report signs of anemia, (fatigue, headache, irritability, faintness, shortness of breath)
- Tell patient to report any changes in breathing or coughing even several months after treatment
- Tell patient that hair may be lost during treatment; a wig or hairpiece may make patient feel better; new hair may be different in color, texture
- Advise patient to avoid vaccinations during treatment; serious reactions may occur
- Teach patient to report signs/symptoms of infection: fever, chills, sore throat; patient should avoid crowds and persons with known infections

Evaluation

Positive therapeutic outcome

- Decreased size and spread of malignancy

aluminum acetate (OTC)

Bluboro Powder, Boropak Powder, Burow's Solution, Domeboro, Modified Burow's Solution, Pedi-Boro Soak Paks

Func. class.: Astringent (topical)

Chem. class.: Aluminum product

Pregnancy category C

Action: Maintains skin acidity, which is protective to skin surface; an astringent

➡ **Therapeutic Outcome:** Soothing of skin irritation, decreased skin inflammation

Uses: Skin irritation, inflammation, athlete's foot, insect bites, poison ivy, eczema, acne, rash, bruises, pruritus (anal)

Dosage and routes

P ***Adult and child:*** TOP apply for 15-30 min, q4-8h (1 : 10-40 sol); gargle use 1 : 10 sol prn

Available forms: Sol packets (1 : 40 sol); tabs for dissolving (1 : 20, 1 : 40 sol); cream ♣

Adverse effects

INTEG: Irritation, increasing inflammation

Contraindications: Tight, occlusive dressing

Precautions: Pregnancy **C**

Pharmacokinetics

Absorption	Not usually absorbed
Distribution	Unknown
Metabolism	Unknown
Excretion	Unknown
Half-life	Unknown

Pharmacodynamics

	TOP
Onset	Immediately
Peak	Unknown
Duration	Unknown

Interactions

Individual drugs

Collagenase: Blocks action of collagenase

Soap: ↓ action of aluminum acetate

NURSING CONSIDERATIONS

Assessment

• Check area of body to receive top application for irritation, rash breaks, dryness, lesions, excoriation, drainage

Nursing diagnoses

✓ Skin integrity, impaired (uses)
✓ Pain (uses)
✓ Knowledge deficit (teaching)

Implementation

Top route

• Mix 1 packet in 1 pt water (1:10-40 warm water); apply wet dressings loosely; do not use precipitate or occlusive dressings; sol is stable for 1 wk at room temperature

• Apply sol and dressings to ⅓ of body at a time; provide bath blanket to prevent chilling to the rest of the body

Patient/family education

• Instruct patient to discontinue use if irritation occurs or becomes worse

• Instruct patient to avoid using near eye area, mucous membranes

• Teach patient or family members on use of sol

Evaluation

Positive therapeutic outcome

• Decreased skin irritation, pain, inflammation

aluminum hydroxide (OTC)

Alterna GEL, Alu-Cap, Alugel ♣, Aluminett, Aluminum Hydroxide, Aluminum Hydroxide Gel, Alu-Tab, Amphojel, concentrated aluminum hydroxide, Nephrox

Func. class.: Antacid-hypophosphatemic

Chem. class.: Aluminum product

Pregnancy category C

Action: Neutralizes gastric acidity, binds phosphates in GI tract; these phosphates are excreted

Uses: Peptic, gastric, duodenal ulcers; hyperphosphatemia in chronic renal failure; reflux esophagitis, hyperacidity

A

Investigational uses: stress ulcer, GI bleeding

Therapeutic Outcome: Decreased acidity, healing of ulcers; decreased phosphate levels in chronic renal failure

Dosage and routes

Adult: SUSP 5-10 ml 1 hr pc, hs; PO 600 mg 1 hr pc, hs, chewed with milk or water

GI bleeding

P ***Infant:*** PO 2-5 ml/dose q1-2h

P ***Child:*** PO 5-15 ml/dose q1-2h

Hyperphosphatemia in renal failure

Adult: Susp 500 mg-2 g bid-qid

Available forms

Caps 475, 500 mg; tabs 300, 500 mg; chewable tabs 600 mg; susp (4%) 600 mg/5 ml; liq 320 mg/5 ml, 600 mg/5 ml

Adverse effects

GI: Constipation, anorexia, ***obstruction,*** fecal impaction

META: Hypophosphatemia, hypercalciuria

Contraindications: Hypersensitivity to this drug or aluminum products, abdominal pain of unknown origin

G **Precautions:** Elderly, fluid restriction, decreased GI motility, GI obstruction, dehydration, renal disease, sodium-restricted diets, pregnancy **C**

Pharmacokinetics

Absorption	Not usually absorbed
Distribution	Widely distributed if absorbed; crosses placenta
Metabolism	Unknown
Excretion	Feces, kidneys (small amounts), breast milk
Half-life	Unknown

Pharmacodynamics

Onset	20-40 min
Peak	½ hr
Duration	½-3 hr

Interactions

Individual drugs

Amphetamine: ↑ levels
Chlorpromazine: ↓ absorption
Isoniazid: ↓ absorption
Mexiletine: ↑ levels
Quinidine: ↑ levels
Salicylate: ↓ levels
Tetracycline: ↓ absorption

NURSING CONSIDERATIONS

Assessment

- Assess pain symptoms: location, duration, intensity, alleviating precipitating factors
- Monitor phosphate levels, since drug is bound in GI system; urinary pH, calcium, electrolytes; hypophosphatemia: anorexia, weakness, fatigue, bone pain, hyperreflexia
- Monitor constipation; increase bulk in diet if needed

Nursing diagnoses

✓ Pain, chronic (uses)
✓ Constipation (adverse reactions)
✓ Knowledge deficit (teaching)

Implementation

- Give laxatives or stool softeners if constipation occurs, G especially elderly
- Give after shaking liq; follow with water to facilitate passage
- Tab may be chewed if patient is unable to swallow; drink 8 oz of water after chewing; or by nasogastric tube if patient unable to swallow
- Give 1 hr before or after other medications to prevent poor absorption

• Give 15 ml 30 min pc and hs (esophagitis)
• May be given as prescribed q1-2 hr and given by gastric tube after diluting with water (peptic ulcer)

Patient/family education
• Instruct patient to increase fluids to 2000 ml/day unless contraindicated
• Instruct patient to avoid phosphate foods (most dairy products, eggs, fruits, carbonated beverages) during drug therapy; to add cheese, corn, pasta, plums, prunes, lentils after drug (hypophosphatemia)
• Instruct patient not to use for prolonged periods if serum phosphate is low or if on a low-sodium diet; CHF patients should check for sodium content and use sodium-reduced products
• Instruct patient that stools may appear white or speckled; constipation may result; to report black tarry stools, which indicate gastric bleeding
• Instruct patient to check with prescriber after 2 wk of self-prescribed antacid use; may be used for 4-6 wk after symptoms subside or as prescribed

Evaluation
Positive therapeutic outcome
• Absence of pain, decreased acidity
• Increased pH of gastric secretions
• Decreased phosphate levels

amantadine (℞)
(a-man'ta-deen)
amantadine HCl, Symadine, Symmetrel
Func. class.: Antiviral, antiparkinsonian agent
Chem. class.: Tricyclic amine
Pregnancy category C

Action: Prevents uncoating of nucleic acid in viral cell, preventing penetration of virus to host; causes release of dopamine from neurons

➔ **Therapeutic Outcome:** Decreased Parkinson's symptoms, decreased symptoms of influenza type A or prevention

Uses: Prophylaxis or treatment of influenza type A, extrapyramidal reactions, parkinsonism, respiratory tract infections

Investigational uses: Neuroleptic malignant syndrome, cocaine dependency, enuresis

Dosage and routes
Influenza type A
P ***Adult and child >12 yr:*** PO 200 mg/day in single dose or divided bid
P ***Child 9-12 yr:*** PO 100 mg bid
P ***Child 1-9 yr:*** PO 4.4-8.8 mg/kg/day divided bid-tid, not to exceed 200 mg/day

Extrapyramidal reaction/ parkinsonism
Adult: PO 100 mg bid, up to 400 mg/day in EPS; give for 1 wk then 100 mg as needed up to 400 mg in parkinsonism

Available forms: Caps 100 mg; syr 50 mg/5 ml

A

Adverse effects

CNS: Headache, dizziness, drowsiness, fatigue, anxiety, psychosis, depression, hallucinations, tremors, ***convulsions***
CV: Orthostatic hypotension, ***CHF***
EENT: Blurred vision
GI: Nausea, vomiting, constipation, dry mouth
GU: Frequency, retention
HEMA: ***Leukopenia***
INTEG: Photosensitivity, dermatitis

Contraindications: Hypersensitivity, lactation, P child <1 yr, eczematic rash

Precautions: Epilepsy, CHF, orthostatic hypotension, psychiatric disorders, hepatic disease, renal disease, peripheral edema, pregnancy **C**

Pharmacokinetics

Absorption	Well absorbed
Distribution	Crosses blood-brain barrier
Metabolism	Not metabolized
Excretion	Kidneys (90%) unchanged, breast milk
Half-life	24 hr

Pharmacodynamics

Onset	48 hr
Peak	2 wk
Duration	Unknown

Interactions

Individual drugs

Atropine: ↑ anticholinergic effects
Disopyramide: ↑ anticholinergic effects
Quinidine: ↑ anticholinergic effects

Drug classifications

Antidepressants, tricylic: ↑ anticholinergic effects
Antihistamines: ↑ anticholinergic effects
Phenothiazines: ↑ anticholinergic effects

NURSING CONSIDERATIONS

Assessment

- Assess for Parkinson's symptoms: tremors, akinesia, rigidity, impaired motor movements; as drug therapy continues, these symptoms should lessen
- Assess for drug toxicity: tremors, convulsions, lability, dysrhythmias; drug should be discontinued and physostigmine given
- Assess for symptoms of influenza A: increased temperature, malaise, aches and pains
- Monitor I&O ratio; report frequency, hesitancy, bowel pattern before, during treatment
- Check for mottling of skin (livedo reticularis), which disappears after several weeks of treatment
- Assess for skin eruptions, photosensitivity after administration of drug
- Monitor respiratory status: rate, character, wheezing, tightness in chest
- Assess for allergies before initiation of treatment, reaction of each medication

Nursing diagnoses

✓ Infection, risk for (uses)
✓ Knowledge deficit (teaching)

Implementation

- Give before exposure to influenza; continue for 10 days after contact
- Give at least 4 hr before hs to prevent insomnia
- Administer after meals for better absorption, to decrease GI symptoms; caps may be opened and mixed with food for easy swallowing

- Give in divided doses to prevent CNS disturbances: headache, dizziness, fatigue, drowsiness
- Store in tight, dry container

Patient/family education

- Teach patient to change body position slowly to prevent orthostatic hypotension
- Teach patient about aspects of drug therapy: the need to report dyspnea, weight gain, dizziness, poor concentration, dysuria, behavioral changes
- Teach patient to avoid hazardous activities if dizziness, blurred vision occur
- Teach patient to take drug exactly as prescribed; parkinsonian crisis may occur if drug is discontinued abruptly; drug should be tapered slowly
- Tell patient to avoid alcohol, OTC medications until discussed with prescriber, serious side effects can occur

Evaluation

Positive therapeutic outcome

- Absence of fever, malaise, cough, dyspnea in influenza A
- Decreased tremors, shuffling gait in Parkinson's disease, extrapyramidal symptoms

Treatment of overdose: Withdraw drug, maintain airway, administer epinephrine, aminophylline, O_2 IV corticosteroids, physostigmine

amifostine (℞)

(a-mi-foss'teen)

Ethyol

Func. class.: Cytoprotective agent for cisplatin

Pregnancy category C

Action: Binds and detoxifies damaging metabolites of cisplatin by converting this drug by aklaline phosphatase in tissue to an active free thiol compound

➔ Therapeutic Outcome: Decreased toxic reaction from cisplatin

Uses: Used to reduce renal toxicity when cisplatin is given in ovarian cancer

Dosage and routes

Adult: **IV** 910 mg/m² qd, within ½ hr before chemotherapy

Available forms: Powder for inj 500 mg/vial with 500 mg mannitol

Adverse effects

CNS: Dizziness, somnolence
CV: Hypotension
EENT: Sneezing
GI: Nausea, vomiting, hiccups
INTEG: Flushing
MISC: Hypocalcemia, rash, chills

Contraindications: Hypersensitivity to mannitol, aminothiol; hypotension, dehydration, lactation

G P Precautions: Elderly, CV disease, pregnancy **C,** children

Pharmacokinetics

Absorption	Complete
Distribution	Unknown
Metabolism	To free thiol compound
Excretion	Unknown
Half-life	8 min

Pharmacodynamics

Unknown

Interactions

Drug classfications

Antihypertensives: ↑ hypotension

NURSING CONSIDERATIONS
Assessment

- Assess fluid status before administration; administer antiemetic prior to administration to prevent severe nausea and vomiting; also, dexamethasone 20 mg **IV** and a serotonin antagonist such as ondanestron or granisetron
- Monitor calcium levels before and during treatment; calcium supplements may be given for low calcium levels
- Monitor blood pressure prior to and q5 min during infusion; if severe hypotension occurs, give **IV** 0.9% NaCl to expand fluid volume, place in Trendelenburg position

Nursing diagnoses

✓ Injury, risk for (uses)
✓ Knowledge deficit (teaching)

Implementation

IV • Give by **IV** intermittent INF after reconstituting with 9.5 ml of sterile 0.9% NaCl, further dilute with 0.9% NaCl to a concentration of 5-40 mg/ml, give at a rate over 15 min within ½ hr of chemotherapy

Additive incompatibilities: Do not mix with other drugs or solutions

Patient/family education

- Teach reason for medication and expected results
- Teach that side effects may cause severe nausea, vomiting, decreased B/P, chills, dizziness, somnolence, hiccups, sneezing

Evaluation

Positive therapeutic outcome

- Absence of renal damage

amikacin (℞)

(am-i-kay'sin)

amikacin sulfate, Amikin

Func. class.: Antibiotic

Chem. class.: Aminoglycoside

Pregnancy category D

Action: Interferes with protein synthesis in bacterial cell by binding to ribosomal subunit, which causes misreading of genetic code; inaccurate peptide sequence forms in protein chain, causing bacterial death

➔ **Therapeutic Outcome:** Bactericidal effects for the following organisms: *Pseudomonas aeruginosa, Escherichia coli, Enterobacter, Acinetobacter, Providencia, Citrobacter, Staphylococcus, Serratia, Proteus*

Uses: Severe systemic infections of CNS, respiratory, GI, urinary tract, bone, skin, soft tissues

Investigational uses: Mycobacterium avium complex (intrathecal or intraventricular)

Dosage and routes
Severe systemic infections

P ***Adult and child:*** **IV** inf 15 mg/kg/day in 2-3 divided doses q8-12h in 100-200 ml D_5W over 30-60 min, not to exceed 1.5 g; decreased dosages are needed in poor renal function as determined by blood levels, renal function studies; IM 15 mg/kg/day in divided doses q8-12h

P ***Neonates:*** **IV** inf 10 mg/kg initially, then 7.5 mg/kg q12h in D_5W over 1-2 hr

Severe urinary tract infections
Adults: IM 250 mg bid
Adults with poor renal function: 7.5 mg/kg initially, then increased as determined by blood levels, renal function studies

Available forms: Inj IM, **IV** 50, 250 mg/ml

Adverse effects
CNS: Confusion, depression, numbness, tremors, ***convulsions,*** muscle twitching, ***neurotoxicity,*** dizziness, vertigo, tinnitus
CV: Hypotension or hypertension, palpitations
EENT: ***Ototoxicity,*** deafness, visual disturbances
GI: Nausea, vomiting, anorexia, increased ALT (SGPT), AST (SGOT), bilirubin, hepatomegaly, ***hepatic necrosis,*** splenomegaly
GU: ***Oliguria, hematuria, renal damage, azotemia, renal failure, nephrotoxicity***
HEMA: ***Agranulocytosis, thrombocytopenia, leukopenia, eosinophilia, anemia***
INTEG: Rash, burning, urticaria, dermatitis, alopecia

Contraindications: Mild to moderate infections, hypersensitivity to aminoglycosides

P ***Precautions:*** Neonates, mild renal disease, pregnancy **D,** myasthenia gravis, lactation, hearing deficits, Parkinson's
G disease, elderly

Pharmacokinetics

Absorption	Well absorbed (IM), complete absorbed (IV)
Distribution	Widely distributed in extracellular fluids, poor in CSF; crosses placenta
Metabolism	Minimal; liver
Excretion	Mostly unchanged (79%) in kidneys
Half-life	2-3 hr; increased in renal disease

Pharmacodynamics

	IM	IV
Onset	Rapid	Rapid
Peak	1-2 hr	1-2 hr

Interactions
Individual drugs
Amphotericin B: ↑ ototoxicity, neurotoxicity, nephrotoxicity
Cisplatin: ↑ ototoxicity, neurotoxicity, nephrotoxicity
Ethacrynic acid: ↑ ototoxicity, neurotoxicity, nephrotoxicity
Furosemide: ↑ ototoxicity, neurotoxicity, nephrotoxicity
Mannitol: ↑ ototoxicity, neurotoxicity, nephrotoxicity
Methoxyflurane: ↑ ototoxicity, neurotoxicity, nephrotoxicity
Polymyxin: ↑ ototoxicity, neurotoxicity, nephrotoxicity
Succinylcholine: ↑ neuromuscular blockade, respiratory depression
Vancomycin: ↑ ototoxicity, neurotoxicity, nephrotoxicity
Drug classifications
Anesthetics: ↑ neuromuscular blockade, respiratory depression
Aminoglycosides: ↑ ototoxicity, neurotoxicity, nephrotoxicity
Nondepolarizing neuromuscular blockers: ↑ neuromuscular blockade, respiratory depression

NURSING CONSIDERATIONS

Assessment

- Assess patient for previous sensitivity reaction
- Assess patient for signs and symptoms of infection, including characteristics of wounds, sputum, urine, stool, WBC >10,000, earache, temp; obtain baseline information and during treatment
- Obtain culture and sensitivity tests before beginning drug therapy to identify if correct treatment has been initiated
- Assess for allergic reactions: rash, urticaria, pruritus
- Identify urine output; if decreasing, notify prescriber (may indicate nephrotoxicity); also notify prescriber of increased BUN and creatinine, urine CrCl <80 ml/min; lower dosage should be given in renal impairment; urinalysis daily for protein, cells, casts
- Monitor blood studies: AST, ALT, CBC, Hct, bilirubin, LDH, alkaline phosphatase; Coombs' test monthly if patient is on long-term therapy
- Monitor electrolytes: potassium, sodium, chloride, magnesium monthly if patient is on long-term therapy
- Assess bowel pattern qd; if severe diarrhea occurs, drug should be discontinued
- Monitor for bleeding: ecchymosis, bleeding gums, hematuria, stool guaiac daily if on long-term therapy
- Assess for overgrowth of infection: perineal itching, fever, malaise, redness, pain, swelling, drainage, rash, diarrhea, change in cough, sputum
- Obtain weight before treatment; calculation of dosage is usually based on ideal body weight, but may be calculated on actual body weight
- Monitor VS during infusion, watch for hypotension, change in pulse
- Assess **IV** site for thrombophlebitis including pain, redness, swelling q30 min; change site if needed; apply warm compresses to discontinued site
- Obtain serum peak, drawn 30-60 min after IV infusion or 60 min after IM injection; trough level drawn just before next dose; blood level should be 2-4 times bacteriostatic level
- Urine pH if drug is used for UTI; urine should be kept alkaline
- Deafness by audiometric testing, ringing, roaring in ears, vertigo; assess hearing before, during, after treatment
- Dehydration: high sp gr, decrease in skin turgor, dry mucous membranes, dark urine
- Vestibular dysfunction: nausea, vomiting, dizziness, headache; drug should be discontinued if severe

Nursing diagnoses

- ✓ Infection, risk for (uses)
- ✓ Diarrhea (side effects)
- ✓ Knowledge deficit (teaching)
- ✓ Injury, risk for (side effects)

Implementation

IM route

- Give deeply in large muscle mass

IV route

- Dilute 500 mg of drug in 100-200 ml of **IV** D_5W, D_5NaCl or 0.9% NaCl and give over ½-1 hr; flush after administration with D_5W or 0.9% NaCl

Syringe compatibilities: Clindamycin, doxapram

Y-site compatibilities: Acyclovir, amifostine, amiodarone, amsacrine, aztreonam, cyclophosphamide, diltiazem, enalamprilat, esmolol, filgrastim, fluconazole, fludarabine, foscarnet, furosemide, idarubicin, IL-2, labetalol, lorazepam, magnesium sulfate, melphalan, midazolam, morphine, ondansetron, paclitaxel, perphenazine, sargramostim, teniposide, thiotepa, TPN #54, #61, #91, vinorelbine, zidovudine

Additive compatibilities: Amobarbital, ascorbic acid inj, bleomycin, calcium chloride, calcium gluconate, cesepime, cefoxitin, chloramphenicol, chlorpheniramine, cimetidine, ciprofloxacin, clindamycin, cloxacillin, colistimethate, dimenhydrinate, diphenhydramine, epinephrine, ergonovine, fluconazole, furosemide, hydraluronidase, hydrocorticose, lincomycin, metaraminol, metronidazole, norepinephrine, pentobarbital, phenobarbital, phytonadione, polymyxin B, prochlorperazine, ranitidine, secobarbital, sodium bicarbonate, succinylcholine, vancomycin, verapamil

Patient/family education

- Teach patient to report sore throat, bruising, bleeding, joint pain; may indicate blood dyscrasias (rare)
- Advise patient to contact prescriber if vaginal itching, loose foul-smelling stools, furry tongue occur; may indicate superinfection

Evaluation

Positive therapeutic outcome

- Absence of signs/symptoms of infection: WBC <10,000, temp WNL; absence of red draining wounds; absence of earache
- Reported improvement in symptoms of infection

Treatment of overdose: Withdraw drug; administer epinephrine, O_2, hemodialysis, **P** exchange transfusion in the newborn; monitor serum levels of drug; may give ticarcillin or carbenicillin

amiloride (℞)

(a-mill'oh-ride)

Amiloride HCl, Midamor

Func. class.: Potassium-sparing diuretic

Chem. class.: Pyrazine

Pregnancy category B

Action: Acts primarily on proximal distal tubule by inhibiting reabsorption of sodium and water and increasing potassium retention and conserving hydrogen ions

➔ **Therapeutic Outcome:** Diuretic and antihypertensive effect while retaining potassium

Uses: Diuretic-induced hypokalemia; used with other agents to treat edema, hypertension

Investigational uses: Cystic fibrosis (INH), lithium-induced polyuria

Dosage and routes

Adult: PO 5 mg qd; may be increased to 10-20 mg qd if needed

Available forms: Tabs 5 mg

Adverse effects

CNS: Headache, dizziness,

fatigue, weakness, paresthesias, tremor, depression, anxiety
CV: Orthostatic hypotension, dysrhythmias, angina
EENT: Loss of hearing, tinnitus, blurred vision, nasal congestion, increased intraocular pressure
ELECT: ***Hyperkalemia***
GI: Nausea, diarrhea, dry mouth, *vomiting, anorexia,* cramps, constipation, abdominal pain, jaundice, bleeding
GU: Polyuria, dysuria, frequency, impotence
HEMA: Aplastic anemia, neutroperia (rare)
INTEG: Rash, pruritus, alopecia, urticaria
RESP: Cough, dyspnea, shortness of breath

Contraindications: Anuria, hypersensitivity, hyperkalemia, impaired renal function

Precautions: Dehydration, pregnancy **B,** diabetes, acidosis, lactation, hepatic disease

Pharmacokinetics

Absorption	Variable (10%-15%)
Distribution	Unknown
Metabolism	Unchanged in urine (50%) in feces (40%)
Excretion	Renal; breast milk
Half-life	6-9 hr

Pharmacodynamics

Onset	2 hr
Peak	6-10 hr
Duration	24 hr

Interactions

Drug classifications

ACE inhibitors: ↑ hyperkalemia
Antihypertensives: ↑ action
Diuretics, potassium-sparing: ↑ hyperkalemia
NSAIDs: ↓ effectiveness of amiloride
Potassium products: ↑ hyperkalemia
Salt substitutes: ↑ hyperkalemia

Food

Potassium foods: ↑ hyperkalemia

Lab test interferences

Interference: GTT

NURSING CONSIDERATIONS

Assessment

- Monitor manifestations of hyperkalemia: *MS:* fatigue, muscle weakness; *CARDIAC:* dysrhythmias, hypotension; *NEURO:* paresthesias, confusion; *RESP:* dyspnea
- Monitor for manifestations of hyponatremia: *CV:* increased B/P, cold, clammy skin, hypovolemia or hypervolemia; *GI:* anorexia, nausea, vomiting, diarrhea, abdominal cramps; *NEURO:* lethargy, increased ICP, confusion, headache, seizures, coma, fatigue, tremors, hyperreflexia
- Monitor for manifestations of hyperchloremia: *NEURO:* weakness, lethargy, coma; *RESP:* deep rapid breathing
- Assess fluid volume status: I&O ratios and record, weight, distended red veins, crackles in lung, color, quality and sp gr of urine, skin turgor, adequacy of pulses, moist mucous membranes, bilateral lung sounds, peripheral pitting edema; dehydration symptoms of decreasing output, thirst, hypotension, dry mouth and mucous membranes should be reported
- Monitor electrolytes: potassium, sodium, calcium, magnesium; also include BUN, ABGs, uric acid, CBC, blood sugar

- Assess B/P before and during therapy with patient lying, standing, and sitting as appropriate; orthostatic hypotension can occur rapidly

Nursing diagnoses

- ✓ Fluid volume deficit (side effects)
- ✓ Fluid volume excess (uses)
- ✓ Knowledge deficit (teaching)

Implementation

- Give in AM to avoid interference with sleep
- With food; if nausea occurs, absorption may be increased

Patient/family education

General

- Teach patient to take medication early in the day to prevent nocturia
- Instruct patient to take with food or milk if GI symptoms of nausea and anorexia occur
- Teach patient to maintain a weekly record of weight and notify prescriber of weight loss >5 lb
- Caution patient that this drug causes an increase in potassium levels, so foods high in potassium should be avoided; refer to dietician for assistance, planning
- Caution patient not to exercise in hot weather or stand for prolonged periods since orthostatic hypotension will be enhanced
- Teach patient not to use alcohol or any OTC medications without prescriber's approval; serious drug reactions may occur
- Emphasize the need to contact prescriber immediately if muscle cramps, weakness, nausea, dizziness, or numbness occurs
- Teach patient to take own B/P and pulse and record
- Advise patient that dizziness and confusion may occur; avoid driving or other hazardous activities if alertness is decreased
- Teach patient to continue taking medication even if feeling better; this drug controls symptoms but does not cure the condition
- Advise patient with hypertension to continue other medical treatment (exercise, weight loss, relaxation techniques, cessation of smoking)

Evaluation

Positive therapeutic outcome

- Prevention of hypokalemia (diuretic use)
- Decreased edema
- Decreased B/P
- Increased diuresis

Treatment of overdose: Lavage if taken orally; monitor electrolytes; administer **IV** fluids; monitor hydration, CV, renal status

amino acid (℞)

(a-mee'noe)

Injection: Aminess, Aminosyn, BranchAmin, NephrAmine, FreAmine HBC, HepatAmine Solution: Aminosyn, Aminosyn II, Aminosyn-PF, FreAmine III, Novamine, ProcalAmine, RenAmin, Travasol, Trophamine

Func. class.: Caloric agent

Chem. class.: Nitrogen product

Pregnancy category C

Action: Needed for anabolism to maintain structure; decreases catabolism, promotes healing

Therapeutic Outcome: Positive nitrogen balance, decreased catabolism

Uses: Hepatic encephalopathy, cirrhosis, hepatitis, nutritional support in cancer trauma, intestinal obstruction, short bowel syndrome, severe malabsorption

Dosage and routes

Amino acid inj

Adult: **IV** 80-120 g/day; 500 ml of amino acids/500 ml D_{50} given over 24 hr

Amino acid solution

Adult: **IV** 1-1.5 g/kg/day titrated to patient's needs

P ***Child:*** **IV** 2-3 g/kg/day titrated to patient's needs

Available forms: Inj **IV** 2.75%, 3.5%, 4.25%, 5%, 5.5%, 6%, 8.5%, 10%, 11.4%, 15% amino acids

Adverse effects

CNS: Dizziness, headache, confusion, ***loss of consciousness***

CV: Hypertension, ***CHF, pulmonary edema***

ENDO: Hyperglycemia, rebound hypoglycemia, electrolyte imbalances, hyperosmolar syndrome, hyperosmolar hyperglycemic nonketotic syndrome, alkalosis, acidosis, hypophosphatemia, hyperammonemia, dehydration, hypocalcemia

GI: Nausea, vomiting, liver fat deposits, abdominal pain

GU: Glycosuria, osmotic diuresis

INTEG: Chills, flushing, warm feeling, rash, urticaria, extravasation necrosis, phlebitis at injection site

Contraindications: Hypersensitivity, severe electrolyte imbalances, anuria, severe liver damage, maple syrup urine disease, PKU

Precautions: Renal disease, P pregnancy **C,** children, diabetes mellitus, CHF

Pharmacokinetics

Absorption	Complete bioavailability
Distribution	Widely distributed
Metabolism	Anabolism
Excretion	Kidney to urea nitrogen
Half-life	Unknown

Pharmacodynamics

Unknown

Interactions

Drug classifications

Diuretics: ↑ negative nitrogen balance

Glucocorticoids: ↑ negative nitrogen balance

Tetracyclines: ↑ negative nitrogen balance

NURSING CONSIDERATIONS

Assessment

- Monitor electrolytes (potassium, sodium, calcium, chloride, magnesium), blood glucose, ammonia, phosphate, ketones; renal, liver function studies: BUN, creatinine, ALT (SGPT), AST (SGOT), bilirubin; urine glucose q6h using Chemstrips, which are not affected by infusion substances; if BUN increases over 15%, therapy may need to be discontinued
- Check injection site for extravasation: redness along vein, edema at site, necrosis, pain; for a hard, tender area
- Monitor respiratory function q4h: auscultate lung fields bilaterally for crackles; monitor respirations for quality, rate,

rhythm that indicates fluid overload
• Monitor temperature q4h for increased fever, indicating infection; if infection is suspected, infusion is discontinued and tubing bottle, catheter tip cultured; blood catheter may be obtained
• Monitor for impending hepatic coma: asterixis, confusion, fetor, lethargy
• Hyperammonemia: nausea, vomiting, malaise, tremors, anorexia, convulsions; increased ammonia, ketone levels may occur

Nursing diagnoses
- Nutrition, less than body requirements (uses)
- Injury, risk for physical (uses, adverse reactions)
- Infection, risk for (adverse reactions)
- Knowledge deficit (teaching)

Implementation
• Give up to 40% protein and dextrose (up to 12.5%) via peripheral vein; stronger solutions require central **IV** administration; TPN only mixed with dextrose to promote protein synthesis
• Use immediately after mixing in pharmacy under strict aseptic technique using laminar flowhood; use infusion pump, in-line filter (0.22 µm) unless mixed with fat emulsion and dextrose (3 in 1)
• Use careful monitoring technique; do not speed up infusion; pulmonary edema, glucose overload will result
• Storage depends on type of solution; consult manufacturer
• Change dressing and IV tubing to prevent infection q24-48h or q5-7 days if transparent dressing is used

Additive compatibility:
Epoetin alpha

Y-*site incompatibility:*
Cephradine

Y-*site compatibilities:*
Aminophylline, amoxicillin, ascorbic acid inj, atracurium, calcium gluconate, cefamandole, cefazolin, cefoperazone, cefotaxime, cefoxitin, ceftazidime, ceftriaxone, cephalothin, cephapirin, chloramphenicol, cimetidine, ciprofloxacin, clindamycin, clonazepam, diazepam, digoxin, dobutamine, dopamine, doxycycline, epinephrine, erythromycin lactobionate, fat emulsion, fluconazole, folic acid, foscarnet, furosemide, gentamicin, haloperidol, heparin, hydrocortisone, idarubicin, IL-2, insulin (regular), isoproterenol, kanamycin, lidocaine, meperidine, methicillin, mezlocillin, miconazole, morphine, moxalactam, multivitamins, nafcillin, netilmicin, norepinephrine, oxacillin, penicillin G potassium, piperacillin, potassium chloride, ranitidine, salbutamol, sargramostim, thiotepa, ticarcillin, tobramycin, urokinase, vancomycin, vecuronium

Patient/family education
• Teach reason for use of amino acids as part of nutrition (TPN)
• Instruct patient to report at once to prescriber if chills, sweating are experienced

Evaluation
Positive therapeutic outcome
• Weight gain
• Decreased jaundice in liver disorders
• Increased LOC

A

aminocaproic acid (℞)

(a-mee-noe-ka-proe'ik)

Amicar, aminocaproic acid

Func. class.: Hemostatic

Chem. class.: Synthetic monoaminocarboxylic acid

Pregnancy category C

Action: Inhibits fibrinolysis by inhibiting plasminogen activator substances

→ Therapeutic Outcome: Decreased fibrinolysis, decreased bleeding, increased clot formation

Uses: Hemorrhage from hyperfibrinolysis, adjunctive therapy in hemophilia, amegakaryocytic thrombocytopenia, hereditary angioneurotic edema

Investigational uses: Prevention of recurrent subarachnoid hemorrhage

Dosage and routes

Adult: PO/**IV** 5-g loading dose, then 1-1.25 g q1h if needed, not to exceed 30 g/day

Available forms: Inj 250 mg/ml; tabs 500 mg; syr 250 mg/ml

Adverse effects

CNS: Headache, dizziness, malaise, fatigue, hallucinations, delirium, psychosis, ***convulsions,*** weakness

CV: ***Dysrhythmias,*** orthostatic hypotension, bradycardia

EENT: Tinnitus, nasal congestion, conjunctival suffusion

GI: Nausea, vomiting, abdominal cramps, diarrhea

GU: Dysuria, frequency, oliguria, ***renal failure,*** ejaculatory failure, menstrual irregularities

HEMA: Thrombosis

INTEG: Rash

Contraindications: Hypersensitivity, abnormal bleeding, postpartum bleeding, DIC, upper urinary tract bleeding, new burns

P Precautions: Neonates/infants, mild or moderate renal disease, hepatic disease, thrombosis, cardiac disease, pregnancy **C**

Pharmacokinetics

Absorption	Well absorbed (PO)
Distribution	Widely distributed
Metabolism	Unknown
Excretion	Kidneys, unchanged
Half-life	Unknown

Pharmacodynamics

	PO/IV
Onset	Unknown
Peak	2 hr
Duration	Unknown

Interactions: None

Lab test interferences

↑ Potassium, ↑ CPK, ↑ AST (SGOT), ↑ aldolase

NURSING CONSIDERATIONS

Assessment

- Monitor I&O ratios if urinary output decreases; notify prescriber and stop drug
- Monitor blood studies: coagulation factors, platelets, protamine coagulation factors, platelets, protamine coagulation test for extravascular clotting, thrombophlebitis; creatinine phosphokinase; check for thromboembolic symptoms (leg pain, redness, positive Homans' sign) edema, dyspnea, chest pain
- Monitor B/P, pulse, respiratory status; watch for increasing B/P and pulse
- Monitor drug level: 0.13

mg/ml is required to decrease fibrinolysis
• Assess for allergy: fever, rash, itching, jaundice
• Monitor myopathy: if weakness, fever, myoglobinemia, or oliguria, discontinue drug; watch for increased CPK, AST (SGOT), aldolase
• Assess for bleeding q15 min: mucous membranes, epistaxis, ecchymosis, petechiae, hematuria, hematemesis
• Monitor neurologic status (LOC, pupils, motor status) in subarachnoid hemorrhage

Nursing diagnoses

✓ Tissue perfusion, altered (uses)
✓ Injury, risk for (uses, adverse reactions)
✓ Cardiac output (adverse reaction)
✓ Knowledge deficit (teaching)

Implementation

IV **IV route**
• Give **IV** after dilution with 4-5 g/250 ml NS, D_5W, LR; give over 1 hr; may give by cont inf after loading dose(s); use inf pump; do not give by direct IV; stabilize catheter to prevent thrombophlebitis

IV **Cont IV**
• May be diluted in 50 ml of diluent and run at 1 g/hr by inf pump
• Store in tight container in cool environment; do not freeze; do not mix with other drugs

Additive compatibility: Netilmicin

Patient/family education

• Instruct patient to report any signs of bleeding (gums, under skin, urine, stools, emesis) or myopathy
• Instruct patient to change position slowly to decrease orthostatic hypotension
• Teach patient proper administration for 8-10 days following dental procedure in hemophilia
• Instruct patient to inform physicians and dentists that drug is being taken

Evaluation

Positive therapeutic outcome
• Decreased bleeding
• Absence of rebleeding (subarachnoid hemorrhage)

aminoglutethimide (℞)

(a-meen-oh-gloo-teth'i-mide)

Cytadren

Func. class.: Antineoplastic, adrenal steroid inhibitor

Chem. class.: Hormone

Pregnancy category D

Action: Acts by inhibiting DNA, RNA, protein synthesis; is derived from *Streptomyces verticillus;* replication is decreased by binding to DNA, which causes strand splitting; phase specific in G_2 and M phases; blocks biosynthesis of all steroid hormones (cortisol, androgens, progestins)

➔ **Therapeutic Outcome:** Decreased spread of malignancy; decreased adrenal hormone in Cushing's syndrome

Uses: Suppression of adrenal function in Cushing's syndrome, metastatic breast cancer, adrenal cancer

Investigational uses: Advanced prostate cancer, metastatic postmenopausal breast cancer

Dosage and routes
Adult: PO 250 mg qid at 6-hr intervals; may increase by 250 mg/day q1-2 wk, not to exceed 2 g/day

Available forms: Tabs 250 mg

Adverse effects
CNS: Drowsiness, dizziness, headache, lethargy
CV: Hypotension, tachycardia
GI: Nausea, vomiting, anorexia, ***hepatotoxicity***
INTEG: Rash, pruritus, hirsutism, *morbilliform skin rash*

Contraindications: Hypersensitivity, hypothyroidism, pregnancy **D**

Precautions: Renal disease, hepatic disease, respiratory disease

Pharmacokinetics

Absorption	Well absorbed
Distribution	Unknown
Metabolism	Liver (50%)
Excretion	Kidneys, unchanged (50%)
Half-life	13 hr initially

Pharmacodynamics

Unknown

Interactions
Individual drugs
Alcohol: ↑ effects of aminoglutethimide
Dexamethasone: ↑ metabolism, ↓ effect of dexamethasone
Digitoxin: ↓ effects of digitoxin
Medroxyprogesterone: ↓ effects of medroxyprogesterone
Theophylline: ↓ effects of theophylline
Warfarin: ↓ effects of warfarin

NURSING CONSIDERATIONS
Assessment
- Monitor renal function studies: BUN, serum uric acid, urine CrCl, electrolytes before, during therapy; I&O ratio; report fall in urine output of 30 ml/hr
- Monitor temperature q4h; may indicate beginning infection
- Monitor liver function tests before, during therapy (bilirubin, AST, ALT, LDH) as needed or monthly; RBC, Hct, Hgb, since these may be decreased
- Monitor inflammation of mucosa, breaks in skin, yellowing of skin and sclera, dark urine, clay-colored stools, itchy skin, abdominal pain, fever, diarrhea
- Assess symptoms indicating severe allergic reaction: rash, pruritus, urticaria, purpuric skin lesions, itching, flushing; if rash develops, drug may need to be discontinued
- Assess for Cushing's syndrome: buffalo hump, moon face, personality changes, hypertension, weakness, hirsutism

Nursing diagnoses
- ✓ Injury, risk for (adverse reactions)
- ✓ Body image disturbance (adverse reactions)
- ✓ Infection, risk for (adverse reactions)
- ✓ Knowledge deficit (teaching)

Implementation
- Give with food or fluids for GI upset
- Give in equal intervals q6h

Patient/family education
- Instruct patient to report side effects
- Advise patient to avoid use

of alcohol, which potentiates this drug

Evaluation

Positive therapeutic outcome

- Prevention of rapid division of malignant cells, postmenopausal cancer, prostate cancer
- Suppression of adrenal function (Cushing's syndrome)

Treatment of overdose: Induce vomiting, provide supportive care

aminophylline (℞)

(am-in-off'i-lin)

Corophyllin ✦, Palaron ✦, Phyllocontin, Truphylline

Func. class.: Bronchodilator

Chem. class.: Xanthine, ethylenediamine

Pregnancy category C

Action: Relaxes smooth muscle of respiratory system by blocking phosphodiesterase, which increases cyclic AMP; increased cyclic AMP alters intracellular calcium ion movements; produces bronchodilatation, increased pulmonary blood flow, relaxation of respiratory tract

➔ **Therapeutic Outcome:** Increased ability to breathe

Uses: Bronchial asthma, bronchospasm, Cheyne-Stokes respirations

Investigational uses: Apnea in infancy for respiratory/myocardial stimulation, Cheyne-Stokes respirations as a respiratory stimulant [P]

Dosage and routes

Adult: PO 500 mg, then 250-500 mg q6-8h; cont **IV** 0.3-0.9 mg/kg/hr (maintenance); REC 500 mg q6-8h

[P] ***Child:*** PO 7.5 mg/kg, then 3-6 mg/kg q6-8h; **IV** 7.5 mg/kg, then 3-6 mg/kg q6-8h injected over 5 min; do not exceed 25 mg/min; may give loading dose of 5.6 mg/kg over ½ hr; cont **IV** 1 mg/kg/hr (maintenance); for [P] children/infants use drug without preservative of alcohol

[P] ***Neonates:*** **IV**/PO 1 mg/kg initially for plasma increases of each 2 μg/ml, then 1 mg/kg q6h

Available forms: Inj **IV**, IM, rec supp 250, 500 mg; oral liq 105 mg/5 ml; tabs 100, 200 mg; con-rel tabs 225 mg

Adverse effects

CNS: Anxiety, restlessness, insomnia, ***dizziness, convulsions,*** headache, lightheadedness, muscle twitching

CV: Palpitations, sinus tachycardia, hypotension, flushing, dysrhythmias, increased respiratory rate

GI: Nausea, vomiting, anorexia, diarrhea, bitter taste, dyspepsia, anal irritation (suppositories), epigastric pain

GU: Urinary frequency

INTEG: Flushing, urticaria, *rec supp (irritation)*

RESP: Increased rate

Contraindications: Hypersensitivity to xanthines, tachydysrhythmias

[G] **Precautions:** Elderly, CHF, cor pulmonale, hepatic disease, active peptic ulcer disease, diabetes mellitus, hyperthyroidism, hypertension, [P] children, pregnancy **C,** glaucoma, prostatic hypertrophy

Pharmacokinetics

Absorption	Well absorbed (PO), slow (PO–ext rel), erratic (rec)
Distribution	Widely distributed; crosses placenta
Metabolism	Liver to caffeine
Excretion	Kidneys
Half-life	3-12 hr, increased in renal disease, CHF

Pharmacodynamics

	PO	PO–EXT REL	IV
Onset	15-60 min	Unknown	Immediate
Peak	1-2 hr	4-7 hr	Infusion's end
Duration	6-8 hr	8-12 hr	6-8 hr

Interactions

Individual drugs

Allopurinol: ↓ metabolism, ↑ toxicity of aminophylline
Carbamazepine: ↑ or ↓ aminophylline levels
Cimetidine: ↓ metabolism, ↑ toxicity of aminophylline
Disulfiram: ↓ metabolism, ↑ toxicity of aminophylline
Erythromycin: ↓ metabolism, ↑ toxicity of aminophylline
Halothane: ↑ risk of dysrhythmias
Interferon: ↓ metabolism, ↑ toxicity of aminophylline
Isoniazid: ↑ or ↓ aminophylline level
Ketoconazole: ↑ metabolism, ↓ effect of aminophylline
Lithium: ↓ effect of lithium
Mexiletine: ↓ metabolism, ↑ toxicity
Phenytoin: ↑ metabolism, ↓ effect of aminophylline
Rifampin: ↑ metabolism, ↓ effect of aminophylline
Thiabendazole: ↓ metabolism, ↑ toxicity

Drug classifications

Barbiturates: ↓ effect of aminophylline
β-Adrenergic blockers: ↓ metabolism, ↑ toxicity
Diuretics, loop: ↑ or ↓ aminophylline levels
Fluoroquinolones: ↓ metabolism, ↑ toxicity
Glucocorticoids: ↓ metabolism, ↑ toxicity
Sympathomimetics: ↑ CNS, CV adverse reactions

Smoking

↑ metabolism, ↓ effect

Food

Caffeinated foods (cola, coffee, tea, chocolate): ↑ CNS, CV, adverse reactions
Charcoal-smoked foods: ↓ effect

Lab test interferences

↑Plasma free fatty acids

NURSING CONSIDERATIONS

Assessment

- Monitor theophylline blood levels (therapeutic level is 10-20 μg/ml); toxicity may occur with small increase above G 20 μg/ml, especially elderly; determine whether theophylline was given recently (24 hr); check for toxicity: nausea, vomiting, anxiety, restlessness, insomnia, tachycardia, dysrhythmias, convulsions; notify prescriber immediately
- Monitor I&O; diuresis will occur; dehydration may result G in elderly or children in whom P diuresis is great
- Monitor respiratory rate, rhythm, depth; auscultate lung fields bilaterally; notify prescriber of abnormalities; check ECG for tachycardia, PVCs, PACs in patients with cardiac problems
- Monitor allergic reactions: rash, urticaria; if these occur, drug should be discontinued, prescriber notified

Nursing diagnoses

- ✓ Airway clearance, ineffective (uses)
- ✓ Activity intolerance (uses)
- ✓ Injury, risk for (uses, adverse reactions)
- ✓ Knowledge deficit (teaching)

Implementation

General

- Give around the clock to maintain blood (theophylline) levels
- If switching from **IV** to PO, give controlled-release dose at time of **IV** infusion discontinuation; if giving tab (immediate release), discontinue **IV** and wait >4 hr

PO route

- Give PO after meals or water to decrease GI symptoms; absorption may be affected with a full glass of water or food
- Do not crush or chew enteric-coated or controlled-release tabs

IV route

- Give **IV** after diluting in 5% dextrose to decrease burning sensation at inj site; only clear solutions; may be diluted for IV inf in 100-200 ml in D_5W, $D_{10}W$, $D_{20}W$, 0.9% NaCl, 0.45% NaCl, LR

Syringe compatibilities: Heparin, metoclopramide, pentobarbital, thiopental

Y-site compatibilities: Amifostine, cimetidine, enalaprilat, esmolol, famotidine, filgrastim, fluconazole, fludarabine, foscarnet, heparin sodium with hydrocortisone sodium succinate, morphine, netilmicin, paclitaxel, pancuronium, potassium chloride, ranitidine, sargramostim, tacrolimus, teniposide, thiotepa, tolazoline, vecuronium, Vit B with C

Y-site incompatibilities: Dobutamine, hydralazine, ondansetron

Additive compatibilities: Amobarbital, bretylium, calcium gluconate, chloramphenicol, cimetidine, dexamethasone, diphenhydramine, dopamine, erythromycin lactobionate, esmolol, floxacillin, flumazenil, furosemide, heparin, hydrocortisone, lidocaine, methyldopate, metronidazole, nitroglycerin, pentobarbital, phenobarbital, potassium chloride, ranitidine, secobarbital, sodium bicarbonate, terbutaline

Additive incompatibilities: Ascorbic acid, bleomycin, cephalothin, cefotaxime, chlorpromazine, cimetidine, clindamycin, codeine, dimenhydrinate, dobutamine, doxorubicin, doxycycline, epinephrine, erythromycin gluceptate, hydralazine, hydroxyzine, insulin, isoproterenol, meperidine, methicillin, morphine, nafcillin, nitroprusside, norepinephrine, oxytetracycline, papaverine, penicillin G, pentazocine, phenobarbital, phenytoin, prochlorperazine, promazine, promethazine, sulfisoxazole, tetracycline, vancomycin

- Avoid IM injection; pain and tissue damage may occur
- Only clear sol; flush **IV** line before dose; store diluted sol for 24 hrs if refrigerated

Rectal route

- Rec dose if patient is unable to take PO; retain rec dose for ½ hour

Patient/family education

- Teach patient to take doses as prescribed, not to skip dose; to check OTC medications, current prescription medications for ephedrine which will increase CNS stimulation; advise patient not to drink alcohol or caffeine products (tea, coffee, chocolate, colas), which will increase action

- Teach patient to avoid hazardous activities; dizziness may occur
- Teach patient if GI upset occurs, to take drug with 8 oz water or food; absorption may be decreased
- Teach patient to remain in bed 15-20 min after rec supp is inserted to prevent removal
- Instruct patient that smoking increases metabolism; dosage may need to be increased
- Teach patient to obtain blood levels of drug every few months to prevent toxicity; not to change brands, since effect may not be the same
- Teach patient to increase fluids to 2 L/day to decrease viscosity of secretions

Evaluation

Positive therapeutic outcome

- Decreased dyspnea
- Respiratory stimulation in infants
- Clear lung fields bilaterally

amiodarone (℞)

(a-mee-o'da-rone)

Cordarone

Func. class.: Antidysrhythmic (Class III)

Chem. class.: Iodinated benzofuran derivative

Pregnancy category C

Action: Prolongs action potential duration and effective refractory period, slows sinus rate with increasing PR and QT intervals, noncompetitive α- and β-adrenergic inhibition

Therapeutic Outcome: Decreased amount and severity of ventricular dysrhythmias

Uses: Severe ventricular tachycardia, supraventricular tachycardia, ventricular fibrillation or atrial fibrillation not controlled by 1st-line agents

Dosage and routes

Adult: PO loading dose 800-1600 mg/day × 1-3 wk; then 600-800 mg/day × 1 mo; maintenance 200-600 mg/day

***Adult:* IV** loading dose (first rapid) 150 mg over the 1st 10 min (15 mg/min), add 3 ml (150 mg) to 100 ml D_5W, infuse 100 mg/ml, then slow 360 mg over the next 6 hr (1 mg/min), add 18 ml (900 mg) to 500 ml D_5W (1.8 mg/ml); maintenance at 540 mg given over the remaining 18 hr (0.5 mg/min), decrease rate of the slow inf to 0.5 mg/min

Available forms: Tabs 200 mg; inj 50 mg/ml

Adverse effects

CNS: Headache, dizziness, involuntary movement, tremors, peripheral neuropathy, malaise, fatigue, ataxia, paresthesias, insomnia

CV: Hypotension, bradycardia, ***sinus arrest, CHF, dysrhythmias, SA node dysfunction***

EENT: Blurred vision, halos, photophobia, ***corneal microdeposits,*** dry eyes

ENDO: Hyperthyroidism or hypothyroidism

GI: Nausea, vomiting, diarrhea, abdominal pain, anorexia, constipation, ***hepatotoxicity***

INTEG: Rash, photosensitivity, blue-gray skin discoloration,

alopecia, spontaneous ecchymosis
MISC: Flushing, abnormal taste or smell, edema, abnormal salivation, coagulation abnormalities
MS: Weakness, pain in extremities
RESP: Pulmonary fibrosis, pulmonary inflammation

Contraindications: Sinus node dysfunction; 2nd, 3rd degree AV block

Precautions: Goiter, Hashimoto's thyroiditis, SN dysfunction, 2nd- or 3rd-degree AV block, electrolyte imbalances, pregnancy **C,** bradycardia, lactation

Pharmacokinetics

Absorption	Slow, variable (PO) up to 65%
Distribution	Body tissues; crosses placenta
Metabolism	Liver
Excretion	Bile, kidney (minimal)
Half-life	15-100 days

Pharmacodynamics

	PO
Onset	1-3 wk
Peak	Unknown
Duration	Up to months

Interactions

Individual drugs

Digoxin: ↑ blood levels,↑ toxicity
Disopyramide: ↑ levels, ↑ toxicity
Flecainide: ↑ levels, ↑ toxicity
Lidocaine: Bradycardia, cardiac arrest
Mexiletine: ↑ levels, ↑ toxicity
Phenytoin: ↑ blood levels
Procainamide: ↑ levels, ↑ toxicity
Quinidine: ↑ levels, ↑ toxicity
Warfarin: ↑ level, ↑ bleeding

Drug classifications

β-Blockers: ↑ dysrhythmias, cardiac arrest
Calcium channel blockers: ↑ dysrhythmias, cardiac arrest

Lab test interference:

↑ T_4

NURSING CONSIDERATIONS

Assessment

- Monitor I&O ratio; monitor electrolytes: potassium, sodium, chloride
- Monitor chest x-ray, thyroid function tests
- Monitor liver function studies: AST (SGOT), ALT (SGPT), bilirubin, alkaline phosphatase
- Monitor ECG continuously to determine drug effectiveness; measure PR, QRS, QT intervals; check for PVCs, other dysrhythmias; monitor B/P continuously for hypotension, hypertension; check for rebound hypertension after 1-2 hr
- Monitor for dehydration or hypovolemia
- Assess for CNS symptoms: confusion, psychosis, numbness, depression, involuntary movements; if these occur, drug should be discontinued
- Assess for hypothyroidism: lethargy, dizziness, constipation, enlarged thyroid gland, edema of extremities, cool, pale skin
- Monitor hyperthyroidism: restlessness, tachycardia, eyelid puffiness, weight loss, frequent urination, menstrual irregularities, dyspnea, warm, moist skin
- Assess for pulmonary toxicity: dyspnea, fatigue, cough, fever, chest pain; drug should be discontinued if these occur

A

• Monitor cardiac rate, respiration: rate, rhythm, character, chest pain, ventricular tachycardia, supraventricular tachycardia or fibrillation
• Assess sight and vision before treatment and throughout therapy; microdeposits on the cornea may cause blurred vision, halos, and photophobia

Nursing diagnoses

✓ Cardiac output, decreased (uses)
✓ Gas exchange, impaired (adverse reactions)
✓ Knowledge deficit (teaching)

Implementation

PO route

• Give reduced dosage slowly with ECG monitoring only
• Give with meals for GI upset

IV **IV route**

Additive compatibilities: Dobutamine, lidocaine, potassium chloride, procainimide, verapamil

Y-site compatibilities: Amikacin, bretylium, clindamycin, dobutamine, dopamine, doxycycline, erythromycin, esmolol, gentamicin, insulin (regular), isoproterenol, labetalol, lidocaine,metaruminol, metronidazole, midazolam, morphine, nitroglycerin, norepinephrine, penicillin G potassium, phentolamine, phenylephrine, potassium chloride, procainamide, tobramycin, vancomycin

Patient/family education

• Instruct patient to report side effects immediately to prescriber
• Instruct patient that skin discoloration is usually reversible but skin may turn bluish on neck, face, arms when used for long periods
• Advise patient that dark glasses may be needed for photophobia
• Instruct patient to use sunscreen and protective clothing to prevent burning associated with photosensitivity
• Instruct patient to take medication as prescribed, not to double doses
• Instruct patient to complete follow-up appointment with health care provider including pulmonary function studies, chest x-ray, ophthalmic examinations

Treatment of overdose: Administer O_2, artificial ventilation, ECG, dopamine for circulatory depression, diazepam or thiopental for convulsions, isoproterenol

amitriptyline (℞)
(a-mee-trip'ti-leen)
amitriptyline HCl, Apo-Amitriptyline ✤, Elavil, Endep, Enovil, Levate ✤, Meravil ✤, Novotriptyn ✤, Rolavil ✤
Func. class.: Antidepressant—tricyclic
Chem. class.: Tertiary amine
Pregnancy category C

Action: Blocks reuptake of norepinephrine, serotonin into nerve endings that increase action of norepinephrine, serotonin in nerve cells

Uses: Major depression

Investigational uses: Chronic pain management, prevention of cluster/migraine headaches

Therapeutic Outcome: Decreased symptoms of depression after 2-3 wk

Dosage and routes

Depression

Adult: PO 30-100 mg hs; may increase to 200 mg qd, not to exceed 300 mg/day; IM 20-30 mg qid, or 80-120 mg hs

P G ***Adolescent/geriatric:*** PO 30 mg/day in divided doses; may be increased to 150 mg/day

Cluster/migraine headaches

Adult: PO 50-150 mg/d

Chronic pain

Adult: PO 75-150 mg/d

Available forms: Tabs 10, 25, 50, 75, 100, 150 mg; inj IM 10 mg/ml; syrup 10 mg/5 ml ✽

Adverse effects

CNS: Dizziness, drowsiness, confusion, headache, anxiety, tremors, stimulation, weakness, insomnia, nightmares, EPS G (elderly), increased psychiatric symptoms

CV: Orthostatic hypotension, ***ECG changes, tachycardia, hypertension,*** palpitations

EENT: Blurred vision, tinnitus, mydriasis, ophthalmoplegia

GI: Diarrhea, dry mouth, nausea, vomiting, ***paralytic ileus,*** increased appetite, cramps, epigastric distress, jaundice, ***hepatitis,*** stomatitis

GU: Retention

HEMA: **Agranulocytosis, thrombocytopenia, eosinophilia, leukopenia**

INTEG: Rash, urticaria, sweating, pruritus, photosensitivity

Contraindications: Hypersensitivity to tricyclic antidepressants, recovery phase of myocardial infarction

Precautions: Suicidal patients, convulsive disorders, prostatic hypertrophy, schizophrenia, psychosis, severe depression, increased intraocular pressure, narrow angle glaucoma, urinary retention, cardiac disease, hepatic/renal disease, hyperthyroidism, electroshock P therapy, elective surgery, child G <12 yr, pregnancy **C,** elderly

Pharmacokinetics

Absorption	Well absorbed
Distribution	Widely distributed; crosses placenta
Metabolism	Liver, extensively
Excretion	Kidneys, breast milk
Half-life	10-50 hr

Pharmacodynamics

	PO/IM
Onset	45 min
Peak	2-12 hr
Duration	Unknown

Interactions

Individual drugs

Alcohol: ↑ CNS depression

Cimetidine: ↑ levels, ↑ toxicity

Clonidine: ↑ hypertension; avoid use

Disulfiram: Organic brain syndrome

Fluoxetine: ↑ levels, ↑ toxicity

Guanethidine: ↓ effects

Drug classifications

Antihypertensives: Blocked response to antihypertensive

MAOI: Hypertensive crisis, convulsions

Barbiturates: ↑ CNS effects

Benzodiazepines: ↑ CNS effects

CNS depressants: ↑ CNS effects

Sympathomimetics, indirect acting: ↓ effects

Oral contraceptives: ↑ effects, toxicity

Smoking
↑ metabolism, ↓ effects
Lab test interferences
↑ Serum bilirubin, ↑ blood glucose, ↑ alkaline phosphatase
↓ VMA, ↓ 5-HIAA
False ↑ urinary catecholamines

NURSING CONSIDERATIONS
Assessment
• Monitor B/P (with patient lying, standing), pulse q4h; if systolic B/P drops 20 mm Hg, hold drug, notify prescriber; take vital signs q4h in patients with cardiovascular disease
• Monitor blood studies: CBC, leukocytes, differential, cardiac enzymes if patient is receiving long-term therapy
• Monitor hepatic studies: AST (SGOT), ALT (SGPT), bilirubin
• Check weight weekly; appetite may increase with drug
• Assess ECG for flattening of T wave, bundle branch block, AV block, dysrhythmias in cardiac patients
• Assess for EPS primarily in G elderly: rigidity, dystonia, akathisia
• Assess mental status: mood, sensorium, affect, suicidal tendencies; increase in psychiatric symptoms: depression, panic
• Monitor urinary retention, constipation; constipation is P more likely to occur in children G or elderly
• Assess for withdrawal symptoms: headache, nausea, vomiting, muscle pain, weakness; do not usually occur unless drug was discontinued abruptly
• Identify alcohol consumption; if alcohol is consumed, hold dose until morning

Nursing diagnoses
✓ Coping, ineffective individual (uses)
✓ Injury, risk for physical (side effects)
✓ Knowledge deficit (teaching)
✓ Noncompliance (teaching)

Implementation
PO route
• Give with food or milk for GI symptoms
• Crush if patient is unable to swallow medication whole
• Give dosage hs if oversedation occurs during day; may G take entire dose hs; elderly may not tolerate once/day dosing
• Store at room temp; do not freeze

Patient/family education
• Teach patient that therapeutic effects may take 2-3 wk
• Instruct patient to use caution in driving or other activities requiring alertness because of drowsiness, dizziness, blurred vision; to avoid rising quickly from sitting to G standing, especially elderly
• Advise patient to avoid alcohol ingestion, other CNS depressants
• Teach patient not to discontinue medication quickly after long-term use; may cause nausea, headache, malaise
• Advise patient to wear sunscreen or large hat, since photosensitivity occurs
• Teach patient to increase fluids, bulk in diet if constipation, urinary retention occur, G especially elderly
• Teach patient to take gum, hard sugarless candy, or frequent sips of water for dry mouth

Evaluation

Positive therapeutic outcome

- Decreased depression
- Absence of suicidal thoughts

Treatment of overdose: ECG monitoring, induce emesis, lavage, activated charcoal, administer anticonvulsant

amlodipine (℞)

(am-loe'di-peen)

Norvasc

Func. class.: Calcium channel blocker, antianginal, antihypertensive

Chem. class.: Dihydropyridine

Pregnancy category C

Action: Inhibits calcium ion influx across cell membrane during cardiac depolarization; produces relaxation of coronary vascular smooth muscle, peripheral vascular smooth muscle; dilates coronary vascular arteries; increases myocardial oxygen delivery in patients with vasospastic angina

➡ **Therapeutic Outcome:** Decreased angina pectoris, dysrhythmias, B/P

Uses: Chronic stable angina pectoris, hypertension, vasospastic angina

Dosage and routes

Angina

Adult: PO 5-10 mg qd

Hypertension

Adult: PO 5 mg qd initially; may increase up to 10 mg/day

Available forms: Tabs 2.5, 5, 10 mg

Adverse effects

CNS: Headache, fatigue, dizziness, anxiety, depression, insomnia, paresthesia, somnolence, asthenia

CV: Dysrhythmia, edema, bradycardia, hypotension, palpitations, syncope, AV block

GI: Nausea, vomiting, diarrhea, gastric upset, constipation, abdominal cramps, flatulence, anorexia

GU: Nocturia, polyuria

INTEG: Rash, pruritus, urticaria, hair loss

MISC: Flushing, nasal congestion, sweating, shortness of breath, sexual difficulties, muscle cramps, cough, weight gain, tinnitus, epistaxis

Contraindications: Sick sinus syndrome, 2nd- or 3rd-degree heart block, hypotension less than 90 mm Hg systolic, hypersensitivity

Precautions: CHF, hypotension, hepatic injury, pregnancy C, lactation, **P** children, renal disease, **G** elderly

Pharmacokinetics	
Absorption	Well absorbed up to 90%
Distribution	Crosses placenta
Metabolism	Liver, extensively
Excretion	Kidneys to metabolites (90%)
Half-life	30-50 hr

Pharmacodynamics	
Onset	Unknown
Peak	6-12 hr
Duration	24 hr

Interactions

Individual drugs

Alcohol: ↑ hypotension

Fentanyl: ↑ hypotension

Drug classifications

Antihypertensives: ↑ hypotension

Nitrates: ↑ hypotension

NURSING CONSIDERATIONS

Assessment

• Assess fluid volume status: I&O ratio and record, weight, distended red veins, crackles in lung, color, quality and specific gravity of urine, skin turgor, adequacy of pulses, moist mucous membranes, bilateral lung sounds, peripheral pitting edema; dehydration symptoms of decreasing output, thirst, hypotension, dry mouth and mucous membranes should be reported
• Monitor B/P and pulse; if B/P drops call prescriber
• Monitor ALT (SGPT), AST (SGOT), bilirubin daily; if these are elevated, hepatotoxicity is suspected
• Monitor if platelets are <150,000/mm^3; drug is usually discontinued and another drug started
• Monitor cardiac status: B/P, pulse, respiration, ECG

Nursing diagnoses

✓ Cardiac output, decreased (uses)
✓ Knowledge deficit (teaching)

Implementation

• Give once a day, with food for GI symptoms

Patient/family education

• Advise patient to avoid hazardous activities until stabilized on drug, dizziness is no longer a problem
• Instruct patient to avoid alcohol and OTC drugs unless directed by prescriber
• Advise patient to comply in all areas of medical regimen: diet, exercise, stress reduction, drug therapy; to notify prescriber of irregular heart beat, shortness of breath, swelling of feet and hands, pronounced dizziness, constipation, nausea, hypotension
• Teach patient to use as directed even if feeling better; may be taken with other cardiovascular drugs (nitrates, β-blockers)
⊘ • Do not open, crush, break, or chew sus rel caps

Evaluation

Positive therapeutic outcome
• Decreased anginal pain
• Decreased B/P

Treatment of overdose:

Defibrillation, β-agonists, **IV** calcium inotropic agents, diuretics, atropine for AV block, vasopressor for hypotension

amobarbital (℞)

(am-oh-bar'bi-tal)
amobarbital sodium,
Amytal, Amytal Sodium,
Amytal Sodium Pulvules
Novamabarb ✦

Func. class.: Sedative/hypnotic barbiturate (intermediate acting) anticonvulsant
Chem. class.: Amylobarbitone

Pregnancy category D

Controlled substance schedule II (USA), schedule G (Canada)

Action: Depresses activity in brain cells primarily in reticular activating system in brainstem; also selectively depresses neurons in posterior hypothalamus, limbic structures; able to decrease seizure activity by inhibition of impulses in CNS; decreases motor activity

➔ **Therapeutic Outcome:** Sedation, anticonvulsant, improved energy

Uses: Sedation, preanesthetic sedation, insomnia, anticonvulsant, adjunct in psychiatry, hypnotic

Dosage and routes

Preanesthetic sedation

P ***Adult and child:*** PO/IM 200 mg 1-2 hr preoperatively

Sedation

Adult: PO 30-50 mg bid or tid; may be 15-120 mg bid-qid

P ***Child:*** PO 2 mg/kg/day in 4 divided doses

Anticonvulsant/psychiatry

Adult: **IV** 65-500 mg given over several min, not to exceed 100 mg/min; not to exceed 1 g

P ***Child less than 6 yr:*** **IV**/IM 3-5 mg/kg over several min

Insomnia

Adult: PO/IM 65-200 mg hs, not to exceed 5 ml in one site

P ***Child:*** IM 3-5 mg/kg hs, not to exceed 5 ml in one site

Available forms: Tabs 30, 50, 100 mg; caps 65, 200 mg; powder for inj 250, 500 mg/vial

Adverse effects

CNS: ***Lethargy, drowsiness,*** G ***hangover,*** dizziness, stimulation P in the elderly and children, lightheadedness, physical dependence, CNS depression, mental depression, slurred speech

CV: Hypotension, bradycardia

GI: Nausea, vomiting, diarrhea, constipation

HEMA: ***Agranulocytosis, thrombocytopenia, megaloblastic anemia*** (long-term treatment)

INTEG: *Rash,* urticaria, pain, abscesses at injection site, ***angioedema,*** thrombophlebitis, ***Stevens-Johnson syndrome***

RESP: ***Depression, apnea, laryngospasm, bronchospasm***

Contraindications: Hypersensitivity to barbiturates, respiratory depression, addiction to barbiturates, severe liver impairment, porphyria

Precautions: Anemia, pregnancy **D**, lactation, hepatic disease, renal disease, hypertension, G elderly, acute/chronic pain

Pharmacokinetics

Absorption	Well absorbed (PO, IM)
Distribution	Widely distributed; crosses placenta
Metabolism	Liver
Excretion	Kidneys
Half-life	16-40 hr

Pharmacodynamics

	PO	IM	IV
Onset	45-60 min	30-45 min	10 min
Peak	Unknown	Unknown	Unknown
Duration	6-8 hr	6-8 hr	3-6 hr

Interactions

Individual drugs

Acebutolol: ↓ effectiveness
Alcohol: ↑ CNS depression
Chloramphenicol: ↓ effectiveness
Doxycycline: ↑ half-life
Griseofulvin: ↓ effectiveness
Metoprolol: ↓ effectiveness
Propranolol: ↓ effectiveness
Quinidine: ↓ effectiveness
Timolol: ↓ effectiveness

Drug classifications

Antidepressants, tricyclics: ↑ CNS depression
Antihistamines: ↑ CNS depression
Estrogens: ↓ effectiveness

Glucocorticoids: ↓ effectiveness
MAOI: ↑ CNS depression
Narcotics: ↑ CNS depression
Oral contraceptives: ↓ effectiveness
Phenothiazines: ↓ CNS depression
Sedatives/hypnotics: ↑ CNS depression
Tricyclics: ↓ effectiveness

Lab test interferences

False ↑ sulfobromophthalein

NURSING CONSIDERATIONS

Assessment

• Mental status: mood, sensorium, affect, memory (long, short), especially elderly; if using as a hypnotic, assess sleep patterns during therapy; drug suppresses REM sleep with dreaming; withdrawal insomnia may occur after short-term use; do not start using drug again, insomnia will improve in 1-3 nights; may experience increased dreaming

• Monitor for respiratory dysfunction: respiratory depression, character, rate, rhythm (when using **IV**); hold drug if respirations are <10/min or if pupils are dilated; also check VS q30 min after parenteral route for 2 hr

• Assess for barbiturate toxicity: hypotension, pulmonary constriction, cold, clammy skin, cyanosis of lips, CNS depression, nausea, vomiting, hallucinations, delirium, weakness, coma, pupillary constriction; mild symptoms may occur in 8-12 hr without drug

• Assess for blood dyscrasias: fever, sore throat, bruising, rash, jaundice, epistaxis (long-term treatment only)

• Assess for pain in postoperative patients; pain threshold is lowered when patients are taking this medication

Nursing diagnoses

- ✓ Sleep pattern disturbance (uses)
- ✓ Injury, risk for (adverse reactions)
- ✓ Knowledge deficit (teaching)
- ✓ Noncompliance (teaching)

Implementation

• Use after removal of cigarettes, to prevent fires; after trying conservative measures for insomnia

PO route

• Give 30 min before hs for expected sleeplessness; on empty stomach for best absorption

IM route

• Reconstitute with sterile water for inj (100 mg/ml); mix by rotating vial; do not shake

• Give in deep muscle mass (gluteal) to minimize irritation to tissues; split inj of >5 ml into 2 since irritation to tissues may occur; reconstitute with sterile water for inj (100 mg/ml); mix by rotating vial, do not shake

IV route

• Reconstitute with sterile water for inj (100 mg/ml); mix by rotating vial; do not shake; may be further diluted with D_5W, $D_{10}W$, $D_{20}W$, D_5/0.9% NaCl, D_5LR, 0.9% NaCl, 3% NaCl, LR; use within 30 min; do not use if cloudy or colored after 5 min of reconstitution

Direct IV route

• Use large vein to prevent extravasation; if extravasation occurs, use moist heat to the area and procaine sol 5% injected into area; give at 100 mg/min or more (adult); 60 P mg/m^2/min (child); give **IV** only with resuscitative equipment available (only by qualified personnel)

Additive compatibilities: Amikacin, aminophylline, sodium bicarbonate

Additive incompatibilities: Cefazolin, cephalothin, cimetidine, chlorpromazine, clindamycin, codeine, diphenhydramine, droperidol, hydroxyzine, regular insulin, levorphanol, meperidine, methadone, morphine, norepinephrine, pentazocine, procaine, streptomycin, tetracycline, vancomycin

Patient/family education

- Teach patient that hangover is common
- Instruct patient that drug is indicated only for short-term treatment of insomnia and is probably ineffective after 2 wk
- Inform patient that physical dependency may result when used for extended time (45-90 days depending on dosage)
- Caution patient to avoid driving or other activities requiring alertness
- Caution patient to avoid alcohol ingestion and CNS depressants; serious CNS depression may result
- Instruct patient not to discontinue medication quickly after long-term use; drug should be tapered over 1 wk
- Emphasize the need to tell all prescribers that a barbiturate is being taken
- Inform patient that withdrawal insomnia may occur after short-term use; do not start using drug again; insomnia will improve in 1-3 nights; may experience increased dreaming
- Inform patient that effects may take 2 nights for benefits to be noticed; teach patient alternate measures to improve sleep: reading, exercise several hours before hs, warm bath, warm milk, TV, self-hypnosis, deep breathing
- Teach patient to make position changes slowly; orthostatic hypotension may occur
- Instruct patient to notify prescriber immediately if bruising or bleeding occurs, which may indicate blood dyscrasias

Evaluation

Positive therapeutic outcome

- Improved sleeping patterns
- Decreased seizure activity
- Improved energy

Treatment of overdose: Lavage, activated charcoal, warming blanket, vital signs, hemodialysis, alkalinize urine; give **IV** volume expanders, **IV** fluids

amoxapine (℞)

(a-mox'a-peen)

amoxapine, Asendin

Func. class.: Antidepressant—tetra

Chem. class.: Dibenzoxazepine derivative, secondary amine

Pregnancy category C

Action: Blocks reuptake of norepinephrine, serotonin into nerve endings, thereby increasing action of norepinephrine, serotonin in nerve cells

➔ Therapeutic Outcome: Decreased symptoms of depression after 2-3 wk

Uses: Depression

Dosage and routes

Adult: PO 50 mg tid; may increase to 100 mg tid on 3rd day of therapy; not to exceed 300 mg/day unless lower doses have been given for at least 2 wk; may be given daily dose hs; not to exceed 600 mg/day in hospitalized patients

G ***Elderly:*** PO 25 mg bid-tid, may increase to 50 mg bid-tid, not to exceed 300 mg/day

Available forms: Tabs 25, 50, 75, 100, 150 mg

Adverse effects

CNS: Dizziness, drowsiness, confusion, headache, anxiety, tremors, stimulation, weakness, insomnia, nightmares, EPS G (elderly), increased psychiatric symptoms, paresthesia, impairment of sexual functioning

CV: Orthostatic hypotension, ECG changes, tachycardia, ***hypertension,*** palpitations

EENT: Blurred vision, tinnitus, mydriasis, ophthalmoplegia

GI: Diarrhea, dry mouth, constipation, nausea, vomiting, ***paralytic ileus,*** increased appetite, cramps, epigastric distress, jaundice, ***hepatitis,*** stomatitis

GU: Retention, ***acute renal failure***

HEMA: ***Agranulocytosis, thrombocytopenia, eosinophilia, leukopenia***

INTEG: Rash, urticaria, sweating, pruritus, photosensitivity

Contraindications: Hypersensitivity to tricyclic antidepressants, recovery phase of myocardial infarction, convulsive disorders, prostatic hypertrophy

Precautions: Suicidal patients, severe depression, increased intraocular pressure, narrow-angle glaucoma, urinary retention, cardiac disease, hepatic disease, hyperthyroidism, electroshock therapy, elective G surgery, elderly, pregnancy **C**

Pharmacokinetics

Absorption	Well absorbed
Distribution	Widely distributed; crosses placenta
Metabolism	Liver, extensively
Excretion	Kidneys, breast milk
Half-life	8 hr

Pharmacodynamics

Onset	1-2 wk
Peak	2-6 wk
Duration	6-12 wk

Interactions

Individual drugs

Alcohol: ↑ CNS depression

Cimetidine: ↑ levels, ↑ toxicity of amoxapine

Clonidine: Severe hypotension; avoid use

Disulfiram: Organic brain syndrome

Fluoxetine: ↑ levels, ↑ toxicity of amoxapine

Guanethidine: ↓ effects of amoxapine

Drug classifications

MAOI: Hypertensive crisis, convulsions

Barbiturates: ↑ effects of amoxapine

Benzodiazepines: ↑ effects of amoxapine

CNS depressants: ↑ effects of amoxapine

Sympathomimetics, indirect acting: ↓ effects of amoxapine

Oral contraceptives: ↑ effects, toxicity of amoxapine

Smoking

↑ metabolism, ↓ effects

Lab test interferences

↑ Serum bilirubin, ↑ blood

glucose, ↑ alkaline phosphatase ↓ VMA, ↓ 5-HIAA
False ↑ Urinary catecholamines

NURSING CONSIDERATIONS
Assessment
- Monitor B/P (with patient lying, standing), pulse q4h; if systolic B/P drops 20 mm Hg hold drug, notify prescriber; take vital signs q4h in patients with cardiovascular disease
- Monitor blood studies: CBC, leukocytes, differential, cardiac enzymes if patient is receiving long-term therapy
- Monitor hepatic studies: AST (SGOT), ALT (SGPT), bilirubin
- Check weight weekly; appetite may increase with drug
- Assess ECG for flattening of T wave, bundle branch block, AV block, dysrhythmias in cardiac patients
- Assess for EPS primarily in G elderly: rigidity, dystonia, akathisia
- Assess mental status: mood, sensorium, affect, suicidal tendencies; increase in psychiatric symptoms: depression, panic
- Monitor urinary retention, constipation; constipation is P more likely to occur in G children and elderly
- Assess for withdrawal symptoms: headache, nausea, vomiting, muscle pain, weakness; do not usually occur unless drug was discontinued abruptly
- Identify alcohol consumption; if alcohol is consumed, hold dose until morning

Nursing diagnoses
✓ Coping, ineffective individual (uses)
✓ Injury, risk for physical (side effects)
✓ Knowledge deficit (teaching)
✓ Noncompliance (teaching)

Implementation
- Give with food or milk for GI symptoms
- Crush if patient is unable to swallow medication whole
- Store at room temp; do not freeze

Patient/family education
- Teach patient that therapeutic effects may take 2-3 wk
- Instruct patient to use caution in driving or other activities requiring alertness because of drowsiness, dizziness, blurred vision; to avoid rising quickly from sitting to standing, G especially elderly
- Teach patient to avoid alcohol ingestion, other CNS depressants
- Teach patient not to discontinue medication quickly after long-term use: may cause nausea, headache, malaise
- Teach patient to wear sunscreen or large hat, since photosensitivity occurs
- Teach patient to increase fluids, bulk in diet if constipation, urinary retention occur, G especially elderly
- Advise patient to take gum, hard sugarless candy, or frequent sips of water for dry mouth

Evaluation
Positive therapeutic outcome
- Decreased depression
- Absence of suicidal thoughts

Treatment of overdose:
ECG monitoring, induce emesis, lavage, activated charcoal, administer anticonvulsant

A

amoxicillin (℞)

(a-mox-i-sill'in)

amoxicillin, Amoxil, Amoxil Pediatric Drops, Apo-Amoxi ✤, Novamoxin ✤, Nu-Amoxi ✤, Polymox, Polymox Drops, Trimox 125, Trimox 250, Trimox 500, Wymox

Func. class.: Broad-spectrum antibiotic

Chem. class.: Aminopenicillin

Pregnancy category B

Action: Interferes with cell wall replication of susceptible organisms by binding to the bacterial cell wall; the cell wall, rendered osmotically unstable, swells and bursts from osmotic pressure

➔ **Therapeutic Outcome:** Bactericidal effects for the following organisms: effective for gram-positive cocci *(Streptococcus pyogenes, S. faecalis, S. pneumoniae)*, gram-negative cocci *(Neisseria gonorrhoeae, N. meningitidis, Escherichia coli)*, gram-negative bacilli *(Haemophilus influenzae, Proteus mirabilis, Salmonella)*

Uses: Infections of respiratory tract, skin, skin structures, genitourinary tract, otitis media, meningitis, septicemia, sinusitis and endocarditis prophylaxis

Investigational uses: Lyme disease, *Chlamydia trachomatis* in pregnancy

Dosage and routes

Systemic infections

Adult: PO 750 mg-1.5 g qd in divided doses q8h

P ***Child:*** PO 20-40 mg/kg/day in divided doses q8h

Gonorrhea/urinary tract infections

Adult: PO 3 g given with 1 g probenecid as a single dose

Chlamydia trachomatis

Adult: PO 500 mg/d × 1 wk

Available forms: Caps 250, 500 mg; chewable tabs 125, 250 mg; powder for oral susp 50mg/ml, 125, 250 mg/5 ml

Adverse effects

CNS: Headache, fever

GI: Nausea, vomiting, diarrhea, increased AST (SGOT), ALT (SPGT), abdominal pain, glossitis, colitis, ***pseudomembranous colitis***

HEMA: Anemia, increased bleeding time, ***bone marrow depression, granulocytopenia***

SYST: ***Anaphylaxis, respiratory distress***

Contraindications: Hypersensitivity to penicillins; P neonates

Precautions: Pregnancy **B**, hypersensitivity to cephalosporins

Pharmacokinetics

Absorption	Well absorbed (90%)
Distribution	Readily in body tissues, fluids, CSF; crosses placenta
Metabolism	Liver (30%)
Excretion	Breast milk, kidney, unchanged (70%)
Half-life	1-1.3 hr

Pharmacodynamics

Onset	½ hr
Peak	2 hr

Interactions

Individual drugs

Aspirin: ↑ amoxicillin levels, ↓ renal excretion

Probenecid: ↑ amoxicillin levels, ↓ renal excretion

Drug classifications

Erythromycins: ↓ antimicrobial effectiveness

Oral anticoagulants: ↑ anticoagulant effects

Oral contraceptives: ↓ contraceptive effectiveness

Tetracyclines: ↓ antimicrobial effectiveness

Lab test interferences

False positive: Urine glucose, urine protein

NURSING CONSIDERATIONS

Assessment

- Assess patient for previous sensitivity reaction to penicillins or other cephalosporins; cross-sensitivity between penicillins and cephalosporins is common
- Assess patient for signs and symptoms of infection, including characteristics of wounds, sputum, urine, stool, WBC >10,000, earache, fever; obtain baseline information and monitor symptoms during treatment
- Obtain C&S before beginning drug therapy to identify if correct treatment has been initiated
- Assess for allergic reactions during treatment: rash, urticaria, pruritus, chills, fever, joint pain; angioedema may occur a few days after therapy begins; epinephrine and resuscitation equipment should be available for anaphylactic reactions
- Identify urine output; if decreasing, notify prescriber (may indicate nephrotoxicity); also, increased BUN, creatinine
- Monitor blood studies: AST (SGOT), ALT (SGPT), CBC, Hct, bilirubin, LDH, alkaline phosphatase, Coombs' test monthly if patient is on long-term therapy
- Monitor electrolytes: potassium, sodium, chloride monthly if patient is on long-term therapy
- Assess bowel pattern qd; if severe diarrhea occurs, notify prescriber; drug should be discontinued; may indicate pseudomembranous colitis
- Monitor for bleeding: ecchymosis, bleeding gums, hematuria, stool guaiac daily if on long-term therapy
- Assess for overgrowth of infection: perineal itching, fever, malaise, redness, pain, swelling, drainage, rash, diarrhea, change in cough, sputum

Nursing diagnoses

✓ Infection, risk for (uses)
✓ Diarrhea (side effects)
✓ Injury, risk for (side effects)
✓ Knowledge deficit (teaching)
✓ Noncompliance (teaching)

Implementation

- Give in even doses around the clock; if GI upset occurs, give with food; drug must be given for 10-14 days to ensure organism death and prevent superinfection; store in tight container
- The caps may be opened and contents taken with fluids
- Shake susp; store in refrigerator for 7-10 days

Patient/family education

- ❗ Teach patient to report sore throat, bruising, bleeding, joint pain; may indicate blood dyscrasias (rare)
- Advise patient to contact prescriber if vaginal itching, loose, foul-smelling stools, furry tongue occur; may indicate superinfection
- Instruct patient to take all medication prescribed for the length of time ordered

Advise patient to notify prescriber of diarrhea with blood or pus, which may indicate pseudomembranous colitis

Evaluation

Positive therapeutic outcome

- Absence of signs/symptoms of infection (WBC <10,000, temp WNL, absence of red draining wounds or earache)
- Reported improvement in symptoms of infection

Treatment of anaphylaxis: Withdraw drug, maintain airway, administer epinephrine, aminophylline, O_2, **IV** corticosteroids

amoxicillin/ clavulanate (℞)

(a-mox-i-sill'in)

Augmentin, Clavulin ♣

Func. class.: Broad-spectrum antibiotic (extended spectrum)

Chem. class.: Aminopenicillin-β-lactamase inhibitor

Pregnancy category B

Action: Interferes with cell wall replication of susceptible organisms; the cell wall, rendered osmotically unstable, swells and bursts from osmotic pressure; combination increases spectrum of activity, β-lactamase resistance

➔ **Therapeutic Outcome:** Bactericidal effects for the following organisms: *Escherichia coli, Proteus mirabilis, Haemophilus influenzae, Streptococcus faecalis, S. pneumoniae;* and β-lactamase–producing organisms: *Neisseria gonorrhoeae, N. meningitis, Shigella, Salmonella, Enterococcus, Streptococcus*

Uses: Infections of respiratory tract, skin, skin structures, genitourinary tract; otitis media, meningitis, septicemia, sinusitis, and endocarditis prophylaxis

Dosage and routes

Adult: PO 250-500 mg q8h depending on severity of infection

P ***Child:*** PO 20-40 mg/kg/day in divided doses q8h

Available forms: Tabs 250, 500, 875 mg/125 mg clavulanate; chewable tabs 125, 200, 250, 400 mg; powder for oral susp 125, 200, 250, 400 mg/5 ml

Adverse effects

CNS: Headache, fever

GI: Nausea, diarrhea, vomiting, increased AST (SGOT), ALT (SGPT), abdominal pain, glossitis, colitis, black tongue, ***pseudomembranous colitis***

GU: **Oliguria, proteinuria, hematuria,** *vaginitis, moniliasis,* ***glomerulonephritis***

HEMA: Anemia, ***bone marrow depression, granulocytopenia, leukopenia, eosinophilia,*** *thrombocytopenic purpura*

META: Hyperkalemia, hypokalemia, alkalosis, hypernatremia

SYST: Anaphylaxis

Contraindications: Hypersen-
P sitivity to penicillins; neonates

Precautions: Pregnancy **B,** hypersensitivity to cephalosporins, lactation

Pharmacokinetics

Absorption	Well absorbed (90%)
Distribution	Readily in body tissues, fluids, CSF; crosses placenta
Metabolism	Liver (30%)
Excretion	Breast milk; kidney, unchanged (70%)
Half-life	1-1.3 hr

Pharmacodynamics

Onset	½ hr
Peak	2 hr

Interactions

Individual drugs

Aspirin: ↑ amoxicillin levels, decreased renal excretion
Probenecid: ↑ amoxicillin levels, decreased renal excretion

Drug classifications

Erythromycins: ↓ antimicrobial effectiveness
Oral anticoagulants: ↑ anticoagulant effects
Oral contraceptives: ↓ contraceptive effectiveness
Tetracyclines: ↓ antimicrobial effectiveness

Lab test interferences

False positive: Urine glucose, urine protein

NURSING CONSIDERATIONS

Assessment

- Assess patient for previous sensitivity reaction to penicillins or other cephalosporins; cross-sensitivity between penicillins and cephalosporins is common
- Assess patient for signs and symptoms of infection, including characteristics of wounds, sputum, urine, stool, WBC >10,000, earache, fever; obtain baseline information and during treatment
- Complete C&S before beginning drug therapy to identify if correct treatment has been initiated
- Assess for allergic reactions: rash, urticaria, pruritus, chills, fever, joint pain; angioedema may occur a few days after therapy begins; epinephrine and resuscitation equipment should be available for anaphylactic reaction
- Identify urine output; if decreasing, notify prescriber (may indicate nephrotoxicity); also, increased BUN, creatinine
- Monitor blood studies: AST (SGOT), ALT (SGPT), CBC, Hct, bilirubin, LDH, alkaline phosphatase, Coombs' test monthly if patient is on long-term therapy
- Monitor electrolytes: potassium, sodium, chloride monthly if patient is on long-term therapy
- Assess bowel pattern qd; if severe diarrhea occurs, drug should be discontinued; may indicate pseudomembranous colitis
- Monitor for bleeding: ecchymosis, bleeding gums, hematuria, stool guaiac daily if on long-term therapy
- Assess for overgrowth of infection: perineal itching, fever, malaise, redness, pain, swelling, drainage, rash, diarrhea, change in cough, sputum

Nursing diagnoses

- ✓ Infection, risk for (uses)
- ✓ Injury, risk for (side effects)
- ✓ Diarrhea (side effects)
- ✓ Knowledge deficit (teaching)
- ✓ Noncompliance (teaching)

Implementation

- Give in even doses around the clock; if GI upset occurs, give with food; drug must be taken for 10-14 days to ensure organism death and prevent superinfection; store in tight container; cap can be opened and mixed with food or liq; chewable tabs should be chewed

- Shake susp, store in refrigerator for 2 wk or 1 wk at room temp

Patient/family education

- Teach patient to report sore throat, bruising, bleeding, joint pain; may indicate blood dyscrasias (rare)
- Advise patient to contact prescriber if vaginal itching, loose, foul-smelling stools occur; may indicate superinfection
- Instruct patient to take all medication prescribed for the length of time prescribed
- Advise patient to notify prescriber of diarrhea with blood or pus, which may indicate pseudomembranous colitis

Evaluation

Positive therapeutic outcome

- Absence of signs/symptoms of infection (WBC <10,000, temp WNL, absence of red draining wounds, earache)
- Reported improvement in symptoms of infection

Treatment of anaphylaxis: Withdraw drug, maintain airway, administer epinephrine, aminophylline, O_2, **IV** corticosteroids

amphetamine (℞)

(am-fet'a-meen)

amphetamine sulfate

Func. class.: Cerebral stimulant

Chem. class.: Amphetamine

Pregnancy category C

Controlled substance schedule II

Action: Increases release of norepinephrine in nerve endings, dopamine in cerebral cortex to reticular activating system; increases CNS, respiratory stimulation, pupillary dilatation, vasoconstriction

Therapeutic Outcome: Increased alertness, decreased fatigue, ability to stay awake (treatment of narcolepsy), increased attention span, decreased hyperactivity (ADHD)

Uses: Narcolepsy, ADHD

Dosage and routes

Narcolepsy

Adult: PO 5-60 mg qd in divided doses

P ***Child >12 yr:*** PO 10 mg qd increasing by 10 mg/day at weekly intervals

P ***Child 6-12 yr:*** PO 5 mg qd increasing by 5 mg/wk, max 60 mg/day

ADHD

P ***Child >6 yr:*** PO 5 mg qd-bid increasing by 5 mg/day at weekly intervals

P ***Child 3-6 yr:*** PO 2.5 mg qd increasing by 2.5 mg/day at weekly intervals

Available forms: Tabs 5, 10 mg; long-acting caps 5, 10 mg

Adverse effects
CNS: Hyperactivity, insomnia, restlessness, talkativeness, dizziness, headache, chills, stimulation, dysphoria, irritability, aggressiveness, tremor, dependence, addiction
CV: Palpitations, tachycardia, hypertension, dysrhythmias, decreased heart rate
GI: Nausea, vomiting, anorexia, dry mouth, diarrhea, constipation, weight loss, metallic taste, cramps
GU: Impotence, change in libido
INTEG: Urticaria

Contraindications: Hypersensitivity to sympathomimetic amines, hyperthyroidism, hypertension, glaucoma, severe arteriosclerosis, drug abuse, cardiovascular disease, anxiety

Precautions: Gilles de la Tourette's syndrome, lactation, P child <6 yr, pregnancy **C**

Pharmacokinetics

Absorption	Well absorbed within 3 hr
Distribution	Widely distributed; crosses placenta; high concentrations in brain
Metabolism	Liver
Excretion	Kidneys: pH dependent, increased pH leads to increased reabsorption; breast milk
Half-life	10-30 hr; increased when urine is alkaline, decreased when urine is acidic

Pharmacodynamics

Onset	½ hr
Peak	1-3 hr
Duration	4-20 hr

Interactions
Individual drugs
Acetazolamide: ↓ excretion, ↑ effect
Ammonium chloride: ↓ effect
Ascorbic acid: ↓ effect
Meperidine: Hypertensive crisis
Sodium bicarbonate: ↓ excretion, ↑ effect
Thyroid: ↑ effects
Drug classifications
Antidepressants, tricyclics: ↑ dysrhythmias
β-Blockers: ↑ hypertension
Cardiac glycosides: ↑ dysrhythmias
MAOI: Hypertensive crisis
Sympathomimetics: ↑ effect
Food
Cranberries/juice: ↑ amphetamine effect

NURSING CONSIDERATIONS
Assessment
- Monitor VS, B/P, since this drug may reverse antihypertensives; check patients with cardiac disease more often for increased B/P
- Monitor CBC, urinalysis; in diabetes blood sugar, urine sugar; insulin changes may be required, since eating will decrease
- Monitor height and weight q3 mo, since growth rate in P children may be decreased; appetite is suppressed, weight loss is common during the first few months of treatment
- Monitor mental status: mood, sensorium, affect, stimulation, insomnia; aggressiveness may occur; depression with crying spells may occur after drug has worn off
- Assess for physical dependency; should not be used for extended time except in ADHD; should be discontinued gradually to prevent withdrawal symptoms
- Assess for narcoleptic symptoms before medication and

after; ability to stay awake should increase significantly

P • In children or adults with ADHD, monitor for improved organizational skills, attention span, attending to tasks, impulse control, socialization, and ability to get along better with others

! • Assess for withdrawal symptoms: headache, nausea, vomiting, muscle pain, weakness; drug tolerance develops after long-term use; dosage should not be increased if tolerance develops; this medication has a high abuse potential

Nursing diagnoses

✓ Thought processes, altered (uses, adverse reactions)
✓ Coping, impaired individual (uses)
✓ Knowledge deficit (teaching)
✓ Family coping, impaired individual (uses)

Implementation

• Give at least 6 hr hs to avoid sleeplessness; titrate to patient's response, lowest dosage should be used to control symptoms
• Use gum, hard candy, frequent sips of water for dry mouth at beginning of treatment; these symptoms tend to lessen with time

Patient/family education

• Advise patient to decrease caffeine consumption (coffee, tea, cola, chocolate), which may increase irritability and stimulation; to avoid OTC preparations unless approved by prescriber; to avoid alcohol ingestion; these may cause serious drug interactions
• Instruct patient to taper off drug over several wks, or depression, increased sleeping, lethargy may occur
• Advise patient to avoid hazardous activities until stabilized on medication
• Instruct patient not to double doses if medication is missed; prescriber may suggest drug holidays (ADHD) during the school year to assess progress and determine continued drug necessity
• Instruct patient/family to notify health care provider if significant side effects occur: tremors, insomnia, palpitations, restlessness, drug changes may be needed
• Inform patient that if dry mouth occurs to use frequent sips of water, sugarless gum, hard candy during beginning therapy; dry mouth lessens with continued treatment
• Tell patient to get needed rest; patients feel more tired at end of day; to give last dose at least 6 hr hs to avoid insomnia

Evaluation

Positive therapeutic outcome

• Decreased activity in ADHD
• Absence of sleeping during day in narcolepsy

Treatment of overdose: Administer fluids, hemodialysis, peritoneal dialysis, antihypertensives for increased B/P; ammonium chloride for increased excretion

amphotericin B

(℞)
(am-foe-ter'i-sin)
Amphotec, amphotericin B, Fungizone IV, Fungizone
Func. class.: Antifungal
Chem. class.: Amphoteric polyene
Pregnancy category B

Action: Increases cell membrane permeability in susceptible organisms by binding sterols in fungal cell membrane; decreases potassium, sodium, and nutrients in cell

Therapeutic Outcome: Fungistatic against histoplasmosis, blastomycosis, coccidioidomycosis, cryptococcosis, aspergillosis, phycomycosis, candidiasis, sporotrichosis

Uses: Treatment of severe, possibly fatal fungal infections (**IV**); treatment of topical fungal infections (top)

Investigational uses: Candiduria (bladder irrigation)

Dosage and routes

P ***Adult and child:*** **IV** inf 1 mg/250 ml D_5W (0.1 mg/ml) over 2-4 hr or 0.25 mg/kg/day over 6 hr; may be increased gradually up to 1 mg/kg/day, not to exceed 1.5 mg/kg; intrathecal 25 μg/0.1 ml diluted in 10-20 ml CSF given by barbotage 2-3 times a wk, gradually increased to 0.5 mg q48-72 hr

Candidal infection of GI tract

Adults: 100 mg PO qid × 2 wk

Candidal oral infection

Adult: 1 loz qid × 7-14 days; allow loz to dissolve slowly in mouth

P ***Adult and child:*** TOP bid-qid for 7-21 days or longer if needed

Available forms: Powder for inj 50, 100 mg; susp for inj 100 mg/20ml; cream, lotion, oint 3%

Adverse effects

CNS: Headache, fever, chills, peripheral nerve pain, paresthesias, peripheral neuropathy, ***convulsions,*** dizziness
EENT: Tinnitus, deafness, diplopia, blurred vision
GI: Nausea, vomiting, anorexia, diarrhea, cramps, ***hemorrhagic gastroenteritis, acute liver failure***
GU: Hypokalemia, axotemia, hyposthenuria, ***renal tubular acidosis,*** nephrocalcinosis, ***permanent renal impairment, anuria, oliguria***
HEMA: Normochromic and normocytic anemia, ***thrombocytopenia, agranulocytosis, leukopenia, eosinophilia,*** hypokalemia, hyponatremia, hypomagnesemia
INTEG: Burning, irritation, pain, necrosis at inj site with extravasation, flushing, dermatitis, skin rash (top route)
MS: ***Arthralgia, myalgia,*** generalized pain, weakness, weight loss

Contraindications: Hypersensitivity, severe bone marrow depression

Precautions: Renal disease, pregnancy **B**

A

Pharmacokinetics

Absorption	Complete bioavailability (IV), rapidly absorbed (top)
Distribution	Body tissues
Metabolism	Liver
Excretion	Kidneys, detectable for several weeks
Half-life	Initial 24-48 hr, terminal 15 days

Pharmacodynamics

	IV	TOP
Onset	Immediate	Unknown
Peak	1-2 hr	Unknown

Interactions

Individual drugs

Mezlocillin: ↑ hypokalemia
Piperacillin: ↑ hypokalemia
Ticarcillin: ↑ hypokalemia

Drug classifications

Diuretics: ↑ nephrotoxicity, hypokalemia
Glucocorticoids: ↑ hypokalemia
Nephrotoxic drugs: ↑ nephrotoxicity

NURSING CONSIDERATIONS

Assessment

IV IV route

• Monitor VS q15-30 min during first inf; note changes in pulse, B/P

• Monitor blood studies: Hgb, Hct, potassium, sodium, calcium, magnesium q2 wk; BUN, creatinine weekly; decreased Hgb, Hct and magnesium are common with increased potassium

• Monitor weight weekly; if weight increases over 2 lb/wk, edema is present; renal damage should be considered

• Monitor for renal toxicity: increasing BUN, serum creatinine; if BUN is >40 mg/dl or if serum creatinine >3 mg/dl, drug may be discontinued or dosage reduced; I&O ratio: watch for decreasing urinary output, change in sp gr; discontinue drug to prevent permanent damage to renal tubules; provide hydration of 2-3 L/day

• Monitor for hepatotoxicity: increasing AST (SGOT), ALT (SGPT), alkaline phosphatase, bilirubin

• Monitor for allergic reaction: dermatitis, rash; drug should be discontinued, antihistamines (mild reaction) or epinephrine (severe reaction) administered; check inj site for thrombophlebitis

• Monitor for hypokalemia: anorexia, drowsiness, weakness, decreased reflexes, dizziness, increased urinary output, increased thirst, paresthesias; if these occur, drug should be decreased or discontinued and potassium administered

Top route

• Monitor for allergic reaction: burning, stinging, swelling, redness

Nursing diagnoses

☑ Infection, risk for (uses)
☑ Injury, risk for physical (adverse reaction)
☑ Knowledge deficit (teaching)

Implementation

Top route

• Provide enough medication to cover lesions completely; do not cover with occlusive dressing; apply liberally and rub thoroughly into affected area; administer after cleansing with soap, water before each application, dry well (as ordered), wear gloves during application

• Store at room temp in dry place

IV IV route

• Give after diluting 50 mg in

10 ml sterile water (no preservatives); shake well, further dilute with 500 ml of D_5W to concentration of 0.1 mg/ml; do not use other diluents or sol; use large needle (20 G); change needle for each step; wear gloves

- Use test dosage of 1 mg/20 ml D_5W; give over 10-30 min; if no reaction, drug is administered as ordered
- Administer **IV** using in-line filter (mean pore diameter >1 µm) using distal veins; check for extravasation, necrosis q8h; use an inf pump; administer over 6 hr; rapid inf may result in circulation collapse; may also be given through central line
- Give drug only after C&S confirm organism, drug needed to treat condition; make sure drug is used in life-threatening infections
- Provide protection from light during infusion; cover with foil
- Store protected from moisture and light; diluted sol is stable for 24 hr at room temp, 1 wk refrigerated

Syringe compatibility: Heparin

Y-site compatibilities: Aldesleukin, diltiazem, tacrolimus, teniposide, thiotepa, zidovudine

Y-site incompatibilities: Enalaprilat, fludarabine, foscarnet, ondansetron

Additive compatibilities: Fluconazole, heparin, hydrocortisone, methylprednisolone, sodium bicarbonate

Patient/family education

Top route

- Teach patient that skin and clothing may become discolored; to use asepsis (hand washing) before, after each application to prevent further infection
- Instruct patient to apply with glove to prevent further infection; not to cover with occlusive dressing; to continue even if condition improves
- Teach patient to avoid use of OTC creams, ointments, lotions, unless directed by prescriber
- Instruct patient to report increased itching, burning, rash, redness; ointment may irritate most hairy areas; to report if condition worsens

IV **IV route**

- Advise patient that long-term therapy may be needed to clear infection (2 wk-3 mo depending on type of infection)
- Teach patient side effects and when to notify prescriber

Evaluation

Positive therapeutic outcome

- Decrease in size, number of lesions (top)
- Decreased fever, malaise, rash
- Negative C&S for infecting organism

ampicillin (℞)
(am-pi-sill'in)
Amcil, Ampicin ♣, Apo-Ampi ♣, D-Amp ♣, Nu-Ampi ♣, NovoAmpicillin ♣, Polycillin, Omnipen, Omnipen-N, Polycillin-N, Supen, Totacillin, Totacillin-N
Func. class.: Broad-spectrum antibiotic
Chem. class.: Aminopenicillin

Pregnancy category B

Action: Interferes with cell wall replication of susceptible organisms; the cell wall, rendered osmotically unstable, swells, bursts from osmotic pressure

➔ **Therapeutic Outcome:** Bactericidal effects for the following organisms: effective for gram-positive cocci *(Streptococcus pyogenes, S. faecalis, S. pneumoniae)*, gram-negative cocci *(Neisseria gonorrhoeae, N. meningitidis)*, gram-negative bacilli *(Haemophilus influenzae, Proteus mirabilis, Salmonella, Shigella, Listeria monocytogenes)*, gram-positive bacilli

Uses: Infections of respiratory tract, skin, skin structures, genitourinary tract; otitis media, meningitis, septicemia, sinusitis, and endocarditis prophylaxis

Dosage and routes
Systemic infections
Adult: PO 250-500 mg q6h or 1-2 g qd in divided doses q6h; **IV**/IM 250-500 mg q6h, (up to 2 g q4h in severe infections) or 2-8 g qd in divided doses q4-6h

P ***Child:*** PO 50-100 mg/kg/day in divided doses q6h; **IV**/IM 100-200 mg/kg/day in divided doses q6h for septicemia or bacterial meningitis

Meningitis
Adult: **IV** 8-14 g/day in divided doses q3-4h × 3 days

P ***Child:*** **IV** 200-300 mg/kg/day in divided doses q3-4h × 3 days

Gonorrhea
Adult: PO 3.5 g given with 1 g probenecid as a single dose or IM/**IV** 500 mg q 8-12 hr × 2 doses

Available forms: Powder for inj 125, 250, 500 mg, 1, 2, 10 g; **IV** inf 500 mg, 1, 2 g; caps 250, 500 mg, powder for oral susp 100/1 ml, 125, 250, 500 mg/5 ml

Adverse effects
CNS: Lethargy, hallucinations, anxiety, depression, twitching, ***coma, convulsions***
GI: Nausea, vomiting, diarrhea
GU: Oliguria, proteinuria, hematuria, *vaginitis, moniliasis,* ***glomerulonephritis***
HEMA: Anemia, increased bleeding time, ***bone marrow depression, granulocytopenia***
INTEG: Rash, urticaria
SYST: Anaphylaxis

Contraindications: Hypersensitivity to penicillins

Precautions: Pregnancy **B**; hypersensitivity to
P cephalosporins; neonates

Pharmacokinetics

Absorption	Moderate, duodenum (35%-50%)
Distribution	Readily in body tissues, fluids, CSF; crosses placenta
Metabolism	Liver (30%)
Excretion	Breast milk; kidney unchanged (70%)
Half-life	50-110 min

Pharmacodynamics

	PO	IM	IV
Onset	Rapid	Rapid	Rapid
Peak	2 hr	1 hr	Infusion's end

Interactions

Individual drugs

Aspirin: ↑ ampicillin levels, ↓ renal excretion

Probenecid: ↑ ampicillin levels, ↓ renal excretion

Drug classifications

Erythromycins: ↓ antimicrobial effectiveness

Oral anticoagulants: ↑ anticoagulant effects

Oral contraceptives: ↓ contraceptive effectiveness

Tetracyclines: ↓ antimicrobial effectiveness

Lab test interferences

False positive: Urine glucose, urine protein

NURSING CONSIDERATIONS

Assessment

- Assess patient for previous sensitivity reaction to penicillins or other cephalosporins; cross-sensitivity between penicillins and cephalosporins is common
- Assess patient for signs and symptoms of infection, including characteristics of wounds, sputum, urine, stool, WBC >10,000, earache, fever; obtain baseline information and during treatment
- Obtain C&S before beginning drug therapy to identify if correct treatment has been initiated
- Assess for allergic reactions: rash, urticaria, pruritus, chills, fever, joint pain; angioedema may occur a few days after therapy begins; epinephrine and resuscitation equipment should be on unit for anaphylactic reaction; also, check for ampicillin rash: pruritic, red, raised
- Identify urine output; if decreasing, notify prescriber (may indicate nephrotoxicity); also, check for increased BUN, creatinine
- Monitor blood studies: AST (SGOT), ALT (SGPT), CBC, Hct, bilirubin, LDH, alkaline phosphatase, Coombs' test monthly if patient is on long-term therapy
- Monitor electrolytes: potassium, sodium, chloride monthly if patient is on long-term therapy
- Assess bowel pattern qd; if severe diarrhea occurs, drug should be discontinued; may indicate pseudomembranous colitis
- Monitor for bleeding: ecchymosis, bleeding gums, hematuria, stool guaiac daily if on long-term therapy
- Assess for overgrowth of infection: perineal itching, fever, malaise, redness, pain, swelling, drainage, rash, diarrhea, change in cough, sputum

Nursing diagnoses

- ✓ Infection, risk for (uses)
- ✓ Injury, risk for (side effects)
- ✓ Diarrhea (side effects)
- ✓ Knowledge deficit (teaching)
- ✓ Noncompliance (teaching)

Implementation

PO route

- Give in even doses around

the clock; if GI upset occurs, give with food; drug must be taken for 10-14 days to ensure organism death and prevent superinfection; store caps in tight container

- Tabs may be crushed or caps opened and mixed with water
- Shake suspension; store in refrigerator for 2 wk or 1 wk at room temp

IM route

- Reconstitute with 125 mg/ 0.9-1.2 ml; 250 mg/0.9-1.9 ml; 500 mg/1.2-1.8 ml; 1 g/2.4-7.4 ml; 2 g/6.8 ml
- Give deep in large muscle mass

IV **IV route**

- Reconstitute with 125 mg/ 0.9-1.2 ml; 250 mg/0.9-1.9 ml; 500 mg/1.2-1.8 ml; 1 g/2.4-7.4 ml; 2 g/6.8 ml
- Give by direct **IV** over 3-5 min in lower dosages (125-500 mg) or over 15 min in higher dosages (1-2 g)
- Give by intermittent inf after diluting with 0.9% NaCl, LR, D_5W, D_5/0.45% NaCl; use 50 ml of sol and dilute to concentration of <30 mg/ml

Syringe incompatibilities: Erythromycin, gentamicin, kanamycin, lincomycin, metoclopramide, oxytetracycline, streptomycin, tetracycline

Syringe compatibilities: Chloramphenicol, colistimethate, heparin, procaine

Y-site incompatibilities: Calcium gluconate, epinephrine, fluconazole, hetastarch, hydromorphone, hydralazine, ondansetron, sargramostim, verapamil, vinorelbine

Y-site compatibilities: Acyclovir, amifostine, allopurinol, aztreonam, cyclophosphamide, enalaprilat, esmolol, famotidine, filgrastim, fludarabine, foscarnet, heparin, hydromorphone, regular insulin, labetalol, magnesium sulfate, melphalan, meperidine, morphine, oflaxacin, perphenazine, phytonadione, potassium chloride, thiotepa, tolazoline, vitamin B with C

Additive incompatibilities: Amikacin, azetreonam, chlorpromazine, dopamine, gentamicin, hydralazine, hydrocortisone, prochlorperazine

Additive compatibilities: Cefotiam, clindamycin, erythromycin, floxacillin, furosemide, tacrolimus, teniposide, theophylline, verapamil

Patient/family education

- Teach patient to report sore throat, bruising, bleeding, joint pain; may indicate blood dyscrasias (rare)
- Advise patient to contact prescriber if vaginal itching, loose, foul-smelling stools, furry tongue occur; may indicate superinfection
- Instruct patient to take all medication prescribed for the length of time ordered
- Advise patient to notify prescriber of diarrhea with blood or pus, which may indicate pseudomembranous colitis
- Tab may be crushed; cap may be opened and mixed with water

Evaluation

Positive therapeutic outcome

- Absence of signs/symptoms of infection (WBC <10,000, temp WNL, absence of red draining wounds, earache)
- Reported improvement in symptoms of infection

Treatment of anaphylaxis: Withdraw drug, maintain airway, administer epinephrine, aminophylline, O_2, **IV** corticosteroids

ampicillin/ sulbactam (℞)

(am-pi-sill'in/sul-bak'tam)

Unasyn

Func. class.: Broad-spectrum antibiotic

Chem. class.: Aminopenicillin

Pregnancy category B (ampicillin)

Action: Interferes with cell wall replication of susceptible organisms; the cell wall, rendered osmotically unstable, swells and bursts from osmotic pressure; this combination extends the spectrum of activity and inhibits β-lactamase that may inactivate ampicillin

➔ Therapeutic Outcome: Bactericidal against *Pneumococcus, Enterococcus, Streptococcus, Escherichia coli, Proteus mirabilis, Neisseria meningitidis, N. gonorrhoeae, Shigella, Salmonella,* and *Haemophilus influenzae organisms;* use only with β-lactamase–producing strain of infection

Uses: Skin and structure infections, intraabdominal infections, gynecologic infections, soft tissue infections, otitis media, sinusitis, meningitis, septicemia

Dosage and routes

Adult: **IV** 1 g ampicillin and 0.5 g sulbactam or 2 g ampicillin, and 1 g sulbactam q6h, not to exceed 4 g/day sulbactam

Available forms: Powder for inj 1.5 g (1 g ampicillin, 0.5 g sulbactam), 3 g (2 g ampicillin, 1 g sulbactam)

Adverse effects

CNS: Lethargy, hallucinations, anxiety, depression, twitching, ***coma, convulsions***

GI: Nausea, vomiting, diarrhea, increased AST (SGOT), ALT (SGPT), abdominal pain, glossitis, colitis

GU: Oliguria, proteinuria, hematuria, *vaginitis, moniliasis,* ***glomerulonephritis***

HEMA: Anemia, increased bleeding time, ***bone marrow depression, granulocytopenia***

SYST: Anaphalaxis

Contraindications: Hypersensitivity to penicillins

Precautions: Pregnancy **B,** hypersensitivity to cephalosporins, **P** neonates

Pharmacokinetics

Absorption	Well absorbed (IM)
Distribution	Readily in body tissues, fluids, CSF; crosses placenta
Metabolism	Liver (10%-50%)
Excretion	Breast milk; kidney unchanged (75%)
Half-life	50-110 min (ampicillin)

Pharmacodynamics

	IM	IV
Onset	Rapid	Immediate
Peak	1 hr	Infusion's end

Interactions

Individual drugs

Aspirin: ↑ ampicillin levels, ↓ renal excretion

Probenecid: ↑ ampicillin levels, ↓ renal excretion

A

Drug classifications
Erythromycins: ↓ antimicrobial effectiveness
Oral anticoagulants: ↑ anticoagulant effects
Oral contraceptives: ↓ contraceptive effectiveness
Tetracyclines: ↓ antimicrobial effectiveness
Lab test interferences
False positive: Urine glucose, urine protein

NURSING CONSIDERATIONS
Assessment
- Assess patient for previous sensitivity reaction to penicillins or cephalosporins; cross-sensitivity between penicillins and cephalosporins is common
- Assess patient for signs and symptoms of infection; including characteristics of wounds, sputum, urine, stool, WBC >10,000, earache, fever; obtain baseline information and during treatment
- Complete C&S before beginning drug therapy to identify if correct treatment has been initiated
- Assess for allergic reactions: rash, urticaria, pruritus, chills, fever, joint pain; angioedema may occur a few days after therapy begins; epinephrine and resuscitation equipment should be on unit for anaphylactic reaction
- Identify urine output; if decreasing, notify prescriber (may indicate nephrotoxicity); also, check for increased BUN, creatinine
- Monitor blood studies: AST (SGOT), ALT (SGPT), CBC, Hct, bilirubin, LDH, alkaline phosphatase, Coombs' test monthly if patient is on long-term therapy
- Monitor electrolytes: potassium, sodium, chloride monthly if patient is on long-term therapy
- Assess bowel pattern qd; if severe diarrhea occurs, drug should be discontinued; may indicate pseudomembranous colitis
- Monitor for bleeding: ecchymosis, bleeding gums, hematuria, stool guaiac daily if on long-term therapy
- Assess for superinfection: perineal itching, fever, malaise, redness, pain, swelling, drainage, rash, diarrhea, change in cough, sputum

Nursing diagnoses
- ✓ Infection, risk for (uses)
- ✓ Diarrhea (adverse reactions)
- ✓ Injury, risk for (adverse reactions)
- ✓ Knowledge deficit (teaching)
- ✓ Noncompliance (teaching)

Implementation
IM route
- Reconstitute by adding 3.2 ml/1.5 g or 6.4 ml/3 g; use sterile water, 0.5% or 2% lidocaine; give within 1 hr of preparation; give deep in large muscle mass
- Give after C&S completed; on empty stomach

IV route
- Give **IV** after diluting 1.5 g/4 ml or more sterile H_2O for inj (375 mg/ml); allow to stand until foaming stops; give directly over 15-30 min; dilute further in 50 ml or more of D_5W, $D_5$10.45% NaCl, 10% invert sugar in water, LR, 6% sodium lactate, isotonic NaCl; administer within 1 hr after reconstitution; give as an intermittent inf over 15-30 min

Y-site incompatibilities:
Idarubicin, ondansetron, sargramostim

Y-site compatibilities: Amifostine, aztreonam, cefepime, enalaprilat, famotidine, filgrastim, fluconazole, heparin, regular insulin, meperidine, morphine, paclitaxel, tacrolimus, teniposide, theophylline, thiotepa

Additive incompatibility: Aminoglycosides

Additive compatibility: Aztreonam

Patient/family education

- Teach patient to report sore throat, bruising, bleeding, joint pain; may indicate blood dyscrasias (rare)
- Advise patient to contact prescriber if vaginal itching, loose, foul-smelling stools, furry tongue occur; may indicate superinfection
- Instruct patient to use another form of contraception other than oral contraceptives

Evaluation

Positive therapeutic outcome

- Absence of signs/symptoms of infection (WBC <10,000, temp WNL, absence of red draining wounds, earache)
- Reported improvement in symptoms of infection

Treatment of overdose: Withdraw drug, maintain airway, administer epinephrine, aminophylline, O_2, **IV** corticosteroids for anaphylaxis

amrinone (℞)

(am'ri-none)

Inocor

Func. class.: Cardiac inotropic agent

Chem. class.: Bipyrimidine derivative

Pregnancy category C

Action: Positive inotropic agent with vasodilator properties; reduces preload and afterload by direct relaxation of vascular smooth muscle; increases myocardial contractility

Therapeutic Outcome: Increased inotropic effect resulting in increased cardiac output

Uses: Short-term management of CHF that has not responded to other medication; can be used with digitalis products

Dosage and routes

Adult: **IV** bol 0.75 mg/kg given over 2-3 min; start inf of 5-10 μg/kg/min; may give another bol 30 min after start of therapy, not to exceed 10 mg/kg total daily dose

Available forms: Inj 5 mg/ml

Adverse effects

CV: Dysrhythmias, hypotension, headache, chest pain
ELECT: Hypokalemia
GI: Nausea, vomiting, anorexia, abdominal pain, ***hepatotoxicity, ascites,*** jaundice, hiccups
HEMA: ***Thrombocytopenia***
INTEG: Allergic reactions, burning at inj site
RESP: Pleuritis, ***pulmonary densities, hypoxemia,*** dyspnea

Contraindications: Hypersensitivity to this drug or

bisulfites, severe aortic disease, severe pulmonic valvular disease, acute MI

Precautions: Lactation, pregnancy **C**, children, renal disease, hepatic disease, atrial flutter/fibrillation, elderly

P G

Pharmacokinetics

Absorption	Complete bioavailability
Distribution	Unknown
Metabolism	Liver, 50%
Excretion	Kidney, metabolites (60%-90%)
Half-life	4-6 hr, increased in CHF

Pharmacodynamics

Onset	2-5 min
Peak	10 min
Duration	Variable

Interactions

Individual drugs

Disopyramide: ↑ hypotension

Drug classifications

Antihypertensives: ↑ hypotension

Cardiac glycosides: ↑ inotropic effect

NURSING CONSIDERATIONS

Assessment

- Monitor manifestations of hypokalemia: *renal:* acidic urine, reduced urine, osmolality, nocturia; *CV:* hypotension, broad T wave, U wave, ectopy, tachycardia, weak pulse; *neuro:* muscle weakness, altered LOC, drowsiness, apathy, lethargy, confusion, depression; *GI:* anorexia, nausea, cramps, constipation, distention, paralytic ileus; *resp:* hypoventilation, respiratory muscle weakness
- Assess fluid volume status: I&O ratio and record, weight, distended red veins, crackles in lung, color, quality and sp gr of urine, skin turgor, adequacy of pulses, moist mucous membranes, bilateral lung sounds, peripheral pitting edema; dehydration symptoms of decreasing output, thirst, hypotension, dry mouth, and mucous membranes should be reported
- Monitor electrolytes: potassium, sodium, calcium, magnesium; also include BUN, blood pH, ABGs
- Monitor B/P and pulse, PCWP, CVP, index, often during infusion; if B/P drops 30 mm Hg, stop infusion and call prescriber
- Monitor ALT (SGPT), AST (SGOT), bilirubin daily; if these are elevated, hepatoxicity is suspected
- If platelets are <150,000/mm^3, drug is usually discontinued and another drug started
- Assess for extravasation: change site q48h

Nursing diagnoses

- ✓ Cardiac output, decreased (uses)
- ✓ Fluid volume excess (uses)
- ✓ Knowledge deficit (teaching)

Implementation

General

- Patients with low potassium levels (hypokalemia) should receive potassium supplements before amrinone administration
- Administer potassium supplements if ordered for potassium levels <3.0 mg/dl

IV route

- Do not mix directly with glucose sol; chemical reaction occurs over 24 hr; precipitate forms if amrinone and furosemide come in contact

Direct IV

- Administer into running dextrose inf through

Y-connector or directly into tubing; may give undiluted over 2-3 min or dilute with NS to concentration of 1-3 mg/ml; run at prescribed rate; another loading dose may be given in 30 min

IV **Cont IV**

• Give after diluting with 0.9%, or 0.45% NaCl (1-3 mg/ml); do not dilute with dextrose sol; decomposition of drug will occur; use inf pump; use sol within 24 hr of dilution; titrate to patient response

Syringe compatibilities: Propranolol, verapamil

Y-site compatibilities: Aminophylline, atropine, bretylium, calcium chloride, cimetidine, digoxin, dobutamine, dopamine, epinephrine, famotidine, hydrocortisone, isoproterenol, lidocaine, metaraminol, methylprednisolone, nitroglycerin, nitroprusside, norepinephrine, phenylephrine, potassium chloride, procainamide, propranolol, verapamil

Y-site incompatibilities: Furosemide, sodium bicarbonate

Patient/family education

• Teach patient reason for medication and expected results

• Instruct patient to make position changes slowly; orthostatic hypotension may occur

• Teach patient signs and symptoms of hypersensitivity reactions and hypokalemia

Evaluation

Positive therapeutic outcome

• Increased cardiac output

• Decreased PCWP, adequate CVP

• Decreased dyspnea, fatigue, edema, ECG

Treatment of overdose: Discontinue drug, support circulation

amyl nitrite (℞)

(am'il nye'trite)

amyl nitrite, Amyl Nitrite Aspirols, Amyl Nitrite Vaporole

Func. class.: Coronary vasodilator (antianginal, antidote for cyanide)

Chem. class.: Nitrite

Pregnancy category X

Action: Relaxes vascular smooth muscle; may dilate coronary blood vessels, resulting in reduced venous return, decreased cardiac output; reduces preload, afterload, which decreases left ventricular end diastolic pressure, systemic vascular resistance; converts hemoglobin to methemoglobin, which is able to bind cyanide

➡ **Therapeutic Outcome:** Decreased amount, severity of angina; prevention of death in cyanide poisoning

Uses: Acute angina pectoris

Investigational uses: Cardiac murmur diagnosis

Dosage and routes

Angina

Adult: INH 0.18-0.3 ml as needed, 1-6 inhalations from 1 cap; may repeat in 3-5 min

Cyanide poisoning

Adult: INH 0.3-ml ampule 15 sec until preparation of sodium nitrite infusion is ready

A

Available forms: INH pearls 0.18, 0.3 ml

Adverse effects

CNS: Headache, dizziness, weakness, syncope

CV: Postural hypotension, ***tachycardia, cardiovascular collapse,*** palpitations

GI: Nausea, vomiting, abdominal pain

INTEG: Flushing, pallor, sweating

MISC: Muscle twitching, ***hemolytic anemia, methemoglobinemia***

Contraindications: Hypersensitivity to nitrites, severe anemia, increased intracranial pressure, hypertension, pregnancy **X**

Precautions: Lactation, P children, drug abuse, head injury, cerebral hemorrhage, hypotension

Pharmacokinetics

Absorption	Well absorbed
Distribution	Widely distributed
Metabolism	Forms methemoglobin
Excretion	Kidneys (33%)
Half-life	1-4 min

Pharmacodynamics

Onset	30 sec
Peak	Unknown
Duration	3-5 min

Interactions

Individual drugs

Acetylcholine: ↓ effects of acetylcholine

Ephedrine: ↓ antianginal effects

Epinephrine: ↑ hypotension

Histamine: ↓ effects of histamine

Norepinephrine: ↓ effects of norepinephrine

Phenylephrine: ↓ antianginal effects

Drug classifications

Antihypertensives: ↑ hypotension

Sympathomimetics: ↓ antianginal effects

NURSING CONSIDERATIONS

Assessment

- Monitor B/P with patient supine and sitting, pulse during treatment until stable
- Monitor for drug tolerance: need for more medication for each attack
- Monitor for postural hypotension, headache during treatment, which are common side effects because of vasodilatation

Nursing diagnoses

✓ Cardiac output, decreased (uses)

✓ Poisoning (uses)

✓ Tissue perfusion, decreased (uses)

✓ Knowledge deficit (teaching)

Implementation

- Give after wrapping, crushing ampule to avoid cuts; order analgesic if headache develops
- Give to patient who is sitting or lying down during treatment; keep head low, use deep breaths, which will decrease dizziness; have patient rest for 15 min
- Store in light-resistant area in cool environment or refrigerate

Patient/family education

- Instruct patient to keep a record of angina attacks and what aggravates condition; prolonged chest pain may indicate MI: seek emergency treatment
- Advise patient that medication may explode in presence of flame; to keep drug out of reach of children and in secure

place, as there is high abuse potential
• Instruct patient to take several deep breaths despite foul odor; to make position changes slowly to prevent orthostatic hypotension

Evaluation

Positive therapeutic outcome
• Relief of chest pain (angina)
• Absence of death (cyanide poisoning)
• Decreased intensity (heart murmur)

anastrozole (℞)
(an-ass-stroh'zole)
Arimidex
Func. class.: Antineoplastic
Chem. class.: Aromatase inhibitor
Pregnancy category C

Action: Lowers serum estradiol concentrations; many breast cancers have strong estrogen receptors

Therapeutic Outcome: Prevention of rapidly growing malignant cells

Uses: Advanced breast carcinoma that has not responded to other therapy in estrogen-receptor-positive patients (usually postmenopausal)

Dosage and routes
Adult: PO 1 mg qd

Available forms: Tab 1 mg

Adverse effects
CNS: Hot flashes, headache, light-headedness, depression, dizziness, confusion, insomnia, anxiety
CV: Chest pain, hypertension, thrombophlebitis
GI: Nausea, vomiting, altered taste; anorexia; diarrhea, constipation, abdominal pain, dry mouth
GU: Vaginal bleeding, pruritus vulvae
HEMA: Thrombocytopenia, leukopenia
INTEG: ***Rash,*** alopecia
MS: Bone pain, myalgia
RESP: Cough, sinusitis

Contraindications: Hypersensitivity

Precautions: Leukopenia, thrombocytopenia, lactation, cataracts, pregnancy **C,** P children, G elderly, liver disease, renal disease

Pharmacokinetics	
Absorption	Adequately absorbed
Distribution	Unknown
Metabolism	Liver
Excretion	Feces, urine
Half-life	50 hr

Pharmacodynamics	
Onset	Unknown
Peak	4-7 hr
Duration	Unknown

Interactions
Lab test interferences
↑ GGT, ↑ AST, ↑ ALT, ↑ alk phosphatase, ↑ cholesterol, ↑ LDL

NURSING CONSIDERATIONS
Assessment
• Monitor CBC, differential, platelet count weekly; withhold drug if WBC is <4000 or platelet count is <75,000; notify prescriber of results; monitor calcium levels (hypercalcemia is common)
• Assess for tumor flare: increase in bone, tumor pain during beginning treatment; give analgesics as ordered to decrease pain
• Assess for bleeding: hematuria, guaiac, bruising or pete-

chiae, mucosa or orifices, q8h; no rec temp

Nursing diagnoses

✓ Injury, risk for (adverse reactions)

✓ Knowledge deficit (teaching)

Implementation

• Give with food or fluids for GI upset; do not break, crush, or chew enteric products; repeat dose may be needed if vomiting occurs

• Store in light-resistant container at room temp

Patient/family education

• Instruct patient to report any complaints, side effects to health care prescriber; if dose is missed, do not double next dose

• Advise patient that vaginal bleeding, pruritus, hot flashes, can occur, and are reversible after discontinuing treatment

• Inform patient about who should be told about tamoxifen therapy

• Advise patient to report vaginal bleeding immediately; that tumor flare—increase in size or tumor, increased bone pain—may occur and will subside rapidly; may take analgesics for pain

• Caution patient to use sunscreen and protective clothing to prevent burns because photosensitivity is common

• Teach patient that hair loss may occur during treatment; a wig or hairpiece may make patient feel better; new hair may be different in color, texture

• Inform patient that rash or lesions are temporary and may become large during beginning therapy

Evaluation

Positive therapeutic outcome

• Decreased spread of malignant cells in breast cancer

anistreplase (APSAC) (℞)

(an-is-tre-plaze′)

Eminase

Func. class.: Thrombolytic enzyme

Chem. class.: Anisolated plasminogen streptokinase activator complex

Pregnancy category C

Action: Promotes thrombolysis by promoting conversion of plasminogen to plasmin; complex is a combination of plasminogen and streptokinase

➔ **Therapeutic Outcome:** Thrombolysis in coronary arteries

Uses: Management of acute MI; although not yet approved, anistreplase will also be used for other conditions requiring thrombolysis: PE, DUT, unclotting arteriovenous shunts

Dosage and routes

Adult: **IV** inj 30 U over 4-5 min as soon as possible after onset of symptoms

Available forms: Powder, lyophilized 30 U/vial

Adverse effects

CNS: Headache, fever, sweating, agitation, dizziness, paresthesia, tremor, vertigo

CV: Hypotension, dysrhythmias, conduction disorders

GI: Nausea, vomiting

HEMA: Decreased Hct, ***GI, GU, intracranial, retroperito-***

neal, surface bleeding, ***thrombocytopenia***
INTEG: Rash, urticaria, phlebitis at site, itching, flushing
MS: Low back pain, arthralgia
RESP: Altered respirations, dyspnea, ***bronchospasm, lung edema***
SYST: ***Anaphylaxis (rare)***

Contraindications: Hypersensitivity, active internal bleeding, intraspinal or intracranial surgery, neoplasms of CNS, severe hypertension, cerebral embolism, thrombosis, hemorrhage

Precautions: Arterial emboli from left side of heart, pregnancy **C,** ulcerative colitis/enteritis, renal disease, hepatic disease, hypocoagulation, COPD, subacute bacterial endocarditis, rheumatic valvular disease, intraarterial diagnostic procedure or surgery (10 days), recent major surgery, hypersensitivity to this drug or streptokinase

Pharmacokinetics	
Absorption	Complete bioavailability
Distribution	Unknown
Metabolism	Binds to plasmin
Excretion	Kidneys
Half-life	105 min

Pharmacodynamics	
Onset	Unknown
Peak	45 min
Duration	Unknown

Interactions
Individual drugs
Aspirin: ↑ bleeding potential
Dipyridamole: ↑ bleeding potential
Heparin: ↑ bleeding potential
Indomethacin: ↑ bleeding potential
Phenylbutazone: ↑ bleeding potential

Drug classifications
Anticoagulants: ↑ bleeding potential
NSAIDs: ↑ bleeding potential
Lab test interferences
↑ PT, ↑ APTT, ↑ TT
↓ Fibrinogen, ↓ plasminogen

NURSING CONSIDERATIONS
Assessment
- Monitor VS, B/P, pulse, respirations, neurologic signs, temp at least q4h, temp >104° F (40° C) or indicators of internal bleeding, cardiac rhythm after intracoronary administration
- Assess for allergy: fever, rash, itching, chills; mild reaction may be treated with antihistamines; hypersensitivity reactions/dyspnea, wheezing, facial swelling should be treated with epinephrine
- Monitor bleeding during 1st hr of treatment (hematuria, hematemesis, bleeding from mucous membranes, epistaxis, ecchymosis); blood studies (Hct, platelets, PTT, PT, TT, APTT) before starting therapy; PT or APTT must be less than 2 × control before starting therapy; TT or PT q3-4h during treatment

Nursing diagnoses
- ✓ Tissue perfusion, decreased (uses)
- ✓ Injury, risk for (uses, adverse reactions)
- ✓ Knowledge deficit (teaching)

Implementation
- Give heparin therapy after thrombolytic therapy is discontinued, TT or APTT less than 2 × control (about 3-4 hr)
- Avoid invasive procedures: inj, rec temp; about 10% of patients have high streptococ-

cal antibody titers, requiring increased loading doses

- Treat fever with acetaminophen
- Provide pressure for 30 sec to minor bleeding sites, 30 min to sites of arterial puncture followed by dressing; inform prescriber if hemostasis not attained; apply pressure dressing
- Give after reconstituting single-dose vial/5 ml sterile water for inj (not bacteriostatic water), and roll (not shake) to enhance reconstitution, try to minimize foaming; give over 2-5 min by direct **IV**, give within ½ hr of reconstitution or discard, do not add other meds to vial or syringe; give within 6 hr of thrombi identification for best results; cryoprecipitate or fresh frozen plasma if bleeding occurs; store powder in refrigerator; use within 30 min after reconstitution

Incompatibilities:
Do not mix with other drugs in sol or syringe

Patient/family education

- Teach patient action of drug and expected outcome; alert patient to possible hypersensitivity reactions and symptoms to report
- Advise patient bed rest is needed during entire course of treatment; handle patient as little as possible during therapy

Evaluation

Positive therapeutic outcome

- Absence of thrombolysis in MI
- Improved ventricular function

antihemophilic factor (AHF) (℞)

(an-tee-hee-moe-fill'ik)

antihemophilic factor, Humate-P, Hemofil M, Koate-HT, Koate-HS, Kogenate, Kryobulin VH ✤, Monoclate, Monoclate P, Profilate OSD, Recombinate

Func. class.: Hemostatic, blood factor

Chem. class.: Factor VIII

Pregnancy category C

Action: Necessary for clotting. Activates factor X in conjunction with activated factor IX; transforms prothrombin to thrombin

→ **Therapeutic Outcome:** Control of hemorrhage or excessive bleeding in factor VIII deficiency

Uses: Hemophilia A, patients with acquired circulating factor VIII inhibitors, factor VIII deficiency

Dosage and routes

Depends on severity of deficiency and level of antihemophilic factor

Massive hemorrhage

P ***Adult/child:*** **IV** 40-50 U/kg, then 20-25 U/kg q8-12h

Bleeding (frank, overt)

P ***Adult/child:*** **IV** 15-25 U/kg, then 8-15 U/kg q8-12h × 4 days

Hemorrhage near vital organs

P ***Adult/child:*** **IV** 15 U/kg, then 8 U/kg q8h × 2 days, then 4 U/kg q8h × 2 days

Minor hemorrhage

P ***Adult/child:*** **IV** 8-10 U/kg/q24 hr × 2-3 days or 8 U/kg q12h × 2 days, then q24h × 2 days

Joint bleeding

P ***Adult/child:*** **IV** 5-10 U/kg q8-12h × 1-2 days

Available forms: Inj 250, 500, 1000, 1500 U/vial (number of units noted on label)

Adverse effects

CNS: Headache, *lethargy, chills, fever, flushing*
CV: Hypotension, tachycardia
GI: Nausea, vomiting, abdominal cramps, jaundice, ***viral hepatitis***
*HEMA: **Thrombosis, hemolysis, AIDS***
INTEG: Rash, flushing, *urticaria,* stinging at inj site
*RESP: **Bronchospasm***

Contraindications: Hypersensitivity, monoclonal antibody–derived factor VIII

P **Precautions:** Neonates/infants, hepatic disease, blood types A, B, AB, pregnancy **C,** factor VIII inhibitor

Pharmacokinetics	
Absorption	Complete availability
Distribution	Plasma
Metabolism	Not metabolized
Excretion	No excretion
Half-life	Biphasic 4 hr, 15 hr

Pharmacodynamics	
Onset	Immediate
Peak	Unknown
Duration	12 hr

Interactions: None

NURSING CONSIDERATIONS

Assessment

- Monitor blood studies (coagulation factors assay by % normal: 5% prevents spontaneous hemorrhage, 30%-50% for surgery, 80%-100% for severe hemorrhage; blood group of patient, donors (if applicable; most factor VIII not from specific blood group donors)
- Monitor I&O, urine color; notify prescriber if urine becomes orange, red; change in urine color signifying hemolytic reaction; patients other than blood type O are more at risk
- Monitor pulse: discontinue infusion if significant increase
- Obtain test for factor VIII inhibitors before starting treatment, may require concomitant antiinhibitor coagulant complex therapy; Hct, Coombs' test with blood types A, B, AB
- Assess for allergy: fever, rash, itching, jaundice, wheezing, tachycardia, nausea, vomiting; give diphenhydramine (Benadryl); continue therapy if reaction is mild, discontinue if severe; notify prescriber
- ! Monitor bleeding at ankles, knees, elbows, other joints; check for rebleeding after 15-30 min

Nursing diagnoses

- ✓ Tissue perfusion altered (uses)
- ✓ Injury, risk for (uses, adverse reactions)
- ✓ Knowledge deficit (teaching)

Implementation

- Administer **IV** slowly; use plastic syringe to reconstitute and administer; do not use glass, drug adheres to glass; use another needle as a vent when reconstituting; rotate gently to mix
- Administer after dilution with warm NS, D_5W, LR; give within 3 hr
- Administer by **IV** inf: give at ≤2 ml/min if concentration exceeds 34 U/ml; or over 3

min if concentration is less than 34 U/ml; filter before using
• Store in refrigerator; do not freeze; after reconstitution, do not refrigerate; give within 3 hr

Additive compatibilities: Do not mix with other drugs in sol or syringe

Patient/family education

• Advise patient to report any signs of bleeding: gums, under skin, urine, stools, emesis; review methods to prevent bleeding; to be checked q2-3 mo for HIV screen
• Instruct patient to avoid salicylates and ibuprofen; increases bleeding tendencies, decreases clotting
• Instruct patient to prepare, administer factor VIII concentrates at first sign of danger
• Instruct patient to advise health professionals of treatment for hemophilia
• Advise patient that immunization for hepatitis B may be given first
• Instruct patient to report hives, urticaria, chest tightness, hypotension; may be monoclonal antibody–derived factor VII; signs of viral hepatitis, AIDS
• Advise patient to carry identification describing disease process, drugs used

Evaluation

Positive therapeutic outcome

• Absence of bleeding
• Prevention of rebleeding

ascorbic acid (vitamin C) (OTC, ℞)

(as-kor'bic)

Ascorbic Acid, Ascorbicap, Ascorbic Acid Caplets, Apo-C ✤, Cecon, Cenolate, Cemill, Cetane, Cevalin, Cevi-Bid, Ce-Vi-Sol, C-Crystals, Cebid Time Celles, Dull-C, Flavorcee, Kamu-Jay ✤, N'ice Vitamin C Drops, Redoxon ✤, Sunkist Vitamin C, Vita-C

Func. class.: Vitamin C, water-soluble vitamin

Pregnancy category A

Action: Needed for wound healing, collagen synthesis, antioxidant, carbohydrate metabolism, protein, lipid synthesis, prevention of infection

Therapeutic Outcome: Replacement and supplementation of vitamin C

Uses: Vitamin C deficiency, scurvy, delayed wound and bone healing, chronic disease, urine acidification, before gastrectomy; increased need: lactation, pregnancy, hyperthyroidism, emotional stress, trauma, burns

Investigational uses: Acidification of urine, common cold prevention

Dosage and routes

Scurvy

Adult: PO/SC/IM/**IV** 100 mg-500 mg qd, then 50 mg or more qd

P ***Child:*** PO/SC/IM/**IV** 100-300 mg qd, then 35 mg or more qd

Wound healing/chronic disease/fracture
Adult: SC/IM/**IV**/PO 200-500 mg qd

P ***Child:*** SC/IM/**IV**/PO 100-200 mg added doses

Urine acidification
Adult: 4-12 g qd in divided doses

Available forms: Tabs 25, 50, 100, 250, 500, 1000, 1500 mg; effervescent tabs 1000 mg; chewable tabs 100, 250, 500 mg; timed release tabs 500, 750, 1000, 1500 mg; timed release caps 500 mg; crystals 4 g/tsp; powder 4 g/tsp; liq 35 mg/0.6 ml; sol 100 mg/ml; syr 20 mg/ml, 500 mg/5 ml; inj SC, IM, **IV** 100, 250, 500 mg/ml

Adverse effects
CNS: Headache, insomnia, dizziness, fatigue, flushing
GI: Nausea, vomiting, diarrhea, anorexia, heartburn, cramps
GU: Polyuria, urine acidification, oxalate or urate renal stones
HEMA: Hemolytic anemia in patients with G6PD

Contraindications: None significant

Precautions: Gout, pregnancy **A**

Pharmacokinetics	
Absorption	Actively absorbed (PO)
Distribution	Widely distributed; crosses placenta
Metabolism	Oxidation
Excretion	Kidneys, inactive; breast milk
Half-life	Unknown

Pharmacodynamics
Unknown

Interaction
Individual drugs
Amphetamine: ↑ excretion in acidic urine
Deferoxamine: ↑ iron toxicity
Mexiletine: ↑ excretion in acidic urine
Primadone: ↑ requirements for vitamin C
Drug classifications
Anticoagulants, oral: ↓ action of anticoagulants
Antidepressants, tricyclic: ↑ excretion in acidic urine
Salicylates: ↑ requirements of vitamin C
Smoking
Smoking decreases vitamin C levels
Lab test interferences
False positive: negatives in glucose tests (Clinitest, Tes-Tape)
False negative: Occult blood (large dose)
↓ Bilirubin, ↓ urine oxalate, ↓ cysteine

NURSING CONSIDERATIONS
Assessment
- Assess nutritional status for inclusion of foods high in vitamin C: citrus fruits, cantaloupe, tomatoes
- Assess for vitamin C deficiency before, during, and after treatment; scurvy (gingivitis, bleeding gums, loose teeth); poor bone development
- Monitor I&O ratio, polyuria; in patients receiving large doses renal stones may occur
- Monitor ascorbic acid levels throughout treatment if continued deficiency is suspected
- Assess inj sites for inflammation, pain, redness

Nursing diagnoses
✓ Nutrition, less than body requirements (uses)

✓ Knowledge deficit (teaching)

Implementation

IV route

- Give undiluted by *direct* **IV** 100 mg over at least 1 min
- Give by intermittent inf after diluting with D_5W, $D_{10}W$, 0.9% NaCl, 0.45% NaCl, LR, Ringer's sol, dextrose/saline, dextrose/Ringer's combinations; temperature will increase pressure in ampules; wrap with gauze before breaking

Syringe incompatibilities: Cefazolin, doxapram

Syringe compatibility: Metoclopramide

Additive incompatibilities: Bleomycin, cephapirin, nafcillin, sodium bicarbonate, warfarin

Additive compatibilities: Amikacin, calcium chloride, calcium gluceptate, calcium gluconate, cephalothin, chloramphenicol, chlorpromazine, colistimethate, cyanocobalamin, diphenhydramine, heparin, kanamycin, methicillin, methyldopate, penicillin G potassium, polymyxin B, prednisolone, procaine, prochlorperazine, promethazine, verapamil

PO route

- Mix **oral sol** with foods or fluids; **ext rel caps** should be swallowed whole
- Do not crush, break, or chew

IM route

- Not to be diluted; give deep in large muscle mass

Patient/family education

- Teach patient necessary foods to be included in diet that are rich in vitamin C: citrus fruits, cantaloupe, tomatoes, chili peppers (red)
- Teach patient that, if oral contraceptives are taken, increased levels of vitamin C are needed; oral contraceptives deplete vitamin C
- Teach patient that smoking decreases vitamin C levels; not to exceed prescribed dose; increases will be excreted in urine, except time release
- Teach patient not to exceed RDA recommended dose, urinary stones may occur
- Teach patient using ascorbic acid for acidification of urine to test urine pH periodically

Evaluation

Positive therapeutic outcome

- Absence of anorexia, irritability, pallor, joint pain, hyperkeratosis, petechiae, poor wound healing
- Reversal of scurvy: bleeding gums, gingivitis, loose teeth

asparaginase (L-asparaginase) (℞)

(a-spar'a-gin-ase)

Elspar, Kidrolase ✦

Func. class.: Antineoplastic

Chem. class.: Escherichia coli enzyme

Pregnancy category D

Action: Indirectly inhibits protein synthesis in tumor cells; without amino acids, DNA, RNA synthesis is halted; asparagine, protein synthesis is halted; G_1 phase of cell cycle specific; a nonvesicant

Therapeutic Outcome: Prevention of rapidly growing malignant cells in leukemia

Uses: Acute lymphocytic leukemia in combination with

other antineoplastics unresponsive to other agents

Investigational uses: Lymphosarcoma, other leukemias

Dosage and routes

In combination

Adult: **IV** 1000 IU/kg/day × 10 days given over 30 min; IM 6000 IU/m^2/day

Sole induction

Adult: **IV** 200 IU/kg/day × 28 days

Available forms: Inj 10,000 IU

Adverse effects

CNS: Neuritis, dizziness, headache, ***coma,*** depression, fatigue, confusion, hallucinations

CV: Chest pain

ENDO: Hyperglycemia

GI: Nausea, vomiting, anorexia, cramps, stomatitis, ***hepatotoxicity, pancreatitis***

GU: Urinary retention, ***renal failure,*** glycosuria, polyuria, azotemia, uric acid neuropathy

HEMA: ***Thrombocytopenia, leukopenia, myelosuppression, anemia, decreased clotting factors***

INTEG: Rash, urticaria, chills, fever

RESP: ***Fibrosis, pulmonary infiltrate***

SYST: ***Anaphylaxis, hypersensitivity***

Contraindications: Hypersensitivity, infants, pregnancy **D,** lactation, pancreatitis

Precautions: Renal disease, hepatic disease

Pharmacokinetics

Absorption	Complete bioavailability (IV)
Distribution	Intravascular spaces
Metabolism	Unknown
Excretion	Reticuloendothelial system
Half-life	8-30 hr (IV), 39-49 hr (IM)

Pharmacodynamics

	IV	IM
Onset	Immediate	Immediate
Peak	14-24 hr	Unknown
Duration	3-5 wk	3-5 wk

Interactions

Individual drugs

Methotrexate: Blocked action of methotrexate

Vincristine: ↑ neurotoxicity

Drug classifications

Hepatotoxic agents: ↑ hepatotoxicity

Glucocorticosteroids: ↑ hyperglycemia

Lab test interferences

↓ Thyroid function tests

↑ BUN

NURSING CONSIDERATIONS

Assessment

- Assess for signs and symptoms of pancreatitis (nausea, vomiting, severe abdominal pain), anaphylaxis (bronchospasm, dyspnea), cyanosis; monitor amylase, glucose
- Assess symptoms indicating severe allergic reaction: rash, pruritus, urticaria, purpuric skin lesions, itching, flushing; joint pain, bronchospasm, hypotension; epinephrine and crash carts should be nearby
- Monitor for frequency of stools, characteristics: cramping, acidosis; signs of dehydration: rapid respirations, poor skin turgor, decreased urine output, dry skin, restlessness, weakness

- Monitor CBC, differential, platelet count weekly; withhold drug if WBC count is <4000/mm^3 or platelet count is <100,000/mm^3, notify prescriber of results; also monitor PT, PTT, and TT, which may be increased
- Monitor pulmonary function tests, chest x-ray studies before, during therapy; chest x-ray film should be obtained q2 wk during treatment
- Monitor renal function studies: BUN, serum uric acid, ammonia urine CrCl, electrolytes before, during therapy
- Check I&O ratio; report fall in urine output of 30/ml/hr
- Monitor temperature q4h; may indicate beginning infection
- Obtain liver function tests before, during therapy (bilirubin, AST [SGOT], ALT [SGPT], LDH) as needed or monthly
- Monitor RBC, Hct, Hgb, since these may be decreased; serum, urine glucose levels
- Assess for bleeding: hematuria, guaiac, bruising or petechiae, mucosa, or orifices q8h
- Assess for dyspnea, rales, nonproductive cough, chest pain, tachypnea fatigue, increased pulse, pallor, lethargy, or swelling around eyes or lips; anaphylaxis may occur
- Assess for yellowing of skin and sclera, dark urine, clay-colored stools, itchy skin, abdominal pain, fever, diarrhea

Nursing diagnoses

- ✓ Injury, risk for (uses, adverse reactions)
- ✓ Body image disturbance (adverse reactions)

Implementation

- Give after intradermal skin testing and desensitization, give 0.1 ml (2 IU) intradermally after reconstituting with 5 ml sterile H_2O or 0.9% NaCl for injection; then add 0.1 ml of reconstituted drug to 9.9 ml diluent (20 IU/ml); observe for 1 hr, check for wheal
- Use allopurinol or sodium bicarbonate to reduce uric acid levels, alkalinization of urine

IV route

- Give by **IV** infusion using 21-, 23-, 25-gauge needle; administer by slow **IV** infusion via Y-tube or 3-way stopcock of flowing D_5W or NS infusion over 30 min after diluting 10,000 IU/5 ml of sterile H_2O or 0.9% NaCl (no preservatives) (2000 IU/ml); use of filter may be necessary if fibers are present

Y-site compatibilities: Methotrexate, sodium bicarbonate

Patient/family education

- Teach patient to report any complaints or side effects to nurse or physician
- Teach patient to report any changes in breathing or coughing

Evaluation

Positive therapeutic response

- Decreased replication of leukemia cells

Treatment of anaphylaxis: Administer epinephrine, diphenhydramine, **IV** corticosteroids

aspirin 🗝 (OTC)
(as'pir-in)
Ancasal ✱, A.S.A., Aspergum, Aspirin ✱, Bayer, Bayer Children's aspirin, Easprin, Ecotrin, Ecotrin Maximum Strength, 8-Hour Bayer Timed Release, Empirin, Entrophen ✱, Genprin, Maximum Bayer, Norwich Extra-Strength, Novasen ✱, Sal-Adult ✱, Sal-Infant ✱, St. Joseph Children's, Supasa ✱, Therapy Bayer, ZORprin
Func. class.: Nonnarcotic analgesic
Chem. class.: Salicylate
Pregnancy category D

Action: Blocks pain impulses in CNS, inhibition of prostaglandin synthesis; antipyretic action results from vasodilatation of peripheral vessels; decreases platelet aggregation

➔ **Therapeutic Outcome:** Decreased pain, inflammation, fever; absence of MI, transient ischemic attacks, thrombosis

Uses: Mild to moderate pain or fever including rheumatoid arthritis, osteoarthritis, thromboembolic disorders, transient ischemic attacks in men, rheumatic fever, post-MI, prophylaxis of MI

Investigational uses: Prevention of cataracts (long-term use)

Dosage and routes

Arthritis

Adult: PO 2.6-5.2 g/day in divided doses q4-6h

P ***Child:*** PO 90-130 mg/kg/day in divided doses q4-6h

Pain/fever

Adult: PO/REC 325-650 mg q4h prn, not to exceed 4 g/day

P ***Child:*** PO/REC 40-100 mg/kg/day in divided doses q4-6h prn

Thromboembolic disorders

Adult: PO 325-650 mg/day or bid

Transient ischemic attacks

Adult: PO 650 mg qid or 325 mg qid

Available forms: Tabs 65, 81, 325, 500, 650, 975 mg; chewable tabs 81 mg; caps 325, 500 mg; cont rel tabs 800 mg; time-release tabs 650 mg; supp 60, 120, 125, 130, 195, 200, 300, 325, 600, 650 mg, 1.2 g; cream; gum 227.5 mg

Adverse effects

CNS: Stimulation, drowsiness, dizziness, confusion, ***convulsion,*** headache, flushing, hallucinations, ***coma***

CV: Rapid pulse, pulmonary edema

EENT: Tinnitus, hearing loss

ENDO: Hypoglycemia, hyponatremia, hypokalemia

GI: Nausea, vomiting, ***GI bleeding,*** diarrhea, heartburn, anorexia, ***hepatitis***

HEMA: ***Thrombocytopenia, agranulocytosis, leukopenia, neutropenia, hemolytic anemia,*** increased pro-time, PTT, bleeding time

INTEG: Rash, urticaria, bruising

RESP: Wheezing, hyperpnea

Contraindications: Hypersensitivity to salicylates, tartrazine (FDC yellow dye #5), GI bleeding, bleeding disorders, P children <12 yr, children with flulike symptoms, pregnancy

D, lactation, vitamin K deficiency, peptic ulcer

Precautions: Anemia, hepatic disease, renal disease, Hodgkin's disease, pre/postoperatively

Pharmacokinetics

Absorption	Well absorbed, small intestine (PO); erratic (enteric); slow (rec)
Distribution	Rapidly, widely distributed; crosses placenta
Metabolism	Liver, extensively
Excretion	Inactive metabolites, kidney; breast milk
Half-life	2-3 hr (low doses); 30 hr (high doses)

Pharmacodynamics

	PO	REC
Onset	15-30 min	Slow
Peak	1-2 hr	4-5 hr
Duration	4-6 hr	6-7 hr

Interactions

Individual drugs

Alcohol: ↑ bleeding
Cefamandole: ↑ bleeding
Furosemide: ↑ toxic effects
Heparin: ↑ bleeding
Insulin: ↑ effects of insulin
Methotrexate: ↑ effects of methotrexate
PABA: ↑ toxic effects
Phenytoin: ↑ effects of phenytoin
Plicamycin: ↑ bleeding
Probenecid: ↓ effects of probenecid
Spironolactone: ↓ effects
Sulfinpyrazone: ↓ effects
Valproic acid: ↑ bleeding
Vancomycin: ↑ ototoxicity

Drug classifications

Antacids: ↓ effects of aspirin
Anticoagulants: ↑ bleeding
Carbonic anhydrase inhibitors: ↑ toxic effects
NSAIDs: ↑ gastric ulcers
Penicillins: ↑ effects of penicillins
Salicylates: ↓ blood sugar levels
Steroids: ↓ effects of aspirin, ↑ gastric ulcers
Sulfonylamides: ↓ effects of sulfonylamides
Urinary acidifiers: ↑ salicylate levels
Urinary alkalizers: ↓ effects of aspirin

Lab test interferences

↑ Coagulation studies, ↑ liver function studies, ↑ serum uric acid, ↑ amylase, ↑CO_2, ↑ urinary protein
↓ Serum potassium, ↓ PBI, ↓ cholesterol
Interference: Urine catecholamines, pregnancy test, urine glucose tests (Clinistix, Tes-Tape)

NURSING CONSIDERATIONS

Assessment

- Monitor liver function studies: AST (SGOT), ALT (SGPT), bilirubin, creatinine if patient is on long-term therapy
- Monitor renal function studies: BUN, urine creatinine if patient is on long-term therapy
- Monitor blood studies: CBC, Hct, Hgb, pro-time if patient is on long-term therapy
- Check I&O ratio; decreasing output may indicate renal failure (long term therapy)
- ! Assess hepatotoxicity: dark urine, clay-colored stools, yellowing of the skin and sclera, itching, abdominal pain, fever, diarrhea if patient is on long-term therapy
- Assess for allergic reactions: rash, urticaria; if these occur, drug may have to be discontinued

- Assess for ototoxicity: tinnitus, ringing, roaring in ears; audiometric testing needed before, after long-term therapy
- Assess for visual changes: blurring, halos; corneal, retinal damage
- Check edema in feet, ankles, legs
- Identify prior drug history; there are many drug interactions
- Monitor pain: location, duration, type, intensity, before dose and 1 hr after
- Monitor musculoskeletal status: ROM before dose
- Identify fever: length of time and related symptoms

Nursing diagnoses

✓ Pain (uses)
✓ Mobility, impaired physical (uses)
✓ Injury, risk for (side effects)
✓ Knowledge deficit (teaching)

Implementation

PO route

- Administer to patient crushed or whole; chewable tab may be chewed
- ⊘ Do not crush enteric product
- Give with food or milk to decrease gastric symptoms; give 30 min before or 2 hr pc; absorption may be slowed
- Give antacids 1-2 hr after enteric products

Patient/family education

- Teach patient to report any symptoms of hepatotoxicity, renal toxicity, visual changes, ototoxicity, allergic reactions, bleeding (long-term therapy)
- Instruct patient to take with 8 oz of water and sit upright for 30 min after dose
- Instruct patient not to exceed recommended dosage; acute poisoning may result
- Advise patient to read label on other OTC drugs; many contain aspirin
- Inform patient that the therapeutic response takes 2 wk (arthritis)
- Teach patient to report tinnitus, confusion, diarrhea, sweating, hyperventilation
- Advise patient to avoid alcohol ingestion; GI bleeding may occur
- Advise patient with allergies that allergic reactions may develop
- Instruct patient to avoid buffered or effervescent products
- P Teach patient not to give to children; Reye's syndrome may develop

Evaluation

Positive therapeutic outcome

- Decreased pain
- Decreased inflammation
- Decreased fever
- Absence of MI
- Absence of transient ischemic attacks, thrombosis

Treatment of overdose: Lavage, activated charcoal, monitor electrolytes, VS

astemizole (℞)

(a-stem'i-zole)

Hismanal

Func. class.: Antihistamine

Chem. class.: H_1-histamine antagonist

Pregnancy category C

Action: Acts on blood vessels, GI, respiratory system by competing with histamine for H_1receptor site; decreases allergic response by blocking pharmacologic effects of histamine; less sedation rate than with other antihistamines; causes increased heart rate, vasodilatation, increased secretions

Therapeutic Outcome: Absence of allergy symptoms and rhinitis

Uses: Rhinitis, allergy symptoms, chronic idiopathic urticaria

Dosage and routes

P ***Adult and child >12 yr:*** PO 10 mg qd; to reduce time to steady state may take 30 mg day 1, 20 mg day 2, followed by 10 mg daily

Available forms: Tabs 10 mg

Adverse effects

CNS: Headache, stimulation, drowsiness, sedation, fatigue, confusion, blurred vision, tinnitus, restlessness, tremors, P paradoxical excitation in G children or elderly

CV: Hypotension, palpitations, bradycardia, tachycardia, ***dysrhythmias*** (rare)

GI: Nausea, diarrhea, abdominal pain, vomiting, constipation

GU: Frequency, dysuria, urinary retention, impotence

HEMA: Hemolytic anemia, thrombocytopenia, leukopenia, agranulocytosis, pancytopenia

INTEG: Rash, eczema, photosensitivity, urticaria

RESP: Thickening of bronchial secretions, dry nose, throat

Contraindications: Hypersen- P sitivity, newborn or premature infants, lactation, severe hepatic disease

Precautions: Pregnancy **C,** G elderly, children, respiratory P disease, narrow angle glaucoma, prostatic hypertrophy, bladder neck obstruction, asthma

Pharmacokinetics

Absorption	Well absorbed
Distribution	Unknown, 97% bound to plasma proteins
Metabolism	Liver, extensively; converted to desmethylastemizole
Excretion	Kidneys
Half-life	Biphasic 3½, 16-23 hr

Pharmacodynamics

Onset	Unknown
Peak	1-2 hr
Duration	Unknown

Interactions

Individual drugs

Alcohol: ↑ CNS depression
Erythromycin: ↑ CV reaction
Itraconazole: ↑ CV reaction
Ketoconazole: ↑ CV reaction

Drug classifications

Anticoagulants, oral: ↓ action
CNS depressants: ↑ CNS depression
MAOI: ↑ anticholinergic effect
Narcotics: ↑ CNS depression
Sedative/hypnotics: ↑ CNS depression

Food

↓ absorption

Lab test interferences

False negative: Skin allergy tests (discontinue antihistamine 3 days before testing)

NURSING CONSIDERATIONS

Assessment

- Assess respiratory status: rate, rhythm, increase in bronchial secretions, wheezing, chest tightness; provide fluids to 2 L/day to decrease secretion thickness
- Monitor I&O ratio: be alert for urinary retention, frequency, dysuria, especially G elderly; drug should be discontinued if these occur

• Monitor CBC during long-term therapy; blood dyscrasias may occur but are rare

Nursing diagnoses

✓ Airway clearance, ineffective (uses)
✓ Injury, risk for (side effects)
✓ Knowledge deficit (teaching)
✓ Noncompliance (teaching, overuse)

Implementation

• Give on an empty stomach 1 hr before or 2 hr pc to facilitate absorption
• Store in tight, light-resistant container

Patient/family education

• Teach all aspects of drug uses; to notify prescriber if confusion, sedation, hypotension occur; to avoid driving or other hazardous activity if drowsiness occurs; to avoid alcohol or other CNS depressants that may potentiate effect
• Instruct patient to take 1 hr before or 2 hr pc to facilitate absorption
• Instruct patient not to exceed recommended dose; dysrhythmias may occur
• Teach patient hard candy, gum, frequent rinsing of mouth may be used for dryness

Evaluation

Positive therapeutic outcome

• Absence of running or congested nose, rashes

Treatment of overdose: Administer ipecac syrup or lavage, diazepam, vasopressors, barbiturates (short acting)

atenolol (℞)

(a-ten'oh-lole)

Apo-Atenolol ✱, atenolol, Novo-Atenolol ✱, Tenormin

Func. class.: Antihypertensive

Chem. class.: β-Blocker; β_1-; β_2-blocker (high doses)

Pregnancy category C

Action: Competitively blocks stimulation of β-adrenergic receptor within vascular smooth muscle; produces negative chronotropic activity, positive inotropic activity (decreases rate of SA node discharge, increases recovery time), slows conduction of AV node, decreases heart rate, decreases O_2 consumption in myocardium; also decreases renin-aldosterone-angiotensin system at high doses, inhibits β_2-receptors in bronchial system at higher doses

➡ **Therapeutic Outcome:** Decreased B/P, heart rate, prevention of angina pectoris, MI

Uses: Mild to moderate hypertension, prophylaxis of angina pectoris, suspected or known MI

Investigational uses: Dysrhythmia, mitral valve prolapse, pheochromocytoma, hypertrophic cardiomyopathy, vascular headaches, thyrotoxicosis, tremors, alcohol withdrawal

Dosage and routes

Adult: **IV** 5 mg; repeat in 10 min if initial dose is well tolerated, then start PO dose 10 min after last **IV** dose

Adult: PO 50 mg qd, increasing q1-2 wk to 100 mg qd; may increase to 200 mg qd for angina

Available forms: Tabs 25, 50, 100 mg; **IV** 5 mg/10 ml

Adverse effects

CNS: Insomnia, fatigue, dizziness, mental changes, memory loss, hallucinations, depression, lethargy, drowsiness, strange dreams, catatonia
CV: Profound hypotension, bradycardia, CHF, cold extremities, postural hypotension, 2nd- or 3rd-degree heart block
EENT: Sore throat, dry burning eyes
ENDO: Increased hypoglycemic response to insulin
GI: Nausea, diarrhea, vomiting, ***mesenteric arterial thrombosis, ischemic colitis***
GU: Impotence
HEMA: Agranulocytosis, thrombocytopenia, purpura
INTEG: Rash, fever, alopecia
RESP: ***Bronchospasm,*** dyspnea, wheezing

Contraindications: Hypersensitivity to β-blockers, cardiogenic shock, 2nd- or 3rd-degree heart block, sinus bradycardia, CHF, cardiac failure

Precautions: Major surgery, pregnancy **C**, lactation, diabetes mellitus, renal disease, thyroid disease, COPD, asthma, well-compensated heart failure

Pharmacokinetics	
Absorption	50%-60% (PO)
Distribution	Crosses placenta; protein binding (5%-15%)
Metabolism	Not metabolized
Excretion	Breast milk, kidneys (50%), feces (50%—unabsorbed drug)
Half-life	6-7 hr

Pharmacodynamics	PO
Onset	1 hr
Peak	2-4 hr
Duration	24 hr

Interactions

Individual drugs

Alcohol: ↑ hypotension (large amounts)
Epinephrine: α-Adrenergic stimulation
Hydralazine: ↑ hypotension, bradycardia
Indomethacin: ↓ antihypertensive effect
Insulin: ↑ hypoglycemia
Methyldopa: ↑ hypotension, bradycardia
Prazosin: ↑ hypotension, bradycardia
Reserpine: ↑ hypotension, bradycardia
Thyroid: ↓ effectiveness of atenolol
Verapamil: ↑ myocardial depression

Drug classifications

Antihypertensives: ↑ hypertension
β_2-Agonist: ↓ bronchodilatation
Cardiac glycosides: ↑ bradycardia
Nitrates: ↑ hypotension
Theophyllines: ↓ bronchodilatation

Lab test interferences

Interference: Glucose insulin tolerance tests

↑ Uric acid, ↑ potassium, ↑ triglyceride, ↑ lipoproteins

NURSING CONSIDERATIONS

Assessment

- Monitor B/P during beginning treatment, periodically thereafter; pulse q4h; note rate, rhythm, quality: apical/radial pulse before administration; notify prescriber of any significant changes (pulse <50 bpm)
- Check for baselines in renal, liver function tests before therapy begins
- Assess for edema in feet, legs daily; monitor I&O, daily weight; check for jugular vein distention, rales bilaterally, dyspnea (CHF)
- Monitor skin turgor, dryness of mucous membranes for hydration status, especially G elderly

Nursing diagnoses

- ✓ Cardiac output, decreased (uses)
- ✓ Injury, risk for physical (side effects)
- ✓ Knowledge deficit (teaching)
- ✓ Noncompliance (teaching)

Implementation

PO route

- Given ac, hs, tablet may be crushed or swallowed whole; give with food to prevent GI upset; reduced dosage in renal dysfunction
- Store protected from light, moisture; place in cool environment

IV IV route

- Give **IV** direct over 5 min or diluted in 10-50 ml D_5W, 0.9% NaCl, and give at prescribed rate

Y-site compatibilities: Meperidine, morphine

Patient/family education

- ! Teach patient not to discontinue drug abruptly; taper over 2 wk; may cause precipitate angina if stopped abruptly
- Teach patient not to use OTC products containing α-adrenergic stimulants (such as nasal decongestants, OTC cold preparations); to avoid alcohol, smoking; to limit sodium intake as prescribed
- Teach patient how to take pulse and B/P at home; advise when to notify prescriber
- Instruct patient to comply with weight control, dietary adjustments, modified exercise program
- Advise patient to carry/wear Medic Alert ID for drugs and allergies; tell patient drug controls symptoms but does not cure
- Caution patient to avoid hazardous activities if dizziness, drowsiness is present
- Teach patient to report symptoms of CHF: difficult breathing, especially on exertion or when lying down, night cough, swelling of extremities or bradycardia, dizziness, confusion, depression, fever
- Teach patient to take drug as prescribed, not to double doses, skip doses; take any missed doses as remembered if at least 6 hr until next dose

Evaluation

Positive therapeutic outcome

- Decreased B/P in hypertension (after 1-2 wk)
- Absence of dysrhythmias
- Absence of MI
- Decreased angina

Treatment of overdose: Lavage, **IV** atropine for bradycardia, **IV** theophylline for bronchospasm, digitalis, O_2, diuretic for cardiac failure, hemodialysis, **IV** glucose for hyperglycemia, **IV** diazepam (or phenytoin) for seizures

atorvastatin (℞)

(at-or'va-sta-tin)

Lipitor

Func. class.: Antihyperlipidemic

Chem. class.: Synthetically derived fermentation product

Pregnancy category X

Action: Inhibits HMG-CoA reductase enzyme, which reduces cholesterol synthesis

➡ **Therapeutic Outcome:** Decreased cholesterol levels and LDLs, increased HDLs

Uses: As an adjunct in primary hypercholesterolemia (types Ia, Ib)

Dosage and routes

Adult: PO 10 mg qd, usual range 10-80, dosage adjustments may be made in 2-4 wk intervals

Available forms: Tabs 10, 20, 40 mg

Adverse effects

CNS: Headache

EENT: Lens opacities

GI: Dyspepsia, flatus, *liver dysfunction,* pancreatitis

INTEG: Rash, pruritus, alopecia

MS: Myalgia

Contraindications: Hypersensitivity, pregnancy **X,** lactation, active liver disease

Precautions: Past liver disease, alcoholism, severe acute infections, trauma, hypotension, uncontrolled seizure disorders, severe metabolic disorders, electrolyte imbalance

Pharmacokinetics

Absorption	Unknown
Distribution	Unknown
Metabolism	Liver
Excretion	Bile, feces, kidneys
Half-life	14 hr

Pharmacodynamics

Unknown

Interactions

Individual drugs

Cholestyramine: ↓ action of atorvastatin

Colestipol: ↓ action of atorvastatin

Cyclosporine: ↑ risk of myopathy

Erythromycin: ↑ risk of myopathy

Gemfibrozil: ↑ risk of myopathy

Niacin: ↑ risk of myopathy

Warfarin: ↑ action

Digoxin: ↑ action

Oral contraceptives: ↑ action

NURSING CONSIDERATIONS

Assessment

- Assess nutrition: fat, protein, carbohydrates; nutritional analysis should be completed by dietician before treatment
- Monitor bowel pattern daily; diarrhea may be a problem
- Monitor triglycerides, cholesterol at baseline and throughout treatment; LDL and VLDL should be watched closely; if increased, drug should be discontinued
- Monitor liver function studies q1-2 mo during the first 1½ yr of treatment; AST (SGOT), ALT (SGPT), liver function tests may be increased
- Monitor renal studies in patients with compromised

renal system: BUN, I&O ratio, creatinine
• Assess eyes with slit lamp before, 1 mo after treatment begins, annually

Nursing diagnoses
✓ Diarrhea (adverse reactions)
✓ Knowledge deficit (teaching)
✓ Noncompliance (teaching)

Implementation
• Give with evening meal; if dosage is increased, take total daily dose with evening meal
• Store in cool environment in airtight, light-resistant container

Patient/family education
• Inform patient that compliance is needed for positive results to occur, not to double doses
• Teach patient that risk factors should be decreased: high-fat diet, smoking, alcohol consumption, absence of exercise
• Advise patient to notify prescriber if the GI symptoms of diarrhea, abdominal or epigastric pain, nausea, vomiting occur; of if chills, fever, sore throat occur
• Advise patient that treatment will take several years
• Advise patient that blood work and eye exam will be necessary during treatment

Evaluation
Positive therapeutic outcome
• Decreased cholesterol levels, serum triglyceride
• Improved ratio of HDLs

atovaquone (℞)
(a-toe'va-kwon)
Mepron
Func. class.: Antiprotozoal
Chem. class.: Aromatic diamide derivative; analog of ubiquinone
Pregnancy category C

Action: Interferes with DNA/RNA synthesis in protozoa, specifically ATP and nucleic acid synthesis

➔ **Therapeutic Outcome:** Antiprotozoal for *Pneumocystis carinii* only

Uses: *Pneumocystis carinii* infections resistant to trimethoprim/sulfamethoxazole (co-trimoxazole)

Dosage and routes
Adult: PO 750 mg with food tid for 21 days

Available forms: Tabs 250 mg

Adverse effects
CNS: Dizziness, headache, anxiety
CV: Hypotension
GI: Nausea, vomiting, diarrhea, anorexia, increased AST (SGOT) and ALT (SGPT), acute pancreatitis, constipation, abdominal pain
HEMA: Anemia, ***leukopenia***
INTEG: Pruritus, urticaria, *rash,* oral monilia
META: Hyperkalemia, hyperglycemia, hyponatremia

Contraindications: Hypersensitivity or history of developing life-threatening allergic reactions to any component of the formulation

Precautions: Blood dyscrasias, hepatic disease, diabetes mellitus, pregnancy **C**, lactation, children, elderly

P G

Pharmacokinetics

Absorption	Poor; increased when taken with fatty foods
Distribution	Unknown
Metabolism	Hepatic recycling
Excretion	Feces, unchanged (94%)
Half-life	2-3 days

Pharmacodynamics

Onset	Unknown
Peak	1-8 hr

Interactions

Drug classifications

Use cautiously with highly protein-bound drugs

Food

↑ absorption of drug, especially fatty foods

NURSING CONSIDERATIONS

Assessment

- Assess for *Pneumocystis carinii:* monitor WBC, bilateral lung sounds, sputum for C&S; these should be checked before, periodically during, and after treatment; after collection of 1st sputum, therapy may begin
- Monitor for symptoms of hyponatremia: *CV:* increased B/P, cold, clammy skin, hypovolemia or hypervolemia; *GI:* anorexia, nausea, vomiting, diarrhea, abdominal cramps; *neuro:* lethargy, increased ICP, confusion, headache, seizures, coma, fatigue, tremors, hyperreflexia
- Monitor for symptoms of hypoglycemia/hyperglycemia in diabetic patients
- Monitor blood studies: blood glucose, CBC, platelets; I&O ratio; ECG for cardiac dysrhythmias, check B/P; liver studies: AST (SGOT), ALT (SGPT)
- Monitor for signs of infection; anemia; monitor bowel pattern before, during treatment
- Monitor respiratory status: rate, character, wheezing, dyspnea
- Assess for dizziness, confusion, hallucination
- Assess for allergies before treatment, reaction of each medication; place allergies on chart; notify all people giving drugs

Nursing diagnoses

- ✓ Infection, risk for (uses)
- ✓ Diarrhea (adverse reactions)
- ✓ Knowledge deficit (teaching)

Implementation

- Give with food (preferably fatty); increased absorption of the drug and higher plasma concentrations will occur; give tid × 3 wks

Patient/family education

- Instruct patient to take with food, preferably fatty foods, to increase plasma concentrations
- Advise patient to take drug exactly as prescribed

Evaluation

Positive therapeutic outcome

- Decreased temperature
- Ability to breathe
- Three negative sputum cultures

atracurium (℞)
(a-tra-cure'ee-um)
Tracrium
Func. class.: Neuromuscular blocker (nondepolarizing)
Chem. class.: Biquaternary ammonium ester
Pregnancy category C

Action: Inhibits transmission of nerve impulses by binding with cholinergic receptor sites, antagonizing action of acetylcholine

➔ Therapeutic Outcome: Skeletal muscle paralysis after anesthesia

Uses: Facilitation of endotracheal intubation; skeletal muscle relaxation during mechanical ventilation, surgery, or general anesthesia

Dosage and routes
Adult: **IV** bol 0.4-0.5 mg/kg, then 0.08-0.10 mg/kg 20-45 min after 1st dose if needed for prolonged procedures

P ***Child 1 mo-2 yr:*** **IV** bol 0.3-0.4 mg/kg

Available forms: Inj 10 mg/ml

Adverse effects
CV: Bradycardia, tachycardia, increased, decreased B/P
EENT: Increased secretions
INTEG: Rash, flushing, pruritus, urticaria
MS: Inadequate or prolonged block
RESP: Prolonged apnea, bronchospasm, cyanosis, respiratory depression

Contraindications: Hypersensitivity

Precautions: Pregnancy **C**, cardiac disease, lactation, P children <2 yr, electrolyte imbalances, dehydration, neuromuscular disease, respiratory disease

Pharmacokinetics

Absorption	Complete bioavailability
Distribution	Extracellular space, crosses placenta
Metabolism	Plasma
Excretion	Unknown
Half-life	Biphasic 2 min, 29 min

Pharmacodynamics

Onset	2 min
Peak	5 min
Duration	20-60 min

Interactions
Individual drugs
Clindamycin: ↑ paralysis
Colistin: ↑ paralysis
Lidocaine: ↑ paralysis
Lithium: ↑ paralysis
Magnesium: ↑ paralysis
Polymyxin B: ↑ paralysis
Procainamide: ↑ paralysis
Quinidine: ↑ paralysis
Succinylcholine: ↑ paralysis
Drug classifications
Aminoglycosides: ↑ paralysis
β-Blockers: ↑ paralysis
Diuretics, potassium-losing: ↑ paralysis
General anesthesia: ↑ paralysis

NURSING CONSIDERATIONS
Assessment
- Assess for electrolyte imbalances (potassium, magnesium); may lead to increased action of this drug
- Monitor vital signs (B/P, pulse, respirations, airway) until fully recovered; rate, depth, pattern of respirations, strength of hand grip
- Monitor I&O ratio; check for urinary retention, frequency, hesitancy

- Assess recovery: decreased paralysis of face, diaphragm, leg, arm, rest of body
- Monitor allergic reactions: rash, fever, respiratory distress, pruritus; drug should be discontinued

Nursing diagnoses

✓ Breathing pattern, ineffective (uses)
✓ Communication, impaired verbal (adverse reactions)
✓ Fear (adverse reactions)

Implementation

- Anesthesiologist should use nerve stimulator to determine neuromuscular blockade
- Give anticholinesterase to reverse neuromuscular blockade
- Give undiluted direct **IV** over 5 min, or diluted in 10-50 ml of D_5W (½ NaCl or NS) and give as an inf at prescribed rate
- Give only by qualified person, usually an anesthesiologist; do not administer IM
- Give only slightly discolored solution
- Store in light-resistant area

Y-site compatibilities: Cefazolin, cefuroxime, cimetidine, dobutamine, dopamine, epinephrine, esmolol, fentanyl, gentamicin, heparin, hydrocortisone, isoproterenol, lorazepam, midazolam, morphine, nitroglycerine, ranitidine, sodium nitroprusside, trimethoprim/sulfamethoxazole, vancomycin

Y-site incompatibility: Diazepam

Additive compatibilities: Bretylium, cimetidine, dobutamine, dopamine, esmolol, gentamicin, isoproterenol, lidocaine, morphine, potassium chloride, procainamide, vancomycin

Additive incompatibilities: Barbiturates, sodium bicarbonate

Syringe compatibilities: Alfantanil, fentanyl, midazolam, sufentanil

Patient/family education

- Provide reassurance if communication is difficult during recovery from neuromuscular blockade
- Provide explanation of all treatments and procedures before beginning

Evaluation

Positive therapeutic outcome

- Paralysis of jaw, eyelid, head, neck, rest of body

Treatment of overdose: Edrophonium or neostigmine, atropine; monitor VS; may require mechanical ventilation

atropine (℞)

(a'troe-peen)

Atropine-1, Atropine Care Ophthalmic, Atropine Sulfate Ophthalmic, atropine sulfate S.O.P., Atropisol Ophthalmic, Isopto Atropine, Atropair, Atro-Pen, I-tropine, Minims Atropine ✦

Func. class.: Anticholinergic parasympatholytic, mydriatic

Chem. class.: Belladonna alkaloid

Pregnancy category C

Action: Blocks acetylcholine at parasympathetic neuroeffector sites; increases cardiac output, heart rate by blocking vagal stimulation in heart; dries secretions, decreases sweating, salivation in low doses; mydriasis, increased heart rate and cycloplegia occur at moderate doses; motility of GI, GU systems at high dose

➔ **Therapeutic Outcome:** Drying of secretions, increased heart rate, cycloplegia, mydriasis

Uses: Bradycardia, bradydysrhythmia, anticholinesterase, insecticide poisoning, blocking cardiac vagal reflexes, decreasing secretions before surgery, antispasmodic with GU and biliary surgery, bronchodilator; opthalmically for cycloplegia, mydriasis

Dosage and routes

Bradycardia/ bradydysrhythmias

Adult: **IV** bol 0.5-1 mg given q3-5 min, not to exceed 2 mg

P ***Child:*** **IV** bol 0.01-0.03 mg/kg up to 0.4 mg or 0.3 mg/m^2; may repeat q4-6h

Insecticide poisoning

P ***Adult and child:*** IM/**IV** 2 mg qh until muscarinic symptoms disappear; may need 6 mg qh

Before surgery

Adult: SC/IM/**IV** 0.4-0.6 mg before anesthesia

P ***Child:*** SC 0.1-0.4 mg 30 min before surgery

Cycloplegic refraction

Adult: OPHTH i-ii gtt of 1% sol 1 hr before exam

P ***Child:*** OPHTH i-ii gtt of 0.5% sol bid-tid for up to 3 days before and 1 hr after exam

GI disorders

Adult: PO 0.3-1.2 mg q4-6h

Available forms: Inj 0.05, 0.1, 0.3, 0.4, 0.5, 0.8, 1 mg/ml; tabs 0.4 mg; tabs soluble 0.4, 0.6 mg; oint 1%; sol (ophth) 0.5%, 1%, 2%

Adverse effects

CNS: Headache, dizziness, involuntary movement, confusion, psychosis, anxiety, coma, flushing, drowsiness, insomnia, weakness

CV: Hypotension, paradoxic bradycardia, angina, PVCs, hypertension, tachycardia, ectopic ventricular beats

EENT: Blurred vision, photophobia, glaucoma, eye pain, pupil dilatation, nasal congestion

GI: Dry mouth, nausea, vomiting, abdominal pain, anorexia, constipation, paralytic ileus, abdominal distention, altered taste

GU: Retention, hesitancy, impotence, dysuria

INTEG: Rash, urticaria, contact dermatitis, dry skin, flushing

MISC: Suppression of lactation, decreased sweating

Contraindications: Hypersensitivity to belladonna alkaloids, angle closure glaucoma, GI obstructions, myasthenia gravis, thyrotoxicosis, ulcerative colitis, prostatic hypertrophy, tachycardia/ tachydysrhythmias, asthma, acute hemorrhage, hepatic disease, myocardial ischemia

Precautions: Pregnancy **C**, renal disease, lactation, CHF, tachydysrhythmias, hyperthyroidism, COPD, hepatic dis-
P ease, child <6 yr, hyperten-
G sion, elderly, intraabdominal

infections, Down's syndrome, spastic paralysis, gastric ulcer

Pharmacokinetics

Absorption	Well absorbed (PO, SC, IM)
Distribution	Crosses blood-brain barrier, placenta
Metabolism	Liver
Excretion	Kidneys, unchanged (70%-90%); breast milk
Half-life	13-40 hr

Pharmacodynamics

	PO	IM/SC	IV	OPHTH
Onset	½ hr	15 min	2-4 min	½ hr
Peak	½-1 hr	30 min	2-4 min	30-60 min
Duration	4-6 hr	4-6 hr	4-6 hr	1-2 wk

Interactions

Individual drugs

Amantadine: ↑ anticholinergic effect
Disopyramide: ↑ anticholinergic effect
Potassium chloride, oral: ↑ GI lesions
Quinidine: ↑ anticholinergic effect

Drug classifications

Antacids: ↓ absorption of atropine
Anticholinergics: ↑ anticholinergic effect
Antidepressants, tricyclic: ↑ anticholinergic effect
Antihistamines: ↑ anticholinergic effect

NURSING CONSIDERATIONS

Assessment

- Monitor I&O ratio; check for urinary retention and daily output in elderly or postoperative patients
- Monitor ECG for ectopic ventricular beats, PVC, tachycardia
- Monitor for bowel sounds; check for constipation; abdominal distention and constipation may occur
- Monitor respiratory status: rate, rhythm, cyanosis, wheezing, dyspnea, engorged neck veins
- Monitor for increased intraocular pressure: eye pain, nausea, vomiting, blurred vision, increased tearing; discontinue use if pain occurs (optic)
- Monitor cardiac rate: rhythm, character, B/P continuously
- Monitor allergic reaction: rash, urticaria

Nursing diagnoses

- ✓ Cardiac output, decreased (uses)
- ✓ Sensory-perceptual alteration: visual (adverse reactions)
- ✓ Constipation (adverse reactions)
- ✓ Knowledge deficit (teaching)

Implementation

IV route

- Give **IV** undiluted or diluted with 10 ml sterile H_2O; give at a rate of 0.6 mg/min; give through Y-tube or 3-way stopcock; do not add to **IV** sol; may cause paradoxic bradycardia lasting 2 min

Syringe compatibilities: Benzquinamide, butorphanol, chlorpromazine, cimetidine, dimenhydrinate, diphenhydramine, droperidol, fentanyl, glycopyrrolate, heparin, hydromorphone, hydroxyzine, meperidine, metoclopramide, midazolam, milrinone, morphine, nalbuphine, pentazocine, prochlorperazine, promazine, promethazine, propiomazine, ranitidine, scopolamine, sufentanil, Vit B with C

Y-site compatibilities: Amrinone, famotidine, heparin, hydrocortisone sodium succinate, nafcillin, potassium chloride

Additive compatibilities: Dobutamine, netilmicin, sodium bicarbonate, verapamil

PO route
- PO 30 min ac
- Give increased bulk, water in diet if constipation occurs (anticholinergic effect)

IM route
- Expect atropine flush 15-20 min after inj; it may occur in P children and is not harmful

Patient/family education
- Advise patient not to perform strenuous activity in high temperatures; heat stroke may result
- Instruct patient to take as prescribed; not to skip doses
- Instruct patient to report change in vision; blurring or loss of sight; trouble breathing; sweating; flushing, chest pain, allergic reactions
- Caution patient not to operate machinery if drowsiness occurs
- Advise patient not to take OTC products without approval of physician

Ophthalmic route
- Teach patient method of instillation: pressure on lacrimal sac for 1 min; do not touch dropper to eye
- Instruct patient that blurred vision will decrease with repeated use of drug; to omit next instillation if side effects are present
- Instruct patient not to perform hazardous tasks until able to see
- Advise patient to wait 5 min to use other drops; not to blink more than usual; use sunglasses to protect eyes

Evaluation

Positive therapeutic outcome
- Decreased dysrhythmias
- Increased heart rate
- Decreased secretions, GI, GU spasms
- Bronchodilatation
- Decrease in inflammation (iritis) or cycloplegic refraction (ophthalmic)

Treatment of overdose: O_2, artificial ventilation, ECG; administer dopamine for circulatory depression; administer diazepam or thiopental for convulsion; assess need for antidysrhythmics

attapulgite (OTC)

(at-a-pull'gite)

Diar Aid, Diasorb, Fowler's Diarrhea Tablets ✤, Hydrated Magnesium Silicate, Kaopectate, Kaopectate Advanced Formula, Kaopectate Maximum Strength, Parepectolin, Rheaban, St. Joseph Antidiarrheal

Func. class.: Antidiarrheal

Chem. class.: Hydrous magnesium aluminum silcate

Pregnancy class C

Action: Decreases gastric motility, water content of stool; adsorbent, demulcent

➔ Therapeutic Outcome: Decreased diarrhea

Uses: Diarrhea (cause undetermined), mild to moderate

Dosage and routes
Adult: PO 60-120 ml (45-90 ml conc) after each loose bowel movement

P *Child >12 yr:* PO 60 ml after each loose bowel movement

P *Child 6-12 yr:* PO 30-60 ml (30 ml conc) after each loose bowel movement

P *Child 3-6 yr:* PO 15-30 ml (15 ml conc) after each loose bowel movement

Available forms: Susp kaolin 0.87 g/5 ml, pectin 43 mg/5 ml; kaolin 0.98 g/5 ml, pectin 21.7 mg/5 ml

Adverse effects
GI: Constipation (chronic use)

Precautions: Pregnancy C

Pharmacokinetics

Absorption	Not absorbed
Distribution	Unknown
Metabolism	Unknown
Excretion	Unknown
Half-life	Unknown

Pharmacodynamics

Unknown

Interactions
All drugs: ↓ action of all other drugs

Nursing diagnoses
✓ Diarrhea (uses)
✓ Constipation (adverse reactions)
✓ Knowledge deficit (teaching)

NURSING CONSIDERATIONS
Assessment
• Assess bowel pattern before, during, and after treatment; check for rebound constipation
• Monitor for dehydration in P children

Implementation
• For 48 hr only after each diarrhea stool

Patient/family education
• Advise patient not to exceed recommended dosage; notify prescriber if symptoms continue
• Instruct patient to shake well before administration

Evaluation
Positive therapeutic outcome
• Decreased diarrhea

auranofin (℞)
(au-ran'oh-fin)
Ridaura
Func. class.: Antiinflammatory (gold)
Chem. class.: Active gold compound (29%)
Pregnancy category C

Action: Antiinflammatory action unknown; may decrease phagocytosis, lysosomal activity or decrease prostaglandin synthesis; decreases concentration of rheumatoid factor, immunoglobulins

➔ **Therapeutic Outcome:** Relief of pain, inflammation, slowing of rheumatoid arthritis resistant to other treatment

Uses: Rheumatoid arthritis unresponsive to other treatment

Investigational uses: SLE, psoriatic arthritis, pemphigus

Dosage and routes
Adult: PO 6 mg qd or 3 mg bid, may increase to 9 mg/day after 3 mo

Available forms: Caps 3 mg

Adverse effects
CNS: Dizziness, confusion, hallucinations, ***seizures***, EEG abnormalities

*GI: **Diarrhea**, abdominal cramping, stomatitis, nausea, vomiting, enterocolitis,* anorexia, flatulence, metallic taste, dyspepsia, jaundice, increased AST (SGOT), ALT (SGPT), glossitis, gingivitis, melena, constipation
GU: ***Proteinuria, hematuria,*** increased BUN, creatinine, vaginitis
HEMA: ***Thrombocytopenia, agranulocytosis, aplastic anemia, leukopenia, eosinophilia, neutropenia***
INTEG: Rash, pruritus, dermatitis, ***exfoliative dermatitis,*** urticaria, alopecia, photosensitivity
MISC: Iritis, corneal ulcers, gold deposits in ocular tissues
RESP: ***Interstitial pneumonitis, fibrosis,*** cough, dyspnea

Contraindications: Hypersensitivity to gold, necrotizing enterocolitis, bone marrow P aplasia, child <6 yr, lactation, pulmonary fibrosis, exfoliative dermatitis, blood dyscrasias, recent radiation therapy, renal/hepatic disease, marked hypertension, uncontrolled CHF

G **Precautions:** Elderly, CHF, diabetes mellitus, allergic conditions, ulcerative colitis, renal disease, liver disease, pregnancy **C**

Pharmacokinetics

Absorption	20%-30%
Distribution	Widely distributed; concentrated in joints
Metabolism	Unknown
Excretion	Kidneys slow (60%-90%); feces (10%-40%); breast milk
Half-life	1 mo (blood); up to 4 mo (tissue)

Pharmacodynamics

Onset	Unknown
Peak	2 hr
Durations	8-16 wk (steady state)

Interactions

Individual drugs

Penicillamine: ↑ toxicity
Radiation: ↑ bone marrow toxicity

Drug classifications

Antineoplastics: ↑ bone marrow toxicity

Lab test interferences

False positive: TB skin test

NURSING CONSIDERATIONS

Assessment

- Assess symptoms of rheumatoid arthritis: pain in joints, stiffness, poor range of motion, inflammation
- Assess respiratory status: dyspnea, wheezing; if respiratory problems occur, drug should be discontinued; pneumonitis, fibrosis may occur
- Monitor urine; hematuria, proteinuria, increased BUN, creatinine may require decrease in dosage or discontinuation of treatment; I&O ratio
- Monitor blood studies: platelets, WBC, eosinophils, granulocytes monthly; drug should be discontinued if platelets <100,000/mm^3, WBC <4000 mm^3, eosinophils >5%, granulocytes <1500 mm^3
- Monitor hepatic test: ALT (SGPT), AST (SGOT), alkaline phosphatase monthly
- Monitor diarrhea stools; if severe, drug should be discontinued
- Assess allergy: rash, dermatitis, pruritus, angioneurotic edema, nitroid reactions; drug should be discontinued if any of these occur

- Assess gold toxicity: decreased Hgb, WBC <4000/mm^3, granulocytes <1500/mm^3, platelets <150,000/mm^3, severe diarrhea, stomatitis, hematuria, rash, itching, proteinuria; drug should be discontinued and dimercaprol (BAL) with glucocorticoids given

Nursing diagnoses

- ✓ Mobility, impaired (uses)
- ✓ Injury, risk for (adverse reactions)
- ✓ Diarrhea (adverse reactions)
- ✓ Knowledge deficit (teaching)

Implementation

- Give bid or may give as single dose qAM with food or drink to prevent GI symptoms
- Do not chew, crush caps

Patient/family education

- Instruct patient that drug must be taken as prescribed to be useful; to obtain lab work monthly; that therapeutic effect may take 3-4 mo; patient should not double or skip doses
- Teach patient that diarrhea is common, but if blood appears in stools or urine, notify prescriber at once; that patient should check for bruising, hematemesis, hematuria, petechiae, bleeding gums, which indicate thrombocytopenia
- Advise patient to report abnormal skin conditions, stomatitis, fatigue, jaundice; may indicate blood dyscrasias; to notify prescriber of sore throat, fever, malaise; infection, gold toxicity: severe diarrhea, stomatitis, rash, itching; to avoid exposure to sunlight or ultraviolet light; to use sunscreen to prevent burns
- Teach patient to use dilute hydrogen peroxide for mild stomatitis, avoid hot spicy foods and food with high acidic content; use soft toothbrush, rinse more frequently, floss daily
- Teach patient that contraception should be used during treatment

Evaluation

Positive therapeutic outcome

- Ability to move joints with less pain
- Absence of stiffness, inflammation in joints

aurothioglucose/gold sodium thiomalate (℞)

(aur-oh-thye-oh-gloo'kose)

Solganal/Myochrysine

Func. class.: Antiinflammatory (gold)

Chem. class.: Active gold compound (50%)

Pregnancy category C

Action: Antiinflammatory action unknown; may decrease phagocytosis, lysosomal activity, prostaglandin synthesis

Therapeutic Outcome: Relief of pain, inflammation; slowing of rheumatoid arthritis

Uses: Rheumatoid arthritis resistant to other treatment, psoriatic arthritis

Dosage and routes

Adult: IM 10 mg; then 25 mg weekly × 2-3 wk; then 50 mg/wk until total of 1 g is administered; then 25-50 mg q3-4 wk if there is improvement without toxicity (aurothioglucose); total of 800 mg-1 g

Adult: IM 10 mg, then 25 mg after 1 wk, then 50 mg weekly for total of 14-20 doses; then 50 mg q2 wk × 4; then 50 mg q3 wk × 4; then 50 mg monthly for maintenance (gold sodium thiomalate)

P ***Child 6-12 yr:*** IM 1 mg/kg/wk × 20 wk, or ¼ of adult dosage (aurothioglucose)

P ***Child <6 yr:*** IM 1 mg/kg/wk × 20 wk, then q3-4 wk if improvement without toxicity (gold sodium thiomalate), not to exceed 2.5 mg

Available forms: Inj 50 mg/ml, 25 mg/ml

Adverse effects

CNS: Dizziness, EEG abnormalities, *encephalitis,* confusion, hallucinations

CV: Bradycardia, rapid pulse

EENT: Iritis, corneal ulcers

GI: Stomatitis, nausea, vomiting, metallic taste, jaundice, ***hepatitis,*** diarrhea, cramping, flatulence

GU: Proteinuria, hematuria, ***nephrosis, tubular necrosis***

HEMA: ***Thrombocytopenia, agranulocytosis, aplastic anemia, leukopenia, eosinophilia, neutropenia***

INTEG: Rash, pruritus, dermatitis, urticaria, alopecia, photosensitivity, ***exfoliative dermatitis, angioedema***

RESP: Interstitial pneumonitis, pharyngitis, ***pulmonary fibrosis***

SYST: ***Anaphylaxis***

Contraindications: Hypersensitivity to gold, SLE, uncontrolled diabetes mellitus, marked hypertension, recent radiation therapy, CHF, lactation, renal disease, liver disease

Precautions: Decreased tolerance in elderly, children, blood dyscrasias, pregnancy **C**

G P

Pharmacokinetics

Absorption	Slow
Distribution	Widely distributed; concentration in joints
Metabolism	Unknown
Excretion	Kidneys, slow (60%-90%); feces (10%-40%); breast milk
Half-life	26 days (blood); up to 4 mo (tissue)

Pharmacodynamics

Onset	Unknown
Peak	4-6 hr
Duration	8-16 wk (steady state)

Interactions

Individual drugs

Penicillamine: ↑ toxicity

Radiation: ↑ bone marrow toxicity

Drug classifications

Antineoplastics: ↑ bone marrow toxicity

Lab test interferences

False positive: TB skin test

NURSING CONSIDERATIONS

Assessment

- Assess symptoms of rheumatoid arthritis: pain in joints, stiffness, poor range of motion, inflammation
- Assess respiratory status: dyspnea, wheezing; if respiratory problems occur, drug should be discontinued; pneumonitis, fibrosis may occur
- Monitor urine; hematuria, proteinuria, increased BUN, creatinine may require decrease in dosage or discontinuation of treatment; I&O ratio
- Monitor blood studies: platelets, WBC, eosinophils, granulocytes monthly; drug should be discontinued if platelets <100,000/mm^3, WBC <4000 mm^3, eosinophils >5%, granulocytes <1500 mm^3

• Monitor hepatic test: ALT (SGPT), AST (SGOT), alkaline phosphatase monthly
• Monitor diarrhea stools; if severe, drug should be discontinued
• Assess allergy: rash, dermatitis, pruritus, angioneurotic edema, nitroid reactions; drug should be discontinued if any of these occur
• Assess gold toxicity: decreased Hgb, WBC <4000/mm^3, granulocytes <1500/mm^3, platelets <150,000/mm^3, severe diarrhea, stomatitis, hematuria, rash, itching, proteinuria; drug should be discontinued and dimercaprol (BAL) with glucocorticoids given

Nursing diagnoses
✓ Mobility, impaired physical (uses)
✓ Injury, risk for (adverse reactions)
✓ Diarrhea (adverse reactions)
✓ Knowledge deficit (teaching)

Implementation
• Give deep IM, never **IV**; slow administration; keep recumbent for 10 min after inj; monitor for transient reaction
• Shake well before giving

Patient/family education
• Teach patient that drug must be taken as prescribed to be useful; to obtain lab work monthly; that therapeutic effect may take 3-4 mo; patient should not double or skip doses
• Instruct patient that diarrhea is common, but if blood appears in stools or urine, notify prescriber at once; that patient should check for bruising, hematemesis, hematuria, petechiae, bleeding gums, which indicate thrombocytopenia
• Tell patient to report abnormal skin conditions, stomatitis, fatigue, jaundice; may indicate blood dyscrasias; to notify prescriber of sore throat, fever, malaise (infection); severe diarrhea, stomatitis, rash, itching (gold toxicity); to avoid exposure to sunlight or ultraviolet light; to use sunscreen to prevent burns
• Teach patient to use dilute hydrogen peroxide for mild stomatitis, avoid hot spicy foods and food with high acidic content; use soft toothbrush, rinse more frequently, floss daily
• Teach patient that contraception should be used during treatment

Evaluation

Positive therapeutic outcome
• Ability to move joints with less pain
• Absence of stiffness, inflammation of joints

azatadine (℞)

(a-za'ta-deen)

Optimine

Func. class.: Antihistamine

Chem. class.: Piperidine H_1-receptor antagonist

Pregnancy category B

Action: Acts on blood vessels, GI, respiratory system by competing with histamine for H_1receptor site; decreases allergic response by blocking histamine; causes increased heart rate, vasodilatation, secretions

Therapeutic Outcome: Absence of allergy symptoms and rhinitis

Uses: Allergy symptoms, rhinitis, allergic dermatoses, nasal allergies

Investigational uses: Cluster headaches, anorexia nervosa (as an appetite stimulant)

Dosage and routes

Adult: PO 1-2 mg bid, not to exceed 4 mg/day

Available forms: Tabs 1 mg

Adverse effects

CNS: Dizziness, drowsiness, poor coordination, fatigue, anxiety, euphoria, confusion, paresthesia, neuritis, sweating, chills

CV: Hypotension, palpitations, tachycardia

EENT: Blurred vision, dilated pupils, tinnitus, nasal stuffiness, dry nose, throat, mouth

GI: Constipation, dry mouth, nausea, vomiting, anorexia, diarrhea

GU: Retention, dysuria, frequency, impotence

*HEMA: **Thrombocytopenia, agranulocytosis, hemolytic anemia***

INTEG: Rash, urticaria, photosensitivity

RESP: Increased thick secretions, wheezing, chest tightness

Contraindications: Hypersensitivity to H_1-receptor antagonist, acute asthma attack, lower respiratory tract disease, P child <12 yr

Precautions: Increased intraocular pressure, renal disease, cardiac disease, bronchial asthma, seizure disorder, stenosed peptic ulcers, hyperthyroidism, prostatic hypertrophy, bladder neck obstruction, pregnancy **B**, G elderly

Pharmacokinetics	
Absorption	Well absorbed
Distribution	Crosses placenta
Metabolism	Liver, extensively
Excretion	Kidneys, unchanged (20%)
Half-life	9-12 hr

Pharmacodynamics	
Onset	15-60 min
Peak	4 hr
Duration	12 hr

Interactions

Individual drugs

Alcohol: ↑ CNS depression

Drug classifications

CNS depressants: ↑ CNS depression

MAOI: ↑ anticholinergic effect

Narcotics: ↑ CNS depression

Sedative/hypnotics: ↑ CNS depression

Lab test interferences

False negative: Skin allergy tests (discontinue antihistamines 3 days before testing)

NURSING CONSIDERATIONS

Assessment

- Assess respiratory status: rate, rhythm, increase in bronchial secretions, wheezing, chest tightness; provide fluids to 2 L/day to decrease secretion thickness
- Monitor I&O ratio: be alert for urinary retention, frequency, dysuria, especially G elderly; drug should be discontinued if these occur
- Monitor CBC during long-term therapy; blood dyscrasias may occur but are rare

Nursing diagnoses

- ✓ Airway clearance, ineffective (uses)
- ✓ Injury, risk for (side effects)
- ✓ Knowledge deficit (teaching)
- ✓ Noncompliance (teaching-overuse)

Implementation
- May give with food to prevent GI upset; absorption is not altered by food
- Store in tight, light-resistant container

Patient/family education
- Teach all aspects of drug uses; to notify prescriber if confusion, sedation, hypotension occur; to avoid driving or other hazardous activity if drowsiness occurs; to avoid alcohol or other CNS depressants that may potentiate effect
- Teach patient to take 1 hr ac or 2 hr pc to facilitate absorption
- Caution patient not to exceed recommended dosage; dysrhythmias may occur
- Teach patient hard candy, gum, frequent rinsing of mouth may be used for dryness

Evaluation
Positive therapeutic outcome
- Absence of running or con gested nose, rashes

Treatment of overdose: Administer ipecac syrup or lavage, diazepam, vasopressors, barbiturates (short acting)

azathioprine (R)

(ay-za-thye'oh-preen)
Imuran
Func. class.: Immunosuppressant
Chem. class.: Purine analog
Pregnancy category D

Action: Produces immunosuppression by inhibiting purine synthesis, DNA, RNA in cells

Therapeutic Outcome: Absence of graft rejection, slowing of rheumatoid arthritis

Uses: Renal transplants to prevent graft rejection, often used with corticosteroids, cytotoxics; refractory rheumatoid arthritis, refractory ITP, glomerulonephritis, nephrotic syndrome, bone marrow transplant

Investigational uses: Myasthenia gravis, chronic ulcerative colitis, Crohn's disease, Behcet's syndrome

Dosage and routes
Prevention of rejection
P ***Adult and child:*** PO, **IV** 3-5 mg/kg/day, then maintenance (PO) of at least 1-2 mg/kg/day

Refractory rheumatoid arthritis
Adult: PO 1/mg/kg/day; may increase dosage after 2 mo by 0.5 mg/kg/day; not to exceed 2.5 mg/kg/day

Available forms: Tabs 50 mg; inj **IV** 100 mg

Adverse effects
GI: Nausea, vomiting, stomatitis, esophagitis, ***pancreatitis, hepatotoxicity, jaundice***
HEMA: Leukopenia, thrombocytopenia, anemia, pancytopenia
INTEG: Rash
MS: Arthralgia, muscle wasting

Contraindications: Hypersensitivity, pregnancy **D**

Precautions: Severe renal disease, severe hepatic disease

Pharmacokinetics

Absorption	Readily (PO)
Distribution	Crosses placenta
Metabolism	Liver to mercap topurine
Excretion	Kidney, minimal
Half-life	3 hr

Pharmacodynamics

	PO	IV
Onset	Unknown	Unknown
Peak	4 hr	Unknown
Duration	Unknown	Unknown

Interactions

Individual drugs

Allopurinol: ↑ toxicity
Cyclosporine: ↑ myelosuppression

Drug classification

Antineoplastics: ↑ myelosuppression

NURSING CONSIDERATIONS

Assessment

- Assess symptoms of rheumatoid arthritis: pain in joints, stiffness, poor range of motion, inflammation
- Monitor blood studies: Hgb, WBC, platelets during treatment monthly; if leukocytes are <3000/mm^3 or platelets <100,000/mm^3, drug should be discontinued or reduced; decreased Hgb level may indicate bone marrow suppression
- Monitor liver function studies: alkaline phosphatase, AST (SGOT), ALT (SGPT), amylase, bilirubin; and for hepatotoxicity: dark urine, jaundice, itching, light-colored stools; drug should be discontinued

Nursing diagnoses

- ✓ Mobility, impaired (uses)
- ✓ Infection, risk for (uses)
- ✓ Knowledge deficit (teaching)

Implementation

PO route

- Give all medications PO if possible, avoiding IM injections, since bleeding may occur
- Give with meals to reduce GI upset; nausea is common
- For several days before transplant surgery, patients should be placed in protective isolation

IV IV route

- Give after diluting 100 mg/10 ml of sterile water for inj; rotate to dissolve; may further dilute with 50 ml or more saline or glucose in saline given over >30 min (intermittent inf)

Sol compatibilities: D_5W, NaCl 0.9%, NaCl 0.45%

Patient/family education

- Teach patient that therapeutic response may take 3-4 mo in rheumatoid arthritis; that drug is needed for life in renal transplant
- Instruct patient to report fever, rash, severe diarrhea, chills, sore throat, fatigue, since serious infections may occur; or clay-colored stools and cramping (hepatotoxicity)
- Advise patient to use contraceptive measures during treatment for 12 wk after ending therapy; drug is teratogenic
- Tell patient to avoid crowds and persons with known infections to reduce risk of infection
- Instruct patient not to use OTC medications without approval of prescriber

Evaluation

Positive therapeutic outcome

- Absence of graft rejection
- Immunosuppression in autoimmune disorders
- Increased joint mobility

without pain in rheumatoid arthritis

azithromycin (℞)

(ay-zi-thro-my'sin)

Zithromax

Func. class.: Antibacterial

Chem. class.: Macrolide (azalide) antibiotic

Pregnancy category B

Action: Binds to 50S ribosomal subunits of susceptible bacteria and suppresses protein synthesis; much greater spectrum of activity than erythromycin

➔ Therapeutic Outcome: Bacteriostatic against the following susceptible organisms: *Moraxella catarrhalis, Streptococcus pneumoniae, S. pyogenes, Staphylococcus aureus, Haemophilus influenzae, Clostridium, Legionella pneumophila, Chlamydia trachomatis, Mycoplasma;* no effect on methicillin-resistant *S. aureus;* P in children: acute otitis media *(H. influenzae, M. catarrhalis, S. pneumoniae) PO;* community-acquired pneumonia *(C. pneumoniae, H. influenzae, M. pneumoniae, S. pneumoniae) PO;* pharyngitis/tonsillitis *(S. pyogenes)*

Uses: Mild to moderate infections of the upper respiratory tract, lower respiratory tract; uncomplicated skin and skin structure infections, nongonococcal urethritis, or cervicitis

Dosage and routes

Adult: PO 500 mg on day 1, then 250 mg qd on days 2-5 for a total dose of 1.5 g; may give a one-time dose of 1 g for chlamydial infections

Available forms: Caps 250 mg; tabs 250, 600 mg; powder for inj 500 mg; powder for oral susp 100 mg/5 ml, 200mg/5 ml, 300 mg/15 ml, 600 mg/15 ml, 900 mg/22.5 ml, 1 gm/packet

Adverse effects

CNS: Dizziness, headache, vertigo, somnolence

CV: Palpitations, chest pain

GI: Nausea, vomiting, diarrhea, ***hepatotoxicity,*** abdominal pain, stomatitis, heartburn, dyspepsia, flatulence, melena, ***cholestatic jaundice***

GU: Vaginitis, moniliasis, nephritis

INTEG: Rash, urticaria, pruritus, photosensitivity

Contraindications: Hypersensitivity to azithromycin or erythromycin

Precautions: Pregnancy **B,** lactation, hepatic/renal/ G cardiac disease, elderly, P children <16 yr

Pharmacokinetics	
Absorption	Rapid, (PO) up to 50%
Distribution	Widely distributed
Metabolism	Unknown, minimal metabolism
Excretion	Unchanged (bile); kidneys, minimal
Half-life	11-70 hr

Pharmacodynamics	
Onset	Unknown
Peak	Unknown
Duration	24 hr

Interactions

Individual drugs

Astemizole: ↑ toxicity

Carbamazepine: ↑ toxicity

Terfenadine: ↑ toxicity

Theophylline: ↑ toxicity

Drug classifications
Aluminum antacids: ↓ peak serum
Anticoagulants, orals: ↑ effect of oral anticoagulants
Magnesium antacids: ↓ levels of azithromycin
Food
↓ absorption
Lab test interferences
False ↑ 17-OHCS/17-KS, ↑ AST (SGOT), ↑ ALT (SGPT)
↓ Folate assay

NURSING CONSIDERATIONS
Assessment
- Assess for signs and symptoms of infection: drainage, fever, increased WBC >10,000 mm^3, urine culture positive, sore throat, sputum culture positive
- Monitor respiratory status: rate, character, wheezing, tightness in chest; discontinue drug if these occur
- Monitor allergies before treatment, reaction of each medication; place allergies on chart, notify all people giving drugs; skin eruptions, itching
- Monitor I&O ratio, renal studies; report hematuria, oliguria in renal disease; check urinalysis, protein, blood
- Monitor liver studies: AST (SGOT), ALT (SGPT), bilirubin, LDH, alkaline phosphatase
- Monitor C&S before drug therapy; drug may be taken as soon as culture is taken; C&S may be repeated after treatment
- Monitor bowel pattern before, during treatment

Nursing diagnoses
✓ Infection, risk for (uses)
✓ Diarrhea (adverse reactions)
✓ Knowledge deficit (teaching)

Implementation
- Provide adequate intake of fluids (2 L) during diarrhea episodes
- Give with a full glass of water; do not give with food; give 1 hr before or 2 hr pc; do not give with fruit juices
- Store at room temperature

Patient/family education
- Instruct patient to report sore throat, black furry tongue, fever, loose foul-smelling stool, vaginal itching, discharge, fatigue; may indicate superinfection
- Caution patient not to take aluminum/magnesium-containing antacids or food simultaneously with this drug; blood levels of azithromycin will be decreased
- Instruct patient to notify prescriber of diarrhea stools, dark urine, pale stools, yellow discoloration of eyes or skin, severe abdominal pain; cholestatic jaundice is a severe adverse reaction
- Teach patient to take at evenly spaced intervals; complete dosage regimen; to notify prescriber if symptoms continue
- Teach patient that if pregnancy is suspected to notify prescriber
- Inform patient that sunburns may occur; wear protective clothing and sunscreen

Evaluation
Positive therapeutic outcome
- C&S negative for infection
- WBC within 5000-10,000 mm^3

A

aztreonam (℞)
(az-tree'oh-nam)
azactam
Func. class.: Misc. antibiotic
Chem. class.: Monobactam
Pregnancy category B

Action: Inhibits organisms by inhibiting bacterial cell wall synthesis, which causes death of organism (bactericidal)

➔ **Therapeutic Outcome:** Bactericidal action against susceptible organisms, specifically gram-negative aerobic organisms: *Escherichia coli, Serratia, Klebsiella, Enterobacter, Haemophilus influenzae, Shigella, Providencia, Salmonella, Neisseria gonorrhoeae, Pseudomonas aeruginosa,* including strains resistant to other drugs

Uses: Urinary tract infection; septicemia; skin, muscle, bone infection and other infections caused by gram-negative organisms

Dosage and routes
Urinary tract infections
Adult: **IV**/IM 500 mg-1 g q8-12h

Systemic infections
Adult: **IV**/IM 1-2 g q8-12h

Severe systemic infections
Adult: **IV**/IM 2 g q6-8h; do not exceed 8 g/day
Continue treatment for 48 hr after negative culture or until patient is asymptomatic

Available forms: Powder for inj 500 mg, 1, 2 g

Adverse effects
CNS: Lethargy, hallucinations, anxiety, depression, twitching, ***coma, convulsions,*** malaise
EENT: Tinnitus, diplopia, nasal congestion
GI: Nausea, vomiting, diarrhea, increased AST (SGOT), ALT (SGPT), abdominal pain, glossitis, colitis
GU: Vaginal candidiasis, vaginitis, breast tenderness
HEMA: Anemia, increased bleeding time, ***bone marrow depression, granulocytopenia***

Contraindications: Hypersensitivity

Precautions: Pregnancy **B,** lactation, children, impaired renal/hepatic function, elderly

P G

Pharmacokinetics

Absorption	Well absorbed (IM)
Distribution	Widely distributed; crosses placenta
Metabolism	Liver, minimal
Excretion	Kidneys, unchanged (65%-75%); breast milk
Half-life	1.7 hr; increased in renal disease

Pharmacodynamics

	IM	IV
Onset	Rapid	Rapid
Peak	1 hr	Infusion's end

Interactions
Drug classifications
Antiinfectives: ↑ antagonist effect
Clindamycin: ↓ action of clindamycin
Furosemide: ↑ levels
Penicillins: ↑ or ↓ action of penicillins
Probenicid: ↑ levels

NURSING CONSIDERATIONS
Assessment
• Assess patient for previous sensitivity reaction to penicillins or cephalosporins; cross-

sensitivity between penicillins, cephalosporins and this drug is common

- Assess patient for signs and symptoms of infection including characteristics of wounds, sputum, urine, stool, WBC >10,000, fever; obtain baseline information before and during treatment
- Complete C&S before beginning drug therapy to identify if correct treatment has been initiated
- Identify urine output; if decreasing, notify prescriber (may indicate nephrotoxicity); also check for increased BUN, creatinine; note color, character, pH of urine if drug is administered for urinary tract infection; output should be 800 ml less than intake; if urine is highly acidic, alkalinization may be needed
- Monitor blood studies: AST (SGOT), ALT (SGPT), CBC, Hct, bilirubin, LDH, alkaline phosphatase, Coombs' test monthly if patient is on long-term therapy
- Monitor electrolytes: potassium, sodium, chloride monthly if patient is on long-term therapy
- Assess bowel pattern daily; if severe diarrhea occurs, drug should be discontinued; may indicate pseudomembranous colitis
- Monitor for bleeding: ecchymosis, bleeding gums, hematuria, stool guaiac daily if on long-term therapy
- Assess for overgrowth of infection; perineal itching, fever, malaise, redness, pain, swelling, drainage, rash, diarrhea, change in cough, sputum

Nursing diagnoses

- ✓ Infection, risk for (uses)
- ✓ Diarrhea (side effects)
- ✓ Injury, risk for (side effects)
- ✓ Knowledge deficit (teaching)
- ✓ Noncompliance (teaching)

Implementation

IM route

- Reconstitute 1 g/3 ml or more of sterile water for inj 0.9% NaCl; may be diluted with 0.5% or 1% lidocaine to prevent pain; give deep in large muscle mass, massage; sol stable 1 wk refrigerated

IV route

- Check for irritation, extravasation, phlebitis daily; change **IV** site q72h
- For direct **IV**, dilute 1 g/10 ml or 2 g/20 ml sterile water for injection, shake, let stand until clear; give over 3-5 min into running **IV**
- For intermittent inf, further dilute with 50-100 ml of D_5W, $D_{10}W$, D_5/0.25% NaCl, D_5/0.45% NaCl, D_5/0.9% NaCl, 0.9% NaCl, D_5/LR, D_5/0.02%, sodium bicarbonate, Ringer's or LR; give over 15-60 min into running **IV**

Syringe compatibility:
Clindamycin

Y-site compatibilities:
Ciprofloxacin, enalaprilat, foscarnet, melphalan, ondansetron, vinorelbine, zidovudine

Y-site incompatibility:
Vancomycin

Additive compatibilities:
Allopurinol, amikacin, aminophylline, amifestine, ampicillin, bleomycin, bumetanide, bupremorphine, butorphanol, calcium gluconate, carboplatin, carmustine, cephalosporins, ciprofloxacin, cisplatin, clinda-

mycin, dacarbazine, diphenhydramine, doxycycline, fluconazole, gentamicin, thiotepa, tobramycin

Additive incompatibilities: Nafcillin, cephradine, metronidazole

Patient/family education

- Teach patient to report sore throat, bruising, bleeding, joint pain; may indicate blood dyscrasias (rare)
- Advise patient to contact prescriber if vaginal itching, loose, foul-smelling stools, furry tongue occur; may indicate superinfection; report itching, rash, pruritus, urticaria
- Instruct patient to take all medication prescribed for the length of time ordered; drug must be taken around the clock to maintain blood levels; do not give medication to others
- Advise patient to notify prescriber of diarrhea with blood or pus

Evaluation

Positive therapeutic outcome

- Absence of signs/symptoms of infection (WBC <10,000, temp WNL, absence of red draining wounds)
- Reported improvement in symptoms of infection

B

baclofen (℞)

(bak'loe-fen)

Alpha-Baclofen ♣, baclofen, Lioresal, Lioresal DS, Lioresal Intrathecal

Func. class.: Skeletal muscle relaxant, central acting

Chem. class.: GABA chlorophenyl derivative

Pregnancy category C

Action: Inhibits synaptic responses in CNS by decreasing GABA, which decreases neurotransmitter function; decreases frequency, severity of muscle spasms

Therapeutic Outcome: Decreased spasticity of muscles

Uses: Spinal cord injury, spasticity in multiple sclerosis

Dosage and routes

Adult: PO 5 mg tid × 3 days, then 10 mg tid × 3 days, then 15 mg tid × 3 days, then 20 mg tid × 3 days, then titrated to response; not to exceed 80 mg/day

Intrathecal: Use implantable intrathecal inf pump; use screening trial of 3 separate bol doses if needed (50 μg/ml, 75 μg/1.5 ml, 100 μg/2 ml); initially double screening dose that produced result and give over 24 hr; increase by 10%-30% q24h only; maintenance: 12-1500 μg/day

Available forms: Tabs 10, 20 mg, Intrathecal sol 10 mg/20 ml (500 μg/ml), 10 mg/5 ml (2000 μg/ml)

Adverse effects

CNS: Dizziness, weakness, fatigue, drowsiness, headache,

disorientation, insomnia, paresthesias, tremors
CV: Hypotension, chest pain, palpitations, edema
EENT: Nasal congestion, blurred vision, mydriasis, tinnitus
GI: Nausea, constipation, vomiting, increased AST (SGOT), alkaline phosphatase, abdominal pain, dry mouth, anorexia
GU: Urinary frequency
INTEG: Rash, pruritus

Contraindications: Hypersensitivity

Precautions: Peptic ulcer disease, renal disease, hepatic disease, stroke, seizure disorder, diabetes mellitus, pregnancy **C**, elderly

Pharmacokinetics	
Absorption	Rapid
Distribution	Widely, crosses placenta
Metabolism	Liver, partially
Excretion	Kidney, unchanged
Half-life	2½-4 hr

Pharmacodynamics	PO
Onset	Unknown
Peak	2-3 hr
Duration	>8 hr

Interactions
Individual drugs
Alcohol: CNS depression
Drug classifications
Antidepressants, tricyclic: ↑ CNS depression
Barbiturates: ↑ CNS depression
Narcotics: ↑ CNS depression
Sedative/hypnotics: ↑ CNS depression
Lab test interferences
↑ AST (SGOT), ↑ alkaline phosphatase, ↑ blood glucose

NURSING CONSIDERATIONS
Assessment
- Monitor B/P, weight, blood sugar, and hepatic function periodically
- Check for increased seizure activity in epilepsy patient; this drug decreases seizure threshold, monitor ECG
- Check I&O ratio; check for urinary retention, frequency, hesitancy
- Allergic reactions: rash, fever, respiratory distress; severe weakness, numbness in extremities
- Assess CNS depression: dizziness, drowsiness, psychiatric symptoms
- Check dosage, as individual titration is required

Nursing diagnoses
✓ Mobility, impaired uses
✓ Injury, risk for (adverse reactions)
✓ Knowledge deficit (teaching)

Implementation
PO route
- Give with meals for GI symptoms; gum, frequent sips of water for dry mouth
- Store in airtight container at room temperature

IV route
- Titration is based on response
- Test dose: 50 mg/ml, give over 1 min or more

Patient/family education
- Advise patient not to discontinue medication quickly; hallucinations, spasticity, tachycardia will occur; drug should be tapered off over 1-2 wk
- Advise patient not to take with alcohol, other CNS depressants
- Caution patient to avoid altering activities while taking this drug; to avoid hazardous

activities if drowsiness or dizziness occurs
- Advise patient to avoid using OTC medication: cough preparations, antihistamines unless directed by prescriber
- Tell patient to increase fluid intake >2 L/day; to take with food

Evaluation

Positive therapeutic outcome
- Decreased pain, spasticity

Treatment of overdose: Induce emesis if conscious patient, lavage, dialysis

beclomethasone (℞)

(be-kloe-meth'a-sone)

Beclodisk ✦, Becloforte Inhaler ✦, Beclovent, Beconase, Beconase AQ Nasal, Beconase Inhalation, Vancenase AQ Nasal, Vancenase Nasal, Vanceril

Func. class.: Synthetic glucocorticoid (long acting)

Chem. class.: Beclomethasone diester

Pregnancy category C

Action: Antiinflammatory; vasoconstrictive properties; also immunosuppressive

➔ **Therapeutic Outcome:** Decreased inflammation and normal immunity

Uses: Seasonal, perennial allergic rhinitis, nasal polyps, chronic steroid-dependent asthma

Dosage and routes

P ***Adult and child >12 yr:*** INSTILL 1-2 sprays in each nostril bid-qid; INH 2-4 puffs tid-qid

P ***Child 6-12 yrs:*** INSTILL 1 spray in each nostril tid; INH 1-2 puffs tid-qid

Available forms: Aero 42 µg/spray (nasal); aero for inh 42 µg/activation; aerosol for nasal inh 0.042%

Adverse effects

CNS: Headache, paresthesia

EENT: Dryness, nasal irritation, burning, sneezing, secretions with blood, nasal ulcerations, ***perforation of nasal septum, candidal infection,*** earache, hoarseness

ENDO: Adrenal suppression

INTEG: Rash, urticaria, pruritus

RESP: Acute status asthmaticus, wheezing

Contraindications: Hypersensitivity, systemic corticosteroid therapy

Precautions: Pregnancy **C**, P children <12, nasal ulcers, recurrent epistaxis

Pharmacokinetics

Absorption	Locally only
Distribution	Not distributed
Metabolism	Minimal
Excretion	Feces
Half-life	3-15 hr

Pharmacodynamics

	INH	NASAL
Onset	10 min	10 min
Peak	Unknown	Unknown
Duration	Unknown	Unknown

NURSING CONSIDERATIONS

Assessment
- Assess adrenal suppression: 17-KS, plasma cortisol for decreased levels, adrenal function periodically for HPA axis suppression
- Check nasal passages during long-term treatment for changes in mucus; check for

burning, stinging; assess for glucocorticoid withdrawal: dizziness, hypotension, fatigue, muscle/joint pain; notify prescriber immediately

• Assess respiratory status: rest, rhythm, characteristics; auscultate lung bilaterally before and throughout treatment

Nursing diagnoses

☑ Airway clearance, ineffective (uses)
☑ Oral mucous membranes, altered (adverse reactions)
☑ Knowledge deficit (teaching)
☑ Noncompliance (teaching)

Implementation

• Use after cleaning aerosol top daily with warm water; dry thoroughly
• Store in cool environment; do not puncture or incinerate container

Patient/family education

• Teach patient to continue using product even if mild nasal bleeding occurs; is usually transient
• Teach patient method of instillation after providing written instructions from manufacturer
• Teach patient to clear nasal passages before administration; use decongestant if needed; shake inhaler, invert, tilt head backward, insert nozzle into nostril, away from septum; hold other nostril closed and depress activator, inhale through nose, exhale through mouth

Evaluate

Positive therapeutic outcome

• Decrease in runny nose, improved symptoms of bronchial asthma

benazepril (℞)

(ben-a′za-pril)
Lotensin
Func. class.: Antihypertensive
Chem. class.: ACE inhibitor
Pregnancy category D

Action: Selectively suppresses renin-angiotensin-aldosterone system; inhibits ACE; prevents conversion of angiotensin I to angiotensin II; results in dilatation of arterial, venous vessels

➔ **Therapeutic Outcome:** Decreased B/P in hypertension

Uses: Hypertension, alone or in combination with thiazide diuretics

Dosage and routes

Adult: PO 10 mg qd initially, then 20-40 mg/day divided bid or qd; **renal impairment:** 5 mg qd with CrCl<30 ml/min/1.73 m^2; increase as needed to maximum of 40 mg/day

Available forms: Tabs 5, 10, 20, 40 mg

Adverse effects

CNS: Anxiety, hypertonia, insomnia, paresthesia, headache, dizziness, fatigue
CV: Hypotension, postural hypotension, syncope, palpitations, angina
GI: Nausea, constipation, vomiting, gastritis, melena
GU: Increased BUN, creatinine, decreased libido, impotence, urinary tract infection
HEMA: Neutropenia, agranulocytosis
INTEG: Angioedema, rash, flushing, sweating

META: Hyperkalemia, hyponatremia
MS: Arthralgia, arthritis, myalgia
RESP: Cough, asthma, bronchitis, dyspnea, sinusitis

Contraindications: Hypersensitivity to ACE inhibitors, P pregnancy **D,** lactation, children

Precautions: Impaired renal/liver function, dialysis patients, hypovolemia, blood dyscrasias, G CHF, COPD, asthma, elderly, bilateral renal artery stenosis

Pharmacokinetics	
Absorption	<40%
Distribution	Unknown; crosses placenta
Metabolism	Liver metabolites; serum protein binding 97%
Excretion	Kidney, breast milk (minimal)
Half-life	10-11 hr (metabolite); increased in renal disease

Pharmacodynamics	
Onset	Unknown
Peak	½-1 hr
Duration	Unknown

Interactions

Individual drugs

Alcohol: ↑ hypotension (large amounts)
Allopurinol: ↑ hypersensitivity
Digoxin: ↑ serum levels
Hydralazine: ↑ toxicity
Indomethacin: ↓ antihypertensive effect
Lithium: ↑ serum levels
Prazosin: ↑ toxicity

Drug classifications

Adrenergic blockers: ↑ hypotension
Antacids: ↓ absorption
Antihypertensives: ↑ hypotension
Diuretics: ↑ hypotension
Diuretics, potassium-sparing: ↑ toxicity
Ganglionic blockers: ↑ hypotension
Potassium supplements: ↑ toxicity
Sympathomimetics: ↑ toxicity

Lab test interferences

False positive: Urine acetone

NURSING CONSIDERATIONS

Assessment

- Monitor blood studies: neutrophils, decreased platelets
- Monitor B/P, check for orthostatic hypotension, syncope; if changes occur, dosage change may be required
- Monitor renal studies: protein, BUN, creatinine; watch for increased levels that may indicate nephrotic syndrome and renal failure; monitor renal symptoms: polyuria, oliguria, frequency, dysuria
- Establish baselines in renal, liver function tests before therapy begins
- Check potassium levels throughout treatment, although hyperkalemia rarely occurs
- Check for edema in feet, legs daily
- Assess for allergic reactions: rash, fever, pruritus, urticaria; drug should be discontinued if antihistamines fail to help

Nursing diagnoses

- ✓ Cardiac output, decreased (uses)
- ✓ Injury, potential for (side effects)
- ✓ Knowledge deficit (teaching)
- ✓ Noncompliance (teaching)

Implementation

PO route

- Store in air-tight container at 86° F (30° C) or less
- Severe hypotension may

occur after 1st dose of this medication; decreased hypotension may be prevented by reducing or discontinuing diuretic therapy 3 days before beginning benazepril therapy
- Give **IV** infusion of 0.9% NaCl (as ordered) to expand fluid volume if severe hypotension occurs

Patient/family education
- Instruct patient not to discontinue drug abruptly; advise patient to tell all persons associated with care
- Teach patient not to use OTC products (cough, cold, allergy) unless directed by prescriber; serious side effects can occur; xanthines such as coffee, tea, chocolate, cola can prevent action of drug
- Emphasize the importance of complying with dosage schedule, even if feeling better; to continue with medical regimen to decrease B/P: exercise, cessation of smoking, decreasing stress, diet modifications
- Emphasize the need to rise slowly to sitting or standing position to minimize orthostatic hypotension; not to exercise in hot weather because increased hypotension can occur
- Teach patient to notify prescriber of mouth sores, sore throat, fever, swelling of hands or feet, irregular heartbeat, chest pain, coughing, shortness of breath
- Caution patient to report excessive perspiration, dehydration, vomiting, diarrhea; may lead to fall in B/P
- Caution patient that drug may cause dizziness, fainting, light-headedness; may occur during 1st few days of therapy; to avoid activities that may be hazardous
- Teach patient how to take B/P; teach normal readings for age group; ensure patient takes own B/P

Evaluation

Positive therapeutic outcome
- Decreased B/P in hypertension

Treatment of overdose: 0.9% NaCl **IV** inf, hemodialysis

benzocaine (Key Drug) (OTC)

(ben′zoe-kane)

Anbesol Maximum Strength, Baby Anbesol, Children's Chloraseptic, Medamint, Orabase Baby, Oracin, Ora-Jel, Oratect, Spec-T Anesthetic, T-Caine, Tyrobenz

Func. class.: Topical local anesthetic

Chem. class.: Ester

Pregnancy category C

Action: Inhibits conduction of nerve impulses from sensory nerves

→ **Therapeutic Outcome:** Absence of pain, irritation

Uses: Oral irritation, sore throat, toothache, cold sore, canker sore, sunburn, minor cuts, insect bites, pain, itching

Dosage and routes

(P) ***Adult and child >12 yr:*** TOP apply to affected area; LOZ suck as needed

Available forms: Cream 1%, 5%; lotion 0.5%, 8%; oint 2%, 5%, 20%; sol 2.1%, 2.5%, 6.3%, 20%; loz 3, 5, 6.25, 10 mg; top aerosol 20%; gel 6.3%, 7.5%, 10%, 20%

Adverse effects
EENT: Itching, irritation in ear
INTEG: Rash, urticaria

Contraindications: Hypersensitivity

Precautions: Pregnancy **C**

Pharmacokinetics

Absorption	Poorly absorbed
Distribution	Unknown
Metabolism	Plasma, liver cholinesterase
Excretion	Unknown
Half-life	Unknown

Pharmacodynamics

	TOP
Onset	Unknown
Peak	1 min
Duration	½-1 hr

Interactions: None

NURSING CONSIDERATIONS
Assessment
- Assess pain: location, duration, characteristics before and after administration
- Assess for infection: redness, drainage, inflammation; this drug should not be used until infection is treated

Nursing diagnoses
✓ Pain (uses)
✓ Knowledge deficit (teaching)

Implementation
- Apply to gums as needed for teething pain
- Use loz for temporary sore throat pain
- Store in tight, light-resistant container; do not freeze, puncture, or incinerate aerosol container

Patient/family education
- Advise patient to avoid contact with eyes
- Caution patient not to use for prolonged periods: use for <1 wk; if condition remains, prescriber should be contacted

Evaluation
Positive therapeutic outcome
- Decreased redness, swelling, pain on affected area

benzquinamide (℞)
(benz-kwin'a-mide)
Emete-Con
Func. class.: Antiemetic
Chem. class.: Benzoquinolizine amide

Pregnancy category C

Action: Acts centrally by blocking chemoreceptor trigger zone, which in turn acts on vomiting center

Therapeutic Outcome: Absence of nausea, vomiting

Uses: To inhibit nausea, vomiting associated with anesthetic

Dosage and routes
Adult: IM 50 mg or 0.5-1 mg/kg; may be repeated in 1 hr, then q3-4h prn; **IV** 25 mg or 0.2-0.4 mg/kg as a one-time dose

Available forms: Inj 50 mg/vial

Adverse effects
CNS: Drowsiness, fatigue, restlessness, tremor, headache, stimulation, dizziness, insomnia, twitching, excitement, nervousness, extrapyramidal symptoms
CV: ***PACs or PVCs, atrial fibrillation,*** hypertension, hypotension
EENT: Dry mouth, blurred vision, hiccups, salivation
GI: Nausea, anorexia
INTEG: Rash, urticaria, fever,

chills, flushing, hives, shivering, sweating, temperature

Contraindications: Hypersensitivity, hypertension

P G **Precautions:** Children, pregnancy C, lactation, elderly

Pharmacokinetics

Absorption	Rapidly (IM) absorbed; completely (IV)
Distribution	Widely distributed
Metabolism	Liver
Excretion	Kidneys, unchanged; feces
Half-life	40 min

Pharmacodynamics

	IM/IV
Onset	15 min
Peak	Unknown
Duration	3-4 hr

Interactions

Individual drugs

Alcohol: ↑ CNS depression

Epinephrine: ↑ hypertension

Drug classifications

Analgesics, narcotics: ↑ CNS depression

Antihistamines: ↑ CNS depression

CNS depressants: ↑ CNS depression

Vasopressors: ↑ hypertension

NURSING CONSIDERATIONS

Assessment

- Monitor vital signs, B/P, I&O; check patients with cardiac disease more often; hypotension, hypertension, dysrhythmias may occur
- Observe for drowsiness; instruct patient not to drive, operate machinery if drowsiness occurs

Nursing diagnoses

✓ Fluid deficit (uses)
✓ Nutrition: Less than body requirements (uses)
✓ Knowledge deficit (teaching)

Implementation

IV **IV route**

- Give after reconstituting 50 mg of drug with 2.2 ml sterile water for inj to a concentration of 25 mg/ml, do not use NaCl; give direct **IV** 25 mg over 30-60 sec by Y-tube or 3-way stopcock; **IV** route may cause dysrhythmias
- Reduce dosage if patient is receiving pressor drugs
- Store inj before, after reconstitution in light-resistant, single-dose container

Y-site compatibility: Foscarnet

Syringe compatibilities: Atropine, droperidol/fentanyl, glycopyrrolate, hydroxyzine, ketamine, meperidine, midazolam, morphine, naloxone, pentazocine, propranolol, scopolamine

Syringe incompatibilities: Chlordiazepoxide, diazepam, pentobarbital, phenobarbital, secobarbital, thiopental

IM route

- Give deep in large muscle mass, aspirate to prevent **IV** administration; deltoid is not preferred area

Patient/family education

- Instruct patient to rise slowly from sitting or recumbent position to minimize orthostatic hypotension; to ask for assistance when ambulating; drowsiness may occur
- Teach patient to use gum, hard candy, or frequent sips of water for dry mouth

Evaluation

Positive therapeutic outcome

- Absence of nausea, vomiting

Treatment of overdose: Supportive care; atropine may be helpful

benztropine (℞)
(benz'troe-peen)
benztropine mesylate,
Cogentin
Func. class.: Cholinergic blocker
Chem. class.: Tertiary amine
Pregnancy category C

Action: Blockade of central acetylcholine receptors in the CNS, neurotransmitters are balanced

Therapeutic Outcome: Decreased involuntary movements

Uses: Parkinsonian symptoms, extrapyramidal symptoms associated with neuroleptic drugs, acute dystonia

Dosage and routes
Drug-induced extrapyramidal symptoms
Adult: IM/**IV** 1-4 mg qd/bid; give PO dose as soon as possible; PO 1-2 mg bid/tid; increase by 0.5 mg q5-6 days
Parkinsonian symptoms
Adult: PO 0.5-1 mg qd; increased 0.5 mg q5-6 days titrated to patient response
Acute dystonic reactions
Adult: IM/**IV** 1-2 mg, may increase to 1-2 mg bid (PO)

Available forms: Tabs 0.5, 1, 2 mg; inj IM, **IV** 1 mg/ml

Adverse effects
CNS: Confusion, anxiety, restlessness, irritability, delusions, hallucinations, headache, sedation, depression, incoherence, dizziness, memory loss
CV: Palpitations, tachycardia, hypotension, bradycardia
EENT: Blurred vision, photophobia, dilated pupils, difficulty swallowing, dry eyes, mydriasis, increased intraocular tension, angle closure glaucoma
GI: Dryness of mouth, constipation, nausea, vomiting, abdominal distress, ***paralytic ileus,*** epigastric distress
GU: Hesitancy, retention, dysuria
INTEG: Rash, urticaria, dermatoses
MISC: Increased temperature, flushing, decreased sweating, hyperthermia, heat stroke, numbness of fingers
MS: Muscular weakness, cramping

Contraindications: Hypersensitivity, narrow angle glaucoma, myasthenia gravis, P GI/GU obstruction, child <3 yr, peptic ulcer, megacolon, prostate hypertrophy

Precautions: Pregnancy **C**, G elderly, lactation, tachycardia, liver, kidney disease, drug abuse history, dysrhythmias, hypotension, hypertension, P psychiatric patients, children

Pharmacokinetics

Absorption	Well (PO, IM), completely (IV) absorbed
Distribution	Unknown
Metabolism	Unknown
Excretion	Unknown
Half-life	Unknown

Pharmacodynamics

	IM/IV	PO
Onset	15 min	1 hr
Peak	Unknown	Unknown
Duration	6-10 hr	6-10 hr

Interactions
Individual drugs
Amantadine: ↑ anticholinergic effects

Digoxin: ↑ levels of digoxin
Levodopa: ↓ levels of levodopa
Haloperidol: ↑ schizophrenic symptoms

Drug classifications
Antacids: ↓ absorption of benzotropine
Antidepressants, tricyclic: ↑ anticholinergic effects
Antihistamines: ↑ anticholinergic effects
Phenothiazines: ↑ anticholinergic effects

NURSING CONSIDERATIONS

Assessment

- Monitor I&O ratio; retention commonly causes decreased urinary output, distention, frequency, incontinence
- Assess for parkinsonism, extrapyramidal symptoms: shuffling gait, muscle rigidity, involuntary movements, pill rolling, muscle spasms, drooling before and during treatment
- Monitor for urinary hesitancy, retention; palpate bladder if retention occurs
- Monitor for constipation, cramping, pain in abdomen, abdominal distention; increase fluids, bulk, exercise if this occurs
- Assess for tolerance over long-term therapy; dosage may have to be increased or changed
- Assess for mental status: affect, mood, CNS depression, worsening of mental symptoms during early therapy
- Assess for benztropine "buzz" or "high," patients may imitate EPS

Nursing diagnoses

✓ Mobility, impaired (uses)
✓ Knowledge deficit (teaching)
✓ Noncompliance (teaching)

Implementation

PO route

- Give with or after meals to prevent GI upset; may give with fluids other than water; hard candy, frequent drinks, gum to relieve dry mouth
- Give hs to avoid daytime drowsiness in patient with parkinsonism
- May be crushed and mixed with food
- Store at room temperature

IM route

- Give in large muscle mass for dystonic symptoms

IV **IV route**

- Give parenteral dose with patient recumbent to prevent postural hypotension; give undiluted 2 mg or less >1 min or more

Syringe compatibilities: Chlorpromazine, fluphenazine, metoclopramide, perphenazine, thiothixene

Y-*site compatibilities:* Fluconazole, tacrolimus

Patient/family education

- Teach patient to use caution in hot weather; drug may increase susceptibility to stroke since perspiration is decreased; patient should remain indoors
- Advise patient not to discontinue this drug abruptly; to taper off over 1 wk to prevent withdrawal symptoms (insomnia, involuntary movements, anxiety, tachycardias)
- Caution patient to avoid driving or other hazardous activities; drowsiness, dizziness may occur
- Teach patient to avoid OTC medication: cough, cold preparations with alcohol, antihistamines unless directed by prescriber; increased CNS depression may occur

• Advise patient to rise from sitting or recumbent position slowly to minimize orthostatic hypotension
• Teach patient to use gum, hard candy, frequent sips of water to decrease dry mouth; if dry mouth continues, saliva substitutes may be prescribed
• Instruct patient that doses should not be doubled, but missed dose may be taken up to 2 hr before next dose

Evaluation

Positive therapeutic outcome

• Absence of involuntary movements (pill rolling, tremors, muscle spasms)

bepridil (℞)

(be'pri-dil)

Vascor

Func. class.: Calcium channel blocker, antianginal, antihypertensive

Chem. class.: Angina

Pregnancy category C

Action: Inhibits calcium ion influx across cell membrane during cardiac depolarization; produces relaxation of coronary vascular smooth muscle, peripheral vascular smooth muscle; dilates coronary vascular arteries; increases myocardial oxygen delivery in patients with vasospastic angina

Therapeutic Outcome: Decreased angina pectoris

Uses: Chronic stable angina, used alone or in combination with propranolol

Dosage and routes

Adult: 200 mg qd, after 10 days may increase dose if needed; max dose 400mg/day

Available forms: Tabs, film-coated, 200, 300, 400 mg

Adverse effects

CNS: Headache, fatigue, drowsiness, dizziness, anxiety, depression, weakness, insomnia, confusion, lightheadedness, nervousness

CV: Dysrhythmia, edema, CHF, bradycardia, hypotension, palpitations, AV block, torsados de pointes

GI: Nausea, vomiting, diarrhea, gastric upset, constipation, increased levels in liver function studies

GU: Nocturia, polyuria

HEMA: Agranulocytosis

Contraindications: Sick sinus syndrome, 2nd- or 3rd-degree heart block, Wolff-Parkinson-White syndrome, hypotension less than 90 mm Hg systolic, cardiogenic shock, history of serious ventricular arrhythmias

Precautions: CHF, hypotension, hepatic injury, pregnancy C, lactation, children, renal disease, IHSS, concomitant β-blocker therapy

Pharmacokinetics	
Absorption	Well absorbed
Distribution	Plasma protein bound (99%), crosses placenta
Metabolism	Liver
Excretion	Urine, feces
Half-life	42 hr

Pharmacodynamics	
Onset	Unknown
Peak	2-3 hr
Duration	Unknown

Interactions

Individual drugs

Fentanyl: ↑ hypotension
Digoxin: ↑ levels of digoxin

Drug classifications
β-Blockers: ↑ adverse reactions
Lab test interferences
↑ Liver function tests, ↑ aminotransferase, ↑ CPK, ↑ LDH

NURSING CONSIDERATIONS
Assessment
- Assess fluid volume status: I&O ratio and record, weight, distended red veins, crackles in lung, color, quality, and sp gr of urine, skin turgor, adequacy of pulses, moist mucous membranes, bilateral lung sounds, peripheral pitting edema
- Assess cardiac status: B/P, pulse, respiration, ECG intervals (PR, QRS, QT), dysrhythmias
- Obtain digoxin levels if cardiac glycosides are given with bepridil

Nursing diagnoses
✓ Cardiac output, decreased (uses)
✓ Knowledge deficit (teaching)

Implementation
- Give once a day, with food for GI symptoms
- ⊘ Do not break, chew, crush tabs

Patient/family education
- Instruct patient to avoid hazardous activities until stabilized on drug and dizziness is no longer a problem
- Instruct patient to limit caffeine consumption; to avoid alcohol and OTC drugs unless directed by prescriber
- Advise patient to comply in all areas of medical regimen: diet, exercise, stress reduction, drug therapy; to notify prescriber of irregular heart beat, shortness of breath, swelling of feet and hands, pronounced dizziness, constipation, nausea, hypotension
- Teach patient to use as directed even if feeling better; may be taken with other cardiovascular drugs (nitrates, β-blockers)

Evaluation
Positive therapeutic outcome
- Decreased anginal pain

Treatment of overdose: Defibrillation, atropine for AV block, vasopressor for hypotension

P beractant (℞)
(ber-ak'tant)
Survanta
Func. class.: Natural lung surfactant
Pregnancy category N/A

Action: Replenishes surfactant and restores surface activity to P the lungs in premature infants

→ Therapeutic Outcome: P Ability of neonate to breathe without assistance

Uses: Prevention and treatment (rescue) of respiratory distress syndrome in premature P infants

Dosage and routes
Intratracheal instill: 4 doses can be administered in the 1st 48 hr of life; give doses no more frequently than q6h; each dose is 100 mg of phospholipids/kg birth weight (4 ml/kg)

Available forms: Susp 25 mg phospholipids/ml in 0.9% NaCl in single-use vials containing 8 ml susp

B

Adverse effects
RESP: Pulmonary air leaks, pulmonary interstitial emphysema, apnea, pulmonary hemorrhage
SYST: Patent ductus arteriosus, intracranial hemorrhage, severe intracranial hemorrhage, necrotizing entercolitis, posttreatment sepsis, posttreatment infection, bradycardia, oxygen desaturation, pallor, vasoconstriction, hypotension, hypertension

Precautions: Bradycardia, rales, infections

Pharmacokinetics	
Absorption	Unknown
Distribution	Lung
Metabolism	Recycled
Excretion	Unknown
Half-life	Unknown

Pharmacodynamics	
Onset	Few min
Peak	Unknown
Duration	Becomes lung associated within hours of administration

Interactions: None

NURSING CONSIDERATIONS
Assessment
- Assess respiratory rate, rhythm, character, chest expansion, color, transcutaneous saturation, ABGs; monitor ECG
- Check endotracheal tube placement before dosing; monitor for apnea after endotracheal administration
- Check for reflux of drug into the endotracheal tube during administration; stop drug administration if this occurs, and if needed increase peak inspiratory pressure on the ventilator by 4-5 cm H_2O until tube is cleared
- P Assess infant for repeat dosing using radiographic confirmation of respiratory distress syndrome; repeat doses should be given as noted above; ventilator settings for repeat doses FIO_2 are decreased by 0.2 or amount to prevent cyanosis; ventilator rate of 30/min; inspiratory time <1 sec; if infant's pretreatment rate was >30, leave unchanged during dosing; resume usual ventilator management after dosing

Nursing diagnoses
✓ Gas exchange, impaired (uses)
✓ Knowledge deficit (teaching)

Implementation
- P Administer after suctioning; give by endotracheal administration only by persons trained in neonatal intubation and ventilation
- Use a no. 5 Fr end-hole catheter inserted into the endotracheal tube with the tip protruding just beyond the end of the endotracheal tube; shorten the catheter before insertion; do not insert the drug into the mainstem bronchus
- P Divide each dose into quarters and administer with infant in different positions
- P Determine the dosing by weight of infant; slowly withdraw the contents into the plastic syringe through a 20-G needle; do not filter or shake; attach the premeasured no. 5 Fr catheter to syringe; fill with drug and discard excess through the catheter so only dose to be given remains in syringe
- P For **prevention dosing,** stabilize, weigh, and intubate the infant; give drug within 15

min of birth if possible; position infant and inj first quarter dose through catheter over 2-3 sec; remove catheter and manually ventilate with O_2 to prevent cyanosis (60 bpm) and sufficient positive pressure to promote adequate air exchange and chest wall excursion

- For **rescue dosing,** give drug as soon as infant is placed on ventilator after birth; immediately before administering dose, change ventilator settings to 60/min, inspiratory time 0.5 sec, FIO_2 l; position infant and inj first quarter through catheter over 2-3 sec; remove catheter; return to mechanical ventilator
- Ventilate infant for >30 sec or until stable after prevention or rescue strategy; reposition for next dose; same procedure for subsequent dosing; do not suction for at least 1 hr after dosing unless airway obstruction is evident; resume ventilator therapy after dosing
- Reduce peak ventilator inspiratory pressures immediately if chest expansion improves substantially after dose
- Reduce in FIO_2 in small, repeated steps when infant becomes pink and transcutaneous oxygen saturation is in excess of 95%; oxygen saturation should remain between 90% and 95%
- Suction all infants before administration to prevent mucus plugging; if endotracheal tube obstruction is suspected, remove the obstruction and replace tube immediately
- Store in refrigerator; protect from light; warm to room temp for >20 min or warm in hand 8 min before giving; do not use artificial warming methods; enter a vial only once; unopened, unused vials that have been warmed to room temp may be rerefrigerated within 8 hr of warming; do not warm and return to refrigerator more than once

Patient/family education

- Explain disease process and purpose of medication to parents; communicate neonate's progress

Evaluation

Positive therapeutic outcome

- Significant improvement in respiratory status (oxygenation, arterial blood gases, WNL)

betamethasone/ betamethasone sodium phosphate/ betamethasone disodium phosphate/ betamethasone acetate/ betamethasone sodium phosphate (℞)

(bay-ta-meth'a-sone)

Beclovent, Beconase AQ Nasal, Beconase Inhalaton ♣, Benisone, Betaderm ♣, betamethasone dipropionate, betamethasone valerate, Betatrex, Beta-Val, Betnelan, Celestone/Alphatrex, Celestone Phosphate, Cel-U-Jec, Diprolene AF/ betamethasone sodium phosphate, Diprosone, Maxivate, Selestoject, Teladar/Diprolene, Uticort, Valisone, Valisone Reduced Strength, Vancenase AQ Nasal, Vancenase Nasal Beta Cort, Vanceril

Func. class.: Corticosteroid, synthetic

Chem. class.: Glucocorticoid, long acting

Pregnancy category C

Action: Decreases inflammation by suppression of migration of polymorphonuclear leukocytes, fibroblasts, reversal of increased capillary permeability and lysosomal stabilization

➔ **Therapeutic Outcome:** Decreased inflammation and normal immunity

Uses: Immunosuppression, severe inflammation, prevention of neonatal respiratory distress syndrome (by administration to mother), chronic asthma, rhinitis (inh); psoriasis, eczema, contact dermatitis, pruritus (top)

Dosage and routes

Adult: PO 0.6-7.2 mg qd; IM/**IV** 0.6-7.2 mg qd in joint or soft tissue (sodium phosphate)

Pregnant adult: IM 12 mg 36-48 hr, before premature delivery, then same dose in 24 hr (betamethasone acetate)

P ***Adult and child:*** Apply top to affected area qid

Adult: INH 2-4 puffs tid-qid; not to exceed 20 inh/day

P ***Child: 6-12 yr:*** INH 1-2 puffs tid-qid; not to exceed 10 inh/ day

P ***Adult and child >12 yr:*** INSTILL 1-2 sprays in each nostril bid-qid

Available forms: Tabs 0.6 mg; syr 0.6 mg/5 ml; inj 3, 4 mg/ml; oint 0.025%, 0.1%; cream 0.025%, 0.01%, 0.1%; lotion 0.025%, 0.1%; gel 0.025%; aero 42 μg/spray

Adverse effects

CNS: Depression, flushing, sweating, headache, ecchymosis, bruising, mood changes
CV: Hypertension, ***circulatory collapse, thrombophlebitis, embolism,*** tachycardia, ***necrotizing angiitis, CHF***
EENT: Fungal infections, increased intraocular pressure, blurred vision
GI: Diarrhea, nausea, abdominal distention, ***GI hemorrhage, increased appetite, pancreatitis***
HEMA: ***Thrombocytopenia***
INTEG: Acne, poor wound

healing, ecchymosis, bruising, petechiae
MS: Fractures, osteoporosis, weakness

Contraindications: Psychosis, hypersensitivity, idiopathic thrombocytopenia, acute glomerulonephritis, amebiasis, fungal infections, nonasthmatic bronchial disease, P child <2 yr, AIDS, TB

Precautions: Pregnancy **C,** diabetes mellitus, glaucoma, osteoporosis, seizure disorders, ulcerative colitis, CHF, myasthenia gravis, renal disease, esophagitis, peptic ulcer

Pharmacokinetics

Absorption	Well absorbed (PO); systemic (top)
Distribution	Crosses placenta
Metabolism	Liver, extensively
Excretion	Kidney, breast milk
Half-life	3-5 hr, adrenal suppression 3-4 days

Pharmacodynamics

	PO	IM	IV	TOP
Onset	1-2 hr	Unknown	Rapid	Unknown
Peak	2 hr	4-8 hr	4-8 hr	Unknown
Duration	3 days	1-1½ days	1-1½ days	Unknown

Interactions
Individual drugs
Amphotericin B: ↑ hypokalemia
Insulin: ↑ need for insulin
Mezlocillin: ↑ hypokalemia
Phenytoin: ↓ action, ↑ metabolism
Rifampin: ↓ action, ↑ metabolism
Ticarcillin: ↑ hypokalemia
Drug classifications
Barbiturates: ↓ action, ↑ metabolism
Diuretics: ↑ hypokalemia
Hypoglycemic agents: ↑ need for hypoglycemic agents
Lab test interferences
↑ Cholesterol, ↑ sodium, ↑ blood glucose, ↑ uric acid, ↑ calcium, ↑ urine glucose
↓ Calcium, ↓ potassium, ↓ T_4, ↓ T_3, ↓ thyroid ^{131}I uptake test, ↓ urine 17-OHCS, ↓ 17-KS, ↓ PBI
False negative: Skin allergy tests

NURSING CONSIDERATIONS
Assessment
Systemic route
- Monitor potassium, blood sugar, urine glucose while on long-term therapy; hypokalemia and hyperglycemia; check weight daily; notify prescriber of weekly gain >5 lb
- Monitor B/P q4h, pulse; notify prescriber if chest pain occurs
- Monitor I&O ratio; be alert for decreasing urinary output and increasing edema
- Check plasma cortisol levels during long-term therapy (normal level: 138-635 nmol/L [SI units] when drawn at 8 AM); adrenal function periodically for HPA axis suppression
- Assess for symptoms of infection: increase temperature, WBC even after withdrawal of medication; drug masks infection symptoms
- Assess for symptoms of potassium depletion: paresthesias, fatigue, nausea, vomiting, depression, polyuria, dysrhythmias, weakness
- Monitor for edema, hypertension, cardiac symptoms
- Assess for mental status: affect, mood, behavioral changes, aggression

B

Top route

• Check temperature; if fever develops, drug should be discontinued

• Assess for systemic absorption: increased temperature, inflammation, irritation

Nursing diagnoses

✓ Infection, risk for (adverse reactions)

✓ Knowledge deficit (teaching)

✓ Noncompliance (teaching)

Implementation

IV **IV route**

• Give **IV** (only sodium phosphate product); give over >1 min; may be given by **IV** inf in compatible sol after shaking susp (parenteral)

• Give titrated dose; use lowest effective dose

Y-site compatibilities: Heparin, hydrocortisone, potassium chloride, Vit B/C

IM route

• Give IM injection deep in large mass, rotate sites, avoid deltoid, use 21-G needle; in one dose in AM to prevent adrenal suppression; avoid SC administration; may damage tissue

PO route

• Give with food or milk to decrease GI symptoms

Inh route

• Give inh with water to decrease possibility of fungal infections; titrated dose; use lowest effective dose

• Use after cleaning aerosol top daily with warm water; dry thoroughly

• Store in cool environment; do not puncture or incinerate container

Top route

• Apply only to affected areas; do not get in eyes; apply medication, then cover with occlusive dressing (only if prescribed), seal to normal skin, change q12h; syst absorption may occur

• Apply only to dermatoses; do not use on weeping, denuded, or infected area

• Cleanse before applying drug; use treatment for a few days after area has cleared

• Store at room temperature

Patient/family education

Systemic route

• Advise patient that long-term therapy may be needed to clear infection (1-2 mo depending on type of infection); that ID as steroid user should be carried; dosage adjustment may be needed

❗• Instruct patient to notify prescriber if therapeutic response decreases; caution patient not to discontinue abruptly; adrenal crisis can result

• Instruct patient to avoid OTC products: salicylates, alcohol in cough products, cold preparations unless directed by prescriber

• Teach patient all aspects of drug usage including cushingoid symptoms

• Teach patient symptoms of adrenal insufficiency: nausea, anorexia, fatigue, dizziness, dyspnea, weakness, joint pain

Top route

• Caution patient to avoid sunlight on affected area; burns may occur

Evaluation

Positive therapeutic outcome

• Ease of respirations, decreased inflammation (systemic)

• Absence of severe itching, patches on skin, flaking (top)

bethanechol ⊶ (℞)

(be-than'e-kol)
bethanechol chloride,
Duvoid, Myotonachol,
Urecholine

Func. class.: Cholinergic stimulant
Chem. class.: Synthetic choline ester

Pregnancy category C

Action: Stimulates muscarinic acetylcholine receptors directly; mimics effects of parasympathetic nervous system stimulation; stimulates gastric motility, micturition

➔ **Therapeutic Outcome:** Absence of continued urinary retention

Uses: Urinary retention (postoperative, postpartum), neurogenic atony of bladder with retention

Dosage and routes
Test dose
Adult: SC 2.5 mg repeated 15-30 min intervals × 4 doses to determine effective dose

Adult: PO 10-50 mg bid-qid; SC 2.5-10 mg tid-qid prn

Available forms: Tabs 5, 10, 25, 50 mg; inj SC 5 mg/ml

Adverse effects
CNS: Dizziness
CV: Hypotension, bradycardia, orthostatic hypotension, reflex tachycardia, ***cardiac arrest, circulatory collapse***
EENT: Miosis, increased salivation, lacrimation, blurred vision
GI: Nausea, bloody diarrhea, belching, vomiting, cramps, fecal incontinence
GU: Urgency
INTEG: Rash, urticaria, flushing, increased sweating
RESP: Acute asthma, dyspnea

Contraindications: Hypersensitivity, severe bradycardia, asthma, severe hypotension, hyperthyroidism, peptic ulcer, parkinsonism, seizure disorders, CAD, coronary occlusion, mechanical obstruction, peritonitis, recent urinary or GI surgery

Precautions: Hypertension, pregnancy **C**, lactation, P child <8 yr, urinary retention

Pharmacokinetics

Absorption	Poorly absorbed (PO); well absorbed (SC)
Distribution	Does not cross blood-brain barrier
Metabolism	Unknown
Excretion	Kidneys
Half-life	Unknown

Pharmacodynamics

	PO	SC
Onset	30-90 min	5-15 min
Peak	1 hr	15-30 min
Duration	1-6 hr	2 hr

Interactions
Individual drugs
Procainamide: ↓ action of bethanechol
Quinidine: ↓ action of bethanechol
Drug classifications
Cholinergics: ↑ action of bethanechol
Ganglionic blockers: ↑ hypotension
Lab test interferences
↑ AST (SGOT), ↑ lipase/amylase, ↑ bilirubin

NURSING CONSIDERATIONS
Assessment
- Monitor B/P, pulse, respirations; observe after parenteral dose for 1 hr
- Check I&O ratio; check for

urinary retention or incontinence; if bladder emptying does not occur, notify prescriber; catheterization may be needed

• Assess for bradycardia, hypotension, bronchospasm, headache, dizziness, convulsions, sweating, cramping, respiratory depression; drug should be discontinued if toxicity occurs; atropine administration

Nursing diagnoses

✓ Urinary elimination, altered patterns (uses)

✓ Injury, risk for (adverse reactions)

✓ Knowledge deficit (teaching)

Implementation

SC route

• Give parenteral dose by SC route; use of IM, **IV** may result in cardiac arrest or cholinergic crisis (diarrhea with blood, cramping, hypotension, circulatory collapse)

• Administer only with atropine sulfate available for cholinergic crisis; give only after all other cholinergics have been discontinued

• Do not use sol with a precipitate, or if discolored

PO route

• Give increased doses if tolerance occurs as prescribed

• To avoid nausea and vomiting, take on an empty stomach; 1 hr ac or 2 hr pc

• Store at room temperature

Patient/family education

• Instruct patient to take drug exactly as prescribed; do not double doses; if dose is missed take within 1 hr of scheduled dose

• Caution patient to make position changes slowly; orthostatic hypotension may occur

• Instruct patient to report cramping, diarrhea with blood, flushing to prescriber

Evaluation

Positive therapeutic outcome

• Absence of urinary retention

• Absence of abdominal distention

Treatment of overdose: Administer atropine 0.6-1.2 mg **IV** or IM (adult)

bicalutamide (℞)

(bi-kal-yut'ah-mide)

Casodex

Func. class.: Antineoplastic

Chem. class.: Nonsteroidal antiandrogen

Pregnancy category X

Action: Competitively inhibits the action to androgens by binding to cytosol androgen receptors in target tissue

Therapeutic Outcome: Prevention of growth of malignant cells

Uses: Prostate cancer in combination with luteinizing hormone-releasing hormone (LHRH) analog

Dosage and routes

Adult: PO 50 mg qd with LHRH

Available forms: Tab 50 mg

Adverse effects

GI: Diarrhea, constipation, nausea, vomiting, increased liver enzyme test

CV: Hot flashes, hypertension

CNS: Dizziness, paresthesia, insomnia

INTEG: Rash, sweating

GU: Nocturia, **hematuria,**

UTI, impotence, gynecomastia, urinary incontinence
MISC: Infection, anemia, dyspnea, bone pain, headache, asthenia, back pain, flu syndrome

Contraindications: Hypersensitivity, pregnancy **X**

Precautions: Renal, hepatic G disease, elderly, lactation

Pharmacokinetics

Absorption	Well absorbed
Distribution	Unknown
Metabolism	Liver
Excretion	Urine, feces
Half-life	Unknown

Pharmacodynamics

Unknown

Interactions

Drug classifications

Anticoagulants: May be displaced from their binding sites

Lab test interferences

↑ AST, ↑ ALT, ↑ bilirubin, ↑ BUN, ↑ creatinine
↓ Hgb, ↓ WBC

NURSING CONSIDERATIONS

Assessment

- Assess for diarrhea, constipation, nausea, vomiting
- Assess for hot flashes, gynecomastia; assure patient that these are common side effects
- Monitor PSA (Prostate Specific Antigen), liver function studies

Nursing diagnoses

✓ Injury, risk for (uses, adverse reactions)
✓ Knowledge deficit (teaching)

Implementation

- Give at same time each day either AM or PM with or without food
- Give only with LHRH treatment

Patient/family education

- Teach patient to recognize and report signs of anemia, hepatotoxicity, renal toxicity

Evaluation

Positive therapeutic outcome

- Decreased tumor size, spread of malignancy

biperiden (℞)

(bye-per′i-den)

Akineton

Func. class.: Cholinergic blocker, antiparkinsonian agent

Pregnancy category C

Action: Centrally acting competitive anticholinergic; blocks cholinergic responses in the CNS

➔ **Therapeutic Outcome:** Decreased involuntary movements

Uses: Parkinsonian symptoms, extrapyramidal symptoms secondary to neuroleptic drug therapy

Dosage and routes

Extrapyramidal symptoms

Adult: PO 2 mg qd-tid; IM/**IV** 2 mg q30 min, if needed, not to exceed 8 mg/24 hr

Parkinsonian symptoms

Adult: PO 2 mg tid-qid; max 16 mg/24 hr

Available forms: Tabs 2 mg; inj IM/**IV** 5 mg/ml (lactate)

Adverse effects

CNS: Confusion, anxiety, restlessness, irritability, delusions, hallucinations, headache,

sedation, depression, incoherence, dizziness, euphoria, tremors, memory loss
CV: Palpitations, tachycardia, postural hypotension, bradycardia
EENT: Blurred vision, photophobia, dilated pupils, difficulty swallowing, mydriasis, increased intraocular tension, angle closure glaucoma
GI: Dryness of mouth, constipation, nausea, vomiting, abdominal distress, ***paralytic ileus***
GU: Hesitancy, retention, dysuria
INTEG: Rash, urticaria, dermatoses
MISC: Increased temperature, flushing, decreased sweating, hyperthermia, heat stroke, numbness of fingers
MS: Weakness, cramping

Contraindications: Hypersensitivity, narrow-angle glaucoma, myasthenia gravis, GI/GU obstruction, megacolon, stenosing peptic ulcers, prostatic hypertrophy

Precautions: Pregnancy **C**, G elderly, lactation, tachycardia, dysrhythmias, liver, kidney disease, drug abuse, hypotension, hypertension, psychiatric patients, P children

Pharmacokinetics

Absorption	Well absorbed (PO, IM)
Distribution	Unknown
Metabolism	Unknown
Excretion	Unknown
Half-life	18-24 hr

Pharmacodynamics

	IM/IV	PO
Onset	15 min	1 hr
Peak	Unknown	Unknown
Duration	6-10 hr	6-10 hr

Interactions

Individual drugs

Amantadine: ↑ anticholinergic effects
Digoxin: ↑ levels of digoxin
Levodopa: ↓ levels of levodopa
Haloperidol: ↑ schizophrenic symptoms

Drug classifications

Antidepressants, tricyclic: ↑ anticholinergic effects
Antihistamines: ↑ anticholinergic effects
Phenothiazines: ↑ anticholinergic effects

NURSING CONSIDERATIONS

Assessment

- Monitor I&O ratio; retention commonly causes decreased urinary output, distention, frequency, incontinence
- Assess for parkinsonism, extrapyramidal symptoms: shuffling gait, muscle rigidity, involuntary movements, pill rolling, muscle spasms, drooling before and during treatment
- Assess patient response if anticholinergics are given
- Monitor for urinary hesitancy, retention; palpate bladder if retention occurs
- Monitor for constipation, cramping, pain in abdomen, abdominal distention; increase fluids, bulk, exercise if this occurs
- Assess for tolerance over long-term therapy; dosage may have to be increased or changed
- Assess for mental status: affect, mood, CNS depression, worsening of mental symptoms during early therapy

Nursing diagnoses

✓ Mobility, impaired (uses)
✓ Knowledge deficit (teaching)

Implementation

PO route

- Give with food or pc to prevent GI upset; may give with fluids other than water; hard candy, frequent drinks, gum to relieve dry mouth
- Give hs to avoid daytime drowsiness in patients with parkinsonism
- Store at room temp

IV **IV route**

- Give parenteral dose with patient recumbent to prevent postural hypotension; give undiluted 2 mg or less over 1 min or more

Patient/family education

- Teach patient to use caution in hot weather; drug may increase susceptibility to heat stroke since perspiration is decreased; patient should remain indoors
- Teach patient not to discontinue this drug abruptly; to taper off over 1 wk to prevent withdrawal symptoms (insomnia, involuntary movements, anxiety, tachycardias)
- Teach patient to avoid driving or other hazardous activities; drowsiness, dizziness may occur
- Teach patient to avoid OTC medication: cough, cold preparations with alcohol, antihistamines unless directed by prescriber; increased CNS depression may occur
- Caution patient to rise from sitting or recumbent position slowly to minimize orthostatic hypotension
- Teach patient to use gum, hard candy, frequent sips of water to decrease dry mouth; if dry mouth continues, saliva substitutes may be prescribed
- Instruct patient that doses should not be doubled, but missed dose may be taken up to 2 hr before next dose

Evaluation

Positive therapeutic outcome

- Absence of involuntary movements (pill rolling, tremors, muscle spasms)

bisacodyl (OTC)

(bis-a-koe'dill)

Apo-Bisacodyl ✤, bisacodyl, Bisacodyl Uniserts, Bisco-Lax, Dulcagen, Dulcolax, Fleet Bisacodyl

Func. class.: Laxative, stimulant

Chem. class.: Diphenylmethane

Pregnancy category C

Action: Acts directly on intestine by increasing motor activity; thought to irritate colonic intramural plexus; increases water in the colon

→ **Therapeutic Outcome:** Decreased constipation

Uses: Short-term treatment of constipation, bowel or rectal preparation for surgery, examination

Dosage and routes

Adult: PO 10-15 mg in PM or AM; may use up to 30 mg for bowel or rec preparation; REC 10 mg; ENEMA 1.25 oz

P ***Child <2 yr:*** REC 5 mg

P ***Child >6 yr:*** PO 5-10 mg

P ***Child >12 yr:*** REC 10 mg

Available forms: Enteric coated tabs 5 mg; rec supp 5, 10 mg

Adverse effects

CNS: Muscle weakness

GI: Nausea, vomiting, anorexia, cramps, diarrhea, rectal burning (supp)
META: Protein-losing enteropathy, alkalosis, hypokalemia, ***tetany,*** electrolyte and fluid imbalances

Contraindications: Hypersensitivity, rectal fissures, abdominal pain, nausea, vomiting, appendicitis, acute surgical abdomen, ulcerated hemorrhoids, acute hepatitis, fecal impaction, intestinal/biliary tract obstruction

Precautions: Pregnancy **C**

Pharmacokinetics

Absorption	Poor
Distribution	Unknown
Metabolism	Liver, minimally
Excretion	Kidneys
Half-life	Unknown

Pharmacodynamics

	PO	REC
Onset	6-10 hr	15-60 min
Peak	Unknown	Unknown
Duration	Unknown	Unknown

Interactions

Drug classifications

Antacids: ↓ of enteric coating of drugs
H_2-blockers: ↑ gastric irritation

NURSING CONSIDERATIONS

Assessment

- Monitor blood, urine electrolytes if used often by patient; check I&O ratio to identify fluid loss
- Assess cramping, rectal bleeding, nausea, vomiting; if these symptoms occur, drug should be discontinued; identify cause of constipation; identify whether fluids, bulk, or exercise missing from lifestyle

Nursing diagnoses

- Constipation (uses)
- Diarrhea (side effects)
- Knowledge deficit (teaching)
- Noncompliance (teaching)

Implementation

PO route

- Give alone with water only for better absorption; do not take within 1 hr of antacids, milk
- Administer in AM or PM (oral dose)
- Do not chew; swallow tabs whole

Rectal route

- Lubricate before insertion, patient should retain for ½ hr

Patient/family education

- Discuss with the patient that adequate fluid and bulk consumption is necessary
- Advise patient that normal bowel movements do not always occur daily
- Teach patient not to use in presence of abdominal pain, nausea, vomiting; tell patient to notify prescriber if constipation unrelieved or if symptoms of electrolyte imbalance occur: muscle cramps, pain, weakness, dizziness, excessive thirst

Evaluation

Positive therapeutic outcome

- Decreased constipation within 3 days

bismuth subsalicylate (OTC)

(bis'meth sub-sa-li'si-late)

Bismtrol, Pepto-Bismol, Pepto-Bismol Maximum Strength, Pink Bismuth

Func. class.: Antidiarrheal

Chem. class.: Salicylate

Pregnancy category C

Action: Inhibits prostaglandin synthesis responsible for GI hypermotility; stimulates absorption of fluid and electrolytes; antimicrobial, antisecretory effects

Therapeutic Outcome: Absence of loose, watery stools

Uses: Diarrhea (cause undetermined); prevention of diarrhea when traveling

Dosage and routes

Adult: PO 30 ml or 2 tabs q30-60 min, not to exceed 8 doses per day for >2 days

P ***Child 10-14 yr:*** PO 15 ml

Available forms: Chewable tabs 262 mg; susp 262 mg/ 15 ml, 524 mg/15 ml

Adverse effects

CNS: Confusion, twitching

EENT: Hearing loss, tinnitus, metallic taste, blue gums

GI: Increased fecal impaction (high doses), dark stools, constipation

HEMA: Increased bleeding time

P **Contraindications:** Child <3 yr; impaction, children, teens with flulike symptoms, hypersensitivity (aspirin)

Precautions: Anticoagulant G therapy, pregnancy **C,** elderly, lactation, gout, diabetes mellitus

Pharmacokinetics

Absorption	Salicylate >90%
Distribution	None
Metabolism	None
Excretion	Feces (unchanged)
Half-life	Unknown

Pharmacodynamics

Onset	1 hr
Peak	2 hr
Duration	4 hr

Interactions

Individual drugs

Aminosalicylic acid: ↑ side effects, ↑ toxicity

Aspirin: ↑ salicylate levels

Tetracycline: ↓ absorption

Drug classifications

Anticoagulants, oral: ↓ effect of anticoagulants

Lab test interferences

Interfere: Radiographic studies of GI system

NURSING CONSIDERATIONS

Assessment

- Monitor skin turgor; dehydration may occur in severe diarrhea; monitor electrolytes (potassium, sodium, chloride) if diarrhea is severe or continues long term
- Assess bowel pattern (frequency, consistency, shape, volume, color) before drug therapy, after treatment; check weight, bowel sounds; identify factors contributing to diarrhea (bacteria, diet, medications, tube feedings)

Nursing diagnoses

- ✓ Diarrhea (uses)
- ✓ Constipation (adverse reactions)
- ✓ Knowledge deficit (teaching)

Implementation

- Shake susp before use; chewable tabs should not be swallowed whole

B

Patient/family education

• Teach patient to stop use if symptoms do not improve within 2 days or become worse, or if diarrhea is accompanied by high fever
• Teach patient to increase fluids for rehydration
• Tell patient to chew or dissolve chewable tabs in mouth; do not swallow whole; shake susp before using
• Tell patient to avoid other salicylates unless directed by prescriber; not to give to P children because of possibility of Reye's syndrome
• Tell patient that stools may turn gray; tongue may darken; impaction may occur in debilitated patients

Evaluation

Positive therapeutic outcome
• Decreased diarrhea

bisoprolol (℞)

(bis-oh'pro-lole)

Zebeta

Func. class.: Antihypertensive

Chem. class.: β_1-Blocker (selective)

Pregnancy category C

Action: Preferentially and competitively blocks stimulation of β_1-adrenergic receptor within cardiac muscle; produces negative chronotropic and inotropic activity (decreases rate of SA node discharge, increases recovery time), slows conduction of AV node, decreases heart rate, which decreases O_2 consumption in myocardium; decreases renin-aldosterone-angiotensin system; inhibits β_2-receptors in bronchial and vascular smooth muscle at high doses

➔ **Therapeutic Outcome:** Decreased B/P, heart rate

Uses: Mild to moderate hypertension

Investigational uses: Angina pectoris, supraventricular tachycardia

Dosage and routes

Hypertension

Adult: PO 2.5-5 mg qd; may increase if necessary to 20 mg once daily; may need to reduce dose in presence of renal or hepatic impairment

Available forms: Tabs 5, 10 mg

Adverse effects

CNS: Vertigo, headache, insomnia, fatigue, dizziness, mental changes, memory loss, hallucinations, depression, lethargy, drowsiness, strange dreams, catatonia, peripheral neuropathy
CV: ***Ventricular dysrhythmias, profound hypotension, bradycardia, CHF,*** cold extremities, postural hypotension, 2nd- or 3rd-degree heart block
EENT: Sore throat, dry burning eyes
ENDO: Increased hypoglycemic response to insulin
GI: Nausea, diarrhea, vomiting, mesenteric arterial thrombosis, ischemic colitis, flatulence, gastritis, gastric pain
GU: Impotence, decreased libido
HEMA: ***Agranulocytosis, thrombocytopenia,*** purpura, ***eosinophilia***
INTEG: Rash, fever, alopecia, pruritus, sweating
MISC: Facial swelling, weight

gain, decreased exercise tolerance
MS: Joint pain, arthralgia
RESP: Bronchospasm, dyspnea, wheezing, cough, nasal stuffiness

Contraindications: Hypersensitivity to β-blockers, cardiogenic shock, heart block (2nd, 3rd degree), sinus bradycardia, CHF, cardiac failure

Precautions: Major surgery, P pregnancy **C,** lactation, children, diabetes mellitus, renal or hepatic disease, thyroid disease, COPD, asthma, well-compensated heart failure, aortic or mitral valve disease, peripheral vascular disease, myasthenia gravis

Pharmacokinetics	
Absorption	Well absorbed
Distribution	Unknown; protein binding (30%)
Metabolism	Liver, inactive metabolites
Excretion	Urine, unchanged (50%)
Half-life	9-12 hr

Pharmacodynamics	
Onset	Unknown
Peak	2-4 hr
Duration	24 hr

Interactions

Individual drugs
Alcohol: (large amounts) ↑ hypotension
Clonidine: Fatal reactions after discontinuing clonidine
Epinephrine: ↑ hypertension, then bradycardia
Flecainide: ↑ effects of both drugs
Haloperidol: ↑ effects of both drugs
Hydralazine: ↑ hypotension, bradycardia
Lidocaine: ↑ lidocaine toxicity
Quinidine: ↑ hypotension, bradycardia
Prazosin: ↑ hypotension, bradycardia
Theophylline: ↓ bronchodilatation

Drug classifications
Barbiturates: ↓ antihypertensive effects
Calcium channel blockers: ↑ hypotension
Contraceptives, oral: ↑ hypotension
Diuretics, loop: ↑ CV effects
MAOI: ↑ bradycardia
Penicillins: ↓ antihypertensive effects
Salicylates: ↓ antihypertensive effects
Sulfonylureas: ↓ hypoglycemic effect

Lab test interferences
↑ AST (SGOT), ↑ ALT (SGPT)
Interference: Glucose/insulin tolerance tests

NURSING CONSIDERATIONS

Assessment

- Monitor B/P during beginning treatment, periodically thereafter; pulse q4h: note rate, rhythm, quality; apical/radial pulse before administration; notify prescriber of any significant changes (pulse <50 bpm)
- Check for baselines in renal, liver function tests before therapy begins
- Assess for edema in feet, legs daily, monitor I&O, daily weight; check for jugular vein distention, rales bilaterally, dyspnea (CHF)
- Monitor skin turgor, dryness of mucous membranes for hydration status, especially G elderly

Nursing diagnoses

- ✓ Cardiac output, decreased (uses)
- ✓ Injury, risk for (side effects)
- ✓ Knowledge deficit (teaching)
- ✓ Noncompliance (teaching)

Implementation

- Give qd; give with food to prevent GI upset; may be crushed
- Store protected from light, moisture; place in cool environment

Patient/family education

- Teach patient not to discontinue drug abruptly; taper over 2 wk; may cause precipitate dysrhythmias if stopped abruptly
- Teach patient not to use OTC products containing α-adrenergic stimulants (such as nasal decongestants, cold preparations); to avoid alcohol, smoking and to limit sodium intake as prescribed
- Teach patient how to take pulse and B/P at home; advise when to notify prescriber
- Instruct patient to comply with weight control, dietary adjustments, modified exercise program
- Tell patient to carry/wear Medic Alert ID to identify drug being taken, allergies; tell patient drug controls symptoms but does not cure
- Caution patient to avoid hazardous activities if dizziness, drowsiness present
- Teach patient to take drug as prescribed, not to double doses, skip doses; take any missed doses as soon as remembered if at least 8 hr until next dose

Evaluation

Positive therapeutic outcome

- Decreased B/P in hypertension (after 1-2 wk)

Treatment of overdose: Lavage, **IV** atropine for bradycardia, **IV** theophylline for bronchospasm, digitalis, O_2, diuretic for cardiac failure, hemodialysis, **IV** glucose for hyperglycemia, **IV** diazepam (or phenytoin) for seizures

bitolterol (℞)

(bye-tole'ter-ole)

Tornalate

Func. class.: β_2-Adrenergic agonist; bronchodilator

Chem. class.: Acid ester of colterol

Pregnancy category C

Action: Causes bronchodilatation by action on β_2-receptors with increased synthesis of cyclic AMP; relaxes bronchial smooth muscle; inhibits mast cell degranulation; stimulates cilia to remove secretions with very little effect on heart rate

Therapeutic Outcome: Ability to breathe without difficulty

Uses: Asthma, bronchospasm

Dosage and routes

P ***Inhaler >12 yr:*** INH 2 puffs; wait 1-3 min before 3rd puff if needed; not to exceed 3 inh q6h or 2 inh q4h

Nebulization

P ***Adult/child >12 yr:*** INH 0.5 ml (1 mg) tid by intermittent flow or 1.25 mg tid by continuous flow

Available forms: Aerosol 0.37 mg/actuation; 0.2% neb sol

Adverse effects

CNS: Tremors, anxiety, insomnia, headache, dizziness, stimulation, restlessness, hallucinations
CV: Palpitations, tachycardia, hypertension, angina, hypotension
EENT: Dry nose, irritation of nose and throat
GI: Heartburn, nausea, vomiting, anorexia
MS: Muscle cramps
RESP: ***Bronchospasm,*** dyspnea

Contraindications: Hypersensitivity to sympathomimetics

Precautions: Lactation, pregnancy **C,** cardiac disorders, hyperthyroidism, diabetes mellitus

Pharmacokinetics	
Absorption	Unknown
Distribution	Unknown
Metabolism	Lungs to active metabolite
Excretion	Unknown
Half-life	Unknown

Pharmacodynamics	
Onset	3-4 min
Peak	½-1 hr
Duration	5-8 hr

Interactions

Drug classifications

β-Adrenergic blockers: Block therapeutic effect
Bronchodilators, aerosol: ↑ action of bronchodilator
MAOI: ↑ chance of hypertensive crisis
Sympathomimetics: ↑ adrenergic side effects

NURSING CONSIDERATIONS

Assessment

• Monitor respiratory function: vital capacity, FEV, ABGs, lung sounds, heart rate, rhythm (baseline)
• Determine client's ability to self-medicate
• Monitor for evidence of allergic reactions; paradoxic bronchospasm; withhold dose; notify prescriber

Nursing diagnoses

✓ Impaired gas exchange (uses)
✓ Airway clearance, ineffective (uses)
✓ Knowledge deficit (teaching)

Implementation

• Give after shaking, exhale, place mouthpiece in mouth, inhale slowly, hold breath, remove, exhale slowly; allow at least 1 min between inh
• Store in light-resistant container; do not expose to temp over 86° F (30° C)

Patient/family education

• Tell patient not to use OTC medications; extra stimulation may occur; to use this medication before other medications and allow at least 5 min between each; to prevent overstimulation
• Teach patient use of inhaler; review package insert with patient; to avoid getting aerosol in eyes; blurring may result; to wash inhaler in warm water daily and dry well; to avoid smoking, smoke-filled rooms, persons with respiratory tract infections
• Teach patient that paradoxic bronchospasm may occur and to stop drug immediately and notify prescriber; to limit caffeine products such as chocolate, coffee, tea, and colas
• Instruct patient on administration of dose; not to use more than prescribed; serious side effects may occur; if taking

regularly and dose is missed, take when remembered; space other doses on new time schedule

Evaluation

Positive therapeutic outcome

- Absence of dyspnea, wheezing after 1 hr
- Improved airway exchange
- Improved ABGs

Treatment of overdose: Administer a β_2-adrenergic blocker

bleomycin (℞)

(blee-oh-mye'sin)

Blenoxane

Func. class.: Antineoplastic, antibiotic

Chem. class.: Glycopeptide

Pregnancy category D

Action: Inhibits synthesis of DNA, RNA, protein; derived from *Streptomyces verticillus;* replication is decreased by binding to DNA, which causes strand splitting; phase specific in the G_2 and M phases; a nonvesicant

Therapeutic Outcome: Prevention of rapidly growing malignant cells

Uses: Cancer of head, neck, penis, cervix, vulva of squamous cell origin, Hodgkin's disease, lymphosarcoma, reticulum cell sarcoma, testicular carcinoma, malignant pleural effusion

Dosage and routes

Adult: SC/**IV**/IM 0.25-0.5 U/kg q1-2 wk or 10-20 U/m^2; then 1 U/day or 5 U/wk; may also be given intraarterially; do not exceed total dose, 400 U in lifetime

Available forms: Powder for inj 15 U, 30 U

Adverse effects

CNS: Fever, chills

CV: Hypotension, peripheral vasoconstriction

GI: Nausea, vomiting, anorexia, stomatitis, weight loss

HEMA: Hypotension, peripheral vasoconstriction

INTEG: Rash, hyperkeratosis, nail changes, alopecia, fever and chills

RESP: ***Fibrosis,*** pneumonitis, wheezing, ***pulmonary toxicity***

SYST: ***Anaphylaxis***

IDIOSYNCRATIC REACTION: Hypotension, confusion, fever, chills, wheezing

Contraindications: Hypersensitivity

Precautions: Renal, hepatic, respiratory disease, pregnancy **D**

Pharmacokinetics

Absorption	Well absorbed (IM, SC, intrapleural, intraperitoneal)
Distribution	Widely distributed
Metabolism	Liver, 30%
Excretion	Kidneys, unchanged (50%)
Half-life	2 hr; ↑ in renal disease

Pharmacodynamics

Unknown

Interactions

Individual drugs

Radiation: ↑ toxicity, bone marrow suppression

Drug classifications

Antineoplastics: ↑ toxicity, bone marrow suppression

NURSING CONSIDERATIONS

Assessment

- Assess buccal cavity q8h for dryness, sores or ulceration, white patches, oral pain, bleeding, dysphagia; obtain prescription for viscous lidocaine (Xylocaine)
- Assess symptoms indicating severe allergic reaction: rash, pruritus, urticaria, purpuric skin lesions, itching, flushing
- Monitor CBC, differential, platelet count weekly; withhold drug if WBC count is <4000/mm^3 or platelet count is <100,000/mm^3; notify prescriber of results if WBC <20,000/mm^3, platelets <150,000/mm^3
- Monitor temp q4h (may indicate beginning of infection)
- Monitor liver function tests before and during therapy (bilirubin, AST [SGOT], ALT [SGPT], LDH) as needed or monthly
- Assess for bleeding: hematuria, stool guaiac, bruising or petechiae, mucosa or orifices q8h; inflammation of mucosa, breaks in skin
- Identify dyspnea, rales, unproductive cough, chest pain, tachypnea
- Identify effects of alopecia on body image; discuss feelings about body changes; if edema in feet, joint pain, stomach pain, shaking present, prescriber should be notified; identify inflammation of mucosa, breaks in skin

Nursing diagnoses

- ✓ Injury, risk for (adverse reactions)
- ✓ Body image disturbance (adverse reactions)
- ✓ Infection, risk for (adverse reactions)
- ✓ Knowledge deficit (teaching)

Implementation

- Avoid contact with skin, very irritating; wash completely to remove
- Give fluids **IV** or PO before chemotherapy to hydrate patient
- Give antacid before oral agent; give antiemetic 30-60 min before giving drug to prevent vomiting and prn and antibiotics for prophylaxis of infection
- Provide liq diet: carbonated beverages, gelatin may be added if patient is not nauseated or vomiting
- Rinsing of mouth tid-qid with water, club soda; brushing of teeth bid-qid with soft brush or cotton-tipped applicators for stomatitis; use unwaxed dental floss

SC/IM route

- Reconstitute with 1-5 ml sterile water for inj; D_5W, 0.9% NaCl

IV route

- Drug should be prepared by experienced personnel using proper precautions
- Two test doses 2-5 U before initial dose; monitor for anaphylaxis
- Give by direct **IV** after reconstituting 15 U or less/5 ml or more of D_5W or 0.9% NaCl; give 15 U or less/10 min through Y-tube or 3-way stopcock initial dose; monitor for anaphylaxis

Intermittent inf

- Administer after diluting

50-100 ml 0.9% NaCl, D_5W and giving at prescribed rate

Syringe compatibilities: Cisplatin, cyclophosphamide, doxorubicin, droperidol, fluorouracil, furosemide, heparin, leucovorin, methotrexate, metoclopramide, mitomycin, vinblastine, vincristine

Y-*site compatibilities:* Allopurinol, amisostine, aztreonam, cisplatin, cyclophosphamide, doxorubicin, droperidol, filgrastim, fludarabine, fluorouracil, heparin, leucovorin, melphalan, methotrexate, metoclopramide, mitomycin, ondansetron, paclitaxel, sargramostim, teniposide, thiotepa, vinblastine, vincristine, vinorelbine

Additive incompatibilities: Aminophylline, ascorbic acid inj, carbenicillin, cefazolin, cephalothin, diazepam, hydrocortisone, methotrexate, mitomycin, nafcillin, penicillin G sodium, terbutaline

Additive compatibilities: Amikacin, cephapirin, dexamethasone, diphenhydramine, fluorouracil, gentamicin, heparin, hydrocortisone, phenytoin, streptomycin, tobramycin, vincristine, vinblastine

Solution compatibilities: D_5W, 0.9% NaCl

Patient/family education

- Teach patient to avoid use of products containing aspirin or ibuprofen, razors, commercial mouthwash; bleeding may occur; to report symptoms of bleeding (hematuria, tarry stools)
- Instruct patient to report signs of anemia (fatigue, headache, irritability, faintness, shortness of breath)
- Instruct patient to report any changes in breathing or coughing even several months after treatment; to avoid crowds and persons with respiratory tract or other infections
- Inform patient that hair may be lost during treatment; a wig or hairpiece may make patient feel better; new hair may be different in color, texture
- Caution patient not to have any vaccinations without the advice of the prescriber; serious reactions can occur
- Advise patient contraception is needed during treatment and for several months after completion of therapy

Evaluation

Positive therapeutic outcome

- Prevention of rapid division of malignant cells

B

bretylium 🗝 (℞)
(bre-til'ee-um)
Bretylate ✤, bretylium tosylate, Bretylol
Func. class.: Antidysrhythmic (Class III)
Chem. class.: Quaternary ammonium compound
Pregnancy category C

Action: After a transient release of norepinephrine, inhibits further release by postganglionic nerve endings; prolongs action potential, duration, and effective refractory period

➡ **Therapeutic Outcome:** Absence of dysrhythmias

Uses: Serious ventricular tachycardia, cardioversion, ventricular fibrillation; for short-term use only

Dosage and routes

Severe ventricular fibrillation

Adult: **IV** bol 5 mg/kg; increase to 10 mg/kg repeated q15 min, up to 30 mg/kg; **IV** inf 1-2 mg/min or give 5-10 mg/kg over 10 min q6h (maintenance)

Ventricular tachycardia

Adult: **IV** inf 500 mg diluted in 50 ml D_5W or NS; infuse over 10-30 min; may repeat in 1 hr; maintain with 1-2 mg/min or 5-10 mg/kg over 10-30 min q6h; IM 5-10 mg/kg undiluted; repeat in 1-2 hr if needed; maintain with same dose q6-8h

Available forms: Inj 50 mg/ml; 1, 2, 4 mg/ml prefilled syringes

Adverse effects

CNS: Syncope, dizziness, confusion, psychosis, anxiety

CV: Hypotension, postural hypotension, bradycardia, angina, PVCs, substernal pressure, transient hypertension, precipitation of angina

GI: Nausea, vomiting

RESP: Respiratory depression

Contraindications: Hypersensitivity, digitalis toxicity, aortic stenosis, pulmonary hypertension, P children

Precautions: Renal disease, pregnancy **C**, lactation, P children

Pharmacokinetics

Absorption	Complete bioavailability (IV)
Distribution	Unknown
Metabolism	Not metabolized
Excretion	Kidneys, unchanged
Half-life	4-17 hr

Pharmacodynamics

	IV	IM
Onset	5 min	½-2 hr
Peak	Infusion's end	Unknown
Duration	6-24 hr	6-24 hr

Interactions

Individual drugs

Caffeine: ↓ effects of adenosine

Carbamazepine: ↑ heart block

Digoxin: ↑ digitalis toxicity

Dopamine: ↑ pressor effects

Norepinephrine: ↑ pressor effects

Drug classifications

Cardiac glycosides: ↑ toxicity

Lab test interferences

↑ Liver function tests

NURSING CONSIDERATIONS

Assessment

• Monitor ECG continuously to determine drug effectiveness; measure PR, QRS, QT intervals; check for PVCs, other dysrhythmias; monitor B/P continuously for hypotension, hypertension; check for rebound hypertension after 1-2 hr

Nursing diagnoses

✓ Cardiac output, decreased (uses)

✓ Gas exchange, impaired (adverse reactions)

✓ Knowledge deficit (teaching)

Implementation

IM route

• Give in large muscle mass, rotate sites to prevent necrosis

IV **IV route**

Direct

• Give **IV** bol undiluted; give 6 mg or less over 1 min; if using an **IV** line, use port near insertion site, flush with normal saline (50 ml)

B

Intermittent inf
• Give by intermittent inf after diluting 500 mg/50 ml or more with 0.9% NaCl, D_5W, D_5/0.45% NaCl, D_5/0.9% NaCl, LR, ⅙ mol/L sodium lactate; run over >8 min
Cont inf
• Give by cont inf diluted in sol; give 1-2 mg/min; use inf site
• Store at room temp; sol should be clear

Additive compatibilities: Aminophylline, atracurium, calcium chloride, calcium gluconate, digoxin, dopamine, esmolol, regular insulin, lidocaine, potassium chloride, quinadine verapamil

Additive incompatibility: Phenytoin

Y-site compatibilities: Amiodarone, amrinone, diltiazem, dobutamine, famotidine, isoproterenol, ranitidine

Evaluation
Positive therapeutic outcome
• Decreased B/P, dysrhythmias, heart rate; normal sinus rhythm

bromocriptine (℞)
(broe-moe-krip'teen)
Parlodel
Func. class.: Antiparkinsonian agent; dopamine receptor agonist; ovulation stimulant
Chem. class.: Ergot alkaloid derivative
Pregnancy category D

Action: Inhibits prolactin release by activating postsynaptic dopamine receptors; activation of striatal dopamine receptors may be reason for improvement in Parkinson's disease

➔ **Therapeutic Outcome:** Decreased involuntary movements in Parkinson's disease; decreased lactation; decreased hormone levels in acromegaly; absence of amenorrhea in hyperprolactinemia

Uses: Female infertility, adjunct with levodopa in Parkinson's disease, prevention of postpartum lactation, amenorrhea caused by hyperprolactinemia, acromegaly

Dosage and routes
Hyperprolactinemic indications
Adult: PO 1.25-2.5 mg with meals; may increase by 2.5 mg q3- 7 days; usual dosage 5-7.5 mg
Acromegaly
Adult: PO 1.25-2.5 mg/day × 3 days hs; may increase by 1.25-2.5 mg q3-7 days; usual range 20-30 mg/day; max 100 mg/day
Postpartum lactation
Adult: PO 2.5 mg qd-tid with meal × 14 or 21 days
Parkinson's disease
Adult: PO 1.25 mg bid with meals; may increase q2-4 wk by 2.5 mg/day; not to exceed 100 mg/day

Available forms: Caps 5 mg; tabs 2.5 mg

Adverse effects
CNS: Headache, depression, restlessness, anxiety, nervousness, confusion, ***convulsions,*** hallucinations, ***dizziness,*** fatigue, drowsiness, abnormal involuntary movements, psychosis

CV: Orthostatic hypotension, decreased B/P, palpitations, extrasystole, ***shock,*** dysrhythmias, bradycardia
EENT: Blurred vision, diplopia, burning eyes, nasal congestion
GI: Nausea, vomiting, anorexia, cramps, constipation, diarrhea, dry mouth, GI hemorrhage
GU: Frequency, retention, incontinence, diuresis
INTEG: Rash on face, arms, alopecia

Contraindications: Hypersensitivity to ergot, severe ischemic disease, pregnancy **D,** severe peripheral vascular disease

Precautions: Lactation, hepatic disease, renal disease, P children, pituitary tumors

Pharmacokinetics	
Absorption	Poorly absorbed
Distribution	Unknown
Metabolism	Liver, completely
Excretion	85%-98% feces
Half-life	4 hr (initial); 50 hr (terminal)

Pharmacodynamics	
Onset	½-1½ hr
Peak	1-3 hr
Duration	8-12 hr

Interactions

Individual drugs

Haloperidol: ↓ levels of bromocriptine
Levodopa: ↑ neurologic effects
Methyldopa: ↓ levels of bromocriptine
Reserpine: ↓ effects of bromocriptine

Drug classifications

Antihistamines: ↑ CNS depression
Antihypertensives: ↑ hypotension
Analgesics, opioid: ↑ CNS depression
Phenothiazines: ↓ levels of bromocriptine
Sedative/hypnotics: ↑ CNS depression
Antidepressants, tricyclics: ↓ levels of bromocriptine

Lab test interferences

↑ Growth hormone, ↑ AST (SGOT), ↑ ALT (SGPT), ↑ CPK, ↑ BUN, ↑ uric acid, ↑ alkaline phosphatase, ↑ GGTP

NURSING CONSIDERATIONS

Assessment

- Assess symptoms of Parkinson's disease (extrapyramidal symptoms): shuffling gait, muscle rigidity, involuntary movements, pill rolling, muscle spasms, drooling before and during treatment
- Assess for symptoms of suppression of lactation: decreasing breast tenderness and discomfort, decreasing milk production
- Monitor B/P; establish baseline, compare with other readings; this drug decreases B/P; patient should remain recumbent for 2-4 hr after first dose; supervise ambulation

Nursing diagnoses

✓ Mobility, impaired (uses)
✓ Knowledge deficit (teaching)

Implementation

- Give with meals or milk to prevent GI symptoms; crush tab if patient has swallowing difficulty
- Give hs so dizziness, orthostatic hypotension do not occur
- Store at room temp in airtight container

Patient/family education

- Advise patient to change position slowly to prevent orthostatic hypotension
- Tabs may be crushed and mixed with food
- Caution patient to use contraceptives during treatment with this drug; pregnancy may occur; to use methods other than oral contraceptives
- Teach patient that therapeutic effect for Parkinson's disease may take 2 mo: galactorrhea, amenorrhea
- Caution patient to avoid hazardous activity if dizziness, drowsiness occurs during treatment start-up
- Advise patient to avoid alcohol and OTC medication unless approved by prescriber
- Teach patients with acromegaly to notify prescriber immediately if severe headache, nausea, vomiting, blurred vision occur; indicates change in enlargement of tumor
- Teach patients using drug for lactation suppression that treatment will last up to 3 wk and breast engorgement with milk production may occur after treatment is discontinued

Evaluation

Positive therapeutic outcome

- Parkinson's disease: decreased dyskinesia, decreased slow movements, decreased drooling
- Decreased breast engorgement with accompanied pain, tenderness
- Acromegly: decreased growth hormone levels

B

brompheniramine (OTC, ℞)

(brome-fen-eer'a-meen)

Bromphen, brompheniramine, Codimal-A, Cophene-B, Dehist, Diamine T.D., Dimetane, Dimetane Extentabs, Histaject, Nasahist-B, ND-Stat

Func. class.: Antihistamine

Chem. class.: Alkylamine, H_1-receptor antagonist

Pregnancy category B

Action: Acts on blood vessels, GI, respiratory system by competing with histamine for H_1-receptor site; decreases allergic response by blocking histamine

➔ Therapeutic Outcome: Absence of allergy symptoms and rhinitis

Uses: Allergy symptoms, rhinitis, allergic dermatoses, nasal allergies, hypersensitivity reactions including blood transfusion reactions, anaphylaxis

Dosage and routes

Adult: PO 4-8 mg tid-qid, not to exceed 36 mg/day; TIME REL 8-12 mg bid-tid, not to exceed 36 mg/day; IM/**IV**/SC 5-20 mg q6-12h, not to exceed 40 mg/day

P ***Child >6 yr:*** PO 2 mg tid-qid, not to exceed 12 mg/day; IM/**IV**/SC 0.5 mg/kg/day divided tid or qid

P ***Child <6 yr:*** 1 mg q4-6h (not to exceed 6 mg/day)

Available forms: Tabs 4, 8, 12 mg; time rel tabs 8, 12 mg; elix 2 mg/5 ml; inj 10, 100 mg/ml

Adverse effects

*CNS: **Dizziness, drowsiness,*** poor coordination, fatigue, anxiety, euphoria, confusion, paresthesia, neuritis

CV: Hypotension, palpitations, tachycardia

EENT: Blurred vision, dilated pupils, tinnitus, nasal stuffiness, dry nose, throat, mouth

GI: Dry mouth, nausea, vomiting, anorexia, constipation, diarrhea

GU: Retention, dysuria, frequency, impotence

*HEMA: **Thrombocytopenia, agranulocytosis, hemolytic anemia***

INTEG: Photosensitivity

RESP: Increased thick secretions, wheezing, chest tightness

Contraindications: Hypersensitivity to H_1-receptor antagonists, acute asthma attack, lower respiratory tract disease, P child <6 yr

Precautions: Increased intraocular pressure, renal disease, cardiac disease, hypertension, bronchial asthma, seizure disorder, stenosed peptic ulcers, hyperthyroidism, prostatic hypertrophy, bladder neck obstruction, pregnancy **B**

Pharmacokinetics

Absorption	Well absorbed (PO, IM)
Distribution	Widely distributed; crosses blood-brain barrier
Metabolism	Liver, extensively
Excretion	Kidneys, metabolite; breast milk (minimal)
Half-life	12-34 hr

Pharmacodynamics

	PO	SC/IM	IV
Onset	15-30 min	30 min	Immediate
Peak	2-5 hr	Unknown	Unknown
Duration	6-12 hr	8-12 hr	8-12 hr

Interactions

Individual drugs

Alcohol: ↑ CNS depression

Drug classifications

CNS depressants: ↑ CNS depression

MAOI: ↑ anticholinergic effect

Narcotics: ↑ CNS depression

Sedative/hypnotics: ↑ CNS depression

Lab test interferences

False negative: Skin allergy tests (discontinue antihistamines before testing)

NURSING CONSIDERATIONS

Assessment

- Assess respiratory status: rate, rhythm, increase in bronchial secretions, wheezing, chest tightness; provide fluids to 2 L/day to decrease secretion thickness
- Monitor I&O ratio: be alert for urinary retention, frequency, dysuria, especially G elderly; drug should be discontinued if these occur
- Monitor CBC during long-term therapy; blood dyscrasias may occur but are rare
- **IV** administration may result in rapid drop in B/P, sweating, G dizziness, especially in elderly

Nursing diagnoses

- ✓ Airway clearance, ineffective (uses)
- ✓ Injury, risk for (side effects)
- ✓ Knowledge deficit (teaching)
- ✓ Noncompliance (teaching, overuse)

Implementation

PO route

- May give with food to prevent GI upset; absorption is not altered by food
- Store in tight, light-resistant container

IV route

- Give undiluted or dilute 10 mg/ml using 0.9% NaCl at a rate of 1 min or more
- May be further diluted in 0.9% NaCl, D_5W; give as intermittent inf at prescribed rate

Patient/family education

- Teach patient all aspects of drug use; to notify prescriber if confusion, sedation, hypotension occur; to avoid driving or other hazardous activity if drowsiness occurs; to avoid alcohol or other CNS depressants that may potentiate effect
- Instruct patient not to exceed recommended dosage; dysrhythmias may occur
- Teach patient hard candy, gum, frequent rinsing of mouth may be used for dryness

Evaluation

Positive therapeutic outcome

- Absence of running or congested nose, rashes

Treatment of overdose: Administer ipecac syrup or lavage, diazepam, vasopressors, barbiturates (short acting)

bumetanide (℞)

(byoo-met'a-nide)

Bumex

Func. class: Loop diuretic

Chem. class.: Sulfonamide derivative

Pregnancy category C

Action: Acts on the ascending loop of Henle in the kidney to inhibit the reabsorption of the electrolytes sodium and chloride, causing excretion of sodium, calcium, magnesium, chloride, water, and some potassium; also decreases reabsorption of sodium and chloride and increases the excretion of potassium in the distal tubule of the kidney; responsible for antihypertensive effect and peripheral vasodilatation

Therapeutic Outcome: Decreased edema in lung tissue and peripherally; decreased B/P

Uses: Edema in congestive heart failure, nephrotic syndrome, ascites caused by hepatic disease, hepatic cirrhosis

Investigational uses: May be used alone or as adjunct with antihypertensives such as spironolactone, triamterene

Dosage and routes

Adult: PO 0.5-2 mg qd; may give 2nd or 3rd dose at 4-5 hr intervals; not to exceed 10 mg/day; may be given on alternate days or intermittently; **IV**/IM 0.5-1 mg/day; may give 2nd or 3rd dose at 2-3 hr intervals; not to exceed 10 mg/day

Available forms: Tabs 0.5, 1, 2 mg; inj 0.25 mg/ml

Adverse effects

CNS: Headache, fatigue, weakness, vertigo, paresthesias
CV: Orthostatic hypotension, chest pain, ECG changes, circulatory collapse
EENT: Ear pain, tinnitus, blurred vision
ELECT: Hypokalemia, hypochlorsemic alkalosis, hypomagnesia, hyperuricemia, hypocalcemia, hyponatremia, metabolic alkalosis
ENDO: Hyperglycemia
GI: Nausea, diarrhea, dry mouth, vomiting, anorexia, cramps, oral and gastric irritations, pancreatitis
GU: Polyuria, ***renal failure,*** *glycosuria*
HEMA: ***Thrombocytopenia, leukopenia, anemia***
INTEG: Rash, pruritus, purpura, urticaria
MS: Cramps, stiffness

Contraindications: Hypersensitivity to sulfonamides, anuria, electrolyte depletion

Precautions: Diabetes mellitus, dehydration, severe renal disease, pregnancy **C**, lactation

Pharmacokinetics

	PO/IM
Absorption	Rapidly, completely absorbed
	PO/IM/IV
Distribution	Crosses placenta
Metabolism	Liver (30%-40%)
Excretion	Breast milk, urine, feces
Half-life	1-1½ hr

Pharmacodynamics

	PO	IM	IV
Onset	½-1 hr	40 min	5 min
Peak	1-2 hr	Unknown	½ hr
Duration	4 hr	4 hr	2-3 hr

Interactions

Individual drugs

Alcohol: ↑ orthostatic hypotension
Cisplatin: ↑ risk of ototoxicity
Ethacrynic acid: Combination may cause ↑ chance of arrhythmias (do not use together)
Indomethacin: ↓ diuretic and antihypertensive effects of bumetanide
Lithium: ↓ renal clearance causing ↑ toxicity
Mezlocillin: ↑ hypokalemia
Probenecid: ↓ effect of bumetanide
Piperacillin: ↑ hypokalemia
Ticarcillin: ↑ hypokalemia

Drug classifications

Aminoglycosides: ↑ ototoxicity
Anticoagulants: ↑ bleeding
Antihypertensives: ↑ antihypertensive effects
Digitalis glycosides: ↑ potassium loss with relating arrhythmias
Glucocorticoids: ↑ hypokalemia

NURSING CONSIDERATIONS

Assessment

- Assess patient for tinnitus, hearing loss, ear pain; periodic testing of hearing is needed when high doses of this drug are given by **IV** route
- Monitor for manifestations of hypokalemia: *Renal:* acidic urine, reduced urine osmolality, nocturia, polyuria, polydipsia; *CV:* hypotension, broad T wave, U wave, ectopy, tachycardia, weak pulse; *Neuro:* muscle weakness, altered LOC, drowsiness, apathy, lethargy, confusion, depression; *GI:* anorexia, nausea, cramps, constipation, distention, paralytic ileus; *Resp:* hypoventila-

tion, respiratory muscle weakness
• Monitor for manifestations of hypocalcemia: *CNS:* personality changes, anxiety, disturbances, depression, psychosis; *GI:* nausea, vomiting, constipation, abdominal pain from muscle spasm; *CV:* decreased contractility, decreased cardiac output, hypotension, lengthened ST segment, prolonged QT interval; *Integ:* scaling eczema, alopecia, hyperpigmentation; *Neuro:* tetany, muscle twitching, cramping, grimacing, seizure, altered deep tendon reflexes, spasm
• Monitor for manifestations of hypomagnesemia: *CNS:* agitation; *Neuro:* muscle twitching, paresthesias, hyperactive reflexes, positive Babinski's reflex, dysphagia, nystagmus, seizures, tetany; *GI:* nausea, vomiting, diarrhea, anorexia, abdominal distention; *CV:* ectopy, tachycardia, broad, flat, or inverted T waves, depressed ST segment, prolonged QT, decreased cardiac output, hypotension
• Monitor for manifestations of hyponatremia: *CV:* increased B/P, cold, clammy skin, hypovolemia or hypervolemia; *GI:* anorexia, nausea, vomiting, diarrhea, abdominal cramps; *Neuro:* lethargy, increased ICP, confusion, headache, seizures, coma, fatigue, tremors, hyperreflexia
• Monitor for manifestations of hyperchloremia: *Neuro:* weakness, lethargy, coma; *Resp:* deep rapid breathing
• Assess fluid volume status: I&O ratio and record, count or weigh diapers as appropriate, distended red veins, crackles in lung, color, quality and sp gr of urine, skin turgor, adequacy of pulses, moist mucous membranes, bilateral lung sounds, peripheral pitting edema; dehydration symptoms of decreasing output, thirst, hypotension, dry mouth and mucous membranes should be reported
• Monitor electrolytes: potassium, sodium, calcium, magnesium; also include BUN, blood pH, ABGs, uric acid, CBC, blood sugar
• Assess B/P before and during therapy with patient lying, standing, and sitting as appropriate; orthostatic hypotension can occur rapidly

Nursing diagnoses

✓ Altered urinary elimination (side effects)
✓ Fluid volume deficit (side effects)
✓ Fluid volume excess (uses)
✓ Knowledge deficit (teaching)

Implementation

• Give in AM to avoid interference with sleep
• Potassium replacement if potassium level is <3.0 mg/dl whole, or use oral solutions; drug may be crushed if patient is unable to swallow

PO route

• With food, if nausea occurs; absorption may be reduced

IV **IV route**

• Do not use solution that is yellow or has a precipitate or crystals

IV **Direct IV**

• Give undiluted through Y-tube on 3-way stopcock; give 20 mg or less/min

Intermittent inf

• May be added to NS, D_5W, $D_{10}W$, $D_{20}W$, invert sugar 10%

in electrolyte #1, LR, sodium lactate ⅙ mol/L; use within 24 hr to ensure compatibility; give through Y-tube or 3-way stopcock; give at 4 mg/min or less; use infusion pump

Y-site compatibilities: Allopurinol, amifostine, aztreonam, cefepime, diltiazem, filgrastim, lorazepam, morphine, teniposide, thiotepa, vinorelbine

Syringe compatibility: Doxapram

Additive compatibilities: Floxacillin, furosemide

Patient/family education

- Teach patient to take the medication early in the day to prevent nocturia
- Instruct the patient to take with food or milk if GI symptoms of nausea and anorexia occur
- Teach patient to maintain weekly record of weight and notify prescriber of weight loss of >5 lb
- Caution the patient that this drug causes a loss of potassium so food rich in potassium should be added to the diet; refer to a dietician for assistance in planning
- Caution the patient not to exercise in hot weather or stand for prolonged periods since orthostatic hypotension will be enhanced
- Teach patient not to use alcohol or any OTC medications without prescriber's approval; serious drug reactions may occur
- Emphasize the need to contact prescriber immediately if muscle cramps, weakness, nausea, dizziness, or numbness occurs
- Teach patient to take own B/P and pulse and record
- Caution the patient that orthostatic hypotension may occur; patient should rise slowly from sitting or reclining positions and lie down if dizziness occurs
- Teach patient to continue taking medication even if feeling better; this drug controls symptoms but does not cure the condition
- Advise the patient with hypertension to continue other medical treatment (exercise, weight loss, relaxation techniques, cessation of smoking)

Evaluation

Positive therapeutic outcome

- Decreased edema
- Decreased B/P
- Increased diuresis

buprenorphine (℞)

(byoo-pre-nor'feen)

Buprenex

Func. class.: Narcotic analgesic

Chem. class.: Opiate, thebaine derivative

Pregnancy category C

Controlled substance schedule V

Action: Inhibits ascending pain pathways in limbic system, thalamus, midbrain, hypothalamus by binding to opiate receptor sites; this alters pain perception and response; generalized CNS depression

➡ **Therapeutic Outcome:** Relief of pain

Uses: Moderate to severe pain

Dosage and routes

Adult: IM/**IV** 0.3-0.6 mg q6h prn; may repeat dose after ½ hr; reduce dosage in elderly

Available forms: Inj 0.3 mg/ml (1 ml vials)

Adverse effects

CNS: Drowsiness, dizziness, confusion, headache, sedation, euphoria
CV: Palpitations, bradycardia, change in B/P
EENT: Tinnitus, blurred vision, miosis, diplopia
GI: Nausea, vomiting, anorexia, constipation, cramps
GU: Increased urinary output, dysuria
INTEG: Rash, urticaria, bruising, flushing, diaphoresis, pruritus
RESP: Respiratory depression

Contraindications: Hypersensitivity, addiction (narcotic)

Precautions: Addictive personality, pregnancy **C,** lactation, increased intracranial pressure, MI (acute), severe heart disease, respiratory depression, hepatic disease, renal disease

Pharmacokinetics

Absorption	Well absorbed (IM)
Distribution	Crosses placenta
Metabolism	Liver, extensively
Excretion	Kidneys, breast milk
Half-life	2½-3½ hr

Pharmacodynamics

	IM	IV
Onset	10-15 min	Immediate
Peak	1 hr	5 min
Duration	4 hr	2-5 hr

Interactions

Individual drugs

Alcohol: ↑ respiratory depression, hypotension, sedation

Drug classifications

Antihistamines: ↑ respiratory depression, hypotension
CNS depressants: ↑ respiratory depression, hypotension
MAOI: Do not use 2 wk before alfentanil
Sedative/hypnotics: ↑ respiratory depression, hypotension

NURSING CONSIDERATIONS

Assessment

- Assess pain characteristics: location, intensity, type before medication administration and following treatment
- Monitor VS after parenteral route; note muscle rigidity, drug history, liver, kidney function tests, respiratory dysfunction: respiratory depression, character, rate, rhythm; notify prescriber if respirations are <10/min
- Monitor CNS changes: dizziness, drowsiness, hallucinations, euphoria, LOC, pupil reaction
- Monitor allergic reactions: rash, urticaria

Nursing diagnoses

- ✓ Pain (uses)
- ✓ Sensory-perceptual alteration: visual, auditory (adverse reactions)
- ✓ Breathing pattern, ineffective (adverse reactions)
- ✓ Knowledge deficit (teaching)

Implementation

- Give by inj (IM, **IV**), only with resuscitative equipment available; give slowly to prevent rigidity

IM route

- Give deep in large muscle mass; rotate sites of inj

IV route

- Give **IV** direct undiluted over 3-5 min; give slowly

Y-site compatibilities: Allopurinol, amifostine, aztreonam, cefepime, filgrastim, melphalan, teniposide, thiotepa, vinorelbine

Syringe compatibility: Midazolam

Additive compatibilities: Atropine, diphenhydramine, droperidol, glycopyrrolate, haloperidol, hydroxyzine, promethazine, scopolamine

Additive incompatibilities: Diazepam, floxacillin, furosemide lorezepam

Patient/family education

- Instruct patient to report any symptoms of CNS changes, allergic reactions
- Caution patients to avoid CNS depressants: alcohol, sedative/hypnotics for at least 24 hr after taking this drug
- Discuss with patient that dizziness, drowsiness, and confusion are common; to avoid getting up without assistance
- Discuss in detail all aspects of the drug
- Instruct patient to change position slowly to prevent orthostatic hypotension
- Teach patient to turn, cough, deep breathe after surgery to prevent atelectasis

Evaluation

Positive therapeutic outcome

- Relief of pain

Treatment of overdose: Narcan 0.2-0.8 **IV**, O_2, **IV** fluids, vasopressors

bupropion (℞)

(byoo-proe'pee-on)

Wellbutrin, Wellbutrin SR, Zyban

Func. class.: Misc. antidepressant

Chem. class.: Amino ketone

Pregnancy category B

Action: Inhibits reuptake of dopamine, serotonin, norepinephrine

➔ **Therapeutic Outcome:** Decreased symptoms of depression after 2-3 wk

Uses: Depression, smoking cessation

Dosage and routes

Adult: PO 100 mg bid initially, then increase after 3 days to 100 mg tid if needed; may increase after 1 mo to 150 mg tid

Smoking cessation:

Adult: PO 150 mg bid, begin with 150 mg qd x 3 days then 300 mg/day continue for 7-12 wk

Available forms: Tabs 75, 100 mg; tabs, sus rel 100, 150 mg

Adverse effects

CNS: Headache, agitation, confusion, ***seizures,*** akathisia, delusions, insomnia, sedation, tremors

CV: Dysrhythmias, hypertension, palpitations, tachycardia, hypotension

EENT: Blurred vision, auditory disturbance

GI: Nausea, vomiting, dry mouth, increased appetite, constipation

GU: Impotence, frequency, retention
INTEG: Rash, pruritus, sweating

Contraindications: Hypersensitivity, seizure disorder, eating disorders

Precautions: Renal and hepatic disease, recent MI, cranial trauma, pregnancy **B,** lactation, P children

Pharmacokinetics

Absorption	Well absorbed; bioavailability poor
Distribution	Unknown
Metabolism	Liver extensively
Excretion	Kidneys
Half-life	14 hr, steady state 1 wk

Pharmacodynamics

Onset	Up to 4 wk
Peak	Unknown
Duration	Unknown

Interactions

Individual drugs

Alcohol: ↑ risk of seizures
Cimetidine: ↑ levels, ↑ toxicity
Levodopa: ↑ adverse reactions
Phenytoin: ↑ toxicity

Drug classifications

Antihistamines: ↑ CNS depression
Barbiturates: ↑ effects
Benzodiazepines: ↑ risk of seizures
CNS depressants: ↑ effects
MAOI: Acute toxicity, convulsions
Phenothiazines: ↑ toxicity

Lab test interferences

↑ serum bilirubin, ↑ blood glucose, ↑ alkaline phosphatase
↓ VMA, ↓ 5-HIAA
False ↑ Urinary catecholamines

NURSING CONSIDERATIONS

Assessment

- Monitor B/P (with patient lying, standing), pulse q4h; if systolic B/P drops 20 mm Hg hold drug, notify prescriber; take vital signs q4h in patients with cardiovascular disease
- Monitor blood studies: CBC, leukocytes, differential, cardiac enzymes if patient is receiving long-term therapy
- Monitor hepatic studies: AST (SGOT), ALT (SGPT), bilirubin if on long-term treatment
- Check weight weekly; appetite may increase with drug
- Assess ECG for flattening of T wave, bundle branch block, AV block, dysrhythmias in cardiac patients
- Assess for EPS primarily in G elderly: rigidity, dystonia, akathisia
- Assess mental status: mood, sensorium, affect, suicidal tendencies; increase in psychiatric symptoms: depression, panic
- Monitor urinary retention, constipation; constipation is P more likely to occur in children G or elderly
- Identify alcohol consumption; if alcohol was consumed, hold dose

Nursing diagnoses

- ✓ Coping, ineffective individual (uses)
- ✓ Injury, risk for (side effects)
- ✓ Knowledge deficit (teaching)
- ✓ Noncompliance (teaching)

Implementation

- Give with food or milk for GI symptoms
- Store at room temp; do not freeze

Patient/family education

- Teach patient that therapeutic effects may take 2-3 wk
- Teach patient to use caution in driving or other activities

requiring alertness because of drowsiness, dizziness, blurred vision; to avoid rising quickly from sitting to standing, G especially elderly

- Teach patient to avoid alcohol ingestion, obtain approval for other drugs
- Teach patient to increase fluids, bulk in diet if constipation, urinary retention occur, G especially elderly
- Teach patient to take gum, hard sugarless candy, or frequent sips of water for dry mouth

Evaluation

Positive therapeutic outcome

- Decrease in depression
- Absence of suicidal thoughts

Treatment of overdose: ECG monitoring, induce emesis, lavage, activated charcoal, administer anticonvulsant

buspirone (℞)

(byoo-spye'rone)

BuSpar

Func. class.: Antianxiety agent

Chem. class.: Azaspirodecanedione

Pregnancy category B

Action: Acts by inhibiting the action of serotonin (5-HT) by binding to serotonin and dopamine receptors; also increases norepinephrine metabolism

Therapeutic Outcome: Decreased anxiety

Uses: Management and short-term relief of anxiety disorders

Dosage and routes

Adult: PO 5 mg tid; may increase by 5 mg/day q2-3 days; not to exceed 60 mg/day

Available forms: Tabs 5, 10 mg

Adverse effects

CNS: Dizziness, headache, depression, stimulation, insomnia, nervousness, lightheadedness, numbness, paresthesia, incoordination, tremors, excitement, involuntary movements, confusion, akathisia

CV: Tachycardia, palpitations, hypotension, hypertension, *CVA, CHF, MI*

EENT: Sore throat, tinnitus, blurred vision, nasal congestion, red, itching eyes, change in taste, smell

GI: Nausea, dry mouth, diarrhea, constipation, flatulence, increased appetite, rectal bleeding

GU: Frequency, hesitancy, menstrual irregularity, change in libido

INTEG: Rash, edema, pruritus, alopecia, dry skin

MISC: Sweating, fatigue, weight gain, fever

MS: Pain, weakness, muscle cramps, spasms

RESP: Hyperventilation, chest congestion, shortness of breath

Contraindications: Hypersensitivity, P child <18 yr

Precautions: Pregnancy **B,** G lactation, elderly, impaired hepatic/renal function

Pharmacokinetics	
Absorption	Rapidly absorbed
Distribution	Unknown
Metabolism	Liver, extensively
Excretion	Feces
Half-life	3 hr

Pharmacodynamics
Unknown

Interactions
Individual drugs
Alcohol: ↑ CNS depression
Trazodone: ↑ ALT (SGPT)
Drug classifications
MAOI: ↑ B/P
Psychotropics: ↑ CNS depression

NURSING CONSIDERATIONS
Assessment
- Assess anxiety reaction: inability to sleep, apprehension, dread, foreboding, or uneasiness related to unidentified source of danger
- Assess for previous drug dependence or tolerance; if patient is drug dependent or tolerant, amount of medication should be restricted
- Monitor B/P (lying, standing), pulse; if systolic B/P drops 20 mm Hg, hold drug, notify prescriber; check I&O; may indicate renal dysfunction
- Monitor mental status: mood, sensorium, affect, sleeping patterns, drowsiness, dizziness, suicidal tendencies

Nursing diagnoses
✓ Anxiety (uses)
✓ Knowledge deficit (teaching)
✓ Noncompliance (teaching)

Implementation
- Give with food or milk for GI symptoms; sugarless gum, hard candy, frequent sips of water for dry mouth
- May be crushed

Patient/family education
- Teach patient that drug may be taken with food; if dose is missed take as soon as remembered; do not double doses
- Caution patient to avoid OTC preparations unless approved by the prescriber; to avoid alcohol ingestion and other psychotropic medications unless prescribed by prescriber; that 1-2 wk of therapy may be required before therapeutic effects occur
- Caution patient to avoid driving and activities requiring alertness, since drowsiness may occur; until medication response is known, tell patient that drowsiness may worsen at beginning of treatment
- Instruct patient not to discontinue medication abruptly after long-term use
- Advise patient to rise slowly or fainting may occur, especially in elderly [G]

Evaluation
Positive therapeutic outcome
- Increased well-being
- Decreased anxiety, restlessness, sleeplessness, dread

Treatment of overdose: Gastric lavage, VS, supportive care

busulfan (℞)
(byoo-sul′fan)
Myleran
Func. class.: Antineoplastic alkylating agent
Chem. class.: Nitrosourea
Pregnancy category D

Action: Changes essential cellular ions to covalent bonding with resultant alkylation; this interferes with normal biologic function of DNA; activity is not phase specific; action is due to myelosuppression

➔ **Therapeutic Outcome:** Prevention of rapid growth of malignant cells in chronic myelocytic leukemia

Uses: Chronic myelocytic leukemia

Dosage and routes

Adult: PO 4-12 mg/day initially until WBC levels fall to 10,000/mm^3; then drug is stopped until WBC levels rise over 50,000/mm^3; then 1-3 mg/day

P ***Child:*** PO 0.06-0.12 mg/kg or 1.8-4.6 mg/m^2/day; dosage is titrated to maintain WBC levels at 20,000/mm^3

Available forms: Tabs 2 mg

Adverse effects

GI: Nausea, vomiting, ***diarrhea, weight loss***

GU: Impotence, sterility, amenorrhea, gynecomastia, ***renal toxicity,*** hyperuremia, adrenal insufficiency–like syndrome

HEMA: ***Thrombocytopenia, leukopenia, pancytopenia, severe bone marrow depression***

INTEG: Dermatitis, hyperpigmentation, alopecia

RESP: ***Irreversible pulmonary fibrosis,*** pneumonitis

OTHER: ***Chromosomal aberrations***

Contraindications: Radiation, chemotherapy, lactation, pregnancy **D** (3rd trimester), blastic phase of chronic myelocytic leukemia, hypersensitivity

Precautions: Childbearing age men and women, leukopenia, thrombocytopenia, anemia, hepatotoxicity, renal toxicity

Pharmacokinetics	
Absorption	Rapidly absorbed
Distribution	Unknown; crosses placenta
Metabolism	Liver, extensively
Excretion	Kidneys, breast milk
Half-life	Unknown

Pharmacodynamics
Unknown

Interactions

Individual drugs

Radiation: ↑ toxicity, bone marrow suppression

Drug classifications

Antineoplastics: ↑ toxicity, bone marrow suppression

Lab test interferences

False positive: Breast, bladder, cervix, lung cytology tests

NURSING CONSIDERATIONS

Assessment

- Monitor CBC, differential, platelet count weekly; withhold drug if WBC is $<4000/mm^3$ or platelet count is $<75,000/mm^3$; notify prescriber of results if WBC $<20,000/mm^3$, platelets $<150,000/mm^3$
- Monitor pulmonary function tests, chest x-ray films before, during therapy; chest film should be obtained q2 wk during treatment; check for dyspnea, rales, nonproductive cough, chest pain, tachypnea
- Assess for increased uric acid levels, swelling, joint pain primarily in extremities; patient should be well hydrated to prevent urate deposits
- Monitor renal function studies: BUN, serum uric acid, urine CrCl before, during therapy; I&O ratio; report fall in urine output of 30 ml/hr; check for decreased hyperuricemia
- Monitor for cold, fever, sore throat (may indicate beginning infection); identify edema in feet, joint or stomach pain, shaking; prescriber should be notified
- Assess for bleeding: hematuria, guaiac, bruising or pete-

chiae, mucosa or orifices q8h; no rectal temps

Nursing diagnoses

✓ Injury, risk for (adverse reactions)
✓ Body image disturbance (adverse reactions)
✓ Infection, risk for (adverse reactions)
✓ Knowledge deficit (teaching)

Implementation

- Give 1 hr before or 2 hr pc to lessen nausea and vomiting or give antacid before oral agent; give drug after evening meal, before bedtime; antiemetic 30-60 min before giving drug to prevent vomiting
- Give either allopurinol or sodium bicarbonate to maintain uric acid levels, alkalinization of urine; increase fluid intake to 2-3 L/day to prevent urate deposits, calculus formation
- Administer antibiotics for prophylaxis of infection; may be prescribed since infection potential is high
- Store in tight container

Patient/family education

- Teach patient to avoid use of products containing aspirin or ibuprofen, razors, commercial mouthwash since bleeding may occur; to report symptoms of bleeding (hematuria, tarry stools)
- Instruct patient to report signs of anemia (fatigue, headache, irritability, faintness, shortness of breath)
- Instruct patient to report any changes in breathing or coughing even several months after treatment; to avoid crowds and persons with respiratory tract or other infections
- Teach patient that hair loss may occur; discuss the use of wigs or hair pieces
- Caution patient not to have any vaccinations without the advice of the prescriber; serious reactions can occur
- Advise patient that contraception is needed during treatment and for several months after the completion of therapy

Evaluation

Positive therapeutic outcome

- Decreased leukocytes to normal limits
- Absence of sweating at night
- Increased appetite, increased weight

butoconazole (Rx)

(byoo-toe-koe'na-zole)

Femstat

Func. class.: Local anti-infective

Chem. class.: Antifungal

Pregnancy category C

Action: Binds sterols in fungal cell membrane, which increases membrane permeability, decreases osmotic resistance

➔ **Therapeutic Outcome:** Fungistatic/fungicidal against susceptible organisms: *Candida* only

Uses: Vulvovaginal infections caused by *Candida* organisms

Dosage and routes

Adult: Intravaginal 1 applicatorful hs × 3 days (nonpregnant), × 6 days (2nd/3rd trimester pregnancy)

Available forms: Vaginal cream 2%

Adverse effects

GU: Rash, stinging, *burning,* vulvovaginal itching, soreness, swelling, discharge, finger itching

Contraindications: Hypersensitivity

Precautions: Pregnancy **C**, lactation

Pharmacokinetics

Absorption	Minimal
Distribution	Unknown
Metabolism	Liver
Excretion	Feces, kidneys
Half-life	Unknown

Pharmacodynamics

Unknown

Interactions: None

NURSING CONSIDERATIONS

Assessment

- Check for allergic reaction: burning, stinging, itching, discharge, soreness

Nursing diagnoses

✓ Skin integrity, impaired (uses)
✓ Infection, risk for (uses)
✓ Knowledge deficit (teaching)

Implementation

Top route

- Administer 1 applicatorful qPM high into the vagina
- Store at room temp in dry place

Patient/family education

- Instruct patient in asepsis (hand washing) before, after each application
- Teach patient to apply with applicator only; to avoid use of any other vaginal product unless directed by prescriber; sanitary napkin may prevent soiling of undergarments
- Instruct patient to abstain from sexual intercourse until treatment is completed; reinfection and irritation may occur
- Instruct patient if symptoms persist to notify prescriber

Evaluation

Positive therapeutic outcome

- Decrease in itching or white discharge (vaginal)

butorphanol (℞)

(byoo-tor'fa-nole)

Stadol, Stadol NS

Func. class.: Narcotic analgesic

Chem. class.: Opiate

Pregnancy category C

Action: Inhibits ascending pain pathways in limbic system, thalamus, midbrain, hypothalamus by binding to opiate receptor sites; this alters pain perception and response

➔ **Therapeutic Outcome:** Relief of pain

Uses: Moderate to severe pain, analgesia during labor, sedation preoperatively

Investigational uses: Migraine headache, pain

Dosage and routes

Adult: IM 1-4 mg q3-4h prn; **IV** 0.5-2 mg q3-4h prn; nasal spray in 1 nostril; may give another in 1-1½ hr; may repeat q3-4h

Available forms: Inj 1, 2 mg/ml; intranasal 10 mg/ml

Adverse effects

CNS: Drowsiness, dizziness, confusion, headache, sedation, euphoria, weakness, hallucinations

CV: Palpitations, bradycardia, change in B/P

EENT: Tinnitus, blurred vision, miosis, diplopia

GI: Nausea, vomiting, anorexia, constipation, cramps
GU: Increased urinary output, dysuria, urinary retention
INTEG: Rash, urticaria, bruising, flushing, diaphoresis, pruritus
RESP: Respiratory depression, pulmonary hypertension

Contraindications: Hypersensitivity, addiction (narcotic), CHF, MI

Precautions: Addictive personality, pregnancy **C,** lactation, increased intracranial pressure, respiratory depression, hepatic disease, renal disease, child <18 yr

Pharmacokinetics

Absorption	Well absorbed (IM, Nasal); complete (IV)
Distribution	Crosses placenta
Metabolism	Liver, extensively
Excretion	Feces (10%-15%); kidneys, unchanged (small amounts)
Half-life	3-4 hr

Pharmacodynamics

	IM	IV	NASAL
Onset	10-30 min	1 min	15 min
Peak	½ hr	5 min	1-2 hr
Duration	3-4 hr	2-4 hr	4-5 hr

Interactions
Individual drugs
Alcohol: ↑ respiratory depression, hypotension, sedation
Drug classifications
Antihistamines: ↑ respiratory depression, hypotension
CNS depressants: ↑ respiratory depression, hypotension
MAOI: Do not use 2 wk before alfentanil
Sedative/hypnotics: ↑ respiratory depression, hypotension
Lab test interferences
↑ Amylase, ↑ lipase

NURSING CONSIDERATIONS
Assessment
- Monitor VS after parenteral route; note muscle rigidity, drug history, liver, kidney function tests, respiratory dysfunction: respiratory depression, character, rate, rhythm; notify prescriber if respirations are <10/min
- Monitor CNS changes: dizziness, drowsiness, hallucinations, euphoria, LOC, pupil reaction
- Monitor allergic reactions: rash, urticaria

Nursing diagnoses
✓ Pain (uses)
✓ Sensory-perceptual alteration: visual, auditory (adverse reactions)
✓ Injury, risk for (adverse reactions)
✓ Knowledge deficit (teaching)

Implementation
- Store in light resistant container at room temp

IM route
- Give deeply in large muscle mass; rotate injection sites

Intranasal
- Give 1 spray in nostril

IV route
- Give **IV** undiluted at a rate of ≤2 mg/>3-5 min; titrate to patient response

Syringe compatibilities: Atropine, chlorpromazine, cimetidine, diphenhydramine, droperidol, fentanyl, hydroxyzine, meperidine, methotrimeprazine, metoclopramide, midazolam, morphine, pentazocine, perphenazine, prochlorperazine, promethazine, scopolamine, thiethylperazine

Syringe incompatibilities: Dimenhydrinate, pentobarbital

Y-site compatibilities: Allopurinol, amifostine, azetreonam, cefepime, enalaprilat, esmolol, filgrastim, fludarabine, labetalol, melphalan, paclitaxel, sargramostim, teniposide, thiotepa, vinorelbine

Patient/family education

- Instruct patient to report any symptoms of CNS changes, allergic reactions; to avoid CNS depressants: alcohol, sedative/hypnotics for at least 24 hr after taking this drug
- Discuss with patient that dizziness, drowsiness, and confusion are common; to avoid getting up without assistance
- Discuss in detail all aspects of the drug

Nasal route

- Teach patient to blow nose to clear both nostrils before using; remove clip and cover, prime before using until spray appears; pump must be reprimed q48h; close nostril with finger and spray once quickly; have patient sniff
- Patient should replace clip and cover after use; caution patient not to shake medication

Evaluation

Positive therapeutic outcome

- Pain relief

Treatment of overdose: Narcan 0.2-0.8 **IV**, O_2, **IV** fluids, vasopressors

calcitonin (human) (℞)

(kal-si-toe'nin)

Cibacalcin, Miacalcin

Func. class.: Parathyroid agents (calcium regulator)

Chem. class.: Polypeptide hormone

Pregnancy category C

Action: Decreases bone resorption, blood calcium levels by direct action on bone, GI system, and kidney; increases deposits of calcium in bones; renal excretion of calcium occurs

➔ Therapeutic Outcome: Lowered calcium level, decreasing symptoms of Paget's disease

Uses: Paget's disease

Dosage and routes

Adult: SC 0.5 mg/day initially; may require 0.5 mg bid × 6 mo, then decrease until symptoms reappear

Available forms: Inj (SC) 0.5 mg/vial

Adverse effects

CNS: Headache, ***tetany,*** chills, weakness, dizziness

CV: Chest pressure

GI: Nausea, diarrhea, vomiting, anorexia, abdominal pain, salty taste, epigastric pain

GU: Diuresis

INTEG: Rash, flushing, pruritus of earlobes, edema of feet

MS: Swelling, tingling of hands

RESP: Dyspnea

Contraindications: Hypersensitivity

Precautions: Renal disease, **P** children, lactation, osteogenic sarcoma, pregnancy **C**

Pharmacokinetics	
Absorption	Completely absorbed
Distribution	Unknown
Metabolism	Rapid; kidneys, tissue, blood
Excretion	Kidneys, inactive metabolite
Half-life	1 hr

Pharmacodynamics	SC
Onset	15 min
Peak	4 hr
Duration	8-24 hr

Interactions: None

NURSING CONSIDERATIONS
Assessment
- Assess for GI symptoms, polyuria, flushing, head swelling, tingling, headache; may indicate hypercalcemia; nervousness, irritability, twitching, seizures, spasm, paresthesia indicate hypocalcemia during beginning of treatment
- Identify nutritional status; check diet for sources of vitamin D (milk, some seafood), calcium (dairy products, dark green vegetables), phosphates
- Monitor BUN, creatinine, uric acid, chloride, electrolytes, urine pH, urinary calcium, magnesium, phosphate, urinalysis (calcium should be kept at 9-10 mg/dl; vitamin D 50-135 IU/dl), alkaline phosphatase baseline and q3-6 mo; check urine sediment for casts throughout treatment
- Assess for increased drug level, since toxic reactions occur rapidly; have calcium chloride or gluconate on hand if calcium level drops too low; check for tetany

Nursing diagnoses
- ✓ Injury, risk for (adverse reactions)
- ✓ Pain, chronic (uses)
- ✓ Knowledge deficit (teaching)

Implementation
- Store at <77° F (25° C); protect from light

SC route
- Give by SC route only; rotate inj sites; use within 6 hr of reconstitution; give hs to minimize nausea, vomiting

Patient/family education
- Teach method of inj if patient will be responsible for self-medication
- Instruct patient to notify prescriber for hypercalcemic relapse: renal calculi, nausea, vomiting, thirst, lethargy, deep bone or flank pain
- Teach patient that warmth and flushing occur and last 1 hr
- Provide a low-calcium diet as prescribed (Paget's disease, hypercalcemia)
- Advise patients with osteoporosis to increase calcium and vitamin D in diet and to continue with moderate exercise to prevent continued bone loss

Evaluation
Positive therapeutic outcome
- Calcium levels 9-10 mg/dl
- Decreasing symptoms of Paget's disease, including pain
- Decreased bone loss in osteoporosis

calcitonin (salmon) (℞)

(kal-si-toe'nin)

Calcimar, Miacalcin

Func. class.: Parathyroid agents (calcium regulator)

Chem. class.: Polypeptide hormone

Pregnancy category C

Action: Decreases bone resorption, blood calcium levels by direct action on bone, GI system, and kidney; increases deposits of calcium in bones; renal excretion of calcium occurs

➡ **Therapeutic Outcome:** Lowered calcium level, decreasing symptoms of Paget's disease

Uses: Paget's disease, hypercalcemia, postmenopausal osteoporosis

Dosage and routes

Postmenopausal osteoporosis

Adult: SC/IM 100 IU/day; nasal 200 IU qd alternating nostrils qd, activate pump before 1st dose

Paget's disease

Adult: SC/IM 100 IU qd; maintenance for Paget's disease 50-100 IU qd or qod

Hypercalcemia

Adult: SC/IM 4 IU/kg q12h, increase to 8 IU/kg q12h if response is unsatisfactory

Available forms: Inj 200 IU/ml; nasal spray 200 IU/activation (0.09 ml/dose)

Adverse effects

CNS: Headache, flushing, *tetany,* chills, weakness, dizziness

GI: Nausea, diarrhea, vomiting, anorexia, abdominal pain, salty taste

GU: Diuresis

INTEG: Rash, pruritus of earlobes, edema of feet

MS: Swelling, tingling of hands

Contraindications: Hypersensitivity, P children, lactation

Precautions: Renal disease, osteoporosis, pernicious anemia, Zollinger-Ellison syndrome, pregnancy **C**

Pharmacokinetics

Absorption	Completely absorbed (IM, SC)
Distribution	Unknown
Metabolism	Rapid; kidneys, tissue, blood
Excretion	Kidneys, inactive metabolite
Half-life	Human 1 hr

Pharmacodynamics

	IM/SC
Onset	15 min
Peak	4 hr
Duration	8-24 hr

Interactions: None

NURSING CONSIDERATIONS

Assessment

- Assess for GI symptoms, polyuria, flushing, head swelling, tingling, headache; may indicate hypercalcemia; nervousness, irritability, twitching, seizures, spasm, paresthesia indicate hypocalcemia during beginning of treatment
- Identify nutritional status; check diet for sources of vitamin D (milk, some seafood), calcium (dairy products, dark green vegetables), phosphates
- Monitor BUN, creatinine, uric acid, chloride, electrolytes, urine pH, urinary calcium, magnesium, phosphate, urinalysis (calcium should be kept

at 9-10 mg/dl; vitamin D 50-135 IU/dl), alkaline phosphatase baseline and q3-6 mo; check urine sediment for casts throughout treatment
• Assess for increased drug level, since toxic reactions occur rapidly; have calcium chloride or gluconate on hand if calcium level drops too low; check for tetany

Nursing diagnoses

✓ Injury, risk for (adverse reactions)
✓ Pain, chronic (uses)
✓ Knowledge deficit (teaching)

Implementation

• Store at <77° F (25° C); protect from light

SC route

• Give by SC route; rotate injection sites; use within 6 hr of reconstitution; give hs to minimize nausea, vomiting

IM route

• Rotate inj site; do not give >2 ml in one site

Patient/family education

• Teach method of injection if patient will be responsible for self-medication
• Instruct patient to notify prescriber for hypercalcemic relapse: renal calculi, nausea, vomiting, thirst, lethargy, deep bone or flank pain
• Teach patient that warmth and flushing occur and last 1 hr
• Provide a low calcium diet as prescribed (Paget's disease, hypercalcemia)
• Advise patients with osteoporosis to increase calcium and vitamin D in diet and to continue with moderate exercise to prevent continued bone loss

Evaluation

Positive therapeutic outcome

• Calcium levels 9-10 mg/dl
• Decreasing symptoms of Paget's disease including pain
• Decreased bone loss in osteoporosis

calcitriol (1,25-dihydroxycholecalciferol) (℞)

(kal-si-tree'ole)

Calcijex, Rocaltrol

Func. class.: Parathyroid agent (calcium regulator)

Chem. class.: Vitamin D hormone

Pregnancy category C

Action: Increases intestinal absorption of calcium, provides calcium for bones, increases renal tubular resorption of phosphate

Therapeutic Outcome: Calcium at normal level

Uses: Hypocalcemia in chronic renal disease, hypoparathyroidism, pseudohypoparathyroidism

Dosage and routes

Hypocalcemia

Adult: PO 0.25 μg qd, may increase by 0.25 μg/day q4-8 wk; maintenance 0.25 μg qod-1 μg qd

Hypoparathyroidism/pseudohypoparathyroidism

P ***Adult and child >1 yr:*** PO 0.25 μg qd; may be increased q2-4 wk; maintenance 0.25-2 μg qd

Available forms: Caps 0.25, 0.5 μg

Adverse effects

CNS: Drowsiness, headache, vertigo, fever, lethargy
GI: Nausea, diarrhea, vomiting, jaundice, anorexia, dry mouth, constipation, cramps, metallic taste
GU: Polyuria, hypercalciuria, hyperphosphatemia, hematuria
MS: Myalgia, arthralgia, decreased bone development

Contraindications: Hypersensitivity, hyperphosphatemia, hypercalcemia, vitamin D toxicity

Precautions: Pregnancy **C**, renal calculi, lactation, CV disease

Pharmacokinetics	
Absorption	Well absorbed
Distribution	To liver, crosses placenta
Metabolism	Liver
Excretion	Bile
Half-life	3-6 hr

Pharmacodynamics	
Onset	2-6 hr
Peak	4 hr
Duration	Up to 5 days

Interactions: None

NURSING CONSIDERATIONS

Assessment

- Assess GI symptoms, polyuria, flushing, head swelling, tingling, headache; may indicate hypercalcemia
- Identify nutritional status; check diet for sources of vitamin D (milk, some seafood), calcium (dairy products, dark green vegetables), phosphates
- Monitor BUN, creatinine, uric acid, chloride, electrolytes, urine pH, urinary calcium, magnesium, phosphate, urinalysis (calcium should be kept at 9-10 mg/dl; vitamin D 50-135 IU/dl), alkaline phosphatase baseline and q3-6 mo
- Assess for increased drug level, since toxic reactions occur rapidly; have calcium chloride on hand if calcium level drops too low; check for tetany

Nursing diagnoses

- ✓ Injury, risk for (adverse reactions)
- ✓ Pain, chronic (uses)
- ✓ Knowledge deficit (teaching)

Implementation

- Give with meals for GI symptoms
- Do not crush or chew caps

Patient/family education

- Teach patient the symptoms of hypercalcemia and about foods rich in calcium
- Advise patient to avoid products with sodium: cured meats, dairy products, cold cuts, olives, beets, pickles, soups, meat tenderizers in chronic renal failure
- Advise patient to avoid products with potassium: oranges, bananas, dried fruit, peas, dark green leafy vegetables, milk, melons, beans in chronic renal failure
- Advise patient to avoid OTC products containing calcium, potassium, or sodium in chronic renal failure
- Instruct patient to avoid all preparations containing Vit D
- Instruct patient to monitor weight weekly

Evaluation

Positive therapeutic outcome

- Calcium levels 9-10 mg/dl

calcium chloride/ calcium gluceptate/ calcium gluconate/ calcium lactate (PO, OTC; IV, ℞)

Func. class.: Electrolyte replacement—calcium product

Pregnancy category C

Action: Cation needed for maintenance of nervous, muscular, skeletal systems, enzyme reactions, normal cardiac contractility, coagulation of blood; affects secretory activity of endocrine, exocrine glands

➔ **Therapeutic Outcome:** Calcium at normal level, absence of increased magnesium, potassium

Uses: Prevention and treatment of hypocalcemia, hypermagnesemia, hypoparathyroidism, neonatal tetany, cardiac toxicity caused by hyperkalemia, lead colic, hyperphosphatemia, vitamin D deficiency

Dosage and routes

Calcium chloride

Adult: **IV** 500 mg-1 g q1-3 days as indicated by serum calcium levels; give at <1 ml/min; IAV 200-800 mg injected in ventricle of heart

P ***Child:*** **IV** 25 mg/kg over several min

Calcium gluceptate

Adult: **IV** 5-20 ml; IM 2-5 ml

P ***Newborn:*** 0.5 ml/100 ml of blood transfused

Calcium gluconate

Adult: PO 0.5-2 g bid-qid; **IV** 0.5-2 g at 0.5 ml/min (10% sol)

P ***Child:*** PO/**IV** 500 mg/kg/day in divided doses

Calcium lactate

Adult: PO 325 mg-1.3 g tid with meals

P ***Child:*** PO 500 mg/kg/day in divided doses

Available forms: Many; check product listings

Adverse effects

CV: Shortened QT, heart block, hypotension, bradycardia, dysrythmias, ***cardiac arrest***

GI: Vomiting, nausea, constipation

HYPERCALCEMIA: Drowsiness, lethargy, muscle weakness, headache, constipation, ***coma***, anorexia, nausea, vomiting, polyuria, thirst

INTEG: Pain, burning at **IV** site, severe venous thrombosis, necrosis, extravasation

Contraindications: Hypercalcemia, digitalis toxicity, ventricular fibrillation, renal calculi

Precautions: Pregnancy **C**, P lactation, children, renal disease, respiratory disease, cor pulmonale, digitalized patient, respiratory failure

Pharmacokinetics

Absorption	Complete bioavailability (IV)
Distribution	Readily extracellular; crosses placenta
Metabolism	Liver
Excretion	Feces (80%), kidney (20%), breast milk
Half-life	Unknown

Pharmacodynamics

	PO	IV
Onset	Unknown	Immediate
Peak	Unknown	Rapid
Duration	Unknown	½-1½ hr

Interactions

Individual drugs

Atenolol: ↓ effects of atenolol
Tetracycline: ↓ absorption of tetracycline (PO)
Verapamil: ↓ effects of verapamil

Drug classifications

Antacids: Milk-alkali syndrome (renal disease)
Cardiac glycosides: ↑ toxicity
Diuretics, thiazide: ↑ hypercalcemia
Fluoroquinolones: ↓ absorption of fluoroquinolones
Iron salts: ↓ absorption of iron

Food

Calcium (dairy products): ↑ hypercalcemia

Lab test interferences

False ↓ Magnesium
↓ 17-OHCS

NURSING CONSIDERATIONS

Assessment

- Monitor ECG for decreased QT and T wave inversion: in hypercalcemia, drug should be reduced or discontinued
- Monitor calcium levels during treatment (9-10 mg/dl is normal level)
- Assess cardiac status: rate, rhythm, CVP, (PWP, PAWP if being monitored directly)

Nursing diagnoses

☑ Injury, risk for (uses, adverse reactions)
☑ Knowledge deficit (teaching)

Implementation

IV **IV route**

- Administer **IV** undiluted or diluted with equal amounts of 0.9% NaCl for inj to a 5% sol; give 0.5-1 ml/min
- Give through small-bore needle into large vein; if extravasation occurs, necrosis will result (**IV**); IM injection may cause severe burning, necrosis, and tissue sloughing; warm sol to body temp before administering
- Provide seizure precautions: padded side rails, decreased stimuli (noise, light); place airway suction equipment, padded mouth gag if calcium levels are low

Syringe compatibilities: Calcium chloride

Milrinone

Y-site compatibilities:

Amrinone, dobutamine, epinephrine, esmolol, morphine, paclitaxel

Additive compatibilities:

Amikacin, ascorbic acid, bretylium, chloramphenicol, dopamine, hydrocortisone, isoproterenol, lidocaine, methicillin, norepinephrine, penicillin G sodium, pentobarbital, phenobarbital, sodium bicarbonate, verapamil, Vit B/C

PO route

- Give PO with or following meals to enhance absorption
- Store at room temp

Patient/family education

- Advise patient to remain recumbent 30 min after **IV** dose
- Caution patient to add food high in vitamin D content; to add calcium-rich foods to diet: dairy products, shellfish, dark green leafy vegetables; decrease oxalate-rich and zinc-rich foods: nuts, legumes, chocolate, spinach, soy
- Advise patient to prevent injuries, avoid immobilization

Evaluation

Positive therapeutic outcome

- Decreased twitching, paresthesias, muscle spasms

• Absence of tremors, convulsions, dysrhythmias, dyspnea, laryngospasm, negative Chvostek's sign, negative Trousseau's sign

calcium polycarbophil (OTC)

(pol-i-kar'boe-fil)

Fiber Norm, Mitrolan

Func. class.: Laxative, bulk-forming

Pregnancy category C

Action: Attracts water, expands in intestine to increase peristalsis; also absorbs excess water in stool; decreases diarrhea

Therapeutic Outcome: Absence of constipation or diarrhea in irritable bowel syndrome

Uses: Constipation, irritable bowel syndrome (diarrhea), acute, nonspecific diarrhea

Dosage and routes

Adult: PO 1 g qd-qid prn, not to exceed 6 g/24 hr

P ***Child 6-12 yr:*** PO 500 mg bid prn, not to exceed 3 g/ 24 hr

P ***Child 3-6 yr:*** PO 500 mg bid prn, not to exceed 1.5 g/24 hr

Available forms: Chewable tabs 500, 625, 1250 mg

Adverse effects

GI: ***Obstruction,*** *abdominal distention, flatus*

Contraindications: Hypersensitivity, GI obstruction

Precautions: Pregnancy **C**

Pharmacokinetics

Absorption	None
Distribution	None
Metabolism	Unknown
Excretion	Feces
Half-life	Not known

Pharmacodynamics

Onset	12-24 hr
Peak	1-3 days
Duration	Unknown

Interactions

Individual drugs

Tetracycline: ↓ absorption of tetracycline

NURSING CONSIDERATIONS

Assessment

• Monitor blood, urine electrolytes if used often by patient; check I&O ratio to identify fluid loss

• Assess cramping, rectal bleeding, nausea, vomiting; if these symptoms occur, drug should be discontinued; identify cause of constipation; identify whether fluids, bulk, or exercise is missing from lifestyle

Nursing diagnoses

✓ Constipation (uses)

✓ Diarrhea (side effects)

✓ Knowledge deficit (teaching)

✓ Noncompliance (teaching)

Implementation

• Give alone for better absorption; give after mixing with water immediately before use; administer with 8 oz water or juice followed by another 8 oz of fluid

• Administer in AM or PM

Patient/family education

• Discuss with the patient that adequate fluid consumption is necessary

• Teach patient that normal

bowel movements do not always occur daily

• Teach patient not to use in presence of abdominal pain, nausea, vomiting; tell patient to notify prescriber if constipation unrelieved or if symptoms of electrolyte imbalance occur: muscle cramps, pain, weakness, dizziness, excessive thirst

Evaluation

Positive therapeutic outcome

• Decreased constipation within 3 days

• Decreased diarrhea in colitis within 1 wk

captopril 🔑 (℞)

(kap'toe-pril)

Capoten

Func. class.: Antihypertensive

Chem. class.: Angiotensin-converting enzyme inhibitor

Pregnancy category C

Action: Selectively suppresses renin-angiotensin-aldosterone system; inhibits ACE; prevents conversion of angiotensin I to angiotensin II; results in dilatation of arterial, venous vessels

➔ **Therapeutic Outcome:** Decreased B/P in hypertension; decreased preload, afterload in CHF

Uses: Hypertension, heart failure unresponsive to conventional therapy, left ventricular dysfunction after MI, diabetic nephropathy

Dosage and routes

Malignant hypertension

Adult: PO 25 mg increasing q2h until desired response; not to exceed 450 mg/day

Hypertension

Initial dose: PO 12.5 mg bid-tid; may increase to 50 mg bid-tid at 1-2 wk intervals; usual range 25-150 mg bid-tid; max 450 mg

CHF

Adult: PO 12.5 mg bid-tid given with a diuretic; may increase to 50 mg bid-tid; after 14 days may increase to 150 mg tid if needed

LVD after MI

Adult: PO 50 mg tid, may begin treatment 3 days after MI; give 6.25 mg as a single dose, then 12.5 mg tid, increase to 25 mg tid for several days, then 50 mg tid

Diabetic nephropathy

Adult: PO 25 mg tid

Available forms: Tabs 12.5, 25, 100 mg

Adverse effects

CNS: Fever, chills

CV: Hypotension, postural hypotension

GI: Loss of taste

GU: Impotence, dysuria, nocturia, ***proteinuria, nephrotic syndrome, acute reversible renal failure,*** polyuria, oliguria, frequency

HEMA: Neutropenia

INTEG: Rash, ***angioedema***

META: Hyperkalemia

RESP: Bronchospasm, dyspnea, cough

Contraindications: Hypersensitivity, pregnancy **C,** lactation, P heart block, children, potassium-sparing diuretics, bilateral renal artery stenosis

Precautions: Dialysis patients, hypovolemia, leukemia, scleroderma, LE, blood dyscrasias, CHF, diabetes mellitus, renal disease, thyroid disease, COPD, asthma

Pharmacokinetics

Absorption	Well absorbed
Distribution	Widely distributed; crosses placenta
Metabolism	Liver (50%)
Excretion	Kidneys, unchanged (50%)
Half-life	1½-2 hr

Pharmacodynamics

Onset	¼-1 hr
Peak	1 hr
Duration	6-12 hr

Interactions

Individual drugs

Alcohol: ↑ hypotension (large amounts)
Allopurinol: ↑ hypersensitivity
Digoxin: ↑ serum levels
Indomethacin: ↓ antihypertensive effect
Lithium: ↑ serum levels
Tetracycline: ↓ absorption of tetracycline

Drug classifications

Antacids: ↓ absorption
Antihypertensives: ↑ hypotension
Diuretics: ↑ hypotension
Diuretics, potassium-sparing: ↑ toxicity
Potassium supplements: ↑ toxicity

Lab test interferences

False positive: Urine acetone

NURSING CONSIDERATIONS

Assessment

- May be crushed and mixed with food
- Monitor blood studies: neutrophils, decreased platelets
- Monitor B/P, check for orthostatic hypotension, syncope; if changes occur, dosage change may be required
- Monitor renal studies: protein, BUN, creatinine; watch for increased levels that may indicate nephrotic syndrome and renal failure; monitor renal symptoms: polyuria, oliguria, frequency, dysuria
- Establish baselines in renal, liver function tests before therapy begins
- Check potassium levels throughout treatment, although hyperkalemia rarely occurs
- Check for edema in feet, legs daily; monitor weight daily
- Assess for allergic reactions: rash, fever, pruritus, urticaria; drug should be discontinued if antihistamines fail to help

Nursing diagnoses

- ✓ Cardiac output, decreased (uses)
- ✓ Injury, risk for (side effects)
- ✓ Knowledge deficit (teaching)
- ✓ Noncompliance (teaching)

Implementation

- Store in air-tight container at 86° F (30° C) or less
- Severe hypotension may occur after 1st dose of this medication; decreasing hypotension may be prevented by reducing or discontinuing diuretic therapy 3 days before beginning benzapril therapy
- Give **IV** inf of 0.9% NaCl (as ordered) to expand fluid volume if severe hypotension occurs

Patient/family education

- Caution patient not to discontinue drug abruptly; advise patient to tell all persons associated with care
- Teach patient not to use OTC products (cough, cold, allergy) unless directed by prescriber; serious side effects can occur; xanthines such as coffee, tea, chocolate, cola can prevent action of drug

• Teach patient importance of complying with dosage schedule, even if feeling better; to continue with medical regimen to decrease B/P: exercise, cessation of smoking, decreasing stress, diet modifications
• Emphasize the need to rise slowly to sitting or standing position to minimize orthostatic hypotension; not to exercise in hot weather or increased hypotension can occur
• Teach patient to notify prescriber of mouth sores, sore throat, fever, swelling of hands or feet, irregular heartbeat, chest pain, coughing, shortness of breath
• Caution patient to report excessive perspiration, dehydration, vomiting, diarrhea; may lead to fall in B/P
• Caution patient that drug may cause dizziness, fainting, lightheadedness; may occur during 1st few days of therapy; to avoid activities that may be hazardous
• Teach patient how to take B/P, and teach normal readings for age group; ensure patient takes regularly

Evaluation

Positive therapeutic outcome
• Decreased B/P in hypertension

Treatment of overdose: 0.9% NaCl **IV** infusion, hemodialysis

carbachol (℞)

(kar'ba-kole)
Carboptic, Isopto carbachol, Miostat
Func. class.: Miotic, cholinergic
Pregnancy category C

Action: Contracts sphincter muscle of iris; causes spasms of ciliary muscle, deepening of anterior chamber

➔ Therapeutic Outcome: Reduction of intraocular pressure

Uses: Miosis in ocular surgery, glaucoma (open angle, narrow angle)

Dosage and routes

Ocular surgery

Adult: INSTILL 0.5 ml (intraocular) of 0.01% sol in anterior chamber of eye (done by physician) for miosis during surgery

Glaucoma

Adult: INSTILL 1-2 gtt (top) of 0.75%-3% sol into eye bid-tid

Available forms: 0.75%, 1.5%, 2.25%, 3.0% sol for top use; 0.01% oph sol

Adverse effects

*CV: **Marked hypotension,*** bradycardia, headache
EENT: Blurred vision, varying degrees of myopia, decreased visual acuity in dim light, slight conjunctival hyperemia, altered distance vision, decreased night vision, eyeache
GI: Nausea, vomiting, abdominal discomfort, diarrhea, salivation
RESP: Asthma attacks

Contraindications: Hypersensitivity; when miosis is undesirable; corneal abrasions

Precautions: Bradycardia, CAD, hyperthyroidism, asthma, pregnancy **C,** obstruction of GI or urinary tract, peptic ulcer, parkinsonism, epilepsy, peritonitis

Pharmacokinetics

Absorption	Minimal
Distribution	Minimal
Metabolism	None
Excretion	Lacrimation
Half-life	Short

Pharmacodynamics

	OPHTHALMIC
Onset	10-20 min (miosis)
Peak	Unknown
Duration	4-8 hr

NURSING CONSIDERATIONS

Assessment

• Assess heart, respiratory rate, B/P; lung sounds, changes in respiratory rate; if these occur, notify prescriber

Nursing diagnoses

✓ Pain (uses)
✓ Sensory-perceptual alteration: visual (uses)
✓ Knowledge deficit (teaching)

Implementation

Ophthalmic route

• Use reconstituted sol immediately; discard unused portion

Patient/family education

• Teach patient to report change in vision, blurring, or loss of sight, trouble breathing, sweating, flushing
• Teach patient method of instillation, including pressure on lacrimal sac for 1 min, and not to touch dropper to eye; use demonstration, return demonstration
• Advise patient that blurred vision will decrease with repeated use of drug
• Caution patient not to drive during first few days of treatment; visual changes may occur including impaired night vision, eye and brow ache

Evaluation

Positive therapeutic outcome

• Decreasing intraocular pressure; miosis during ocular surgery

carbamazepine (℞)

(kar-ba-maz'e-peen)

Apo-Carbamazepine ✦, Epitol, Mazepine ✦, Tegretol, Tegretol-XR

Func. class.: Anticonvulsant

Chem. class.: Iminostilbene derivative

Pregnancy category C

Action: Inhibits nerve impulses by limiting influx of sodium ions across cell membrane in motor cortex

➔ **Therapeutic Outcome:** Absence of seizures; decreased trigeminal neuralgia pain

Uses: Tonic-clonic, complex-partial, mixed seizures; trigeminal neuralgia

Investigational uses: Diabetes insipidus, bipolar disorder, neurogenic pain

Dosage and routes

Seizures

P ***Adult and child >12 yr:*** PO 200 mg bid; may be increased by 200 mg/day in divided doses q6-8h; maintenance 800-1200 mg/day; maximum 1200 mg/day; adjustment is needed to minimum dose to control seizures; ext rel give bid

P ***Child <12 yr:*** PO 10-20 mg/kg day in 3-4 divided doses

Trigeminal neuralgia

Adult: PO 100 mg/bid; may increase 100 mg q12h until pain subsides; not to exceed 1.2 g/day; maintenance is 200-400 mg bid

Available forms: Chewable tabs 100 mg; tabs 200 mg; oral susp 100 mg/5 ml; ext rel 100, 200, 400 mg

Adverse effects

CNS: Drowsiness, dizziness, confusion, fatigue, ***paralysis,*** headache, hallucinations

CV: ***Hypertension, CHF,*** hypotension, aggravation of CAD

EENT: Tinnitus, dry mouth, blurred vision, diplopia, nystagmus, conjunctivitis

GI: Nausea, constipation, diarrhea, anorexia, vomiting, abdominal pain, stomatitis, glossitis, increased liver enzymes, ***hepatitis***

GU: Frequency, retention, albuminuria, glycosuria, impotence

HEMA: ***Thrombocytopenia, agranulocytosis, leukocytosis, neutropenia, aplastic anemia, eosinophilia,*** increased protime

INTEG: Rash, ***Stevens-Johnson syndrome,*** urticaria

RESP: Pulmonary hypersensitivity (fever, dyspnea, pneumonitis)

Contraindications: Hypersensitivity to carbamazepine or tricyclic antidepressants, bone marrow depression, concomitant use of MAOIs

Precautions: Glaucoma, hepatic disease, renal disease, cardiac disease, psychosis, P pregnancy **C**, lactation, child <6 yr

Pharmacokinetics

Absorption	Slow; completely absorbed
Distribution	Widely distributed
Metabolism	Extensively, liver
Excretion	Kidneys
Half-life	14-16 hr or more

Pharmacodynamics

Onset	2-4 day
Peak	4-8 hr
Duration	Unknown

Interactions

Individual drugs

Acetaminophen: ↑ metabolism, ↓ action

Diltiazem: ↑ toxicity

Doxycycline: ↓ half-life

Haloperidol: ↓ serum levels, ↓ therapeutic efficacy

Phenobarbital: ↑ effects

Phenytoin: ↑ and ↓ plasma levels, ↓ carbamazepine plasma levels

Lithium: ↑ CNS toxicity

Theophylline: ↓ effect of theophylline, carbamazepine

Valproic acid: ↓ plasma levels, ↑ half-life of carbamazepine

Verapamil: ↑ toxicity

Drug classifications

Barbiturates: ↓ serum levels of carbamazepine

Nondepolarizing muscle relaxants: Resistance to or reversal of effects of these agents

Posterior pituitary hormones: Potentiates antidiuretic effects

Succinimides: ↓ plasma levels

Lab test interferences

↓ Thyroid function tests

NURSING CONSIDERATIONS

Assessment

- Monitor liver function tests (AST [SGOT], ALT [SGOT]) and urine function tests, BUN, urine protein periodically during treatments
- Check blood levels during treatment; therapeutic level 6-12 μg/ml
- Assess for blood dyscrasias: fever, sore throat, bruising, rash, jaundice, epistaxis (long-term treatment only)
- Assess seizure activity including type, location, duration, and character; provide seizure precaution

Nursing diagnoses

✓ Injury, risk for (side effects)
✓ Knowledge deficit (teaching)

Implementation

- Give with food for GI symptoms
- Chew tab: tell patient to chew, not swallow whole

Patient/family education

- Teach patient to carry Medic Alert ID stating patient's name, drugs taken, condition, prescriber's name, phone number
- Caution patient to avoid driving, other activities that require alertness until stabilized on medication
- Teach patient not to discontinue medication quickly after long-term use
- Teach patient to use a nonhormonal type of contraception to prevent harm to the fetus
- Advise patient to use sunscreen to prevent burns
- Teach patient to take exactly as prescribed, do not double or omit doses

Evaluation

Positive therapeutic outcome

- Decreased seizure activity

Treatment of overdose: Lavage, vital signs

carbidopa-levodopa (℞)

(kar-bi-doe'pa lee-voe-doe'pa)

carbidopa/levodopa, Sinemet, Sinemet CR

Func. class.: Antiparkinsonism agent

Chem. class.: Catecholamine

Pregnancy category C

Action: Decarboxylation of levodopa to periphery is inhibited by carbidopa; more levodopa is made available for transport to brain and conversion to dopamine in the brain

➔ **Therapeutic Outcome:** Absence of involuntary movements

Uses: Parkinsonism

Dosage and routes

Adult: PO 3-6 tabs of 25 mg carbidopa/250 mg levodopa qd in divided doses, not to exceed 8 tabs/day; SUS REL 1 tab bid at intervals of not less than 6 hr; usual dosage 2-8 tabs/day at intervals of 4-8 hr

Available forms: Tabs 10/100, 25/100, 25 mg carbidopa/250 mg levodopa; sus rel tabs 50 mg/200 mg (carbidopa/levodopa)

Adverse effects

CNS: Involuntary choreiform movements, hand tremors, fatigue, headache, anxiety,

twitching, numbness, weakness, confusion, agitation, insomnia, nightmares, psychosis, hallucination, hypomania, severe depression, dizziness
CV: Orthostatic hypotension, tachycardia, hypertension, palpitation
EENT: Blurred vision, diplopia, dilated pupils
GI: Nausea, vomiting, anorexia, abdominal distress, dry mouth, flatulence, dysphagia, bitter taste, diarrhea, constipation
HEMA: Hemolytic anemia, leukopenia, agranulocytosis
INTEG: Rash, sweating, alopecia
MISC: Urinary retention, incontinence, weight change, dark urine

Contraindications: Hypersensitivity, narrow-angle glaucoma, undiagnosed skin lesions

Precautions: Renal disease, cardiac disease, hepatic disease, respiratory disease, MI with dysrhythmias, convulsions, peptic ulcer, pregnancy **C**

Pharmacokinetics

Absorption	Well absorbed (PO); sus rel dose slow
Distribution	Widely distributed
Metabolism	Liver, extensively
Excretion	Kidneys, metabolites
Half-life	Levodopa (1 hr); carbidopa (1-2 hr)

Pharmacodynamics

	PO	PO-SUS REL
Onset	Unknown	Unknown
Peak	1 hr	2½ hr
Duration	6-24 hr	Unknown

Interactions

Individual drugs

Metoclopramide: ↑ effects of levodopa
Papaverine: ↓ effects of levodopa
Pyridoxine: ↓ effects of levodopa

Drug classifications

Antacids: ↑ effects of levodopa
Anticholinergics: ↓ effects of levodopa
Antidepressants, tricyclics: ↑ hypotension
Benzodiazepines: ↓ effects of levodopa
Hydantoins: ↓ effects of levodopa
MAOI: Hypertensive crisis

Lab test interferences

False positive: Urine ketones
False negative: Urine glucose
False ↑ Uric acid, ↑ urine protein
↓ VMA, ↓ BUN, ↓ creatinine

NURSING CONSIDERATIONS

Assessment

- Monitor I&O ratio; retention commonly causes decreased urinary output, distention, frequency, incontinence; palpate bladder if retention occurs
- Assess for parkinsonism, shuffling gait, muscle rigidity, involuntary movements, pill rolling, muscle spasms, drooling before and during treatment
- Monitor for constipation, cramping, pain in abdomen, abdominal distention; increase fluids, bulk, exercise if this occurs
- Assess for tolerance over long-term therapy; dose may have to be increased or changed
- Assess for mental status: affect, mood, CNS depression, worsening of mental symptoms during early therapy

Nursing diagnoses
✓ Physical mobility, impaired (uses)
✓ Knowledge deficit (teaching)

Implementation
PO route
- Give drug until NPO before surgery; check with prescriber for continuing drug
- Adjust dosage depending on patient response
- Give with meals or pc to prevent GI symptoms; limit protein taken with drug
- Give only after MAOIs have been discontinued for 2 wk; if previously on levodopa, discontinue for at least 8 hr before change to levodopa-carbidopa
- Controlled-release tabs should be swallowed whole, not crushed or chewed

Patient/family education
- Teach patient to change positions slowly to prevent orthostatic hypotension
- Teach patient to report side effects: twitching, eye spasms, grimacing, protrusion of tongue, personality changes that indicate overdose
- Instruct patient to use drug exactly as prescribed; if drug is discontinued abruptly, parkinsonian crisis may occur; do not double doses; take missed dose as soon as remembered up to 2 hr before next dose
- Teach patient that urine, sweat may darken and is harmless
- Advise patient to use physical activities to maintain mobility and lessen spasms
- Instruct patient that OTC medications should not be used unless approved by prescriber
- Advise patient that drowsiness, dizziness are common; to avoid hazardous activities until response is known
- Explain that sips of water, hard candy, or gum may lessen dry mouth
- Teach patient to take with meals to prevent GI symptoms; to limit protein intake, which impairs drug's absorption

Evaluation
Positive therapeutic outcome
- Decrease in akathisia
- Improved mood
- Decreased involuntary movements

C

carboplatin (℞)
(kar'boe'pla-tin)
Paraplatin
Func. class.: Antineoplastic alkylating agent
Chem. class.: Platinum coordination compound
Pregnancy category D

Action: Produces interstrand DNA cross-links and to a lesser extent DNA-protein cross-links; activity is not cell cycle phase specific

➔ Therapeutic Outcome: Prevention of rapidly growing malignant cells

Uses: Palliative treatment of ovarian carcinoma recurrent after treatment with other antineoplastic agents, including cisplatin

Dosage and routes
(single agent)

Adult: **IV** inf 360 mg/m^2 given over 15 min on day 1 q4 wk; do not repeat single intermittent courses until neutrophil count is >2000/mm^3 and platelet count is >100,000/mm³

Available forms: Inj 50, 150, 450 mg/vial

Adverse effects

CNS: ***Convulsions, central neurotoxicity,*** peripheral neuropathy
CV: Cardiac abnormalities
EENT: Tinnitus, hearing loss, ***vestibular toxicity***
GI: Severe nausea, vomiting, diarrhea, weight loss
GU: ***Renal tubular damage,*** renal insufficiency, impotence, sterility, amenorrhea, gynecomastia
HEMA: ***Thrombocytopenia, leukopenia, pancytopenia, neutropenia,*** anemia, bleeding
INTEG: Alopecia, dermatitis, rash, erythema, pruritus, urticaria
META: Hypomagnesemia, hypocalcemia, hypokalemia, hyponatremia, hyperuremia
RESP: Mucositis

Contraindications: Hypersensitivity to this drug, platinum products, mannitol; severe bone marrow depression, significant bleeding, pregnancy **D**

Precautions: Radiation therapy with 1 mo, chemotherapy with 1 mo, lactation, liver disease

Pharmacokinetics

Absorption	Complete
Distribution	Unknown
Metabolism	Liver
Excretion	Kidneys
Half-life	Initial 1-2 hr; postdistribution 2½-6 hr; increased in renal disease

Pharmacodynamics

Onset	½ hr
Peak	Unknown
Duration	4-6 hr

Interactions

Individual drugs

Radiation: ↑ toxicity, bone marrow suppression

Drug classifications

Aminoglycosides: ↑ nephrotoxicity
Antineoplastics: ↑ toxicity, bone marrow suppression
Bone marrow–suppressing drugs: ↑ bone marrow suppression
Diuretics, loop: ↑ ototoxicity

Lab test interferences

False positive: Breast, bladder, cervix, lung, cytology tests

NURSING CONSIDERATIONS

Assessment

- Monitor CBC, differential, platelet count weekly; withhold drug if WBC count is <4000/mm³ or platelet count is <100,000/mm³; notify prescriber of results if WBC <20,000/mm³, platelets <150,000/mm³
- Monitor renal function studies: BUN, creatinine, serum uric acid, urine CrCl before and during therapy; I&O ratio; report fall in urine output to <30 ml/hr
- Monitor temp q4h (may indicate beginning of infection)
- Monitor liver function tests before and during therapy (bilirubin, AST [SGOT], ALT [SGPT], LDH) as needed or monthly; note yellowing of skin or sclera, dark urine, clay-colored stools, itchy skin, abdominal pain, fever, diarrhea
- Assess for bleeding: hema-

turia, stool guaiac, bruising or petechiae, mucosa or orifices q8h; inflammation of mucosa, breaks in skin

- Identify dyspnea, rales, unproductive cough, chest pain, tachypnea
- Identify effects of alopecia on body image; discuss feelings about body changes

Nursing diagnoses

- ✓ Injury, risk for (adverse reactions)
- ✓ Body image disturbance (adverse reactions)
- ✓ Infection, risk for (adverse reactions)
- ✓ Knowledge deficit (teaching)

Implementation

- Antiemetic 30-60 min before giving drug to prevent vomiting, and prn
- Administer antibiotics for prophylaxis of infection

IV IV route

- Give **IV** after diluting 10 mg/ml of sterile water for inj, D_5W, NS (10 mg/ml); then further dilute with the same sol 1-4 mg/ml; give over 15 min or more (intermittent inf)
- Give **IV** inf over 5-6 hr; do not use needles or **IV** administration sets containing aluminum; may cause precipitate
- Store protected from light at room temp; reconstituted sol is stable for 8 hr at room temp

Y-site compatibilities: Allopurinol, amifostine, aztreonam, cefepime, filgrastim, fludarabine, granisetron, melphalan, ondansetron, paclitaxel, sargramostim, teniposide, thiotepa, vinorelbine

Additive compatibilities: Ifosfamide, ifosfamide/etoposide

Additive incompatibilities: Fluorouracil, mesna

Solution compatibilities: D_5/0.2% NaCl, D_5/0.45% NaCl, D_5/0.9% NaCl, 0.9% NaCl, D_5W, sterile water for inj

Solution incompatibility: Sodium bicarbonate

Patient/family education

- Teach patient to avoid use of products containing aspirin or ibuprofen, razors, commercial mouthwash, since bleeding may occur; to report symptoms of bleeding (hematuria, tarry stools)
- Instruct patient to report signs of anemia (fatigue, headache, irritability, faintness, shortness of breath)
- Instruct patient to report any changes in breathing or coughing even several months after treatment; to avoid crowds and persons with respiratory tract or other infections
- Advise patient that hair may be lost during treatment; a wig or hairpiece may make patient feel better; new hair may be different in color, texture
- Caution patient not to have any vaccinations without the advice of the prescriber; serious reactions can occur
- Teach patient that contraception is needed during treatment and for several months after the completion of therapy

Evaluation

Positive therapeutic outcome

- Prevention of rapid division of malignant cells

C

carboprost (℞)

(kar'boe-prost)

Hemabate, Prostin/15M ❋

Func. class.: Oxytocic

Chem. class.: Prostaglandin

Pregnancy category C

Action: Stimulates uterine contractions, causing complete abortion in approximately 16 hr

➔ **Therapeutic Outcome:** Loss of fetus; decreased postpartum bleeding

Uses: Abortion between 13-20 wk gestation; postpartum hemorrhage

Dosage and routes

Adult: IM 250 μg, then 250 μg q1½-3½ hr, may increase to 500 μg if no response, not to exceed 12 mg total dose

Available forms: Inj 250 μg/ml

Adverse effects

CNS: Fever, chills, headache

GI: Nausea, vomiting, diarrhea

Contraindications: Hypersensitivity, severe hepatic disease, severe renal disease, PID, respiratory disease, cardiac disease

Precautions: Asthma, anemia, jaundice, diabetes mellitus, convulsive disorders, past uterine surgery, pregnancy **C**

Pharmacokinetics	
Absorption	Well absorbed (nasal)
Distribution	Widely distributed (extracellular fluid)
Metabolism	Liver—rapidly
Excretion	Kidneys
Half-life	3-9 min

Pharmacodynamics	
Onset	Unknown
Peak	16 hr
Duration	Unknown

Interactions

Drug classifications

Oxytocics: ↑ effects

NURSING CONSIDERATIONS

Assessment

- Monitor B/P, pulse; watch for change that may indicate hemorrhage
- Monitor respiratory rate, rhythm, depth; notify physician of abnormalities
- For length, duration of contraction; notify physician of contractions lasting over 1 min or absence of contractions
- Assess for incomplete abortion, pregnancy must be terminated by another method; drug is teratogenic

Nursing diagnoses

✓ Knowledge deficit (teaching)

Implementation

- Give IM in deep muscle mass; rotate injection sites if additional doses are given
- Have crash cart available on unit

Patient/family education

- Advise patient to report increased blood loss, abdominal cramps, increased temperature or foul-smelling lochia
- Teach methods of comfort control and pain control

Evaluation

Positive therapeutic outcome

- Loss of fetus

carisoprodol (℞)

(kar-i-soe-proe'dole)

carisoprodol, Rela, Sodol, Soma, Soprodol, Soridol

Func. class.: Skeletal muscle relaxant, central acting

Chem. class.: Meprobamate congener

Pregnancy category C

Action: Depresses CNS by blocking interneuronal activity in descending reticular formation of spinal cord, producing sedation

Therapeutic Outcome: Relaxation of skeletal muscles

Uses: Relieving pain, stiffness in musculoskeletal disorders

Dosage and routes

P ***Adult and child >12 yr:*** PO 350 mg tid-qid

Available forms: Tabs 350 mg

Adverse effects

CNS: Dizziness, weakness, drowsiness, headache, tremor, depression, insomnia, ataxia, irritability

CV: Postural hypotension, tachycardia

EENT: Diplopia, temporary loss of vision

GI: Nausea, vomiting, hiccups, epigastric discomfort

INTEG: Rash, pruritus, fever, facial flushing

Contraindications: Hypersensitivity, child <12 yr, intermittent porphyria

Precautions: Renal disease, hepatic disease, addictive personality, pregnancy **C,** elderly

Pharmacokinetics

Absorption	Well absorbed
Distribution	Crosses placenta
Metabolism	Liver, partially
Excretion	Kidney, unchanged; breast milk
Half-life	8 hr

Pharmacodynamics

Onset	½ hr
Peak	Unknown
Duration	4-6 hr

Interactions

Individual drugs

Alcohol: ↑ CNS depression

Drug classifications

Antidepressants, tricyclic: ↑ CNS depression

Barbiturates: ↑ CNS depression

Narcotics: ↑ CNS depression

Sedative/hypnotics: ↑ CNS depression

Lab test interferences

↑ AST (SGOT), ↑ alkaline phosphatase, ↑ blood glucose

NURSING CONSIDERATIONS

Assessment

- Monitor ROM, atrophy, stiffness, and pain in muscles; assess throughout treatment
- Assess for idiosyncratic reaction with a few min or hr of administration (disorientation, restlessness, weakness, blurred vision); patient should be reassured that reaction is temporary
- Check for allergic reactions: rash, fever

Nursing diagnoses

- ✓ Mobility, impaired uses
- ✓ Injury, risk for (adverse reactions)
- ✓ Knowledge deficit (teaching)

Implementation

PO route

- Give with meals for GI symptoms

• Have patient use gum, frequent sips of water for dry mouth
• Store in tight container at room temp

Patient/family education
• Caution patient not to take with alcohol, other CNS depressants
• Advise patient to avoid altering activities while taking this drug
• Caution patient to avoid hazardous activities if drowsiness or dizziness occurs
• Caution patient to avoid using OTC medication such as cough preparations, antihistamines, unless directed by prescriber

Evaluation
Positive therapeutic outcome
• Decreased pain, spasticity

Treatment of overdose: Induce emesis of conscious patient, lavage, dialysis

carmustine (BCNU) (℞)
(kar-mus'teen)
BiCNU, BCNU
Func. class.: Antineoplastic alkylating agent
Chem. class.: Nitrosourea
Pregnancy category D

Action: Alkylates DNA, RNA; inhibits enzymes that allow synthesis of amino acids in proteins; also responsible for cross-linking DNA strands; activity is not cell cycle phase specific

➡ **Therapeutic Outcome:** Prevention of rapidly growing malignant cells

Uses: Brain tumors such as glioblastoma, medulloblastoma, astrocytoma; multiple myeloma, Hodgkin's disease, other lymphomas; GI, breast, bronchogenic, and renal carcinomas

Dosage and routes
Adult: **IV** 75-100 mg/m² over 1-2 hr × 2 days or 200 mg/m² × 1 dose q6-8 wk; if leukocytes fall below 2000 or platelets below 75,000, only 50% of dose should be given; water: 8 inserted into resection cavity

Available forms: Powder for inj 100 mg

Adverse effects
GI: Nausea, vomiting, anorexia, stomatitis, hepatotoxicity
GU: Azotemia, ***renal failure***
HEMA: ***Thrombocytopenia, leukopenia, myelosuppression, anemia***
INTEG: Burning, hyperpigmentation at inj site, alopecia
RESP: ***Fibrosis, pulmonary infiltrate***

Contraindications: Hypersensitivity, leukopenia, thrombocytopenia

Precautions: Pregnancy **D**

Pharmacokinetics	
Absorption	Completely absorbed
Distribution	Readily penetrates CSF
Metabolism	Liver, rapid
Excretion	Kidneys, breast milk
Half-life	Unknown

Pharmacodynamics
Unknown

Interactions
Individual drugs
Phenytoin: ↑ metabolism, ↓ effect
Radiation: ↑ toxicity, bone marrow suppression

Drug classifications
Antineoplastics: ↑ toxicity, bone marrow suppression
Bone marrow–suppressing drugs: ↑ bone marrow suppression
Live vaccines: ↑ adverse reactions, ↓ antibody reaction

NURSING CONSIDERATIONS

Assessment

- Assess buccal cavity q8h for dryness, sores or ulceration, white patches, pain, bleeding, dysphagia; obtain prescription for viscous lidocaine (Xylocaine)
- Assess symptoms indicating severe allergic reaction: rash, pruritus, urticaria, purpuric skin lesions, itching, flushing; drug should be discontinued
- Monitor CBC, differential, platelet count weekly; withhold drug if WBC count is <4000/mm^3 or platelet count is <100,000/mm^3; notify prescriber of results if WBC <20,000/mm^3, platelets <150,000/mm^3
- Monitor renal function studies: BUN, creatinine, urine CrCl before and during therapy; I&O ratio; report fall in urine output to <30 ml/hr
- Monitor temp q4h (may indicate beginning of infection)
- Monitor liver function tests before and during therapy (bilirubin, AST [SGOT], ALT [SGPT], LDH) as needed or monthly; note yellowing of skin or sclera, dark urine, clay-colored stools, itchy skin, abdominal pain, fever, diarrhea; hepatotoxicity can be serious and fatal
- Assess for bleeding: hematuria, stool guaiac, bruising or petechiae, mucosa or orifices q8h; inflammation of mucosa, breaks in skin
- Identify effects of alopecia on body image; discuss feelings about body changes

Nursing diagnoses

- ✓ Injury, risk for (adverse reactions)
- ✓ Body image disturbance (adverse reactions)
- ✓ Infection, risk for (adverse reactions)
- ✓ Knowledge deficit (teaching)

Implementation

- Administer after diluting 100 mg/3 ml ethyl alcohol (provided); then further dilute 27 ml sterile water for inj; then dilute with 100-500 ml 0.9% NaCl or D_5W; give over 1 hr or more; reduce rate if discomfort is felt
- Give fluids **IV** or PO before chemotherapy to hydrate patient
- Provide antiemetic 30-60 min before giving drug to prevent vomiting, and prn; antibiotics for prophylaxis of infection
- Provide liq diet (carbonated beverages); gelatin may be added if patient is not nauseated or vomiting

Additive incompatibility: Sodium bicarbonate

Y-*site compatibilities:* Amifostine, aztreonam, cefepime, filgrastim, fludarabine, melphalan, ondansetron, sargramostim, teniposide, thiotepa, vinorelbine

Patient/family education

- Teach patient to avoid use of products containing aspirin or ibuprofen, razors, commercial mouthwash, since bleeding may occur; to report symptoms of bleeding (hematuria, tarry stools)

- Instruct patient to report signs of anemia (fatigue, headache, irritability, faintness, shortness of breath)
- Advise patient that hair may be lost during treatment; a wig or hair piece may make patient feel better; new hair may be different in color, texture
- Caution patient not to have any vaccinations without the advice of the prescriber; serious reactions can occur
- Advise patient that contraception is needed during treatment and for several months after completion of therapy; drug has teratogenic properties

Evaluation

Positive therapeutic outcome

- Prevention of rapid division of malignant cells

carteolol (℞)

(kar-tee′oe-lole)

Cartrol, Ocupress

Func.class.: Antihypertensive

Chem. class.: Nonselective β-blocker

Pregnancy category C

Action: Produces fall in B/P without reflex tachycardia or significant reduction in heart rate through mixture of alpha-blocking, beta-blocking effects and intrinsic sympathomimetic activity; elevated plasma renins are reduced; decreased intraocular pressure in glaucoma and intraocular hypertension

➡ Therapeutic Outcome: Decreased B/P, heart rate; decreased intraocular pressure

Uses: Mild to moderate hypertension; oph intraocular hypertension, open-angle glaucoma

Dosage and routes

Adult: PO 2.5 mg qd initially; may gradually increase to desired response, max 10 mg/day oph i gtt bid

Available forms: Tabs 2.5, 5 mg; oph sol 1%

Adverse effects

CNS: Dizziness, mental changes, drowsiness, fatigue, headache, catatonia, depression, anxiety, nightmares, paresthesia, lethargy, insomnia, decreased concentration

CV: Orthostatic hypotension, ***bradycardia, CHF, chest pain, ventricular dysrhythmias, AV block, peripheral vascular insufficency,*** palpitations

EENT: Tinnitus, visual changes, sore throat, double vision, dry, burning eyes

GI: Nausea, vomiting, diarrhea, dry mouth, flatulence, constipation, anorexia

GU: Impotence, dysuria, ejaculatory failure, urinary retention

HEMA: ***Agranulocytosis, thrombocytopenic purpura (rare)***

INTEG: Rash, alopecia, urticaria, pruritus, fever

MS: Joint pain, arthralgia, muscle cramps, pain

OTHER: Facial swelling, decreased exercise tolerance, weight change, Raynaud's disease

RESP: ***Bronchospasm,*** dyspnea, wheezing, nasal stuffiness, pharyngitis

Contraindications: Hypersensitivity to β-blockers, cardiogenic shock, heart block (2nd or 3rd degree), sinus bradycardia, CHF, bronchial asthma

Precautions: Major surgery, pregnancy **C,** lactation, diabetes mellitus, renal disease, thyroid disease, COPD, well-compensated heart failure, nonallergic bronchospasm

Pharmacokinetics

Absorption	80%-90%
Distribution	Unknown; protein binding 23%-30%
Metabolism	Liver to active metabolite
Excretion	Kidneys, unchanged (50%-75%)
Half-life	Carteolol (6-8 hr); metabolite (8-12 hr); ↑ renal disease

Pharmacodynamics

	PO	OPH
Onset	Unknown	Unknown
Peak	1-3 hr	Unknown
Duration	Unknown	Unknown

Interactions
Individual drugs
Alcohol: ↑ hypotension (large amounts)
Epinephrine: α-Adrenergic stimulation
Hydralazine: ↑ hypotension, bradycardia
Indomethacin: ↓ antihypertensive effect
Insulin: ↑ hypoglycemia
Prazosin: ↑ hypotension, bradycardia
Reserpine: ↑ hypotension, bradycardia
Thyroid: ↓ effectiveness of carteolol
Verapamil: ↑ myocardial depression
Drug classifications
Antihypertensives: ↑ hypertension
β_2-Agonists: ↓ bronchodilatation
Cardiac glycosides: ↑ bradycardia
Theophyllines: ↓ bronchodilatation
Lab test interferences
False ↑ Urinary catecholamines

NURSING CONSIDERATIONS
Assessment
- Monitor B/P during beginning treatment, periodically thereafter; pulse q4h; note rate, rhythm, quality: apical/radial pulse before administration; notify prescriber of any significant changes (pulse <50 bpm)
- Check for baselines in renal, liver function tests before therapy begins
- Assess for edema in feet, legs daily; monitor I&O, daily weight; check for jugular vein distention and rales bilaterally, dyspnea (CHF)
- Monitor skin turgor, dryness of mucous membranes for hydration status, especially G elderly

Nursing diagnoses
- ✓ Cardiac output, decreased (uses)
- ✓ Injury, risk for (side effects)
- ✓ Knowledge deficit (teaching)
- ✓ Noncompliance (teaching)

Implementation
PO route
- Give ac, hs; tab may be crushed or swallowed whole; give with food to prevent GI upset; reduce dosage in renal dysfunction
- Store protected from light, moisture; placed in cool environment

Ophthalmic route
- Give bid, one drop in each eye

Patient/family education

• Teach patient not to discontinue drug abruptly; taper over 2 wk; may cause precipitate dysrhythmias, hypertension if stopped abruptly

• Teach patient not to use OTC products containing α-adrenergic stimulants (such as nasal decongestants, cold preparations); to avoid alcohol, smoking and to limit sodium intake as prescribed

• Teach patient how to take pulse and B/P at home; advise when to notify prescriber

• Instruct patient to comply with weight control, dietary adjustments, modified exercise program

• Advise patient to carry/wear Medic Alert ID to identify drug being taken, allergies; tell patient drug controls symptoms but does not cure

• Caution patient to avoid hazardous activities if dizziness, drowsiness present

• Teach patient to report symptoms of CHF; difficult breathing, especially on exertion or when lying down, night cough, swelling of extremities or bradycardia, dizziness, confusion, depression, fever

• Teach patient to take drug as prescribed, not to double doses, skip doses; take any missed doses as soon as remembered if at least 4 hr until next dose

• Teach patient method of instillation for ophthalmic route

Evaluation

Positive therapeutic outcome

• Decreased B/P in hypertension (after 1-2 wk)

• Lessened intraocular pressure in glaucoma

Treatment of overdose: Lavage, **IV** atropine for bradycardia; **IV** theophylline for bronchospasm, digitalis, O_2, diuretic for cardiac failure; hemodialysis, **IV** glucose for hyperglycemia; **IV** diazepam (or phenytoin) for seizures

carvedilol (℞)

(kar-veh'dee-lol)

Coreg

Func. class.: α/β blocker

Pregnancy category C

Action: A mixture of nonselective β-blocking and α-blocking activity; decreases cardiac output, exercise-induced tachycardia, reflex orthostatic tachycardia; causes reduction in peripheral vascular resistance and vasodilation

Therapeutic Outcome: Decreased B/P in hypertension

Uses: Essential hypertension alone or in combination with other antihypertensives, CHF

Investigational uses: Angina pectoris, idiopathic cardiomyopathy

Dosage and routes

Essential hypertension

Adult: PO 6.25 mg bid × 7-14 if tolerated well, then increase to 12.5 mg bid × 7-14 days if tolerated well, may be increased if needed to 25 mg bid, max 50 mg qd

Congestive heart failure

Adult: PO 12.5-50 mg bid

Angina pectoris

Adult: PO 25-50 mg bid

Idiopathic cardiomyopathy
Adult: PO 6.25-25 mg bid

Available forms: Tabs 3.125, 6.25, 12.5, 25 mg

Adverse effects
CNS: Dizziness, somnolence, insomnia, ataxia, hypesthesia, paresthesia, vertigo, depression
GI: Diarrhea, abdominal pain
CV: Bradycardia, postural hypotension, dependent edema, peripheral edema, ***AV block, extrasystoles,*** hypertension, hypotension, palpitations, peripheral ischemia
RESP: Rhinitis, pharyngitis, dyspnea
MISC: Fatigue, injury, back pain, UTI, viral infection, hypertriglyceridemia, ***thrombocytopenia***

Contraindications: Hypersensitivity, bronchial asthma, class IV decompensated cardiac failure, 2nd or 3rd degree heart block, cardiogenic shock, severe bradycardia

Precautions: Cardiac failure, hepatic injury, peripheral vascular disease, anesthesia, major surgery, diabetes mellitus, G thyrotoxicosis, elderly, P pregnancy (C), lactation, children, emphysema, chronic bronchitis, renal disease

Pharmacokinetics

Absorption	Readily and extensively absorbed
Distribution	>98% bound to plasma proteins
Metabolism	Extensively liver
Excretion	Via bile into feces
G **Half-life**	Terminal half-life 5-9 hrs, increased in the elderly, hepatic disease

Pharmacodynamics

Unknown

Interactions
Individual drugs
Cimetidine: ↑ levels of carvedilol
Clonidine: ↑ heart rate, B/P
Digoxin: ↑ concentrations of digoxin
Reserpine: ↑ hypotension, bradycardia
Rifampin: ↓ levels of carvedilol
Drug classifications
Antidiabetic agents: ↑ hypoglycemia

NURSING CONSIDERATIONS
Assessment
- Monitor renal studies including protein, BUN, creatinine; watch for increased levels that may indicate nephrotic syndrome; obtain baselines in renal and liver function studies before beginning treatment
- Monitor I&O, weight daily
- Monitor B/P during beginning treatment and periodically thereafter, pulse q4h, note rate, rhythm, quality
- Monitor apical/radial pulse before administration; notify prescriber of significant changes
- Assess for edema in feet and legs daily

Nursing diagnoses
✓ Cardiac output, decreased (uses)
✓ Injury, risk for (adverse reactions)
✓ Knowledge deficit (teaching)
✓ Noncompliance (teaching)

Implementation
- Give PO ac, hs; tablets may be crushed or swallowed whole, give with food to ↓ orthostatic hypotension
- Administer reduced dosage in renal dysfunction

Patient/family education
- Tell patient to comply with dosage schedule even if feeling better
- Teach patient to rise slowly to sitting or standing position to minimize orthostatic hypotension
- Encourage patient to report bradycardia, dizziness, confusion, depression, fever
- Teach patient to take pulse at home; advise when to notify prescriber
- Encourage patient not to discontinue drug abruptly

Evaluation
Positive therapeutic outcome
- Decreased B/P

cascara sagrada/ cascara sagrada aromatic fluid extract/ cascara sagrada fluid extract (OTC)

(kas-kar'a)
Func. class.: Laxative
Chem. class.: Anthraquinone
Pregnancy category C

Action: Direct chemical irritation in colon; increases propulsion of stool; increases fluid in colon

Therapeutic Outcome: Decreased constipation; removal of bowel contents before surgery or diagnostic tests

Uses: Constipation; bowel or rectal preparation for surgery or examination

Dosage and routes
Adult: PO 325 mg hs; fluid 1 ml qd; aromatic fluid 5 ml qd
P ***Child 2-12 yr:*** PO/fluid/aromatic fluid ½ adult dose
P ***Child <2 yr:*** PO/fluid/aromatic fluid ¼ adult dose

Available forms: Powder, tabs 325 mg; oral sol

Adverse effects
GI: ***Nausea, vomiting, anorexia, cramps, diarrhea***
META: Hypocalcemia, enteropathy, alkalosis, hypokalemia, ***tetany***

Contraindications: Hypersensitivity, GI bleeding, obstruction, CHF, lactation, abdominal pain, nausea/vomiting, appendicitis, acute surgical abdomen, alcoholics (aromatic fluid extract)

Precautions: Pregnancy **C**

Pharmacokinetics	
Absorption	Minimal
Distribution	Unknown
Metabolism	Liver, minimally
Excretion	Kidneys, feces
Half-life	Not known

Pharmacodynamics	
Onset	6-12 hr
Peak	Unknown
Duration	Unknown

Interactions
Individual drugs
Digitalis: ↓ absorption
Nitrofurantoin: ↓ absorption
Drug classifications
Antibiotics: ↓ absorption
Oral anticoagulants: ↓ absorption
Salicylates: ↓ absorption
Tetracyclines: ↓ absorption

NURSING CONSIDERATIONS
Assessment
- Monitor blood, urine electrolytes if drug used often by patient; check I&O ratio to identify fluid loss

- Assess cramping, rectal bleeding, nausea, vomiting; if these symptoms occur, drug should be discontinued; identify cause of constipation; identify whether fluids, bulk, or exercise is missing from lifestyle

Nursing diagnoses

✓ Bowel elimination, altered: constipation (uses)
✓ Bowel elimination, altered: diarrhea (side effects)
✓ Knowledge deficit (teaching)
✓ Noncompliance (teaching)

Implementation

- Give alone with water only for better absorption; do not administer with food; do not take within 1 hr of antacids, milk, or cimetidine
- Do not crush; swallow tabs whole
- Give in AM or PM (oral dose); evacuation will occur 6-12 hr later

Patient/family education

- Discuss with the patient that adequate fluid consumption is necessary
- Teach patient that normal bowel movements do not always occur daily
- Teach patient not to use in presence of abdominal pain, nausea, vomiting; tell patient to notify prescriber if constipation unrelieved or if symptoms of electrolyte imbalance occur: muscle cramps, pain, weakness, dizziness, excessive thirst

Evaluation

Positive therapeutic outcome

- Decreased constipation in 6-12 hr
- Removal of bowel contents

cefaclor (Rx)

(sef'a-klor)

Ceclor, Ceclor CD

Func. class.: Antibiotic

Chem. class.: Cephalosporin (2nd generation)

Pregnancy category B

Action: Inhibits bacterial cell wall synthesis, which renders cell wall osmotically unstable, leading to cell death by binding to cell wall membrane

Therapeutic Outcome: Bactericidal effects for the following: gram-negative bacilli *Haemophilus influenzae, Escherichia coli, Proteus mirabilis, Klebsiella,* gram-positive organisms *Streptococcus pneumoniae, Staphylococcus,* beta-hemolytic; Streptococci, anaerobes, bacteroides sp.

Uses: Upper and lower respiratory tract, urinary tract, skin infections; otitis media; increased bone, joint, gynecologic infections; septicemia

Dosage and routes

Adult: PO 250-500 mg q8h, not to exceed 4 g/day or 375-500 mg q12h × 7-10 days

P ***Child >1 mo:*** PO 20-40 mg/kg/qd in divided doses q8h, or total daily dose may be divided and given q12h, not to exceed 1 g/day

Acute bacterial exacerbations of chronic bronchitis or acute bronchitis

Adult: 500 mg/12h × 1 wk (ext rel)

Pharyngitis/tonsilitis

Adult: 375 mg/12h × 10 days (ext rel)

Available forms: Caps 250, 500 mg; oral susp 125, 187, 250, 375 mg/5 ml, tabs, ext rel 375, 500 mg

Adverse effects

CNS: Headache, dizziness, weakness, paresthesia, fever, chills

GI: Nausea, vomiting, ***diarrhea, anorexia,*** pain, glossitis, bleeding; increased AST (SGOT), ALT (SGPT), bilirubin, LDH, alkaline phosphatase; abdominal pain, ***pseudomembranous colitis***

GU: ***Proteinuria,*** vaginitis, pruritus, candidiasis, increased BUN, ***nephrotoxicity, renal failure***

HEMA: ***Leukopenia, thrombocytopenia, agranulocytosis,*** anemia, ***neutropenia, lymphocytosis, eosinophilia, pancytopenia, hemolytic anemia***

INTEG: Rash, urticaria, dermatitis

RESP: Dyspnea

SYST: ***Anaphylaxis***

Contraindications: Hypersensitivity to cephalosporins, P infants <1 mo

Precautions: Hypersensitivity to penicillins, pregnancy **B,** lactation, renal disease

Pharmacokinetics

Absorption	Well absorbed
Distribution	Widely distributed; crosses placenta
Metabolism	Not metabolized
Excretion	Unchanged by kidneys (60%-80%); enters breast milk
Half-life	36-54 min; increased in renal disease

Pharmacodynamics

Onset	15 min
Peak	½-1 hr

Interactions

Individual drugs

Probenecid: ↓ excretion of drug and increased blood levels

Sulfinpyrazone: ↑ toxicity

Vancomycin: ↑ toxicity

Drug classifications

Aminoglycosides: ↑ toxicity

Lab test interferences

False ↑ Creatinine (serum urine), false ↑ urinary 17-KS

False positive: Urinary protein, direct Coombs' test, urine glucose

Interference: Cross-matching

NURSING CONSIDERATIONS

Assessment

- Assess patient for previous sensitivity reaction to penicillins or other cephalosporins; cross-sensitivity between penicillins and cephalosporins is common
- Assess patient for signs and symptoms of infection including characteristics of wounds, sputum, urine, stool, WBC >10,000, earache, fever; obtain baseline information and during treatment
- Obtain C&S before beginning drug therapy to identify if correct treatment has been initiated
- Assess for allergic reactions: rash, urticaria, pruritus, chills, fever, joint pain; angioedema may occur a few days after therapy begins; epinephrine, resuscitation equipment should be on unit for anaphylactic reaction
- Identify urine output; if decreasing, notify prescriber (may indicate nephrotoxicity); also check for increased BUN, creatinine
- Monitor blood studies: AST (SGOT), ALT (SGPT), CBC, Hct, bilirubin, LDH, alkaline

phosphatase, Coombs' test monthly if patient is on long-term therapy

- Monitor electrolytes: potassium, sodium, chloride monthly if patient is on long-term therapy
- Assess bowel pattern qd; if severe diarrhea occurs, drug should be discontinued; may indicate pseudomembranous colitis
- Monitor for bleeding: ecchymosis, bleeding gums, hematuria, stool guaiac daily if on long-term therapy
- Assess for overgrowth of infection: perineal itching, fever, malaise, redness, pain, swelling, drainage, rash, diarrhea, change in cough, sputum

Nursing diagnoses

- ✓ Infection, risk for (uses)
- ✓ Diarrhea (side effects)
- ✓ Fluid volume deficit, risk for (side effects)
- ✓ Injury, risk for (side effects)
- ✓ Knowledge deficit (teaching)
- ✓ Noncompliance (teaching)

Implementation

- Give in even doses around the clock; if GI upset occurs, give with food; drug must be given for 10-14 days to ensure organism death and prevent superinfection
- Shake suspension, refrigerate, discard after 2 wks
- Do not crush, cut, or chew ext rel tabs

Patient/family education

- Teach patient to report sore throat, bruising, bleeding, joint pain; may indicate blood dyscrasias (rare)
- Advise patient to contact prescriber if vaginal itching, loose, foul-smelling stools, furry tongue occur; may indicate superinfection
- Instruct patient to take all medication prescribed for the length of time ordered
- Advise patient to notify prescriber of diarrhea with blood or pus, which may indicate pseudomembranous colitis

Evaluation

Positive therapeutic outcome

- Absence of signs/symptoms of infection (WBC <10,000, temp WNL, absence of red draining wounds, earache)
- Reported improvement in symptoms of infection
- Negative C&S

Treatment of anaphylaxis: Epinephrine, antihistamines, resuscitate if needed

cefadroxil (℞)

(sef-a-drox'ill)

Cefadroxil, Duricef

Func. class.: Antibiotic

Chem. class.: Cephalosporin (1st generation)

Pregnancy category B

Action: Inhibits bacterial cell wall synthesis, rendering cell wall osmotically unstable, leading to cell death by binding to cell wall membrane

Therapeutic Outcome: Bactericidal effects for the following: gram-negative bacilli *Escherichia coli, Proteus mirabilis, Klebsiella (UTI only)*; gram-positive organisms *Streptococcus pneumoniae, S. pyogenes, Staphylococcus aureus*

Uses: Upper, lower respiratory tract, urinary tract, skin infections; otitis media; tonsillitis, pharyngitis; particularly for UTI

Dosage and routes

Adult: PO 1-2 g qd or in divided doses q12h; give a loading dose of 1 g initially; dosage reduction indicated in renal impairment (CrCl <50 ml/min)

P ***Child:*** 30 mg/kg/day or in divided doses

Available forms: Caps 500 mg; tabs 1 g; oral susp 125, 250, 500 mg/5 ml

Adverse effects

CNS: Headache, dizziness, weakness, paresthesia, fever, chills

GI: Nausea, vomiting, ***diarrhea, anorexia,*** pain, glossitis, bleeding; increased AST (SGOT), ALT (SGPT), bilirubin, LDH, alkaline phosphatase; abdominal pain, ***pseudomembranous colitis***

GU: ***Proteinuria,*** vaginitis, pruritus, candidiasis, increased BUN, ***nephrotoxicity, renal failure***

HEMA: ***Leukopenia, thrombocytopenia, agranulocytosis,*** anemia, ***neutropenia, lymphocytosis, eosinophilia, pancytopenia, hemolytic anemia***

INTEG: Rash, urticaria, dermatitis, ***anaphylaxis***

RESP: Dyspnea

Contraindications: Hypersensitivity to cephalosporins,
P infants <1 mo

Precautions: Hypersensitivity to penicillins, pregnancy **B,** lactation, renal disease

Pharmacokinetics

Absorption	Well absorbed
Distribution	Widely distributed; crosses placenta
Metabolism	Not metabolized
Excretion	Unchanged by kidneys; enters breast milk
Half-life	1½-2 hr

Pharmacodynamics

	PO
Onset	Rapid
Peak	1½-2 hr

Interactions

Individual drugs

Probenecid: ↓ excretion of drug and ↑ blood levels

Vancomycin: ↑ toxicity

Drug classifications

Aminoglycosides: ↑ toxicity

Lab test interferences

False ↑ Creatinine (serum urine), false ↑ urinary 17-KS

False positive: Urinary protein, direct Coombs' test, urine glucose

Interference: Cross-matching

NURSING CONSIDERATIONS

Assessment

- Assess patient for previous sensitivity reaction to penicillins or other cephalosporins; cross-sensitivity between penicillins and cephalosporins is common
- Assess patient for signs and symptoms of infection including characteristics of wounds, sputum, urine, stool, WBC >10,000, earache, fever; obtain baseline information and during treatment
- Obtain C&S before beginning drug therapy to identify if correct treatment has been initiated
- Assess for allergic reactions: rash, urticaria, pruritus, chills, fever, joint pain; angioedema may occur a few days after

therapy begins; epinephrine and resuscitation equipment should be available for anaphylactic reaction

- Identify urine output; if decreasing, notify prescriber (may indicate nephrotoxicity); also check for increased BUN, creatinine
- Monitor blood studies: AST (SGOT), ALT (SGPT), CBC, Hct, bilirubin, LDH, alkaline phosphatase, Coombs' test monthly if patient is on long-term therapy
- Monitor electrolytes: potassium, sodium, chloride monthly if patient is on long-term therapy
- Assess bowel pattern qd; if severe diarrhea occurs, drug should be discontinued; may indicate pseudomembranous colitis
- Monitor for bleeding: ecchymosis, bleeding gums, hematuria, stool guaiac daily if on long-term therapy
- Assess for superinfection: perineal itching, fever, malaise, redness, pain, swelling, drainage, rash, diarrhea, change in cough, sputum

Nursing diagnoses

- ✓ Infection, risk for (uses)
- ✓ Diarrhea (side effects)
- ✓ Fluid volume deficit, risk for (side effects)
- ✓ Injury, risk for (side effects)
- ✓ Knowledge deficit (teaching)
- ✓ Noncompliance (teaching)

Implementation

- Give in even doses around the clock; if GI upset occurs, give with food; drug must be given for 10-14 days to ensure organism death and prevent superinfection
- Shake suspension, refrigerate, discard after 2 wks

Patient/family education

- Teach patient to report sore throat, bruising, bleeding, joint pain; may indicate blood dyscrasias (rare)
- Advise patient to contact prescriber if vaginal itching, loose, foul-smelling stools, furry tongue occur; may indicate superinfection
- Instruct patient to take all medication prescribed for the length of time ordered
- Advise patient to notify prescriber of diarrhea with blood or pus, which may indicate pseudomembranous colitis

Evaluation

Positive therapeutic outcome

- Absence of signs/symptoms of infection (WBC <10,000, temp WNL, absence of red draining wounds, earache)
- Reported improvement in symptoms of infection
- Negative C&S

Treatment of anaphylaxis: Epinephrine, antihistamines, resuscitate if needed

cefamandole (℞)

(sef-a-man'dole)

Mandol

Func. class.: Antibiotic

Chem. class.: Cephalosporin (2nd generation)

Pregnancy category B

Action: Inhibits bacterial cell wall synthesis, rendering cell wall osmotically unstable, leading to cell death by binding to cell wall membrane

➔ **Therapeutic Outcome:** Bactericidal effects for the following: gram-negative anarobes *Bacteroides sp.*,

Clostridium sp., Fusobacterium sp., Peptococcus sp., Peptostreptococcus sp., Haemophilus influenzae, Escherichia coli, Proteus mirabilis, Klebsiella; gram-positive organisms *S. pneumoniae, Streptococcus pyogenes, Staphylococcus aureus;* organisms *Enterobacter sp., Morganella morganii, Proteus vulgaris, Provencia rettgeris*

Uses: Upper, lower respiratory tract, urinary tract, skin infections; peritonitis, septicemia, surgical prophylaxis

Dosage and routes

Adult: IM/**IV** 500 mg-1 g q4-8h; may give up to 2 g q4h for severe infections

P ***Child >1 mo:*** IM/**IV** 50-100 mg/kg/day in divided doses q4-8h, not to exceed adult dose

Dosage reduction indicated in renal impairment (CrCl <50 ml/min)

Available forms: Inj 500 mg, 1, 2, 10 g

Adverse effects

CNS: Headache, dizziness, weakness, paresthesia, fever, chills

*GI: **Nausea, vomiting, diarrhea, anorexia,*** pain, glossitis, bleeding; increased AST (SGOT), ALT (SGPT), bilirubin, LDH, alkaline phosphatase; abdominal pain, pseudomembranous colitis

*GU: **Proteinuria,*** vaginitis, pruritus, candidiasis, increased BUN, ***nephrotoxicity, renal failure***

*HEMA: **Leukopenia, thrombocytopenia, agranulocytosis,*** anemia, ***neutropenia, lymphocytosis, eosinophilia, pancytopenia, hemolytic anemia,*** bleeding, ***hypoprothrombinemia***

INTEG: Rash, urticaria, dermatitis

RESP: Dyspnea

*SYST: **Anaphylaxis***

Contraindications: Hypersensitivity to cephalosporins, P infants <1 mo

Precautions: Hypersensitivity to penicillins, pregnancy **B,** lactation, renal disease

Pharmacokinetics

Absorption	Well absorbed
Distribution	Widely distributed; crosses placenta
Metabolism	Not metabolized
Excretion	Unchanged by kidneys (60%-80%); enters breast milk
Half-life	½-1½ hr

Pharmacodynamics

	IM	IV
Onset	Rapid	Immediate
Peak	½-2 hr	Infusion's end

Interactions

Individual drugs

Probenecid: ↓ excretion of drug and ↑ blood levels

Vancomycin: ↑ toxicity

Drug classifications

Aminoglycosides: ↑ toxicity

Anticoagulants: ↑ bleeding

Thrombolytics: ↑ bleeding

Lab test interferences

False ↑ Urinary 17-KS

False positive: Urinary protein, direct Coombs', urine glucose

Interference: Cross-matching

NURSING CONSIDERATIONS

Assessment

- Assess patient for previous sensitivity reaction to penicillins or other cephalosporins; cross-sensitivity between penicillins and cephalosporins is common
- Assess patient for signs and symptoms of infection includ-

ing characteristics of wounds, sputum, urine, stool, WBC >10,000, earache, fever; obtain baseline information and during treatment

- Obtain C&S before beginning drug therapy to identify if correct treatment has been initiated
- Assess for allergic reactions: rash, urticaria, pruritus, chills, fever, joint pain; angioedema may occur a few days after therapy begins; epinephrine and resuscitation equipment should be available for anaphylactic reaction
- Identify urine output; if decreasing, notify prescriber (may indicate nephrotoxicity); also check for increased BUN, creatinine
- Monitor blood studies: AST (SGOT), ALT (SGPT), CBC, Hct, bilirubin, LDH, alkaline phosphatase, Coombs' test monthly if patient is on long-term therapy
- Monitor electrolytes: potassium, sodium, chloride monthly if patient is on long-term therapy
- Assess bowel pattern qd; if severe diarrhea occurs, drug should be discontinued; may indicate pseudomembranous colitis
- Monitor for bleeding: ecchymosis, bleeding gums, hematuria, stool guaiac daily if on long-term therapy
- Assess for superinfection: perineal itching, fever, malaise, redness, pain, swelling, drainage, rash, diarrhea, change in cough, sputum

Nursing diagnoses

✓ Infection, risk for (uses)
✓ Injury, risk for (side effects)
✓ Diarrhea (side effects)
✓ Knowledge deficit (teaching)
✓ Noncompliance (teaching)

Implementation

IM route

- Reconstitute with 3 ml sterile or bacteriostatic water for inj, 0.9% NaCl, or 0.5%-2.0% lidocaine HCl; give deep in large muscle mass; massage; check for redness, abscess at inj site

IV route

- Check for irritation, extravasation, phlebitis daily; change site q72h
- Direct **IV**: Dilute each g of drug with 10 ml of D_5W, 0.9% NaCl, or sterile water for inj; give over 5 min
- For intermittent inf further dilute with 100 ml of D_5W, $D_{10}W$, D_5/0.25% NaCl, D_5/0.45% NaCl, D_5/0.9% NaCl, D_5 LR, 0.9% NaCl; give over 15-30 min; may be refrigerated up to 96 hr or 24 hr at room temp
- For cont inf dilute with 500-1000 ml of above solutions; give over prescribed rate

Y-site incompatibilities: Amiodarone, hetastarch

Y-site compatibilities: Acyclovir, cyclophosphamide, hydromorphone, magnesium sulfate, meperidine, morphine, perphenazine

Syringe incompatibilities: Cimetidine, gentamicin, tobramycin

Syringe compatibility: Heparin

Additive incompatibilities: Aminoglycosides, calcium gluceptate, calcium gluconate, cimetidine, gentamicin

Additive compatibilities: Clindamycin, floxacillin, furosemide, metronidazole, or verapamil

Patient/family education

- Teach patient to report sore throat, bruising, bleeding, joint pain; may indicate blood dyscrasias (rare)
- Advise patient to contact prescriber if vaginal itching, loose, foul-smelling stools, furry tongue occur; may indicate superinfection
- Instruct patient to take all medication prescribed for the length of time ordered
- Advise patient to notify prescriber of diarrhea with blood or pus, which may indicate pseudomembranous colitis

Evaluation

Positive therapeutic outcome

- Absence of signs/symptoms of infection (WBC <10,000, temp WNL, absence of red draining wounds, earache)
- Reported improvement in symptoms of infection
- Negative C&S

Treatment of anaphylaxis: Epinephrine, antihistamines, resuscitate if needed

cefazolin (℞)

(sef-a'zoe-lin)

Ancef, cefazolin sodium, Kefzol, Zolicef

Func. class.: Antibiotic

Chem. class.: Cephalosporin (1st generation)

Pregnancy category B

Action: Inhibits bacterial cell wall synthesis, rendering cell wall osmotically unstable, leading to cell death

➔ Therapeutic Outcome: Bactericidal effects for the following: gram-negative organisms *Enterobacter sp., Haemophilus influenzae, Escherichia coli, Proteus mirabilis, Klebsiella;* gram-positive organisms *Streptococcus pneumoniae, S. pyogenes, Staphlyococcus aureus*

Uses: Upper, lower respiratory tract, urinary tract, skin infections; bone, joint, biliary, genital infections; endocarditis, surgical prophylaxis, septicemia

Dosage and routes

Life-threatening infections

Adult: IM/**IV** 1-1.5 g q6h

P ***Child >1 mo:*** IM/**IV** 100 mg/kg in 3-4 equal doses

Mild/moderate infections

Adult: IM/**IV** 250 mg-1 g q8h

P ***Child >1 mo:*** IM/**IV** 25-50 mg/kg in 3-4 equal doses

Dosage reduction indicated in renal impairment (CrCl <50 ml/min)

Available forms: Inj 250, 500 mg, 1, 5, 10 g

Adverse effects

CNS: Headache, dizziness, weakness, paresthesia, fever, chills

GI: Nausea, vomiting, *diarrhea, anorexia,* pain, glossitis, bleeding; increased AST (SGOT), ALT (SGPT), bilirubin, LDH, alkaline phosphatase; abdominal pain, oral candidiasis, ***pseudomembranous colitis***

GU: ***Proteinuria,*** vaginitis, pruritus, candidiasis, increased BUN, ***nephrotoxicity, renal failure***

HEMA: ***Leukopenia, thrombocytopenia, agranulocytosis,***

anemia, ***neutropenia, lymphocytosis, eosinophilia, pancytopenia, hemolytic anemia***
INTEG: Rash, urticaria, dermatitis,
SYST: ***Anaphylaxis***

Contraindications: Hypersensitivity to cephalosporins, P infants <1 mo

Precautions: Hypersensitivity to penicillins, pregnancy **B**, lactation, renal disease

Pharmacokinetics

Absorption	Well absorbed
Distribution	Widely distributed; crosses placenta
Metabolism	Not metabolized
Excretion	Unchanged by kidneys; enters breast milk
Half-life	1½-2½ hr

Pharmacodynamics

	IM	IV
Onset	Rapid	10 min
Peak	1-2 hr	Infusion's end

Interactions
Individual drugs
Probenecid: ↓ excretion of drug and ↑ blood levels
Vancomycin: ↑ toxicity
Drug classifications
Aminoglycosides: ↑ toxicity, ↑ nephrotoxicity
Lab test interferences
False ↑ Urinary 17-KS
False positive: Urinary protein, direct Coombs', urine glucose
Interference: Cross-matching

NURSING CONSIDERATIONS
Assessment
- Assess patient for previous sensitivity reaction to penicillins or other cephalosporins; cross-sensitivity between penicillins and cephalosporins is common
- Assess patient for signs and symptoms of infection including characteristics of wounds, sputum, urine, stool, WBC >10,000, earache, fever; obtain baseline information and during treatment
- Obtain C&S before beginning drug therapy to identify if correct treatment has been initiated
- Assess for allergic reactions: rash, urticaria, pruritus, chills, fever, joint pain; angioedema may occur a few days after therapy begins; epinephrine and resuscitation equipment should be available for anaphylactic reaction
- Identify urine output; if decreasing, notify prescriber (may indicate nephrotoxicity); also check for increased BUN, creatinine
- Monitor blood studies: AST (SGOT), ALT (SGPT), CBC, Hct, bilirubin, LDH, alkaline phosphatase, Coombs' test monthly if patient is on long-term therapy
- Monitor electrolytes: potassium, sodium, chloride monthly if patient is on long-term therapy
- Assess bowel pattern qd; if severe diarrhea occurs, drug should be discontinued; may indicate pseudomembranous colitis
- Monitor for bleeding: ecchymosis, bleeding gums, hematuria, stool guaiac daily if on long-term therapy
- Assess for overgrowth of infection: perineal itching, fever, malaise, redness, pain, swelling, drainage, rash, diarrhea, change in cough, sputum

Nursing diagnoses
- ✓ Infection, risk for (uses)
- ✓ Diarrhea (side effects)
- ✓ Injury, risk for (side effects)

- ✓ Knowledge deficit (teaching)
- ✓ Noncompliance (teaching)

Implementation

IM route

- Reconstitute 250-500 mg of drug with 2 ml sterile or bacteriostatic water for inj, or 0.9% NaCl; reconstitute 1 g of drug with 2.5 ml; give deep in large muscle mass, massage

IV route

- Check for irritation, extravasation, phlebitis daily, change site q72h
- For direct **IV** dilute in 10 ml of sterile water for injection; give over 5 min
- For intermittent inf dilute reconstituted sol (500 mg or 1 mg) in 50-100 ml D_5W, $D_{10}W$, D_5/0.25% NaCl, D_5/0.45% NaCl, D_5/0.9% NaCl, D_5/LR, or LR, 0.9% NaCl; give over 30-60 min; may be refrigerated up to 96 hr or stored 24 hr at room temp

Y-site incompatibilities: Amiodarone, hetastarch, hydromorphone, idarubicin, vinorelbine tartrate

Y-site compatibilities: Acyclovir, allopurinol, amifostine, atracurium, aztreonam, calcium gluconate, cyclophosphamide, diltiazem, enalaprilat, esmolol, famotidine, filgrastim, fluconazole, fludarabine, foscarnet, heparin, labetalol, lidocaine, magnesium sulfate, melphalan, meperidine, midazolam, morphine, multivitamins, ondansetron, perphenazine, pancuronium, regular insulin, sargramostim, tacrolimus, teniposide, theophylline, thiotepa, vecuronium, vitamin B complex with C

Syringe incompatibilities: Ascorbic acid injection, cimetidine, lidocaine, vitamin B complex with C

Syringe compatibilities: Heparin, vitamin B complex

Additive incompatibilities: Amikacin, amobarbital, bleomycin, calcium gluceptate, calcium gluconate, colistimethate, erythromycin, kanamycin, oxytetracycline, pentobarbital, polymyxin B, tetracycline

Additive compatibilities: Aztreonam, clindamycin, famotidine, fluconazole, metronidazole, verapamil

Patient/family education

- Teach patient to report sore throat, bruising, bleeding, joint pain; may indicate blood dyscrasias (rare)
- Advise patient to contact prescriber if vaginal itching, loose, foul-smelling stools, furry tongue occur; may indicate superinfection
- Advise patient to notify prescriber of diarrhea with blood or pus, which may indicate pseudomembranous colitis

Evaluation

Positive therapeutic outcome

- Absence of signs/symptoms of infection (WBC <10,000, temp WNL, absence of red draining wounds, earache)
- Reported improvement in symptoms of infection
- Negative C&S

Treatment of anaphylaxis: Epinephrine, antihistamines, resuscitate if needed

C

cefepime (℞)
(sef′e-peem)
Maxipime
Func. class.: Broad-spectrum antibiotic
Chem. class.: Cephalosporin (3rd generation)
Pregnancy category B

Action: Inhibits bacterial cell wall synthesis, rendering cell wall osmotically unstable, leading to cell death

➔ **Therapeutic Outcome:** Bactericidal effects for the following: gram-negative bacilli, *Escherichia coli, Proteus, Klebsiella;* gram-positive organisms *Streptococcus pneumoniae, S. pyogenes, Staphylococcus aureus*

Uses: Lower respiratory tract, urinary tract, skin, bone, gonococcal infections; septicemia, peritonitis

Dosage and routes
Urinary tract infections (mild to moderate)
Adult: IM/**IV** 0.5-1g q12h × 7-10 days
Urinary tract infections (severe)
Adult: **IV** 2 g q12h × 10 days
Pneumonia (moderate to severe)
Adult: **IV** 1-2 g q12h × 10 days

Available forms: Powder for inj 500 mg, 1, 2g

Adverse effects
CNS: Headache, dizziness, weakness, paresthesia, fever, chills
GI: Nausea, vomiting, diarrhea, anorexia, pain, glossitis, bleeding; increased AST (SGOT), ALT (SGPT), bilirubin, LDH, alkaline phosphatase; abdominal pain
GU: Proteinuria, vaginitis, pruritus, candidiasis, increased BUN; ***nephrotoxicity, renal failure***
HEMA: Leukopenia, thrombocytopenia, agranulocytosis, anemia, *neutropenia, lymphocytosis, eosinophilia, pancytopenia, hemolytic anemia*
INTEG: Rash, urticaria, dermatitis, thrombophlebitis
SYST: Anaphylaxis

Contraindications: Hypersensitivity to cephalosporins;
P infants <1 mo

Precautions: Hypersensitivity to penicillins, pregnancy **B,** lactation, renal disease

Pharmacokinetics

Absorption	Well absorbed (IM)
Distribution	Widely distributed; crosses placenta
Metabolism	Not metabolized
Excretion	Kidneys, unchanged; enters breast milk
Half-life	2 hr; increased in renal disease

Pharmacodynamics

	IM	IV
Onset	Rapid	Immediate
Peak	79 mins	Infusion's end

Interactions
Individual drugs
Probenecid: ↓ excretion of drug and ↑ blood levels
Vancomycin: ↑ toxicity
Drug classifications
Aminoglycosides: ↑ toxicity
Lab test interferences
False ↑ Creatinine (serum urine), false ↑ urinary 17-KS
False positive: Urinary protein, direct Coombs' test, urine glucose
Interference: Cross-matching

NURSING CONSIDERATIONS
Assessment
- Assess patient for previous sensitivity reaction to penicillins or other cephalosporins; cross-sensitivity between penicillins and cephalosporins is common
- Assess patient for signs and symptoms of infection including characteristics of wounds, sputum, urine, stool, WBC >10,000, fever; obtain baseline information and during treatment
- Obtain C&S before beginning drug therapy to identify if correct treatment has been initiated
- Assess for allergic reactions: rash, urticaria, pruritus, chills, fever, joint pain; angioedema may occur a few days after therapy begins; epinephrine and resuscitation equipment should be on unit for anaphylactic reaction
- Identify urine output; if decreasing, notify prescriber (may indicate nephrotoxicity); also check for increased BUN, creatinine
- Monitor blood studies: AST (SGOT), ALT (SGPT), CBC, Hct, bilirubin, LDH, alkaline phosphatase, Coombs' test monthly if patient is on long-term therapy
- Monitor electrolytes: potassium, sodium, chloride, monthly if patient is on long-term therapy
- Assess bowel pattern qd; if severe diarrhea occurs, drug should be discontinued; may indicate pseudomembranous colitis
- Monitor for bleeding: ecchymosis, bleeding gums, hematuria, stool guaiac daily if on long-term therapy
- Assess for overgrowth of infection: perineal itching, fever, malaise, redness, pain, swelling, drainage, rash, diarrhea, change in cough, sputum

Nursing diagnoses
- ✓ Infection, risk for (uses)
- ✓ Injury, risk for (side effects)
- ✓ Diarrhea (side effects)
- ✓ Knowledge deficit (teaching)

Implementation
IM route
- Reconstitute 1 g/2 ml of sterile water for inj; may be diluted with 0.5% or 1% lidocaine to prevent pain; give deep in large muscle mass, massage

IV IV route
- Check for irritation, extravasation, phlebitis daily; change site q72h
- For intermittent inf dilute with 50-100 ml of D_5W, give over 30 min
- *Solution compatibilities:* 0.9% NaCl, D_5, 0.5, 1.0% lidocaine, bacteriostatic water for inj with parabens/benzyl alcohol

Patient/family education
- Teach patient to report sore throat, bruising, bleeding, joint pain; may indicate blood dyscrasias (rare)
- Advise patient to contact prescriber if vaginal itching, loose foul-smelling stools, furry tongue occur; may indicate superinfection
- Advise patient to notify prescriber of diarrhea with blood or pus, may indicate pseudomembranous colitis

Evaluation
Positive therapeutic outcome
- Absence of signs/symptoms of infection (WBC <10,000, temp WNL, absence of red draining wounds)

• Reported improvement in symptoms of infection

Treatment of anaphylaxis: Epinephrine, antihistamines, resuscitate if needed

cefixime (℞)

(sef-icks'ime)

Suprax

Func. class: Broad-spectrum antibiotic

Chem. class: Cephalosporin (3rd generation)

Pregnancy category B

Action: Inhibits bacterial cell wall synthesis, rendering cell wall osmotically unstable, leading to cell death

Therapeutic Outcome: Bactericidal effects of the following: *Escherichia coli, Proteus mirabilis, Streptococcus pyogenes, Haemophilus influenzae, Moraxella catarrhalis, S. pneumoniae*

Uses: Uncomplicated UTI, pharyngitis and tonsillitis, otitis media, acute bronchitis, and acute/exacerbations of chronic bronchitis

Dosage and routes

Adult: PO 400 mg qd as a single dose or 200 mg q12h

P ***Child >50 kg or >12 years:*** PO use adult dosage

P ***Child <50 kg or <12 years:*** PO 8 mg/kg/day as a single dose or 4 mg/kg/day q12h

Available forms: Tabs 200, 400 g; powder for oral susp 100 mg/5 ml

Adverse effects

CNS: Headache, dizziness, paresthesia, fever, chills, lethargy, fatigue, confusion

GI: Nausea, vomiting, *diarrhea,* anorexia, pain, glossitis, bleeding; increased AST (SGOT), ALT (SGPT), bilirubin, LDH, alkaline phosphatase; heartburn, dysgeusia, flatulence, ***pseudomembranous colitis***

GU: ***Proteinuria,*** vaginitis, pruritus, increased BUN, ***nephrotoxicity, renal failure, pyuria, dysuria***

HEMA: ***Leukopenia, thrombocytopenia, agranulocytosis,*** anemia, ***neutropenia, lymphocytosis, eosinophilia, pancytopenia, hemolytic anemia***

INTEG: Rash, urticaria, ***exfoliative dermatitis***

RESP: ***Bronchospasm,*** dyspnea, tight chest

SYST: ***Anaphylaxis***

Contraindications: Hypersensitivity to cephalosporins, P infants <6 mo

Precautions: Hypersensitivity to penicillins, pregnancy **B,** lactation, renal disease

Pharmacokinetics

Absorption	40%-50% (PO: tab)
Distribution	Widely distributed
Metabolism	Not metabolized
Excretion	Kidneys, unchanged (50%); bile (10%); enters breast milk
Half-life	3-4 hr, increased in renal disease

Pharmacodynamics

Onset	15-30 min
Peak	1-2 hr

Interactions

Individual drugs

Probenecid: ↓ excretion of drug and ↑ blood levels

Vancomycin: ↑ toxicity

Drug classifications

Aminoglycosides: ↑ toxicity

Lab test interferences

False ↑ Creatinine (serum urine), false ↑ urinary 17-KS

False positive: Urinary protein, direct Coombs' test, urine glucose

Interference: Cross-matching

NURSING CONSIDERATIONS

Assessment

- Assess patient for previous sensitivity reaction to penicillins or other cephalosporins; cross-sensitivity between penicillins and cephalosporins is common
- Assess patient for signs and symptoms of infection including characteristics of wounds, sputum, urine, stool, WBC >10,000, earache, fever; obtain baseline information and during treatment
- Obtain C&S before beginning drug therapy to identify if correct treatment has been initiated
- Assess for allergic reactions: rash, urticaria, pruritus, chills, fever, joint pain; angioedema may occur a few days after therapy begins; epinephrine and resuscitation equipment should be available for anaphylactic reaction
- Identify urine output; if decreasing, notify prescriber (may indicate nephrotoxicity); also check for increased BUN, creatinine
- Monitor blood studies: AST (SGOT), ALT (SGPT), CBC, Hct, bilirubin, LDH, alkaline phosphatase, Coombs' test monthly if patient is on long-term therapy
- Monitor electrolytes: potassium, sodium, chloride monthly if patient is on long-term therapy
- Assess bowel pattern qd; if severe diarrhea occurs, drug should be discontinued; may indicate pseudomembranous colitis
- Monitor for bleeding: ecchymosis, bleeding gums, hematuria, stool guaiac daily if on long-term therapy
- Assess for overgrowth of infection: perineal itching, fever, malaise, redness, pain, swelling, drainage, rash, diarrhea, change in cough, sputum

Nursing diagnoses

✓ Infection, risk for (uses)
✓ Diarrhea (side effects)
✓ Injury, risk for (side effects)
✓ Knowledge deficit (teaching)
✓ Noncompliance (teaching)

Implementation

- Give in even doses around the clock; if GI upset occurs, give with food; drug must be given for 10-14 days to ensure organism death and prevent superinfection
- Shake suspension

Patient/family education

- Teach patient to report sore throat, bruising, bleeding, joint pain; may indicate blood dyscrasias (rare)
- Advise patient to contact prescriber if vaginal itching, loose, foul-smelling stools, furry tongue occur; may indicate superinfection
- Instruct patient to take all medication prescribed for the length of time ordered
- Advise patient to notify prescriber of diarrhea with blood or pus, which may indicate pseudomembranous colitis

Evaluation

Positive therapeutic outcome

- Absence of signs/symptoms of infection (WBC <10,000, negative, temp WNL, absence

of red draining wounds, earache)
- Reported improvement in symptoms of infection
- Negative C&S

Treatment of anaphylaxis: Epinephrine, antihistamines, resuscitate if needed

cefmetazole (℞)
(sef-met′a-zole)
Zefazone
Func. class.: Broad-spectrum antibiotic
Chem. class.: Cephalosporin (2nd generation)
Pregnancy category B

Action: Inhibits bacterial cell wall synthesis, rendering cell wall osmotically unstable, leading to cell death

Therapeutic Outcome: Bactericidal effects for the following: anaerobes, including *Clostridium, Bacteroides sp., Fusobacterium sp.;* gram-negative organisms *Morganella morganii, Haemophilus influenzae, Escherichia coli, Proteus, Klebsiella, Bacteroides fragilis;* gram-positive organisms *Streptococcus pneumoniae, S. pyogenes, Staphylococcus aureus*

Uses: Infections of lower respiratory tract, urinary tract, skin, bone; intraabdominal infections

Dosage and routes
Adult: **IV** 2 g divided q6-12h × 5-14 days

Available forms: Powder for inj 1, 2 g/vial

Adverse effects
CNS: Headache, dizziness, paresthesia, fever, chills, lethargy, fatigue, confusion
GI: Nausea, vomiting, diarrhea, anorexia, pain, glossitis, bleeding; increased AST (SGOT), ALT (SGPT), bilirubin, LDH, alkaline phosphatase; heartburn, flatulence
*GU: **Proteinuria,*** vaginitis, pruritus, candidiasis, increased BUN, ***nephrotoxicity, renal failure***
*HEMA: **Leukopenia, thrombocytopenia, agranulocytosis,*** anemia, ***neutropenia, lymphocytosis, eosinophilia, pancytopenia, hemolytic anemia***
INTEG: Rash, urticaria, ***exfoliative dermatitis,*** thrombophlebitis ***angioedema,*** erythema, pruritus
*SYST: **Anaphylaxis***

Contraindications: Hypersensitivity to cephalosporins, P infants <1 mo

Precautions: Hypersensitivity to penicillins, pregnancy **B,** lactation, renal disease

Pharmacokinetics

Absorption	Complete
Distribution	Widely distributed; crosses placenta
Metabolism	Not metabolized
Excretion	Kidneys, unchanged (85%); enters breast milk
Half-life	½-2 hr, increased in renal disease

Pharmacodynamics

Onset	Rapid
Peak	Infusion's end

Interactions
Individual drugs
Alcohol: Disulfiram reaction if ingested within 48-72 hr of cephalosporin
Plicamycin: ↑ bleeding

Probenecid: ↓ excretion of drug and ↑ blood levels
Sulfinpyrazone: ↑ toxicity
Valproic acid: ↑ bleeding
Vancomycin: ↑ toxicity

Drug classifications

Aminoglycosides: ↑ toxicity
Anticoagulants: ↑ bleeding
Thrombolytics: ↑ bleeding

Lab test interferences

False ↑ Creatinine (serum urine), false ↑ urinary 17-KS
False positive: Urinary protein, direct Coombs' test, urine glucose
Interference: Cross-matching

NURSING CONSIDERATIONS

Assessment

- Assess patient for previous sensitivity reaction to penicillins or other cephalosporins; cross-sensitivity between penicillins and cephalosporins is common
- Assess patient for signs and symptoms of infection including characteristics of wounds, sputum, urine, stool, WBC >10,000, earache, fever; obtain baseline information and during treatment
- Obtain C&S before beginning drug therapy to identify if correct treatment has been initiated
- Assess for allergic reactions: rash, urticaria, pruritus, chills, fever, joint pain; angioedema may occur a few days after therapy begins; epinephrine and resuscitation equipment should be available for anaphylactic reaction
- Identify urine output; if decreasing, notify prescriber (may indicate nephrotoxicity); also check for increased BUN, creatinine
- Monitor blood studies: AST (SGOT), ALT (SGPT), CBC, Hct, bilirubin, LDH, alkaline phosphatase, Coombs' test monthly if patient is on long-term therapy
- Monitor electrolytes: potassium, sodium, chloride monthly if patient is on long-term therapy
- Assess bowel pattern qd; if severe diarrhea occurs, drug should be discontinued; may indicate pseudomembranous colitis
- Monitor for bleeding: ecchymosis, bleeding gums, hematuria, stool guaiac daily if on long-term therapy
- Assess for overgrowth of infection: perineal itching, fever, malaise, redness, pain, swelling, drainage, rash, diarrhea, change in cough, sputum

Nursing diagnoses

✓ Infection, risk for (uses)
✓ Diarrhea (side effects)
✓ Injury, risk for (side effects)
✓ Knowledge deficit (teaching)
✓ Noncompliance (teaching)

Implementation

- Check for irritation, extravasation, phlebitis daily; change site q72h
- For intermittent inf, reconstitute with sterile, bacteriostatic water for inj or 0.9% NaCl; may be further diluted with 0.9% NaCl, LR, D_5W (1-20 mg/ml); give over 30-60 min; may be refrigerated for 1 week or stored 24 hr at room temp

Additive compatibilities:
Famotidine, clindamycin, KCI

Patient/family education

- Teach patient to report sore throat, bruising, bleeding, joint pain, may indicate blood dyscrasias (rare)
- Advise patient to contact

prescriber if vaginal itching, loose, foul-smelling stools, furry tongue occur; may indicate superinfection
• Advise patient to notify prescriber of diarrhea with blood or pus, which may indicate pseudomembranous colitis

Evaluation

Positive therapeutic outcome
• Absence of signs/symptoms of infection (WBC <10,000, temp WNL, absence of red draining wounds)
• Reported improvement in symptoms of infection
• Negative C&S

Treatment of anaphylaxis: Epinephrine, antihistamines, resuscitate if needed

cefonicid (℞)
(se-fon′i-sid)
Monocid
Func. class.: Antibiotic
Chem. class.: Cephalosporin (2nd generation)
Pregnancy category B

Action: Inhibits bacterial cell wall synthesis, rendering cell wall osmotically unstable, leading to cell death

Therapeutic Outcome: Bactericidal effects for the following: gram-negative organisms *Morganella morganii, Proteus vulgaris, Providencia vettger, Haemophilus influenzae, Escherichia coli, Proteus mirabilis, Klebsiella;* gram-positive organisms *Streptococcus pneumoniae, S. pyogenes, Staphylococcus aureus*

Uses: Lower respiratory tract, urinary tract, skin, bone, joint infections; otitis media, peritonitis, septicemia, preoperative prophylaxis

Dosage and routes

Life-threatening infections

Adult: IM/**IV** bol or inf 1-2 g/24 hr; divide in 2 doses if giving 2 g

Dosage reduction indicated in renal impairment

Available forms: Inj 500 mg, 1, 10 g

Adverse effects

CNS: Headache, dizziness, weakness, paresthesia, fever, chills

GI: Nausea, vomiting, diarrhea, anorexia, pain, glossitis, ***bleeding;*** increased AST (SGOT), ALT (SGPT), bilirubin, LDH, alkaline phosphatase; abdominal pain, ***Pseudomembranous colitis***

GU: ***Proteinuria,*** vaginitis, pruritus, candidiasis, increased BUN, ***nephrotoxicity, renal failure***

HEMA: ***Leukopenia, thrombocytopenia, agranulocytosis,*** anemia, ***neutropenia, lymphocytosis, eosinophilia, pancytopenia, hemolytic anemia***

INTEG: Rash, urticaria, dermatitis

SYST: ***Anaphylaxis***

Contraindications: Hypersensitivity to cephalosporins, infants <1 mo

Precautions: Hypersensitivity to penicillins, pregnancy **B,** lactation, renal disease

Pharmacokinetics

Absorption	Well absorbed (IM)
Distribution	Widely distributed; crosses placenta
Metabolism	Not metabolized
Excretion	Kidneys, unchanged; enters breast milk
Half-life	4½ hr; increased in renal disease

Pharmacodynamics

	IM	IV
Onset	Rapid	5 min
Peak	1 hr	Infusion's end

Interactions

Individual drugs

Probenecid: ↓ excretion of drug and ↑ blood levels
Vancomycin: ↑ toxicity

Drug classifications

Aminoglycosides: ↑ toxicity

Lab test interferences

False ↑ Creatinine (serum urine), false ↑ urinary 17-KS
False positive: Urinary protein, direct Coombs' test, urine glucose
Interference: Cross-matching

NURSING CONSIDERATIONS

Assessment

- Assess patient for previous sensitivity reaction to penicillins or other cephalosporins; cross-sensitivity between penicillins and cephalosporins is common
- Assess patient for signs and symptoms of infection including characteristics of wounds, sputum, urine, stool, WBC >10,000, earache, fever; obtain baseline information and during treatment
- Obtain C&S before beginning drug therapy to identify if correct treatment has been initiated
- Assess for allergic reactions: rash, urticaria, pruritus, chills, fever, joint pain; angioedema may occur a few days after therapy begins; epinephrine and resuscitation equipment should be available for anaphylactic reaction
- Identify urine output; if decreasing, notify prescriber (may indicate nephrotoxicity); also check for increased BUN, creatinine
- Monitor blood studies: AST (SGOT), ALT (SGPT), CBC, Hct, bilirubin, LDH, alkaline phosphatase, Coombs' test monthly if patient is on long-term therapy
- Monitor electrolytes: potassium, sodium, chloride monthly if patient is on long-term therapy
- Assess bowel pattern qd; if severe diarrhea occurs, drug should be discontinued; may indicate pseudomembranous colitis
- Monitor for bleeding: ecchymosis, bleeding gums, hematuria, stool guaiac daily if on long-term therapy
- Assess for overgrowth of infection: perineal itching, fever, malaise, redness, pain, swelling, drainage, rash, diarrhea, change in cough, sputum

Nursing diagnoses

- ✓ Infection, risk for (uses)
- ✓ Injury, risk for (side effects)
- ✓ Diarrhea (side effects)
- ✓ Knowledge deficit (teaching)
- ✓ Noncompliance (teaching)

Implementation

IM route

- Reconstitute 500 mg/2 ml of sterile water for inj (220 mg/ml) or 1000 mg/2.5 ml (325 mg/ml)
- Give deep in large muscle mass, massage

IV IV route

- Check for irritation, extrava-

sation, phlebitis daily; change site q72h
- For direct **IV** give over 5 min
- For intermittent inf reconstituted sol should be further diluted in 50-100 ml D_5W, $D_{10}W$, D_5/LR, D_5/0.25% NaCl, D_5/0.45% NaCl, D_5/0.9% NaCl, 0.9% NaCl; or Ringer's, LR; give over 30 min; may be refrigerated up to 96 hr or stored 24 hr at room temp

Y-site incompatibilities: Hetastarch, sargramostim

Y-site compatibilities: Acyclovir, amifostine, aztreonam, teniposide, thiotepa

Additive incompatibility: Aminoglycosides

Additive incompatibility: Clindamycin

Patient/family education
- Teach patient to report sore throat, bruising, bleeding, joint pain; may indicate blood dyscrasias (rare)
- Advise patient to contact prescriber if vaginal itching, loose, foul-smelling stools, furry tongue occur; may indicate superinfection
- Advise patient to notify prescriber of diarrhea with blood or pus, which may indicate pseudomembranous colitis

Evaluation

Positive therapeutic outcome
- Absence of signs/symptoms of infection (WBC <10,000, temp WNL, absence of red draining wounds, earache)
- Reported improvement in symptoms of infection
- Negative C&S

Treatment of anaphylaxis: Epinephrine, antihistamines, resuscitate if needed

cefoperazone (℞)
(sef-oh-per'a-zone)
Cefobid
Func. class.: Broad-spectrum antibiotic
Chem. class.: Cephalosporin (3rd generation)
Pregnancy category B

Action: Inhibits bacterial cell wall synthesis, rendering cell wall osmotically unstable, leading to cell death

Therapeutic Outcome: Bactericidal effects for the following: gram-negative organisms *Acinetobacter, Morganella morganii, Neisseria gonorrhea, Proteus vulgaris;* gram-positive organisms *Staphylococci, Streptococci, Streptococci* (beta-hemolytic), *Streptococci pneumoniae, Haemophilus influenzae, Escherichia coli, Proteus mirabilis, Klebsiella, Enterobacter, Serratia, Citrobacter, Providencia, Pseudomonas aeruginosa;* anaerobes *Bacteroides, Clostridium, Eubacterium, Fusobacterium, Peptococcus, Peptostreptococcus*

Uses: Lower respiratory tract, urinary tract, skin, bone infections; bacterial septicemia, peritonitis, pelvic inflammatory disease (PID), endometritis

Dosage and routes
Decrease dose in hepatic/biliary disease

Mild/moderate infections
Adult: IM/**IV** 1-2 g q12h or 2-4 g/day in divided doses q8-12h

Severe infections
Adult: IM/**IV** 6-12 g/day divided in 2-4 equal doses

Available forms: Inj 1, 2 g

Adverse effects

CNS: Headache, dizziness, weakness, paresthesia, fever, chills

*GI: **Nausea, vomiting, diarrhea, anorexia,*** pain, glossitis, ***bleeding;*** increased AST (SGOT), ALT (SGPT), bilirubin, LDH, alkaline phosphatase; abdominal pain, ***pseudomembranous colitis***

*GU: **Proteinuria,*** vaginitis, pruritus, candidiasis, increased BUN, ***nephrotoxicity, renal failure***

*HEMA: **Leukopenia, thrombocytopenia, agranulocytosis,*** anemia, ***neutropenia, lymphocytosis, eosinophilia, pancytopenia, hemolytic anemia, bleeding, hypoprothrombinemia***

INTEG: Rash, urticaria, dermatitis

RESP: Dyspnea

*SYST: **Anaphylaxis***

Contraindications: Hypersensitivity to cephalosporins, P infants <1 mo

Precautions: Hypersensitivity to penicillins, pregnancy **B,** lactation, hepatic disease

Pharmacokinetics

Absorption	Well absorbed (IM)
Distribution	Widely distributed; crosses placenta
Metabolism	Not metabolized
Excretion	Bile; enters breast milk
Half-life	2 hr

Pharmacodynamics

	IM	IV
Onset	Rapid	5 min
Peak	1-2 hr	Infusion's end

Interactions

Individual drugs

Probenecid: ↓ excretion of drug and ↑ blood levels

Vancomycin: ↑ toxicity

Drug classifications

Aminoglycosides: ↑ toxicity

Anticoagulants: ↑ bleeding

Thrombolytics: ↑ bleeding

Lab test interferences

False ↑ Creatinine (serum urine), false ↑ urinary 17-KS

False positive: Urinary protein, direct Coombs' test, urine glucose

Interference: Cross-matching

NURSING CONSIDERATIONS

Assessment

- Assess patient for previous sensitivity reaction to penicillins or other cephalosporins; cross-sensitivity between penicillins and cephalosporins is common
- Assess patient for signs and symptoms of infection including characteristics of wounds, sputum, urine, stool, WBC >10,000, fever; obtain baseline information and during treatment
- Obtain C&S before beginning drug therapy to identify if correct treatment has been initiated
- Assess for allergic reactions: rash, urticaria, pruritus, chills, fever, joint pain; angioedema may occur a few days after therapy begins; epinephrine and resuscitation equipment should be available for anaphylactic reaction
- Identify urine output; if decreasing, notify prescriber (may indicate nephrotoxicity); also check for increased BUN, creatinine
- Monitor blood studies: AST (SGOT), ALT (SGPT), CBC, Hct, bilirubin, LDH, alkaline phosphatase, Coombs' test monthly if patient is on long-term therapy
- Monitor electrolytes: potas-

sium, sodium, chloride monthly if patient is on long-term therapy

• Assess bowel pattern qd; if severe diarrhea occurs, drug should be discontinued; may indicate pseudomembranous colitis

• Monitor for bleeding: ecchymosis, bleeding gums, hematuria, stool guaiac daily if on long-term therapy

• Assess for overgrowth of infection: perineal itching, fever, malaise, redness, pain, swelling, drainage, rash, diarrhea, change in cough, sputum

Nursing diagnoses

✓ Infection, risk for (uses)
✓ Injury, risk for (side effects)
✓ Diarrhea (side effects)
✓ Knowledge deficit (teaching)

Implementation

IM route

• Reconstitute 1 g/2.8 ml of sterile or bacteriostatic water for inj, or 2 g/5.4 ml; may be diluted further with 1 ml or 1.8 ml of 2% lidocaine to prevent pain; give deep in large muscle mass, massage

IV **IV route**

• Check for irritation, extravasation, phlebitis daily; change site q72h

• For intermittent inf, reconstituted sol should be further diluted 1 g/20-40 ml of 0.9% NaCl, D_5W, D_5/0.9% NaCl, D_5/LR, or LR; give over 15-30 min; may be refrigerated up to 96 hr or stored 24 hr at room temp

• For cont inf, final concentration is 2-25 mg/ml give at prescribed rate

Y-site incompatibilities: Gentamicin, hetastarch, labetalol, meperidine, ondansetron, perphenazine, sargramostim, tobramycin, vinorelbine tartrate

Y-site compatibilities: Acyclovir, allopurinol, aztreonam, cyclophosphamide, enalaprilat, esmolol, famotidine, foscarnet, fludarabine, hydromorphone, magnesium sulfate, melphalan, morphine, teniposide, thiotepa

Syringe incompatibility: Doxapram

Syringe compatibility: Heparin

Additive incompatibility: Aminoglycosides

Additive compatibilities: Cimetidine, clindamycin, furosemide

Patient/family education

• Teach patient to report sore throat, bruising, bleeding, joint pain, may indicate blood dyscrasias (rare)

• Advise patient to contact prescriber if vaginal itching, loose, foul-smelling stools, furry tongue occur; may indicate superinfection

• Advise patient to notify prescriber of diarrhea with blood or pus, which may indicate pseudomembranous colitis

Evaluation

Positive therapeutic outcome

• Absence of signs/symptoms of infection (WBC <10,000, temp WNL, absence of red draining wounds, pelvic pain)

• Reported improvement in symptoms of infection

• Negative C&S

Treatment of anaphylaxis: Epinephrine, antihistamines, resuscitate if needed

cefotetan (℞)

(sef'oh-tee-tan)

Cefotan

Func. class.: Broad-spectrum antibiotic

Chem. class.: Cephalosporin (2nd generation)

Pregnancy category B

Action: Inhibits bacterial cell wall synthesis, which renders cell osmotically unstable, leading to cell death

Therapeutic Outcome: Bactericidal effects for the following: gram-negative organisms *Haemophilus influenzae, Escherichia coli, Enterobacter aerogenes, Proteus mirabilis, Klebsiella, Morganella morganii, Proteus vulgaris, Providencia, Enterobacter, Salmonella, Shigella, Acinetobacter, Bacteroides fragilis, Neisseria, Serratia;* gram-positive organisms *Streptococcus pneumoniae, S. pyogenes, Staphylococcus aureus;* anaerobes *Bacteroides, Clostridium, Fusobacterium, Peptococcus, Peptostreptococcus*

Uses: Serious upper or lower respiratory tract, urinary tract, gynecologic, skin, bone, joint, gonococcal, intraabdominal infections

Dosages and routes

Reduce dose in renal disease

Adult: **IV**/IM 1-2g q12h × 5-10 days

Perioperative prophylaxis

Adult: **IV** 1-2 g ½-1 hr before surgery

Available forms: Inj 1, 2, 10 g

Adverse effects

CNS: Headache, dizziness, weakness, paresthesia, fever, chills

GI: Nausea, vomiting, diarrhea, anorexia, pain, glossitis, ***bleeding;*** increased AST (SGOT), ALT (SGPT), bilirubin, LDH, alkaline phosphatase; *pseudomembranous colitis*

GU: Proteinuria, vaginitis, pruritus, candidiasis, increased BUN, *nephrotoxicity, renal failure*

HEMA: Leukopenia, thrombocytopenia, agranulocytosis, anemia, *neutropenia, lymphocytosis, eosinophilia, pancytopenia, hemolytic anemia*

INTEG: Rash, urticaria, dermatitis

RESP: Dyspnea

SYST: Anaphylaxis

Contraindications: Hypersensitivity to cephalosporins, P children

Precautions: Hypersensitivity to penicillins, pregnancy **B,** lactation, renal disease

Pharmacokinetics

Absorption	Well absorbed (IM)
Distribution	Widely distributed; crosses placenta
Metabolism	Not metabolized
Excretion	Kidneys, unchanged; enters breast milk
Half-life	5 hr; increased in renal disease

Pharmacodynamics

	IM	IV
Onset	Rapid	Immediate
Peak	1-3 hr	Infusion's end

Interactions

Individual drugs

Probenecid: ↓ excretion of drug and ↑ blood levels

Vancomycin: ↑ toxicity

Drug classifications
Aminoglycosides: ↑ toxicity
Anticoagulants: ↑ bleeding
Thrombolytics: ↑ bleeding
Lab test interferences
False ↑ Creatinine (serum urine), ↑ false urinary 17-KS
False positive: Urinary protein, direct Coombs' test, urine glucose
Interference: Cross-matching

NURSING CONSIDERATIONS
Assessment
- Assess patient for previous sensitivity reaction to penicillins or other cephalosporins; cross-sensitivity between penicillins and cephalosporins is common
- Assess patient for signs and symptoms of infection including characteristics of wounds, sputum, urine, stool, WBC >10,000, fever; obtain baseline information and during treatment
- Obtain C&S before beginning drug therapy to identify if correct treatment has been initiated
- Assess for allergic reactions: rash, urticaria, pruritus, chills, fever, joint pain; angioedema may occur a few days after therapy begins; epinephrine and resuscitation equipment should be available for anaphylactic reaction
- Identify urine output; if decreasing, notify prescriber (may indicate nephrotoxicity); also check for increased BUN, creatinine
- Monitor blood studies: AST (SGOT), ALT (SGPT), CBC, Hct, bilirubin, LDH, alkaline phosphatase, Coombs' test monthly if patient is on long-term therapy
- Monitor electrolytes: potassium, sodium, chloride monthly if patient is on long-term therapy
- Assess bowel pattern qd; if severe diarrhea occurs, drug should be discontinued; may indicate pseudomembranous colitis
- Monitor for bleeding: ecchymosis, bleeding gums, hematuria, stool guaiac daily if on long-term therapy
- Assess for overgrowth of infection: perineal itching, fever, malaise, redness, pain, swelling, drainage, rash, diarrhea, change in cough, sputum

Nursing diagnoses
✓ Infection, risk for (uses)
✓ Injury, risk for (side effects)
✓ Diarrhea (side effects)
✓ Knowledge deficit (teaching)

Implementation
IM route
- Reconstitute 1 g/2ml or 2 g/3 ml of sterile or bacteriostatic water for inj; may be diluted with 0.5% of 1% lidocaine to prevent pain; give deep in large muscle mass, massage

IV **IV route**
- May be stored 96h refrigerated or 24h room temp
- Check for irritation, extravasation, phlebitis daily; change site q72h
- For direct **IV** dilute in 1 g/10 ml or more and give over 5 min
- For intermittent inf further dilute in 50-100 ml of 0.9% NaCl or D_5W; give over 3-5 min; discontinue primary line while running intermittent inf

Y-site compatibilities: Allopurinol, amifostine, aztreonam, diltiazem, famotidine, filgrastim, fluconazole, fludarabine, heparin, regular insulin, melphalan, meperidine, morphine, paclitaxel, sargramostim, tacrolimus, teniposide, theophylline, thiotepa

Syringe incompatibility: Doxapram

Additive incompatibilities: Aminoglycosides, tetracyclines, heparin

Patient/family education

- Teach patient to report sore throat, bruising, bleeding, joint pain; may indicate blood dyscrasias (rare)
- Advise patient to contact prescriber if vaginal itching, loose, foul-smelling stools, furry tongue occur; may indicate superinfection
- Advise patient to notify prescriber of diarrhea with blood or pus, which may indicate pseudomembranous colitis

Evaluation

Positive therapeutic outcome

- Absence of signs/symptoms of infection (WBC <10,000, temp WNL, absence of red draining wounds)
- Reported improvement in symptoms of infection
- Negative C&S

Treatment of anaphylaxis: Epinephrine, antihistamines, resuscitate if needed

cefoxitin (℞)

(se-fox'i-tin)

Mefoxin

Func. class.: Broad-spectrum antibiotic

Chem. class.: Cephalosporin (2nd generation)

Pregnancy category B

Action: Inhibits bacterial cell wall synthesis, rendering cell wall osmotically unstable, leading to cell death

Therapeutic Outcome: Bactericidal effects for the following: gram-negative bacilli *Haemophilus influenzae, Escherichia coli, Proteus, Klebsiella, Providencia, Neisseria gonorrhoeae;* gram-positive organisms *Streptococcus pneumoniae, S. pyogenes, Staphylococcus aureus;* anaerobes including *Clostridium, Bacteroides, Peptococcus, Peptostreptococcus*

Uses: Lower respiratory tract, urinary tract, skin, bone, gynecologic, gonococcal infections; septicemia, peritonitis

Dosage and routes

Adult: IM/**IV** 1-2 g q6-8h; dosage reduction indicated in renal impairment (CrCl <50 ml/min)

Uncomplicated gonorrhea

Adult: 2 g IM as single dose with 1 g PO probenecid at same time

Severe infections

Adult: IM/**IV** 2 g q4h

P ***Child ≥3 mo:*** IM/**IV** 80-160 mg/kg/day divided q4-6h; max 12 g/day

Available forms: Powder for inj 1, 2, 10 g

Adverse effects

CNS: Headache, dizziness, weakness, paresthesia, fever, chills

GI: Nausea, vomiting, diarrhea, anorexia, pain, glossitis, ***bleeding***; increased AST (SGOT), ALT (SGPT), bilirubin, LDH, alkaline phosphatase; abdominal pain

*GU: **Proteinuria***, vaginitis, pruritus, candidiasis, increased BUN, ***nephrotoxicity, renal failure***

*HEMA: **Leukopenia, thrombocytopenia, agranulocytosis***, anemia, ***neutropenia, lymphocytosis, eosinophilia, pancytopenia, hemolytic anemia***

INTEG: Rash, urticaria, dermatitis, thrombophlebitis

*SYST: **Anaphylaxis***

Contraindications: Hypersensitivity to cephalosporins; P infants <3 mo

Precautions: Hypersensitivity to penicillins, pregnancy **B**, lactation, renal disease

Pharmacokinetics

Absorption	Well absorbed (IM)
Distribution	Widely distributed; crosses placenta
Metabolism	Not metabolized
Excretion	Kidneys, unchanged; enters breast milk
Half-life	½-1 hr; increased in renal disease

Pharmacodynamics

	IM	IV
Onset	Rapid	Immediate
Peak	½ hr	Infusion's end

Interactions

Individual drugs

Probenecid: ↓ excretion of drug and ↑ blood levels

Vancomycin: ↑ toxicity

Drug classifications

Aminoglycosides: ↑ toxicity

Lab test interferences

False ↑ Creatinine (serum urine), false ↑ urinary 17-KS

False positive: Urinary protein, direct Coombs' test, urine glucose

Interference: Cross-matching

NURSING CONSIDERATIONS

Assessment

- Assess patient for previous sensitivity reaction to penicillins or other cephalosporins; cross-sensitivity between penicillins and cephalosporins is common
- Assess patient for signs and symptoms of infection including characteristics of wounds, sputum, urine, stool, WBC >10,000, fever; obtain baseline information and during treatment
- Obtain C&S before beginning drug therapy to identify if correct treatment has been initiated
- Assess for allergic reactions: rash, urticaria, pruritus, chills, fever, joint pain; angioedema may occur a few days after therapy begins; epinephrine and resuscitation equipment should be on unit for anaphylactic reaction
- Identify urine output; if decreasing, notify prescriber (may indicate nephrotoxicity); also check for increased BUN, creatinine
- Monitor blood studies. AST (SGOT), ALT (SGPT), CBC, Hct, bilirubin, LDH, alkaline phosphatase, Coombs' test monthly if patient is on long-term therapy
- Monitor electrolytes: potassium, sodium, chloride monthly if patient is on long-term therapy
- Assess bowel pattern qd; if

severe diarrhea occurs, drug should be discontinued; may indicate pseudomembranous colitis

- Monitor for bleeding: ecchymosis, bleeding gums, hematuria, stool guaiac daily if on long-term therapy
- Assess for overgrowth of infection: perineal itching, fever, malaise, redness, pain, swelling, drainage, rash, diarrhea, change in cough, sputum

Nursing diagnoses

- ✓ Infection, risk for (uses)
- ✓ Injury, risk for (side effects)
- ✓ Diarrhea (side effects)
- ✓ Knowledge deficit (teaching)

Implementation

IM route

- Reconstitute 1 g/2 ml of sterile water for inj; may be diluted with 0.5% or 1% lidocaine to prevent pain; give deep in large muscle mass, massage

IV **IV route**

- Check for irritation, extravasation, phlebitis daily; change site q72h
- For direct **IV**, dilute 1 g/10 ml or 2 g/20 ml sterile water for inj; shake, let stand until clear; give over 3-5 min
- For intermittent inf further dilute with 50-100 ml of D_5W, $D_{10}W$, D_5/0.25% NaCl, D_5/0.45% NaCl, D_5/0.9% NaCl, 0.9% NaCl, D_5/LR, D_5/0.02%, sodium bicarbonate, Ringer's, or LR; give over 15-30 min; may store 96h refrigerated or 24h room temp
- For cont inf dilute in 500-1000 ml; give at prescribed rate

Y-site incompatibility: Hetastarch

Y-site compatibilities: Acyclovir, amifostine, aztreonam, cyclophosphamide, diltiazem, famotidine, fluconazole, foscarnet, hydromorphone, magnesium sulfate, meperidine, morphine, ondansetron, perphenazine, teniposide, thiotepa

Additive compatibilities: Amikacin, cimetidine, clindamycin, gentamicin, kanamycin, multivitamins, sodium bicarbonate, tobramycin, verapamil, vitamin B complex with C

Additive incompatibility: Aztreonam

Syringe compatibility: Heparin, insulin

Patient/family education

- Teach patient to report sore throat, bruising, bleeding, joint pain; may indicate blood dyscrasias (rare)
- Advise patient to contact prescriber if vaginal itching, loose, foul-smelling stools, furry tongue occur; may indicate superinfection
- Advise patient to notify prescriber of diarrhea with blood or pus, which may indicate pseudomembranous colitis

Evaluation

Positive therapeutic outcome

- Absence of signs/symptoms of infection (WBC <10,000, temp WNL, absence of red draining wounds)
- Reported improvement in symptoms of infection
- Negative C&S

Treatment of anaphylaxis: Epinephrine, antihistamines, resuscitate if needed

cefpodoxime (℞)
(sef-poe-docks'eem)
Vantin
Func. class.: Antibiotic
Chem. class.: Cephalosporin (3rd generation)
Pregnancy category B

Action: Inhibits bacterial cell synthesis, which renders cell wall osmotically unstable, leading to cell death

Therapeutic Outcome: Bactericidal effects for the following: gram-negative organisms *Neisseria gonorrhoeae, Haemophilus influenzae, Escherichia coli, Proteus mirabilis, Klebsiella;* gram-positive organisms *Streptococcus pneumoniae, S. pyogenes, Staphylococcus aureus*

Uses: Upper and lower respiratory tract, urinary tract, skin infections; otitis media, sexually transmitted diseases

Dosage and routes

P Adult and child ≥13 yr

Pneumonia: 200 mg q12h × 14 days

Uncomplicated gonorrhea: 200 mg single dose

Skin and skin structure: 400 mg q12h × 7-14 days

Pharyngitis and tonsillitis: 100 mg q12h × 10 days

Uncomplicated UTI: 100 mg q12h × 7 days; dosing interval increased in presence of severe renal impairment

P Child (5 mo-12 yr):

Acute otitis media: 5 mg/kg q12h × 10 days

Pharyngitis/tonsillitis: 5 mg/kg q12h (max 100 mg/dose or 200 mg/day) × 5-10 days

Reduce dose in renal disease

Available forms: Tabs 100, 200 mg; granules for susp 50 mg, 100 mg/5 ml

Adverse effects

CNS: Headache, dizziness, lethargy, fatigue, paresthesia, fever, chills
GI: Nausea, vomiting, diarrhea, anorexia, pain, glossitis, ***bleeding;*** increased AST (SGOT), ALT (SGPT), bilirubin, LDH, alkaline phosphatase
GU: ***Proteinuria,*** vaginitis, pruritus, candidiasis, increased BUN, nephrotoxicity, renal failure
HEMA: Leukopenia, thrombocytopenia, agranulocytosis, anemia, neutropenia, lymphocytosis, eosinophilia, pancytopenia, hemolytic anemia
INTEG: Rash, urticaria, dermatitis
RESP: Dyspnea
SYST: ***Anaphylaxis***

Contraindications: Hypersensitivity to cephalosporins; P infants <5 mo

Precautions: Hypersensitivity to penicillins, pregnancy **B**, lactation, renal disease

Pharmacokinetics

Absorption	Well absorbed (PO)
Distribution	Widely distributed; crosses placenta
Metabolism	Not metabolized
Excretion	Kidneys, unchanged; enters breast milk
Half-life	2-3 hr, increased in renal disease

Pharmacodynamics	
	PO
Onset	Unknown
Peak	Unknown

Interactions

Individual drugs

Probenecid: ↓ excretion of drug and ↑ blood levels
Vancomycin: ↑ toxicity

Drug classifications

Aminoglycosides: ↑ toxicity
Anticoagulants: ↑ bleeding
Erythromycins: ↓ effects
Tetracyclines: ↓ effects
Thrombolytics: ↑ bleeding

Lab test interferences

False ↑ Creatinine (serum urine), false ↑ urinary 17-KS
False positive: Urinary protein, direct Coombs' test, urine glucose
Interference: Cross-matching

NURSING CONSIDERATIONS

Assessment

- Assess patient for previous sensitivity reaction to penicillins or other cephalosporins; cross-sensitivity between penicillins and cephalosporins is common
- Assess patient for signs and symptoms of infection including characteristics of wounds, sputum, urine, stool, WBC >10,000, earache, fever; obtain baseline information and during treatment
- Obtain C&S before beginning drug therapy to identify if correct treatment has been initiated
- Assess for allergic reactions: rash, urticaria, pruritus, chills, fever, joint pain; angioedema may occur a few days after therapy begins; epinephrine and resuscitation equipment should be available for anaphylactic reaction
- Identify urine output; if decreasing, notify prescriber (may indicate nephrotoxicity); also check for increased BUN, creatinine
- Monitor blood studies: AST (SGOT), ALT (SGPT), CBC, Hct, bilirubin, LDH, alkaline phosphatase, Coombs' test monthly if patient is on long-term therapy
- Monitor electrolytes: potassium, sodium, chloride monthly if patient is on long-term therapy
- Assess bowel pattern qd; if severe diarrhea occurs, drug should be discontinued; may indicate pseudomembranous colitis
- Monitor for bleeding: ecchymosis, bleeding gums, hematuria, stool guaiac daily if on long-term therapy
- Assess for overgrowth of infection: perineal itching, fever, malaise, redness, pain, swelling, drainage, rash, diarrhea, change in cough, sputum

Nursing diagnoses

✓ Infection, risk for (uses)
✓ Diarrhea (side effects)
✓ Injury, risk for (side effects)
✓ Knowledge deficit (teaching)
✓ Noncompliance (teaching)

Implementation

IM route

- Reconstitute 1 g/2 ml or 2 g/3 ml of sterile or bacteriostatic water for inj; may be diluted with 0.5% or 1% lidocaine to prevent pain; give deep in large muscle mass, massage

IV **IV route**

- Check for irritation, extravasation, phlebitis daily; change site q72h

- For direct **IV** dilute in 1 g/10 ml or more and give over 5 min
- For intermittent inf further dilute in 50-100 ml of 0.9% NaCl or D_5W; give over 3-5 min; discontinue primary line while running intermittent inf

Y-site compatibilities: Famotidine, fluconazole, fludarabine, regular insulin, meperidine, morphine, sargramostim

Syringe incompatibility: Doxapram

Additive incompatibility: Aminoglycosides, tetracyclines, heparin

Patient/family education

- Teach patient to report sore throat, bruising, bleeding, joint pain; may indicate blood dyscrasias (rare)
- Advise patient to contact physician if vaginal itching, loose, foul-smelling stools, furry tongue occur; may indicate superinfection
- Advise patient to notify prescriber of diarrhea with blood or pus, which may indicate pseudomembranous colitis

Evaluation

Positive therapeutic outcome

- Absence of signs/symptoms of infection (WBC <10,000, temp WNL, absence of red draining wounds, earache)
- Reported improvement in symptoms of infection
- Negative C&S

Treatment of anaphylaxis: Epinephrine, antihistamines, resuscitate if needed

cefprozil (℞)

(sef-pro'zil)

Cefzil

Func. class.: Antibiotic

Chem. class.: Cephalosporin (2nd generation)

Pregnancy category B

Action: Inhibits bacterial cell wall synthesis, which renders cell wall osmotically unstable, leading to cell death

→ **Therapeutic Outcome:** Bactericidal effects for the following: gram-negative bacilli *Haemophilus influenzae, Escherichia coli;* gram-positive organisms *Streptococcus pneumoniae, S. pyogenes, Staphylococcus aureus*

Uses: Upper and lower respiratory tract, urinary tract, skin infections; otitis media

Dosage and routes

Upper respiratory tract infections

Adult: PO 500 mg qd ×10 days

P ***Child (6 mo-12 yr):*** PO 15mg/kg q12h × 10 days

Lower respiratory tract infections

Adult: PO 500 mg q12h × 10 days

Skin/skin structure infections

Adult: PO 250-500mg q12h × 10 days

Reduce dose in renal disease

Available forms: Tabs 250, 500 mg; susp 125, 250 mg/5 ml

Adverse effects

CNS: Headache, dizziness,

C

lethargy, fatigue, paresthesia, fever, chills
GI: Nausea, vomiting, diarrhea, anorexia, pain, glossitis, ***bleeding;*** increased AST (SGOT), ALT (SGPT), bilirubin, LDH, alkaline phosphatase
GU: ***Proteinuria,*** vaginitis, pruritus, candidiasis, increased BUN, nephrotoxicity, renal failure
HEMA: ***Leukopenia, thrombocytopenia, agranulocytosis, anemia, neutropenia, lymphocytosis, eosinophilia, pancytopenia, hemolytic anemia***
INTEG: Rash, urticaria, dermatitis
RESP: Dyspnea
SYST: ***Anaphylaxis***

Contraindications: Hypersensitivity to cephalosporins; P infants

Precautions: Hypersensitivity to penicillins, pregnancy **B,** lactation, renal disease

Pharmacokinetics

Absorption	Well absorbed (PO)
Distribution	Widely distributed; crosses placenta
Metabolism	Not metabolized
Excretion	Kidneys, unchanged; enters breast milk
Half-life	1-1½ hr; increased in renal disease

Pharmacodynamics

	PO
Onset	Unknown
Peak	Unknown

Interactions

Individual drugs

Probenecid: ↓ excretion of drug and ↑ blood levels
Vancomycin: ↑ toxicity

Drug classifications

Aminoglycosides: ↑ toxicity
Anticoagulants: ↑ bleeding
Thrombolytics: ↑ bleeding

Lab test interferences

False ↑ Creatinine (serum urine), false ↑ urinary 17-KS
False positive: Urinary protein, direct Coombs' test, urine glucose
Interference: Cross-matching

NURSING CONSIDERATIONS

Assessment

- Assess patient for previous sensitivity reaction to penicillins or other cephalosporins; cross-sensitivity between penicillins and cephalosporins is common
- Assess patient for signs and symptoms of infection including characteristics of wounds, sputum, urine, stool, WBC >10,000, earache, fever; obtain baseline information and during treatment
- Obtain C&S before beginning drug therapy to identify if correct treatment has been initiated
- Assess for allergic reactions: rash, urticaria, pruritus, chills, fever, joint pain; angioedema may occur a few days after therapy begins; epinephrine and resuscitation equipment should be available for anaphylactic reaction
- ❗ Identify urine output; if decreasing, notify prescriber (may indicate nephrotoxicity); also check for increased BUN, creatinine
- Monitor blood studies: AST (SGOT), ALT (SGPT), CBC, Hct, bilirubin, LDH, alkaline phosphatase, Coombs' test monthly if patient is on long-term therapy
- Monitor electrolytes: potassium, sodium, chloride monthly if patient is on long-term therapy

• Assess bowel pattern qd; if severe diarrhea occurs, drug should be discontinued; may indicate pseudomembranous colitis
• Monitor for bleeding: ecchymosis, bleeding gums, hematuria, stool guaiac daily if on long-term therapy
• Assess for overgrowth of infection: perineal itching, fever, malaise, redness, pain, swelling, drainage, rash, diarrhea, change in cough, sputum

Nursing diagnoses

✓ Infection, risk for (uses)
✓ Diarrhea (side effects)
✓ Injury, risk for (side effects)
✓ Knowledge deficit (teaching)
✓ Noncompliance (teaching)

Implementation

IM route

• Reconstitute 1 g/2 ml or 2 g/3 ml of sterile or bacteriostatic water for inj; may be diluted with 0.5% or 1% lidocaine to prevent pain; give deep in large muscle mass, massage

IV **IV** route

• Check for irritation, extravasation, phlebitis daily, change site q72h
• For direct **IV** dilute 1 g/10 ml or more and give over 5 min
• For intermittent inf further dilute in 50-100 ml of 0.9% NaCl or D_5W; give over 3-5 min; discontinue primary line while running intermittent infusion

Y-site compatibilities: Famotidine, fluconazole, fludarabine, regular insulin, meperidine, morphine, sargramostim

Syringe incompatibility: Doxapram

Additive incompatibilities: Aminoglycosides, tetracyclines, heparin

Patient/family education

• Teach patient to report sore throat, bruising, bleeding, joint pain; may indicate blood dyscrasias (rare)
• Advise patient to contact prescriber if vaginal itching, loose, foul-smelling stools, furry tongue occur; may indicate superinfection
• Advise patient to notify prescriber of diarrhea with blood or pus, which may indicate pseudomembranous colitis

Evaluation

Positive therapeutic outcome

• Absence of signs/symptoms of infection (WBC <10,000, temp WNL, absence of red draining wounds, earache)
• Reported improvement in symptoms of infection
• Negative C&S

Treatment of anaphylaxis: Epinephrine, antihistamines, resuscitate if needed

ceftazidime (℞)

(sef'ta-zi-deem)

Ceptaz, Fortaz, Pentacef, Tazicef, Tazidine

Func. class.: Broad-spectrum antibiotic

Chem. class.: Cephalosporin (3rd generation)

Pregnancy category B

Action: Inhibits bacterial cell wall synthesis, which renders cell osmotically unstable, leading to cell death

➔ **Therapeutic Outcome:** Bactericidal effects for the

following: gram-negative organisms: *Haemophilus influenzae, Escherichia coli, Enterobacter aerogenes, Proteus mirabilis, Klebsiella, Citrobacter, Enterobacter, Pseudomonas aeruginosa, Shigella, Acinetobacter, Bacteroides fragilis, Neisseria;* gram-positive organisms *Streptococcus pneumoniae, S. pyogenes, Staphylococcus aureus*

Uses: Serious upper or lower respiratory tract, urinary tract, skin, gynecologic, bone, joint, intraabdominal infections; septicemia, meningitis

Dosage and routes
Adult: **IV**/IM 1-2 g q8-12h × 5-10 days

P ***Children:*** **IV** 30-50 mg/kg/q8h, not to exceed 6 g/day

P ***Neonates:*** **IV** 30 mg/kg q12h

Reduce dose in renal disease

Available forms: Inj 1, 2 g

Adverse effects
CNS: Headache, dizziness, weakness, paresthesia, fever, chills
GI: Nausea, vomiting, diarrhea, anorexia, metallic taste, pain, glossitis, ***bleeding;*** increased AST (SGOT), ALT (SGPT), bilirubin, LDH, alkaline phosphatase; ***Pseudomembranous colitis***
GU: ***Proteinuria,*** vaginitis, pruritus, candidiasis, increased BUN, ***nephrotoxicity, renal failure***
HEMA: ***Leukopenia, thrombocytopenia, agranulocytosis,*** anemia, ***neutropenia, lymphocytosis, eosinophilia, pancytopenia, hemolytic anemia***
INTEG: Rash, urticaria, dermatitis
RESP: Dyspnea
SYST: ***Anaphylaxis***

Contraindications: Hypersensitivity to cephalosporins

Precautions: Hypersensitivity to penicillins, pregnancy **B,** lactation, renal disease

Pharmacokinetics

Absorption	Well absorbed (IM)
Distribution	Widely distributed; crosses placenta
Metabolism	Not metabolized
Excretion	Kidneys, unchanged; enters breast milk
Half-life	½-1 hr; increased in renal disease

Pharmacodynamics

	IM	IV
Onset	Rapid	Immediate
Peak	1 hr	Infusion's end

Interactions
Individual drugs
Probenecid: ↓ excretion of drug and ↑ blood levels
Vancomycin: ↑ toxicity
Drug classifications
Aminoglycosides: ↑ toxicity
Erythromycins: ↓ effects
Tetracyclines: ↓ effects
Lab test interferences
False ↑ Creatinine (serum urine), false ↑ urinary 17-KS
False positive: Urinary protein, direct Coombs' test, urine glucose
Interference: Cross-matching

NURSING CONSIDERATIONS
Assessment

- Assess patient for previous sensitivity reaction to penicillins or other cephalosporins; cross-sensitivity between penicillins and cephalosporins is common
- Assess patient for signs and symptoms of infection includ-

ing characteristics of wounds, sputum, urine, stool, WBC >10,000, temperature; obtain baseline information and during treatment

- Obtain C&S before beginning drug therapy to identify if correct treatment has been initiated
- Assess for allergic reactions: rash, urticaria, pruritus, chills, fever, joint pain; angioedema may occur a few days after therapy begins; epinephrine and resuscitation equipment should be available for anaphylactic reaction
- Identify urine output; if decreasing, notify prescriber (may indicate nephrotoxicity); also check for increased BUN, creatinine
- Monitor blood studies: AST (SGOT), ALT (SGPT), CBC, Hct, bilirubin, LDH, alkaline phosphatase, Coombs' test monthly if patient is on long-term therapy
- Monitor electrolytes: potassium, sodium, chloride monthly if patient is on long-term therapy
- Assess bowel pattern qd; if severe diarrhea occurs, drug should be discontinued; may indicate pseudomembranous colitis
- Monitor for bleeding: ecchymosis, bleeding gums, hematuria, stool guaiac daily if on long-term therapy
- Assess for overgrowth of infection: perineal itching, fever, malaise, redness, pain, swelling, drainage, rash, diarrhea, change in cough, sputum

Nursing diagnoses

✓ Infection, risk for (uses)
✓ Injury, risk for (side effects)
✓ Diarrhea (side effects)
✓ Knowledge deficit (teaching)

Implementation

IM route

- Reconstitute 500 mg/1.5 ml or 1 g/3 ml of sterile or bacteriostatic water for inj; may be diluted with 0.5% or 1% lidocaine to prevent pain; give deep in large muscle mass, massage

IV **IV route**

- Check for irritation, extravasation, phlebitis daily; change site q72h
- For direct **IV** dilute 500 mg/5 ml or 1 g/10 ml sterile water for inj; give over 3-5 min; do not use sol with benzyl alcohol for neonates P
- For intermittent inf further dilute 1 g/10 ml or more 0.9% NaCl, D_5W, $D_{10}W$, D_5/0.25% NaCl, D_5/0.45% NaCl, D_5/ 0.9% NaCl, or LR; give over 30-60 min
- Store for 96h refrigerated, 24h room temp

Y-site incompatibilities: Amsacrine, fluconazole, sargramostim, idarubicin

Y-site compatibilities: Acyclovir, allopurinol, amifostine, aztreonam, ciprofloxacin, diltiazem, enalaprilat, esmolol, famotidine, filgrastim, fludarabine, foscarnet, granisetron, heparin, hydromorphone, labetalol, meperidine, melphalan, morphine, ondansetron, paclitaxel, rantidine, tacrolimus, teniposide, theophylline, thiotepa, vinorelbine tartrate, zidovudine

Additive incompatibilities: Aminoglycosides, sodium bicarbonate

Additive compatibilities: Ciprofloxacin, clindamycin,

fluconazole, metronidazole, ofloxacin,

Patient/family education

• Teach patient to report sore throat, bruising, bleeding, joint pain; may indicate blood dyscrasias (rare)
• Advise patient to contact prescriber if vaginal itching, loose, foul-smelling stools, furry tongue occur; may indicate superinfection
• Advise patient to notify prescriber of diarrhea with blood or pus, which may indicate pseudomembranous colitis

Evaluation

Positive therapeutic outcome

• Absence of signs/symptoms of infection (WBC <10,000, temp WNL, absence of red draining wounds, earache)
• Reported improvement in symptoms of infection
• Negative C&S

Treatment of anaphylaxis: Epinephrine, antihistamines, resuscitate if needed

ceftibuten (℞)

(sef-ti-byoo'tin)

Cedax

Func. class.: Antibiotic

Chem. class.: Cephalosporin

Pregnancy category B

Action: Inhibits bacterial cell wall synthesis, which renders cell wall osmotically unstable, leading to cell death

Therapeutic Outcome: Bactericidal effects for the following: gram-negative bacilli *Haemophilus influenzae, Escherichia coli;* gram-positive organisms *Streptococcus pneumoniae, S. pyogenes, Staphylococcus aureus*

Uses: Upper and lower respiratory tract infections; otitis media

Dosage and routes

Adult: PO 400 mg qd × 10 days

P ***Child*** 6 mo-12 yr: PO 9 mg/kg qd × 10 days

Available forms: Caps 400 mg; susp 90, 180 mg/5 ml

Adverse effects

CNS: Headache, dizziness, lethargy, fatigue, paresthesia, fever, chills

GI: Nausea, vomiting, diarrhea, anorexia, pain, glossitis, bleeding, increased AST (SGOT), ALT (SGPT), bilirubin, LDH, alkaline phosphatase

GU: Proteinuria, vaginitis, pruritus, candidiasis; increased BUN; nephrotoxicity, renal failure

HEMA: ***Leukopenia, thrombocytopenia, agranulocytosis, anemia, neutropenia, lymphocytosis, eosinophilia, pancytopenia, hemolytic anemia***

INTEG: Rash, urticaria, dermatitis

RESP: Dyspnea

SYST: Anaphylaxis

Contraindications: Hypersensitivity to cephalosporins; P infants

Precautions: Hypersensitivity to penicillins, pregnancy **B,** lactation, renal disease

Pharmacokinetics	
Absorption	Well absorbed
Distribution	Widely distributed; crosses placenta
Metabolism	Not metabolized
Excretion	Kidneys, unchanged; enters breast milk
Half-life	1-1½ hr; increased in renal disease

Pharmacodynamics

Onset	Unknown
Peak	Unknown

Interactions
Individual drugs
Probenecid: ↓ excretion of drug and ↑ blood levels
Vancomycin: ↑ toxicity
Drug classifications
Aminoglycosides: ↑ toxicity
Anticoagulants: ↑ bleeding
Thrombolytics: ↑ bleeding
Lab test interferences
False ↑ Creatinine (serum urine), false ↑ urinary 17-KS
False positive: Urinary protein, direct Coombs' test, urine glucose
Interference: Cross-matching

NURSING CONSIDERATIONS
Assessment
- Assess patient for previous sensitivity reaction to penicillins or other cephalosporins; cross-sensitivity between penicillins and cephalosporins is common
- Assess patient for signs and symptoms of infection including characteristics of wounds, sputum, urine, stool, WBC >10,000, earache, fever; obtain baseline information and during treatment
- Obtain C&S before beginning drug therapy to identify if correct treatment has been initiated
- Assess for allergic reactions: rash, urticaria, pruritus, chills, fever, joint pain; angioedema may occur a few days after therapy begins; epinephrine and resuscitation equipment should be available for anaphylactic reaction
- Identify urine output; if decreasing, notify prescriber (may indicate nephrotoxicity); also check for increased BUN, creatinine
- Monitor blood studies: AST (SGOT), ALT (SGPT), CBC, Hct, bilirubin, LDH, alkaline phosphatase, Coombs' test monthly if patient is on long-term therapy
- Monitor electrolytes: potassium, sodium, chloride monthly if patient is on long-term therapy
- Assess bowel pattern qd; if severe diarrhea occurs, drug should be discontinued; may indicate pseudomembranous colitis
- Monitor for bleeding: ecchymosis, bleeding gums, hematuria, stool guaiac daily if on long-term therapy
- Assess for overgrowth of infection; perineal itching, fever, malaise, redness, pain, swelling, drainage, rash, diarrhea, change in cough, sputum

Nursing diagnoses
- ✓ Infection, risk for (uses)
- ✓ Diarrhea (side effects)
- ✓ Injury, risk for (side effects)
- ✓ Knowledge deficit (teaching)
- ✓ Noncompliance (teaching)

Implementation
- Administer for 10 days to ensure organism death, prevent superimposed infection
- Administer after C&S

Patient/family education
- Teach patient to report sore throat, bruising, bleeding, joint pain; may indicate blood dyscrasias (rare)
- Advise patient to contact prescriber if vaginal itching, loose foul-smelling stools, furry tongue occur; may indicate superinfection
- Advise patient to notify prescriber of diarrhea with

blood or pus, may indicate pseudomembranous colitis

Evaluation

Positive therapeutic outcome

- Absence of signs/symptoms of infection (WBC <10,000, temp WNL, absence of red draining wounds, earache)
- Reported improvement in symptoms of infection

Treatment of anaphylaxis: Epinephrine, antihistamines, resuscitate if needed

ceftizoxime (℞)

(sef-ti-zox'eem)

Cefizox

Func. class.: Broad-spectrum antibiotic

Chem. class.: Cephalosporin (3rd generation)

Pregnancy category B

Action: Inhibits bacterial cell wall synthesis, which renders cell wall osmotically unstable, leading to cell death

➔ **Therapeutic Outcome:** Bactericidal effects for the following: gram-negative organisms *Haemophilus influenzae, Escherichia coli, Enterobacter aerogenes, Proteus mirabilis, Klebsiella, Acinetobacter, Neisseria gonorrhea, Providencia rettgeri, Pseudomonas aeruginosa, Serratia, Enterobacter;* gram-positive organisms *Streptococcus pneumoniae, S. pyogenes, Staphylococcus aureus;* anaerobes *Bacteroides, Peptococcus, Peptostreptococcus*

Uses: Serious lower respiratory tract, urinary tract, skin, intraabdominal infections; septicemia, meningitis; bone, joint infections; pelvic inflammatory disease (PID) caused by *Neisseria gonorrhoeae*

Dosage and routes

Reduce dose in renal disease

Adult: IM/**IV** 1-2 g q8-12h; may give up to 2 g q4h in life-threatening infections

Child <6 mo: IM/**IV** 50 mg/kg q6-8h, max is adult dose

Pelvic inflammatory disease

Adult: **IV** 2 g q8h; may increase to 2 g q4h in severe infections

Available forms: Inj 500 mg, 1, 2 g/100 ml piggyback, 50 ml/5% D_5

Adverse effects

CNS: Headache, dizziness, paresthesia, fever

GI: Nausea, vomiting, diarrhea, anorexia, pain, glossitis, ***bleeding;*** increased AST (SGOT), ALT (SGPT), bilirubin, LDH, alkaline phosphatase; abdominal pain, ***pseudomembranous colitis***

GU: ***Proteinuria,*** vaginitis, pruritus, candidiasis

HEMA: ***Leukopenia, thrombocytopenia, agranulocytosis,*** anemia, ***neutropenia, eosinophilia, hemolytic anemia***

INTEG: Rash, urticaria, dermatitis

RESP: Dyspnea

SYST: ***Anaphylaxis***

Contraindications: Hypersensitivity to cephalosporins, P infants <1 mo

Precautions: Hypersensitivity to penicillins, pregnancy **B,** lactation, renal disease

Pharmacokinetics	
Absorption	Well absorbed (IM)
Distribution	Widely distributed; crosses placenta
Metabolism	Not metabolized
Excretion	Kidneys, unchanged; enters breast milk
Half-life	1½-2 hr; increased in renal disease

Pharmacodynamics	IM	IV
Onset	Rapid	Immediate
Peak	1 hr	Infusion's end

Interactions

Individual drugs

Probenecid: ↓ excretion of drug and ↑ blood levels

Vancomycin: ↑ toxicity

Drug classifications

Aminoglycosides: ↑ toxicity

Lab test interferences

False ↑ Creatinine (serum urine), false ↑ urinary 17-KS

False positive: Urinary protein, direct Coombs' test, urine glucose

Interference: Cross-matching

NURSING CONSIDERATIONS

Assessment

- Assess patient for previous sensitivity reaction to penicillins or other cephalosporins; cross-sensitivity between penicillins and cephalosporins is common
- Assess patient for signs and symptoms of infection including characteristics of wounds, sputum, urine, stool, WBC >10,000, fever; obtain baseline information and during treatment
- Obtain C&S before beginning drug therapy to identify if correct treatment has been initiated
- Assess for allergic reactions: rash, urticaria, pruritus, chills, fever, joint pain; angioedema may occur a few days after therapy begins; epinephrine and resuscitation equipment should be on unit for anaphylactic reaction
- Identify urine output; if decreasing, notify prescriber (may indicate nephrotoxicity); also check for increased BUN, creatinine
- Monitor blood studies: AST (SGOT), ALT (SGPT), CBC, Hct, bilirubin, LDH, alkaline phosphatase, Coombs' test monthly if patient is on long-term therapy
- Monitor electrolytes: potassium, sodium, chloride monthly if patient is on long-term therapy
- Assess bowel pattern qd; if severe diarrhea occurs, drug should be discontinued; may indicate pseudomembranous colitis
- Monitor for bleeding: ecchymosis, bleeding gums, hematuria, stool guaiac daily if on long-term therapy
- Assess for overgrowth of infection: perineal itching, fever, malaise, redness, pain, swelling, drainage, rash, diarrhea, change in cough, sputum

Nursing diagnoses

- ✓ Infection, risk for (uses)
- ✓ Diarrhea (side effects)
- ✓ Injury, risk for (side effects)
- ✓ Knowledge deficit (teaching)
- ✓ Noncompliance (teaching)

Implementation

IM route

- Reconstitute 250 mg/0.9 ml, 500 mg/1.8 ml, 1 g/3.6 ml, 2 g/7.2 ml; may be diluted with 0.5% or 1% lidocaine to prevent pain; give deep in large muscle mass, massage

IV IV route

- Check for irritation, extravasation, phlebitis daily; change site q72h

• For intermittent inf reconstitute 250 mg/2.4 ml, 500 mg/4.8 ml, 1 gm/9.6 mg/2 gm/19.2 ml sterile water for inj, D_5W, or 0.9% NaCl; do not use sol with benzyl alcohol for neonates; may be further diluted in 50-100 ml D_5W, $D_{10}W$, 0.9% NaCl, or LR; give over 30-60 min

• May store 96h refrigerated, 24h room temp

Y-site compatibilities: Acyclovir, allopurinol, amifostine, aztreonam, enalaprilat, esmolol, famotidine, fludarabine, foscarnet, hydromorphone, labetalol, melphalan, meperidine, morphine, ondansetron, sargramostim, teniposide, thiotepa, vinorelbine

Additive incompatibility: Aminoglycosides

Additive compatibilities: Clindamycin, metronidazole

Patient/family education

• Teach patient to report sore throat, bruising, bleeding, joint pain; may indicate blood dyscrasias (rare)

• Advise patient to contact prescriber if vaginal itching, loose, foul-smelling stools, furry tongue occur; may indicate superinfection

• Advise patient to notify prescriber of diarrhea with blood or pus, which may indicate pseudomembranous colitis

Evaluation

Positive therapeutic outcome

• Absence of signs/symptoms of infection (WBC <10,000, temp WNL, absence of red draining wounds)

• Reported improvement in symptoms of infection

• Negative C&S

Treatment of anaphylaxis: Epinephrine, antihistamines, resuscitate if needed

ceftriaxone (℞)

(sef-try-ax'one)

Rocephin

Func. class.: Broad spectrum antibiotic

Chem. class.: Cephalosporin (3rd generation)

Pregnancy category B

Action: Inhibits bacterial cell wall synthesis, which renders cell wall osmotically unstable, leading to cell death

Uses: Serious lower respiratory tract, urinary tract, skin, gonococcal, intraabdominal infections; septicemia, meningitis; bone, joint infections

Therapeutic Outcome: Bactericidal effects on the following: gram-negative organisms *Haemophilus influenzae, Escherichia coli, Enterobacter aerogenes, Proteus mirabilis, Klebsiella, Citrobacter, Enterobacter, Pseudomonas aeruginosa, Neisseria, Serratia;* gram-positive organisms *Streptococcus pneumoniae, S. pyogenes, Staphylococcus aureus;* anaerobes *Bacteroides*

Dosage and routes

Adult: IM/**IV** 1-2 g qd, max 2 g q12h

Child: IM/**IV** 50-75 mg/kg/day in equal doses q12h

Uncomplicated gonorrhea
Adult: 250 mg IM as single dose

Dosage reduction may be indicated in severe renal impairment (CrCl <50 ml/min)

Meningitis
P ***Adult and child:*** IM/**IV** 100 mg/kg/day in equal doses q12h, max 4 g/day

Surgical prophylaxis
Adult: **IV** 1 g ½-2 hr preop

Available forms: Inj 250, 500 mg, 1, 2, 10 g

Adverse effects
CNS: Headache, dizziness, weakness, paresthesia, fever, chills
GI: Nausea, vomiting, diarrhea, anorexia, pain, glossitis, ***bleeding;*** increased AST (SGOT), ALT (SGPT), bilirubin, LDH, alkaline phosphatase; abdominal pain, ***pseudomembranous colitis***
GU: ***Proteinuria,*** vaginitis, pruritus, candidiasis, increased BUN, ***nephrotoxicity, renal failure***
HEMA: ***Leukopenia, thrombocytopenia, agranulocytosis,*** anemia, ***neutropenia, lymphocytosis, eosinophilia, pancytopenia, hemolytic anemia***
INTEG: Rash, urticaria, dermatitis
RESP: Dyspnea
SYST: ***Anaphylaxis***

Contraindications: Hypersensitivity to cephalosporins,
P infants <1 mo

Precautions: Hypersensitivity to penicillins, pregnancy **B,** lactation, renal disease

Pharmacokinetics

Absorption	Well absorbed
Distribution	Widely distributed; crosses placenta; enters CSF
Metabolism	Liver
Excretion	Kidneys, partly
Half-life	5-8 hr

Pharmacodynamics

	IM	IV
Onset	Rapid	Immediate
Peak	1 hr	Infusion's end

Interactions
Individual drugs
Probenecid: ↓ excretion of drug and ↑ blood levels
Vancomycin: ↑ toxicity
Drug classifications
Aminoglycosides: ↑ toxicity
Lab test interferences
False ↑ Creatinine (serum urine), false ↑ urinary 17-KS
False positive: Urinary protein, direct Coombs' test, urine glucose
Interference: Cross-matching

NURSING CONSIDERATIONS
Assessment
- Assess patient for previous sensitivity reaction to penicillins or other cephalosporins; cross-sensitivity between penicillins and cephalosporins is common
- Assess patient for signs and symptoms of infection including characteristics of wounds, sputum, urine, stool, WBC >10,000, fever; obtain baseline information and during treatment
- Obtain C&S before beginning drug therapy to identify if correct treatment has been initiated
- Assess for allergic reactions: rash, urticaria, pruritus, chills, fever, joint pain; angioedema may occur a few days after

therapy begins; epinephrine and resuscitation equipment should be available for anaphylactic reaction

- Identify urine output; if decreasing, notify prescriber (may indicate nephrotoxicity); also check for increased BUN, creatinine
- Monitor blood studies: AST (SGOT), ALT (SGPT), CBC, Hct, bilirubin, LDH, alkaline phosphatase, Coombs' test monthly if patient is on long-term therapy
- Monitor electrolytes: potassium, sodium, chloride monthly if patient is on long-term therapy
- Assess bowel pattern qd; if severe diarrhea occurs, drug should be discontinued; may indicate pseudomembranous colitis
- Monitor for bleeding: ecchymosis, bleeding gums, hematuria, stool guaiac daily if on long-term therapy
- Assess for overgrowth of infection: perineal itching, fever, malaise, redness, pain, swelling, drainage, rash, diarrhea, change in cough, sputum

Nursing diagnoses

- ✓ Infection, risk for (uses)
- ✓ Injury, risk for (side effects)
- ✓ Diarrhea (side effects)
- ✓ Knowledge deficit (teaching)

Implementation

IM route

- Reconstitute 250 mg/0.9 ml, 500 mg/1.8 ml, 1 g/3.6 ml, 2 g/7.2 ml; may be diluted with 0.5% or 1% lidocaine to prevent pain; give deep in large muscle mass, massage

IV route

- Check for irritation, extravasation, phlebitis daily; change site q72h
- For intermittent inf reconstitute 250 mg/2.4 ml, 500 mg/4.8 ml, 1 g/9.6 ml/2 g/19.2 ml sterile water for inj, D_5W, 0.9% NaCl; do not use sol with benzyl alcohol for neonates; may be further diluted in 50-100 ml D_5W, $D_{10}W$, 0.9% NaCl; or LR; give over 30-60 min
- Store for 96h refrigerated, 24h room temp

Y-site incompatibilities: Amsacrine, fluconazole, vancomycin

Y-site compatibilities: Acyclovir, allopurinol, amifostine, aztreonam, diltiazem, fludarabine, foscarnet, heparin, melphalan, meperidine, methotrexate, morphine, paclitaxel, sargramostim, tacrolimus, teniposide, theophylline, thiotepa, vinorelbine, zidovudine

Additive incompatibilities: Aminoglycosides, clindamycin

Additive compatibilities: Amino acids or sodium bicarbonate, metronidazole

Patient/family education

- Teach patient to report sore throat, bruising, bleeding, joint pain; may indicate blood dyscrasias (rare)
- Advise patient to contact prescriber if vaginal itching, loose, foul-smelling stools, furry tongue occur; may indicate superinfection
- Advise patient to notify prescriber of diarrhea with blood or pus, which may indicate pseudomembranous colitis

Evaluation

Positive therapeutic outcome

- Absence of signs/symptoms of infection (WBC <10,000,

temp WNL, absence of red draining wounds)
- Reported improvement in symptoms of infection
- Negative C&S

Treatment of anaphylaxis: Epinephrine, antihistamines, resuscitate if needed

cephalexin (℞)

(sef-a-lex'in)

Apo-Cephalex ✤, Keftab, Biocef, cephalexin, Ceporex ✤, Keflex, Novolexin ✤

Func. class.: Antibiotic

Chem. class.: Cephalosporin (1st generation)

Pregnancy category B

Action: Inhibits bacterial cell wall synthesis, rendering cell wall osmotically unstable, leading to cell death

Therapeutic Outcome: Bactericidal effects of the following: gram-negative organisms *Haemophilus influenzae, Escherichia coli, Proteus mirabilis, Klebsiella;* gram-positive organisms *Streptococcus pneumoniae, S. pyogenes, Staphylococcus aureus*

Uses: Upper, lower respiratory tract, urinary tract, skin, bone infections; otitis media

Dosage and routes

Adult: PO 250-500 mg q6h

P ***Child:*** PO 25-50 mg/kg/day in 4 equal doses

Moderate skin infections

500 mg q12h

Severe infections

Adult: PO 500 mg-1 g q6h

P ***Child:*** PO 50-100 mg/kg/day in 4 equal doses

Dosage reduction indicated in renal impairment (CrCl <50 ml/min)

Available forms: Caps 250, 500 mg; tabs 250, 500, 1000 mg; oral susp 125, 250 mg/5 ml

Adverse effects

CNS: Headache, dizziness, weakness, paresthesia, fever, chills

GI: Nausea, vomiting, diarrhea, anorexia, pain, glossitis, ***bleeding;*** increased AST (SGOT), ALT (SGPT), biliru bin, LDH, alkaline phosphatase; abdominal pain, ***pseudomembranous colitis***

GU: ***Proteinuria,*** vaginitis, pruritus, candidiasis, increased BUN, ***nephrotoxicity, renal failure***

HEMA: ***Leukopenia, thrombocytopenia, agranulocytosis,*** anemia, ***neutropenia, lymphocytosis, eosinophilia, pancytopenia, hemolytic anemia***

INTEG: Rash, urticaria, dermatitis

RESP: Dyspnea

SYST: ***Anaphylaxis***

Contraindications: Hypersensitivity to cephalosporins,
P infants <1 mo

Precautions: Hypersensitivity to penicillins, pregnancy **B**, lactation, renal disease

Pharmacokinetics	
Absorption	Well absorbed
Distribution	Widely distributed; crosses placenta
Metabolism	Not metabolized
Excretion	Kidneys, unchanged; enters breast milk
Half-life	½-1 hr; increased in renal disease

Pharmacodynamics

Onset	15-30 min
Peak	1 hr

Interactions
Individual drugs
Probenecid: ↓ excretion of drug and ↑ blood levels
Vancomycin: ↑ toxicity
Drug classifications
Aminoglycosides: ↑ toxicity, ↑ nephrotoxicity
Lab test interferences
False ↑ Creatinine (serum urine), false ↑ urinary 17-KS
False positive: Urinary protein, direct Coombs' test, urine glucose
Interference: Cross-matching

NURSING CONSIDERATIONS
Assessment
- Assess patient for previous sensitivity reaction to penicillins or other cephalosporins; cross-sensitivity between penicillins and cephalosporins is common
- Assess patient for signs and symptoms of infection including characteristics of wounds, sputum, urine, stool, WBC >10,000, earache, fever; obtain baseline information and during treatment
- Obtain C&S before beginning drug therapy to identify if correct treatment has been initiated
- Assess for allergic reactions: rash, urticaria, pruritus, chills, fever, joint pain; angioedema may occur a few days after therapy begins; epinephrine and resuscitation equipment should be available for anaphylactic reaction
- ❗ Identify urine output; if decreasing, notify prescriber (may indicate nephrotoxicity); also check for increased BUN, creatinine
- Monitor blood studies: AST (SGOT), ALT (SGPT), CBC, Hct, bilirubin, LDH, alkaline phosphatase, Coombs' test monthly if patient is on long-term therapy
- Monitor electrolytes: potassium, sodium, chloride monthly if patient is on long-term therapy
- Assess bowel pattern qd; if severe diarrhea occurs, drug should be discontinued; may indicate pseudomembranous colitis
- Monitor for bleeding: ecchymosis, bleeding gums, hematuria, stool guaiac daily if on long-term therapy
- Assess for overgrowth of infection: perineal itching, fever, malaise, redness, pain, swelling, drainage, rash, diarrhea, change in cough, sputum

Nursing diagnoses
- ✓ Infection, risk for (uses)
- ✓ Injury, risk for (side effects)
- ✓ Diarrhea (side effects)
- ✓ Knowledge deficit (teaching)
- ✓ Noncompliance (teaching)

Implementation
- ⊘ Advise not to crush or chew caps
- Give in even doses around the clock; if GI upset occurs, give with food; drug must be taken for 10-14 days to ensure organism death and prevent superinfection
- Shake suspension, refrigerate, discard after 2 wks

Patient/family education
- Teach patient to report sore throat, bruising, bleeding, joint pain; may indicate blood dyscrasias (rare)
- Advise patient to contact prescriber if vaginal itching,

loose, foul-smelling stools, furry tongue occur; may indicate superinfection

- Instruct patient to take all medication prescribed for the length of time ordered
- Advise patient to notify prescriber of diarrhea with blood or pus, which may indicate pseudomembranous colitis

Evaluation

Positive therapeutic outcome

- Absence of signs/symptoms of infection (WBC <10,000, temp WNL, absence of red draining wounds, earache)
- Reported improvement in symptoms of infection
- Negative C&S

Treatment of anaphylaxis: Epinephrine, antihistamines, resuscitate if needed

cephalothin (℞)

(sef-a'loe-thin)

cephalothin sodium, Ceporacin ✱, Keflin Neutral

Func. class.: Broad-spectrum antibiotic

Chem. class.: Cephalosporin (1st generation)

Pregnancy category B

Action: Inhibits bacterial cell wall synthesis, rendering cell wall osmotically unstable and leading to cell death by binding to the cell wall membrane

➔ Therapeutic Outcome: Bactericidal effects for the following: gram-negative bacilli *Haemophilus influenzae, Escherichia coli, Proteus mirabilis, Klebsiella, Salmonella, Shigella;* gram-positive organisms *Streptococcus pneumoniae, S. pyogenes, Staphylococcus aureus*

Uses: Lower respiratory tract, urinary tract, skin and bone infections; septicemia, endocarditis; bacterial peritonitis

Dosage and routes

Adult: IM/**IV** 500 mg-1 g q4-6h

P ***Child:*** IM/**IV** 14-27 mg/kg q4h or 20-40 mg/kg q6h

Dosage reduction indicated in renal impairment (CrCl <50 ml/min)

Uncomplicated gonorrhea

2 g IM as single dose

Severe infections

Adult: IM/**IV** 1-2 g q4h

Child: IM/**IV** 80-160 mg/kg/day in divided doses q6h

Available forms: Powder for inj 1, 2, 20 g; frozen **IV** 20, 40 mg/ml

Adverse effects

CNS: Headache, dizziness, weakness, paresthesia, fever, chills

GI: Nausea, vomiting, diarrhea, anorexia, pain, glossitis, ***bleeding;*** increased AST (SGOT), ALT (SGPT), bilirubin, LDH, alkaline phosphatase; abdominal pain, ***pseudomembranous colitis***

GU: ***Proteinuria,*** vaginitis, pruritus, candidiasis, increased BUN, ***nephrotoxicity, renal failure***

HEMA: ***Leukopenia, thrombocytopenia, agranulocytosis,*** anemia, ***neutropenia, lymphocytosis, eosinophilia, pancytopenia, hemolytic anemia***

INTEG: Rash, urticaria, dermatitis

RESP: Dyspnea

SYST: ***Anaphylaxis***

Contraindications: Hypersensitivity to cephalosporins

Precautions: Hypersensitivity to penicillins, pregnancy **B**, lactation, renal disease

Pharmacokinetics

Absorption	Well absorbed
Distribution	Widely distributed; crosses placenta
Metabolism	Not metabolized
Excretion	Kidneys, unchanged; enters breast milk
Half-life	½-1 hr

Pharmacodynamics

	IM	IV
Onset	Rapid	Immediate
Peak	½ hr	Infusion's end

Interactions

Individual drugs

Probenecid: ↓ excretion of drug and ↑ blood levels

Vancomycin: ↑ toxicity

Drug classifications

Aminoglycosides: ↑ toxicity, ↑ nephrotoxicity

Lab test interferences

False ↑ Creatinine (serum urine), false ↑ urinary 17-KS

False positive: Urinary protein, direct Coombs' test, urine glucose

Interference: Cross-matching

NURSING CONSIDERATIONS

Assessment

- Assess patient for previous sensitivity reaction to penicillins or other cephalosporins; cross-sensitivity between penicillins and cephalosporins is common
- Assess patient for signs and symptoms of infection including characteristics of wounds, sputum, urine, stool, WBC >10,000, fever; obtain baseline information and during treatment
- Obtain C&S before beginning drug therapy to identify if correct treatment has been initiated
- Assess for allergic reactions: rash, urticaria, pruritus, chills, fever, joint pain; angioedema may occur a few days after therapy begins; epinephrine and resuscitation equipment should be available for anaphylactic reaction
- Identify urine output; if decreasing, notify prescriber (may indicate nephrotoxicity); also check for increased BUN, creatinine
- Monitor blood studies: AST (SGOT), ALT (SGPT), CBC, Hct, bilirubin, LDH, alkaline phosphatase, Coombs' test monthly if patient is on long-term therapy
- Monitor electrolytes: potassium, sodium, chloride monthly if patient is on long-term therapy
- Assess bowel pattern qd; if severe diarrhea occurs, drug should be discontinued; may indicate pseudomembranous colitis
- Monitor for bleeding: ecchymosis, bleeding gums, hematuria, stool guaiac daily if on long-term therapy
- Assess for overgrowth of infection: perineal itching, fever, malaise, redness, pain, swelling, drainage, rash, diarrhea, change in cough, sputum

Nursing diagnoses

- ✓ Infection, risk for (uses)
- ✓ Injury, risk for (side effects)
- ✓ Diarrhea (side effects)
- ✓ Knowledge deficit (teaching)

Implementation

IM route

- Reconstitute 1 g/4 ml sterile water for inj; give deep in large muscle mass and massage

• IM route not preferred; causes intense pain and induration

IV route

• Check for irritation, extravasation, phlebitis daily; change site q72h

• For direct **IV** dilute 1 g/10 ml or more sterile water for inj, D_5W, 0.9% NaCl; give over 3-5 min

• For intermittent inf, reconstitute 1-2 mg/50 ml sterile water for inj, D_5W, $D_{10}W$, D_5/LR, D_5/0.9% NaCl, 0.9% NaCl; may be further diluted in 50-100 ml D_5W, $D_{10}W$, 0.9% NaCl, or LR; give over 15-30 min

• For cont inf may be diluted in 500-1000 ml and run at prescribed rate; may use hydrocortisone 10-25 mg added to inf containing 4-6 g or more of cephalothin to decrease the incidence of thrombophlebitis

• Store refrigerated 96h, room temp 24h

Y-site incompatibility:
Hetastarch

Y-site compatibilities:
Cyclophosphamide, famotidine, heparin, hydromorphone, magnesium sulfate, meperidine, morphine, multivitamins, perphenazine, potassium chloride, vitamin B complex with C

Syringe incompatibility:
Metoclopramide

Syringe compatibility:
Cimetidine

Additive incompatibilities:
Aminoglycosides, amikacin, aminophylline, amobarbital, bleomycin, calcium chloride, calcium gluceptate, calcium gluconate, colistimethate, diphenhydramine, doxorubicin, erythromycin, gentamicin, kanamycin, oxytetracycline, pentobarbital, penicillin G sodium, phenobarbital, polymyxin B, prochlorperazine, tetracycline

Additive compatibilities:
Ascorbic acid, chloramphenicol, clindamycin, fluorouracil, hydrocortisone, isoproterenol, magnesium sulfate, metaraminol, methicillin, methotrexate, potassium chloride, prednisolone, procaine, sodium bicarbonate, vit B/C

Patient/family education

• Teach patient to report sore throat, bruising, bleeding, joint pain; may indicate blood dyscrasias (rare)

• Advise patient to contact prescriber if vaginal itching, loose, foul-smelling stools, furry tongue occur; may indicate superinfection

• Advise patient to notify prescriber of diarrhea with blood or pus, which may indicate pseudomembranous colitis

Evaluation

Positive therapeutic outcome

• Absence of signs/symptoms of infection (WBC <10,000, temp WNL, absence of red draining wounds)

• Reported improvement in symptoms of infection

• Negative C&S

Treatment of anaphylaxis:
Epinephrine, antihistamines, resuscitate if needed

cephapirin (℞)
(sef-a-pye'rin)
Cefadyl, cephapirin sodium
Func. class.: Broad spectrum antibiotic
Chem. class.: Cephalosporin (1st generation)
Pregnancy category B

Action: Inhibits bacterial cell wall synthesis, rendering cell wall osmotically unstable, leading to cell death

Therapeutic Outcome: Bactericidal effects for the following: gram-negative bacilli *Haemophilus influenzae, Escherichia coli, Proteus mirabilis, Klebsiella;* gram-positive organisms *Streptococcus pneumoniae, S. viridans, Staphylococcus aureus*

Uses: Lower respiratory tract, urinary tract, skin infections; septicemia, endocarditis, bacterial peritonitis

Dosage and routes
Adult: IM/**IV** 500 mg-1 g q4-6h
P ***Child:*** IM/**IV** 10-20 mg/ kg, q6h
Dosage reduction indicated in renal impairment (CrCl <50 ml/min)

Available forms: Powder for inj 500 mg, 1, 2, 20 g; IV only 1, 2, 4 g

Adverse effects
CNS: Headache, dizziness, weakness, paresthesia, fever, chills
GI: Nausea, vomiting, diarrhea, anorexia, pain, glossitis, ***bleeding;*** increased AST (SGOT), ALT (SGPT), bilirubin, LDH, alkaline phosphatase; abdominal pain, ***pseudomembranous colitis***
GU: ***Proteinuria,*** vaginitis, pruritus, candidiasis, increased BUN, ***nephrotoxicity, renal failure***
HEMA: ***Leukopenia, thrombocytopenia, agranulocytosis,*** anemia, ***neutropenia, lymphocytosis, eosinophilia, pancytopenia, hemolytic anemia***
INTEG: Rash, urticaria, dermatitis
RESP: Dyspnea
SYST: ***Anaphylaxis***

Contraindications: Hypersensitivity to cephalosporins, P infants <1 mo

Precautions: Hypersensitivity to penicillins, pregnancy **B,** lactation, renal disease

Pharmacokinetics	
Absorption	Well absorbed
Distribution	Widely distributed; crosses placenta
Metabolism	Not metabolized
Excretion	Kidneys, unchanged; enters breast milk
Half-life	½-1 hr

Pharmacodynamics	IM	IV
Onset	Rapid	Immediate
Peak	½ hr	Infusion's end

Interactions
Individual drugs
Probenecid: ↓ excretion of drug and ↑ blood levels
Vancomycin: ↑ toxicity
Drug classifications
Aminoglycosides: ↑ toxicity
Lab test interferences
False ↑ Creatinine (serum urine), false ↑ urinary 17-KS
False positive: Urinary protein, direct Coombs' test, urine glucose
Interference: Cross-matching

C

NURSING CONSIDERATIONS

Assessment

- Assess patient for previous sensitivity reaction to penicillins or other cephalosporins; cross-sensitivity between penicillins and cephalosporins is common
- Assess patient for signs and symptoms of infection including characteristics of wounds, sputum, urine, stool, WBC >10,000, fever; obtain baseline information and during treatment
- Obtain C&S before beginning drug therapy to identify if correct treatment has been initiated
- Assess for allergic reactions: rash, urticaria, pruritus, chills, fever, joint pain; angioedema may occur a few days after therapy begins; epinephrine and resuscitation equipment should be available for anaphylactic reaction
- Identify urine output; if decreasing, notify prescriber (may indicate nephrotoxicity); also check for increased BUN, creatinine
- Monitor blood studies: AST (SGOT), ALT (SGPT), CBC, Hct, bilirubin, LDH, alkaline phosphatase, Coombs' test monthly if patient is on long-term therapy
- Monitor electrolytes: potassium, sodium, chloride monthly if patient is on long-term therapy
- Assess bowel pattern qd; if severe diarrhea occurs, drug should be discontinued; may indicate pseudomembranous colitis
- Monitor for bleeding: ecchymosis, bleeding gums, hematuria, stool guaiac daily if on long-term therapy
- Assess for overgrowth of infection: perineal itching, fever, malaise, redness, pain, swelling, drainage, rash, diarrhea, change in cough, sputum

Nursing diagnoses

- ✓ Infection, risk for (uses)
- ✓ Injury, risk for (side effects)
- ✓ Diarrhea (side effects)
- ✓ Knowledge deficit (teaching)

Implementation

IM route

- Reconstitute 1-2 g/1-2 ml of sterile water for inj; give deep in large muscle mass and massage

IV route

- Check for irritation, extravasation, phlebitis daily; change site q72h
- For intermittent inf, reconstitute 250 mg/2.4 ml, 500 mg/4.8 ml, 1 g/9.6 ml, 2 gm/19.2 ml sterile water for inj, D_5W, 0.9% NaCl; do not use sol with benzyl alcohol for neonates; may be further diluted in 50-100 ml D_5W, $D_{10}W$, 0.9% NaCl, or LR; give over 30-60 min
- Store refrigerated 96h, room temp 24h

Y-site compatibilities: Acyclovir, cyclophosphamide, famotidine, heparin, hydrocortisone, hydromorphone, magnesium sulfate, meperidine, morphine, multivitamins, perphenazine, potassium chloride, vitamin B complex with C

Additive incompatibilities: Aminoglycosides, amikacin, ascorbic acid, epinephrine, gentamicin, kanamycin, mannitol, norepinephrine, oxytetracycline, phenytoin, tetracycline, thiopental

Additive compatibilities: Bleomycin, calcium chloride, calcium gluconate, chloramphenicol, diphenhydramine, ergonovine maleate, heparin, hydrocortisone, metaraminol, oxacillin, penicillin G potassium, pentobarbital, phenobarbital, phytonadione, potassium chloride, sodium bicarbonate, succinylcholine, verapamil, warfarin, vitamin B complex

Patient/family education

• Teach patient to report sore throat, bruising, bleeding, joint pain; may indicate blood dyscrasias (rare)

• Advise patient to contact prescriber if vaginal itching, loose, foul-smelling stools, furry tongue occur; may indicate superinfection

• Advise patient to notify prescriber of diarrhea with blood or pus, which may indicate pseudomembranous colitis

Evaluation

Positive therapeutic outcome

• Absence of signs/symptoms of infection (WBC <10,000, temp WNL, absence of red draining wounds)

• Reported improvement in symptoms of infection

• Negative C&S

Treatment of anaphylaxis: Epinephrine, antihistamines, resuscitate if needed

cephradine (℞)

(sef'ra-deen)

cephradine, Velosef

Func. class.: Antibiotic

Chem. class.: Cephalosporin (1st generation)

Pregnancy category B

Action: Inhibits bacterial cell wall synthesis, rendering cell wall osmotically unstable, leading to cell death by binding to cell wall membrane

➡ Therapeutic Outcome: Bactericidal effects for the following: gram-negative bacilli *Haemophilus influenzae, Escherichia coli, Proteus mirabilis, Klebsiella;* gram-positive organisms *Streptococcus pneumoniae, S. pyogenes, Staphylococcus aureus*

Uses: Serious respiratory tract, urinary tract, skin infections; otitis media

Dosage and routes

Adult: IM/**IV** 500 mg-1 g q4-6h; not to exceed 8 g/day; PO 250 mg-1 g q6-12h

P ***Child >1 yr:*** IM/**IV** 12-25 mg/kg q6h or 50-100 mg/kg/day q6h; PO 6-12 mg/kg q6h or 25-50 mg/kg/day q6-12h

Available forms: Powder for inj 250, 500 mg, 1 g; caps 250, 500 mg; oral susp 125, 250 mg/5 ml

Adverse effects

CNS: Headache, dizziness, weakness, paresthesia, fever, chills

GI: Nausea, vomiting, diarrhea, anorexia, pain, glossitis, ***bleeding;*** increased AST (SGOT), ALT (SGPT), bilirubin, LDH, alkaline phos-

phatase, abdominal pain, ***pseudomembranous colitis***
GU: ***Proteinuria,*** vaginitis, pruritus, candidiasis, increased BUN, ***nephrotoxicity, renal failure***
HEMA: ***Leukopenia, thrombocytopenia, agranulocytosis,*** anemia, ***neutropenia, lymphocytosis, eosinophilia, pancytopenia, hemolytic anemia***
INTEG: Rash, urticaria, dermatitis
RESP: Dyspnea
SYST: ***Anaphylaxis***

Contraindications: Hypersensitivity to cephalosporins, P infants <1 mo

Precautions: Hypersensitivity to penicillins, pregnancy **B,** P lactation, renal disease, children

Pharmacokinetics

Absorption	Well absorbed
Distribution	Widely distributed; crosses placenta
Metabolism	Not metabolized
Excretion	Kidneys, unchanged; enters breast milk
Half-life	1-2 hr

Pharmacodynamics

	PO/IM	IV
Onset	Rapid	Immediate
Peak	1 hr	Infusion's end

Interactions
Individual drugs
Probenecid: ↓ excretion of drug and ↑ blood levels
Vancomycin: ↑ toxicity
Drug classifications
Aminoglycosides: ↑ toxicity
Lab test interferences
False ↑ Creatinine (serum urine), false ↑ urinary 17-KS
False positive: Urinary protein, direct Coombs' test, urine glucose
Interference: Cross-matching

NURSING CONSIDERATIONS
Assessment
- Assess patient for previous sensitivity reaction to penicillins or other cephalosporins; cross-sensitivity between penicillins and cephalosporins is common
- Assess patient for signs and symptoms of infection including characteristics of wounds, sputum, urine, stool, WBC >10,000, earache, fever; obtain baseline information and during treatment
- Obtain C&S before beginning drug therapy to identify if correct treatment has been initiated
- Assess for allergic reactions: rash, urticaria, pruritus, chills, fever, joint pain; angioedema may occur a few days after therapy begins; epinephrine and resuscitation equipment should be available for anaphylactic reaction
- Identify urine output; if decreasing, notify prescriber (may indicate nephrotoxicity); also check for increased BUN, creatinine
- Monitor blood studies: AST (SGOT), ALT (SGPT), CBC, Hct, bilirubin, LDH, alkaline phosphatase, Coombs' test monthly if patient is on long-term therapy
- Monitor electrolytes: potassium, sodium, chloride monthly if patient is on long-term therapy
- Assess bowel pattern qd; if severe diarrhea occurs, drug should be discontinued; may indicate pseudomembranous colitis
- Monitor for bleeding: ecchymosis, bleeding gums, hematuria, stool guaiac daily if on long-term therapy

• Assess for overgrowth of infection: perineal itching, fever, malaise, redness, pain, swelling, drainage, rash, diarrhea, change in cough, sputum

Nursing diagnoses

- ☑ Infection, risk for (uses)
- ☑ Diarrhea (side effects)
- ☑ Knowledge deficit (teaching)
- ☑ Noncompliance (teaching)(PO)
- ☑ Injury, risk for (side effects)

Implementation

PO route

• May be given with food for GI symptoms

• When giving susp, shake well; refrigerate unused portion

IM route

• Reconstitute 250 mg/1.2 ml, 500 mg/ml, 1 g/4 ml sterile or bacterostatic water for inj; give deep in large muscle mass, massage

IV **IV route**

• Check for irritation, extravasation, phlebitis daily; change q72h

• Direct **IV** route 250-500 mg/5 ml sterile water, 0.9% NaCl, D_5W, or 1 g/10 ml, 2 g/20 ml; give over 3-5 min

• For intermittent inf, dilute 1 g/10 ml or more sterile water for inj, D_5W, $D_{10}W$, or D_5/0.9% NaCl; give over 3060 min

• Store refrigerated 96h, room temp 24h

Additive incompatibilities: Other antibiotics, calcium salts, D_5W, epinephrine, lidocaine, Ringer's or LR sol, NormosolR, NaCl, TPN #61, tetracycline

Patient/family education

• Teach patient to report sore throat, bruising, bleeding, joint pain; may indicate blood dyscrasias (rare)

• Advise patient to contact prescriber if vaginal itching, loose, foul-smelling stools, furry tongue occur; may indicate superinfection

• Instruct patient to take all medication prescribed for the length of time ordered

• Advise patient to notify prescriber of diarrhea with blood or pus, which may indicate pseudomembranous colitis

Evaluation

Positive therapeutic outcome

• Absence of signs/symptoms of infection (WBC <10,000, temp WNL, absence of red draining wounds, earache)

• Reported improvement in symptoms of infection

• Negative C&S

Treatment of anaphylaxis: Epinephrine, antihistamines, resuscitate if needed

cetirizine (℞)

(se-tear'i-zeen)

Zyrtec

Func. class: Antihistamine

Chem. class.: H_1 histamine antagonist

Pregnancy category C

Action: Acts on blood vessels, GI, respiratory system by competing with histamine for H_1-receptor site; decreases allergic response by blocking pharmacologic effects of histamine; less sedation rate than with other antihistamines; causes increased heart rate, vasodilatation, increased secretions

Therapeutic Outcome: Absence of allergy symptoms and rhinitis

Uses: Rhinitis, allergy symptoms

Dosage and routes

P ***Adult and child >12 yr:*** PO 5-10 mg qd

Available forms: Tabs 5, 10 mg

Adverse effects

CNS: Headache, stimulation, drowsiness, sedation, fatigue, confusion, blurred vision, tinnitus, restlessness, tremors, P parodoxical excitation in G children or elderly

CV: Hypotension, palpitations, bradycardia, tachycardia, *dysrhythmias* (rare)

GI: Nausea, diarrhea, abdominal pain, vomiting, constipation

GU: Frequency, dysuria, urinary retention, impotence

HEMA: Hemolytic anemia, thrombocytopenia, leukopenia, agranulocytosis, pancytopenia

INTEG: Rash, eczema, photosensitivity, urticaria

RESP: Thickening of bronchial secretions; dry nose, throat

Contraindications: Hypersen- P sitivity, newborn or premature infants, lactation, severe hepatic disease

G **Precautions:** Pregnancy **C**, P elderly, children, respiratory disease, narrow-angle glaucoma, prostatic hypertrophy, bladder neck obstruction, G asthma, elderly

Pharmacokinetics	
Absorption	Well absorbed
Distribution	Unknown
Metabolism	Liver
Excretion	Kidneys
Half-life	Unknown

Pharmacodynamics	
Onset	Unknown
Peak	1-2 hr
Duration	Unknown

C

Interactions

Individual drugs

Alcohol: ↑ CNS depression
Erythromycin: ↑ CV reaction
Itraconazole: ↑ CV reaction
Ketoconazole: ↑ CV reaction
Procarbazine: ↑ CNS depression

Drug classifications

Anticoagulants, oral: ↓ action
CNS depressants: ↑ CNS depression
MAOI: ↑ anticholinergic effect
Narcotics: ↑ CNS depression
Sedative/hyponotics: ↑ CNS depression

Food

↓ absorption

Lab test interferences

False negative: Skin allergy tests (discontinue antihistamine 3 days before testing)

NURSING CONSIDERATIONS

Assessment

- Assess respiratory status: rate, rhythm; increase in bronchial secretions, wheezing, chest tightness; provide fluids to 2 L/day to decrease secretion thickness
- Monitor I&O ratio: be alert for urinary retention, frequency, dysuria, especially G elderly; drug should be discontinued if these occur
- Monitor CBC during long-term therapy; blood dyscrasias may occur but are rare

Nursing diagnoses

✓ Airway clearance, ineffective (uses)
✓ Injury, risk for (side effects)
✓ Knowledge deficit (teaching)

☑ Noncompliance (teaching overuse)

Implementation

- Give on an empty stomach 1 hr before or 2 hr pc to facilitate absorption
- Store in tight, light-resistant container

Patient/family education

- Teach all aspects of drug uses; to notify prescriber if confusion, sedation, hypotension occur; to avoid driving or other hazardous activity if drowsiness occurs; to avoid alcohol or other CNS depressants that may potentiate effect
- Instruct patient to take 1 hr before or 2 hr pc to facilitate absorption
- Instruct patient not to exceed recommended dose; dysrhythmias may occur
- Teach patient hard candy, gum, frequent rinsing of mouth may be used for dryness

Evaluation

Positive therapeutic outcome

- Absence of running or congested nose, rashes

Treatment of overdose: Administer ipecac syrup or lavage diazepam, vasopressors, barbiturates (short acting)

chloral hydrate (℞)

(klor'al hye'drate)

Aquachloral Supprettes, chloral hydrate, Noctec, Novochlorhydrate ♣

Func. class.: Sedative/hypnotic

Chem. class.: Chloral derivative

Pregnancy category C

Controlled substance schedule IV (USA), schedule F (Canada)

Action: Reduced to product trichloroethanol, which produces mild cerebral depression, causing sleep; generalized CNS depression

➔ **Therapeutic Outcome:** Ability to sleep, sedation

Uses: Sedation, insomnia, preoperative reduction of anxiety

Dosage and routes

Sedation

Adult: PO/rec 250 mg tid pc

P ***Child:*** PO 8 mg/kg tid, not to exceed 500 mg tid

Insomnia

Adult: PO/rec 500 mg-1g 30 min before hs

P ***Child:*** PO/rec 50 mg/kg in one dose

Available forms: Caps 250, 500 mg; syr 250, 500 mg/5 ml; supp 325, 500, 650 mg

Adverse effects

CNS: Drowsiness, dizziness, stimulation, nightmares, ataxia, hangover (rare), lightheadedness, headache, paranoia

CV: Hypotension, ***dysrhythmias***

GI: Nausea, vomiting, flatu-

lence, diarrhea, unpleasant taste, ***gastric necrosis***
HEMA: ***Eosinophilia, leukopenia***
INTEG: Rash, urticaria, ***angioedema,*** fever, purpura, eczema
RESP: ***Depression***

Contraindications: Hypersensitivity to this drug or triclofos, severe renal disease, severe hepatic disease, GI disorders (oral forms), gastritis

Precautions: Severe cardiac disease, depression, suicidal individuals, asthma, intermittent porphyria, pregnancy **C**, G lactation, elderly

Pharmacokinetics

Absorption	Well absorbed (PO, rec)
Distribution	Widely distributed; crosses placenta
Metabolism	Liver to trichloroethanol
Excretion	Kidneys (inactive metabolite), feces, breast milk
Half-life	8-10 hr; active metabolite

Pharmacodynamics

	PO	REC
Onset	½-1 hr	Slow
Peak	Unknown	Unknown
Duration	4-8 hr	4-6 hr

Interactions
Individual drugs
Alcohol: ↑ CNS depression
Fluoxetine: ↑ action
Furosemide: ↑ diaphoresis, flushing
Propoxyphene: ↑ action
Drug classification
Analgesics, opioid: ↑ CNS depression
Anticoagulants, oral: ↑ action of anticoagulants
Antidepressants: ↑ CNS depression
Antihistamines: ↑ CNS depression
Sedative/hypnotics: ↑ CNS depression
Lab test interferences
Interferences: Urine catecholamines, urinary 17-OHCS
False positive: Urine glucose (copper sulfate test)

NURSING CONSIDERATIONS
Assessment

- Assess patient's sleep pattern and note physical (sleep apnea, obstructed airway, pain/discomfort, urinary frequency) and psychologic (fear, anxiety) circumstances that interrupt sleep
- Assess patient's bedtime routine, presleep cues/props
- Assess potential for abuse; this drug may lead to physical and psychologic dependency; amount of drug should be limited
- Monitor blood studies: Hct, Hgb, RBCs, serum folate (if on long-term therapy), protime in patients receiving anticoagulants since action of anticoagulant may be increased
- Monitor mental status: mood, sensorium, affect, memory (long, short)
- Monitor physical dependency: more frequent requests for medication, shakes, anxiety, pinpoint pupils
- Monitor respiratory dysfunction: respiratory depression, character, rate, rhythm; hold drug if respirations are <10/min or if pupils are dilated (rare)
- Assess for blood dyscrasias: fever, sore throat, bruising, rash, jaundice, epistaxis (rare)
- Assess previous history of substance abuse, cardiac disease, or gastritis

Nursing diagnoses
- ✓ Sleep pattern disturbance (uses)
- ✓ Anxiety (uses)
- ✓ Knowledge deficit (teaching)
- ✓ Noncompliance (teaching)

Implementation
General
- Regulate environmental stimuli (light, noise, temperature), remove foods and fluids that interfere with sleep
- Place side rails up after giving medication for hypnotic; remove cigarettes/matches from patient's environment to prevent fires

PO route
- Give ½-1 hr before hs for sleeplessness; give on empty stomach with full glass of water or juice for best absorption and to decrease corrosion (do not chew); after meals to decrease GI symptoms if used for sedation; dilute syr in 4 oz water or juice
- ⊘ Do not crush, chew caps

Rectal route
- Store supp in dark container, in refrigerator; remove outer wrapper before insertion

Patient/family education
- Caution patient to avoid driving and other activities requiring alertness; to avoid alcohol ingestion or CNS depressants; serious CNS depression may result plus tachycardia, flushing, headache, hypotension
- Instruct patient not to discontinue medication quickly after long-term use; drug should be tapered over 1-2 wk; that effects may take 2 nights for benefits to be noticed; withdrawal symptoms include tremors, anxiety, hallucinations, delirium
- Teach patient alternate measures to improve sleep (reading, exercise several hours before hs, warm bath, warm milk, TV, self-hypnosis, deep breathing)
- Instruct the patient about factors that contribute to sleep pattern disturbances (lifestyle, shift work, long work hours, environmental factors, frequent napping)
- Teach patient to take drug as prescribed, not to double doses

Evaluation
Positive therapeutic outcome
- Ability to sleep at night
- Decreased amount of early morning awakening if taking drug for insomnia
- Sedation

Treatment of overdose: Lavage, activated charcoal; monitor electrolytes, vital signs

chlorambucil (Rx)
(klor-am'byoo-sil)

Leukeran

Func. class.: Antineoplastic alkylating agent

Chem. class.: Nitrogen mustard

Pregnancy category D

Action: Alkylates DNA, RNA; inhibits enzymes that allow synthesis of amino acids in proteins; activity is not cell cycle phase specific

➔ **Therapeutic Outcome:** Prevention of rapidly growing malignant cells

Uses: Chronic lymphocytic leukemia, Hodgkin's disease, other lymphomas, macroglobulinemia, nephrotic syndrome, breast carcinoma, choreocarcinoma, ovarian carcinoma

Dosage and routes

Adult: PO 0.1-0.2 mg/kg/day × 3-6 wk initially, then 2-6 mg/day; maintenance 0.2 mg/kg × 2-4 wk; course may be repeated at 2-4 wk intervals

P ***Child:*** PO 0.1-0.2 mg/kg/day in divided doses or 4.5 mg/m²/day as 1 dose or in divided doses

Available forms: Tabs 2 mg

Adverse effects

P *CNS:* ***Convulsions in children***
GI: Nausea, vomiting, diarrhea, weight loss, ***hepatoxicity, jaundice***
GU: Hyperuremia
HEMA: ***Thrombocytopenia, leukopenia, pancytopenia*** (prolonged use), ***permanent bone marrow depression***
INTEG: Alopecia (rare), dermatitis, rash
RESP: ***Fibrosis, pneumonitis***

Contraindications: Radiation therapy within 1 mo, chemotherapy within 1 mo, thrombocytopenia, smallpox vaccination, pregnancy (1st trimester) **D**

Precautions: *Pneumococcus* vaccination

Pharmacokinetics

Absorption	Rapidly, completely absorbed
Distribution	Crosses placenta
Metabolism	Liver, extensively
Excretion	Kidneys
Half-life	2 hr

Pharmacodynamics

Unknown

Interactions

Individual drugs

Radiation: ↑ toxicity, bone marrow suppression

Drug classifications

Antineoplastics: ↑ toxicity, bone marrow suppression

Bone marrow–suppressing drugs: ↑ bone marrow suppression

Live vaccines: ↑ adverse reactions, ↓ antibody reaction

Lab test interferences

↑ Uric acid

NURSING CONSIDERATIONS

Assessment

- Monitor CBC, differential, platelet count weekly; withhold drug if WBC is <4000 or platelet count is <75,000; notify prescriber of results if WBC <20,000/mm³, platelets <50,000/mm³
- Monitor pulmonary function tests, chest x-ray films before, during therapy; chest film should be obtained q2 wk during treatment; check for dyspnea, rales, unproductive cough, chest pain, tachypnea
- Assess for increased uric acid levels, swelling, joint pain primarily in extremities; patient should be well hydrated to prevent urate deposits
- Monitor renal function studies: BUN, serum uric acid, urine CrCl before, during therapy; I&O ratio; report fall in urine output of 30 ml/hr; monitor for decreased hyperuricemia
- Monitor for cold, fever, sore throat (may indicate beginning infection); identify edema in feet, joint, stomach pain, shaking; prescriber should be notified
- Assess for bleeding: hematuria, guaiac, bruising or pete-

chiae, mucosa or orifices q8h, no rec temp

Nursing diagnoses

✓ Injury, risk for (adverse reactions)
✓ Body image disturbance (adverse reactions)
✓ Infection, risk for (adverse reactions)
✓ Knowledge deficit (teaching)

Implementation

• Give 1 hr ac or 2 hr pc to lessen nausea and vomiting or antacid before oral agent, give drug after evening meal, before hs; antiemetic 30-60 min before giving drug to prevent vomiting
• Give either allopurinol or sodium bicarbonate to maintain uric acid levels, alkalinization of urine; increase fluid intake to 2-3 L/day to prevent urate deposits, calculus formation
• Use of antibiotics for prophylaxis of infection may be prescribed, since infection potential is high
• Store in tight container

Patient/family education

• Teach patient to avoid use of products containing aspirin or ibuprofen, razors, commercial mouthwash, since bleeding may occur; to report symptoms of bleeding (hematuria, tarry stools)
• Instruct patient to report signs of anemia (fatigue, headache, irritability, faintness, shortness of breath)
• Instruct patient to report any changes in breathing or coughing even several mo after treatment; to avoid crowds and persons with respiratory tract or other infections
• Advise patient hair loss is common; discuss the use of wigs or hair pieces
• Caution patient not to have any vaccinations without the advice of the prescriber; serious reactions can occur
• Advise patient contraception is needed during treatment and for several months after the completion of therapy

Evaluation

Positive therapeutic outcome

• Decreased size of tumor
• Decreased spread of malignancy
• Improved blood values
• Absence of sweating at night
• Increased appetite, increased weight

chloramphenicol (℞)

(klor-am-fen′i-kole)

Ak-Chlor, Chloro-fab chlorophe, Econochlor, chloramphenicol, chloramphenicol sodium succinate, Chloromycetin Kapseals, Chloromycetin Sodium Succinate, Chloromycetin Palmitate, Novochlorocap ♣, Fenicol ♣, Ocu-Chlor, Ophthochlor Pentamycetin ♣, Sopamycetin ♣, Spectro-Chlor

Func. class.: Antibacterial/antirickettsial

Chem. class.: Dichloroacetic acid derivative

Pregnancy category C

Action: Binds to 50S ribosomal subunit, which interferes with or inhibits protein synthesis

Therapeutic Outcome: Bactericidal for *H. influenzae, S. typhi, Rickettsia, Neisseria, Mycloplasma*

Uses: Meningitis, bacteremia, abdominal, skin, soft tissue infections; local infections of skin, ear, eye

Dosage and routes

Adult: PO/**IV** 12.5 mg/kg q6h, not to exceed 4 g/day

P ***Children and infants >2 wk:*** **IV**/PO 12 mg/kg q6h or 2.5 mg/kg q2hr

P ***Infants <2 wk and premature:*** **IV**/PO 6.25 mg/kg q6h

P ***Adult and child:*** Ophth 1-2 gtt of sol or ointment q 3-6 mo; otic 2-3 gtt bid or tid; top 1% cream tid or qid

P ***Premature infants and neonates:*** **IV**/PO 25 mg/kg/day in divided doses q6h

Available forms: Inj **IV** 100 mg/ml in 1 g vial; caps 250, 500 mg; oral susp 150 mg/5 ml; ophth ointment 10 mg/g; ophth sol 25 mg/15 ml, 5 mg/ml; top cream 1%; otic sol 0.5%

Adverse effects

CNS: Headache, *depression,* confusion
CV: Gray syndrome in newborns: failure to feed, pallor, cyanosis, abdominal distention, irregular respiration, vasomotor collapse
EENT: Optic neuritis, blindness
GI: Nausea, vomiting, diarrhea, abdominal pain, xerostomia, glossitis, colitis, pruritus ani
HEMA: Anemia, bone marrow depression, thrombocytopenia, aplastic anemia, granulocytopenia, leukopenia (rare)
INTEG: Itching, urticaria, contact dermatitis, rash

Contraindications: Hypersensitivity, severe renal disease, severe hepatic disease, minor infections

Precautions: Hepatic disease, P renal disease, infants, children, bone marrow depression (drug-induced), pregnancy **C**, lactation

Pharmacokinetics

Absorption	Well (PO) Completely (IV)
Distribution	Wide
Metabolism	Liver
Excretion	Kidneys, unchanged
Half-life	1½-4 hr

Pharmacodynamics

	PO	IV	TOP	OPH	OTIC
Onset	15 min	Rapid	Unkn	Unkn	Unkn
Peak	1-2 hr	Inf end	Unkn	Unkn	Unkn

Interactions

Individual drugs

Chlorpromide: ↑ action of chlorpromide
Dicumarol: ↑ action of dicumarol
Folic acid: ↓ action of folic acid
Iron: ↑ action of iron
Phenobarbital: ↑ action of phenobarbital
Phenytoin: ↑ action of phenytoin
Tolbutamide: ↑ action of tolbutamide
Vitamin B_{12}: ↓ action of vitamin B_{12}

Drug classifications

Anticoagulants: ↑ prothrombin time
Barbiturates: ↑ levels of chloramphenicol
Penicillins: synergism

NURSING CONSIDERATIONS

Assessment

- Assess patient for previous sensitivity reaction to other antiinfectives; cross-sensitivity between penicillins and cephalosporins is common
- Assess patient for signs and symptoms of infection including characteristics of wounds, sputum, urine, stool, WBC >10,000, fever; obtain baseline information and during treatment
- Perform C&S testing before starting drug therapy to identify if correct treatment has been initiated
- Monitor blood studies: platelets q2 days, CBC
- Assess bowel pattern qd; if severe diarrhea occurs, drug should be discontinued
- Monitor for bleeding: ecchymosis, bleeding gums, hematuria, stool guaiac daily if on long-term therapy
- Assess for overgrowth of infection: perineal itching, fever, malaise, redness, pain, swelling, drainage, rash, diarrhea, change in cough, sputum

Nursing diagnoses

✓ Infection, risk for (uses)
✓ Diarrhea (adverse reaction)
✓ Injury, risk for (side effects)
✓ Knowledge deficit (teaching)
✓ Noncompliance (teaching)

Implementation

Top route

- Wash hands, clean area to be treated with soap and water before application

Ophthalmic route

- Apply a small amount of ointment in lower lid
- Have patient tilt head back before application

IV **IV route**

- Give after diluting 1 g/10 ml of sterile H_2O for inj or D_5W (10% sol); give >1 min
- May be further diluted in 50-100 ml of D_5W; give through Y-tube, 3-way stopcock, or additive inf set; run over ½-1 hr reconstituted solution at room temp for up to 30 days

Syringe compatibility: Heparin

Y-site incompatibility: Fluconazole

Y-site compatibilities: Acyclovir, cyclophosphamide, enalaprilat, esmolol, foscarnet, hydromorphone, labetalol, magnesium sulfate, meperidine, morphine, perphenazine, tacrolimus

Additive compatibilities: Amikacin, aminophylline, ascorbic acid, calcium chloride/gluconate, cephalothin, cephapirin, corticotropin, cyanocobalamin, dimenhydrinate, dopamine, ephedrine, heparin, hydrocortisone, kanamycin, lidocaine, magnesium sulfate, metaraminol, methicillin, pentobarbital, potassium chloride, sodium bicarbonate, vancomycin

PO route

- Give oral form on empty stomach with full glass of water
- ⊘ Do not crush or chew caps
- Store cap in airtight container at room temp

Patient/family education

- Teach patient all aspects of drug therapy; need to complete entire course of medication to ensure organism death (10-14 days); culture may be taken after complete course of medication
- Advise patient to report sore throat, fever, fatigue, unusual

bleeding, or bruising; could indicate bone marrow depression (may occur weeks or months after termination of drug)

- Tell patient that drug must be taken at regular intervals around clock to maintain blood levels

Evaluation

Positive therapeutic outcome

- Decreased symptoms of infection

chlordiazepoxide (℞)

(klor-dye-az-e-pox'ide)

Apo-Chlordiazepoxide ♣, chlordiazepoxide HCl, Libritabs, Librium, Medilium ♣, Mitran, Novopoxide ♣, Resposans-10, Solium ♣

Func. class.: Antianxiety

Chem. class.: Benzodiazepine

Pregnancy category D

Controlled substance schedule IV

Action: Potentiates the actions of GABA, an inhibitory neurotransmitter, especially in the limbic system reticular formation, which depresses the CNS

➔ **Therapeutic Outcome:** Decreased anxiety, successful alcohol withdrawal, relaxation

Uses: Short-term management of anxiety, acute alcohol withdrawal, preoperative relaxation

Dosage and routes

Mild anxiety

Adult: PO 5-10 mg tid-qid

P ***Child >6 yr:*** 5 mg bid-qid, not to exceed 10 mg bid-tid

Severe anxiety

Adult: PO 20-25 mg tid-qid

Preoperatively

Adult: PO 5-10 mg tid-qid on day before surgery; IM 50-100 mg 1 hr before surgery

Alcohol withdrawal

Adult: PO/IM/**IV** 50-100 mg, not to exceed 300 mg/day

Available forms: Caps 5, 10, 25 mg; tabs 5, 10, 25 mg; powder for IM inj 100 mg

Adverse effects

CNS: Dizziness, drowsiness, confusion, headache, anxiety, tremors, stimulation, fatigue, depression, insomnia, hallucinations

CV: Orthostatic hypotension, ***ECG changes, tachycardia,*** hypotension

EENT: Blurred vision, tinnitus, mydriasis

GI: Constipation, dry mouth, nausea, vomiting, anorexia, diarrhea

INTEG: Rash, dermatitis, itching

Contraindications: Hypersensitivity to benzodiazepines, narrow-angle glaucoma,
P psychosis, pregnancy **D,** child <18 yr

P **Precautions:** Elderly, debilitated, hepatic disease, renal disease

Pharmacokinetics

Absorption	Well absorbed (PO); slow, erratic (IM)
Distribution	Widely distributed; crosses placenta, blood-brain barrier
Metabolism	Liver extensively
Excretion	Kidneys, breast milk
Half-life	5-30 hr

Pharmacodynamics

	PO	IM	IV
Onset	30 min	15-30 min	1-5 min
Peak	½ hr	Unknown	Unknown
Duration	4-6 hr	Unknown	Up to 1 hr

Interactions

Individual drugs

Alcohol: ↑ CNS depression
Cimetidine: ↑ action of cimetidine
Disulfiram: ↑ action of disulfiram
Fluoxetine: ↑ action of fluoxetine
Isoniazid: ↑ action of isoniazid
Ketoconazole: ↑ action of ketoconazole
Levodopa: ↓ action of levodopa
Metoprolol: ↑ action of metoprolol
Propoxyphene: ↑ action of propoxyphene
Propranolol: ↑ action
Rifampin: ↓ action of chlordiazepoxide
Theophylline: ↓ sedative effects
Valproic acid: ↑ action of valproic acid

Drug classifications

Analgesics, opioid: ↑ CNS depression
Antidepressants: ↑ CNS depression
Antihistamines: ↑ CNS depression
Barbiturates: ↓ effect of chlordiazepoxide
Contraceptives, oral: ↑ effect of contraceptive

Lab test interferences

↑ AST (SGOT)/ALT (SGPT), serum bilirubin
False ↑ 17-OHCS
Decrease: RAIU

NURSING CONSIDERATIONS

Assessment

- Assess anxiety reaction: inability to sleep, apprehension, dread, foreboding, or uneasiness related to unidentified source of danger
- Assess for previous drug dependence or tolerance; if drug dependent or tolerant, amount of medication should be restricted
- Monitor B/P (with patient lying, standing), pulse; if systolic B/P drops 20 mm Hg, hold drug, notify prescriber
- Monitor blood studies: CBC during long-term therapy; blood dyscrasias have occurred rarely
- Monitor hepatic studies: AST (SGOT), ALT (SGPT), bilirubin, creatinine, LDH, alkaline phosphatase
- Monitor mental status: mood, sensorium, affect, sleeping patterns, drowsiness, dizziness, suicidal tendencies

Nursing diagnoses

✓ Anxiety (uses)
✓ Knowledge deficit (teaching)
✓ Noncompliance (teaching)

Implementation

PO route

- Give with food or milk for GI symptoms, crushed if patient unable to swallow medication whole; do not open capsules; provide sugarless gum, hard candy, frequent sips of water for dry mouth

IM route

- Reconstitute with diluent provided (2 ml); agitate slowly, do not shake; give deep in large muscle mass to prevent severe pain; do not use IM diluent for **IV** route

IV **IV route**

- Reconstitute 100 mg/5 ml

sterile water for inj or 0.9% NaCl; give over at least 1 min to prevent cardiac arrest, apnea, bradycardia

Y-site compatibilities: Heparin, hydrocortisone, potassium chloride, vitamin B with C

Solution compatibilities: D_5W, 0.9% NaCl

Patient/family education

- Instruct patient that drug may be taken with food; if dose is missed take as soon as remembered; do not double doses
- Tell patient to avoid OTC preparations unless approved by prescriber; to avoid alcohol ingestion or other psychotropic medications unless directed by a prescriber
- Caution patient to avoid driving and activities requiring alertness, since drowsiness may occur; until medication response is known, tell patient that drowsiness may worsen at beginning of treatment
- Instruct patient not to discontinue medication abruptly after long-term use, drug should be tapered over 1 wk
- Caution patient to rise slowly or fainting may occur, especially in elderly

Evaluation

Positive therapeutic outcome

- Increased well being
- Decreased anxiety, restlessness, sleeplessness, dread
- Successful alcohol withdrawal

Treatment of overdose: Lavage, VS, supportive care

chloroquine (℞)

(klor'oh-kwin)

Aralen HCl, Aralen Phosphate, chloroquine phosphate, Novochloroquine ✦

Func. class.: Antimalarial

Chem. class.: Synthetic 4-aminoquinoline derivative

Pregnancy category C

Action: Inhibits parasite replications, transcription of DNA to RNA by forming complexes with DNA of parasite

Therapeutic Outcome: Decreased symptoms of malaria, amebiasis

Uses: Malaria caused by *Plasmodium vivax, P. malariae, P. ovale, P. falciparum* (some strains), amebiasis

Dosage and routes

Malaria suppression

Adult and child: PO 5 mg/kg/wk on same day of week, not to exceed 500 mg; treatment should begin 1-2 wk before exposure and for 8 wk after; if treatment begins after exposure, 600 mg for adult and 10 mg/kg for children in 2 divided doses 6 hr apart

Extraintestinal amebiasis

Adult: IM 200-250 mg qd (HCl) up to 12 days, then 1 g (phosphate) qd × 2 days, then 500 mg qd × 2-3 wk

Child: IM/PO 10 mg/kg qd (HCl) × 2-3 wk, not to exceed 300 mg/day

Available forms: Tabs 250, 500 mg; inj IM 50 mg/ml

Adverse effects

CNS: Headache, stimulation,

fatigue, ***convulsion,*** psychosis
CV: Hypotension, ***heart block, asystole with syncope,*** ECG changes
EENT: Blurred vision, corneal changes, retinal changes, difficulty focusing, tinnitus, vertigo, deafness, photophobia, corneal edema
GI: Nausea, vomiting, anorexia, diarrhea, cramps
HEMA: ***Thrombocytopenia, agranulocytosis, hemolytic anemia, leukopenia***
INTEG: Pruritus, pigmentary changes, skin eruptions, lichen planus–like eruptions, eczema, ***exfoliative dermatitis***

Contraindications: Hypersensitivity, retinal field changes, porphyria

Precautions: Pregnancy **C**, [P] children, blood dyscrasias, severe GI disease, neurologic disease, alcoholism, hepatic disease, G6PD deficiency, psoriasis, eczema, lactation, porphyria

Pharmacokinetics

Absorption	Well absorbed
Distribution	Widely
Metabolism	Liver
Excretion	Kidneys, feces
Half-life	3-5 days

Pharmacodynamics

	PO	IM
Onset	Rapid	Rapid
Peak	1-6 hr	45-60 min
Duration	6-8 hr	Unknown

Interactions
Individual drugs
Cimetidine: ↓ absorption
Kaolin: ↓ absorption
Drug classifications
Antacids, aluminum: ↓ absorption

NURSING CONSIDERATIONS
Assessment
- Monitor liver studies weekly: ALT (SGPT), AST (SGOT), bilirubin; renal status: before exposure, monthly thereafter: BUN, creatinine, output, sp gr, urinalysis
- Assess mental status often: affect, mood, behavioral changes; psychosis may occur
- Assess hepatic status: decreased appetite, jaundice, dark urine, fatigue

Nursing diagnoses
✓ Infection, risk for (uses)
✓ Diarrhea (side effects)
✓ Knowledge deficit (teaching)
✓ Noncompliance (teaching)
✓ Injury, risk for (side effects)

Implementation
PO route
- Give with meals to decrease GI symptoms; better to take on empty stomach 1 hr ac or 2 hr pc
- Give antiemetic if vomiting occurs
- Give after C&S is completed; monthly to detect resistance

IM route
- Give IM after aspirating to prevent inj into bloodstream

Patient/family education
- Advise patient that compliance with dosage schedule, duration is necessary
- Instruct patient that scheduled appointments must be kept or relapse may occur
- Caution patient to avoid alcohol while taking drug
- Instruct diabetic to use blood glucose monitor to obtain correct result
- Teach patient to report weakness, fatigue, loss of appetite, nausea, vomiting, yellowing of skin or eyes, tingling/numbness of hands/feet

- Advise patient that urine may turn rust brown color
- Instruct patient to use sunglasses in bright sunlight to prevent photophobia

Evaluation

Positive therapeutic outcome

- Decreased symptoms of malaria

chlorothiazide (℞)

(klor-oh-thye′a-zide)

Diurigen, Diuril, Diuril Sodium, Diurigen

Func. class.: Diuretic, antihypertensive

Chem. class.: Thiazide; sulfonamide derivative

Pregnancy category B

Action: Acts on the distal tubule and thick ascending limb of the loop of Henle in the kidney, increasing excretion of sodium, water, chloride, magnesium, potassium and bicarbonate

➔ **Therapeutic Outcome:** Decreased BP, decreased edema in tissues, peripherally, diuresis

Uses: Edema in congestive heart failure, nephrotic syndrome; may be used alone or as adjunct with antihypertensives; also for edema in corticosteroids, estrogen therapy

Dosage and routes

Edema, hypertension

Adult: PO/**IV** 50 mg-2 g qd in 2 divided doses

Diuresis

P ***Child >6 mo:*** PO 20 mg/kg/day in 2 divided doses

P ***Child <6 mo:*** PO 30 mg/kg/day in 2 divided doses

Available forms: Tabs 250, 500 mg; oral susp 250 mg/5 ml; inj 500 mg

Adverse effects

CNS: Drowsiness, paresthesia, anxiety, depression, headache, *dizziness, fatigue, weakness, fever, insomnia*

CV: Irregular pulse, orthostatic hypotension, palpitations, volume depletion

EENT: Blurred vision

ELECT: Hypokalemia, hypercalcemia, hyponatremia, hypochloremia, hypophosphatemia, hypomagnesemia, hyperlipidemia

GI: Nausea, vomiting, anorexia, constipation, diarrhea, cramps, pancreatitis, GI irritation, ***hepatitis***

GU: Frequency, polyuria, ***uremia,*** glucosuria, hematuria

HEMA: ***Aplastic anemia, hemolytic anemia, leukopenia, agranulocytosis, thrombocytopenia, neutropenia***

INTEG: Rash, urticaria, purpura, photosensitivity, alopecia

META: Hyperglycemia, *hyperuricemia,* hypomagnesemia, increased creatinine, BUN

Contraindications: Hypersensitivity to thiazides or sulfonamides, anuria, renal decompensation, pregnancy **B,** lactation, hepatic coma

Precautions: Hypokalemia, renal disease, hepatic disease, gout, COPD, LE, diabetes G mellitus, elderly, hyperlipidemia

Pharmacokinetics

	PO
Absorption	GI tract (10%-20%)
Distribution	Extracellular spaces; crosses placenta
Metabolism	Liver
Excretion	Urine, unchanged; breast milk
Half-life	1-2 hr

Pharmacodynamics

	PO	IV
Onset	2 hr	15 min
Peak	4 hr	½ hr
Duration	6-12 hr	2 hr

Interactions

Individual drugs

Allopurinol: ↑ toxicity
Cholestyramine: ↓ absorption of chlorothiazide
Colestipol: ↓ absorption of chlorothiazide
Diazoxide: ↑ hyperglycemia, hyperuricemia, hypotension
Digitalis: ↑ toxicity
Indomethacin: ↓ hypotensive response
Lithium:↑ toxicity
Mezlocillin: ↑ hypokalemia
Piperacillin: ↑ hypokalemia
Ticarcillin: ↑ hypokalemia

Drug classifications

Anticoagulants: ↓ effects
Antidiabetics: ↓ effect of antidiabetic agent
Antihypertensives: ↑ antihypertensive effect
Glucocorticoids: ↑ hypokalemia
NSAIDS: ↓ hypotension
Nondepolarizing skeletal muscle relaxants: ↑ toxicity
Sulfonylureas: ↓ effect of sulfonylurea

Food

Food: ↑ absorption

Lab test interferences

False negative: Phentolamine and tyramine tests
Interference: Urine steroid tests
↑ BSP retention, calcium, amylase, parathyroid test
↓ PBI, ↓ PSP

NURSING CONSIDERATIONS

Assessment

- Assess glucose in urine if patient is diabetic
- Monitor improvement in CVP q8h
- Check for rashes, temp elevation qd
- G Assess for confusion, especially in elderly; take safety precautions if needed
- Monitor manifestations of hypokalemia; *renal:* acidic urine, reduced urine, osmolality, nocturia; *CV:* hypotension, broad T wave, U wave, ectopy, tachycardia, weak pulse; *neuro:* muscle weakness, altered LOC, drowsiness, apathy, lethargy, confusion, depression; *GI:* anorexia, nausea, cramps, constipation, distention, paralytic ileus; *resp:* hypoventilation, respiratory muscle weakness
- Monitor for manifestations of hypomagnesemia; *CNS:* agitation, muscle twitching, paresthesias, hyperactive reflexes, positive Babinski reflex, dysphagia, nystagmus, seizures, tetany; *GI:* nausea, vomiting, diarrhea, anorexia, abdominal distention; *CV:* ectopy, tachycardia, broad, flat, or inverted T waves, depressed ST segment, prolonged QT, decreased cardiac output, hypotension
- Monitor for manifestations of hyponatremia: *CV:* increased B/P, cold, clammy skin, hypovolemia or hypervolemia; *GI:* anorexia, nausea, vomiting, diarrhea, abdominal cramps;

neuro: lethargy, increased ICP, confusion, headache, seizures, coma, fatigue, tremors, hyperreflexia

- Monitor for manifestations of hyperchloremia: *neuro:* weakness, lethargy, coma; *resp:* coma, deep rapid breathing
- Assess fluid volume status: I&O ratios and record, count or weigh diapers as appropriate, weight, distended red veins, crackles in lung, color, quality and sp gr of urine, skin turgor, adequacy of pulses, moist mucous membranes, bilateral lung sounds, peripheral pitting edema; dehydration symptoms of decreasing output, thirst, hypotension, dry mouth and mucous membranes should be reported
- Monitor electrolytes: potassium, sodium, calcium, magnesium; also include BUN, blood pH, ABGs, uric acid, CBC, blood sugar
- Assess BP before and during therapy with patient lying, standing, and sitting as appropriate; orthostatic hypotension can occur rapidly

Nursing diagnoses

- ✓ Altered urinary elimination (adverse reactions)
- ✓ Fluid volume deficit
- ✓ Fluid volume excess (uses)
- ✓ Knowledge deficit (teaching)

Implementation

- Give in AM to avoid interference with sleep
- Potassium replacement if potassium level is 3.0
- Give whole, or use oral sol; drug may be crushed if patient is unable to swallow

PO route

- Give with food; if nausea occurs, absorption may be increased

IV IV route

- Do not use solution that is yellow, has a precipitate, or crystals
- Administer **IV** after diluting 0.5 g/18 ml or more of sterile water for inj; may be diluted further with dextrose or NaCl: give over 5 min; sol is stable at room temp for 24 hr

Additive incompatibilities: Blood, blood products, amikacin, chlorpromazine, codeine, hydralazine, insulin, levorphanol, methadone, morphine, multivitamins, norepinephrine, polymyxin B, procaine, prochlorperazine, promazine, promethazine, streptomycin, tetracycline, triflupromazine, vancomycin

Additive compatibilities: Cimetidine, lidocaine, nafcillin, sodium bicarbonate

Patient/family education

- Teach patient to take the medication early in the day to prevent nocturia
- Instruct patient to take with food or milk if GI symptoms of nausea and anorexia occur
- Teach patient to maintain a weekly record of weight and notify prescriber of weight loss >5 lb
- Caution patient that this drug causes a loss of potassium, so food rich in potassium should be added to the diet; refer to a dietician for assistance in planning
- Caution patient not to exercise in hot weather or stand for prolonged periods, since orthostatic hypotension will be enhanced; to use sunscreen to prevent burning
- Teach patient not to use alcohol or any OTC medications without prescriber's

approval; serious drug reactions may occur

- Emphasize the need to contact prescriber immediately if muscle cramps, weakness, nausea, dizziness, or numbness occurs
- Teach patient to take own B/P and pulse and record
- Caution patient that orthostatic hypotension may occur; patient should rise slowly from sitting or reclining positions and lie down if dizziness occurs
- Teach patient to continue taking medication even if feeling better; this drug controls symptoms but does not cure the condition
- Advise the patient with hypertension to continue other medical treatment (exercise, weight loss, relaxation techniques, cessation of smoking)

Evaluation

Positive therapeutic outcome

- Decreased edema
- Decreased B/P
- Increased diuresis

Treatment of overdose: Lavage if taken orally, monitor electrolytes; administer dextrose in saline; monitor hydration, CV, renal status

chlorpheniramine

(OTC, ℞)
(klor-fen-ir'a-meen)
Aller-Chlor, Allergy, Chlo-Amine, Chlor-100, Chlorate, chlorpheniramine maleate, Chlor-Pro, Chlor-Pro 10, Chlorspan-12, Chlortab-B, Chlortab-4, Chlor-Trimeton, Chlor-Trimeton Repetabs, PediaCare Allergy Formula, Pfeiffer's Allergy, Phenetron, Telachlor, Teldrin

Func. class.: Antihistamine
Chem. class.: Alkylamine, H_1-receptor antagonist

Pregnancy category B

Action: Acts on blood vessels, GI, respiratory system by competing with histamine for H_1-receptor site; decreases allergic response by blocking histamine

Therapeutic Outcome: Absence of allergy symptoms and rhinitis

Uses: Allergy symptoms, rhinitis, allergic dermatoses, nasal allergies, hypersensitive reactions including blood transfusion reactions, anaphylaxis

Dosage and routes

Adult: PO 2-4 mg tid-qid, not to exceed 36 mg/day; time rel 8-12 mg bid-tid, not to exceed 36 mg/day; IM/**IV**/SC 5-40 mg/day

P ***Child 6-12 yr:*** PO 2 mg q4-6h, not to exceed 12 mg/day; sus rel 8 mg hs or qd; sus rel not recommended for child P <6 yr

P ***Child 2-5 yr:*** PO 1 mg q4-6h, not to exceed 4 mg/day

Available forms: Chewable tabs 2 mg; tabs 4 mg; time-rel tabs 8, 12 mg; time-rel caps 8, 12 mg; syr 2 mg/5 ml; inj 10, 100 mg/ml

Adverse effects

CNS: Dizziness, drowsiness, poor coordination, fatigue, anxiety, euphoria, confusion, paresthesia, neuritis

EENT: Blurred vision, dilated pupils, tinnitus, nasal stuffiness, dry nose, throat, mouth

GI: Dry mouth, nausea, anorexia, diarrhea

GU: Retention, dysuria, frequency

HEMA: Thrombocytopenia, agranulocytosis, hemolytic anemia

INTEG: Photosensitivity

RESP: Increased thick secretions, wheezing, chest tightness

Contraindications: Hypersensitivity to H_1-receptor antagonists, acute asthma attack, lower respiratory tract disease

Precautions: Increased intraocular pressure, renal disease, cardiac disease, hypertension, bronchial asthma, seizure disorder, stenosed peptic ulcers, hyperthyroidism, prostatic hypertrophy, bladder neck obstruction, pregnancy **B**, G elderly

Pharmacokinetics

Absorption	Well absorbed (PO, SC, IM, IV)
Distribution	Widely distributed; crosses blood-brain barrier
Metabolism	Liver, mostly
Excretion	Kidneys, metabolite; breast milk (minimal)
Half-life	12-15 hr

Pharmacodynamics

	PO	SC	IM	IV
Onset	15-30 min	Unknown	Unknown	Immediate
Peak	1-2 hr	Unknown	Unknown	Unknown
Duration	6-12 hr	6-12 hr	6-12 hr	6-12 hr

Interactions

Individual drugs

Alcohol: ↑ CNS depression

Atropine: ↑ anticholinergic reactions

Disopyramide: ↑ anticholinergic reactions

Haloperidol: ↑ anticholinergic reactions

Quinidine: ↑ anticholinergic reactions

Drug classifications

Antidepressants: ↑ anticholinergic reactions

Antihistamines: ↑ anticholinergic reactions

CNS depressants: ↑ CNS depression

MAOI: ↑ anticholinergic effect

Narcotics: ↑ CNS depression

Phenothiazines: ↑ anticholinergic reactions

Sedative/hypnotics: ↑ CNS depression

Lab test interferences

False negative: Skin allergy tests (discontinue antihistamines 3 days before testing)

NURSING CONSIDERATIONS

Assessment

- Assess respiratory status: rate, rhythm, increase in bronchial secretions, wheezing, chest tightness; provide fluids to 2 L/day to decrease secretion thickness
- Monitor I&O ratio: be alert for urinary retention, frequency, dysuria, especially G elderly; drug should be discontinued if these occur

• **IV** administration may result in rapid drop in B/P, sweating, G dizziness, especially in elderly

Nursing diagnoses

✓ Airway clearance, ineffective (uses)
✓ Injury, risk for (side effects)
✓ Knowledge deficit (teaching)
✓ Noncompliance (teaching, overuse)

Implementation

PO route

• May give with food to decrease GI upset; chewable tabs should be chewed and not swallowed whole; caps, time rel tabs should be swallowed whole

• Do not open or chew time rel tabs

• Store in tight, light-resistant container

SC/IM route

• Use only 20 mg/ml and 100 mg/ml strengths; does not need to be reconstituted or diluted

IV route

Give undiluted by direct **IV** (10 mg/ml strength only); administer 10 mg over 1 min or more

Additive incompatibilities: Calcium chloride, kanamycin, norepinephrine, pentobarbital

Additive compatibility: Amikacin

Patient/family education

• Teach all aspects of drug uses; to notify prescriber if confusion, sedation, hypotension occur; to avoid driving and other hazardous activity if drowsiness occurs; to avoid alcohol and other CNS depressants that may potentiate effect

• Teach patient not to exceed recommended dosage; dysrhythmias may occur

• Advise patient hard candy, gum, frequent rinsing of mouth may be used for dryness

Evaluation

Positive therapeutic outcome

• Absence of running or congested nose, rashes

Treatment of overdose: Administer ipecac syrup or lavage, diazepam, vasopressors, barbiturates (short acting)

chlorpromazine

(℞)

(klor-proe'ma-zeen)

chlorpromazine HCl, Chlorpromanyl ♣, Ormazine, Thorazine, Thorazine Spansules

Func. class.: Antipsychotic/neuroleptic

Chem. class.: Phenothiazine, aliphatic

Pregnancy category C

Action: Depresses cerebral cortex, hypothalamus, limbic system, which control activity aggression; blocks neurotransmission produced by dopamine at synapse; exhibits a strong α-adrenergic, anticholinergic blocking action; mechanism for antipsychotic effects is unclear

Therapeutic Outcome: Decreased signs and symptoms of psychosis; control of nausea, vomiting, intractable hiccups, decreased anxiety preoperatively

Uses: Psychotic disorders, mania, schizophrenia, anxiety, intractable hiccups, nausea, vomiting, preoperative relaxation, acute intermittent porphyria, behavioral problems in P children

Dosage and routes

Psychiatry

Adult: PO 10-50 mg q1-4h initially, then increase up to 2 g/day if necessary

Adult: IM 10-50 mg q1-4h

P ***Child:*** PO 0.25 mg/lb q4-6h or 0.5 mg/kg

P ***Child:*** IM 0.25 mg/lb q6-8h or 0.5 mg/kg

P ***Child:*** Rec 0.5 mg/lb q6-8h or 1 mg/kg

Nausea and vomiting

Adult: PO 10-25 mg q4-6h prn; IM 25-50 mg q3h prn; rec 50-100 mg q6-8h prn, not to exceed 400 mg/day

P ***Child:*** PO 0.25 mg/lb q4-6h prn; IM 0.25 mg/lb q6-8h prn not to exceed 40 mg/day (<5 yr) or 75 mg/day (5-12 yr); rec 0.5 mg/lb q6-8h prn

Adult: **IV** 25-50 mg qd-qid

P ***Child:*** **IV** 0.55 mg/kg q6-8h

Intractable hiccups

Adult: PO 25-50 mg tid-qid; IM 25-50 mg (used only if PO dose does not work); **IV** 25-50 mg in 500-1000 ml saline (only for severe hiccups)

Available forms: Tabs 10, 25, 50, 100, 200 mg; time rel caps 30, 75, 150, 200, 300 mg; syr 10 mg/5 ml; conc 30, 100 mg/ml; supp 25, 100 mg; inj 25 mg/ml

Adverse effects

CNS: ***Neuroleptic malignant syndrome,*** *extrapyramidal symptoms: pseudoparkinsonism, akathisia, dystonia, tardive dyskinesia,* seizures, *headache*

CV: Orthostatic hypotension, hypertension, ***cardiac arrest,*** ECG changes, ***tachycardia***

EENT: Blurred vision, glaucoma, dry eyes

GI: Dry mouth, nausea, vomiting, anorexia, constipation, diarrhea, jaundice, weight gain

GU: Urinary retention, urinary frequency, enuresis, impotence, amenorrhea, gynecomastia, breast engorgement

HEMA: Anemia, ***leukopenia, leukocytosis, agranulocytosis***

INTEG: Rash, photosensitivity, dermatitis

RESP: ***Laryngospasm,*** dyspnea, ***respiratory depression***

Contraindications: Hypersensitivity, circulatory collapse, liver damage, cerebral arteriosclerosis, coronary disease, severe hypertension/hypotension, blood dyscrasias, P coma, child <2 yr, brain damage, bone marrow depression, alcohol and barbiturate withdrawal

Precautions: Pregnancy **C**, lactation, seizure disorders, hypertension, hepatic disease, G cardiac disease, elderly

Pharmacokinetics

Absorption	Variable (PO); well absorbed (IM)
Distribution	Widely distributed; crosses placenta
Metabolism	Liver, GI mucosa extensively
Excretion	Kidneys
Half-life	30 hr

Pharmacodynamics

	PO	REC	IM	IV
Onset	½1 hr	12 hr	Unkn	Rapid
Peak	Unkn	Unkn	Unkn	Unkn
Duration	4-6 hr*	3-4 hr	4-8 hr	Unkn

*Duration PO ext rel is 10-12 hr.

Interactions

Individual drugs

Alcohol: ↑ effects of both drugs, oversedation

Aluminum hydroxide: ↓ absorption
Bromocriptine: ↓ antiparkinsonian activity
Disopyramide: ↑ anticholinergic effects
Epinephrine: ↑ toxicity
Guanethidine: ↓ antihypertensive response
Levodopa: ↓ antiparkinsonian activity
Lithium: ↓ chlorpromazine levels, ↑ extrapyramidal symptoms, masking of lithium toxicity
Magnesium hydroxide: ↓ absorption
Norepinephrine: ↓ vasoresponse, ↑ toxicity
Phenobarbital: ↓ effectiveness, ↑ metabolism

Drug classifications
Antacids: ↓ absorption
Anticholinergics: ↑ anticholinergic effects
Antidepressants: ↑ CNS depression
Antidiarrheals, adsorbent: ↓ absorption
Antihistamines: ↑ CNS depression
Antihypertensives: ↑ hypotension
Antithyroid agents: ↑ agranulocytosis
Barbiturate anesthetics: ↑ CNS depression
β-Adrenergics: ↑ effects of both drugs
General anesthetics: ↑ CNS depression
MAOI: ↑ CNS depression
Narcotics: ↑ CNS depression
Sedative/hypnotics: ↑ CNS depression

Lab test interferences
↑ Liver function tests, ↑ cardiac enzymes, ↑ cholesterol, ↑ blood glucose, ↑ prolactin, ↑ bilirubin, ↑ PBI, ↑ cholinesterase I, ↑ alkaline phosphatase, ↑ leukocytes, ↑ granulocytes, ↑ platelets
↓ Hormones (blood and urine)
False positive: Pregnancy tests, PKU, urine bilirubin
False negative: Urinary steroids, 17-OHCS

NURSING CONSIDERATIONS
Assessment

- Assess mental status: orientation, mood, behavior, presence of hallucinations, and type before initial administration and monthly; this drug should significantly reduce psychotic behavior
- Check for swallowing of PO medication; check for hoarding or giving of medication to other patients
- Monitor I&O ratio; palpate bladder if low urinary output occurs, especially in elderly; urinalysis recommended before, during prolonged therapy
- Monitor bilirubin, CBC, liver function studies monthly
- Assess affect, orientation, LOC, reflexes, gait, coordination, sleep pattern disturbances
- Monitor B/P with patient sitting, standing, and lying; take pulse and respirations q4h during initial treatment; establish baseline before starting treatment; report drops of 30 mm Hg; obtain baseline ECG, Q wave, and T wave changes
- Check for dizziness, faintness, palpitations, tachycardia on rising; severe orthostatic hypotension is common
- Identify for neuroleptic malignant syndrome: hyperpyrexia, muscle rigidity, increased CPK, altered mental status; drug should be discontinued
- Assess for extrapyramidal symptoms including akathisia (inability to sit still, no pattern

to movements), tardive dyskinesia (bizarre movements of the jaw, mouth, tongue, extremities), pseudoparkinsonism (rigidity, tremors, pill rolling, shuffling gate); an antiparkinsonian drug should be prescribed
- Assess for constipation, urinary retention daily; if these occur, increase bulk, water in diet

Nursing diagnoses
- ✓ Thought processes, altered (uses)
- ✓ Coping, ineffective individual (uses)
- ✓ Knowledge deficit (teaching)
- ✓ Noncompliance (teaching)

Implementation

PO route
- Give drug in liquid form mixed in glass of juice or cola if hoarding is suspected
- Give decreased dosage in elderly, since metabolism is slowed
- Give with full glass of water, milk; or give with food to decrease GI upset
- Do not crush, break or chew time rel caps
- Store in tight, light-resistant container, oral sol in amber bottle

Rec route
- Give after placing in refrigerator for 30 min if too soft to insert; this route is used for nausea, vomiting, hiccups

IM route
- Inject in deep muscle mass; do not give SC; may be diluted with 0.9% NaCl, 2% procaine as prescribed; do not administer sol with a precipitate

IV route
- Give by direct **IV** by diluting with 0.9% NaCl to a concentration of 1 mg/1 ml; administer at a rate of 1 mg/2 min
- Give by cont inf after diluting 50 mg/500-1000 ml of D_5W, $D_{10}W$, 0.9% NaCl, 0.45% NaCl, LR, Ringer's or combinations (used for intractable hiccups)

Syringe incompatibilities: Cimetidine, dimenhydrinate, heparin, pentobarbital, thiopental

Syringe compatibilities: Atropine, butorphanol, diphenhydramine, doxapram, droperidol, fentanyl, glycopyrrolate, hydromorphone, hydroxyzine, meperidine, metoclopramide, midazolam, pentazocine, perphenazine, prochlorperazine, promazine, promethazine, scopolamine

Y-site compatibilities: Heparin, hydrocortisone, ondansetron, potassium chloride, thiotepa

Additive incompatibilities: Aminophylline, amphotericin B, ampicillin, chloramphenicol, chlorothiazide, methicillin, methohexital, penicillin G, phenobarbital

Additive compatibilities: Ascorbic acid, ethacrynate, netilmicin

Patient/family education
- Teach patient to use good oral hygiene; frequent rinsing of mouth, sugarless gum for dry mouth
- Caution patient to avoid hazardous activities until drug response is determined; dizziness, blurred vision may occur
- Inform patient that orthostatic hypotension occurs often and to rise from sitting or lying position gradually, to remain lying down after IM injection for at least 30 min; tell patient

to avoid hot tubs, hot showers, tub baths, since hypotension may occur; tell patient that in hot weather heat stroke may occur; take extra precautions to stay cool

- Advise patient to avoid abrupt withdrawal of this drug, or extrapyramidal symptoms may result; drug should be withdrawn slowly
- Teach patient to avoid OTC preparations (cough, hay fever, cold) unless approved by prescriber, since serious drug interactions may occur; avoid use with alcohol, CNS depressants, since increased drowsiness may occur
- Caution patient to use sunscreen and sunglasses to prevent burns
- Teach patient about extrapyramidal symptoms and necessity of meticulous oral hygiene, since oral candidiasis may occur
- Instruct patient to take antacids 2 hr before or after taking this drug
- Instruct patient to report sore throat, malaise, fever, bleeding, mouth sores; if these occur, CBC should be drawn and drug discontinued
- Teach that urine may turn pink or red
- Teach patient to use contraceptive measures

Evaluation

Positive therapeutic outcome

- Decrease in emotional excitement, hallucinations, delusions, paranoia
- Reorganization of patterns of thought, speech

Treatment of overdose: Lavage if orally ingested; provide airway, *do not induce vomiting or use epinephrine*

chlorpropamide (℞)

(klor-proe'pa-mide)

Apo-chlorpropamide ✤, Chloronase ✤, Chlorpropamide, Diabinese, Novopropamide ✤

Func. class.: Antidiabetic, oral

Chem. class.: Sulfonylurea (1st generation)

Pregnancy category C

Action: Causes functioning β-cells in pancreas to release insulin, leading to drop in blood glucose levels; may improve insulin binding to insulin receptors or increase the number of insulin receptors with prolonged administration; may also reduce basal hepatic glucose secretion; not effective if patient lacks functioning β-cells

➔ Therapeutic Outcome: Decreased blood glucose levels in diabetes mellitus

Uses: Stable adult-onset diabetes mellitus (type II; NIDDM)

Dosage and routes

Adult: PO 100-250 mg qd initially, then 100-500 mg maintenance according to response; not to exceed 750 mg/day

Available forms: Tabs 100, 250 mg scored

Adverse effects

CNS: Headache, weakness, dizziness, drowsiness, tinnitus, fatigue, vertigo

ENDO: Hypoglycemia, hyponatremia

GI: Hepatotoxicity, cholestatic jaundice, nausea, vomiting, diarrhea, heartburn

HEMA: Leukopenia, thrombo-

cytopenia, agranulocytosis, ***aplastic anemia, pancytopenia, hemolytic anemia***
INTEG: Rash, allergic reactions, pruritus, urticaria, eczema, photosensitivity, erythema

Contraindications: Hypersensitivity to sulfonylureas, P juvenile or brittle diabetes, pregnancy **C,** renal failure

G **Precautions:** Elderly, cardiac disease, thyroid disease, renal disease, hepatic disease, severe hypoglycemic reactions

Pharmacokinetics	
Absorption	Well absorbed
Distribution	Bile
Metabolism	Liver to metabolites
Excretion	Kidneys, unchanged
Half-life	36 hr

Pharmacodynamics	
Onset	1 hr
Peak	3-6 hr
Duration	24 hr

Interactions
Individual drugs
Cimetidine: ↑ hypoglycemia
Chloramphenicol: ↑ hypoglycemia
Diazoxide: ↓ effect of both drugs
Guanethidine: ↑ hypoglycemia
Insulin: ↑ hypoglycemia
Methyldopa: ↑ hypoglycemia
Phenobarbital: ↓ action of chlorpropamide
Phenytoin: ↓ action of chlorpropamide
Rifampin: ↓ action of chlorpropamide
Drug classifications
Anticoagulants, oral: ↑ hypoglycemia
Calcium channel blockers: ↓ action of chlorpropamide
Corticosteroids: ↓ action of chlorpropamide
Diuretics, thiazide: ↓ action of chlorpropamide
Estrogens: ↓ action of chlorpropamide
MAOI: ↑ hypoglycemia
NSAIDs: ↑ hypoglycemia
Oral contraceptives: ↓ action of chlorpropamide
Phenothiazines: ↓ action of chlorpropamide
Salicylates: ↑ hypoglycemia
Sulfonamides: ↑ hypoglycemia
Sympathomimetics: ↓ action of chlorpropamide
Thyroid agents: ↓ action of chlorpropamide

NURSING CONSIDERATIONS
Assessment
- Assess for hypoglycemic reactions (sweating, weakness, dizziness, anxiety, tremors, hunger) and hyperglycemic reactions; can occur soon pc
- Monitor CBC (baseline, q3mo) during treatment; check liver function tests periodically (AST [SGOT], LDH) and renal studies (BUN, creatinine) during treatment

Nursing diagnoses
- ✓ Nutrition, altered: more than body requirements (uses)
- ✓ Nutrition altered: less than body requirements (adverse reactions)
- ✓ Knowledge deficit (teaching)
- ✓ Noncompliance (teaching)
- ✓ Injury, risk for physical (adverse reactions)

Implementation
- Conversion from other oral hypoglycemic agents or insulin dosage of <40 U/day may be made without gradual dosage change; patients taking insulin of >40 U/day convert gradu-

ally by receiving oral hypoglycemic and 50% of previous insulin dosage for 3-5 days; monitor serum or urine glucose and ketones tid during conversion
• Give drug 30 min before breakfast; if large dose is required, may be divided into two; give with meals to decrease GI upset and provide best absorption
• Give tabs crushed and mixed with meal or fluids for patients with difficulty swallowing
• Store in tight container in cool environment

Patient/family education
• Teach patient to check for symptoms of cholestatic jaundice: dark urine, pruritus, yellow sclera; if these occur, prescriber should be notified
• Teach patient to use capillary blood glucose test or Chemstrip tid
• Teach patient symptoms of hypoglycemia and hyperglycemia and what to do about each
• Instruct patient that drug must be continued daily; explain consequence of discontinuing drug abruptly
• Teach patient to take drug in morning to prevent hypoglycemic reactions at night
• Caution patient to avoid OTC medications unless they are prescribed
• Teach patient that diabetes is lifelong illness; that this drug is not a cure
• Teach patient that all food included in diet plan must be eaten to prevent hypoglycemia
• Advise patient to carry Medic Alert ID for emergency purposes; carry a glucagon emergency kit

Evaluation
Positive therapeutic outcome
• Decrease in polyuria, polydipsia, polyphagia; clear sensorium, absence of dizziness, stable gait

Treatment of overdose: Glucose 25g **IV**, via dextrose 50% sol, 50 ml or 1 mg glucagon

chlorthalidone (℞)

(klor-tha'li-doan)
Apo-Chlorthalidone ✤, Novothalidone ✤, Uridon ✤, Hygroton, Thalitone
Func. class.: Diuretic, antihypertensive
Chem. class.: Thiazide-like phthalimindine derivative
Pregnancy category B

Action: Acts on the distal tubule and thick ascending limb of the loop of Henle in the kidney, increasing excretion of sodium, water, chloride, magnesium, potassium, and bicarbonate

Therapeutic Outcome: Decreased B/P, decreased edema in lung tissues and peripherally, diuresis

Uses: Edema in congestive heart failure, nephrotic syndrome; may be used alone or as adjunct with antihypertensives; also for edema in corticosteroid estrogen therapy

Dosage and routes
Adult: PO 25-200 mg/day or 200 mg every other day
P ***Child:*** PO 2 mg/kg 3 times a wk

Available forms: Tabs 15, 25, 50, 100 mg

Adverse effects

CNS: Paresthesia, headache, *dizziness, fatigue, weakness,* fever

ELECT: Hypokalemia, hypercalcemia, hyponatremia, hypochloremia, hypomagnesemia

EENT: Blurred vision

GI: Nausea, vomiting, anorexia, constipation, diarrhea, cramps, pancreatitis, GI irritation, ***hepatitis***

GU: Frequency, polyuria, ***uremia,*** glucosuria

HEMA: Aplastic anemia, leukopenia, agranulocytosis, thrombocytopenia, neutropenia

INTEG: Rash, urticaria, purpura, photosensitivity

META: Hyperglycemia, hyperuricemia, increased creatinine, BUN

Contraindications: Hypersensitivity to thiazides or sulfonamides, anuria, renal decompensation, lactation

Precautions: Hypokalemia, renal disease, hepatic disease, gout, COPD, LE, diabetes mellitus, elderly, pregnancy **B,** hyperlipidemia

G

Pharmacokinetics	
Absorption	Well absorbed
Distribution	Extracellular spaces; crosses placenta
Metabolism	Liver
Excretion	Urine, unchanged (30%-60%)
Half-life	40 hr

Pharmacodynamics	
Onset	2 hr
Peak	6 hr
Duration	24-72 hr

Interactions

Individual drugs

Allopurnol: ↑ toxicity
Amphotericin B: ↑ hypokalemia
Cholestyramine: ↓ absorption of chlorothalidone
Colestipol: ↓ absorption of chlorothalidone
Diazoxide: ↑ hyperglycemia, hyperuricemia, hypotension
Digitalis: ↑ toxicity
Indomethacin: ↓ hypotensive response
Lithium: ↑ toxicity
Mezlocillin: ↑ hypokalemia
Piperacillin: ↑ hypokalemia
Ticarcillin: ↑ hypokalemia

Drug classifications

Anticoagulants: ↓ effects of antidiabetics
Antidiabetics: ↓ effect of antidiabetic agent
Antigout agents: ↓ effects of antidiabetics
Antihypertensives: ↑ antihypertensive effect
Nitrates: ↑ hypotension
Nondepolarizing skeletal muscle relaxants: ↑ toxicity
Glucocorticoids: ↑ hypokalemia
Sulfonylureas: ↓ effect of sulfonylurea

Food

↑ absorption

Lab test interferences

↑ BSP retention, ↑ triglycerides, ↑ calcium, ↑ amylase
↓ PBI, ↓ PSP

NURSING CONSIDERATIONS

Assessment

• Monitor manifestations of hypokalemia; *CV:* hypotension, broad T wave, U wave, ectopy, tachycardia, weak pulse; *GI:* anorexia, nausea, cramps, constipation, distention, paralytic ileus; *Neuro:* muscle weakness, altered LOC, drowsiness,

C

apathy, lethargy, confusion, depression; *Renal:* acidic urine, reduced urine, osmolality, nocturia; *Resp:* hypoventilation, respiratory muscle weakness

- Monitor for manifestations of hypomagnesemia; *CNS:* agitation, muscle twitching, paresthesias, hyperactive reflexes, positive Babinski reflex, dysphagia, nystagmus seizures, tetany; *CV:* ectopy, tachycardia, broad, flat or inverted T waves, depressed ST segment, prolonged QT, decreased cardiac output, hypotension; *GI:* nausea, vomiting, diarrhea, anorexia, abdominal distention
- Monitor for manifestations of hyponatremia; *CV:* increased B/P, cold, clammy skin, hypovolemia or hypervolemia; *GI:* anorexia, nausea, vomiting, diarrhea, abdominal cramps; *Neuro:* lethargy, increased ICP, confusion, headache, seizures, coma, fatigue, tremors, hyperreflexia
- Monitor for manifestations of hyperchloremia; *Neuro:* weakness, lethargy, coma; *Resp:* coma, deep rapid breathing
- Assess fluid volumes status: I&O ratios and record, count or weigh diapers as appropriate, weight, distended red veins, crackles in lung, color, quality and sp gr of urine, skin turgor, adequacy of pulses, moist mucous membranes, bilateral lung sounds, peripheral pitting edema; dehydration symptoms of decreasing output, thirst, hypotension, dry mouth, and mucous membranes should be reported
- Monitor electrolytes: potassium, sodium, calcium, magnesium; also include BUN, blood pH, ABGs, uric acid, CBC, blood sugar
- Assess B/P before and during therapy with patient lying, standing, and sitting as appropriate; orthostatic hypotension can occur rapidly

Nursing diagnoses

✓ Altered urinary elimination (side effect)
✓ Fluid volume deficit (adverse reactions)
✓ Fluid volume excess (uses)
✓ Knowledge deficit (teaching)

Implementation

- Give in AM to avoid interference with sleep
- Provide potassium replacement if potassium level is 3.0 mg/dl; give whole, or use oral solutions lightly; drug may be crushed if patient is unable to swallow
- Give with food; if nausea occurs, may crush tab and mix with fluids or applesauce for swallowing

Patient/family education

General

- Teach patient to take the medication early in the day to prevent nocturia
- Instruct patient to take with food or milk if GI symptoms of nausea and anorexia occur
- Teach patient to maintain weekly record of weight and notify prescriber of weight loss >5 lb
- Caution patient that this drug causes a loss of potassium, so food rich in potassium should be added to the diet; refer to a dietician for assistance in planning
- Caution the patient not to exercise in hot weather or stand for prolonged periods, since orthostatic hypotension

will be enhanced; to use sunscreen to prevent burns

- Teach patient not to use alcohol, or any OTC medications without prescriber's approval; serious drug reactions may occur
- Emphasize the need to contact prescriber immediately if muscle cramps, weakness, nausea, dizziness, or numbness occurs
- Teach patient to take own B/P and pulse and record
- Caution patient that orthostatic hypotension may occur; patient should rise slowly from sitting or reclining positions and lie down if dizziness occurs
- Teach patient to continue taking medication even if feeling better; this drug controls symptoms but does not cure the condition
- Advise patient with hypertension to continue other medical treatment (exercise, weight loss, relaxation techniques, cessation of smoking)

Evaluation

Positive therapeutic outcome

- Decreased edema
- Decreased B/P
- Increased diuresis

Treatment of overdose: Lavage if taken orally, monitor electrolytes; administer dextrose in saline; monitor hydration, CV, renal status

cholestyramine

🔑 (℞)

(koe-less-tear'a-meen)

Cholybar, Questran, Questran Light

Func. class.: Antilipemic

Chem. class.: Bile acid sequestrant

Pregnancy category C

Action: Absorbs, combines with bile acids to form an insoluble complex that is excreted through feces; loss of bile acids lowers cholesterol levels

➔ Therapeutic Outcome: Decreasing cholesterol levels and low-density lipoproteins, decreased pruritus

Uses: Primary hypercholesterolemia, pruritus associated with biliary obstruction, diarrhea caused by excess bile acid, xanthomas

Dosage and routes

Adult: PO 4 g ac and hs, not to exceed 32 g/day

P ***Child:*** PO 240 mg/kg/day in 3 divided doses; administer with food or drink

Available forms: Powder 4 g cholestyramine of 9 g or 5 g powder

Adverse effects

CNS: Headache, dizziness, drowsiness, vertigo, tinnitus

GI: Constipation, abdominal pain, nausea, fecal impaction, hemorrhoids, flatulence, vomiting, steatorrhea, peptic ulcer

HEMA: Decreased vitamin A, D, K, red cell folate content, ***hyperchloremic acidosis, bleeding,*** decreased pro-time

INTEG: Rash, irritation of perianal area, tongue, skin
MS: Muscle, joint pain

Contraindications: Hypersensitivity, biliary obstruction

Precautions: Pregnancy **C**, P lactation, children

Pharmacokinetics

Absorption	Not absorbed
Distribution	Not distributed
Metabolism	Not metabolized
Excretion	Binds with bile acids, feces
Half-life	Unknown

Pharmacodynamics

Onset	24-48 hr
Peak	1-3 wk
Duration	2-4 wk

Interactions

Individual drugs

Acetaminophen: ↓ absorption
Amiodarone: ↓ absorption
Methotrexate: ↓ absorption
Naproxen: ↓ absorption
Phenylbutazone: ↓ absorption
Piroxican: ↓ absorption
Propranolol: ↓ absorption
Thyroid: ↓ absorption
Ursodiol: ↓ absorption

Drug classifications

Anticoagulants, oral: ↓ absorption
Cardiac glycosides: ↓ absorption
Diuretics, thiazide: ↓ absorption
Vitamins A,D,E,K: ↓ absorption

Lab test interferences

↑ Liver function studies, ↑ chlorine, ↑ PO_4

NURSING CONSIDERATIONS

Assessment

- Assess nutrition: fat, protein, carbohydrates, nutritional analysis should be completed by dietician
- Assess skin integrity after patient has been receiving drug; itching, pruritus often occur from bile deposits on skin
- Monitor cardiac glycoside level if both drugs are being administered; cardiac glycoside levels will be decreased
- Monitor for signs of vitamin A, D, E, K deficiency; serum cholesterol, triglyceride levels, electrolytes if on extended therapy
- Monitor bowel pattern daily; increase bulk, water in diet if constipation develops

Nursing diagnoses

✓ Constipation (adverse reactions)
✓ Knowledge deficit (teaching)
✓ Noncompliance (teaching)

Implementation

- Give drug ac, hs; give all other medications 1 hr before cholestyramine or 4 hr after cholestyramine to avoid poor absorption; do not take dry; mix drug with applesauce or stir into beverage (2-6 oz); let stand for 2 min; avoid inhaling powder
- Provide supplemental doses of vitamin A, D, E, K, if levels are low

Patient/family education

- ❗ Teach patient symptoms of hypoprothrombinemia: bleeding mucous membranes, dark tarry stools, hematuria, petechiae; report immediately
- Teach patient importance of compliance, since toxicity may result if doses are missed; not to discontinue suddenly
- Teach patient that risk factors should be decreased: high-fat diet, smoking, alcohol consumption, absence of exercise

• Have patient mix drug with 6 oz of milk, water, fruit juice; do not mix with carbonated beverages; rinse glass to make sure all medication is taken or may mix drug in applesauce; allow to stand for 2 min before mixing

Evaluation

Positive therapeutic outcome

• Decreased cholesterol level (hyperlipidemia)

• Decreased diarrhea, pruritus (excess bile acids)

choline salicylate (℞)

(koe'leen sa-lis'ih-late)

Arthropan, Teejel ✤

Func. class.: Nonnarcotic analgesic

Chem. class.: Salicylate

Pregnancy category C

Action: Blocks pain impulses in CNS that occur in response to inhibition of prostaglandin synthesis; antipyretic action results from inhibition of hypothalamic heat-regulating center to produce vasodilatation to allow heat dissipation

➔ **Therapeutic Outcome:** Decreased pain, inflammation, fever

Uses: Mild to moderate pain or fever including arthritis, juvenile rheumatoid arthritis

Dosage and routes

Arthritis

P ***Adult and child >12 yrs:*** PO 870-1740 mg qid; max 6 times a day

Pain/fever

Adult: PO 870 mg q3-4h prn

P ***Child 3-6 yr:*** PO 105-210 mg q4h prn

Available forms: Liq 870 mg/5 ml

Adverse effects

CNS: Stimulation, drowsiness, dizziness, confusion, ***convulsion,*** headache, flushing, hallucinations, ***coma***

CV: Rapid pulse, pulmonary edema

EENT: Tinnitus, hearing loss

ENDO: Hypoglycemia, hyponatremia, hypokalemia

GI: Nausea, vomiting, GI bleeding, diarrhea, heartburn, anorexia, ***hepatitis***

HEMA: ***Thrombocytopenia, agranulocytosis, leukopenia, neutropenia, hemolytic anemia,*** increased pro-time

INTEG: Rash, urticaria, bruising

RESP: Wheezing, hyperpnea

Contraindications: Hypersensitivity to salicylates, GI bleeding, bleeding disorders, P children <3 yr, vitamin K deficiency, children with flulike symptoms

Precautions: Anemia, hepatic disease, renal disease, Hodgkin's disease, pregnancy **C**, lactation

Pharmacokinetics

Absorption	Well absorbed
Distribution	Widely distributed; crosses placenta
Metabolism	Liver, extensively
Excretion	Kidney, active metabolites; breast milk
Half-life	2-3 hr (low doses); 30 hr (high doses)

Pharmacodynamics

Onset	15-30 min
Peak	1-3 hr
Duration	3-6 hr

Interactions

Individual drugs

Alcohol: ↑ bleeding

Cefamandole: ↑ bleeding
Furosemide: ↑ toxic effects
Heparin: ↑ bleeding
Insulin: ↑ effects
Methotrexate: ↑ effects
PABA: ↑ toxic effects
Phenytoin: ↑ effects
Plicamycin: ↑ bleeding
Probenecid: ↓ effects
Spironolactone: ↓ effects
Sulfinpyrazone: ↓ effects
Valproic acid: ↑ effects, ↑ bleeding
Vancomycin: ↑ ototoxicity

Drug classifications

Antacids: ↓ effects of choline salicylate
Anticoagulants: ↑ effects
Carbonic anhydrase inhibitors: ↑ toxic effects
NSAIDs: ↑ gastric ulcers
Penicillins: ↑ effects
Salicylates: ↓ blood sugar levels
Steroids: ↓ effects of choline salicylate, ↑ gastric ulcers
Sulfonylamides: ↓ effects
Urinary acidifiers: ↑ salicylate levels
Urinary alkalizers: ↓ effects of choline salicylate

Lab test interferences

↑ Coagulation studies, ↑ liver function studies, ↑ serum uric acid, ↑ amylase, ↑ CO_2, ↑ urinary protein
↓ Serum potassium, ↓ PBI, ↓ cholesterol
Interference: Urine catecholamines, pregnancy test, urine glucose tests (Clinistix, Tes-Tape)

NURSING CONSIDERATIONS

Assessment

- Monitor pain: location, duration, type, intensity, prior to dose and 1 hr after
- Monitor musculoskeletal status: ROM before dose
- Identify fever, length of time and related symptoms
- Monitor liver function studies: AST (SGOT), ALT (SGPT), bilirubin, creatinine if patient is on long-term therapy
- Monitor renal function studies: BUN, urine creatinine if patient is on long-term therapy
- Monitor blood studies: CBC, Hct, Hgb, pro-time if patient is on long-term therapy
- Check I&O ratio; decreasing output may indicate renal failure (long-term therapy)
- ❗ Assess hepatotoxicity: dark urine, clay-colored stools, yellowing of the skin and sclera, itching, abdominal pain, fever, diarrhea if patient is on long-term therapy
- Assess for allergic reactions: rash, urticaria; if these occur, drug may have to be discontinued
- Assess for ototoxicity: tinnitus, ringing, roaring in ears; audiometric testing needed before, after long-term therapy
- Assess for visual changes: blurring, halos; corneal, retinal damage
- Check edema in feet, ankles, legs
- Identify prior drug history; there are many drug interactions

Nursing diagnoses

- ✓ Pain (uses)
- ✓ Mobility, impaired physical (uses)
- ✓ Knowledge deficit (teaching)
- ✓ Injury, risk for (side effects)

Implementation

- Administer to patient crushed or whole
- Give with food or milk to decrease gastric symptoms;

give 30 min ac or 2 hr pc; absorption may be slowed
- Give antacids 1-2 hr after enteric products

Patient/family education
- Teach patient to report any symptoms of hepatotoxicity, renal toxicity, visual changes, ototoxicity, allergic reactions, bleeding (long-term therapy)
- Advise patient to take with 8 oz of water and sit upright for 30 min after dose
- Caution patient not to exceed recommended dosage; acute poisoning may result
- Caution patient to read label on other OTC drugs; many contain aspirin products
- Inform patient that the therapeutic response takes 2 wk (arthritis)
- Teach patient to report tinnitus, confusion, diarrhea, sweating, hyperventilation
- Caution patient to avoid alcohol ingestion; GI bleeding may occur
- Teach patient that patients who have allergies may develop allergic reactions
- Caution patient to avoid buffered or effervescent products
- Teach patient not to give to children; Reye's syndrome may develop

Evaluation

Positive therapeutic outcome
- Decreased pain
- Decreased inflammation
- Decreased fever
- Increased mobility

Treatment of overdose: Lavage, activated charcoal, monitor electrolytes, VS

ciclopirox (℞)
(sye-kloe-peer'ox)
Loprox
Func. class.: Local antiinfective
Chem. class.: Antifungal
Pregnancy category B

Action: Interferes with fungal cell membrane, which increases permeability, leaking of cell nutrients

Therapeutic Outcome: Fungistatic/fungicidal against susceptible organisms causing tinea pedis, tinea cruris, tinea corporis, tinea versicolor

Uses: Tinea cruris, tinea corporis, tinea pedis, tinea versicolor, cutaneous candidiasis

Dosage and routes
Adult and child >10 yr: Top rub into affected area bid for 2 wks

Available forms: Cream, lotion 1%

Adverse effects
INTEG: Rash, urticaria, stinging, burning, pruritus, pain

Contraindications: Hypersensitivity

Precautions: Pregnancy **B**, lactation, child <10 yr

Pharmacokinetics	
Absorption	Minimal
Distribution	Unknown
Metabolism	Liver
Excretion	Feces, kidneys
Half-life	2 hr

Pharmacodynamics
Unknown

Interactions: None

NURSING CONSIDERATIONS

Assessment

- Assess skin for fungal infections: peeling, dryness, itching before and throughout treatment
- Monitor for allergic reaction: burning, stinging, swelling, redness, dermatitis, rash; drug should be discontinued, antihistamines (mild reaction)

Nursing diagnoses

✓ Skin integrity, impaired (uses)
✓ Infection, risk for (uses)
✓ Knowledge deficit (teaching)

Implementation

- Apply enough medication to cover lesions completely
- Clean with soap, water before each application; dry well
- Store at room temp in dry place

Patient/family education

- Tell patient to apply with glove to prevent further infection; not to cover with occlusive dressings
- Teach patient proper hygiene: hand-washing technique, nail care, use of concomitant top agents if prescribed
- Advise patient to avoid use of OTC creams, ointments, lotions unless directed
- Teach patient to use hand washing before, after each application
- Teach patient to change socks and shoes once a day during treatment of tinea pedis
- Instruct patient to report to prescriber if infection persists or returns or if blisters, burning, oozing, swelling occurs

Evaluation

Positive therapeutic outcome

- Decrease in size, number of lesions

cidofovir (℞)

(si-doh-foh'veer)
Vistide
Func. class.: Antiviral
Chem. class.: Nucleotide analog
Pregnancy category C

Action: Suppresses cytomegalovirus (CMV) replication by selective inhibition of viral DNA synthesis

➔ Therapeutic Outcome: Decreased symptoms of CMV

Uses: CMV retinitis in patients with AIDS

Dosage and routes

Dilute in 100 ml 0.9% saline sol before administration; probenecid must be given PO 2 g 3 hr prior to the cidofovir infusion and 1 g at 2 and 8 hr after ending the cidofovir infusion; give 1 L of 0.9% saline sol **IV** with each INF of cidovovir, give saline INF over 1-2 hr period immediately prior to cidofovir; patient should be given a second L if the patient can tolerate the fluid load second L given at time of cidofovir or immediately afterward and should be given over a 1-3 hr period

Induction

Adult: IV Inf 5 mg/kg given over 1 hr at a constant rate qwk × 2 consecutive wk

Maintenance

Adult: IV Inf 5 mg/kg given over 1 hr q2 wk

Available forms: Inj

Adverse effects

CNS: Fever, chills, *coma,* confusion, abnormal thought, dizziness, bizarre dreams,

headache, psychosis, tremors, somnolence, paresthesia
CV: Dysrhythmias, hypertension/hypotension
EENT: Retinal detachment in CMV retinitis
GI: Abnormal LFTs, nausea, vomiting, anorexia, diarrhea, abdominal pain, *hemorrhage*
GU: Hematuria, increased creatinine, BUN
HEMA: ***Granulocytopenia, thrombocytopenia, irreversible neutropenia, anemia,*** *eosinophilia*
INTEG: Rash, alopecia, pruritus, urticaria, pain at inj site, phlebitis
RESP: Dyspnea

Contraindications: Hypersensitivity to acyclovir or this drug

Precautions: Preexisting cytopenias, renal function impairment, pregnancy **C,** lactation, children <6 mo, elderly, platelet count <25,000/mm^3

Pharmacokinetics

Unknown

Pharmacodynamics

Unknown

NURSING CONSIDERATIONS

Assessment

- Obtain culture before treatment is initiated; cultures of blood, urine, and throat may all be taken; CMV is not confirmed by this method; the diagnosis is made by an ophth exam
- Monitor kidney, liver function, increased hemopoietic studies and BUN; serum creatinine, AST (SGOT), ALT (SGPT), creatinine, AST (SGOT), ALT (SGPT), creatinine clearance, A-G ratio, baseline and drip treatment, blood counts should be done q2wk; watch for decreasing graunlocytes, Hgb; if low, therapy may have to be discontinued and restarted after hematologic recovery; blood transfusions may be required
- Assess for GI symptoms: severe nausea, vomiting, diarrhea, severe symptoms may necessitate discontinuing drug
- Assess electrolytes and minerals: calcium, phosphorous, magnesium, sodium, potassium; watch closely for tetany during first administration
- Assess for symptoms of blood dyscrasias (anemia, granulocytopenia); bruising, fatigue, bleeding, poor healing
- Assess allergic reactions: flushing, rash, urticaria, pruritus
- Assess for leukopenia, neutropenia, thrombocytopenia: WBCs, platelets q2d during 2 ×/day dosing and qwk thereafter; check for leukopenias, with qd WBC count in patients with prior leukopenia, with other nucleoside analogs, or for whom leukopenia counts are <1000 cells/mm^3 at start of treatment
- Monitor serum creatinine or creatinine clearance at least q2wk

Nursing diagnoses

✓ Infection, risk for (uses)

Implementation

- Mix under strict aseptic conditions using gloves, gown and mask, and using precautions for antineoplastics
- Give slowly; do not give by bolus **IV**, **IV**, SC inj
- Use diluted sol within 12 hr, do not refrigerate or freeze; do not use sol with particulate matter or discoloration

Patient/family education
- Advise to notify prescriber if sore throat, swollen lymph nodes, malaise, fever occur, may indicate other infections
- Advise to report perioral tingling, numbness in extremities, and paresthesias
- Teach that serious drug interactions may occur if OTC products are ingested; check first with prescriber
- Teach that drug is not a cure, but will control symptoms
- Advise that regular ophth exams must be continued
- Advise that major toxicities may necessitate discontinuing drug
- Advise to use contraception during treatment and that infertility may occur; men should use barrier contraception for 90 days after treatment

Evaluation
Positive therapeutic outcome
- Decreased symptoms of CMV

Treatment of overdose: Discontinue drug; use hemodialysis, and increase hydration

cimetidine 🔑 (℞, OTC)

(sye-met'i-deen)
Apo-Cimetidine ✤, Novocimetine ✤, Peptol ✤, Tagamet
Func. class.: H_2-receptor antagonist
Chem. class.: Imidazole derivative
Pregnancy category B

Action: Inhibits histamine at H_2-receptor site in the gastric parietal cells, which inhibits gastric acid secretion

➡ Therapeutic Outcome: Healing of duodenal or gastric ulcers; prevention of duodenal ulcers; decreases symptoms of gastroesophageal reflux disease (GERD) and Zollinger-Ellison syndrome

Uses: Short-term treatment of duodenal and gastric ulcers and maintenance; management of GERD and Zollinger-Ellison syndrome

Investigational uses: Prevention of aspiration pneumonitis, stress ulcers, upper GI bleeding

Dosage and routes
Treatment of active ulcers
P ***Adult and child:*** PO 300 mg qid with meals, hs × 8 wk or 400 mg bid, 800 mg hs; after 8 wk give hs dose only; **IV** bol 300 mg/20 ml 0.9% NaCl over 1-2 min q6h; **IV** inf 300 mg/50 ml D_5W over 15-20 min; IM 300 mg q6h, not to exceed 2400 mg

Prophylaxis of duodenal ulcer
P ***Adult and child >16 yr:*** 400 mg hs

GERD
Adult: PO 800-1600 mg/day in divided doses

Hypersecretory conditions (Zollinger-Ellison syndrome)
Adult: PO/IM/**IV** 300-600 mg q6h; may increase to 12 g/day if needed

Upper GI bleeding prophylaxis
Adult: **IV** 50 mg/hr; lowered in renal disease

Aspiration pneumonitis prophylaxis
Adult: IM/**IV** 300 mg IM 1 hr before anesthesia, then 300 mg **IV** q4h until patient is alert

Available forms: Tabs 100, 200, 300, 400, 800 mg; liq 300 mg/5 ml; inj 300 mg/2 ml, 300 mg/50 ml 0.9% NaCl

Adverse effects

CNS: Confusion, headache, depression, dizziness, anxiety, weakness, psychosis, tremors, ***convulsions***

CV: Bradycardia, tachycardia

GI: Diarrhea, abdominal cramps, ***paralytic ileus, jaundice***

GU: Gynecomastia, galactorrhea, impotence, increase in BUN, creatinine

HEMA: ***Agranulocytosis, thrombocytopenia, neutropenia, aplastic anemia, increase in pro-time***

INTEG: Urticaria, rash, alopecia, sweating, flushing, ***exfoliative dermatitis***

Contraindications: Hypersensitivity

Precautions: Pregnancy **B**, P lactation, child <16 yr, organic brain syndrome, hepatic disease, renal disease, G elderly

Pharmacokinetics

Absorption	Well absorbed (PO, IM); completely absorbed (IV)
Distribution	Widely distributed; crosses placenta
Metabolism	Liver (30%)
Excretion	Kidneys, unchanged (70%); breast milk
Half life	1½-2 hr; increased in renal disease

Pharmacodynamics

	PO	IV/IM
Onset	½ hr	10 min
Peak	45-90 min	½ hr
Duration	4-5 hr	4-5 hr

Interactions

Individual drugs

Carmustine: ↑ toxicity
Flecainide: ↑ toxicity
Indomethacin: ↓ absorption of cimetidine
Ketoconazole: ↓ absorption of cimetidine
Lidocaine: ↑ toxicity
Metoclopramide: ↓ absorption of cimetidine
Metoprolol: ↑ toxicity
Procainamide: ↑ toxicity
Propranolol: ↑ toxicity
Quinidine: ↑ toxicity
Succinylcholine: ↑ toxicity
Tocainamide: ↓ absorption of tocainamide

Drug classifications

Analgesics, narcotic: ↑ toxicity
Antacids: ↓ absorption of cimetidine
Anticholinergics: ↓ absorption of cimetidine
Anticoagulants, oral: ↑ toxicity
Antidepressants, tricyclic: ↑ toxicity
Benzodiazepines: ↑ toxicity
Iron salts: ↓ absorption of iron salts
Phenytoins: ↑ toxicity
Tetracyclines: ↓ absorption of tetracyclines
Theophyllines: ↑ toxicity

Smoking

↓ effectiveness

Lab test interferences

↑ Alkaline phosphatase, ↑ AST (SGOT), ↑ creatinine
False positive: Gastric bleeding test, skin allergy tests

NURSING CONSIDERATIONS

Assessment

- Assess patient with ulcers or suspected ulcers: epigastric or abdominal pain, hematemesis, occult blood in stools, blood in gastric aspirate before and/or throughout treatment; monitor gastric pH (5 or > should be maintained)
- Monitor I&O ratio, BUN,

creatinine, CBC with differential monthly

Nursing diagnoses

- ✓ Pain (uses)
- ✓ Knowledge deficit (teaching)

Implementation

PO route

- Give with meals for lengthened drug effect; antacids 1 hr before or 1 hr after cimetidine

IV **IV route**

- Give by direct **IV** after diluting 300 mg/20 ml of normal saline for inj; give over 2 min or more
- Give intermittent **IV** by diluting 300 mg/50 ml of D_5W; run over 15-20 min
- Give by cont inf after using total daily dose (900 mg) diluted in 100-1000 ml D_5W given over 24 hr
- Store diluted sol at room temp up to 48 hr

Syringe compatibilities: Atropine, butorphanol, cephalothin, diazepam, diphenhydramine, doxapram, droperidol, fentanyl, glycopyrrolate, heparin, hydromorphone, hydroxyzine, lorazepam, meperidine, midazolam, morphine, nafcillin, nalbuphine, penicillin G sodium, pentazocine, perphenazine, prochlorperazine, promazine, promethazine, scopolamine

Syringe incompatibilities: Cefamandole, cefazolin, chlorpromazine, pentobarbital, secobarbital

Y-site compatibilities: Acyclovir, amifostine, aminophylline, amrinone, atracurium, cisplatin, cyclophosphamide, cytarabine, diltiazem, doxorubicin, enalaprilat, esmolol, filgrastim, foscarnet, granisetron, haloperidol heparin, hetastarch, idarubicin, labetalol, melphalan, midazolam, ondansetron, paclitaxel, pancuronium, thiotepa, tolazoline, vecuronium, vinorelbine, zidovudine

Y-site incompatibility: Amsacrine

Additive compatibilities: Acetazolamide, amikacin, aminophylline, cefoxitin, chlorothiazide, clindamycin, colistimethate, dexamethasone, digoxin, epinephrine, erythromycin, ethacrynate, floxacillin, flumazenil, furosemide, gentamicin, insulin, isoproterenol, lidocaine, lincomycin, metaraminol, methylprednisolone, norepinephrine, penicillin G potassium, phytonadione, polymyxin B, potassium chloride, protamine, quinidine, tacrolimus, tetracycline, verapamil, vitamin B complex

Additive incompatibility: Amphotericin B

Patient/family education

- Advise patient that any gynecomastia or impotence that develops is reversible after treatment is discontinued
- Caution patient to avoid driving, other hazardous activities until stabilized on this medication; drowsiness or dizziness may occur
- Advise patient to avoid black pepper, caffeine, alcohol, harsh spices, extremes in temp of food; tell patient to avoid OTC preparations: aspirin, cough, cold preparations; condition may worsen
- Advise patient that smoking decreases the effectiveness of the drug; smoking cessation should be considered
- Teach patient that drug must

be continued for prescribed time to be effective and taken exactly as prescribed; doses are not to be doubled; to take missed dose when remembered up to 1 hr before next dose
• Instruct patient to report bruising, fatigue, malaise; blood dyscrasias may occur
• Have patient report to prescriber immediately any diarrhea, black tarry stools, sore throat, dizziness, confusion, or delirium

Evaluation
Positive therapeutic outcome
• Decreased pain in abdomen
• Healing of ulcers
• Absence of gastroesophageal reflux
• Gastric pH of 5 or >

ciprofloxacin (℞)
(sip-ro-floks'a-sin)
Ciloxin, Cipro, Cipro IV
Func. class.: Urinary anti-infectives
Chem. class.: Fluoroquinolone antibacterial
Pregnancy category C

Action: Interferes with conversion of intermediate DNA fragments into high-molecular-weight DNA in bacteria; DNA gyrase inhibitor

Therapeutic Outcome: Bactericidal action against the following: gram-positive organisms *Staphylococcus epidermidis,* methicillin-resistant strains of *S. aureus, Streptococcus pyogenes, S. pneumoniae;* gram-negative organisms *Escherichia coli, Klebsiella* species, *Enterobacter, Salmonella, Shigella, Proteus vulgaris, Providencia stuartii, P. retgeri, Morganella morganii, Pseudomonas aeruginosa, Serratia, Haemophilus, Acinetobacter, Neisseria gonorrhoeae, meningitidis, Branhamella catarrhalis, Yersinia, Vibrio, Brucella, Campylobacter, Aeromonas*

Uses: Adult urinary tract infections (including complicated); lower respiratory, skin, bone, joint infections; infectious diarrhea; conjunctivitis, corneal ulcers (ophthalmic)

Dosage and routes

Uncomplicated urinary tract infections
Adult: PO 250 mg q12h; **IV** 200 mg q12h

Complicated/severe urinary tract infections
Adult: PO 500 mg q12h; **IV** 400 mg q12h

Respiratory, bone, skin, joint infections
Adult: PO 500 mg q12h

Corneal ulcers, conjunctivitis
Adult: Ophth 1-2 gtts q15-30 min until infection is controlled, then 1-2 gtts 4-6 times daily

Available forms: Tabs 250, 500, 750, mg; 200 mg/100 ml D_5, 400 mg/200 ml D_5; 200, 400 mg vial; oph sol

Adverse effects
CNS: Headache, dizziness, fatigue, insomnia, depression, restlessness
GI: Nausea, constipation, increased ALT (SGPT), AST (SGOT), flatulence, insomnia, heartburn, vomiting, diarrhea, oral candidiasis, dysphagia
INTEG: Rash, pruritus, urticaria, photosensitivity, flushing, fever, chills
MS: Blurred vision, tinnitus

Contraindications: Hypersensitivity to quinolones

Precautions: Pregnancy **C**, P lactation, children, renal disease

Pharmacokinetics

Absorption	Well absorbed (75%) (PO)
Distribution	Widely distributed
Metabolism	Liver (15%)
Excretion	Kidneys (40%-50%)
Half-life	3-4 hr; increased in renal disease

Pharmacodynamics

	PO	IV
Onset	Rapid	Immediate
Peak	1 hr	Infusion's end

Interactions

Individual drugs

Caffeine: ↓ effect of ciprofloxacin
Cyclosporine: ↑ nephrotoxicity
Nitrofurantoin: ↓ effectiveness
Probenecid: ↑ blood levels
Sucralfate: ↓ absorption of ciprofloxacin
Theophylline: ↑ toxicity
Warfarin: ↑ warfarin effect
Zinc sulfate: ↓ absorption of ciprofloxacin

Drug classifications

Antacids: ↓ absorption of ciprofloxacin
Anticoagulants, oral: ↑ effect of anticoagulants
Antineoplastics: ↓ ciprofloxacin levels
Iron salts: ↓ absorption of ciprofloxacin

Lab test interferences

↑ AST (SGOT), ↑ ALT (SGPT), ↑ BUN, ↑ creatinine, ↑ alkaline phosphatase

NURSING CONSIDERATIONS

Assessment

- Assess patient for previous sensitivity reaction
- Assess patient for signs and symptoms of infection including characteristics of wounds, sputum, urine, stool, WBC >10,000, fever; obtain baseline information before and during treatment
- Obtain C&S before beginning drug therapy to identify if correct treatment has been initiated
- Assess for allergic reactions: rash, urticaria, pruritus, chills, fever, joint pain; may occur a few days after therapy begins; epinephrine and resuscitation equipment should be available for anaphylactic reaction
- Identify urine output; if decreasing, notify prescriber (may indicate nephrotoxicity); also check for increased BUN, creatinine
- Monitor blood studies: AST (SGOT), ALT (SGPT), CBC, Hct, bilirubin, LDH, alkaline phosphatase, Coombs' test monthly if patient is on long-term therapy
- Monitor electrolytes: potassium, sodium, chloride monthly if patient is on long-term therapy
- Assess bowel pattern qd; if severe diarrhea occurs, drug should be discontinued
- Monitor for bleeding: ecchymosis, bleeding gums, hematuria, stool guaiac daily if on long-term therapy
- Assess for overgrowth of infection: perineal itching, fever, malaise, redness, pain, swelling, drainage, rash, diarrhea, change in cough, sputum

Nursing diagnoses
- ✓ Infection, risk for (uses)
- ✓ Diarrhea (side effects)
- ✓ Injury, risk for (side effects)
- ✓ Knowledge deficit (teaching)
- ✓ Noncompliance (teaching)

Implementation

PO route
- Give around the clock to maintain proper blood levels

IV **IV route**
- Check for irritation, extravasation, phlebitis daily
- For intermittent inf, dilute to 1-2 mg/ml of D_5W, 0.9% NaCl; give over 60 min; it will remain stable under refrigeration for 2 wks

Y-site incompatibilities: Heparin, mezlocillin

Y-site compatibilities: Amifostine, aztreonam, ceftazidime, lorazepam, midazolam, piperacillin, thiotepa, tobramycin

Additive compatibilities: Amikacin, aztreonam, ceftazidime, gentamicin, metronidazole, piperacillin, tobramycin

Additive incompatibilities: Aminophylline, amoxicillin, clindamycin, floxacillin, mezlocillin

Patient/family education
- Teach patient to report sore throat, bruising, bleeding, joint pain; may indicate blood dyscrasias (rare)
- Advise patient to contact prescriber if vaginal itching, loose, foul-smelling stools, furry tongue occur; may indicate superinfection; report itching, rash, pruritus, urticaria
- Instruct patient to take all medication prescribed for the length of time ordered; drug must be taken around the clock to maintain blood levels; do not give medication to others
- Advise patient to notify prescriber of diarrhea with blood or pus

Evaluation

Positive therapeutic outcome
- Absence of signs/symptoms of infection (WBC <10,000, temp WNL, absence of red draining wounds)
- Reported improvement in symptoms of infection

cisapride (℞)

(siss′a-pride)

Propulsid

Func. class.: Cholinergic, gastrointestinal (antireflex)

Pregnancy category C

Action: Enhances response to acetylcholine at the myenteric plexus; the strength of esophageal and sphincter pressure are increased

➔ **Therapeutic Outcome:** Absence of heartburn

Uses: Treatment of heartburn associated with gastroesophageal reflux

Dosage and routes

Adult: PO 10 mg qid at least 15 min ac and hs; may increase to 20 mg; elderly may need higher dosage

Available forms: Tabs 10, 20 mg

Adverse effects

CNS: Headache, sleeplessness, anxiety, nervousness, pain, fever

GI: Diarrhea, constipation, nausea, anorexia, abdominal pain, flatulence, dyspepsia

GU: UTI, frequency
INTEG: Pruritus, rash
RESP: Rhinitis, sinusitis, coughing

Contraindications: Hypersensitivity; GI hemorrhage, obstruction, perforation

P G **Precautions:** Pregnancy **C**, lactation, children, elderly

Pharmacokinetics	
Absorption	Rapidly absorbed PO
Distribution	Unknown
Metabolism	Liver, extensively
Excretion	Breast milk, kidneys
Half-life	6-12 hr

Pharmacodynamics	
Onset	½-1 hr
Peak	1 hr
Duration	Unknown

Interactions
Individual drugs
Alcohol: ↑ sedation
Cimetidine: ↑ levels of cisapride
Digoxin: ↑ or ↓ effects
Erythromycin: life-threatening dysrhythmias
Itraconazole: ↑ inhibition of cisapride metabolism; do not use together
Ketoconazole: ↑ inhibition of cisapride metabolism; do not use together
Miconazole: ↑ inhibition of cisapride metabolism; do not use together
Ranitidine: GI absorption is increased
Troleandomycin: ↑ inhibition of cisapride metabolism; do not use together
Warfarin: ↑ effects of warfarin
Drug classifications
Anticholinergics: ↓ effects of cisapride
Anticonvulsants: ↑ drug effects
Benzodiazepines: ↑ sedation

NURSING CONSIDERATIONS
Assessment
- Assess patient for GI complaints: nausea, vomiting, anorexia, constipation; check for decreasing heartburn

Nursing diagnoses
✓ Pain, acute (uses)
✓ Pain, chronic (uses)
✓ Knowledge deficit (teaching)

Implementation
- Give before meals for better absorption and hs

Patient/family education
- Advise patient to avoid alcohol and other CNS depressants that will enhance sedating properties of this drug
- Warn patient to take exactly as prescribed

Evaluation
Positive therapeutic outcome
- Absence of heartburn

Treatment of overdose: Lavage or activated charcoal, general support

cisatracurium (℞)
(sis-a-tra-cyoor′ee-um)
Nimbex
Func. class.: Neuromuscular blocker (nondepolarizing)
Pregnancy category B

Action: Inhibits transmission of nerve impulses by binding with cholinergic receptor sites, antagonizing action of acetylcholine

➔ **Therapeutic Outcome:** Paralysis of body for administration of anesthesia

Uses: Facilitation of endotracheal intubation, skeletal muscle relaxation during mechanical ventilation surgery, or general anesthesia

Dosage and routes

Adult: **IV** 0.15 and 0.2 mg/kg depending on desired time to intubate and length of surgery: use peripheral nerve stimulation to evaluate dosage

Child 2-12 yr: **IV** 0.1 mg/kg over 5-10 sec with halothane or opioid anesthesia

Available forms: Inj 2, 10 mg/ml

Adverse effects

CV: Bradycardia, tachycardia; increased, decreased B/P
EENT: Increased secretions
RESP: Prolonged apnea, bronchospasm, cyanosis, respiratory depression
INTEG: Rash, flushing, pruritus, urticaria

Contraindications: Hypersensitivity

Precautions: Pregnancy **B,** cardiac disase, lactation, children <2 yr electrolyte imbalances, dehydration, neuromuscular disease, respiratory disease

Pharmacokinetics	
Unknown	

Pharmacodynamics	
Onset	1-3 min
Peak	2-5 min
Duration	Unknown

Interactions

Drug classifications

Aminoglycosides: ↑ neuromuscular blockade
Antibiotics, polymix: ↑ neuromuscular blockade
Analgesics, narcotic: ↑ neuromuscular blockade
Tetracyclines: ↑ neuromuscular blockade

Individual drugs

Clindamycin: ↑ neuromuscular blockade
Lincomycin: ↑ neuromuscular blockade
Lithium: ↑ neuromuscular blockade
Isoflurane: ↑ neuromuscular blockade
Theophylline: ↑ dysrhythmias

NURSING CONSIDERATIONS

Assessment

- Assess for electrolyte imbalances (K, Mg), may lead to increased action of this drug
- Assess vital signs (B/P, pulse, respirations, airway) until fully recovered; rate, depth, pattern of respirations; strength of handgrip
- Assess I&O ratio; check for urinary retention, frequency, hesitancy
- Assess recovery: decreased paralysis of face, diaphragm, legs, arms, rest of body
- Assess allergic reactions: rash, fever, respiratory distress, pruritus; drug should be discontinued

Nursing diagnoses

✓ Breathing pattern, ineffective (uses)
✓ Communication, impaired (adverse reactions)
✓ Knowledge deficit (teaching)

Implementation

IV route

- Use nerve stimulator by anesthesiologist to determine neuromuscular blockade
- Give anticholinesterase to reverse neuromuscular blockade
- Give by slow **IV** only by qualified person, do not administer IM
- Store in light-resistant area
- Reassure if communication is

difficult during recovery from neuromuscular blockage

Evaluation

Positive therapeutic outcome

- Paralysis of jaw, eyelid, head, neck, rest of body

Treatment of overdose: Endrophonium or neostigmine, atropine, monitor VS; mechanical ventilation

cisplatin (℞)

(sis'pla-tin)

Platinol, Platinol-AQ

Func. class.: Antineoplastic alkylating agent

Chem. class.: Inorganic heavy metal

Pregnancy category D

Action: Alkylates DNA, RNA; inhibits enzymes that allow synthesis of amino acids in proteins; activity is not cell cycle phase specific

➔ Therapeutic Outcome: Prevention of rapidly growing malignant cells

Uses: Advanced bladder cancer; adjunctive in metastatic testicular cancer and metastatic ovarian cancer; head, neck, esophageal, prostatic, lung, and cervical cancer; lymphoma

Dosage and routes

Testicular cancer

Adult: **IV** 20 mg/m^2 qd × 5 days, repeat q3 wk for 3 cycles or more, depending on response

Bladder cancer

Adult: **IV** 50-70 mg/m^2 q3-4 wk

Ovarian cancer

Adult: **IV** 100 mg/m^2 q4 wk or 50 mg/m^2 q3 wk with doxorubicin therapy; mix with 2 L of NaCl and 37.5 g mannitol over 6 hr

Available forms: Inj **IV** 10, 50 mg

Adverse effects

CNS: Convulsions, peripheral neuropathy

CV: Cardiac abnormalities

EENT: Tinnitus, hearing loss, vestibular toxicity

GI: Severe nausea, vomiting, diarrhea, weight loss

GU: Renal tubular damage, renal insufficiency, impotence, sterility, amenorrhea, gynecomastia, hyperuremia

HEMA: Thrombocytopenia, leukopenia, pancytopenia

INTEG: Alopecia, dermatitis

META: Hypomagnesemia, hypocalcemia, hypokalemia, hypophosphatemia

RESP: Fibrosis

SYST: Hypersensitivity reaction

Contraindications: Radiation therapy within 1 mo, chemotherapy within 1 mo, thrombocytopenia, smallpox vaccination

Precautions: Pneumococcal vaccination, pregnancy **D**

Pharmacokinetics

Absorption	Complete bioavailability
Distribution	Widely distributed
Metabolism	Liver
Excretion	Kidneys
Half-life	30 hr

Pharmacodynamics

Unknown

Interactions

Individual drugs

Radiation: ↑ toxicity, bone marrow suppression

Drug classifications

Aminoglycosides: ↑ nephrotoxicity

Antineoplastics: ↑ toxicity, bone marrow suppression
Bone marrow–suppressing drugs: ↑ bone marrow suppression
Diuretics, loop: ↑ ototoxicity
Lab test interferences
False positive: Breast, bladder, cervix, lung, cytology tests

NURSING CONSIDERATIONS
Assessment
- Monitor CBC, differential, platelet count weekly; withhold drug if WBC count is <4000/mm^3 or platelet count is <100,000/mm^3; notify prescriber of results if WBC <20,000/mm^3, platelets <150,000/mm^3
- Monitor renal function studies: BUN, creatinine, serum uric acid, urine CrCl before and during therapy; I&O ratio; report fall in urine output to <30 ml/hr
- Monitor temp q4h (may indicate beginning of infection)
- Monitor liver function tests before and during therapy (bilirubin, AST [SGOT], ALT [SGPT], LDH) as needed or monthly; note yellowing of skin or sclera, dark urine, clay-colored stools, itchy skin, abdominal pain, fever, diarrhea
- Assess for increased uric acid levels, swelling, joint pain primarily in extremities; patient should be well hydrated to prevent urate deposits
- Assess for bleeding: hematuria, stool guaiac, bruising or petechiae, mucosa or orifices q8h; note inflammation of mucosa, breaks in skin
- Identify dyspnea, rales, nonproductive cough, chest pain, tachypnea
- Identify effects of alopecia on body image; discuss feelings about body changes
- Identify edema in feet, joint pain, stomach pain, shaking; prescriber should be notified

Nursing diagnoses
- ✓ Injury, risk for (adverse reactions)
- ✓ Body image disturbance (adverse reactions)
- ✓ Infection, risk for (adverse reactions)
- ✓ Knowledge deficit (teaching)

Implementation
- Hydrate patient with 1-2 L of fluids over 8-12 hr before treatment
- Give epinephrine for hypersensitivity reaction; antiemetic 30-60 min before giving drug to prevent vomiting, and prn; allopurinol or sodium bicarbonate to maintain uric acid level, alkalinization of urine; antibiotics for prophylaxis of infection; diuretic (furosemide 40 mg **IV**) or mannitol after infusion
- After diluting 10 mg/10 ml or 50 mg/50 ml sterile water for inj; withdraw prescribed dose, dilute ½ dose with 1000 ml D_5 0.2 NaCl or D_5 0.45 NaCl with 37.5 g mannitol; **IV** inf is given over 3-4 hr; use a 0.45 μm filter; total dose 2000 ml over 6-8 hr; check site for irritation, phlebitis; do not use equipment containing aluminum

Y-site compatibilities:
Allopurinol, aztreonam, bleomycin, cyclophosphamide, doxapram, doxorubicin, droperidol, famotidine, filgrastim, fludarabine, fluorouracil, furosemide, granisetron, heparin, leucovorin, melphalan, methotrexate, metoclopramide, mitomycin, morphine,

ondansetron, paclitaxel, sargramostim, vinblastine, vincristine, vinorelbine

Syringe compatibilities: Bleomycin, cyclophosphamide, doxapram, doxorubicin, droperidol, fluorouracil, furosemide, heparin, leucovorin, methotrexate, metoclopramide, mitomycin, vinblastine, vincristine

Additive incompatibilities: Fluorouracil, mesna, thiotepa

Additive compatibilities: Cyclophosphamide with etoposide, etoposide, etoposide with floxuridine, floxuridine, floxuridine with leucovorin, hydroxyzine, ifosfamide, ifosfamide with etoposide, leucovorin, magnesium sulfate, mannitol, ondansetron

Solution incompatibilities: Sodium bicarbonate 5%, 0.1% NaCl, water

Solution compatibilities: D_5/0.225% NaCl, D_5/0.45% NaCl, D_5/0.9% NaCl, D_5/0.45% NaCl with mannitol 1.875%, D_5/0.33% NaCl with mannitol 1.875%, D_5/0.33% NaCl with KCl 20 mEq and mannitol 1.875%, 0.9% NaCl, 0.45% NaCl, 0.3% NaCl, 0.225% NaCl, water

Patient/family education

• Teach patient to avoid use of products containing aspirin or ibuprofen, razors, commercial mouthwash, since bleeding may occur; to report symptoms of bleeding (hematuria, tarry stools)

• Instruct patient to report signs of anemia (fatigue, headache, irritability, faintness, shortness of breath)

• Instruct patient to report any changes in breathing or coughing even several months after treatment; to avoid crowds and persons with respiratory tract or other infections

• Advise patient that hair may be lost during treatment; a wig or hair piece may make patient feel better; new hair may be different in color, texture

• Tell patient not to have any vaccinations without the advice of the prescriber; serious reactions can occur

• Caution patient contraception is needed during treatment and for several months after the completion of therapy

Evaluation

Positive therapeutic outcome

• Prevention of rapid division of malignant cells

clarithromycin (℞)

(clare-i-thro-mye'sin)

Biaxin

Func. class.: Antibacterial

Chem. class.: Macrolide antibiotic

Pregnancy category C

Action: Binds to 50S ribosomal subunits of susceptible bacteria and suppresses protein synthesis

➔ Therapeutic Outcome: Bactericidal action against the following: *Streptococcus pneumoniae, Mycoplasma pneumoniae, Corynebacterium diphtheriae, Bordetella pertussis, Listeria monocytogenes, Haemophilus influenzae, S. pyogenes, Staphylococcus aureus, M. avium (mac),* complex infections in AIDS patients, M. intracellulare, *H. pylori* in combination with omeprazole

Uses: Mild to moderate infections of the upper respiratory tract, lower respiratory tract; uncomplicated skin and skin structure infections

Dosage and routes
Adult: PO 250-500 mg bid × 7-14 days

Child: PO 15 mg/kg/day divided q12h × 10 days

H. pylori infection
Adult: PO 500 mg qd plus omeprazole 2 × 20 mg q AM (day 1-14) then omeprazole 20 mg q AM (days 15-28)

Available forms: Tabs 250, 500 mg; granules for oral susp 125 mg/5 ml, 250 mg/5 ml

Adverse effects
GI: Nausea, vomiting, diarrhea, ***hepatotoxicity,*** abdominal pain, stomatitis, heartburn, anorexia, abnormal taste
GU: Vaginitis, moniliasis
INTEG: Rash, urticaria, pruritus
MISC: Headache

Contraindications: Hypersensitivity

Precautions: Pregnancy **C,** lactation, hepatic/renal disease

Pharmacokinetics

Absorption	50%
Distribution	Widely distributed
Metabolism	Liver
Excretion	Kidneys, unchanged (20%-30%)
Half-life	4-6 hr

Pharmacodynamics

Onset	Unknown
Peak	2 hr

Interactions
Individual drugs:
Bromocriptine: ↑ effects of bromocriptine
Carbamazepine: ↑ toxicity, from ↑ levels of carbamazepine
Cisapride: ↑ dysrhythmias
Clindamycin: ↓ action of clindamycin
Cyclosporine: ↑ effects of cyclosporine
Digoxin: ↑ blood levels of digoxin
Disopyramide: ↑ effects of disopyramide
Hexobarbital: ↑ effect
Lovastatin: ↑ effect
Phenytoin: ↑ effect
Pimozide: ↑ effect
Theophylline: ↑ toxicity from ↑ levels of theophylline
Triazolam: ↑ effects of triazolam
Valproate: ↑ effect
Zidovudine: ↑ or ↓ action
Drug classifications
Oral anticoagulants: ↑ effects of oral anticoagulants
Lab test interferences
False ↑ 17-OHCS/17-KS, false ↑ AST (SGOT), false ↑ ALT (SGPT), BUN, creatinine, LDH, total bilirubin
↓ Folate assay

NURSING CONSIDERATIONS
Assessment
- Assess patient for signs and symptoms of infection including characteristics of wounds, sputum, urine, stool, WBC >10,000, earache, fever; obtain baseline information before and during treatment
- Obtain C&S before beginning drug therapy to identify if correct treatment has been initiated
- Monitor blood studies: AST (SGOT), ALT (SGPT), CBC, Hct, bilirubin, LDH, alkaline phosphatase, Coombs' test

monthly if patient is on long-term therapy
• Assess bowel pattern qd; if severe diarrhea occurs, drug should be discontinued
• Assess for overgrowth of infection: perineal itching, fever, malaise, redness, pain, swelling, drainage, rash, diarrhea, change in cough, sputum

Nursing diagnoses

✓ Infection, risk for (uses)
✓ Diarrhea (side effects)
✓ Knowledge deficit (teaching)
✓ Noncompliance (teaching)

Implementation

• Give in equal doses in each 24-hr period to maintain proper blood levels

Patient/family education

• Advise patient to contact physician if vaginal itching, loose, foul-smelling stools, furry tongue occur; may indicate superinfection
• Instruct patient to take all medication prescribed for the length of time ordered

Evaluation

Positive therapeutic outcome

• Absence of signs/symptoms of infection (WBC <10,000, temp WNL, absence of red draining wounds)
• Reported improvement in symptoms of infection

clemastine (℞)

(klem'as-teen)
Tavist, Tavist-1
Func. class.: Antihistamine
Chem. class.: Ethanolamine derivative, H_1-receptor antagonist
Pregnancy category B

Action: Acts on blood vessels, GI, respiratory system by competing with histamine for H_1-receptor site; decreases allergic response by blocking histamine

➔ **Therapeutic Outcome:** Absence of allergy symptoms and rhinitis

Uses: Allergy symptoms, rhinitis, allergic dermatoses, nasal allergies, hypersensitive reactions including blood transfusion reactions, anaphylaxis

Dosage and routes

P ***Adult and child >12 yr:*** PO 1.34-2.68 mg bid-tid, not to exceed 8.04 mg/day

Available forms: Tabs 1.34, 2.68 mg; syr 0.67 mg/ml

Adverse effects

CNS: Dizziness, drowsiness, poor coordination, fatigue, anxiety, euphoria, confusion, paresthesia, neuritis, paradoxic P excitement (child)
CV: Hypotension, palpitations, tachycardia
EENT: Blurred vision, dilated pupils, tinnitus, nasal stuffiness, dry nose, throat, *mouth*
GI: Constipation, dry mouth, nausea, vomiting, anorexia, diarrhea
GU: Retention, dysuria, frequency
HEMA: Thrombocytopenia,

agranulocytosis, hemolytic anemia
INTEG: Rash, urticaria, photosensitivity, sweating
RESP: Increased thick secretions, wheezing, chest tightness

Contraindications: Hypersensitivity to H_1-receptor antagonists, acute asthma attack, lower respiratory tract disease

Precautions: Increased intraocular pressure, renal disease, cardiac disease, hypertension, bronchial asthma, seizure disorder, stenosed peptic ulcers, hyperthyroidism, prostatic hypertrophy, bladder neck obstruction, pregnancy **B**, G elderly

Pharmacokinetics

Absorption	Well absorbed
Distribution	Widely distributed
Metabolism	Liver, extensively
Excretion	Kidneys, breast milk (high)
Half-life	Unknown

Pharmacodynamics

Onset	15-60 min
Peak	1-2 hr
Duration	12 hr

Interactions

Individual drugs

Alcohol: ↑ CNS depression

Drug classifications

CNS depressants: ↑ CNS depression
MAOI: ↑ anticholinergic effect
Narcotics: ↑ CNS depression
Sedative/hypnotics: ↑ CNS depression

Lab test interferences

False negative: Skin allergy tests (discontinue antihistamines 3 days before testing)

NURSING CONSIDERATIONS

Assessment

- Assess respiratory status: rate, rhythm, increase in bronchial secretions, wheezing, chest tightness; provide fluids to 2 L/day to decrease secretion thickness
- Monitor I&O ratio: be alert for urinary retention, frequency, dysuria, especially G elderly; drug should be discontinued if these occur

Nursing diagnoses

- ✓ Airway clearance, ineffective (uses)
- ✓ Injury, risk for (side effects)
- ✓ Knowledge deficit (teaching)
- ✓ Noncompliance (teaching, overuse)

Implementation

- May give with food to decrease GI upset
- ⊘ Do not crush or chew caps
- Store in tight, light-resistant container

Patient/family education

- Teach all aspects of drug uses; to notify prescriber if confusion, sedation, hypotension occur; to avoid driving and other hazardous activity if drowsiness occurs; to avoid alcohol and other CNS depressants that may potentiate effect
- Instruct patient to take 1 hr ac or 2 hr pc to facilitate absorption
- Caution patient not to exceed recommended dosage; dysrhythmias may occur
- Teach patient hard candy, gum, frequent rinsing of mouth may be used for dryness
- Tell patient if EENT or CNS symptoms occur (blurred vision, severe dry mouth, dry throat, confusion, dizziness, poor coordination, euphoria), prescriber should be notified

Evaluation
Positive therapeutic outcome
- Absence of running or congested nose, rashes

Treatment of overdose: Administer ipecac syrup or lavage, diazepam, vasopressors, barbiturates (short acting)

clindamycin (℞)

(klin-da-mye'sin)

Cleocin HCl, clindamycin HCl, Dalacin C ✦, Cleocin Pediatric, Cleocin phosphate, clindamycin phosphate

Func. class.: Antibacterial lincosamide

Chem. class.: Lincomycin derivative

Pregnancy category B

Action: Binds to 50S subunit of bacterial ribosomes; suppresses protein synthesis

→ **Therapeutic Outcome:** Absence of infection

Uses: Infections caused by staphylococci, streptococci, *Rickettsia, Fusobacterium, Actinomyces, Peptococcus, Clostridium*

Dosage and routes

Adults: PO 150-450 mg q6hr; IM/**IV** 300 mg q6-12hr, not to exceed 4800 mg/day

PID: Adult **IV** 600 mg q6h plus gentamicin

Vaginal route

Adult: 5 g applicatorful at bedtime × 1 wk

Topical route

Adult: Sol 1% apply bid

P ***Child >1 mo:*** PO 8-20 mg/kg/day in divided doses q6-8hr; IM/**IV** 15-40 mg/kg/day in divided doses q6-8hr in 3-4 equal doses

Available forms: Inj 150-300 mg/ml; caps 75, 150, 300 mg; oral sol 75 mg/ml; top 1% lotion, soap, solution, gel; vag 2% cream

Adverse effects

EENT: Rash, urticaria, pruritus, erythema, pain, abscess at injection site

GI: Nausea, vomiting, abdominal pain, diarrhea, ***pseudomembranous colitis,*** *anorexia, weight loss*

GU: Increased AST (SGOT), ALT (SGPT), bilirubin, alk phosphatase, jaundice, *vaginitis,* urinary frequency

HEMA: Leukopenia, eosinophilia, agranulocytosis, thrombocytopenia, polyarthritis

Contraindications: Hypersensitivity to this drug or lincomycin, ulcerative colitis/enteritis, G infants <1 mo

Precautions: Renal disease, G liver disease, GI disease, elderly, pregnancy **B,** lactation, tartrazine sensitivity

Pharmacokinetics

Absorption	Well absorbed (PO, IM), minimal (top)
Distribution	Widely distributed; crosses placenta
Metabolism	Liver, extensively
Excretion	Kidneys, breast milk
Half-life	2½ hr

Pharmacodynamics

	PO	IM	IV	TOP	VAG
Onset	Rapid	Rapid	Rapid	Rapid	Rapid
Peak	½-1 hr	1½ hr	Infusion's end	Unknown	Unknown

Interactions
Individual drugs
Chloramphenicol: ↓ action of chloramphenicol
Erythromycin: ↓ action of erythromycin
Drug classifications
Nondepolarizing muscle relaxants: ↑ neuromuscular blockade
Lab test interferences
↑ Alk phosphatase, ↑ bilirubin, ↑ CPK, ↑ AST (SGOT), ↑ ALT (SGPT)

NURSING CONSIDERATIONS
Assessment
• Assess any patient with compromised renal system; drug is excreted slowly in poor renal system function; toxicity may occur rapidly
• Assess patient for signs and symptoms of infection including characteristics of wounds, sputum, urine, stool, WBC >10,000, fever; obtain baseline information before and during treatment
• Complete culture and sensitivity testing before beginning drug therapy; this will identify if correct treatment has been initiated
• Assess for allergic reactions: rash, urticaria, pruritus, chills, fever, joint pain; may occur a few days after therapy begins; epinephrine and resuscitation equipment should be available in case of an anaphylactic reaction
• Identify urine output; if decreasing, notify prescriber (may indicate nephrotoxicity); also look for increased BUN and creatinine levels
• Monitor blood studies: AST (SGOT), ALT (SGPT), CBC, Hct, bilirubin, LDH, alk phosphatase, Coombs' test monthly if patient is on long-term therapy
• Monitor electrolytes: potassium, sodium, chloride monthly if patient is on long-term therapy
• Assess bowel pattern qd; if severe diarrhea occurs, drug should be discontinued; may indicate pseudomembranous colitis
• Monitor for bleeding: ecchymosis, bleeding gums, hematuria, stool guaiac daily if on long-term therapy
• Assess for overgrowth of infection: perineal itching, fever, malaise, redness, pain, swelling, drainage, rash, diarrhea, change in cough, sputum

Nursing diagnoses
✓ Infection, risk for (uses)
✓ Diarrhea (adverse reactions)
✓ Injury, risk for (adverse reactions)
✓ Knowledge deficit (teaching)
✓ Noncompliance (teaching)

Implementation
PO route
• Give with 8 oz of water; give with meals for GI symptoms
• Shake liquids well
• Do not refrigerate oral preparations; stable at room temperature for 2 wks
⊘ • Do not crush, chew caps
IM route
• If more than 600 mg must be given, divide into two injections
• Give deeply in large muscle mass; rotate sites
IV **IV route**
• Give by infusion only; do not administer bolus dose; dilute 300 mg or more/50 ml or more of D_5W, NS
• May be further diluted in greater amounts of D_5W, 0.9% NaCl and given as a cont inf in

acute pelvic inflammatory disease (PID); give first dose 10 mg/min over ½ hr, then 0.75 mg/min; increased rates may be used to keep serum blood levels higher; run over >10 min; no more than 120 mg in a 1 hr inf

Syringe compatibilities: Amikacin, aztreonam, gentamicin, heparin

Syringe incompatibility: Tobramycin

Y-site incompatibility: Idarubicin

Y-site compatibilities: Amifostine, cyclophosphamide, enalaprilat, esmolol, foscarnet, hydromorphone, labetolol, magnesium sulfate, melphalan, meperidine, midazolam, morphine, multivitamins, odansetron, perphenazine, thiotepa, vinorelbine, zidovudine

Additive compatibilities Amikacin, ampicillin, aztreonam, cefamandole, cefazolin, cefepine, cefonicid, cefoperazone, cefotaxime, cimetidine, fluconazole, heparin, hydrocortisone, kanamycin, methylplednisolone, metoclopramide, metronidazole, netilmicin, ofloxacin, penicillin G, pipercillin, potassium chloride, sodium bicarbonate, tobramycin, verapamil, vit B/C

Additive incompatibility: Ciprofloxacin

Top route

- Avoid contact with eyes, mucous membranes, and open cuts during topical application; if accidental contact occurs, rinse with cool water
- Wash affected areas with warm water and soap, rinse, pat dry before application

Patient/family education

- Tell patient to take oral drug with full glass of water; may take with food if GI symptoms occur; antiperistaltic drugs may worsen diarrhea
- Teach patient aspects of drug therapy: need to complete entire course of medication to ensure organism death (10-14 days); culture may be taken after medication course has been completed
- Advise patient to report sore throat, fever, fatigue; may indicate superimposed infection
- Advise patient that drug must be taken at equal intervals around clock to maintain blood levels

Evaluation

Positive therapeutic outcome

- Decreased temperature, negative C&S

Treatment of hypersensitivity: Withdraw drug; maintain airway; administer epinephrine, aminophylline, O_2, **IV** corticosteroids

clofazimine (℞)

(kloe-faz′i-meen)

Lamprene

Func. class.: Leprostatic

Pregnancy category C

Action: Inhibits mycobacterial growth, binds to mycobacterial DNA; exerts antiinflammatory properties in controlling leprosy reactions

➔ **Therapeutic Outcome:** Decreased infection of leprosy

Uses: Lepromatous leprosy, dapsone-resistant leprosy, lepromatous leprosy complicated by erythema nodosum leprosum

Dosage and routes

Erythema nodosum leprosum

Adult: PO 100-200 mg qd × 3 mo, then taper dosage to 100 mg when disease is controlled; do not exceed 200 mg/day

Dapsone-resistant leprosy

Adult: PO 100 mg/day in combination with at least one other antileprosy drug × 3 yr, then 100 mg qd clofazimine only

Available forms: Caps 50, 100 mg

Adverse effects

CNS: Dizziness, headache, fatigue, drowsiness

EENT: Pigmentation of cornea and conjunctiva, drying, burning, itching, irritation

GI: Diarrhea, nausea, vomiting, abdominal pain, intolerance, ***GI bleeding, obstruction,*** anorexia, constipation, ***hepatitis,*** jaundice

INTEG: Pink or brown discoloration, dryness, pruritus, rash, photosensitivity, acne, monilial cheilosis

MISC: Discolored urine, feces, sputum, sweat

Precautions: Pregnancy **C**, P lactation, children, abdominal pain, diarrhea, depression

Pharmacokinetics	
Absorption	Partially
Distribution	Crosses placenta
Metabolism	Liver
Excretion	Feces, bile
Half-life	70 days

Pharmacodynamics
Unknown

Interactions

Individual drugs

Alcohol: ↑ toxicity
Carbamazepine: ↑ toxicity
Cycloserine: ↑ toxicity
Ethionamide: ↑ toxicity
Rifampin: ↑ toxicity

Drug classifications

Antacids, aluminum: ↓ absorption

NURSING CONSIDERATIONS

Assessment

- Perform liver studies weekly: ALT (SGPT), AST (SGOT), bilirubin
- Monitor renal status: before initiation of therapy, then monthly: BUN, creatinine, output, sp gr, urinalysis
- Assess mental status often: affect, mood, behavioral changes; psychosis may occur
- Monitor hepatic status: decreased appetite, jaundice, dark urine, fatigue

Nursing diagnoses

✓ Infection, risk for (uses)
✓ Diarrhea (side effects)
✓ Injury, risk for (side effects)
✓ Knowledge deficit (teaching)

Implementation

- Give with meals to decrease GI symptoms
- Provide antiemetic if vomiting occurs
- ⊘ Do not crush, chew caps

Patient/family education

- Teach patient that compliance with dosage schedule, duration is necessary
- Teach patient that scheduled appointments must be kept or relapse may occur
- Caution patient to avoid alcohol while taking drug
- Teach diabetic patients to use blood glucose monitor to obtain correct result
- Advise patient to report

weakness, fatigue, loss of appetite, nausea, vomiting, yellowing of skin or eyes, tingling/numbness of hands/feet

Evaluation

Positive therapeutic outcome

- Decreased symptoms of leprosy

clomiphene (℞)

(kloe'mi-feen)

Clomid, clomiphene citrate, Milophene, Serophene

Func. class.: Ovulation stimulant

Chem. class.: Nonsteroidal antiestrogenic

Pregnancy category X

Action: Increases LH, FSH release from the pituitary, which increase maturation of ovarian follicle, ovulation, development of corpus luteum

➔ **Therapeutic Outcome:** Pregnancy

Uses: Female infertility (ovulatory failure)

Dosage and routes

Adult: PO 50-100 mg qd × 5 days or 50-100 mg qd beginning on day 5 of cycle; may be repeated until conception occurs or 3 cycles of therapy have been completed

Available forms: Tabs 50 mg

Adverse effects

CNS: Headache, depression, restlessness, anxiety, nervousness, fatigue, insomnia, dizziness, flushing

CV: Vasomotor flushing, phlebitis, ***deep vein thrombosis***

EENT: Blurred vision, diplopia, photophobia

GI: Nausea, vomiting, constipation, abdominal pain, bloating

GU: Polyuria, frequency, birth defects, spontaneous abortions, multiple ovulation, breast pain, oliguria, abnormal uterine bleeding

INTEG: Rash, dermatitis, urticaria, alopecia

Contraindications: Hypersensitivity, pregnancy **X,** hepatic disease, undiagnosed uterine bleeding, uncontrolled thyroid or adrenal dysfunction, intracranial lesion, ovarian cysts

Precautions: Hypertension, depression, convulsions, diabetes mellitus

Pharmacokinetics

Absorption	Well distributed
Distribution	Unknown
Metabolism	Liver, extensively
Excretion	Feces
Half-life	5 days

Pharmacodynamics

Unknown

Interactions: None

Lab test interferences

↑ FSH/LH, ↑ BSP, ↑ thyroxine, ↑ TBG

NURSING CONSIDERATIONS

Assessment

- Determine liver function tests before therapy: AST (SGOT), ALT (SGPT), alkaline phosphatase
- Monitor serum progesterone, urinary excretion of pregnanediol to identify occurrence of ovulation
- Pelvic examination should be done to determine ovarian size, cervical condition
- Endometrial biopsy may be done in women over 35 to rule out endometrial carcinoma

Nursing diagnoses

✓ Sexual dysfunction (uses)
✓ Knowledge deficit (teaching)

Implementation

- Give after discontinuing estrogen therapy
- Give at same time qd to maintain drug level; begin on 5th day of menstrual cycle

Patient/family education

- Advise patient that multiple births are common after drug is taken
- Instruct patient to notify prescriber if low abdominal pain occurs; may indicate ovarian cyst, cyst rupture
- Teach patient if dose is missed, double at next time; if more than one dose is missed, call prescriber
- Instruct patient that response usually occurs 4-10 days after last day of treatment
- Teach patient method for taking, recording basal body temp to determine whether ovulation has occurred; if ovulation can be determined (there is a slight decrease in temp, then a sharp increase for ovulation), to attempt coitus 3 days before and qod until after ovulation
- Teach patient if pregnancy is suspected, to notify prescriber immediately

Evaluation

Positive therapeutic outcome

- Fertility

clomipramine (℞)

(klom-ip′ra-meen)

Anafranil

Func. class.: Tricyclic antidepressant

Chem. class.: Tertiary amine

Pregnancy category C

Action: Potent inhibitor of serotonin uptake; also increases dopamine metabolism

➔ **Therapeutic Outcome:** Decreased signs and symptoms of obsessive-compulsive disorder, decreased depression

Uses: Depression, dysphoria, anxiety, agoraphobia and other phobias, obsessive-compulsive disorder

Dosage and routes

Obsessive-compulsive disorder

Adult: PO 25 mg hs; increase gradually over 4 wk to a dosage of 75-300 mg/day in divided doses

P ***Child 10-18 yr:*** PO 25-50 mg/day gradually increased; not to exceed 200 mg/day

Depression

Adult: PO 50-150 mg/day in a single or divided dose

Anxiety/agoraphobia

Adult: PO 25-75 mg/day

Available forms: Caps 25, 50, 75 mg

Adverse effects

CNS: Dizziness, tremors, mania, ***seizures,*** aggressiveness

CV: Hypotension, tachycardia, ***cardiac arrest***

ENDO: Galactorrhea, hyperprolactinemia

GI: Constipation, dry mouth, nausea, dyspepsia

GU: Delayed ejaculation, anorgasmy, retention
HEMA: Agranulocytosis, neutropenia, pancytopenia
INTEG: Diaphoresis
META: Hyponatremia

Contraindications: Hypersensitivity

Precautions: Seizures, suicidal patients, G elderly, pregnancy **C**

Pharmacokinetics

Absorption	Well absorbed
Distribution	Widely distributed
Metabolism	Liver, extensively
Excretion	Kidneys, breast milk
Half-life	21 hr parent compound; 36 hr metabolite

Pharmacodynamics

Unknown

Interactions

Individual drugs

Alcohol: ↑ CNS depression
Cimetidine: ↑ levels, ↑ toxicity
Clonidine: Severe hypertension; avoid use
Disulfiram: Delirium
Fluoxetine: ↑ levels, ↑ toxicity
Guanethidine: ↓ effects

Drug classifications

MAOI: Hypertensive crisis, convulsions
Barbiturates: ↑ effects
Benzodiazepines: ↑ effects
CNS depressants: ↑ effects
Sympathomimetics, indirect-acting: ↓ effects
Oral contraceptives: ↑ effects, toxicity

Smoking

↑ metabolism, ↓ effects

Lab test interferences

↑ Serum bilirubin, ↑ blood glucose, ↑ alkaline phosphatase
↓ VMA, ↓ 5-HIAA
False ↑ Urinary catecholamines

NURSING CONSIDERATIONS

Assessment

- Monitor B/P (with patient lying, standing), pulse q4h; if systolic B/P drops 20 mm Hg hold drug, notify prescriber; take vital signs q4h in patients with cardiovascular disease
- Monitor blood studies: CBC, leukocytes, differential, cardiac enzymes if patient is receiving long-term therapy
- Monitor hepatic studies: AST (SGOT), ALT (SGPT), bilirubin
- Check weight weekly; appetite may increase with drug
- Assess ECG for flattening of T wave, bundle branch block, AV block, dysrhythmias in cardiac patients
- Assess for EPS primarily in G elderly: rigidity, dystonia, akathisia
- Assess mental status: mood, sensorium, affect, suicidal tendencies; increase in psychiatric symptoms: depression, panic
- Monitor urinary retention, constipation; constipation is P more likely to occur in children G or elderly
- Assess for withdrawal symptoms: headache, nausea, vomiting, muscle pain, weakness; do not usually occur unless drug was discontinued abruptly
- Identify alcohol consumption; if alcohol is consumed, hold dose until morning

Nursing diagnoses

- ✓ Coping, ineffective individual (uses)
- ✓ Injury, risk for physical (side effects)
- ✓ Knowledge deficit (teaching)
- ✓ Noncompliance (teaching)

Implementation

• Give with food or milk for GI symptoms
• Do not crush, chew caps
• Store at room temp; do not freeze

Patient/family education

• Teach patient that therapeutic effects may take 2-3 wk
• Teach patient to use caution in driving or other activities requiring alertness because of drowsiness, dizziness, blurred vision; to avoid rising quickly from sitting to standing, especially elderly
• Teach patient to avoid alcohol ingestion, other CNS depressants
• Teach patient not to discontinue medication quickly after long-term use: may cause nausea, headache, malaise
• Teach patient to wear sunscreen or large hat, since photosensitivity occurs
• Teach patient to increase fluids, bulk in diet if constipation, urinary retention occur, especially elderly
• Teach patient to take gum, hard sugarless candy, or frequent sips of water for dry mouth

Evaluation

Positive therapeutic outcome
• Decrease in depression
• Absence of suicidal thoughts

Treatment of overdose:

ECG monitoring, induce emesis, lavage, activated charcoal, administer anticonvulsant

clonazepam (℞)

(kloe-na'zi-pam)
Klonopin, Rivotril ♣, Rivotril
Func. class.: Anticonvulsant
Chem. class.: Benzodiazepine derivative
Pregnancy category C
Controlled substance schedule IV

Action: Inhibits spike, wave formation in absence seizures (petit mal), decreases amplitude, frequency, duration, spread of discharge in minor motor seizures

Therapeutic Outcome
Decreased frequency, severity of seizures

Uses: Absence, atypical absence, akinetic, myoclonic seizures, Lennox-Gastaut syndrome

Investigational uses: Parkinsonian dysarthrias, acute mania, adjunct in schizophrenia, neuralgias, multifocal tic disorders

Dosage and routes

Adult: PO not to exceed 1.5 mg/day in 3 divided doses; may be increased 0.5-1 mg q3 days until desired response; not to exceed 20 mg/day

Child <10 yr or 30 kg: PO 0.01-0.03 mg/kg/day in divided doses q8h, not to exceed 0.05 mg/kg/day; may be increased 0.25-0.5 mg q3 days until desired response; not to exceed 0.1-0.2 mg/kg/day

Available forms: Tabs 0.5, 1, 2 mg

Adverse effects
CNS: Drowsiness, dizziness, confusion, behavioral changes, tremors, insomnia, headache, suicidal tendencies, slurred speech
CV: Palpitations, bradycardia
EENT: Increased salivation, nystagmus, diplopia, abnormal eye movements
GI: Nausea, constipation, polyphagia, anorexia, xerostomia, diarrhea, gastritis, sore gums
GU: Dysuria, enuresis, nocturia, retention
HEMA: Thrombocytopenia, leukocytosis, eosinophilia
INTEG: Rash, alopecia, hirsutism
RESP: Respiratory depression, dyspnea, congestion

Contraindications: Hypersensitivity to benzodiazepines, acute narrow-angle glaucoma

Precautions: Open-angle glaucoma, chronic respiratory disease, pregnancy **C,** renal/ hepatic disease, **G** elderly

Pharmacokinetics

Absorption	Well absorbed
Distribution	Crosses blood-brain barrier, placenta
Metabolism	Liver
Excretion	Kidneys
Half life	18-50 hr

Pharmacodynamics

Onset	½-1 hr
Peak	1-2 hr
Duration	6-12 hr

Interactions
Individual drugs
Alcohol: ↑ CNS depression
Carbamazepine: ↓ effectiveness
Cimetidine: ↓ metabolism, ↑ action
Disulfiram: ↓ metabolism, ↑ action
Fluoxetine: ↓ metabolism, ↑ action
Isoniazid: ↓ metabolism, ↑ action
Ketoconazole: ↓ metabolism, ↑ action
Levodopa: ↓ effectiveness
Metoprolol: ↓ metabolism, ↑ action
Phenytoin: ↑ levels, ↓ clonazepam levels
Propranolol: ↓ metabolism, ↑ action
Propoxyphene: ↓ metabolism, ↑ action
Valproic acid: ↑ seizures
Drug classifications
Antidepressants: ↑ CNS depression
Anticonvulsants: ↑ CNS depression
Antihistamines: ↑ CNS depression
Barbiturates: ↑ CNS depression, ↓ effect of clonazepam
General anesthetics: ↑ CNS depression
Hypnotics: ↑ CNS depression
Oral contraceptives: ↓ metabolism, ↑ action
Narcotics: ↑ CNS depression
Sedatives: ↑ CNS depression
Lab test interferences
↑ AST (SGOT), ↑ alkaline phosphatase

NURSING CONSIDERATIONS
Assessment
- Assess mental status: mood, sensorium, affect, memory (long, short), especially **G** elderly
- Assess for blood dyscrasias: fever, sore throat, bruising, rash, jaundice, epistaxis (long-term treatment only)
- Assess seizure activity including type, location, duration, and character; provide seizure precaution

- Assess renal studies: urinalysis, BUN, urine creatinine
- Monitor blood studies: RBC, Hct, Hgb, reticulocyte counts weekly for 4 wk then monthly
- Monitor hepatic studies: ALT (SGPT), AST (SGOT), bilirubin, creatinine
- Monitor drug levels during initial treatment
- Assess for signs of physical withdrawal if medication suddenly discontinued
- Assess eye problems: need for ophthalmic examinations before, during, after treatment (slit lamp, fundoscopy, tonometry)
- Assess allergic reaction: red raised rash; if this occurs, drug should be discontinued
- Monitor for toxicity: bone marrow depression, nausea, vomiting, ataxia, diplopia, cardiovascular collapse

Nursing diagnoses

✓ Injury, risk for (side effects)
✓ Knowledge deficit (teaching)

Implementation

- Give on empty stomach for best absorption

Patient/family education

- Teach patient to carry ID card or Medic Alert bracelet stating patient's name, drugs taken, condition, physician's name, phone number
- Caution patient to avoid driving, other activities that require alertness
- Caution patient to avoid alcohol ingestion or CNS depressants; increased sedation may occur
- Teach patient not to discontinue medication quickly after long-term use; taper off over several weeks

Evaluation

Positive therapeutic outcome

- Decreased seizure activity

Treatment of overdose: Lavage, activated charcoal, VS, monitor electrolytes

clonidine (℞)

(klon'i-deen)

Apo-clonidine ✤, Catapres, Catapres-TTS, clonidine HCl, Dixarit ✤, Nu-clonidine ✤

Func. class.: Antihypertensive

Chem. class.: Central α-adrenergic agonist

Pregnancy category C

Action: Inhibits sympathetic vasomotor center in CNS, which reduces impulses in sympathetic nervous system; B/P, pulse rate, cardiac output decreased

➔ **Therapeutic Outcome:** Decreased B/P in hypertension

Uses: Mild to moderate hypertension; used alone or in combination

Investigational uses: Narcotic withdrawal, prevention of vascular headaches, treatment of menopausal symptoms, dysmenorrhea, attention deficit disorder

Dosage and routes

Hypertension

Adult: PO/trans 0.1 mg bid, then increase by 0.1 mg/day or 0.2 mg/day until desired response; range 0.2-0.8 mg/day in divided doses

Opioid withdrawal

Adult: PO 0.3-1.2 mg/day;

decreased dosage given over several days

Severe pain

Adult: Cont epidural Inf 30 μg/hr

Available forms: Tabs 0.1, 0.2, 0.3 mg; trans sys 2.5, 5, 7.5 mg delivering 0.1, 0.2, 0.3 mg/24 hr, respectively; inj 100 μg/ml

Adverse effects

CNS: Drowsiness, sedation, headache, fatigue, nightmares, insomnia, mental changes, anxiety, depression, hallucinations, delirium

CV: Orthostatic hypotension, palpitations, ***CHF,*** ECG abnormalities

EENT: Taste change, parotid pain

ENDO: Hyperglycemia

GI: Nausea, vomiting, malaise, constipation, dry mouth

GU: Impotence, dysuria, *nocturia,* gynecomastia

INTEG: Rash, alopecia, facial pallor, pruritus, hives, edema, burning papules, excoriation (trans patches)

MS: Muscle, joint pain, leg cramps

Contraindications: Hypersensitivity

Precautions: MI (recent), diabetes mellitus, chronic renal failure, Raynaud's disease, thyroid disease, depression, COPD, child <12 (patches), asthma, pregnancy **C**, lactation, elderly

Pharmacokinetics

Absorption	Well absorbed (PO, trans)
Distribution	Widely distributed; crosses blood-brain barrier
Metabolism	Liver, extensively
Excretion	Kidneys, unchanged (30%)
Half-life	12-16 hr

Pharmacodynamics

	PO	TRANS
Onset	½-1 hr	3 days
Peak	2-4 hr	Unknown
Duration	8 hr	8 hr (after removal)

Interactions

Individual drugs

Alcohol: ↑ CNS depression

Drug classifications

Amphetamines: ↓ hypotensive effects

Anesthetics: ↑ CNS depression

Antidepressants, tricyclic: ↓ hypotensive effects

β-Blockers: ↑ bradycardia

Cardiac glycosides: ↑ bradycardia

Diuretics: ↑ hypotensive effects

Hypnotics: ↑ CNS depression

Narcotics: ↑ CNS depression

Nitrates: ↑ hypotensive effects

Sedatives: ↑ CNS depression

Lab test interferences

↑ Blood glucose

↓ VMA, ↓ catecholamines, ↓ aldosterone

NURSING CONSIDERATIONS

Assessment

- Perform blood studies: neutrophils, decreased platelets
- Perform renal studies: protein, BUN, creatinine; watch for increased levels that may indicate nephrotic syndrome: polyuria, oliguria, frequency
- Monitor baselines in renal, liver function tests before

therapy begins; check potassium levels, although hyperkalemia rarely occurs
- Check dipstick of urine for protein qd in first morning specimen; if protein is increased, a 24-hr urinary protein should be collected
- Monitor B/P, pulse if the drug is being used for hypertension; notify prescriber of changes
- Assess for narcotic withdrawal in patients receiving the drug for opioid withdrawal, including fever, diarrhea, nausea, vomiting, cramps, insomnia, shivering, dilated pupils, weakness
- Check for edema in feet, legs daily; monitor I&O; check for decreasing output
- Note allergic reaction: rash, fever, pruritus, urticaria; drug should be discontinued if antihistamines fail to help
- Note allergic reaction from patches: rash, urticaria, angioedema; should not continue to use
- Assess for symptoms of CHF: edema, dyspnea, wet rales, B/P, weight gain
- Monitor for retinal degeneration: periodic eye exam

Nursing diagnoses

- ✓ Injury, potential for physical (side effects)
- ✓ Knowledge deficit (teaching)
- ✓ Noncompliance (teaching)

Implementation

PO route

- PO: give last dose at hs

Trans route

- Apply patch weekly; remove old patch and wash off residue; apply to site without hair; best absorption over chest or upper arm; rotate sites with each application; clean site before application; apply firmly, especially around edges
- Store patches in cool environment, tabs in tight container

Patient/family education

- Instruct patient not to discontinue drug abruptly, or withdrawal symptoms may occur: anxiety, increased B/P, headache, insomnia, increased pulse, tremors, nausea, sweating
- Caution patient not to use OTC (cough, cold, or allergy) products unless directed by prescriber
- Caution patient to avoid sunlight or wear sunscreen, protective clothing if in sunlight; photosensitivity may occur
- Teach patient to comply with dosage schedule even if feeling better; drug controls symptoms, does not cure
- Caution patient to change position slowly, to rise slowly to sitting or standing position to minimize orthostatic hypotension, especially elderly [G]
- Instruct patient to notify physician of mouth sores, sore throat, fever, swelling of hands or feet, irregular heartbeat, chest pain, signs of angioedema, increased weight
- Teach patient about excessive perspiration, dehydration, vomiting; diarrhea may lead to fall in B/P; consult prescriber if these occur
- Tell patient that drug may cause dizziness, fainting; lightheadedness may occur during 1st few days of therapy; use hard candy, saliva product, or frequent rinsing of mouth for dry mouth

• Advise patient that compliance is necessary; not to skip or stop drug unless directed by prescriber
• Teach patient that drug may cause skin rash or impaired perspiration
• Teach patient that response may take 2-3 days if drug is given trans; instruct on administration of patch; return demonstration
• Teach patient to avoid hazardous activities, since drug may cause drowsiness, dizziness
• Teach patient to administer 1 hr ac

Evaluation

Positive therapeutic outcome
• Decrease in B/P in hypertension
• Decrease in withdrawal symptoms
• Decrease in vascular headaches
• Decrease in dysmenorrhea
• Decrease in menopausal symptoms

Treatment of overdose: Supportive treatment; administer tolazoline, atropine, dopamine prn

clorazepate (℞)
(klor-az′e-pate)
Apo-clorazepate ♣, clorazepate dipotassium, Gen-Xene, Tranxene, Tranxene-SD, Tranxene-SD Half Strength
Func. class.: Antianxiety, anticonvulsant
Chem. class.: Benzodiazepine
Pregnancy category D
Controlled substance schedule IV

Action: Potentiates the actions of GABA, especially in limbic system, reticular formation has anticonvulsant effects

➔ Therapeutic Outcome: Decreased anxiety, restlessness, insomnia

Uses: Anxiety, acute alcohol withdrawal, adjunct in seizure disorders

Dosage and routes

Anxiety
Adult: PO 15-60 mg/day

Alcohol withdrawal
Adult: PO 30 mg then day 1, 30-60 mg in divided doses; day 2, 45-90 mg in divided doses; day 3, 22.5-45 mg in divided doses; day 4, 15-30 mg in divided doses; then reduce daily dose to 7.5-15 mg

Seizure disorders
P ***Adult and child >12 yr:*** PO 7.5 mg tid; may increase by 7.5 mg/wk or less, not to exceed 90 mg/day

P ***Child 9-12 yr:*** PO 7.5 mg bid; may increase by 7.5 mg/wk or less, not to exceed 60 mg/day

Available forms: Caps 3.75, 7.5, 15 mg; tabs 3.75, 7.5, 15

mg; single-dose tab 11.25, 22.5 mg

Adverse effects

CNS: Dizziness, drowsiness, confusion, headache, anxiety, tremors, stimulation, fatigue, depression, insomnia, hallucinations, lethargy
CV: Orthostatic hypotension, ***ECG changes, tachycardia,*** hypotension
EENT: Blurred vision, tinnitus, mydriasis
GI: Constipation, dry mouth, nausea, vomiting, anorexia, diarrhea
INTEG: Rash, dermatitis, itching

Contraindications: Hypersensitivity to benzodiazepines, narrow-angle glaucoma, psy-
P chosis, pregnancy **D,** child <18 yr

G **Precautions:** Elderly, debilitated, hepatic disease, renal disease

Pharmacokinetics	
Absorption	Well absorbed
Distribution	Widely distributed; crosses placenta
Metabolism	Liver
Excretion	Kidneys, breast milk
Half-life	30-100 hr

Pharmacodynamics	
Onset	15 min
Peak	1-2 hr
Duration	4-6 hr

Interactions

Individual drugs

Alcohol: ↑ effects of clorazepate
Cimetidine: ↑ effects of clorazepate
Disulfiram: ↑ effects of clorazepate
Valproic acid: ↓ effects of clorazepate

Drug classifications

CNS depressants: ↑ effects of clorazepate
MAOI: ↑ effects of clorazepate
Oral contraceptives: ↑ effects of clorazepate

Lab test interferences

↑ AST (SGOT)/ALT (SGPT), ↑ serum bilirubin
↓ RAIU
False ↑ 17-OHCS

NURSING CONSIDERATIONS

Assessment

- Monitor B/P (with patient lying, standing), pulse; if systolic B/P drops 20 mm Hg, hold drug, notify prescriber
- Monitor blood studies: CBC during long-term therapy; blood dyscrasias have occurred rarely
- Monitor hepatic studies: AST (SGOT), ALT (SGPT), bilirubin, creatinine, LDH, alkaline phosphatase
- Monitor I&O; may indicate renal dysfunction
- Monitor mental status: mood, sensorium, affect, sleeping pattern, drowsiness, dizziness, physical dependency; withdrawal symptoms: headache, nausea, vomiting, muscle pain, weakness after long-term use; suicidal tendencies

Nursing diagnoses

✓ Coping, ineffective individual (uses)
✓ Knowledge deficit (teaching)
✓ Noncompliance (teaching)

Implementation

- Give with food or milk for GI symptoms
- ⊘ Do not chew, crush caps
- Use sugarless gum, hard candy, frequent sips of water for dry mouth
- Check to see PO medication has been swallowed

Patient/family education

• Teach patient that drug may be taken with food
• Teach patient not to use for everyday stress or longer than 4 mo, unless directed by a prescriber; not to take more than prescribed amount; may be habit forming
• Caution patient to avoid OTC preparations unless approved by a prescriber
• Caution patient to avoid driving, activities that require alertness; drowsiness may
G occur, especially in elderly
• Advise patient to avoid alcohol ingestion or other psychotropic medications, unless prescribed
• Advise patient not to discontinue medication abruptly after long-term use
• Advise patient to rise slowly or fainting may occur
• Teach patient that drowsiness may worsen at beginning of treatment

Evaluation

Positive therapeutic outcome

• Decreased anxiety, restlessness
• Decreased seizure activity

Treatment of overdose: Lavage, VS, supportive care, flumazenil

cloxacillin (℞)

(klox-a-sill'in)

Apo-Cloxi ✤, Bactopen ✤, cloxacillin sodium, Cloxapen, Novo-cloxin ✤, Orbenin ✤, Tegopen

Func. class.: Broad-spectrum antibiotic
Chem. class.: Penicillinase-resistant penicillin

Pregnancy category B

Action: Interferes with cell wall replication of susceptible organisms; the cell wall, rendered osmotically unstable, swells, bursts from osmotic pressure

➔ **Therapeutic Outcome:** Bactericidal effects for the following: gram-positive cocci *Staphylococcus aureus, S. epidermis,* penicillinase-producing staphylococci

Uses: Penicillinase-producing staphylococci, streptococci; respiratory tract, skin, skin structure infections; sinusitis

Dosage and routes

Adult: PO 1-4 g/day in divided doses q6h or 250 mg-1 g q6h

P ***Child:*** PO 50-100 mg/kg in divided doses q6h

Available forms: Caps 250, 500 mg; powder for oral susp 125 mg/5 ml

Adverse effects

CNS: Lethargy, hallucinations, anxiety, depression, muscle twitching, ***coma, convulsions***
GI: Nausea, vomiting, diarrhea, increased AST (SGOT), ALT (SGPT), abdominal pain, glossitis, ***pseudomembranous*** colitis

GU: ***Oliguria, proteinuria,*** hematuria, *vaginitis, moniliasis,* ***glomerulonephritis***
HEMA: Anemia, increased bleeding time, ***bone marrow depression, granulocytopenia***
SYST: Anaphylaxis

Contraindications: Hypersensitivity to penicillins; neonates, P severe renal, hepatic disease

Precautions: Pregnancy **B,** hypersensitivity to cephalosporins

Pharmacokinetics

Absorption	Moderate (35%-60%)
Distribution	Widely distributed;crosses placenta
Metabolism	Liver (up to 22%)
Excretion	Breast milk; kidneys, unchanged (30%-45%)
Half-life	0.5-1.1 hr, increased in hepatic/renal disease

Pharmacodynamics

Onset	½ hr
Peak	½-2 hr

Interactions

Individual drugs

Probenecid: ↑ cloxacillin levels, ↓ renal excretion

Drug classifications

Oral anticoagulants: ↑ anticoagulant effects

Food

Food, carbonated drinks, citrus fruit juices: ↓ absorption

Lab test interferences

False positive: Urine glucose, urine protein

NURSING CONSIDERATIONS

Assessment

- Assess patient for previous sensitivity reaction to penicillins or other cephalosporins; cross-sensitivity between penicillins and cephalosporins is common
- Assess patient for signs and symptoms of infection including characteristics of wounds, sputum, urine, stool, WBC >10,000, fever; obtain baseline information and during treatment
- Obtain C&S before beginning drug therapy to identify if correct treatment has been initiated
- Assess for allergic reactions: rash, urticaria, pruritus, chills, fever, joint pain may occur a few days after therapy begins; epinephrine and resuscitation equipment should be available for anaphylactic reaction
- ! Identify urine output; if decreasing, notify prescriber (may indicate nephrotoxicity); also check for increased BUN, creatinine
- Monitor blood studies: AST (SGOT), ALT (SGPT), CBC, Hct, bilirubin, LDH, alkaline phosphatase, Coombs' test monthly if patient is on long-term therapy
- Monitor electrolytes: potassium, sodium, chloride monthly if patient is on long-term therapy
- Assess bowel pattern qd; if severe diarrhea occurs, drug should be discontinued; may indicate pseudomembranous colitis
- Monitor for bleeding: ecchymosis, bleeding gums, hematuria, stool guaiac daily if on long-term therapy
- Assess for overgrowth of infection: perineal itching, fever, malaise, redness, pain, swelling, drainage, rash, diarrhea, change in cough, sputum

Nursing diagnoses

- ✓ Infection, risk for (uses)
- ✓ Diarrhea (side effects)

C

- ☑ Injury, risk for (side effects)
- ☑ Knowledge deficit (teaching)
- ☑ Noncompliance (teaching)

Implementation

- Give in even doses around the clock; if GI upset occurs, give with food; drug must be given for 10-14 days to ensure organism death and prevent superinfection; store in airtight container
- Do not crush, chew caps
- Shake susp; store in refrigerator for 2 wk, 1 wk at room temp

Patient/family education

- Teach patient to report sore throat, bruising, bleeding, joint pain; may indicate blood dyscrasis (rare)
- Advise patient to contact prescriber if vaginal itching, loose, foul-smelling stools, furry tongue occur; may indicate superinfection
- Instruct patient to take all medications prescribed for the length of time ordered
- Advise patient to notify prescriber of diarrhea with blood or pus, which may indicate pseudomembranous colitis

Evaluation

Positive therapeutic outcome

- Absence of signs/symptoms of infection (WBC <10,000, temp WNL, absence of red, draining wounds)
- Reported improvement in symptoms of infection

Treatment of anaphylaxis: Withdraw drug, maintain airway, administer epinephrine, aminophylline, O_2, **IV** corticosteroids

clozapine (℞)

(kloz'a-peen)

Clozaril

Func. class.: Antipsychotic

Chem. class.: Tricyclic dibenzodiazepine derivative

Pregnancy category B

Action: Interferes with dopamine receptor binding with lack of extrapyramidal symptoms and tardive dyskinesia; also acts as an adrenergic, cholinergic, histaminergic, serotonergic antagonist

Therapeutic Outcome: Decreased psychotic behavior

Uses: Management of psychotic symptoms in schizophrenic patients for whom other antipsychotics have failed

Dosage and routes

Adult: PO 25 mg qd or bid; may increase by 25-50 mg/day; normal range 300-450 mg/day after 2 wk; do not increase dosage more than 2 times/wk; do not exceed 900 mg/day; use lowest dosage to control symptoms

Available forms: Tabs 25, 100 mg

Adverse effects

CNS: Sedation, salivation, dizziness, headache, tremors, sleep problems, akinesia, fever, ***seizures****, sweating, akathisia, confusion, fatigue, insomnia, depression, slurred speech, anxiety,* ***neuroleptic malignant syndrome***

CV: Tachycardia, hypotension, hypertension, chest pain, ECG changes

GI: Drooling or excessive salivation, constipation, nausea,

abdominal discomfort, vomiting, diarrhea, anorexia
GU: Urinary abnormalities, incontinence, ejaculation dysfunction, frequency, urgency, retention
HEMA: Leukopenia, neutropenia, agranulocytosis, eosinophilia
MS: Weakness; pain in back, neck, legs; spasm
RESP: Dyspnea, nasal congestion, throat discomfort

Contraindications: Hypersensitivity, myeloproliferative disorders, severe granulocytopenia, CNS depression, coma, narrow-angle glaucoma

Precautions: Pregnancy **B,** P lactation, children <16, hepatic, renal, cardiac disease, seizures, prostatic enlargement, G elderly

Pharmacokinetics

Absorption	Well absorbed
Distribution	Widely distributed; crosses blood-brain barrier, placenta; 95% bound to plasma proteins
Metabolism	Liver
Excretion	Kidneys, feces (metabolites)
Half-life	8-12 hr

Pharmacodynamics

Onset	Unknown
Peak	Steady state 2½ hr
Duration	4-12 hr

Interactions

Individual drugs

Alcohol: ↑ effects of both drugs, oversedation
Digoxin: ↑ plasma concentration of digoxin
Warfarin: ↑ plasma concentrations

Drug classifications

Antacids: ↓ absorption
Anticholinergics: ↑ anticholinergic effects
Antidepressants: ↑ CNS depression
Antihistamines: ↑ CNS depression
Antihypertensives: ↑ hypotension
Antineoplastics: ↑ bone marrow suppression

Lab test interferences

↑ Liver function tests, ↑ cardiac enzymes, ↑ cholesterol, ↑ blood glucose, ↑ prolactin, ↑ bilirubin, ↑ PBI, ↑ cholinesterase, ^{131}I
False positive: Pregnancy tests, PKU
False negative: Urinary steroids, 17-OHCS

NURSING CONSIDERATIONS

Assessment

- Assess mental status: orientation, mood, behavior, presence of hallucinations, and type before initial administration and monthly; this drug should significantly reduce psychotic behavior
- Check for swallowing of PO medication; check for hoarding or giving of medication to other patients
- Monitor I&O ratio, palpate bladder if low urinary output G occurs, especially in elderly; urinalysis recommended before, during prolonged therapy
- Monitor bilirubin, CBC, liver function studies monthly
- Assess affect, orientation, LOC, reflexes, gait, coordination, sleep pattern disturbances
- Monitor B/P with patient sitting, standing, and lying; take pulse and respirations q4h during initial treatment; establish baseline before starting treatment; report drops of 30 mm Hg

• Check for dizziness, faintness, palpitations, tachycardia on rising
• Identify for neuroleptic malignant syndrome: hyperpyrexia, muscle rigidity, increased CPK, altered mental status; drug should be discontinued
• Assess for extrapyramidal symptoms including akathisia (inability to sit still, no pattern to movements), tardive dyskinesia (bizarre movements of the jaw, mouth, tongue, extremities), pseudoparkinsonism (rigidity, tremors, pill rolling, shuffling gate)
• Assess for constipation, urinary retention daily; if these occur, increase bulk, water in diet

Nursing diagnoses

☑ Thought processes, altered (uses)
☑ Coping, ineffective individual (uses)
☑ Knowledge deficit (teaching)
☑ Noncompliance (teaching)

Implementation

G • Decrease dosage in elderly since metabolism is slowed
• Give with full glass of water, milk; or give with food to decrease GI upset
• Store in tight, light-resistant container; oral sol in amber bottle

Patient/family education

• Teach patient to use good oral hygiene; frequent rinsing of mouth, sugarless gum for dry mouth
• Caution patient to avoid hazardous activities until drug response is determined
• Inform patient that orthostatic hypotension occurs often and to rise from sitting or lying position gradually
• Caution patient to avoid hot tubs, hot showers, tub baths, since hypotension may occur
• Teach patient to avoid OTC preparations (cough, hay fever, cold) unless approved by prescriber, since serious drug interactions may occur; avoid use with alcohol, CNS depressants; increased drowsiness may occur
• Teach patient about extrapyramidal symptoms and necessity of meticulous oral hygiene, since oral candidiasis may occur
• Teach patient to report sore throat, malaise, fever, bleeding, mouth sores; if these occur, CBC should be drawn and drug discontinued
• Advise patient that in hot weather, heat stroke may occur; take extra precautions to stay cool

Evaluation

Positive therapeutic outcome

• Decrease in emotional excitement, hallucinations, delusions, paranoia
• Reorganization of patterns of thought, speech

Treatment of anaphylaxis: Withdraw drug, maintain airway

codeine 🔑 (℞)

(koe'deen)
Paveral ✱, Codeine
Narcotic analgesics
Func. class.: Opiate, phenanthrene derivative
Pregnancy category C
Controlled substance schedule II, III, IV, V
(depends on route)

Action: Depresses pain impulse transmission at the spinal cord level by interacting with opioid receptors, decreases cough reflex, GI motility

➔ **Therapeutic Outcome:** Pain relief, decreased cough, decreased diarrhea depending on route

Uses: Moderate to severe pain, nonproductive cough

Investigational uses: Diarrhea

Dosage and routes

Pain

Adult: PO 15-60 mg q4h prn; IM/SC 15-60 mg q4h prn

P ***Child:*** PO 3 mg/kg/day in divided doses q4h prn

Cough

Adult: PO 10-20 mg q4-6h, not to exceed 120 mg/day

P ***Child:*** PO 1-1.5 mg/kg/day in 4 divided doses, not to exceed 60 mg/day

Diarrhea

Adult: PO 30 mg; may repeat qid prn

Available forms: Inj 15, 30, 60 mg/ml; tabs 15, 30, 60 mg; oral sol 10mg/5 ml ♣, 15 mg/5 ml

Adverse effects

CNS: Drowsiness, sedation, dizziness, agitation, dependency, lethargy, restlessness

CV: Bradycardia, palpitations, orthostatic hypotension, tachycardia

GI: Nausea, vomiting, anorexia, constipation

GU: Urinary retention

INTEG: Flushing, rash, urticaria

RESP: Respiratory depression, respiratory paralysis

Contraindications: Hypersensitivity to opiates, respiratory depression, increased intracranial pressure, seizure disorders, severe respiratory disorders

G **Precautions:** Elderly, cardiac dysrhythmias, pregnancy **C**

Pharmacokinetics

Absorption	Complete (IM)
Distribution	Widely distributed; crosses placenta
Metabolism	Liver, extensively
Excretion	Kidneys (up to 15%), breast milk
Half-life	3-4 hr

Pharmacodynamics

	PO	IM	SC
Onset	30-45 min	15-30 min	15-30 min
Peak	1-2 hr	30-60 min	Unknown
Duration	4 hr	4 hr	4 hr

Interactions

Individual drugs

Alcohol: ↑ respiratory depression, hypotension, ↑ sedation

Nalbuphine: ↓ analgesia

Pentazocine: ↓ analgesia

Drug classifications

Antihistamines: ↑ respiratory depression, hypotension

CNS depressants: ↑ respiratory depression, hypotension

MAOI: Use with caution

Phenothiazines: ↑ respiratory depression, hypotension

Sedative/hypnotics: ↑ respiratory depression, hypotension

Lab test interferences

↑ Amylase, ↑ lipase

NURSING CONSIDERATIONS

Assessment

- Assess pain: intensity, type, aleviating factors
- Monitor VS after parenteral route; note muscle rigidity, drug history, liver, kidney function tests, respiratory dysfunction: respiratory depression, character, rate,

rhythm; notify prescriber if respirations are <10/min
• Monitor CNS changes: dizziness, drowsiness, hallucinations, euphoria, LOC, pupil reaction
• Monitor allergic reactions: rash, urticaria

Nursing diagnoses
✓ Pain (uses)
✓ Sensory perceptual alteration: visual, auditory (adverse reactions)
✓ Breathing pattern, ineffective (adverse reactions)
✓ Knowledge deficit (teaching)

Implementation
• Give with antiemetic if nausea, vomiting occur
• Administer when pain is beginning to return, determine dosage interval by patient response; continuous dosing of medication is more effective given prn; explain analgesic effect
• Medication should be slowly withdrawn after long-term use to prevent withdrawal symptoms
• Store in light-resistant container at room temp

PO route
• May be given with food or milk to lessen GI upset

IM/SC route
• Do not give if cloudy, or a precipitate has formed

Syringe compatibilities: Glycopyrrolate, hydroxyzine

Additive incompatibilities: Aminophylline, amobarbital, chlorothiazide, heparin, methicillin, pentobarbital, phenobarbital, phenytoin, secobarbital, thiopental

Patient/family education
• Teach patient to report any symptoms of CNS changes, allergic reactions; to avoid CNS depressants: alcohol, sedative/hypnotics for at least 24 hr after taking this drug
• Discuss with patient that dizziness, drowsiness, and confusion are common
• Advise patient to avoid getting up without assistance
• Discuss in detail all aspects of the drug

Evaluation
Positive therapeutic outcome
• Decreased pain
• Decreased cough

Treatment of overdose: Narcan 0.2-0.8 **IV**, O_2, **IV** fluids, vasopressors

colchicine (℞)
(kol'chi-seen)
Func. class.: Antigout agent
Chem. class.: Colchicum autumnale alkaloid
Pregnancy category C

Action: Inhibits microtubule formation of lactic acid in leukocytes, which decreases phagocytosis and inflammation in joints

Therapeutic Outcome: Decreased pain, inflammation of joints

Uses: Gout, gouty arthritis (prevention, treatment); to arrest progression of neurologic disability in multiple sclerosis

Dosage and routes
Prevention
Adult: PO 0.5-1.8 mg qd depending on severity; **IV** 0.5-1 mg qd-bid

Treatment

Adult: PO 0.5-1.2 mg, then 0.5-1.2 mg q1h, until pain decreases or side effects occur; **IV** 2 mg, then 0.5 mg q6h, not to exceed 4 mg/24 hr

Available forms: Tabs 0.5, 0.6 mg; inj **IV** 1 mg/2 ml

Adverse effects

GI: Nausea, vomiting, anorexia, malaise, metallic taste, cramps, peptic ulcer, diarrhea
GU: Hematuria, ***oliguria, renal damage***
HEMA: Agranulocytosis, thrombocytopenia, aplastic anemia, pancytopenia
INTEG: Chills, dermatitis, pruritus, purpura, erythema
MISC: Myopathy, alopecia, reversible azoospermia, peripheral neuritis

Contraindications: Hypersensitivity; serious GI, renal, hepatic, cardiac disorders; blood dyscrasias

Precautions: Severe renal disease, blood dyscrasias, pregnancy **C,** hepatic disease,
G elderly, lactation,
P children

Pharmacokinetics

Absorption	Well absorbed
Distribution	WBCs
Metabolism	Deacetylates in liver
Excretion	Feces (metabolites/active drug)
Half-life	20 min

Pharmacodynamics

	PO
Onset	Unknown
Peak	½-2 hr
Duration	Unknown

Interactions

Individual drugs

Vitamin B_{12}: ↓ action of vitamin B_{12}

Drug classifications

Acidifiers: ↓ action of colchicine
Alkalinizers: ↑ action of colchicine
CNS depressants: ↑ action of CNS depressants
Sympathomimetics: ↑ action of sympathomimetics

Lab test interferences

↑ Alkaline phosphatase, ↑ AST (SGOT)/ALT (SGPT)
False positive: RBC, Hgb

NURSING CONSIDERATIONS

Assessment

- Assess pain and mobility of joints
- Monitor I&O ratio; observe for decrease in urinary output; CBC, platelets, reticulocytes before, during therapy (q 3 mo): Coombs' test to determine Coombs' negative hemolytic anemia

Nursing diagnoses

✓ Pain, chronic (uses)
✓ Immobility, impaired (uses)
✓ Knowledge deficit (teaching)

Implementation

PO route

- Give on empty stomach (1 hr ac or 2 hr pc) for better absorption

IV **IV route**

- Give **IV** undiluted or diluted 1 mg/10-20 ml normal saline or sterile water for inj; give over 2-5 min

Patient/family education

- Teach patient to increase fluids to 3-4 L/day
- Caution patient to avoid alcohol, OTC preparations that contain alcohol; skin rashes have occurred
- Instruct patient to report any pain, redness, or hard area, usually in legs
- Teach patient importance of

complying with medical regimen; bone marrow depression may occur

Evaluation

Positive therapeutic outcome

- Decreased stone formation on x-ray
- Decreased pain in kidney region
- Absence of hematuria
- Decreased pain in joints

colestipol (℞)

(koe-les′ti-pole)

Colestid

Func. class.: Antilipemic

Chem. class.: Bile sequestrant, resin exchange agent

Pregnancy category B

Action: Absorbs, combines with bile acids to form an insoluble complex that is excreted through feces; loss of bile acids lowers cholesterol levels

Therapeutic Outcome: Decreasing cholesterol levels and low-density lipoproteins, decreased pruritus

Uses: Primary hypercholesterolemia, xanthomas, digitalis toxicity, pruritus due to biliary obstruction, diarrhea due to bile acids

Dosage and routes

Adult: PO 15-30 g/day in 2-4 divided doses; 2-8 tabs/day

Available forms: Granules 5 g packets, tabs 1 g

Adverse effects

GI: Constipation, abdominal pain, nausea, fecal impaction, hemorrhoids, flatulence, vomiting, steatorrhea, peptic ulcer

HEMA: Decreased vitamin A, D, E, K, red folate content; ***hyperchloremic acidosis, bleeding, decreased pro-time***

INTEG: Rash, irritation of perianal area, tongue, skin

Contraindications: Hypersensitivity, biliary obstruction

Precautions: Pregnancy **B**, P lactation, children, bleeding disorders

Pharmacokinetics

Absorption	Not absorbed
Distribution	Not distributed
Metabolism	Not metabolized
Excretion	Binds with bile acids, feces
Half-life	Unknown

Pharmacodynamics

Unknown

Interactions

Individual drugs

Acetaminophen: ↓ absorption of acetominophen

Amiodarone: ↓ absorption of amiodarone

Methotrexate: ↓ absorption of methotrexate

Naproxen: ↓ absorption of naproxen

Phenylbutazone: ↓ absorption of phenylbutazone

Piroxicam: ↓ absorption of piroxicam

Propranolol: ↓ absorption of propanolol

Thyroid: ↓ absorption of thyroid

Ursodiol: ↓ absorption of ursodiol

Drug classifications

Anticoagulants, oral: ↓ absorption

Cardiac glycosides: ↓ absorption

Diuretics, thiazide: ↓ absorption

Vitamins A,D,E,K: ↓ absorption

Lab test interferences

↑ Liver function studies, ↑ Cl, ↑ PO_4

NURSING CONSIDERATIONS

Assessment

- Assess nutrition: fat, protein, carbohydrates; nutritional analysis should be completed by dietician
- Assess skin integrity after patient has been receiving drug; itching, pruritus often occur from bile deposits on skin
- Monitor cardiac glycoside level, if both drugs are being administered; cardiac glycoside levels will be decreased
- Monitor for signs of vitamin A, D, E, K deficiency; check serum cholesterol, triglyceride levels, electrolytes if on extended therapy
- Monitor bowel pattern daily; increase bulk, water in diet if constipation develops

Nursing diagnoses

✓ Constipation (adverse reactions)
✓ Knowledge deficit (teaching)
✓ Noncompliance (teaching)

Implementation

- Give drug ac, hs; give all other medications 1 hr before or 4 hr after colestipol to avoid poor absorption; give drug mixed with applesauce or stirred into beverage (2-6 oz); do not take dry, let stand for 2 min
- Provide supplemental doses of vitamins A, D, E, K, if levels are low
- ⊘ Tabs should be swallowed whole; do not crush, chew

Patient/family education

- Teach patient symptoms of hypoprothrombinemia: bleeding mucous membranes, dark, tarry stools, hematuria, petechiae; report immediately
- Teach patient importance of compliance, since toxicity may result if doses are missed; not to discontinue suddenly
- Teach patient that risk factors should be decreased: high-fat diet, smoking, alcohol consumption, absence of exercise
- Tell patient to mix drug with 6 oz of milk, water, fruit juice; may be mixed with carbonated beverages; rinse glass to make sure all medication is taken or may mix drug in applesauce; allow to stand for 2 min before mixing

Evaluation

Positive therapeutic outcome

- Decreased cholesterol level (hyperlipidemia)
- Decreased diarrhea, pruritus (excess bile acids)

colfosceril (℞)

(kole-foss'er-ill)

Exosurf Neonatal

Func. class.: Synthetic lung surfactant

Chem. class.: Dipalmitoylphosphatidylcholine (DPPC)

Pregnancy category N/A

Action: Surfactant maintains lung inflation and prevents collapse by lowering surface tension

➔ Therapeutic Outcome: Ability to breathe without assistance

Uses: Treatment of respiratory

distress syndrome (RDS) in premature infants

Dosage and routes

Prophylactic treatment

Endotracheally: 5 ml/kg as soon as possible after birth and repeat doses 12 and 24 hr later to infants remaining on mechanical ventilation

Rescue treatment

Endotracheally: Administer in two half doses of 5 ml/kg doses; give initial dose after treatment of RDS, then second dose in 12 hr

Available forms: 10 ml/vial with sterile water for inj and 5 endotracheal tube adapters

Adverse effects

RESP: Apnea, pulmonary hemorrhage, pulmonary air leak, congenital pneumonia
SYST: Nonpulmonary fatal infections

Precautions: Congenital anomalies, prophylactic treatment

Pharmacokinetics	
Absorption	Unknown
Distribution	All lobes, alveolar spaces, distal airways
Metabolism	90% of alveolar phospholipids are recycled
Excretion	Unknown
Half-life	Alveolar-12 hr

Pharmacodynamics	
Onset	Immediate
Peak	Unknown
Duration	12 hr

Interactions: None

NURSING CONSIDERATIONS

Assessment

- Assess respiratory rate, rhythm, character; chest expansion, color, transcutaneous saturation, ABGs
- Monitor endotracheal tube placement before dosing; for apnea after endotracheal administration
- Check for reflux of drug into the endotracheal tube during administration; stop drug administration if this occurs, and, if needed, increase peak inspiratory pressure on the ventilator by 4-5 cm H_2O until tube is cleared

Nursing diagnoses

✓ Impaired gas exchange (uses)
✓ Breathing patterns ineffective (uses)

Implementation

- Infants should be suctioned before administration
- Give after selecting an adapter size that corresponds to the diameter of the endotracheal tube, insert the adapter into the tube by twisting, connect the breathing circuit to the adapter, remove the cap from the adapter sideport, and attach the syringe to the sideport; after dose is completed, remove the syringe and recap the sideport
- Administer after reconstituting each vial with 8 ml preservative-free sterile water for inj, fill a 10-12 ml syringe with 8 ml preservative-free sterile water for inj, using an 18-19 G needle; allow the vacuum in the vial to draw the liquid into the vial; aspirate the 8 ml out of the vial into the syringe while maintaining the vacuum and then release the syringe plunger; repeat the aspiration and release until adequately mixed; draw the dose required into the syringe from below the froth in the vial; do not use if large particles are present
- Administer by endotracheal

administration only by persons trained in neonatal intubation and ventilation
- Provide reduction in peak ventilator inspiratory pressures immediately if chest expansion improves substantially after dose
- Provide reduction in F_{IO_2} in small, repeated steps when infant becomes pink and transcutaneous oxygen saturation is in excess of 95%; oxygen saturation should remain between 90% and 95%
- Perform suctioning of all infants before administration to prevent mucous plugging; if endotracheal tube obstruction is suspected, remove the obstruction and replace tube immediately
- Store at room temp in dry place

Evaluation
Positive therapeutic outcome
- Decreased respiratory distress

corticotropin (℞)
(kor-ti-koe-troe'pin)
ACTH, Acthar, corticotropin, ACTH-40, ACTH-80, Duracton ✱, H.P. Acthar Gel
Func. class.: Pituitary hormone
Chem. class.: Adrenocorticotropic hormone
Pregnancy category C

Action: Stimulates adrenal cortex to produce, secrete corticosterone, cortisol; suppresses adrenal function (chronic use); potent mineralocorticoid

➔ **Therapeutic Outcome:** Increased production of adrenal steroids in adrenal insufficiency

Uses: Testing adrenocortical function, treatment of adrenal insufficiency caused by administration of corticosteroids (long term), multiple sclerosis

Dosage and routes
Testing of adrenocortical function
Adult: IM/SC up to 80 U in divided doses; **IV** 10-25 U in 500 ml D_5W given over 8 hr

Inflammation
Adult: SC/IM 40 U in 4 divided doses (aqueous) or 40 U q12-24h (gel/repository form)

Available forms: Inj 25, 40 U/vial; repository inj 40, 80/ml

Adverse effects
CNS: ***Convulsions,*** dizziness, euphoria, insomnia, headache, mood swings, behavioral changes, depression, psychosis
EENT: Cataracts, glaucoma
ENDO: Cushingoid symptoms, diabetes mellitus, antibody formation, growth retardation in children, menstrual irregularities
GI: Nausea, vomiting, ***peptic ulcer perforation,*** pancreatitis, distention, ulcerative esophagitis
GU: Water, sodium retention, hypokalemia
INTEG: Impaired wound healing, rash, urticaria, hirsutism, petechiae, ecchymoses, sweating, acne, hyperpigmentation
MS: Weakness, osteoporosis, compression fractures, muscle atrophy, steroid myopathy, myalgia, arthralgia

Contraindications: Hypersensitivity, scleroderma, osteoporosis, CHF, peptic ulcer disease, hypertension, systemic fungal infections, smallpox vaccination, recent surgery, ocular herpes simplex, primary adrenocortical insufficiency/hyperfunction

Precautions: Pregnancy **C**, lactation, latent TB, hepatic disease, hypothyroiditis, childbearing-age women, psychiatric diagnosis, myasthenia gravis, acute gouty arthritis

Pharmacokinetics

Absorption	Rapidly absorbed (IM, SC)
Distribution	Widely distributed to tissues
Metabolism	Unknown
Excretion	Unknown
Half-life	<20 min

Pharmacodynamics

	IM (gelatin repository)	IV
Onset	Unknown	Unknown
Peak	3-12 hr	1 hr
Duration	Up to 3 days	Unknown

Interactions

Individual drugs

Amphotericin B: ↑ hypokalemia
Insulin: ↑ need for insulin
Mezlocillin: ↑ hypokalemia
Phenobarbital: ↓ effectiveness of corticotropin
Phenytoin: ↓ effectiveness of corticotropin
Piperacillin: ↑ hypokalemia
Rifampin: ↓ effectiveness of corticotropin
Ticarcillin: ↑ hypokalemia

Drug classifications

Diuretics, potassium depleting: ↑ hypokalemia
Live virus vaccines: ↓ antibody reactions
Oral contraceptive: Blocked metabolism of corticotropin

NURSING CONSIDERATIONS

Assessment

- Monitor I&O ratio, weight weekly; report gain over 5 lb/wk
- Obtain 2-hr postprandial chest x-ray, serum potassium, 17-KS, 17-OHCS, cortisol, during long-term treatment
- Assess for dependent edema, moon face, pulmonary edema, cerebral edema; monitor baseline ECG, B/P, chest x-ray, GTT, pulse
- Assess for increased stress in patient's life that may require increased corticosteroids; assess for infection which drug may mask
- Assess for mental status: affect, mood, increased aggressiveness, irritability; a change in mental status may require decreased steroids; changes can be extreme
- P Identify growth rate of child; growth suppression may occur frequently
- P Identify hypoadrenalism in neonates if drug was given during pregnancy
- Identify allergic reaction: rash, urticaria, fever, nausea, vomiting, dyspnea; drug should be discontinued immediately; administer epinephrine 1:1000

Nursing diagnoses

- ✓ Infection, risk for (adverse reactions)
- ✓ Injury, risk for (adverse reactions)
- ✓ Knowledge deficit (teaching)

Implementation

- Give diet with decreased sodium, increased potassium for dependent edema; increase

protein in diet for nitrogen loss before giving; give deep IM using 21 G needle, massage, rotate sites; injection is painful
• Store unused portion in refrigerator; use within 24 hr

IV route
• Give by direct **IV**: give over 2 min; dilute 25 U/1 ml sterile water or normal saline or 40 U/2 ml
• Give by intermittent inf: dilute 10-25 U/500 ml D_5W, 0.9% NaCl, D_5/0.9% NaCl, or LR; give over 8 hr; or 40 U/12-48 hr
• Store unused portion in refrigerator; use within 24 hr

Additive incompatibilities:
Aminophylline, sodium bicarbonate

Additive compatibilities:
Calcium gluconate, chloramphenicol, cytarabine, dimenhydrinate, erythromycin gluceptate, heparin, hydrocortisone, methicillin, norepinephrine, oxytetracycline, penicillin G potassium, potassium chloride, tetracycline, vancomycin

Patient/family education
• Caution patient to avoid vaccinations during drug treatment; tell patient to notify anyone involved in medical or dental care that this drug is being taken
• Teach patient to maintain adequate hydration up to 2 L/day unless contraindicated
• Advise patient to avoid OTC products: salicylates, products with alcohol
• Teach patient not to discontinue medication abruptly; adrenal crisis may occur; drug should be tapered off over several wk; teach patient that drug does not cure condition, only decreases symptoms
• Teach patient to wear Medic Alert ID specifying steroid therapy
• Instruct patient to notify prescriber of infection: increased temp, sore throat, muscular pain

Evaluation

Positive therapeutic outcome
• Absence of inflammation, pain
• Increased muscle strength in multiple sclerosis

cortisone (℞)

(kor'ti-sone)
Cortone Acetate
Func. class.: Corticosteroid, synthetic
Chem. class.: Short-acting glucocorticoid
Pregnancy category C

Action: Decreases inflammation by suppression of migration of polymorphonuclear leukocytes, fibroblasts, reversal of increased capillary permeability, and lysosomal stabilization; suppresses adrenal function with long-term use

Therapeutic Outcome: Replacement of cortisol in adrenal insufficiency

Uses: Inflammation, severe allergy, adrenal insufficiency, collagen disorders, respiratory and dermatologic disorders

Dosage and routes
Adult: PO/IM 25-300 mg qd or q2 days, titrated to patient response

Available forms: Tabs 5, 10, 25 mg; inj 50 mg/ml

Adverse effects
CNS: Depression, flushing, sweating, headache, mood changes
CV: Hypertension, ***circulatory collapse, thrombophlebitis, embolism,*** tachycardia, ***necrotizing angiitis, CHF,*** edema
EENT: Fungal infections, increased intraocular pressure, blurred vision
GI: Diarrhea, nausea, abdominal distention, ***GI hemorrhage,*** increased appetite, ***pancreatitis***
HEMA: ***Thrombocytopenia***
INTEG: Acne, poor wound healing, ecchymosis, bruising, petechiae
MS: Fractures, osteoporosis, weakness

Contraindications: Psychosis, hypersensitivity, idiopathic thrombocytopenia, acute glomerulonephritis, amebiasis, fungal infections, nonasthmatic bronchial disease, child <2 yr, AIDS, TB

Precautions: Pregnancy **C,** diabetes mellitus, glaucoma, osteoporosis, seizure disorders, ulcerative colitis, CHF, myasthenia gravis, renal disease, esophagitis, peptic ulcer

Pharmacokinetics

Absorption	Slowly IM
Distribution	Widely, crosses placenta
Metabolism	Liver
Excretion	Unknown
Half-life	½ hr

Pharmacodynamics

	PO	IM
Onset	Unknown	Unknown
Peak	2 hr	20-48 hr
Duration	1½ days	1½ days

Interactions
Individual drugs
Amphotericin B: ↑ hypokalemia
Insulin: ↑ need for insulin
Mezlocillin: ↑ hypokalemia
Phenobarbital: ↓ effectiveness of cortisone
Phenytoin: ↓ effectiveness of cortisone
Drug classifications
Contraceptives, oral: Blocked metabolism of cortisone
Lab test interferences
↑ Cholesterol, ↑ sodium, ↑ blood glucose, ↑ uric acid, ↑ calcium, ↑ urine glucose
↓ Calcium, ↓ potassium, ↓ T_4, ↓ T_3, ↓ thyroid ^{131}I uptake test, ↓ urine 17-OHCS, ↓ 17-KS, ↓ PBI
False negative: Skin allergy tests

NURSING CONSIDERATIONS
Assessment
- Assess for adrenal insufficiency symptoms: weakness, nausea, vomiting, confusion, anxiety, restlessness, decreased B/P, weight loss; check before and during treatment
- Monitor potassium, blood sugar, urine glucose for patient on long-term therapy; hypokalemia and hyperglycemia can occur
- Check B/P, pulse q4h; notify prescriber if chest pain occurs
- Monitor I&O ratio and weight daily; be alert for decreasing urinary output and increasing edema with bilateral rales, dyspnea, weight gain
- Monitor plasma cortisol levels during long-term therapy (normal level: 138-635 nmol/L if drawn at 8 AM)
- Assess for symptoms of infection: increased temp, WBC even after withdrawal of medication; drug masks symptoms of infection
- Monitor for potassium

depletion: paresthesias, fatigue, nausea, vomiting, depression, polyuria, dysrhythmias, weakness, edema, hypertension, cardiac symptoms, weight daily; notify prescriber of weekly gain >5 lb
- Assess for mental changes: affect, mood, behavioral changes, aggression; depression, psychoses may occur

Nursing diagnoses
- ✓ Infection, risk for (adverse reactions)
- ✓ Injury, risk for (adverse reactions)
- ✓ Knowledge deficit (teaching)

Implementation

IM route
- Give after shaking susp (parenteral); titrate dose; use lowest effective dosage
- Give IM inj deep in large muscle mass; rotate sites; avoid deltoid; use a 21 G needle
- Administer in 1 dose in AM to prevent adrenal suppression; avoid SC administration; damage may be done to tissue; do not give **IV**

PO route
- Administer with food or milk to decrease GI symptoms

Patient/family education
- Advise patient that ID as steroid user should be carried at all times
- Instruct patient to notify prescriber if therapeutic response decreases; dosage adjustment may be needed; teach not to discontinue this medication abruptly or adrenal crisis can result; teach all aspects of drug usage, including cushingoid symptoms
- Caution patient to avoid OTC products: salicylates, potassium, alcohol in cough products, cold preparations unless directed by prescriber
- Teach patient symptoms of adrenal insufficiency: nausea, anorexia, fatigue, dizziness, dyspnea, weakness, joint pain, tarry stools, bruising, blurred vision
- Advise patient to avoid persons with known infections; report probable infection rapidly; drug masks infection
- Caution patient that diet modification is necessary if on long-term treatment: increased calcium, potassium, and protein; also low sodium and carbohydrates

Evaluation

Positive therapeutic outcome
- Ease of respirations, decreased inflammation

C

cosyntropin (℞)
(koe-sin-troe'pin)
Cortrosyn, Synacthen ♣, Tetracosactrin
Func. class.: Pituitary hormone
Chem. class.: Synthetic polypeptide
Pregnancy category C

Action: Stimulates adrenal cortex to produce, secrete corticosterone, cortisol; suppresses adrenal function (chronic use); potent mineralocorticoid

➔ **Therapeutic Outcome:** Increased production of adrenal steroids

Uses: Testing adrenocortical function

Dosage and routes

P ***Adult and child >2 yr:*** IM/

IV 0.25-1 mg between blood sampling

P *Child <2 yr:* IM/**IV** 0.125 mg

Available forms: Inj 0.25 mg/vial

Adverse effects

INTEG: Rash, urticaria, pruritus, flushing

*SYST: **Anaphylaxis***

Contraindications: Hypersensitivity

Precautions: Pregnancy **C**

Pharmacokinetics	
Absorption	Rapidly absorbed
Distribution	Widely distributed to tissues
Metabolism	Unknown
Excretion	Unknown
Half-life	15 min

Pharmacodynamics	
Onset	5 min
Peak	1 hr
Duration	2-4 hr

Interactions

Drug classifications

Estrogens: Blocks metabolism

Glucocorticoids: Altered test results

NURSING CONSIDERATIONS

Assessment

- Identify allergic reaction: rash, urticaria, fever, nausea, vomiting, dyspnea; drug should be discontinued immediately; administer epinephrine 1:1000

Nursing diagnosis

✓ Knowledge deficit (teaching)

Implementation

- Store at room temp for 24 hr or refrigerate for 3 wk

IV **IV route**

Direct IV

- Give after reconstituting 250 μg/1 ml 0.9% NaCl over 2 min

Intermittent inf

Further dilute in D_5W or normal saline; run 40 μg/hr over 4-8 hr as an inf; remains stable for 12 hr at room temp

Patient/family education

- Explain that drug is used for determining type of adrenocortical insufficiency

Evaluation

Positive therapeutic outcome

- Diagnosis of adrenocortical insufficiency (primary, secondary)

cyclobenzaprine (℞)

(sye-kloe-ben′za-preen)

cyclobenzaprine HCl, Cycloflex, Flexeril

Func. class.: Skeletal muscle relaxant, central acting

Chem. class.: Tricyclic amine salt

Pregnancy category B

Action: Unknown; may be related to antidepressant effects

➔ **Therapeutic Outcome:** Relaxation of skeletal muscle

Uses: Adjunct for relief of muscle spasm and pain in musculoskeletal conditions

Dosage and routes

Adult: PO 10 mg tid × 1 wk, not to exceed 60 mg/day × 3 wk

Available forms: Tabs 10 mg

Adverse effects

CNS: Dizziness, weakness, drowsiness, headache, tremor, depression, insomnia, confusion, paresthesia

CV: Postural hypotension, tachycardia, dysrhythmias

EENT: Diplopia, temporary loss of vision
GI: Nausea, vomiting, hiccups, dry mouth
GU: Urinary retention, frequency, change in libido
INTEG: Rash, pruritus, fever, facial flushing, sweating

Contraindications: Acute recovery phase of MI, dysrhythmias, heart block, CHF, hypersensitivity, child <12 yr, intermittent porphyria, thyroid disease

Precautions: Renal disease, hepatic disease, addictive personality, pregnancy **B**, elderly

Pharmacokinetics	
Distribution	Well
Metabolism	Liver, partially
Excretion	Kidney (unchanged)
Half-life	1-3 days

Pharmacodynamics	
Onset	1 hr
Peak	3-8 hr
Duration	12-24 hr

Interactions
Individual drugs
Alcohol: ↑ CNS depression
Drug classifications
Antidepressants, tricyclic: ↑ CNS depression
Antihistamines: ↑ CNS depression
Barbiturates: ↑ CNS depression
MAOI: Do not use within 14 days
Narcotics: ↑ CNS depression
Sedative/hypnotics: ↑ CNS depression

NURSING CONSIDERATIONS
Assessment
- Monitor ECG in epileptic patients; poor seizure control has occurred in patients taking this drug
- Check for allergic reactions: rash, fever, respiratory distress
- Check for severe weakness, numbness, in extremities
- Assess for CNS depression: dizziness, drowsiness, psychiatric symptoms

Nursing diagnoses
✓ Physical mobility, impaired uses
✓ Injury, risk for (adverse reactions)
✓ Knowledge deficit (teaching)

Implementation
- Give with meals for GI symptoms
- Store in airtight container at room temp

Patient/family education
- Teach patient not to discontinue medication quickly; insomnia, nausea, headache, spasticity, tachycardia will occur; drug should be tapered off over 1-2 wk
- Caution patient not to take with alcohol, other CNS depressants
- Advise to avoid altering activities while taking this drug
- Caution patient to avoid hazardous activities if drowsiness/dizziness occurs
- Caution patient to avoid using OTC medication: cough preparations, antihistamines, unless directed by prescriber
- Teach patient to use gum, frequent sips of water for dry mouth

Evaluation
Positive therapeutic outcome
- Decreased pain, spasticity; muscle spasms of acute, painful musculoskeletal conditions are generally short term; long-term therapy is seldom warranted

Treatment of overdose: Empty stomach with emesis, gastric lavage, then administer activated charcoal; use anticonvulsants if indicated; monitor cardiac function

cyclophosphamide

🔑 (℞)

(sye-kloe-foss'fa-mide)

Cytoxan, Neosar, Procytox ♣

Func. class.: Antineoplastic alkylating agent

Chem. class.: Nitrogen mustard

Pregnancy category D

Action: Alkylates DNA, RNA; inhibits enzymes that allow synthesis of amino acids in proteins; is also responsible for cross-linking DNA strands; activity is not cell cycle phase specific

➔ **Therapeutic Outcome:** Prevention of rapidly growing malignant cells

Uses: Hodgkin's disease, lymphomas, leukemia, multiple myeloma, neuroblastoma, retinoblastoma, Ewing's sarcoma, cancer of female reproductive tract, lung, prostate

Dosage and routes

Adult: PO initially 1-5 mg/ kg over 2-5 days; maintenance 1-5 mg/kg; **IV** initially 40-50 mg/kg in divided doses over 2-5 days; maintenance 10-15 mg/kg q7-10 days, or 3-5 mg/kg q3 days

P ***Child:*** PO/**IV** 2-8 mg/kg or 60-250 mg/m^2 in divided doses × 6 or more days; maintenance **IV** 10-15 mg/kg q7-10 days or 30 mg/kg q3-4 wk; or PO 2-5 mg/kg 2×/wk dose should be reduced by half when bone marrow suppression occurs

Available forms: Powder for inj **IV** 100, 200, 500 mg, 1, 2 g; tabs 25, 50 mg

Adverse effects

CNS: Headache, dizziness

CV: ***Cardiotoxicity*** (high doses)

ENDO: Syndrome of inappropriate antidiuretic hormone (SIADH)

GI: Nausea, vomiting, diarrhea, weight loss, colitis, ***hepatotoxicity***

GU: ***Hemorrhagic cystitis, hematuria, neoplasms, amenorrhea, azoospermia, sterility, ovarian fibrosis***

HEMA: ***Thrombocytopenia, leukopenia, pancytopenia, myelosuppression***

INTEG: Alopecia, dermatitis

RESP: ***Fibrosis***

Contraindications: Lactation, pregnancy **D**

Precautions: Radiation therapy

Pharmacokinetics

Absorption	Well absorbed (PO)
Distribution	Widely distributed; crosses placenta, blood-brain barrier (50%)
Metabolism	Liver to active drug
Excretion	Kidneys, unchanged (30%)
Half-life	4-6½ hr

Pharmacodynamics

Unknown

Interactions

Individual drugs

Allopurinol: ↑ bone marrow suppression

Doxorubicin: ↑ cardiotoxicity

Phenobarbital: ↑ toxicity

Radiation: ↑ toxicity, bone marrow suppression
Rifampin: ↑ toxicity, bone marrow suppression
Succinylcholine: ↑ neuromuscular blockade

Drug classifications

Aminoglycosides: ↑ nephrotoxicity
Anticoagulants, oral: ↑ bleeding
Antineoplastics: ↑ toxicity, bone marrow suppression
Bone marrow–suppressing drugs: ↑ bone marrow suppression
Diuretics, loop: ↑ ototoxicity
Live virus vaccines: ↓ antibody reaction

Lab test interferences

↑ Uric acid
False positive: Pap test
False negative: PPD, mumps trichophytin, *Candida*
↓ Pseudocholinesterase

NURSING CONSIDERATIONS

Assessment

- Assess symptoms indicating severe allergic reaction: rash, pruritus, urticaria, purpuric skin lesions, itching, flushing
- Assess for tachypnea, ECG changes, dyspnea, edema, fatigue
- Monitor CBC, differential, platelet count weekly; withhold drug if WBC count is <4000/mm^3 or platelet count is <75,000/mm^3; notify prescriber of results
- Monitor renal function studies: BUN, creatinine, serum uric acid, urine CrCl before and during therapy; I&O ratio; report fall in urine output to <30 ml/hr
- Monitor temp q4h (may indicate beginning of infection)
- Monitor liver function tests before and during therapy (bilirubin, AST [SGOT], ALT [SGPT], LDH) as needed or monthly; note yellowing of skin or sclera, dark urine, clay-colored stools, itchy skin, abdominal pain, fever, diarrhea
- Assess for bleeding: hematuria, stool guaiac, bruising or petechiae, mucosa or orifices q8h
- Identify dyspnea, rales, unproductive cough, chest pain, tachypnea
- Identify effects of alopecia on body image; discuss feelings about body changes
- Identify edema in feet, joint pain, stomach pain, shaking; prescriber should be notified
- Identify inflammation of mucosa, breaks in skin

Nursing diagnoses

- ✓ Injury, risk for (adverse reactions)
- ✓ Body image disturbance (adverse reactions)
- ✓ Infection, risk for (adverse reactions)
- ✓ Knowledge deficit (teaching)

Implementation

- Give fluids **IV** or PO before chemotherapy to hydrate patient
- Give antacid before oral agent, pc PM, before hs; antiemetic 30-60 min before giving drug to prevent vomiting, and prn; antibiotics for prophylaxis of infection
- Give top or syst analgesics for pain; give in AM so drug can be eliminated before hs

IV route

- Give **IV** after diluting 100 mg/5 ml of sterile or bacteriostatic water; shake; let stand until clear; may be further diluted in up to 250 ml D_5 0.9% NaCl, D_5/0.9% NaCl,

0.45% NaCl, LR, Ringer's; give 100 mg or less/min through 3-way stopcock of glucose or saline inf
• Use 21, 23, 25 G needle; check site for irritation, phlebitis

Y-site compatibilities: Amifostine, amikacin, ampicillin, azlocillin, bleomycin, cefamandole, cefazolin, cefoperazone, ceforanide, cefotaxime, cefoxitin, cefuroxime, cephalothin, cephapirin, chloramphenicol, cisplatin, clindamycin, doxorubicin, doxycycline, droperidol, erythromycin, fludarabine, fluorouracil, furosemide, gentamicin, granisetron, heparin, idarubicin, kanamycin, leucovorin, melphalan, methotrexate, metoclopramide, metronidazole, mezlocillin, minocycline, mitomycin, moxalactam, nafcillin, ondansetron, oxacillin, paclitaxel, penicillin G potassium, piperacillin, sargramostim, tetracycline, thiotepa, ticarcillin, ticarcillin-clavulanate, tobramycin, trimethoprim-sulfamethoxazole, vancomycin, vinblastine, vincristine, vinorelbine

Syringe compatibilities: Bleomycin, cisplatin, doxapram, doxorubicin, droperidol, fluorouracil, furosemide, heparin, leucovorin, metoclopramide, methotrexate, mitomycin, mitoxantrone, vinblastine, vincristine

Additive compatibilities: Cisplatin with etoposide, hydroxyzine, methotrexate, methotrexate with fluorouracil, ondansetron

Solution compatibilities: Amino acids 4.25%/D_{25}, D_5/0.9% NaCl, D_5W, 0.9% NaCl

Patient/family education
• Teach patient to avoid use of products containing aspirin or ibuprofen, razors, commercial mouthwash, since bleeding may occur; to report symptoms of bleeding (hematuria, tarry stools)
• Instruct patient to report signs of anemia (fatigue, headache, irritability, faintness, shortness of breath)
• Teach patient to report any changes in breathing or coughing even several months after treatment
• Advise patient that hair may be lost during treatment; a wig or hair piece may make patient feel better; new hair may be different in color, texture
• Teach patient not to have any vaccinations without the advice of the prescriber; serious reactions can occur
• Advise patient contraception is needed during treatment and for several months after the completion of therapy

Evaluation

Positive therapeutic outcome
• Prevention of rapid division of malignant cells
• Increased appetite, increased weight

cyclosporine (℞)
(sye-kloe-spor'een)
Ciclosporin, Cyclosporin A, Sandimmune
Func. class.: Immunosuppressant
Chem. class.: Fungus-derived peptide
Pregnancy category C

Action: Produces immunosuppression by inhibiting T lymphocytes

Therapeutic Outcome: Absence of transplant rejection

Uses: Organ transplants to prevent rejection

Dosage and routes

Adult and child: PO 15 mg/kg several hours before surgery, daily for 2 wk; reduce dosage by 2.5 mg/kg/wk to 5-10 mg/kg/day; **IV** 5-6 mg/kg several hours before surgery; daily, switch to PO form as soon as possible

Available forms: Oral sol 100 mg/ml; inj 50 mg/ml

Adverse effects

CNS: Tremors, headache
GI: Nausea, vomiting, diarrhea, *oral Candida, gum hyperplasia,* ***hepatotoxicity,*** pancreatitis
GU: Albuminuria, hematuria, proteinuria, renal failure
INTEG: Rash, acne, *hirsutism*

Contraindications: Hypersensitivity

Precautions: Severe renal disease, severe hepatic disease, pregnancy **C**

Pharmacokinetics

Absorption	Poorly absorbed (PO)
Distribution	Crosses placenta
Metabolism	Liver to mercaptopurine
Excretion	Kidney, minimal
Half-life	Biphasic 1.2 hr, 25 hr

Pharmacodynamics

	PO
Onset	Unknown
Peak	4 hr
Duration	Unknown

Interactions

Individual drugs

Amphotericin B: ↑ action of cyclosporine
Cimetidine: ↑ action of cyclosporine
Ketoconazole: ↑ action of cyclosporine
Phenytoin: ↓ action of cyclosporine
Rifampin: ↓ action of cyclosporine

NURSING CONSIDERATIONS

Assessment

- Monitor renal studies: BUN, creatinine at least monthly during treatment, 3 mo after treatment
- Monitor liver function studies: alk phosphatase, AST, ALT, bilirubin
- Monitor drug blood levels during treatment
- Assess for hepatotoxicity: dark urine, jaundice, itching, light-colored stools; drug should be discontinued

Nursing diagnoses

- ✓ Mobility, impaired (uses)
- ✓ Infection, risk for (uses)
- ✓ Knowledge deficit (teaching)

Implementation

PO route

- Give with meals for GI upset or drug placed in chocolate milk
- Do not crush, chew caps

- Give with oral antifungal for *Candida* infections

IV **IV route**

- Give IV after diluting each 50 mg/20-100 ml of normal saline or D_5W; run over 2-6 hr; use an infusion pump, glass inf bottles only

Y-site compatibility:
Sargramostim

Sol compatibilities:
D_5W, NaCl 0.9%

- Give for several days before transplant surgery
- Give with corticosteroids

Patient/family education

- Advise patient to report fever, rash, severe diarrhea, chills, sore throat, fatigue, since serious infections may occur; also to report clay-colored stools, cramping (may indicate hepatotoxicity)
- Caution patient to use contraceptive measures during treatment and for 12 wk after ending therapy; drug is teratogenic
- Caution patient to avoid crowds and persons with known infections to reduce risk of infection

Evaluation

Positive therapeutic outcome

- Absence of graft rejection

cyproheptadine (℞)

(si-proe-hep'ta-deen)
cyproheptadine HCl, Periactin, PMS-Cyproheptadine ✦, Vimicon ✦

Func. class.: Antihistamine, H_1-receptor antagonist
Chem. class.: Piperidine

Pregnancy category B

Action: Acts on blood vessels, GI, respiratory system by competing with histamine for H_1-receptor site; decreases allergic response by blocking histamine; blocks serotonin to increase appetite and relieve vascular headaches

➔ **Therapeutic Outcome:** Absence of allergy symptoms and rhinitis

Uses: Allergy symptoms, rhinitis, pruritus, cold urticaria

Investigational uses: Appetite stimulant, management of vascular headache

Dosage and routes

Adult: PO 4 mg tid-qid, not to exceed 0.5 mg/kg/day

P ***Child 7-14 yr:*** PO 4 mg bid-tid, not to exceed 16 mg/day

P ***Child 2-6 yr:*** PO 2 mg bid-tid, not to exceed 12 mg/day

Available forms: Tabs 4 mg; syr 2 mg/5 ml

Adverse effects

CNS: Dizziness, drowsiness, poor coordination, fatigue, anxiety, euphoria, confusion, paresthesia, neuritis
CV: Hypotension, palpitations, tachycardia
EENT: Blurred vision, dilated

pupils; tinnitus; nasal stuffiness; dry nose, throat, mouth
GI: Constipation, dry mouth, nausea, vomiting, anorexia, diarrhea, weight gain
GU: Retention, dysuria, frequency, increased appetite
INTEG: Rash, urticaria, photosensitivity
RESP: Increased thick secretions, wheezing, chest tightness

Contraindications: Hypersensitivity to H_1-receptor antagonist, acute asthma attack, lower respiratory tract disease

Precautions: Increased intraocular pressure, renal disease, cardiac disease, hypertension, bronchial asthma, seizure disorder, stenosed peptic ulcers, hyperthyroidism, prostatic hypertrophy, bladder neck obstruction, pregnancy **B,** G elderly

Pharmacokinetics	
Absorption	Well absorbed
Distribution	Unknown
Metabolism	Liver, complete
Excretion	Kidneys
Half-life	Unknown

Pharmacodynamics	
Onset	15-60 min
Peak	1-2 hr
Duration	8 hr

Interactions
Individual drugs
Alcohol: ↑ CNS depression
Drug classifications
CNS depressants: ↑ CNS depression
MAOI: ↑ anticholinergic effect
Narcotics: ↑ CNS depression
Sedative/hypnotics: ↑ CNS depression
Lab test interferences
False negative: Skin allergy tests (discontinue antihistamine 3 days before testing)

NURSING CONSIDERATIONS
Assessment
- Assess respiratory status: rate, rhythm, increase in bronchial secretions, wheezing, chest tightness; provide fluids to 2 L/ day to decrease secretion thickness
- Monitor I&O ratio: be alert for urinary retention, frequency, dysuria, especially G elderly; drug should be discontinued if these occur; monitor food intake, weight if using as an appetite stimulant

Nursing diagnoses
✓ Airway clearance, ineffective (uses)
✓ Injury, risk for (side effects)
✓ Knowledge deficit (teaching)
✓ Noncompliance (teaching, overuse)

Implementation
- May give with food to decrease GI upset
- Syrup may be used for patients with difficulty swallowing or P children
- Store in tight, light-resistant container

Patient/family education
- Teach all aspects of drug uses; tell patient to notify prescriber if confusion, sedation, hypotension occur; to avoid driving and other hazardous activity if drowsiness occurs; to avoid alcohol and other CNS depressants that may potentiate effect
- Caution patient not to exceed recommended dosage; dysrhythmias may occur
- Teach patient hard candy, gum, frequent rinsing of mouth may be used for dryness

Evaluation

Positive therapeutic outcome

- Absence of running or congested nose, rashes

Treatment of overdose: Administer ipecac syrup or lavage, diazepam, vasopressors, barbiturates (short acting)

cytarabine (℞)

(sye-tare'a-been)

Ara-C, cytarabine, Cytosar ✤, Cytosar-U, Tarabine PFS

Func. class.: Antineoplastic, antimetabolite

Chem. class.: Pyrimidine nucleoside

Pregnancy category C

Action: Competes with physiologic substrate of DNA synthesis, thus interfering with cell replication in the S phase of the cell cycle (before mitosis)

➔ Therapeutic Outcome: Prevention of rapidly growing malignant cells

Uses: Acute myelocytic leukemia, acute lymphocytic leukemia, chronic myelocytic leukemia, and in combination for non-Hodgkin's lymphomas in P children

Dosage and routes

Acute myelocytic leukemia

Adult: **IV** inf 200 mg/m²/day × 5 days; IT 30 mg/m² q4 days, then another dose every 1-4 days × 4 days; SC 1 mg/kg 1-2 ×/wk (maintenance)

In combination

P ***Child:*** **IV** inf 100 mg/m²/day × 5-10 days

Available forms: Inj 100, 500 mg, 1, 2 g

Adverse effects

CNS: Neuritis, dizziness, headache, personality changes, ataxia, mechanical dysphasia, ***coma***

CV: Chest pain, ***cardiopathy***

CYTARABINE SYNDROME: Fever, myalgia, bone pain, chest pain, rash, conjunctivitis, malaise (6-12 hr after administration)

EENT: Sore throat, conjunctivitis

GI: Nausea, vomiting, anorexia, diarrhea, stomatitis, ***hepatotoxicity,*** abdominal pain, hematemesis, ***GI hemorrhage***

GU: Urinary retention, ***renal failure, hyperuricemia***

HEMA: Thrombophlebitis, bleeding, ***thrombocytopenia, leukopenia, myelosuppression, anemia***

INTEG: Rash, fever, freckling, cellulitis

RESP: ***Pneumonia,*** dyspnea

Contraindications: Hypersensitivity, P infants, pregnancy (1st trimester)

Precautions: Renal disease, hepatic disease, pregnancy **C**

Pharmacokinetics

Absorption	Complete
Distribution	Widely distributed; crosses blood-brain barrier, placenta
Metabolism	Liver, extensively
Excretion	Kidneys
Half-life	1-3 hr

Pharmacodynamics

Unknown

Interactions

Individual drugs

Cyclophosphamide: ↑ cardiotoxicity, CHF

Radiation: ↑ toxicity, bone marrow suppression

Drug classifications
Antineoplastics: ↑ toxicity, bone marrow suppression

NURSING CONSIDERATIONS
Assessment
• Assess buccal cavity q8h for dryness, sores or ulceration, white patches, pain, bleeding, dysphagia; obtain prescription for viscous lidocaine (Xylocaine)
• Assess symptoms indicating severe allergic reaction: rash, pruritus, urticaria, purpuric skin lesions, itching, flushing
• Assess tachypnea, dyspnea, edema, fatigue; identify dyspnea, rales, unproductive cough, chest pain, tachypnea
• Monitor CBC, differential, platelet count weekly; withhold drug if WBC count is <4000/mm^3 or platelet count is <75,000/mm^3
• Assess for increased uric acid levels, swelling, joint pain primarily in extremities; patient should be well hydrated to prevent urate deposits
• Monitor renal function studies: BUN, creatinine, serum uric acid, urine CrCl before and during therapy; I&O ratio; report fall in urine output to <30 ml/hr
• Monitor temp q4h (may indicate beginning of infection)
• Monitor liver function tests before and during therapy (bilirubin, AST [SGOT], ALT [SGPT], LDH) as needed or monthly; note yellowing of skin or sclera, dark urine, clay-colored stools, itchy skin, abdominal pain, fever, diarrhea
• Assess for bleeding: hematuria, stool guaiac, bruising or petechiae, mucosa or orifices q8h
• Identify edema in feet, joint pain, stomach pain, shaking; prescriber should be notified
• Identify inflammation of mucosa, breaks in skin

Nursing diagnoses
✓ Injury, risk for (adverse reactions)
✓ Body image disturbance (adverse reactions)
✓ Infection, risk for (adverse reactions)
✓ Knowledge deficit (teaching)

Implementation
• Avoid contact with skin; very irritating; wash completely to remove
• Give fluids **IV** or PO before chemotherapy to hydrate patient
• Give antiemetic 30-60 min before giving drug to prevent vomiting, and prn; antibiotics for prophylaxis of infection
• Give top or syst analgesics for pain
• Give in AM so drug can be eliminated before hs
• Provide liquid diet: carbonated beverages; gelatin may be added if patient is not nauseated or vomiting
• Provide rinsing of mouth tid-qid with water, club soda; brushing of teeth bid-qid with soft brush or cotton-tipped applicators for stomatitis; use unwaxed dental floss
• Give **IV** direct after diluting 100 mg/5 ml of sterile water for inj; give by direct IV over 1-3 min through free-flowing tubing

IV inf
• May be further diluted in 50-100 ml normal saline or D_5W and given over 30 min to 24 hr depending on dosage

Syringe compatibility: Metoclopramide

Y-site compatibilities: Amifostine, amsacrine, aztreonam, cefepime, chlorpromazine, cimetidine, dexamethasone, diphenhydramine, fludarabine, granisetron, ondansetron, sargramostim, thiotepa

Additive incompatibilities: Carbenicillin, fluorouracil, heparin, regular insulin, nafcillin, oxacillin, penicillin G sodium

Additive compatibilities: Corticotropin, daunorubicin with etoposide, hydroxyzine, lincomycin, methotrexate, potassium chloride, prednisolone, ondansetron, sodium bicarbonate, vincristine

Solution compatibilities: Amino acids, 4.25%/D_{25}, D_5/LR, D_5/0.2% NaCl, D_5/0.9% NaCl, D_{10}/0.9% NaCl, D_5W, invert sugar 10% in electrolyte #1, Ringer's LR, 0.9% NaCl, sodium lactate 1/6 mol/L, TPN #57

Intrathecal route

- Reconstitute with 0.9% NaCl (preservative free) or other compatible sol; to prevent contamination use immediately; discard unused portions if any

SC/IM route

- Reconstitute 100 mg/5 ml or 500 mg/10 ml with bacteriostatic water for inj with benzyl alcohol 0.9%; do not use sol with precipitate; stable for 48 hr

Patient/family education

- Advise patient that contraceptive measures are recommended during therapy
- Teach patient to avoid use of products containing aspirin or ibuprofen, razors, commercial mouthwash, since bleeding may occur; to report symptoms of bleeding (hematuria, tarry stools)
- Advise patient to report signs of anemia (fatigue, headache, irritability, faintness, shortness of breath)
- Instruct patient to report any changes in breathing or coughing even several months after treatment; to avoid crowds and persons with respiratory tract or other infections
- Caution patient not to have any vaccinations without the advice of the prescriber; serious reactions can occur

Evaluation

Positive therapeutic outcome

- Prevention of rapid division of malignant cells

dacarbazine (DTIC) (℞)

(da-kar'ba-zeen)

DTIC-Dome

Func. class.: Antineoplastic misc agent

Chem. class.: Imidazole

Pregnancy category C

Action: Alkylates DNA, RNA; inhibits enzymes that allow synthesis of amino acids in proteins; also responsible for cross-linking DNA strands; activity is not cell cycle phase specific

➔ **Therapeutic Outcome:** Prevention of rapidly growing malignant cells

Uses: Hodgkin's disease, sarcomas, neuroblastoma, malignant melanoma

Investigational uses: Metastatic sarcoma

Dosage and routes

Adult: **IV** 2-4.5 mg/kg or 70-160 mg/m² qd × 10 days; repeat q4 wk depending on response or 250 mg/m² qd × 5 days; repeat q3 wk

Available forms: Inj 100, 200 mg

Adverse effects

CNS: Facial paresthesia, flushing, fever, malaise
GI: Nausea, anorexia, vomiting, ***hepatotoxicity***
HEMA: ***Thrombocytopenia, leukopenia,*** anemia
INTEG: Alopecia, dermatitis, pain at inj site

Contraindications: Lactation

Precautions: Radiation therapy, pregnancy (1st trimester) **C**

Pharmacokinetics

Absorption	Complete bioavailability (IV)
Distribution	Widely distributed; concentrates in liver
Metabolism	Liver (50%, 5% protein bound)
Excretion	Kidneys, unchanged (50%)
Half-life	Initial 35 min, terminal 5 hr

Pharmacodynamics

Unknown

Interactions

Individual drugs
Phenobarbital: ↑ toxicity
Phenytoin: ↑ metabolism, ↓ effect
Radiation: ↑ toxicity, bone marrow suppression
Drug classifications
Aminoglycosides: ↑ nephrotoxicity
Antineoplastics: ↑ toxicity, bone marrow suppression
Bone marrow–suppressing drugs: ↑ bone marrow suppression
Diuretics, loop: ↑ ototoxicity
Live vaccines: ↑ adverse reactions, ↓ antibody reaction

NURSING CONSIDERATIONS

Assessment

- Assess symptoms indicating severe allergic reaction: rash, pruritus, urticaria, purpuric skin lesions, itching, flushing; drug should be discontinued
- Monitor CBC, differential, platelet count weekly; withhold drug if WBC count is <4000/mm³ or platelet count is <100,000/mm³
- Monitor renal function studies: BUN, creatinine, urine CrCl before and during therapy; I&O ratio, report fall in urine output to <30 ml/hr
- Monitor temp q4h (may indicate beginning of infection)
- Monitor liver function tests before and during therapy (bilirubin, AST [SGOT], ALT [SGPT], LDH) as needed or monthly; note yellowing of skin or sclera, dark urine, clay-colored stools, itchy skin, abdominal pain, fever, diarrhea; hepatoxicity can be serious and fatal
- Assess for bleeding: hematuria, stool guaiac, bruising or petechiae, mucosa or orifices q8h; check for inflammation of mucosa, breaks in skin
- Identify effects of alopecia on body image; discuss feelings about body changes

Nursing diagnoses

- ✓ Injury, risk for (adverse reactions)
- ✓ Body image disturbance (adverse reactions)

✓ Infection, risk for (adverse reactions)
✓ Knowledge deficit (teaching)

Implementation

- Give fluids **IV** or PO before chemotherapy to hydrate patient
- Give antiemetic 30-60 min before giving drug to prevent vomiting, and prn; antibiotics for prophylaxis of infection
- Provide liquid diet: carbonated beverages; gelatin may be added if patient is not nauseated or vomiting
- After diluting 100 mg/9.9 ml of sterile water for inj (10 mg/ml), give by direct **IV** over 1 min through Y-tube or 3-way stopcock
- May be further diluted in 50-250 ml of D_5W or normal saline for inj and given over 30 min
- Watch for extravasation; give 3-5 ml of mixture of 4 ml sodium thiosulfate 10% plus 5 ml sterile water SC as prescribed

Y-site compatibilities: Amifostine, aztreonam, filgrastim, fludarabine, granisetron, melphalan, ondansetron, paclitaxel, sargramostim, teniposide, thiotepa, vinorelbine

Additive incompatibilities: Hydrocortisone sodium succinate, cysteine

Additive compatibilities: Bleomycin, carmustine, cyclophosphamide, cytarabine, dactinomycin, doxorubicin, fluorouracil, mercaptopurine, methotrexate, vinblastine

Patient/family education

- Teach patient to avoid use of products containing aspirin or ibuprofen, razors, commercial mouthwash, since bleeding may occur; to report symptoms of bleeding (hematuria, tarry stools)
- Instruct patient to report signs of anemia (fatigue, headache, irritability, faintness, shortness of breath)
- Advise patient that hair may be lost during treatment; a wig or hair piece may make patient feel better; new hair may be different in color, texture
- Caution patient not to have any vaccinations without the advice of prescriber; serious reactions can occur
- Advise patient contraception is needed during treatment and for several months after the completion of therapy; drug has teratogenic properties

Evaluation

Positive therapeutic outcome

- Prevention of rapid division of malignant cells

dactinomycin (℞)

(dak-ti-noe-mye'sin)

actinomycin D, Cosmegen

Func. class.: Antineoplastic, antibiotic

Pregnancy category C

Action: Inhibits DNA, RNA, protein synthesis; derived from *Streptomyces parvulus;* replication is decreased by binding to DNA, which causes strand splitting; cell cycle nonspecific; a vesicant

➡ **Therapeutic Outcome:** Prevention of rapidly growing malignant cells, immunosuppression

Uses: Sarcomas, melanomas, trophoblastic tumors in women, testicular cancer,

Wilms' tumor, rhabdomyosarcoma

Dosage and routes

Adult: **IV** 500 µg/m²/day × 5 days; stop drug for 2-4 wk; then repeat cycle

P ***Child:*** **IV** 15 µg/kg/day × 5 days, not to exceed 500 µg/day; stop drug until bone marrow recovery, then repeat cycle

Available forms: Inj 0.5 mg/vial

Adverse effects

CNS: Malaise, fatigue, lethargy, fever

EENT: Cheilitis, dysphagia, esophagitis

GI: Nausea, vomiting, anorexia, stomatitis, ***hepatotoxicity,*** abdominal pain, diarrhea

HEMA: ***Thrombocytopenia, leukopenia, aplastic anemia***

INTEG: Rash, alopecia, pain at inj site, folliculitis, acne, desquamation, ***extravasation***

MS: Myalgia

Contraindications: Hypersensitivity, herpes infections, child P <6 months

Precautions: Renal disease, hepatic disease, pregnancy **C**, lactation, bone marrow suppression

Pharmacokinetics	
Absorption	Complete bioavailability
Distribution	Widely distributed; crosses placenta
Metabolism	Unknown
Excretion	Bile; feces, unchanged (50%); kidneys (10%)
Half-life	36 hr

Pharmacodynamics

Unknown

Interactions

Individual drugs

Radiation: ↑ toxicity, bone marrow suppression

Drug classifications

Antineoplastics: ↑ toxicity, bone marrow suppression

Bone marrow–suppressing drugs: ↑ bone marrow suppression

Live virus vaccines: ↓ antibody reaction

Lab test interferences

↑ Uric acid

NURSING CONSIDERATIONS

Assessment

- Assess buccal cavity q8h for dryness, sores or ulceration, white patches, pain, bleeding, dysphagia; obtain prescription for viscous lidocaine (Xylocaine)
- Assess symptoms indicating severe allergic reaction: rash, pruritus, urticaria, purpuric skin lesions, itching, flushing; drug should be discontinued
- Monitor CBC, differential, platelet count weekly; withhold drug if WBC count is <4000/mm³ or platelet count is <100,000/mm³; notify prescriber of results if WBC <20,000/mm³, platelets <150,000/mm³
- Monitor renal function studies: BUN, creatinine, serum uric acid, urine CrCl before and during therapy; I&O ratio; report fall in urine output to <30 ml/hr
- Monitor temp q4h (may indicate beginning of infection)
- Monitor liver function tests before and during therapy (bilirubin, AST [SGOT], ALT [SGPT], LDH) as needed or monthly; note yellowing of skin or sclera, dark urine, clay-

colored stools, itchy skin, abdominal pain, fever, diarrhea
• Assess for bleeding: hematuria, stool guaiac, bruising or petechiae, mucosa or orifices q8h; check for inflammation of mucosa, breaks in skin
• Identify effects of alopecia on body image; discuss feelings about body changes

Nursing diagnoses

✓ Injury, risk for (adverse reactions)
✓ Body image disturbance (adverse reactions)
✓ Oral mucous membranes, altered (adverse reactions)
✓ Infection, risk for (adverse reactions)
✓ Knowledge deficit (teaching)

Implementation

• Provide antacid before oral agent; give drug pc PM, before hs; antiemetic 30-60 mins before giving drug to prevent vomiting, and prn; antibiotics for prophylaxis of infection
• Provide liquid diet: carbonated beverages; gelatin may be added if patient is not nauseated or vomiting
• Help patient rinse mouth tid-qid with water, club soda, brush teeth bid-qid with soft brush or cotton-tipped applicators for stomatitis, use unwaxed dental floss
• Drug should be prepared by experienced personnel using proper precautions
• Give after diluting 0.5 mg/ 1.1 ml of sterile water for inj without preservative; use 2.2 ml (0.25 mg/ml), give by direct **IV** at 0.5 mg or less/min through Y-tube or 3 way stopcock of inf in progress

Intermittent inf

• May be further diluted in 50 ml D_5W or normal saline for inf; run over 10-15 min
• Give hydrocortisone, sodium thiosulfate to infiltration area, and ice compress after stopping inf
• Store in darkness in cool environment

Y-site compatibilities:

Allopurinol, amifostine, aztreonam, cefepime, fludarabine, melphalan, ondansetron, sargramostim, teniposide, thiotepa, vinorelbine

Patient/family education

• Teach patient to avoid use of products containing aspirin or ibuprofen, razors, commercial mouthwash, since bleeding may occur; to report symptoms of bleeding (hematuria, tarry stools)
• Instruct patient to report signs of anemia (fatigue, headache, irritability, faintness, shortness of breath)
• Advise patient that hair may be lost during treatment; a wig or hair piece may make patient feel better; new hair may be different in color, texture
• Caution patient not to have any vaccinations without the advice of the prescriber, serious reactions can occur
• Advise patient that contraception is needed during treatment and for several months after the completion of therapy

Evaluation

Positive therapeutic outcome

• Prevention of rapid division of malignant cells

danaparoid (℞)

(dan-a-pair′oid)
orgaran
Func. class.: Anticoagulant
Chem. class.: Low molecular weight heparin
Pregnancy category C

Action: Prevents conversion of fibrinogen to fibrin and prothrombin to thrombin by enhancing inhibitory effects of antithrombin III

Therapeutic Outcome: Absence of deep vein thrombosis

Uses: Prevention of vein thrombosis in hemodialysis, stroke, elective surgery for malignancy or total hip replacement, hip fracture surgery

Dosage and routes

Prevention of venous thrombosis/elective surgery
Adult: SC 750 anti-Xa units bid × 7-10 days

Hip fracture surgery
Adult: SC 750 anti-Xa units bid until postoperative days 10-12 has been effective

Hemodialysis
***Adult:* IV** 2400-4800 anti-Xa units given predialysis

Available forms: Inj ampules 750 anti-Xa units in 0.6 ml H_2O for injection

Adverse effects

SYST: Hypersensitivity, hemorrhage
HEMA: Thrombocytopenia
INTEG: Rash

Contraindications: Hypersensitivity to this drug, sulfites; hemophilia, leukemia with bleeding; thrombocytopenia purpura; cerebrovascular hemorrhage, cerebral aneurysm, severe hypertension, other severe cardiac disease

Precautions: Hypersensitivity to heparin, elderly, pregnancy **C,** hepatic disease, severe renal disease, blood dyscrasias, subacute bacterial endocarditis, acute nephritis, lactation, child, recent childbirth, peptic ulcer disease, pericarditis, pericardial effusion, recent lumbar puncture, vasculitis, other diseases where bleeding is possible

Pharmacokinetics

Absorption	Unknown
Distribution	Unknown
Metabolism	Unknown
Excretion	Kidneys
Half-life	2-3 hr

Pharmacodynamics

Onset	Unknown
Peak	4 hr
Duration	Unknown

Interactions

Individual drugs
Aspirin: ↑ risk of bleeding

Drug classifications
Anticoagulants, oral: ↑ risk of bleeding
Platelet inhibitors: ↑ risk of bleeding
Salicylates: ↑ risk of bleeding

NURSING CONSIDERATIONS

Assessment

- Monitor blood studies (Hct, occult blood in stools) during treatment since bleeding can occur; aPTT, ACT, antifactor Xa test, platelets
- Assess for bleeding gums, petechiae, ecchymosis, black tarry stools, hematuria, epistaxis, decrease in Hct, B/P; may indicate bleeding, possible hemorrhage; notify prescriber immediately, drug should be discontinued

• Assess for hypersensitivity: fever, skin rash, urticaria; notify prescriber immediately
• Assess for needed dosage change q1-2wk; dose may need to be decreased if bleeding occurs

Nursing diagnoses

✓ Tissue perfusion, altered (uses)
✓ Injury, risk for (adverse reactions)
✓ Knowledge deficit (teaching)

Implementation

SC route

• Have patient sit or lie down; SC inj may be around the navel in a U-shape, upper outer side of thigh or upper outer quadrangle of the buttocks; rotate inj sites
• Changing needles is not recommended

Patient/family education

• Advise to avoid OTC preparations that may cause serious drug interactions unless directed by prescriber; may contain aspirin, other anticoagulants
• Advise to use soft-bristle toothbrush to avoid bleeding gums, avoid contact sports, use electric razor, avoid IM injection
• Advise to report any signs of bleeding: gums, under skin, urine, stools; unusual bruising

Evaluation

Positive therapeutic outcome

• Absence of deep vein thrombosis

Treatment of overdose: Protamine sulfate 1% given **IV**; 1 mg protamine/100 anti-Xa IU of Fragmin given

danazol (℞)
(da'na-zole)
Cyclomen ✤, danazol, Danocrine
Func. class.: Androgen, hormone
Chem. class.: α-Ethinyl testosterone derivative
Pregnancy category C

Action: Atrophy of endometrial tissue; decreases FSH, LH, which are controlled by pituitary; this leads to amenorrhea/anovulation; has weak androgen, anabolic activity

➔ **Therapeutic Outcome:** Decreased pain and nodules/fibrocystic breast disease; correction in hereditary angioedema; atrophy of endometrial tissue (ectopic)

Uses: Endometriosis, prevention of hereditary angioedema, fibrocystic breast disease

Dosage and routes

Endometriosis

Adult: PO initial dose 500 mg bid, then decrease to 400 mg bid × 3-9 mo

Fibrocystic breast disease

Adult: PO 100-400 mg qd in 2 divided doses × 2-6 mo

Hereditary angioedema

Adult: PO 200 mg bid-tid until desired response, then decrease dose to 100 mg at 1-3 mo intervals

Available forms: Caps 50, 100, 200 mg

Adverse effects

CNS: Dizziness, headache, fatigue, tremors, paresthesias, flushing, sweating, anxiety,

lability, insomnia, carpal tunnel syndrome
CV: Increased B/P
EENT: Conjunctival edema, nasal congestion
ENDO: Abnormal GTT
GI: Nausea, vomiting, constipation, weight gain, ***cholestatic jaundice***
GU: Hematuria, amenorrhea, atrophic vaginitis, decreased libido, decreased breast size, clitoral hypertrophy, testicular atrophy
INTEG: Rash, acneiform lesions, oily hair and skin, flushing, sweating, acne vulgaris, alopecia, hirsutism
MS: Cramps, spasms

Contraindications: Severe renal disease, severe cardiac disease, severe hepatic disease, hypersensitivity, genital bleeding (abnormal)

Precautions: Migraine headaches, seizure disorders, pregnancy **C**

Pharmacokinetics

Absorption	GI absorption
Distribution	Unknown
Metabolism	Liver
Excretion	Kidneys
Half-life	4½ hr

Pharmacodynamics

Unknown

Interactions

Individual drugs
Cyclosporine: ↑ risk of toxicity
Insulin: ↓ effects of insulin
Oxyphenbutazone: ↑ effects of oxyphenbutazone
Drug classifications
Adrenal steroids: ↑ edema
Anticoagulants: ↑ pro-time
Oral hypoglycemics: ↑ effects of hypoglycemics

Lab test interferences
↑ Cholesterol
↓ Cholesterol, ↓ T_4, ↓ T_3, ↓ thyroid ^{131}I uptake test, ↓ 17-KS, ↓ PBI
Interferences: GTT

NURSING CONSIDERATIONS

Assessment

- Assess for lower abdominal (endometrial) pain before and throughout treatment to identify if treatment is effective
- Monitor potassium, blood sugar, urine glucose while patient is on long-term therapy
- Assess breast for fibrocystic nodules; check for pain, tenderness before therapy and throughout to identify if treatment is effective
- Monitor weight daily; notify prescriber if weekly weight gain is >5 lb; I&O ratio; be alert for decreasing urinary output, increasing edema, hypertension, cardiac symptoms, jaundice
- Assess for mental status: affect, mood, behavioral changes, aggression, sleep disorders, depression; change may be extreme
- Assess for signs of virilization: deepening of voice, decreased libido, facial hair (may not be reversible)

Nursing diagnoses

- ✓ Infection, risk for (adverse reactions)
- ✓ Injury, risk for (adverse reactions)
- ✓ Knowledge deficit (teaching)

Implementation

- Store in airtight container at room temp
- Provide ROM exercise for patients who are immobile
- Give with food or milk to decrease GI symptoms

D

• Do not crush, chew caps

Patient/family education

• Teach patient to notify prescriber if therapeutic response decreases; advise that endometriosis tends to recur after drug is discontinued; not to discontinue medication abruptly but to taper over several weeks

• Advise patient that alternate contraceptive measures are needed during treatment; amenorrhea may occur with higher dosages

• Teach patient to report menstrual irregularities; that amenorrhea usually occurs but menstruation resumes 2-3 mo after termination of therapy; that drug should induce anovulation; reversible within 60-90 days after drug is discontinued

• Teach patient about routine breast self-exam technique, to report any increase in nodule size

• Instruct patient to report masculinization: deepening voice, facial hair growth, body hair growth

Evaluation

Positive therapeutic outcome

• Decreased pain in endometriosis

• Decreased size, pain in fibrocystic breast disease

• Decreased signs of angioedema (hereditary)

dantrolene (℞)

(dan'troe-leen)

Dantrium, Dantrium Intravenous

Func. class.: Skeletal muscle relaxant, direct acting

Chem. class.: Hydantoin

Pregnancy category C

Action: Interferes with intracellular release from the sarcoplasmic reticulum of calcium necessary to initiate contraction; slows catabolism in malignant hyperthermia

Therapeutic Outcome: Decreased muscle spasticity; absence of malignant hyperthermia

Uses: Spasticity in multiple sclerosis, stroke, spinal cord injury, cerebral palsy, prevention and treatment of malignant hyperthermia

Dosage and routes

Spasticity

Adult: PO 25 mg/day; may increase by 25-100 mg bid-qid, not to exceed 400 mg/day × 1 wk

P ***Child:*** PO 1 mg/kg/day given in divided doses bid-tid; may increase gradually, not to exceed 100 mg qid

Malignant hyperthermia

P ***Adult and child:*** **IV** 1 mg/kg; may repeat to total dose of 10 mg/kg; PO 4-8 mg/kg/day in 4 divided doses × 3 days to prevent further hyperthermia

Prevention of malignant hyperthermia

P ***Adult and child:*** PO 4-8 mg/kg/day in 3-4 divided

doses × 1-2 days before procedures; give last dose 4 hr preoperatively

Available forms: Caps 25, 50, 100 mg; powder for inj 20 mg/vial

Adverse effects

CNS: Dizziness, weakness, fatigue, drowsiness, headache, disorientation, insomnia, paresthesias, tremors

CV: Hypotension, chest pain, palpitations

EENT: Nasal congestion, blurred vision, mydriasis

GI: Nausea, constipation, vomiting, increased AST (SGOT) and alkaline phosphatase, abdominal pain, dry mouth, anorexia, hepatitis

GU: Urinary frequency, nocturia, impotence, crystalluria

HEMA: Eosinophilia

INTEG: Rash, pruritus, photosensitivity

Contraindications: Hypersensitivity, compromised pulmonary function, active hepatic disease, impaired myocardial function

Precautions: Peptic ulcer disease, renal disease, hepatic disease, stroke, seizure disorder, diabetes mellitus, pregnancy **C**, elderly

Pharmacokinetics

Absorption	PO (30%-35%)
Distribution	Unknown
Metabolism	Liver, extensively
Excretion	Kidney
Half-life	9 hr

Pharmacodynamics

	PO	IV
Onset	Unknown	Immediate
Peak	5 hr	5 hr
Duration	Dose related	Dose related

Interactions

Individual drugs

Alcohol: ↑ CNS depression

Verapamil: ↑ hyperkalemia

Drug classifications

Antidepressants, tricyclic: ↑ CNS depression

Antihistamines: ↑ CNS depression

Barbiturates: ↑ CNS depression

Estrogens: ↑ hepatotoxicity

Narcotics: ↑ CNS depression

Sedative/hypnotics: ↑ CNS depression

NURSING CONSIDERATIONS

Assessment

- Monitor I&O ratio; check for urinary retention, frequency, hesitancy, especially elderly
- Monitor ECG in epileptic patients; poor seizure control has occurred with patients taking this drug; assess for increased seizure activity in epilepsy patient
- Monitor hepatic function by frequent determination of AST (SGOT), ALT (SGPT), renal function studies, CBC
- Assess for allergic reactions: rash, fever, respiratory distress
- Monitor for severe weakness, numbness in extremities
- Assess for CNS depression: dizziness, drowsiness, psychiatric symptoms
- Assess for signs of hepatotoxicity: jaundice, yellow sclera, pain in abdomen, nausea, fever; drug should be discontinued if these signs and symptoms occur

Nursing diagnoses

- ✓ Pain, chronic (uses)
- ✓ Physical mobility, impaired (uses)
- ✓ Injury, risk for (adverse reactions)

✓ Knowledge deficit (teaching)

Implementation

PO route

• Give with meals for GI symptoms; capsules may be opened and mixed with liquid; patient should drink after mixing

• Store in airtight container at room temp

IV **IV route**

• Administer **IV** after reconstituting 20 mg/60 ml sterile water for inj without bacteriostatic agent (333 μg/ml); shake until clear; give by rapid **IV** push through Y-tube or 3-way stopcock; follow by prescribed doses immediately; assess site for extravasation, phlebitis

• Protect diluted sol from light; use reconstituted sol within 6 hr

Patient/family education

• Notify prescriber of abdominal pain, jaundiced sclera, clay-colored stools, change in color of urine; rash, itching occur

• Caution patient not to take with alcohol, other CNS depressants; severe CNS depression can occur; avoid using OTC medication: cough preparations, antihistamines, unless directed by prescriber

• Tell patient that if improvement does not occur within 6 wk, prescriber may discontinue

• Advise patient to avoid altering activities while taking this drug

• Caution patient to avoid hazardous activities if drowsiness, dizziness, blurred vision occurs; wait several days to identify patient response to medication

• Teach patient to use sunscreen, protective clothing for photosensitivity

• Instruct patient to take medication as prescribed; do not double doses; take dose if missed within 1 hr of scheduled time

Evaluation

Positive therapeutic outcome

• Decreased pain, spasticity

• Absence or decreased symptoms of malignant hyperthermia

Treatment of overdose: Induce emesis of conscious patient; lavage, dialysis

daunorubicin (℞)

(daw-noe-roo'bi-sin)

Cerubidine

Func. class.: Antineoplastic, antibiotic

Chem. class.: Anthracycline glycoside

Pregnancy category D

Action: Inhibits DNA synthesis, primarily; derived from *Streptomyces coeruleorubidus;* replication is decreased by binding to DNA, which causes strand splitting; cell cycle specific (S phase); a vesicant

➔ **Therapeutic Outcome:** Prevention of rapidly growing malignant cells; immunosuppression

Uses: Myelogenous, monocytic leukemia, acute nonlymphocytic leukemia, Ewing's sarcoma, Wilms' tumor, neuroblastoma, rhabdomyosarcoma

Dosage and routes

Single agent

Adult: **IV** 60 mg/m^2/day × 3-5 day q4 wk

In combination
***Adult:* IV** 45 mg/m^2/day × 3 days, then 2 days of subsequent courses with cytosine arabinoside

Available forms: Inj 20 mg powder/vial

Adverse effects
CNS: Fever, chills
*CV: **Dysrhythmias, CHF, pericarditis, myocarditis,*** peripheral edema
*GI: Nausea, vomiting, anorexia, mucositis, **hepatotoxicity***
GU: Impotence, sterility, amenorrhea, gynecomastia, hyperuricemia
*HEMA: **Thrombocytopenia, leukopenia, anemia***
*INTEG: Rash, **extravasation**,* dermatitis, reversible alopecia, cellulitis, thrombophlebitis at inj site

Contraindications: Hypersensitivity, pregnancy (1st trimester) **D**, lactation, syst infections, cardiac disease

Precautions: Renal, hepatic disease, gout, bone marrow suppression

Pharmacokinetics

Absorption	Complete
Distribution	Widely distributed; crosses placenta
Metabolism	Liver, extensively
Excretion	Biliary (40%-50%)
Half-life	18½ hr

Pharmacodynamics

Unknown

Interactions
Individual drugs
Cyclophosphamide: ↑ cardiotoxicity, CHF
Radiation: ↑ toxicity, bone marrow suppression
Drug classifications
Antineoplastics: ↑ toxicity, bone marrow suppression
Lab test interferences
↑ Uric acid

NURSING CONSIDERATIONS
Assessment

- Assess buccal cavity q8h for dryness, sores or ulceration, white patches, pain, bleeding, dysphagia; obtain prescription for viscous lidocaine (Xylocaine)
- Assess symptoms indicating severe allergic reaction: rash, pruritus, urticaria, purpuric skin lesions, itching, flushing; drug should be discontinued
- Assess tachypnea, ECG changes, dyspnea, edema, fatigue
- Monitor CBC, differential, platelet count weekly; withhold drug if WBC count is <4000/mm^3 or platelet count is <100,000/mm^3; notify prescriber of results if WBC <20,000/mm^3, platelets <150,000/mm^3
- Assess for increased uric acid levels, swelling, joint pain primarily in extremities; patient should be well hydrated to prevent urate deposits
- Monitor renal function studies: BUN, creatinine, serum uric acid, urine CrCl before and during therapy; I&O ratio; report fall in urine output to <30 ml/hr
- Monitor temp q4h (may indicate beginning of infection)
- Monitor liver function tests before and during therapy (bilirubin, AST [SGOT], ALT [SGPT], LDH) as needed or monthly; note yellowing of skin or sclera, dark urine, clay-colored stools, itchy skin,

abdominal pain, fever, diarrhea; hepatoxicity can be severe

• Assess for bleeding: hematuria, stool guaiac, bruising or petechiae, mucosa or orifices q8h; check for inflammation of mucosa, breaks in skin

• Identify effects of alopecia on body image; discuss feelings about body changes

Nursing diagnoses

✓ Injury, risk for (adverse reactions)

✓ Cardiac output, decreased (adverse reactions)

✓ Body image disturbance (adverse reactions)

✓ Infection, risk for (adverse reactions)

✓ Knowledge deficit (teaching)

Implementation

• Avoid contact with skin; very irritating; wash completely to remove

• Give fluids **IV** or PO before chemotherapy to hydrate patient; give antiemetic 30-60 min before giving drug to prevent vomiting, and prn; antibiotics for prophylaxis of infection

• Provide liquid diet: carbonated beverages; gelatin may be added if patient is not nauseated or vomiting

• Help patient rinse mouth tid-qid with water, club soda, brush teeth bid-qid with soft brush or cotton-tipped applicators for stomatitis, use unwaxed dental floss

• Drug should be prepared by experienced personnel using proper precautions

• Give **IV** after diluting 20 mg/4 ml sterile water for inj (5 mg/ml); rotate; further dilute in 10-15 ml normal saline; give over 3-5 min by direct IV through Y-tube or 3-way stopcock of inf of D_5W or 0.9% NaCl

Intermittent inf route

• Dilute further in 50-100 ml 0.9% NaCl, LR, D_5W; give over 15 min (50 ml), 30 min (100 ml)

Y-site incompatibility: Fludarabine

Y-site compatibilities: Amifostine, filgrastim, melphalan, methotrexate, ondansetron, thiotepa, vinorelbine

Additive incompatibilities: Dexamethasone, heparin

Additive compatibilities: Cytarabine with etoposide, hydrocortisone; not recommended for admixing

Solution compatibilities: $D_{3.3}$/0.3% NaCl, D_5W, Normosol R, Ringer's, 0.9% NaCl

Patient/family education

• Teach patient to avoid use of products containing aspirin or ibuprofen, razors, commercial mouthwash, since bleeding may occur; to report symptoms of bleeding (hematuria, tarry stools)

• Instruct patient to report signs of anemia (fatigue, headache, irritability, faintness, shortness of breath)

• Advise patient that hair may be lost during treatment; a wig or hair piece may make patient feel better; new hair may be different in color, texture

• Caution patient not to have any vaccinations without the advice of the prescriber; serious reactions can occur

• Advise patient that contraception is needed during treatment and for several months after the completion of therapy

Evaluation

Positive therapeutic outcome

- Prevention of rapid division of malignant cells

deferoxamine (℞)

(de-fer-ox'a-meen)

Desferal

Func. class.: Heavy metal antagonist

Chem. class.: Chelating agent

Pregnancy category C

Action: Binds iron ions (ferric ions) to form water-soluble complex that is removed by kidneys

Therapeutic Outcome: Excretion of excess iron and aluminum

Uses: Acute, chronic iron intoxication, hemochromatosis, hemosiderosis

Dosage and routes

Acute iron toxicity

P ***Adult and child:*** IM/**IV** 1 g; then 500 mg q4h × 2 doses; then 500 mg q4-12h × 2 doses, not to exceed 15 mg/kg/hr or 6 g/24 hr

Chronic iron toxicity

P ***Adult and child:*** IM 500 mg-1 g/day plus **IV** inf 2 g given by separate line with each blood transfusion, not to exceed 15 mg/kg/hr or 6 g/24 hr; SC 1-2 g over 8-24 hr by SC infusion pump

Available forms: Powder for inj 500 mg/vial

Adverse effects

CNS: Flushing, ***shock following rapid IV administration***

CV: Hypotension, tachycardia

EENT: Blurred vision, cataracts, decreased healing, *ototoxicity*

GI: Diarrhea, abdominal cramps

GU: Dysuria, pyelonephritis, red urine

INTEG: Urticaria, erythema, pruritus, pain at inj site, fever

MS: Leg cramps

SYST: ***Anaphylaxis***

Contraindications: Hypersensitivity, anuria, severe renal disease

Precautions: Pregnancy **C**, P lactation, child <3 yr

Pharmacokinetics

Absorption	Well absorbed (IM, SC); completely absorbed (IV)
Distribution	Widely distributed
Metabolism	Plasma enzymes
Excretion	Kidneys, unchanged; chelated, excess iron removed by feces and bile (33%-35%)
Half-life	1 hr

Pharmacodynamics

Unknown

Interactions: None

NURSING CONSIDERATIONS

Assessment

- Assess for poisoning: type of iron agent, time, amount ingested, acute or chronic
- Assess for acute iron toxicity: acute early symptoms (nausea, vomiting, abdominal cramping, bloody diarrhea); acute late symptoms (metabolic acidosis, coma, shock)
- Assess vision and hearing periodically; ototoxicity may occur
- Check VS during **IV** administration; watch for dropping B/P, urine color (urine may turn red), rash, urticaria; if

these occur, drug should be discontinued; resuscitation equipment should be available for anaphylaxis

- Monitor I&O, renal function studies: BUN, creatinine, CrCl, serum iron levels

Nursing diagnoses

☑ Poisoning (uses)
☑ Knowledge deficit (teaching)

Implementation

IV route

- Give **IV** (used for shock) after diluting 500 mg/2 ml water for inj; when dissolved, must be further diluted with D_5W, LR, or 0.9% NaCl; run at <15 mg/kg/hr; 2 g/1000 ml usually given over 24 hr; to be used only for short time; IM is preferred route
- Administer only when epinephrine 1:1000 is available for anaphylaxis

IM route

- Give IM after diluting with 2 ml sterile water for inj per 500 mg of drug; rotate inj sites; give deep in large muscle mass; rotate sites

SC route

- Use abdominal SC tissue by inf pump for 8-24 hr/ treatment; use only for chronic iron toxicity

Patient/family education

- Teach patient that urine may turn red; this is not blood but iron excretion
- Caution patient to avoid vitamin C preparations including multivitamins unless approved by prescriber
- Instruct patient that tests are required after treatment for chronic iron toxicity including blood, hearing, and eye tests; stress the importance of follow-up

Evaluation

Positive therapeutic outcome

- Decreased symptoms of heavy metal intoxication

desmopressin (℞)

(des-moe-press'in)

DDAVP, Stimate

Func. class.: Pituitary hormone

Chem. class.: Synthetic antidiuretic hormone

Pregnancy category B

Action: Promotes reabsorption of water by action on renal tubular epithelium in the kidney; causes smooth muscle constriction and increase in plasma factor VIII levels, which increases platelet aggregation resulting in vasopressor effect; similar to vasopressor

Therapeutic Outcome: Prevention of nocturnal enuresis, decreased bleeding in hemophilia A, von Willebrand's disease type 1, control and stabilization of water in diabetes insipidus

Uses: Hemophilia A, von Willebrand's disease type 1, nonnephrogenic diabetes insipidus, symptoms of polyuria/polydipsia caused by pituitary dysfunction, nocturnal enuresis

Dosage and routes

Primary nocturnal enuresis

Child ≥6 yr: Intranasal 20 μg (0.2m) HS, may increase to 40 μg

Diabetes insipidus

Adult: Intranasal 0.1-0.4 mg qd in divided doses (1-4 sprays with pump); **IV**/SC 0.2-0.4 mg qd in two divided doses

P ***Child 3 mo to 12 yr:*** Intranasal 0.05-0.3 mg qd or in divided doses bid

Hemophilia/von Willebrand's disease

P ***Adult and child:*** **IV** 0.3 μg/kg in NaCl over 15-30 min; may repeat if needed

Nocturnal enuresis (primary)

P ***Child 6 yr or more:*** 10 μg in each nostril at hs

Available forms: Intranasal 0.01 mg/ml; inj 4 μg/ml; tabs 0.1, 0.2 mg

Adverse effects

CNS: Drowsiness, headache, lethargy, flushing

CV: Increased B/P

EENT: Nasal irritation, congestion, rhinitis

GI: Nausea, heartburn, cramps

GU: Vulval pain

SYST: Anaphylaxsis **IV**

Contraindications: Hypersensitivity, nephrogenic diabetes insipidus

Precautions: Pregnancy **B**, CAD, lactation, hypertension

Pharmacokinetics

Absorption	Nasal (up to 20%)
Distribution	Unknown
Metabolism	Unknown
Excretion	Unknown; breast milk
Half-life	8 min (initial), 76 min (terminal)

Pharmacodynamics

	INTRANASAL	IV/SC
Onset	1 hr	Rapid
Peak	1-2 hr	15-30 min
Duration	8-20 hr	3 hr

Interactions

Individual drugs

Alcohol: ↓ response of desmopressin

Carbamazepine: ↑ response of desmopressin

Chlorpropamide: ↑ response of desmopressin

Clofibrate: ↑ response of desmopressin

Demeclocycline: ↓ response of desmopressin

Epinephrine (large doses): ↓ response of desmopressin

Heparin: ↓ response of desmopressin

Lithium: ↓ response of desmopressin

Norepinephrine: ↓ response of desmopressin

NURSING CONSIDERATIONS

Assessment

- Monitor I&O ratio, urine osmolality, sp gr, weight daily; check for edema in extremities; if water retention is severe, diuretic may be prescribed; check pulse, B/P when giving drug **IV** or SC
- Assess for water intoxication: lethargy, behavioral changes, disorientation, neuromuscular excitability, dehydration, poor skin turgor, severe thirst, dry skin, tachycardia
- Assess intranasal use: nausea, congestion, cramps, headache; usually decreased with decreased dosage
- Monitor for enuresis during treatment (nocturnal enuresis)
- Assess for allergic reaction including anaphylaxsis (**IV** route)
- Assess for nasal mucosa changes: congestion, edema, discharge, scarring (nasal route)
- Monitor urine volume osmolality and plasma osmolality (diabetes insipidus)
- Monitor factor VIII coagulant activity before using for hemostasis

Nursing diagnoses

✓ Fluid volume deficit (uses)
✓ Fluid volume excess (side effects)
✓ Knowledge deficit (teaching)

Implementation

- Store in refrigerator or cool environment

IV route

Direct IV

- Give undiluted over 1 min in diabetes insipidus or **IV** for hemophilia

Intermittent inf

- Give single dose diluted in 50 ml of 0.9% NaCl (adult and child >10 kg); a single dose/10 ml as an **IV** inf over 15-30 min in von Willebrand's disease or hemophilia A

Patient/family education

- Use demonstration, return demonstration to teach technique for nasal instillation: draw medication into tube, insert tube into nostril to instill drug and blow on other end to deliver sol into nasal cavity; rinse after use
- Teach patient to notify prescriber of dyspnea, vomiting, cramping, drowsiness, headache, nasal congestion
- Caution patient to avoid OTC products (cough, hay fever), since these preparations may contain epinephrine and decrease drug response; do not use with alcohol
- Advise patient to wear Medic Alert ID or other identification specifying disease and medication used
- Advise patient if dose is missed, take when remembered up to 1 hr before next dose; do not double doses

Evaluation

Positive therapeutic outcome

- Absence of severe thirst
- Decreased urine output, osmolality
- Absence of bleeding (hemophilia)

dexamethasone/ dexamethasone acetate/dexamethasone sodium phosphate (℞)

(dex-a-meth'a-sone)

Aeroseb-Dex, Dalalone, Dalalone D.P., Dalalone L.A., Decaderm, Decadron-LA, Decadron Phosphate, Decadron Phosphate Respihaler, Decaject, Decaject-L.A., Decaspray, Dexacen LA-8, Dexacen-4, Dexamethasone Acetate, Dexamethasone Sodium Phosphate, Dexasone, Dexasone L.A., Dexone, Dexone LA, Hexadrol Phosphate, Solurex, Solurex LA

Func. class.: Corticosteroid

Chem. class.: Glucocorticoid, long-acting

Pregnancy category C

Action: Decreases inflammation by suppression of migration of polymorphonuclear leukocytes, fibroblasts, reversal of increased capillary permeability and lysosomal stabilization

Uses: Inflammation, allergies, neoplasms, cerebral edema, septic shock, collagen disorders

Dosage and routes

Inflammation

Adult: PO 0.25-4 mg bid-qid, IM 4-16 mg q1-3 wk (acetate)

Shock
Adult: IV 1-6 mg/kg or 40 mg q2-6h (phosphate)

Cerebral edema
Adult: IV 10 mg, then 4-6 mg IM q6h × 2-4 days, then taper over 1 wk

Child: PO 0.2 mg/kg/day in divided doses

Available forms: Tabs 0.25, 0.5, 0.75, 1, 1.5, 3, 4, 6 mg; inj acetate 8, 16 mg/ml; inj phosphate 4, 10 mg/ml; elix 0.5 mg/5 ml; oral sol 0.5 mg/5 ml, 0.5 mg/1 ml

Adverse effects
INTEG: Acne, poor wound healing, ecchymosis, petechiae
CNS: Depression, flushing, sweating, headache, mood changes
CV: Hypertension, ***circulatory collapse, thrombophlebitis, embolism,*** tachycardia, edema
HEMA: Thrombocytopenia
MS: Fractures, osteoporosis, weakness
GI: Diarrhea, nausea, abdominal distention, ***GI hemorrhage,*** *increased appetite,* ***pancreatitis***
EENT: Fungal infections, increased intraocular pressure, blurred vision

Contraindications: Psychosis, hypersensitivity, idiopathic thrombocytopenia, acute glomerulonephritis, amebiasis, fungal infections, nonasthmatic bronchial disease, child <2 yr, AIDS, TB

Precautions: Pregnancy (C), lactation, diabetes mellitus, glaucoma, osteoporosis, seizure disorders, ulcerative colitis, CHF, myasthenia gravis, renal disease, peptic ulcer, esophagitis

Pharmacokinetics

Absorption	Unknown
Distribution	Unknown
Metabolism	Liver
Excretion	Kidneys
Half-life	3-4½ hr

Pharmacodynamics

	PO	IM
Onset	Unknown	Unknown
Peak	1-2 hr	8 hr
Duration	2⅓ days	6 days

Interactions
Individual drugs
Cholestyramine: ↓ action of Dexamethasone
Colestipol: ↓ action of Dexamethasone
Rifampin: ↓ action of Dexamethasone
Ephedrine: ↓ action of Dexamethasone
Phenytoin: ↓ action of Dexamethasone
Theophylline: ↓ action of Dexamethasone
Neostigmine: ↓ effects of neostigmine
Isoniazid: ↓ effects of isoniazid
Sometrem: ↓ effects of sometrem
Alcohol: ↑ side effects
Indomethacin: ↑ side effects
Amphotericin B: ↑ side effects
Digoxin: ↑ side effects
Cyclosporine: ↑ side effects
Ketoconazole: ↑ side effects

Drug classifications
Barbiturates: ↓ action of dexamethasone
Antacids: ↓ action of dexamethasone
Anticoagulants: ↓ effects of anticoagulants
Anticonvulsants: ↓ effects of anticonvulsants

Antidiabetics: ↓ effects of antidiabetics
Toxoids/Vaccines: ↓ effects of toxoids/vaccines
Anticholinesterases: ↓ effects of anticholinesterases
Salicylates: ↓ effects of salicylates
Diuretics: ↑ side effects
Estrogens: ↑ action of dexamethasone
Contraceptives, oral: ↑ action of dexamethasone
Antibiotics, macrolide: ↑ action of dexamethasone

Lab test interferences
↑ Cholesterol, ↑ Na, ↑ blood glucose, ↑ uric acid, ↑ Ca, ↑ urine glucose
↓ Ca, ↓ K, ↓ T_4, ↓ T_3, ↓ thyroid ^{131}I uptake test, ↓ urine 17-OHCS, ↓ 17-KS, ↓ PBI
False negative: Skin allergy tests

NURSING CONSIDERATIONS

Assessment

- Monitor K, blood sugar, urine glucose while on long-term therapy; hypokalemia and hyperglycemia
- Monitor weight daily; notify prescriber of weekly gain >5 lb
- Monitor B/P q4h, pulse; notify prescriber of chest pain
- Monitor I&O ratio; be alert for decreasing urinary output, increasing edema
- Monitor plasma cortisol levels during long-term therapy (normal: 138-635 nmol/L SI units when drawn at 8 AM)
- Assess infection: fever, WBC even after withdrawal of medication; drug masks infection
- Assess potassium depletion: paresthesias, fatigue, nausea, vomiting, depression, polyuria, dysrhythmias, weakness
- Assess edema, hypertension, cardiac symptoms
- Assess mental status: affect, mood, behavioral changes, aggression

Nursing diagnoses

✓ Infection, risk for (adverse reaction)
✓ Knowledge deficit (teaching)
✓ Mobility, impaired (uses)

Implementation

IV IV route

- IV undiluted direct over 1 min or less or diluted with NS or D_5W and give as an IV inf at prescribed rate
- After shaking suspension (parenteral); do not give suspension IV
- Titrated dose; use lowest effective dose

Additive compatibilities:
Aminophylline, bleomycin, cimetidine, floxacillin, furosemide, lidocaine, nafcillin, netilmicin, ondansetron, prochlorperazine, ranitidine, verapamil

Syringe compatibilities:
Metoclopramide, ranitidine, sufentanil

Y-site compatibilities:
Acyclovir, allopurinol, amsacrine, aztreonam, cefepime, cisplatin, cyclophosphamide, cytarabine, doxorubicin, famotidine, filgrastim, fluconazole, fludarabine, foscarnet, heparin, melphalan, meperidine, morphine, ondansetron, paclitaxel, potassium chloride, sargramostim, sodium bicarbonate, sufentanil, tacrolimus, teniposide, theophylline, vinorelbine, vit B/C, zidovudine

IM route

- IM inj deeply in large muscle mass; rotate sites; avoid deltoid; use 21G needle

- In one dose in AM to prevent adrenal suppression; avoid SC administration, may damage tissue

PO route

- Give with food or milk to decrease GI symptoms
- Provide assistance with ambulation in patient with bone tissue disease to prevent fractures

Patient/family education

- Advise that ID as steroid user should be carried
- Teach to notify prescriber if therapeutic response decreases; dosage adjustment may be needed
- Teach not to discontinue abruptly or adrenal crisis can result
- Teach to avoid OTC products: salicylates, alcohol in cough products, cold preparations unless directed by prescriber
- Teach patient all aspects of drug usage, including cushingoid symptoms
- Teach symptoms of adrenal insufficiency: nausea, anorexia, fatigue, dizziness, dyspnea, weakness, joint pain

Evaluation

Positive therapeutic outcome
Ease of respirations, decreased inflammation

dextroamphetamine (℞)

(dex-troe-am-fet′a-meen)
Dexedrine, Dexedrine Spansules, dextroamphetamine sulfate, Ferndex, Oxydess II, Spancap #1

Func. class.: Cerebral stimulant
Chem. class.: Amphetamine

Pregnancy category C
Controlled substance schedule II

Action: Increases release of norepinephrine, dopamine in cerebral cortex to reticular activating system

Therapeutic Outcome: Increased alertness, decreased fatigue, ability to stay awake (narcolepsy); increased attention span, decreased hyperactivity (ADHD)

Uses: Narcolepsy, attention deficit disorder with hyperactivity

Dosage and routes

Narcolepsy

Adult: PO 5-60 mg qd in divided doses

P ***Child >12 yr:*** PO 10 mg qd increasing by 10 mg/day at weekly intervals

P ***Child 6-12 yr:*** PO 5 mg qd increasing by 5 mg/wk (max 60 mg/day)

ADHD

P ***Child >6 yr:*** PO 5 mg qd-bid increasing by 5 mg/day at weekly intervals

P ***Child 3-6 yr:*** PO 2.5 mg qd increasing by 2.5 mg/day at weekly intervals

Available forms: Tabs 5, 10 mg; sus rel caps 5, 10, 15 mg; elix 5 mg/5 ml

Adverse effects

CNS: Hyperactivity, insomnia, restlessness, talkativeness, dizziness, headache, chills, stimulation, dysphoria, irritability, aggressiveness, tremor, dependence, addiction

CV: Palpitations, tachycardia, hypertension, decrease in heart rate, dysrhythmias

GI: Anorexia, dry mouth, diarrhea, constipation, weight loss, metallic taste

GU: Impotence, change in libido

INTEG: Urticaria

Contraindications: Hypersensitivity to sympathomimetic amines, hyperthyroidism, hypertension, glaucoma, severe arteriosclerosis, drug abuse, cardiovascular disease, anxiety

Precautions: Gilles de la Tourette's disorder, pregnancy C, lactation, P child <3 yr

Pharmacokinetics	
Absorption	Well absorbed
Distribution	Widely distributed; crosses placenta
Metabolism	Liver
Excretion	Kidneys, pH dependent: increased pH, increased reabsorption
Half-life	10-30 hr; increased when urine is alkaline

Pharmacodynamics	
Onset	½ hr
Peak	1-3 hr
Duration	4-10 hr

Interactions

Individual drugs

Acetazolamide: ↓ excretion, ↑ effect
Ammonium chloride: ↓ effect
Ascorbic acid: ↓ effect
Meperidine: Hypertensive crisis
Sodium bicarbonate: ↓ excretion, ↑ effect
Thyroid: ↑ effects

Drug classifications

Antidepressants, tricyclics: ↑ dysrhythmias
β-Blockers: ↑ hypertension
Cardiac glycosides: ↑ dysrhythmias
MAOI: Hypertensive crisis
Sympathomimetics: ↑ effect

NURSING CONSIDERATIONS

Assessment

- Monitor VS, B/P, since this drug may reverse antihypertensives; check patients with cardiac disease more often for increased B/P
- Monitor CBC, urinalysis; for diabetic patients monitor blood sugar, urine sugar; insulin changes may be required, since eating will decrease
- Monitor height and weight q3 mo since growth rate in P children may be decreased; appetite is suppressed so weight loss is common during the first few months of treatment
- Monitor mental status: mood, sensorium, affect, stimulation, insomnia; aggressiveness may occur; depression with crying spells may occur after drug has worn off
- Assess for physical dependency; should not be used for ex tended time except in ADHD; dosage should be decreased gradually to prevent withdrawal symptoms
- Assess for narcoleptic symptoms before medication and after; ability to stay awake should increase significantly
- P In children or adults with ADHD, monitor for improved

organizational skills, attention span, attending to tasks, impulse control, socialization, and ability to get along better with others

• Assess for withdrawal symptoms: headache, nausea, vomiting, muscle pain, weakness; drug tolerance develops after long-term use; dosage should not be increased if tolerance develops; this medication has a high abuse potential

Nursing diagnoses

✓ Thought processes, altered (uses, adverse reactions)
✓ Coping, impaired individual (uses)
✓ Family coping, impaired individual (uses)
✓ Knowledge deficit (teaching)

Implementation

• Give at least 6 hr before hs to avoid sleeplessness; titrate to patient's response; lowest dosage should be used to control symptoms

• Give gum, hard candy, frequent sips of water for dry mouth at beginning of treatment; these symptoms tend to lessen with time

⊘ • Do not crush, chew sus rel forms

Patient/family education

• Advise patient to decrease caffeine consumption (coffee, tea, cola, chocolate), which may increase irritability and stimulation; to avoid OTC preparations unless approved by prescriber; to avoid alcohol ingestion; these may cause serious drug interactions

• Caution patient to taper off drug over several weeks, or depression, increased sleeping, lethargy may occur

• Caution patient to avoid hazardous activities until patient is stabilized on medication

• Instruct patient not to double doses if medication is missed; prescriber may suggest drug holidays (ADHD) during the school year to assess progress and determine continued drug necessity

• Instruct patient/family to notify prescriber if significant side effects occur: tremors, insomnia, palpitations, restlessness, drug changes may be needed

• Inform patient that if dry mouth occurs to use frequent sips of water, sugarless gum, hard candy during beginning therapy; dry mouth lessens with continued treatment

• Advise patient to get needed rest; patients will feel more tired at end of day; to give last dose at least 6 hr before hs to avoid insomnia

Evaluation

Positive therapeutic outcome

• Decreased activity in ADHD
• Absence of sleeping during day in narcolepsy

Treatment of overdose:

Administer fluids, hemodialysis, peritoneal dialysis, antihypertensives for increased B/P; ammonium chloride for increased excretion

D

dextromethorphan (OTC)

(dex-troe-meth-or'fan)

Balminil DM ✱, Benylin DM, Broncho-Grippol-DM ✱, Children's Hold, Delsym, Dextromethorphan, DM Syrup ✱, Hold DM, Koffex ✱, Neo-DM ✱, Ornex-DM ✱, Pertussin, Pertussin ES, Robidex ✱, Robitussin Cough Calmers, Robitussin Pediatric, Sedatuss ✱, St. Joseph Cough Suppressant, Sucrets Cough Control, Suppress, Trocal, Vicks Formula 44

Func. class.: Antitussive, nonnarcotic

Chem. class.: Levorphanol derivative

Pregnancy category C

Action: Depresses cough center in medulla by direct effect related to levorphanol

➔ **Therapeutic Outcome:** Absence of cough

Uses: Nonproductive cough carried by minor respiratory tract infections or irritants that might be inhaled

Dosage and routes

Adult: PO 10-20 mg q4h, or 30 mg q6-8h, not to exceed 120 mg/day; sus rel liq 60 mg bid, not to exceed 120 mg/day

P ***Child 6-12 yr:*** PO 5-10 mg q4h; sus rel liq 30 mg bid, not to exceed 60 mg/day

P ***Child 2-6 yr:*** PO 2.5-5 mg q4h, or 7.5 mg q6-8h, not to exceed 30 mg/day

Available forms: Loz 2.5, 5 mg; sol 3.5. 5, 7.5, 10, 15 mg/5 ml; syr 15 mg/15 ml, 10 mg/5 ml; sus action liq 30 mg/5 ml

Adverse effects

CNS: Dizziness

GI: Nausea

Contraindications: Hypersensitivity, asthma/emphysema, productive cough

Precautions: Nausea/vomiting, increased temp, persistent headache, pregnancy **C**

Pharmacokinetics

Absorption	Rapid (PO); slow (sus rel)
Distribution	Unknown
Metabolism	Liver
Excretion	Kidneys
Half-life	Unknown

Pharmacodynamics

	PO	PO-SUS
Onset	15-30 min	Unknown
Peak	Unknown	Unknown
Duration	3-6 hr	12 hr

Interactions

Individual drugs

Alcohol: ↑ CNS depression

Drug classifications

Analgesics: ↑ CNS depression

Antihistamines: ↑ CNS depression

Antidepressants: ↑ CNS depression

MAOI: ↑ hypotension, hyperpyrexia

NURSING CONSIDERATIONS

Assessment

- Assess cough: type, frequency, character including sputum; provide adequate hydration to 2 L/day to decrease viscosity of secretions

Nursing diagnoses

✓ Airway clearance, ineffective (uses)

✓ Knowledge deficit (teaching)

Implementation
• Administer decreased dosage to elderly patients; their metabolism may be slowed; do not provide water within 30 min of administration because it dilutes drug
• Shake susp before administration

Patient/family education
• Caution patient to avoid driving or other hazardous activities until stabilized on this medication; may cause drowsiness, dizziness in some individuals
• Advise patient to avoid smoking, smoke-filled rooms, perfumes, dust, environmental pollutants, cleaners, which increase cough; may use gum, hard candy to prevent dry mouth
• Advise patient to avoid alcohol or other CNS depressants while taking this medication; drowsiness will be increased
• Caution patient that any cough lasting over a few days should be assessed by prescriber

Evaluation
Positive therapeutic outcome
• Absence of dry, irritating cough

dextrose (D-glucose) (℞)
Glucose, Glutose, Insta-Glucose, Insulin Reaction
Func. class.: Caloric agent
Pregnancy category D

Action: Needed for adequate utilization of amino acids; decreases protein, nitrogen loss; prevents ketosis

Therapeutic Outcome: Provides calories, prevents severe hypoglycemia

Uses: Increases intake of calories; increases fluids in patients unable to take adequate fluids, calories orally; 2.5%-11.5% forms provide calories, increased hydration; 20%-70% forms used to treat severe hypoglycemia

Investigational uses: Varicose veins, acute alcohol intoxication

Dosage and routes
Adult and child: **IV**, depends on individual requirements

Available forms: Inj **IV** 2.5%, 5%, 10%, 20%, 40%, 50%, 60%, 70%, oral gel 40%; chewable tabs 5 g

Adverse effects
CNS: Confusion, ***loss of consciousness,*** dizziness
CV: Hypertension, ***CHF, pulmonary edema***
ENDO: Hyperglycemia, rebound hypoglycemia, hyperosmolar syndrome, hyperglycemic nonketolytic syndrome
GU: Glycosuria, osmotic diuresis
INTEG: Chills, flushing, warm feeling, rash, urticaria, extravasation necrosis

Contraindications: Hyperglycemia, delirium tremens, hemorrhage (cranial/spinal), CHF

Precautions: Renal, liver, cardiac disease, diabetes mellitus

Pharmacokinetics	
Absorption	Well absorbed (PO); completely absorbed (IV)
Distribution	Widely distributed
Metabolism	Unknown
Excretion	Unknown
Half-life	Unknown

Pharmacodynamics

	IV	PO
Onset	Immediate	Rapid
Peak	Immediate	Rapid
Duration	Immediate	Rapid

Interactions

Individual drugs

Insulin: ↑ need for insulin

Drug classifications

Corticosteroids: Cautiously administer fluids

Hypoglycemics, oral: ↑ need for hypoglycemic

NURSING CONSIDERATIONS

Assessment

- Assess I&O, skin turgor, edema, electrolytes (potassium, sodium, calcium, chloride, magnesium), blood glucose, ammonia, phosphate
- Monitor inj site for extravasation: redness along vein, edema at site, necrosis, pain, hard tender area; site should be changed immediately
- Monitor temp q4h for increased fever, indicating infection; if infection suspected, inf is discontinued and tubing, bottle, catheter tip cultured
- Monitor serum glucose in patients receiving hypertonic glucose 5% and over
- Assess nutritional status: calorie count by dietician; GI system function

Nursing diagnoses

✓ Nutrition: less than body requirements (uses)

✓ Fluid volume excess (adverse reactions)

✓ Knowledge deficit (teaching)

Implementation

PO route

- Oral glucose preparations (gel, chewable tabs) are to be used for conscious patients only; serum blood glucose should be monitored after first oral dose; if glucose has not increased by 20 mg/100 ml in 20-30 min, dose should be repeated and serum glucose checked again

IV **IV route**

- Give only protein (4%) and dextrose (up to 12.5%) via peripheral vein; stronger sol requires central **IV** administration
- May be given undiluted via prepared sol; give 10% sol (5 ml/15 sec), 20% sol (1000 ml/3 hr or more), 50% sol (500 ml/30-60 min); too rapid **IV** administration may cause fluid overload and hyperglycemia
- After changing **IV** catheter, change dressing q24h with aseptic technique

Patient/family education

- Teach patient reason for dextrose infusion
- Provide literature and information on when and how to use oral products for hypoglycemia
- Review hypoglycemia/ hyperglycemia symptoms
- Review blood glucose monitoring procedure

Evaluation

Positive therapeutic outcome

- Increased weight
- Blood glucose level at normal limits for patient
- Adequate hydration

dezocine (℞)
(dez'oh-seen)
Dalgan
Func. class.: Narcotic agonist-antagonist analgesic
Chem. class.: Opioid, synthetic
Pregnancy category C

Action: Inhibits ascending pain pathways in limbic system, thalamus, midbrain, hypothalamus by binding to opiate receptor sites, which alters pain perception and response

➔ **Therapeutic Outcome:** Relief of moderate, severe pain

Uses: Moderate to severe pain

Dosage and routes
Adult: IM 5-20 mg q3-6h, not to exceed 120 mg/day; **IV** 2.5-10 mg q2-4h

Available forms: Inj 5, 10, 15 mg single-dose vials, multiple dose 10 mg/ml

Adverse effects
CNS: Drowsiness, dizziness, confusion, sedation, anxiety, headache, depression, delirium, sleep disturbances, dependency
CV: Hypotension, pulse irregularity, hypertension, chest pain, pallor, edema, thrombophlebitis
EENT: Blurred vision, slurred speech, diplopia
GI: Nausea, vomiting, anorexia, constipation, cramps, abdominal pain, dry mouth, diarrhea
GU: Urinary frequency, hesitancy, retention
INTEG: Inj site reactions, pruritus, rash, swelling, chills
RESP: ***Respiratory depression,*** hiccups

Contraindications: Hypersensitivity

Precautions: Addictive personality, pregnancy **C,** lactation, increased intracranial pressure, respiratory depression, hepatic disease, renal disease, P child <18 yr, G elderly, biliary surgery, COPD, sulfite sensitivity

Pharmacokinetics

Absorption	Completely absorbed (IM, IV)
Distribution	Not known
Metabolism	Liver, extensively
Excretion	Kidneys
Half-life	1½-7 hr

Pharmacodynamics

	IM	IV
Onset	½ hr	10 min
Peak	1-2 hr	30 min
Duration	2-4 hr	2-4 hr

Interactions
Individual drugs
Alcohol: ↑ respiratory depression, hypotension, sedation
Cimetidine: ↑ recovery
Erythromycin: ↑ recovery
Nalbuphine: ↓ analgesia
Pentazocine: ↓ analgesia
Drug classifications
Antihistamines: ↑ respiratory depression, hypotension
CNS depressants: ↑ respiratory depression, hypotension
MAOI: Do not use 2 wk before dezocine
Phenothiazines: ↑ respiratory depression, hypotension
Sedative/hypnotics: ↑ respiratory depression, hypotension

NURSING CONSIDERATIONS
Assessment
- Assess respiratory status: respiratory depression, character, rate, rhythm; notify prescriber if respirations are <12/min; note CV status,

bradycardia, syncope; monitor ECG continuously
• Assess pain: location, intensity, duration, alleviating factors

Nursing diagnoses

✓ Pain (uses)
✓ Sensory-perceptual alteration: visual, auditory (adverse reactions)
✓ Breathing pattern, ineffective (adverse reactions)
✓ Knowledge deficit (teaching) (preoperatively)

Implementation

IM route
• Give deeply in large muscle mass; rotate sites; do not give SC

IV **IV route**
• Give undiluted ≤5 mg over 2-3 min

Patient/family education
• Caution patients to avoid CNS depressants: alcohol, sedative/hypnotics for at least 24 hr after taking this drug
• Discuss with patient that dizziness, drowsiness, and confusion are common; to avoid getting up without assistance
• Advise patient to make position changes to lessen orthostatic hypotension

Evaluation

Positive therapeutic outcome
• Decreased pain perception

Treatment of overdose: Narcan 0.2-0.8 **IV**, O_2, **IV** fluids, vasopressors

diazepam ⊶ (℞)

(dye-az'e-pam)
diazepam, diazepam, Diastat, Dizac, Diazemuls ✤, Intensol, D-Tran ✤, E-Pam ✤, Meval ✤, Novodipam ✤, Stress-Pam ✤, Valium, Valrelease, Vazepam, Vivol ✤, Zetran
Func. class.: Antianxiety
Chem. class.: Benzodiazepine

Pregnancy category D
Controlled substance schedule IV

Action: Potentiates the actions of GABA, especially in limbic system, reticular formation; enhances presympathetic inhibition, inhibits spinal polysynaptic afferent paths

Therapeutic Outcome: Decreased anxiety, restlessness, insomnia

Uses: Anxiety, acute alcohol withdrawal, adjunct in seizure disorders; preoperative skeletal muscle relaxation; rectally for acute repetitive seizures

Investigational uses: Panic attacks

Dosage and routes

Anxiety/convulsive disorders
Adult: PO 2-10 mg tid-qid; ext rel 15-30 mg qd
P ***Child >6 mo:*** PO 1-2.5 mg tid-qid

Tetanic muscle spasms
P ***Child <5 yr:*** IM/**IV** 5-10 mg q3-4h prn
P ***Infants >30 days:*** IM/**IV** 1-2 mg q3-4h prn

Status epilepticus
Adult: **IV** bol 5-20 mg, 2

mg/min; may repeat q5-10 min, not to exceed 60 mg; may repeat in 30 min if seizures reappear

P ***Child:*** **IV** bol 0.1-0.3 mg/kg (1 mg/min over 3 min); may repeat q15 min × 2 doses

Available forms: Tabs 2, 5, 10 mg; ext rel caps 15 mg; inj, emulsified 5 mg/ml; oral sol 5 mg/5 ml, 5 mg/ml

Adverse effects

CNS: Dizziness, drowsiness, confusion, headache, anxiety, tremors, stimulation, fatigue, depression, insomnia, hallucinations

CV: Orthostatic hypotension, ***ECG changes, tachycardia,*** hypotension

EENT: Blurred vision, tinnitus, mydriasis

GI: Constipation, dry mouth, nausea, vomiting, anorexia, diarrhea

INTEG: Rash, dermatitis, itching

Contraindications: Hypersensitivity to benzodiazepines, narrow-angle glaucoma, psychosis, pregnancy **D**

G **Precautions:** Elderly, debilitated, hepatic disease, renal disease

Pharmacokinetics

Absorption	Rapid (PO); erratic (IM)
Distribution	Widely distributed; crosses blood-brain barrier, placenta
Metabolism	Liver, extensively
Excretion	Kidneys, breast milk
Half-life	20-80 hr

Pharmacodynamics

	PO	IM	IV
Onset	½ hr	15 min	5 min
Peak	1-2 hr	½-1½ hr	15 min
Duration	2-3 hr	1-1½ hr	15 min

Interactions

Individual drugs

Alcohol: ↑ CNS depression

Cimetidine: ↓ effect of diazepam

Disulfiram: ↓ effect of diazepam

Isoniazid: ↓ effect of diazepam

Propranolol: ↓ effect of diazepam

Rifampin: ↓ effect of diazepam

Valproic acid: ↓ effect of diazepam

Drug classifications

CNS depressants: ↑ CNS depression

Narcotic analgesics: ↓ effects of diazepam

Oral contraceptives: ↓ effects of diazepam

Lab test interferences

↑ AST (SGOT)/ALT (SGPT), ↑ serum bilirubin

False ↑ 17-OHCS

↓ RAIU

NURSING CONSIDERATIONS

Assessment

- Assess degree of anxiety; what precipitates anxiety and whether drug controls symptoms; other signs of anxiety: dilated pupils, inability to sleep, restlessness, inability to focus
- Assess for alcohol withdrawal symptoms, including hallucinations (visual, auditory), delirium, irritability, agitation, fine to coarse tremors
- Monitor B/P (with patient

lying, standing), pulse, respiratory rate; if systolic B/P drops 20 mm Hg, hold drug, notify prescriber; monitor respirations q5-15 min if given **IV**
• Monitor blood studies: CBC during long-term therapy; blood dyscrasias have occurred (rarely)
• Monitor for seizure control; type, duration, and intensity of convulsions; what precipitates seizures
• Monitor hepatic studies: AST (SGOT), ALT (SGPT), bilirubin, creatinine, LDH, alkaline phosphatase
• Assess mental status: mood, sensorium, affect, sleeping pattern, drowsiness, dizziness, suicidal tendencies, and ability of drug to control these symptoms; check for tolerance, withdrawal symptoms: headache, nausea, vomiting, muscle pain, weakness after long-term use

Nursing diagnoses

✓ Anxiety (uses)
✓ Injury, risk of (uses, adverse reactions)
✓ Coping, ineffective individual (uses)
✓ Knowledge deficit (teaching)
✓ Noncompliance (teaching)

Implementation

PO route

• Give with food or milk for GI symptoms; crush tab if patient is unable to swallow medication whole; do not crush ext rel caps; use sugarless gum, hard candy, frequent sips of water for dry mouth
• Reduce narcotic dosage by ⅓ if given concomitantly with diazepam
• Check to see PO medication has been swallowed

IV **IV route**

• Administer **IV** into large vein; do not dilute or mix with any other drug; give **IV** 5 mg or less/1 min or total dose
P over 3 min or more (children, infants); cont inf is not recommended
• Check **IV** site for thrombosis or phlebitis, which may occur rapidly

Additive compatibilities:
Netilmicin, verapamil

Y-site incompatibilities:
Hydromorphone, fluconazole, foscarnet, heparin, pancuronium, potassium chloride, vecuronium, vitamin B with C

Y-site compatibilities:
Dobutamine, nafcillin, quinidine, sufentanil

Syringe incompatibilities:
Benzquinamide, doxapram, glycopyrrolate, heparin, nalbuphine

Syringe compatibility:
Cimetidine

Patient/family education

• Advise patient that drug may be taken with food; that drug is not to be used for everyday stress or used longer than 4 mo unless directed by prescriber; take no more than prescribed amount; may be habit forming
• Caution patient to avoid OTC preparations unless approved by a prescriber; to avoid alcohol, other psychotropic medications unless prescribed; not to discontinue medication abruptly after long-term use
• Inform patient to avoid driving, activities that require alertness; drowsiness may occur; to rise slowly or fainting
G may occur, especially in elderly
• Inform patient that drowsi-

ness may worsen at beginning of treatment

Evaluation

Positive therapeutic outcome

- Decreased anxiety, restlessness, insomnia

Treatment of overdose: Lavage, VS, supportive care, flumazenil

diazoxide (℞)

(dye-az-ox'ide)

Hyperstat IV, Proglycem

Func. class.: Hyperglycemic

Chem. class.: Vasodilator

Pregnancy category C

Action: Decreases release of insulin from β-cells in pancreas, resulting in an increase in blood glucose; relaxes vascular smooth muscle (peripheral arterioles)

Therapeutic Outcome: Decreased B/P, increased blood glucose

Uses: Hypoglycemia caused by hyperinsulinism; emergency treatment of hypertension

Dosage and routes

Hypoglycemia

P ***Adult and child:*** PO 3-8 mg/kg/day in 2-3 divided doses q8-12h

P ***Infants and neonates:*** PO 8-15 mg/kg/day in 2-3 divided doses 8-12h

Hypertension

P ***Adult and child:*** **IV** 1-3 mg/kg q5-15 min, max 150 mg/dose

Available forms: Caps 50 mg; oral susp 50 mg/ml; inj 15 mg/ml, 300 mg/20 ml

Adverse effects

CNS: Headache, weakness, malaise, anxiety, dizziness, insomnia, paresthesia

CV: Tachycardia, palpitations, hypotension, transient hypertension

EENT: Diplopia, cataracts, ring scotoma, subconjunctival hemorrhage, lacrimation

GI: Nausea, vomiting, anorexia, abdominal pain, transient loss of taste, diarrhea

GU: Reversible nephrotic syndrome, decreased urinary output, hematuria

HEMA: ***Thrombocytopenia, leukopenia,*** eosinophilia, decreased Hgb, Hct

INTEG: Increased hair growth or loss of scalp hair, rash, dermatitis, herpes

META: Hyperuricemia, sodium/fluid retention, ketoacidosis, hyperglycemia, azotemia

Contraindications: Hypersensitivity to this drug or thiazides, functional hypoglycemia

Precautions: Pregnancy **C,** lactation, renal disease, diabetes mellitus, CV disease, gout

Pharmacokinetics

Absorption	Well absorbed (PO); completely absorbed (IV)
Distribution	Crosses blood-brain barrier, placenta
Metabolism	Liver (50%)
Excretion	Kidney, unchanged (50%)
Half-life	20-36 hr

Pharmacodynamics

	PO	IV
Onset	1 hr	1-2 min
Peak	8-12 hr	5 min
Duration	8 hr	3-12 hr

Interactions

Individual drugs

Coumadin: ↑ effects

Drug classifications
Diuretics, thiazides: ↑ hyperglycemia
Hydantoins: ↓ anticonvulsant effect
Sulfonylureas: ↑ hyperglycemia

NURSING CONSIDERATIONS
Assessment
- Assess for allergies to sulfonamide; cross-sensitivity may occur
- Assess B/P q5 min until stabilized
- Monitor electrolytes, blood studies: potassium, sodium, chloride, carbon dioxide, CBC, serum glucose
- Monitor weight daily, I&O; edema in feet, legs daily; check skin turgor, dryness of mucous membranes for hydration status
- Assess for rales, dyspnea, orthopnea; peripheral edema, fatigue, weight gain, jugular vein distention (congestive heart failure)
- Assess for signs of hyperglycemia: acetone breath, increased urinary output, severe thirst, lethargy, dizziness

Nursing diagnoses
✓ Cardiac output, decreased (adverse reactions)
✓ Injury, risk for (side effects)
✓ Knowledge deficit (teaching)

Implementation
PO route
- Shake susp before using
- Store protected from light and heat

IV **IV route**
- Give by direct **IV** over 30 sec or less; may repeat q5-15 min until desired response; do not administer dark solution
- Give to patient in recumbent position; keep in that position for 1 hr after

Syringe compatibility:
Heparin

Y-site incompatibilities:
Hydralazine, propranolol

Evaluation
Positive therapeutic outcome
- Decreased B/P in hypertension

Treatment of overdose:
Administer levarterenol, dopamine, or norepinephrine for hypotension, dialysis

diclofenac (℞)
(dye-kloe′fen-ak)
Cataflam, Voltaren, Voltaren SR ✽
Func. class.: Nonsteroidal antiinflammatory
Chem. class.: Phenylacetic acid
Pregnancy category B

Action: Inhibits prostaglandin synthesis by decreasing enzyme needed for biosynthesis; analgesic, antiinflammatory, antipyretic properties

➔ **Therapeutic Outcome:** Decreased pain, inflammation

Uses: Acute, chronic rheumatoid arthritis, osteoarthritis, ankylosing spondylitis, analgesia, primary dysmenorrhea, ophthalmic: to decrease inflammation after cataract extraction

Dosage and routes
Osteoarthritis
Adult: PO 100-125 mg/day in 2-3 divided doses; after therapeutic response occurs, decrease to least amount to control symptoms

Rheumatoid arthritis
Adult: PO 150-200 mg/day in 2-4 divided doses; after therapeutic response decrease to lowest amount to control symptoms
Ankylosing spondylitis
Adult: PO 100-125 mg/day in 4-5 divided doses; give 25 mg qid and 25 mg hs if needed
Analgesia/primary dysmenorrhea
Adult: PO 50 mg tid, max 150 mg/day (potassium product only)
After cataract surgery
Adult: Ophth i gtt qid × 2 wk beginning 24 hr after surgery

Available forms: Enteric coated tabs 25, 50, 75 mg, tabs 50 mg potassium; ophth sol 1%

Adverse effects
CNS: Dizziness, drowsiness, fatigue, tremors, confusion, insomnia, anxiety, depression, nervousness, paresthesia, muscle weakness
CV: **CHF**, tachycardia, peripheral edema, palpitations, dysrhythmias, hypotension, hypertension, fluid retention
EENT: Tinnitus, hearing loss, blurred vision
GI: Nausea, anorexia, vomiting, diarrhea, ***jaundice, cholestatic hepatitis,*** constipation, flatulence, cramps, dry mouth, peptic ulcer, GI bleeding
GU: Nephrotoxicity: dysuria, hematuria, oliguria, azotemia, cystitis, UTI
HEMA: Blood dyscrasias, epistaxis, bruising
INTEG: Purpura, rash, pruritus, sweating, erythema, petechiae, photosensitivity, alopecia
RESP: Dyspnea, hemoptysis, pharyngitis, ***bronchospasm, laryngeal edema,*** rhinitis, shortness of breath

Contraindications: Hypersensitivity to aspirin, iodides, other NSAIDs, asthma

Precautions: Pregnancy **B** 1st, 2nd trimester, lactation, P children, bleeding disorders, GI disorders, cardiac disorders, hypersensitivity to other antiinflammatory agents

Pharmacokinetics

Absorption	Well absorbed (PO, ophth)
Distribution	Crosses placenta; 90% bound to plasma proteins
Metabolism	Liver (50%)
Excretion	Breast milk
Half-life	1-2 hr

Pharmacodynamics

	PO	OPHTH
Onset	Unknown	Unknown
Peak	2-3 hr	Unknown
Duration	Unknown	Unknown

Interactions
Individual drugs
Acetaminophen (long-term use): ↑ renal reactions
Alcohol: ↑ adverse reactions
Aspirin: ↓ effectiveness, ↑ adverse reactions
Coumadin: ↑ anticoagulant effects
Digoxin: ↑ toxicity, ↑ levels
Insulin: ↓ insulin effect
Lithium: ↑ toxicity
Methotrexate: ↑ toxicity
Phenytoin: ↑ toxicity
Probenecid: ↑ toxicity
Sulfonylurea: ↑ toxicity
Drug classifications
Anticoagulants: ↑ risk of bleeding
Antihypertensives: ↓ effect of antihypertensives
Antineoplastics: ↑ risk of hematologic toxicity

β-Blockers: ↑ antihypertension
Cephalosporins: ↑ risk of bleeding
Glucocorticoids: ↑ adverse reactions
Hypoglycemics: ↓ hypoglycemic effect
Diuretics: ↓ effectiveness of diuretics
NSAIDs: ↑ adverse reactions
Potassium supplements: ↑ adverse reactions
Radiation: ↑ risk of hematologic toxicity
Sulfonamides: ↑ toxicity

NURSING CONSIDERATIONS

Assessment

- Assess for pain of rheumatoid arthritis, osteoarthritis, ankylosing spondylitis; check ROM, inflammation of joints, characteristics of pain
- Assess ophth patients for pain, inflammation, redness, swelling
- Monitor blood counts during therapy; watch for decreasing platelets; if low, therapy may need to be discontinued, restarted after hematologic recovery; and for blood dyscrasias (thrombocytopenia): bruising, fatigue, bleeding, poor healing

Nursing diagnoses

- ✓ Pain (uses)
- ✓ Mobility, impaired physical (uses)
- ✓ Injury, risk for (side effects)
- ✓ Knowledge deficit (teaching)

Implementation

PO route

- Administer with food or milk to decrease gastric symptoms;
- Do not crush, dissolve, or chew enteric coated or sus rel caps

Ophth route

- Administer with patient recumbent or tilting head back; pull down on lower lid; when conjunctival sac is exposed, instill 1 drop; wait a few minutes before instilling other drops

Patient/family education

- Teach patient that drug must be continued for prescribed time to be effective; to avoid aspirin, alcoholic beverages
- Caution patient to report bleeding, bruising, fatigue, malaise, since blood dyscrasia do occur
- Instruct patient to use caution when driving; drowsiness, dizziness may occur
- Teach patient to take with a full glass of water to enhance absorption; do not crush, break, or chew

Evaluation

Positive therapeutic outcome

- Decreased pain in arthritic conditions
- Decreased inflammation in arthritic conditions
- Decreased ocular irritation

dicloxacillin (℞)

(dye-klox-a-sill'in)
dicloxacillin sodium, Dycill, Dynapen, Pathocil
Func. class.: Broad-spectrum antibiotic
Chem. class.: Penicillinase-resistant penicillin
Pregnancy category B

Action: Interferes with cell wall replication of susceptible organisms; osmotically unstable cell wall swells, bursts from osmotic pressure

Therapeutic Outcome: Bactericidal effects for the following: gram-positive cocci *Staphylococcus aureus, Streptococcus pyogenes, S. viridans, S. faecalis, S. bovis, S. pneumoniae;* infections caused by penicillinase-producing *Staphylococcus* organisms

Uses: Penicillinase-producing staphylococci, streptococci; respiratory tract, skin, skin structure infections; sinusitis

Dosage and routes

Adult: PO 0.5-4 g/day in divided doses q6h

P ***Child:*** PO 12.5-25 mg/kg in divided doses q6h, max 4 g/d

Available forms: Caps 125, 250, 500 mg; powder for oral susp 62.5 mg/5 ml

Adverse effects

CNS: Lethargy, hallucinations, anxiety, depression, twitching, ***coma, convulsions***

GI: Nausea, vomiting, diarrhea, increased AST (SGOT), ALT (SGPT), abdominal pain, glossitis, pseudomembranous colitis

*GU: **Oliguria, proteinuria, hematuria, vaginitis, moniliasis, glomerulonephritis***

HEMA: Anemia, increased bleeding time, ***bone marrow depression, granulocytopenia***

*SYST: **Anaphylaxis***

Contraindications: Hypersensitivity to penicillins; neonates

Precautions: Hypersensitivity to cephalosporins, pregnancy **B,** severe renal or hepatic disease

Pharmacokinetics	
Absorption	Rapid, incomplete (35%-75%)
Distribution	Widely distributed; crosses placenta
Metabolism	Liver (6%-10%)
Excretion	Kidneys, unchanged (60%); breast milk
Half-life	½-1 hr, increased in hepatic renal disease

Pharmacodynamics	
Onset	½ hr
Peak	½-2 hr

Interactions

Individual drugs

Probenecid: ↑ dicloxacillin levels, ↓ renal excretion

Drug classifications

Oral anticoagulants: ↑ anticoagulant effects

Food

Food, carbonated drinks, citrus fruit juices: ↓ absorption

Lab test interferences

False positive: Urine glucose, urine protein

NURSING CONSIDERATIONS

Assessment

- Assess patient for previous sensitivity reaction to penicillins or other cephalosporins; cross-sensitivity between penicillins and cephalosporins is common
- Assess patient for signs and symptoms of infection including characteristics of wounds, sputum, urine, stool, WBC >10,000, fever; obtain baseline information and during treatment
- Obtain C&S before beginning drug therapy to identify if correct treatment has been initiated
- Assess for allergic reactions: rash, urticaria, pruritus, chills, fever, joint pain may occur a

few days after therapy begins; epinephrine and resuscitation equipment should be available for anaphylactic reaction

- Identify urine output; if decreasing, notify prescriber (may indicate nephrotoxicity); check for increased BUN, creatinine
- Monitor blood studies: AST (SGOT), ALT (SGPT), CBC, Hct, bilirubin, LDH, alkaline phosphatase, Coombs' test monthly if patient is on long-term therapy
- Monitor electrolytes: potassium, sodium, chloride monthly if patient is on long-term therapy
- Assess bowel pattern qd; if severe diarrhea occurs, drug should be discontinued; may indicate pseudomembranous colitis
- Monitor for bleeding: ecchymosis, bleeding gums, hematuria, stool guaiac daily if on long-term therapy
- Assess for overgrowth of infection: perineal itching, fever, malaise, redness, pain, swelling, drainage, rash, diarrhea, change in cough, sputum

Nursing diagnoses

- ✓ Infection, risk for (uses)
- ✓ Diarrhea (side effects)
- ✓ Knowledge deficit (teaching)
- ✓ Noncompliance (teaching)
- ✓ Injury, risk for (side effects)

Implementation

- Give in even doses around the clock; if GI upset occurs, give with food; drug must be given for 10-14 days to ensure organism death and prevent superinfection; store in airtight container
- Do not crush, chew caps
- Shake susp; store in refrigerator for 2 wk or 1 wk at room temp

Patient/family education

- Teach patient to report sore throat, bruising, bleeding, joint pain; may indicate blood dyscrasias (rare)
- Advise patient to contact prescriber if vaginal itching, loose, foul-smelling stools, furry tongue occur; may indicate superinfection
- Instruct patient to take all medication prescribed for the length of time ordered
- Advise patient to notify prescriber of diarrhea with blood or pus, which may indicate pseudomembranous colitis

Evaluation

Positive therapeutic outcome

- Absence of signs/symptoms of infection (WBC <10,000, temp WNL, absence of red draining wounds)
- Reported improvement in symptoms of infection

Treatment of anaphylaxis: Withdraw drug, maintain airway, administer epinephrine, aminophylline, O_2, **IV** corticosteroids

didanosine (ddI, dideoxyinosine) (℞)

(dye-dan'oh-seen)

Videx, DDL, dideoxyinosine

Func. class.: Antiviral

Chem. class.: Synthetic purine nucleoside of deoxyadenosine

Pregnancy category B

Action: Nucleoside analog incorporating into cellular DNA by viral reverse transcriptase, thereby terminating the cellular DNA chain that prevents viral replication

Therapeutic Outcome: Antiviral against the retroviruses, primarily HIV

Uses: Advanced HIV, or AIDS, infections in adults and P children who have been unable to use zidovudine or who have not responded to treatment

Dosage and routes

Adult: >75 kg, PO 300 mg tabs or 375 mg buffered powder bid; 50-74 kg, 200 mg tabs or 250 mg buffered powder bid; 35-49 kg, 125 mg tabs or 167 mg buffered powder bid

P ***Child:*** 1.1-1.4 m^2, PO 100 mg tabs or 125 mg pedi powder bid; 0.8-1 m^2, 75 mg tabs or 94 mg pedi powder bid; 0.5-0.7 m^2, 50 mg tabs or 62 mg pedi powder bid; <0.4 m^2, 25 mg tabs or 31 mg pedi powder bid

Available forms: Buffered chewable/dispersable tabs 25, 50, 100, 150 mg; buffered powder for oral sol 100, 167, 250, 375 mg; pedi powder for oral sol 2, 4 g

Adverse effects

CNS: ***Peripheral neuropathy, seizures,*** confusion, anxiety, hypertonia, abnormal thinking, asthenia, insomnia, *CNS depression,* pain, dizziness, chills, fever

CV: Hypertension, vasodilatation, dysrhythmia, syncope, CHF, palpitations

EENT: Ear pain, otitis, photophobia, visual impairment

GI: ***Pancreatitis,*** diarrhea, nausea, vomiting, abdominal pain, constipation, stomatitis, dyspepsia, liver abnormalities, flatulence, taste perversion, dry mouth, oral thrush, melena, increased ALT (SGPT), AST (SGOT), alkaline phosphatase, amylase

GU: Increased bilirubin, uric acid

HEMA: ***Leukopenia, granulocytopenia, thrombocytopenia, anemia***

INTEG: Rash, pruritus, alopecia, ecchymosis, hemorrhage, petechiae, sweating

MS: Myalgia, arthritis, myopathy, muscular atrophy

RESP: Cough, pneumonia, dyspnea, asthma, epistaxis, hypoventilation, sinusitis

Contraindications: Hypersensitivity

Precautions: Renal, hepatic disease, pregnancy **B,** lactation, P children, sodium-restricted diets, elevated amylase, preexistent peripheral neuropathy

Pharmacokinetics	
Absorption	Rapidly absorbed (up to 40%)
Distribution	Unknown
Metabolism	Not metabolized
Excretion	Kidneys (55%)
Half-life	0.8-1.6 hr, shorter in children

Pharmacodynamics	
Onset	Unknown
Peak	Up to 1 hr
Duration	Unknown

Interactions

Individual drugs

Atropine: ↑ anticholinergic effects

Dapsone: ↓ absorption of dapsone

Disopyramide: ↑ anticholinergic effects

Ketoconazole: ↓ absorption of ketoconazole

Quinidine: ↑ anticholinergic effects

Drug classifications
Antidepressants, tricyclic: ↑ anticholinergic effects
Antihistamines: ↑ anticholinergic effects
Fluoroquinolones: ↓ absorption of fluoroquinolones
Phenothiazines: ↑ anticholinergic effects
Tetracyclines: ↓ absorption of tetracyclines

Food
↓ absorption when used with food

NURSING CONSIDERATIONS

Assessment

- Assess for peripheral neuropathy: tingling or pain in hands and feet, distal numbness; if these occur during therapy drug may be decreased or discontinued
- Assess for pancreatitis: abdominal pain, nausea, vomiting, elevated liver enzymes; drug should be discontinued, since condition can be fatal
- P Assess children by dilated retinal examination q6mo to rule out retinal depigmentation
- Monitor CBC, differential, platelet count monthly; withhold drug if WBC is <4000 or platelet count is <75,000; notify prescriber of results
- Monitor renal function studies: BUN, serum uric acid, urine CrCl before, during therapy; these may be elevated throughout treatment
- Monitor temp q4h; may indicate beginning infection
- Monitor liver function tests before, during therapy (bilirubin, AST (SGOT), ALT (SGPT), amylase, alkaline phosphatase) as needed or monthly

Nursing diagnoses

✓ Infection, risk for (uses)
✓ Injury, risk for (adverse reactions)
✓ Knowledge deficit (teaching)

Implementation

- Give on empty stomach, 1 hr ac or 2 hr pc, q12h; food decreases effectiveness of drug
- Patient should chew tabs; may be crushed and mixed with water
- Pedi powder for oral sol should be prepared in the pharmacy; shake before using
- Packets for oral sol must be mixed with ½ glass of water; stir until dissolved

Patient/family education

- Advise patient to take on empty stomach; not to take dapsone at same time as DDL; to use exactly as prescribed
- Instruct patient to report signs of infection: increased temp, sore throat, flu symptoms; to avoid crowds and those with known infections
- Instruct patient to report signs of anemia: fatigue, headache, faintness, shortness of breath, irritability
- Instruct patient to report bleeding; avoid use of razors and commercial mouthwash
- Advise patient that hair may be lost during therapy; a wig or hair piece may make patient feel better (rare)
- Caution patient to avoid OTC products and other medications without approval of prescriber
- Teach patient not to have any sexual contact without use of a condom; needles should not be shared; blood from infected individual should not come in contact with another's mucous membranes

Evaluation
Positive therapeutic outcome
- Absence of opportunistic infection, symptoms of HIV

dienestrol (℞)
(dye-en-ess'trole)
D V, Ortho Dienestrol
Func. class.: Estrogen
Chem. class.: Nonsteroidal synthetic estrogen
Pregnancy category X

Action: Needed for adequate functioning of female reproductive system and maintenance of secondary sex characteristics; it affects release of pituitary gonadotropins, inhibits ovulation, promotes adequate calcium use in bone structures; reduces cholesterol, protein synthesis, sodium, and water

➔ Therapeutic Outcome: Decreased vaginal, vulval itching, dryness, redness, inflammation in postmenopausal women

Uses: Atrophic vaginitis, kraurosis vulvae

Dosage and routes
Adult: Vag cream 1-2 applications qd × 2 wk, then ½ dose × 2 wk, then 1 application

Available forms: Vag cream 0.01%

Adverse effects
CNS: Dizziness, headache, migraines, depression
CV: Hypotension, thrombophlebitis, edema, ***thromboembolism, stroke, pulmonary embolism, MI***
EENT: Contact lens intolerance, increased myopia, astigmatism
GI: Nausea, vomiting, diarrhea, anorexia, pancreatitis, cramps, constipation, increased appetite, increased weight, ***cholestatic jaundice***
GU: Amenorrhea, cervical erosion, breakthrough bleeding, dysmenorrhea, vaginal candidiasis, breast changes
INTEG: Rash, urticaria, acne, hirsutism, alopecia, oily skin, seborrhea, purpura, melasma
META: Folic acid deficiency, hypercalcemia, hyperglycemia

Contraindications: Breast cancer, thromboembolic disorders, reproductive cancer, genital bleeding (abnormal, undiagnosed), pregnancy **X**

Precautions: Hypertension, asthma, blood dyscrasias, gallbladder disease, CHF, diabetes mellitus, bone disease, depression, migraine headache, convulsive disorders, hepatic disease, renal disease, family history of cancer of the breast or reproductive tract

Pharmacokinetics

Absorption	Through mucous membranes
Distribution	Widely distributed, crosses placenta
Metabolism	Liver
Excretion	Kidneys
Half-life	Unknown

Pharmacodynamics
Unknown

Interactions
Individual drugs
Phenylbutazone: ↓ action of phenylbutazone
Rifampin: ↓ action of rifampin
Drug classifications
Anticoagulants: ↓ action of anticoagulants

D

Anticonvulsants: ↓ action of chlorotrianisene
Antidepressants, tricyclic: ↑ toxicity
Barbiturates: ↓ action of dienestrol
Corticosteroids: ↑ action of corticosteroids
Oral hypoglycemics: ↓ action of hypoglycemics

NURSING CONSIDERATIONS

Assessment

- Monitor urine glucose in patient with diabetes; increased urine glucose may occur
- Monitor weight daily; notify prescriber if weekly weight gain is >5 lb; if increased, diuretic may be ordered; monitor I&O ratio; be alert for decreasing urinary output and increasing edema; check for hypertension, cardiac symptoms, jaundice
- Monitor B/P q4h; watch for increase caused by water and sodium retention
- Obtain liver function studies, including AST (SGOT), ALT (SGPT), bilirubin, alkaline phosphatase
- Assess mental status: affect, mood and behavioral changes, aggression, occur frequently

Nursing diagnoses

✓ Sexual dysfunction (uses)
✓ Injury, risk for physical (side effects)
✓ Knowledge deficit (teaching)

Implementation

- Use at bedtime for better absorption

Patient/family education

- Teach patient how to fill applicator and insert cream; patient should lie down for 30 min after application; use of a sanitary napkin is recommended
- Instruct patient to weigh weekly, report gain >5 lb; demonstrate how to check for peripheral edema
- Advise female patient to report breast lumps, vaginal bleeding, edema, jaundice, dark urine, clay-colored stools, dyspnea, headache, blurred vision, abdominal pain, numbness, stiffness, or pain in legs, chest; male to report impotence or gynecomastia
- Caution patient to check with prescriber before using OTC drugs
- Instruct patient to stop using drug and report to prescriber if pregnancy is suspected

Evaluation

Positive therapeutic outcome

- Decreased signs and symptoms of atrophic vaginitis including itching, inflammation, redness

diethylstilbestrol (℞)

(dye-eth-il-stil-bess'trole)
DES, diethylstilbestrol, Honvol ✦, Stilphostrol
Func. class.: Estrogen
Chem. class.: Nonsteroidal synthetic estrogen
Pregnancy category X

Action: Needed for adequate functioning of female reproductive system; it affects release of pituitary gonadotropins, inhibits ovulation, promotes adequate calcium use in bone structures; responsible for maintenance of water and secondary sex characteristics; lowers cholesterol, retention of water and sodium

➡ **Therapeutic Outcome:** Decreased vaginal, vulval itching, dryness, redness, inflammation; decreased spread of malignant cells

Uses: Postmenopausal breast cancer, prostatic cancer

Dosage and routes

Prostatic cancer

Adult: PO 1-3 mg qd, then1 mg qd; PO 50-200 mg tid (diphosphate); IM 5 mg 2 times/wk, then 4 mg 2 times/wk; **IV** 0.25-1 g qd × 5 days, then 1-2 times/wk

Breast cancer (postmenopausal)

Adult: PO 15 mg qd

Available forms: Tabs 1, 5 mg; diethylstilbestrol diphosphate tabs 50 mg; inj 0.25 g

Adverse effects

CNS: Dizziness, headache, migraines, depression

CV: Hypotension, thrombophlebitis, edema, ***thromboembolism, stroke, pulmonary embolism, MI***

EENT: Contact lens intolerance, increased myopia, astigmatism

GI: Nausea, vomiting, diarrhea, anorexia, pancreatitis, cramps, constipation, increased appetite, increased weight, ***cholestatic jaundice***

GU: Amenorrhea, cervical erosion, breakthrough bleeding, dysmenorrhea, vaginal candidiasis, breast changes, *gynecomastia, testicular atrophy, impotence*

INTEG: Rash, urticaria, acne, hirsutism, alopecia, oily skin, seborrhea, purpura, melasma

META: Folic acid deficiency, hypercalcemia, hyperglycemia

Contraindications: Breast cancer, thromboembolic disorders, reproductive cancer, genital bleeding (abnormal, undiagnosed), pregnancy **X**

Precautions: Hypertension, asthma, blood dyscrasias, gallbladder disease, CHF, diabetes mellitus, bone disease–blocking agents

Pharmacokinetics

Absorption	Well absorbed
Distribution	Widely distributed; crosses placenta
Metabolism	Liver
Excretion	Kidneys
Half-life	Unknown

Pharmacodynamics

Unknown

Interactions

Individual drugs

Phenylbutazone: ↓ action of phenylbutazone

Rifampin: ↓ action of diethylstilbestrol

Drug classifications

Anticoagulants: ↓ action of anticoagulants

Antidepressants, tricyclic: ↑ toxicity

Barbiturates: ↓ action of diethylstilbestrol

Corticosteroids: ↑ action of diethylstilbestrol

Oral hypoglycemics: ↓ action of hypoglycemics

Lab test interferences

↑ BSP retention test, ↑ PBI, ↑ T_4, ↑ serum sodium, ↑ platelet aggregation, ↑ thyroxine-binding globulin (TBG), ↑ prothrombin, ↑ factors VII, VIII, IX, X, ↑ triglycerides

↓ Serum folate, ↓ serum triglyceride, ↓ T_3 resin uptake test, ↓ GTT, ↓ antithrombin III, ↓ pregnanediol, ↓ metyrapone test

False positive: LE prep, ANA

NURSING CONSIDERATIONS

Assessment

- Monitor urine glucose in patient with diabetes; increased urine glucose may occur; check weight daily; notify prescriber if weekly weight gain is >5 lb; if increased, diuretic may be ordered; monitor I&O ratio; be alert for decreasing urinary output and increasing edema
- Monitor B/P q4h; watch for increase caused by water and sodium retention; check liver function studies, including AST (SGOT), ALT (SGPT), bilirubin, alkaline phosphatase
- Assess edema, hypertension, cardiac symptoms, jaundice
- Assess mental status: affect, mood, behavioral changes, aggression

Nursing diagnoses

✓ Sexual dysfunction (uses)
✓ Injury, risk for physical (teaching)

Implementation

PO route

- Give titrated dosage; provide food or milk to decrease GI symptoms
- Give in one dose in AM for prostatic cancer

IV route

- Give IV after diluting in 300 mg of dextrose or saline inj; give at a rate of 1-2 ml/min × 15 min; may increase rate to complete inf 1 hr after starting

Patient/family education

- Instruct patient to weigh weekly, report gain >5 lb
- Teach female patient to report breast lumps, vaginal bleeding, edema, jaundice, dark urine, clay-colored stools, dyspnea, headache, blurred vision, abdominal pain, numbness, stiffness, or pain in legs, chest pain; male to report impotence or gynecomastia
- Advise patient to check with prescriber before using OTC drugs; to take medication as prescribed; do not double doses; if dose is missed take as soon as remembered

Evaluation

Positive therapeutic outcome

- Decrease in tumor size in prostatic cancer, breast cancer

digitoxin (℞)

(di-ji-tox'in)

Crystodigin, digitoxin

Func. class.: Antidysrhythmic, cardiac glycoside, cardiotonic

Chem. class.: Digitalis preparation

Pregnancy category C

Action: Inhibits sodium-potassium ATPase, which makes more calcium available for contractile proteins, resulting in increased cardiac output

Therapeutic Outcome: Positive inotropic and negative chronotropic effect

Uses: Rapid digitalization in CHF, atrial fibrillation, atrial flutter, atrial tachycardia

Dosage and routes

P ***Adult and child >12 yr:*** PO 1.2-1.6 mg initially; give in divided doses over 24 hr; then 150 μg qd; rapid loading dose 0.6 mg, then 0.4 mg, then 0.2 mg q4-6h; slow loading dose 0.2 mg bid x 4 days, then maintenance

Maintenance dose: 0.05-0.3 mg/qd, usual 0.15 mg qd

Child <1 yr: 0.045 mg/Kg

Child 1-2 yr: 0.04 mg/Kg

Child >2 yr: 0.03 mg/Kg (0.75 mg/m^2)

Maintenance: 10% of digitalizing dose

Available forms: Tabs 50, 100, 150, 200 μg

Adverse effects

CNS: Headache, drowsiness, apathy, confusion, disorientation, fatigue, depression, hallucinations

CV: Dysrhythmias, hypotension, bradycardia, AV block

EENT: Blurred vision, yellow-green halos, photophobia, diplopia

GI: Nausea, vomiting, anorexia, abdominal pain, diarrhea

MS: Muscular weakness

Contraindications: Hypersensitivity to digitalis, ventricular fibrillation, ventricular tachycardia, carotid sinus syndrome, 2nd- or 3rd-degree heart block

Precautions: Hepatic disease, acute MI, AV block, hypokalemia, hypomagnesemia, sinus node disease, lactation, severe respiratory disease, hypothyroidism, elderly, pregnancy C

G

Pharmacokinetics

Absorption	Complete
Distribution	Widely distributed, 90-97% protein binding
Metabolism	Liver
Excretion	Kidneys
Half-life	5-7 days

Pharmacodynamics

Onset	1-4 hr
Peak	4-12 hr
Duration	14-21 days

Interactions

Individual drugs

Amiodarone: ↑ levels of digitoxin

Colestipol: ↓ effects digitoxin

Cholestyramine: ↓ effects digitoxin

Diltiazem: ↑ levels of digitoxin

Piperacillin: ↑ hypokalemia

Quinidine: ↑ toxicity digitoxin

Rifampin: ↓ effects digitoxin

Spironolactone: ↑↓ blood levels

Succinylcholine: ↑ toxicity

Thyroid: ↓ level of digitoxin

Ticarcillin: ↑ hypokalemia

Drug classifications

Adrenergics: ↑ toxicity

Barbiturates: ↓ effects digitoxin

Diuretics, thiazide: ↑ hypokalemia, hypomagnasemia

Hydantoins: ↓ effects digitoxin

Thioamines: ↑ toxicity digitoxin

Lab test interferences

↑ CPK

NURSING CONSIDERATIONS

Assessment

- Check apical pulse for 1 min before giving drug; if pulse <60 in adult or <90 in an infant, take again in 1 hr; if <60 in adult, call prescriber; note rate, rhythm, character (P)
- Monitor electrolytes: potassium, sodium, chloride, magnesium, calcium; renal function studies: BUN, creatinine; blood studies: ALT (SGPT), AST (SGOT), bilirubin, Hct, Hgb before initiating treatment and periodically thereafter
- Monitor I&O ratio, daily weight; check skin turgor, lung sounds, peripheral edema
- Monitor drug levels (therapeutic level 9-25 ng/ml)

Nursing diagnoses
- ✓ Cardiac output, decreased (uses)
- ✓ Impaired gas exchange (adverse reactions)
- ✓ Knowledge deficit (teaching)

Implementation
- Give PO with or without food; tabs may be crushed and mixed with food/fluids for swallowing difficulty
- Give potassium supplements if ordered for potassium levels <3 mEq/L, or give foods high in potassium: bananas, orange juice

Patient/family education
- Instruct patient not to stop drug abruptly; teach all aspects of drug; to take exactly as ordered; to keep tabs in container protected from light
- Teach patient to avoid OTC medications, since many adverse drug interactions may occur; do not take antacid or cold products at same time
- Emphasize the importance of notifying prescriber of any loss of appetite, lower stomach pain, diarrhea, weakness, drowsiness, headache, blurred or yellow vision, rash, depression, toxicity
- Teach patient toxic symptoms of this drug and when to notify prescriber
- Advise patient to report shortness of breath, difficulty breathing, weight gain, edema, persistent cough
- Advise patient to carry ID with diagnosis and medication used

Evaluation

Positive therapeutic outcome
- Decreased weight, edema, pulse, respiration, rales
- Increased urine output
- Serum digitoxin level (9-25 ng/ml)

Treatment of overdose: Discontinue drug; administer potassium; monitor ECG, administer an adrenergic blocking agent, digoxin immune Fab

digoxin 🔑 (℞)

(di-jox'in)

digoxin, Lanoxicaps, Lanoxin, Novodigoxin ✤

Func. class.: Antidysrhythmic, cardiac glycoside

Chem. class.: Digitalis preparation

Pregnancy category C

Action: Inhibits sodium-potassium ATPase, which makes more calcium available for contractile proteins, resulting in increased cardiac output

➔ **Therapeutic Outcome:** Decreased edema, pulse, respiration, rales

Uses: Rapid digitalization in CHF, atrial fibrillation, atrial flutter, atrial tachycardia; cardiogenic shock, paroxysmal atrial tachycardia

Dosage and routes

Adult: **IV** 0.5 mg given >5 min (loading dose); then PO/**IV** 0.125-0.5 mg qd in divided doses q4-6h as needed

G ***Elderly:*** PO 0.125 mg qd maintenance; under weight elderly: 0.0625 mg qd or 0.125 qod

P ***Child >2 yr:*** PO 0.02-0.04 mg/kg divided q8h over 24 hr (loading dose); maintenance 0.006-0.012 mg/kg qd in divided doses q12h; **IV** loading dose 0.015-0.035 mg/kg over >5 min

P ***Child 1 mo-2 yr:*** **IV** 0.03-0.05 mg/kg in divided doses over >5 min (loading dose); change to PO as soon as possible; PO 0.035-0.06 mg/kg divided in 3 doses over 24 hr; maintenance 0.01-0.02 mg/kg in divided doses q12h

P ***Neonates:*** **IV** loading dose 0.02-0.03 mg/kg over >5 min in divided doses q4-8h; change to PO as soon as possible; PO loading dose 0.035 mg/kg divided q8h over 24 hr (loading dose); maintenance 0.01 mg/kg in divided doses q12h

P ***Premature infants:*** **IV** 0.015-0.025 mg/kg divided in 3 doses over 24 hr, given >5 min (loading dose); maintenance 0.003-0.009 mg/kg in divided doses q12h

Available forms: Caps 50, 100, 200 µg; elix 50 µg/ml; tabs 125, 250, 500 µg; inj 100, 250 µg/ml; pedi inj 100 µg/ml

Adverse effects

CNS: Headache, drowsiness, apathy, confusion, disorientation, fatigue, depression, hallucinations

CV: ***Dysrhythmias, hypotension***, bradycardia, ***AV block***

EENT: Blurred vision, yellow-green halos, photophobia, diplopia

GI: Nausea, vomiting, anorexia, abdominal pain, diarrhea

Contraindications: Hypersensitivity to digitalis, ventricular fibrillation, ventricular tachycardia, carotid sinus syndrome, 2nd- or 3rd-degree heart block

Precautions: Renal disease, acute MI, AV block, severe respiratory disease, hypothyroidism, G elderly, pregnancy **C**, sinus nodal disease, lactation, hypokalemia

Pharmacokinetics

Absorption	Unknown
Distribution	Widely distributed; 20%-25% protein bound
Metabolism	Liver, small amount; also intestinal bacteria
Excretion	Urine
Half-life	1½ days

Pharmacodynamics

	PO	IV
Onset	½-1½ hr	5-30 min
Peak	2-6 hr	1-5 hr
Duration	After steady state	6-8 days

Interactions

Individual drugs

Amiodarone: ↑ digoxin levels, bradycardia
Amphotericin B: ↑ hypokalemia, toxicity
Calcium IV: ↑ risk of fatal dysrhythmias, digoxin toxicity
Carbenicillin: ↑ hypokalemia
Charcoal: ↓ levels of digoxin by absorption
Diltiazem: ↑ blood levels
Piperacillin: ↑ hypokalemia
Propafenone: ↑ digoxin levels, toxicity
Quinidine: ↑ toxicity, digoxin levels
Rifampin: ↓ digoxin effects
Spironolactone: ↑ blood levels of digoxin
Succinylcholine: ↑ toxicity of both
Thyroid: ↓ level of digoxin
Ticarcillin: ↑ hypokalemia
Verapamil: ↑ blood levels of digoxin, ↓ positive inotropic effect

Drug classifications
Adrenergics: ↑ toxicity
Antacids: ↓ digoxin absorption
Barbiturates: ↓ effects of digoxin
β-Blockers: ↑ bradycardia
Calcium channel blockers: ↑ digoxin levels, toxicity
Diuretics, thiazide: ↑ hypokalemia, toxicity
Hydantoins: ↓ effects of digoxin
Thioamines: ↑ toxicity of digoxin

Lab test interferences
↑ CPK

NURSING CONSIDERATIONS

Assessment

- Assess and document apical pulse for 1 min before giving drug; if pulse for 1 min before giving drug; if pulse <60 in **P** adult or <90 in an infant or is significantly different, take again in 1 hr; if <60 in adult, call prescriber; note rate, rhythm, character
- Monitor electrolytes: potassium, sodium, chloride, magnesium, calcium; renal function studies: BUN, creatinine; other blood studies: ALT (SGPT), AST (SGOT), bilirubin, Hct, Hgb drug levels (therapeutic level 0.5-2 ng/ml) before initiating treatment and periodically thereafter
- Monitor I&O ratio, daily weights; monitor turgor, lung sounds, edema
- Monitor cardiac status: apical pulse, character, rate, rhythm; resolution of atrial dysrhythmias by ECG; if tachydysrhythmia develops, hold drug; delay cardioversion while drug levels are determined
- Monitor ECG continuously during parenteral loading doses and for patients with suspected toxicity; provide hemodynamic monitoring for patients with heart failure or administer multiple cardiac drugs

Nursing diagnoses

- ✓ Cardiac output, decreased (uses)
- ✓ Impaired gas exchange (adverse reactions)
- ✓ Knowledge deficit (teaching)

Implementation

- Do not give at same time as antacids or other drugs that decrease absorption

PO route

- Give PO with or without food; may crush tabs
- Give potassium supplements if ordered for potassium levels <3, or give foods high in potassium: bananas, orange juice

IV **IV route**

- Give **IV** undiluted or 1 ml of drug/4 ml sterile water, D_5, or NS; give over >5 min through Y-tube or 3-way stopcock; during digitalization close monitoring is necessary
- Store protected from light

Y-site compatibilities:
Amrinone, ciprofloxacin, diltiazem, famotidine, meperidine, midazolam, milrinone, morphine, potassium chloride, tacrolimus, vitamin B with C

Y-site incompatibilities:
Fluconazole, foscarnet

Additive compatibilities:
Bretylium, cimetidine, floxacillin, furosemide, lidocaine, ranitidine, verapamil

Additive incompatibility:
Dobutamine

Syringe compatibilities:
Heparin, milrinone

Syringe incompatibility:
Doxapram

Patient/family education

- Caution patient to avoid OTC medications including cough, cold, allergy preparations, antacids, since many adverse drug interactions may occur; do not take antacid at same time
- Instruct patient to notify prescriber of any loss of appetite, lower stomach pain, diarrhea, weakness, drowsiness, headache, blurred or yellow-green vision, rash, depression; teach toxic symptoms of this drug and when to notify prescriber
- Advise patient to maintain a sodium-restricted diet as ordered; to take potassium supplements as ordered to prevent toxicity
- Instruct patient to report shortness of breath, difficulty breathing, weight gain, edema, persistent cough
- Teach patient purpose of drug is to regulate the heart's functioning
- Teach patient that as outpatient to check and record pulse for 1 min before taking dose; if there is a change of >15 bpm from usual pulse, prescriber should be notified
- Teach patient to take medication at the same time each day, take missed doses within 12 hr; do not double doses; notify prescriber if doses are missed for 2 days or more
- Advise patient to carry ID describing dosage and reason for digoxin

Evaluation

Positive therapeutic outcome

- Decreased weight, edema, pulse, respiration, rales
- Increased urine output
- Serum digoxin level 0.5-2 ng/ml

Treatment of overdose: Discontinue drug, administer potassium, monitor ECG, administer an adrenergic blocking agent, digoxin immune Fab

D

digoxin immune Fab (ovine) (℞)

(di-jox'in)

Digibind

Func. class.: Antidote, digoxin specific

Pregnancy category C

Action: Antibody fragments bind to free digoxin to reverse digoxin toxicity by not allowing digoxin to bind to sites of action

➔ Therapeutic Outcome: Correction of digoxin toxicity

Uses: Reversal of life-threatening digoxin or digitoxin toxicity, including severe bradycardia, ventricular tachycardia/fibrillation, severe hypertension

Dosage and routes

Digoxin toxicity

Adult: **IV** dose (mg) = dose ingested (mg) x serum digoxin conc x 5.6 x wt in kg ÷ 1000; if ingested amount is unknown, give 800 mg **IV**; if digoxin liquid caps, **IV** or digoxin used, do not multiply ingested dose by 0.8; Digitoxin body load in mg = serum digitoxin conc x 0.56 x wt in kg ÷ 1000

Available forms: Inj 38 mg/vial (binds 0.5 mg digoxin or digitoxin)

Adverse effects
*CV: **Worsening of CHF**, ventricular rate increase, **atrial fibrillation**, low cardiac output*
INTEG: Hypersensitivity, allergic reactions, facial swelling, redness
META: Hypokalemia
RESP: Impaired respiratory function, rapid respiratory rate

Contraindications: Mild digoxin toxicity, hypersensitivity

P **Precautions:** Children, lactation, cardiac disease, renal disease, pregnancy **C**

Pharmacokinetics	
Absorption	Complete
Distribution	Widely distributed into plasma, interstitial fluids
Metabolism	Unknown
Excretion	Kidneys
Half-life	Biphasic (14-20 hr); increased in renal disease

Pharmacodynamics	
Onset	30 mins (variable)
Peak	Unknown
Duration	Unknown

Interactions
Individual drugs
Digitoxin: ↓ effect of digitoxin
Digoxin: ↓ effect of digoxin
Lanatoside C: ↓ effect of lanatoside
Lab test interferences
Interference: Immunoassay (digoxin)

NURSING CONSIDERATIONS
Assessment
- Assess for hypokalemia: ST depression, flat T waves, presence of U wave, ventricular dysrhythmias
- Obtain information on previous allergies: previous exposure to sheep (ovine) proteins; scratch test may be performed before use of this product; hypersensitive reactions are more common in persons with previous exposure
- Monitor vital signs before, throughout, and after infusion
- Monitor heart rate, B/P q10 min during inf and after it is complete until stabilized; hemodynamic monitoring is used for unstable or hypotensive patients; check potassium levels until toxicity is resolved
- Assess for oxygen or perfusion deficit: hypotension, chest pain, dizziness, loss of consciousness
- Assess respiratory status: auscultate lung fields for bibasilar crackles in patients with advanced CHF

Nursing diagnoses
✓ Injury, risk for (uses)
✓ Knowledge deficit (teaching)

Implementation
- Give after diluting 40 mg/ 4 ml of sterile water (10 mg/ ml), mix gently; may be further diluted with 0.9% NaCl; sol should be clear, colorless
- Give by bol if cardiac arrest is imminent or **IV** over 30 min using a 0.22 μm filter
- Store reconstituted sol for up to 4 hr in refrigerator

Patient/family education
- Teach that purpose of medication is to bind excess digoxin and reduce high blood levels
- Instruct patients to report fever, chills, itching, sweating, dyspnea
- Advise other prescribers that this medication has been used previously

Evaluation

Positive therapeutic outcome

- Correction of digoxin toxicity
- Digoxin blood levels 0.5-2 ng/ml
- Digitoxin blood level 9-25 ng/ml

dihydrotachysterol (℞)

(dye-hye-droh-tak-iss'ter-ole)

DHT, DHT Intensol, Hytakerol

Func. class.: Parathyroid agent (calcium regulator)

Chem. class.: Vitamin D analog

Pregnancy category C

Action: Increases intestinal absorption of calcium, increases renal tubular absorption of phosphorus; is able to regulate calcium levels by regulation of calcitonin, parathyroid hormone

➔ Therapeutic Outcome: Prevention of continued calcium loss in bones

Uses: Renal osteodystrophy, hypoparathyroidism, pseudohypoparathyroidism, familial hypophosphatemia, postoperative tetany

Investigational uses: Renal osteodystrophy

Dosage and routes

Hypophosphatemia

P ***Adult and child:*** PO 0.5-2 mg qd; maintenance 0.3-1.5 mg qd

Hypoparathyroidism/ pseudohypoparathyroidism

Adult: PO 0.8-2.4 mg qd × 4 days, maintenance 0.2-2 mg qd regulated by serum calcium levels

P ***Child:*** PO 1-5 mg qd 1 wk, maintenance 0.2-1 mg qd regulated by serum calcium levels

Renal osteodystrophy

Adult: PO 0.1-0.25 mg qd, then 0.2-1 mg/day

Available forms: Tab 0.125, 0.2, 0.4 mg; cap 0.125 mg; oral sol 0.2, 0.25 mg/5 ml

Adverse effects

CNS: Drowsiness, headache, vertigo, fever, lethargy

EENT: Tinnitus

GI: Nausea, diarrhea, vomiting, jaundice, anorexia, dry mouth, constipation, cramps, metallic taste

GU: ***Polyuria,*** hypercalciuria, hyperphosphatemia, ***hematuria***

MS: Myalgia, arthralgia, decreased bone development

Contraindications: Hypersensitivity, renal disease, hyperphosphatemia, hypercalcemia

Precautions: Pregnancy **C,** renal calculi, lactation, CV disease

Pharmacokinetics	
Absorption	Well absorbed
Distribution	Liver, fat
Metabolism	Liver
Excretion	Feces (inactive, active metabolites)
Half-life	Unknown

Pharmacodynamics	
Onset	2 wk
Peak	2 wk
Duration	2 wk

Interactions

Individual drugs

Cholestyramine: ↓ absorption of dihydrotachysterol

Colestipol: ↓ absorption of dihydrotachysterol
Mineral oil: ↓ absorption of dihydrotachysterol
Phenytoin: ↓ effect of dihydrotachysterol
Verapamil: ↑ dysrhythmias

Drug classifications

Barbiturates: ↓ effect of dihydrotachysterol
Calcium supplements: ↑ hypercalcemia
Cardiac glycosides: ↑ dysrhythmias
Corticosteroids: ↓ effect of dihydrotachysterol
Diuretics, thiazide: ↑ hypercalcemia

Lab test interferences

False ↑ Cholesterol

NURSING CONSIDERATIONS

Assessment

- Monitor BUN, urinary calcium, AST (SGOT), ALT (SGPT), cholesterol, alkaline phosphatase, creatinine, uric acid, chloride, magnesium, electrolytes, urine pH, phosphate; may increase calcium; should be kept at 9-10 mg/dl; keep vitamin D at 50-135 IU/dl, phosphate at 70 mg/dl; these tests should be checked before and throughout treatment
- Monitor for increased blood level, since toxic reaction may occur rapidly
- Monitor for dry mouth, metallic taste, polyuria, bone pain, muscle weakness, headache, fatigue, tinnitus, change in LOC, irregular pulse, dysrhythmias, increased respirations, anorexia, nausea, vomiting, cramps, diarrhea, constipation; may indicate hypercalcemia; if these occur, discontinue drug, give laxatives, low-calcium diet
- Monitor renal status: decreased urinary output (oliguria, anuria), edema in extremities, weight gain >5 lb, periorbital edema
- Assess nutritional status; check diet for sources of vitamin D (milk, some seafood), calcium (dairy products, dark green vegetables); phosphates (dairy products) must be avoided

Nursing diagnoses

✓ Nutrition: Less than body requirements (uses)
✓ Knowledge deficit (teaching)

Implementation

- ⃠ Do not crush, chew caps
- May be increased q4 wk depending on blood level; give with meals for GI symptoms
- Store in tight, light-resistant containers at room temp
- Restrict sodium, potassium if required
- Restriction of fluids may be required for chronic renal failure

Patient/family education

- Teach symptoms of hypercalcemia and when to report symptoms to prescriber
- Teach patient about foods rich in calcium, vitamin D; provide list of calcium-rich foods; renal failure patients are given a renal diet
- Caution patient not to double doses, take exactly as prescribed

Evaluation

Positive therapeutic outcome

- Prevention of bone deficiencies
- Calcium, phosphorus at normal levels

diltiazem (℞)
(dil-tye'a-zem)
Apo-Diltiaz ✤, Cardizem, Cardizem SR, Cardizem CD, diltiazem, Dilacor-XR, Tiamate
Func. class.: Calcium channel blocker, antianginal
Chem. class.: Benzothiazepine
Pregnancy category C

Action: Inhibits calcium ion influx across cell membrane during cardiac depolarization, produces relaxation of coronary vascular smooth muscle, dilates coronary arteries, slows SA/AV node conduction times, dilates peripheral arteries

➔ **Therapeutic Outcome:** Decreased angina pectoris, dysrhythmias, B/P

Uses
Oral: Angina pectoris due to coronary insufficiency, hypertension, vasospasm

Parenteral: Atrial fibrillation, flutter

Investigational use: Raynaud's syndrome

Dosage and routes
Adult: PO 30 mg qid, increasing dose gradually to 180-360 mg/day in divided doses or 60-120 mg bid; may increase to 240-360 mg/day

***Adult* IV**: 0.25 mg/kg over bol 2 min initially, then 0.35 mg/kg may be given after 15 min; if no response, may give cont inf 5-15 mg/hr for up to 24 hr

Adult: PO 180-240 mg (Cardizem CD) qd

Available forms: Tab 30, 60, 90, 120 mg; tab ext rel 120, 180, 240 mg; caps sus rel 60, 90, 120, 180, 240, 300 mg; inj **IV** 5 mg/ml (5, 10 ml)

Adverse effects
CNS: Headache, fatigue, drowsiness, dizziness, depression, weakness, insomnia, tremor, paresthesia
CV: Dysrhythmia, edema
CHF: Bradycardia, hypotension, palpitations, heart block, peripheral edema, angina
GI: Nausea, vomiting, diarrhea, gastric upset, constipation, increased liver function studies
GU: Nocturia, polyuria, ***acute renal failure***
INTEG: Rash, pruritus, flushing, photosensitivity

Contraindications: Sick sinus syndrome, 2nd- or 3rd-degree heart block, hypotension less than 90 mm Hg systolic, acute MI, pulmonary congestion

Precautions: CHF, hypotension, hepatic injury, pregnancy **P** C, lactation, children, renal disease

Pharmacokinetics

Absorption	Well absorbed
Distribution	Not known
Metabolism	Liver, extensively
Excretion	Metabolites (96%)
Half-life	3½-9 hr

Pharmacodynamics

	PO	PO-SUS REL	IV
Onset	½ hr	Unknown	Unknown
Peak	2-3 hr	Unknown	Unknown
Duration	6-8 hr	12 hr	Unknown

Interactions
Individual drugs
Alcohol: ↑ hypotension

Carbamazepine: ↑ toxicity
Digoxin: ↑ digoxin levels, bradycardia, CHF
Phenobarbital: ↓ effectiveness
Phenytoin: ↓ effectiveness
Propranolol: ↑ toxicity
Drug classifications
Antihypertensives: ↑ hypotension
β-Adrenergic blockers: ↑ bradycardia, CHF
Nitrates: ↑ nitrates

NURSING CONSIDERATIONS

Assessment

- Assess fluid volume status: I&O ratio and record, weight, distended red veins, crackles in lung, color, quality, and sp gr of urine, skin turgor, adequacy of pulses, moist mucous membranes, bilateral lung sounds, peripheral pitting edema; dehydration symptoms of decreasing output, thirst, hypotension, dry mouth and mucous membranes should be reported
- Monitor B/P and pulse, PCWP, CVP often during infusion; if B/P drops 30 mm Hg, stop inf and call prescriber
- Monitor ALT (SGOT), AST (SGPT), bilirubin daily; if these are elevated, hepatotoxicity is suspected
- If platelets are <150,000/mm^3, drug is usually discontinued and another drug started
- Assess for extravasation: change site q48h

Nursing diagnoses

✓ Cardiac output, decreased (uses)
✓ Knowledge deficit (teaching)

Implementation

PO route

- Give with meals for GI symptoms; may be crushed and mixed with food/fluids for swallowing difficulty
- Do not chew or crush sus rel caps
- Store in airtight container at room temp

IV route

- Give direct **IV** undiluted over 2 min
- For continuous inf dilute 125 mg/100 ml, (1.25 mg/ml) or 250 mg/250 ml, (1 mg/ml) or 250 mg/500 ml (0.5 mg/ml) of D_5W, 0.9% NaCl, D_5/0.45% NaCl; give 10 mg/hr; may increase by 5 mg/hr to 15 mg/hr; may continue inf up to 24 hr

Y-site compatibilities: Albumin, amikacin, amphotericin B, aztreonam, bretylium, bumetanide, cefazolin, cefotaxime, cefotetan, cefoxitin, ceftazidime, ceftriaxone, cefuroxime, cimetidine, ciprofloxacin, clindamycin, digoxin, dobutamine, dopamine, doxycycline, epinephrine, erythromycin, esmolol, fluconazole, gentamicin, hetastarch, lidocaine, lorazepam, meperidine, metoclopramide, metronidazole, morphine, multivitamins, nitroglycerin, norepinephrine, nitroprusside, oxacillin, penicillin G Potassium, pentamidine, piperacillin, potassium chloride, potassium phosphates, procainamide ranitidine, theophylline, ticarcillin, tobramycin, vancomycin

Patient/family education

- Caution patient to avoid hazardous activities until stabilized on drug and dizziness is no longer a problem
- Instruct patient to limit caffeine consumption; to avoid alcohol and OTC drugs unless directed by prescriber
- Tell patient to comply in all areas of medical regimen; diet,

exercise, stress reduction, drug therapy; to notify prescriber of irregular heart beat, shortness of breath, swelling of feet and hands, pronounced dizziness, constipation, nausea, hypotension

• Teach patient to use as directed even if feeling better; may be taken with other cardiovascular drugs (nitrates, β-blockers)

Evaluation

Positive therapeutic outcome

• Decreased anginal pain
• Decreased B/P
• Absence of dysrhythmias

Treatment of overdose: Defibrillation, atropine for AV block, vasopressor for hypotension

dimenhydrinate (OTC, ℞)

(dye-men-hye'dri-nate)

Calm-X, dimenhydrinate, Dimentabs, Dinate, Dommanate, Dramamine, Dramanate, Dramocen, Dramoject, Dymenate, Gravol ✦, Hydrate, Marmine, Nauseal ✦, Nauseatol ✦, Nico-Vert, Novodimenate ✦, Travamine ✦, Triptone Caplets, Wehamine

Func. class.: Antiemetic, antihistamine, anticholinergic

Chem. class.: H_1-receptor antagonist, ethanolamine derivative

Pregnancy category B

Action: Vestibular stimulator is decreased; anticholinergic, antiemetic, antihistamine response

➔ **Therapeutic Outcome:** Absence of motion sickness

Uses: Motion sickness, nausea, vomiting

Dosage and routes

Adult: PO 50-100 mg q4h; rec 100 mg qd or bid; IM/**IV** 50 mg as needed

P ***Child:*** IM/PO 5 mg/kg divided in 4 equal doses

Available forms: Tab 50 mg; inj 50 mg/ml; liq 12.5 mg/4 ml; supp 50, 100 mg; chew tab 50 mg; cap 50 mg

Adverse effects

CNS: Drowsiness, restlessness, headache, dizziness, insomnia, confusion, nervousness, tingling, vertigo; hallucinations and ***convulsions*** in young P children

CV: Hypertension, hypotension, palpitations

EENT: Dry mouth, blurred vision, diplopia, nasal congestion, photosensitivity

GI: Nausea, anorexia, diarrhea, vomiting, constipation

INTEG: Rash, urticaria, fever, chills, flushing

Contraindications: Hypersensitivity to narcotics, shock

P G **Precautions:** Children, cardiac dysrhythmias, elderly, asthma, pregnancy **B,** prostatic hypertrophy, bladder neck obstruction, narrow-angle glaucoma, stenosing peptic ulcer, pyloroduodenal obstruction

Pharmacokinetics

Absorption	Well absorbed (PO, IM)
Distribution	Unknown; crosses placenta
Metabolism	Liver
Excretion	Kidneys, breast milk
Half-life	Unknown

Pharmacodynamics

	PO	IM	IV
Onset	15-60 min	30 min	Immediate
Peak	1-2 hr	1-2 hr	Unknown
Duration	4-6 hr	4-6 hr	4-6 hr

Interactions

Individual drugs

Alcohol: ↑ CNS depression
Atropine: ↑ anticholinergic reactions
Disopyramide: ↑ anticholinergic reactions
Haloperidol: ↑ anticholinergic reactions
Quinidine: ↑ anticholinergic reactions

Drug classifications

Antidepressants: ↑ anticholinergic reactions
Antihistamines: ↑ anticholinergic reactions
CNS depressants: ↑ CNS depression
MAOIs: ↑ anticholinergic effect
Narcotics: ↑ CNS depression
Phenothiazines: ↑ anticholinergic reactions
Sedative/hypnotics: ↑ CNS depression

Lab test interferences

False negative: Skin allergy tests (discontinue antihistamines 3 days before testing)

NURSING CONSIDERATIONS

Assessment

- Assess for signs of toxicity to other drugs or masking of symptoms of disease (brain tumor, intestinal obstruction); monitor GI symptoms including nausea, vomiting, abdominal pain, increased bowel sounds
- Monitor VS, B/P; check patients with cardiac disease more often
- Monitor I&O; check for dehydration (poor skin turgor, increased sp gr, tachycardia, severe thirst) especially in the G elderly

Nursing diagnoses

✓ Injury, risk for (side effects)
✓ Knowledge deficit (teaching)

Implementation

PO route

- Tab may be swallowed whole, chewed, or allowed to dissolve; give 1-2 hr before activity that may cause motion sickness; use measuring device for liq for correct dosing

IM route

- Give IM injection in large muscle mass; aspirate to avoid IV administration; massage

IV **IV route**

- Give **IV** directly after diluting 50 mg/10 ml or NaCl inj; give 50 mg or less over 2 min

Syringe incompatibilities: Butorphanol, chlorpromazine, glycopyrrolate, hydroxyzine, midazolam, pentobarbital, prochlorperazine, promazine, promethazine, thiopental

Syringe compatibilities: Atropine, diphenhydramine, droperidol, fentanyl, heparin, meperidine, metoclopramide, morphine, pentazocine, perphenazine, ranitidine, scopolamine

Y-site incompatibilities: Aminophylline, heparin, hydrocortisone sodium succinate, hydroxyzine, phenobarbital, phenytoin, prednisolone, prochlorperazine, promazine, promethazine

Additive compatibilities: Amikacin, calcium gluconate, chloramphenicol, corticotropin, erythromycin, heparin, hydroxyzine, methicillin, norepinephrine, oxytetracycline, penicillin G potassium, pentobarbital, phenobarbital, potassium chloride, prochlorperazine, vancomycin, vitamin B with C

Additive incompatibilities: Tetracycline, thiopental

Patient/family education

- Teach all aspects of drug uses; to notify prescriber if confusion, sedation, hypotension occur; to avoid driving and other hazardous activity if drowsiness occurs; to avoid alcohol and other CNS depressants that may potentiate effect
- Tell patient not to exceed recommended dosage
- Inform patient hard candy, gum, frequent rinsing of mouth may be used for dryness
- Advise patient that a false negative result may occur with skin testing; these procedures should not be scheduled until 4 days after discontinuing use
- Caution patient to avoid hazardous activities, activities requiring alertness; dizziness may occur; instruct patient to request assistance with ambulation
- Caution patient to avoid alcohol, other CNS depressants when taking this medication; response will be increased

Evaluation

Positive therapeutic outcome

- Absence of motion sickness
- Absence of nausea, vomiting

dimercaprol (℞)

(dye-mer-cap′role)

BAL in Oil, British Anti-Lewisite ✱, Dimercaptopropanol

Func. class.: Heavy metal antagonist

Chem. class.: Chelating agent (dithiol compound)

Pregnancy category D

Action: Binds ions from arsenic, gold, mercury, lead, copper to form water-soluble complex removed by kidneys

➔ **Therapeutic Outcome:** Excretion of heavy metals and prevention of damage and death

Uses: Arsenic, gold, mercury, lead poisoning; adjunct in severe lead poisoning with encephalopathy

Dosage and routes

Severe gold/arsenic poisoning

Adult: IM 3 mg/kg q4h x 2 days; then qid x 1 day; then bid x 10 days

Mild gold/arsenic poisoning

Adult: IM 2.5 mg/kg qid x 2 days; then bid x 1 day; then qd x 10 days

Acute lead poisoning

Adult: IM 4 mg/kg; then q4h with edetate calcium disodium 12.5 mg/kg IM; not to exceed 5 mg/kg/dose

Mercury poisoning

Adult: IM 5 mg/kg; then 2.5 mg/kg/day or bid x 10 days

Available forms: Inj IM 100 mg/ml

Adverse effects

CNS: Headache, paresthesia,

D

anxiety, tremors, ***convulsions, shock***
CV: Hypertension, tachycardia
EENT: Rhinorrhea, throat pain or constriction, lacrimation
GI: Nausea, vomiting, salivation
GU: Burning sensation in penis, ***nephrotoxicity***
INTEG: Urticaria, erythema, pruritus, pain at inj site, fever, burning of lips, mouth, throat
SYST: ***Anaphylaxis,*** metabolic acidosis

Contraindications: Hypersensitivity, anuria, hepatic insufficiency, poisoning with other metals, severe renal disease, P child <3 yr, pregnancy **D**

Precautions: Hypertension, lactation G6PD deficiency

Pharmacokinetics	
Absorption	Well absorbed
Distribution	Widely distributed
Metabolism	Liver (50%)
Excretion	Unknown
Half-life	Unknown

Pharmacodynamics	
Onset	Unknown
Peak	Unknown
Duration	4 hr

Interactions
Individual drugs
Cadmium: ↑ toxicity
Iron: ↑ toxicity
Selenium: ↑ toxicity
Uranium: ↑ toxicity
Urine alkalinizers: ↓ nephrotoxicity
Food
Alkalinergics: ↓ nephrotoxicity
Lab test interferences
↓ ^{131}I uptake

NURSING CONSIDERATIONS
Assessment
- Assess for poisoning: type of agent, time ingested, amount ingested
- Assess for acute toxicity: gold, lead, arsenic
- Check B/P, pulse, tachycardia may occur
- Monitor I&O, kidney function studies: BUN, creatinine, CrCl, serum iron levels
- Assess for allergic reactions: rash, urticaria; if these occur, drug should be discontinued
- Check temperature q4hr; P drug may cause fever in children, as well as burning sensation of mouth, lips, eyes, thoat

Nursing diagnoses
✓ Poisoning (uses)
✓ Knowledge deficit (teaching)

Implementation
- Give within 2 hr of ingestion; have antihistamine available for allergic reaction
- Wash hands immediately if sol comes in contact with skin; dermatitis can occur
- Rotate inj sites; give deeply in large muscle mass

Patient/family education
- Explain all aspects of drug administration including purpose for medication
- Advise patient to notify prescriber of adverse reactions: constriction in throat, burning of lips, mouth; tell patient that IM route is painful

Evaluation
Positive therapeutic outcome
- Decreased symptoms of heavy metal intoxication

dinoprostone (℞)

(dye-noe-prost′one)

Cervidil, Prepidil, Prostin E_2

Func. class.: Oxytocic, abortifacient

Chem. class.: Prostaglandin E_2

Pregnancy category N/A

Action: Stimulates uterine contractions similar to labor by myometrium stimulation, causing abortion; acts within 30 hr for complete abortion; GI smooth muscle stimulation, effacement, dilatation of the cervix

➔ **Therapeutic Outcome:** Beginning of labor, fetal expulsion

Uses: Abortion during 2nd trimester, benign hydatidiform mole, expulsion of uterine contents in fetal deaths to 28 wk, missed abortion, cervical effacement and dilatation in term pregnancy when they have not occurred spontaneously

Dosage and routes

Adult: Vag supp 20 mg; repeat q3-5h until abortion occurs; max dose is 240 mg

Adult: Gel; warm to room temperature; choose correct length shielded catheter (10 or 20mm), fill catheter by pushing plunger; patient remain recumbent for 15-30 min

Adult: Insert 10 mg; remove upon onset of active labor or 12 hr insertion

Available forms: Vag supp 20 mg; gel 0.5 mg/3 g (prefilled syringe); vag insert 10 mg; gel 0.5 mg

Adverse effects

CNS: Headache, dizziness, chills, fever

CV: Hypotension

EENT: Blurred vision

GI: Nausea, vomiting, diarrhea

GU: Vaginitis, vaginal pain, vulvitis, vaginismus

INTEG: Rash, skin color changes

MS: Leg cramps, joint swelling, weakness

Insert: Uterine hyperstimulation, fever, nausea, vomiting, diarrhea, abdominal pain

Gel: Uterine contractile abnormality, GI side effects, back pain, fever; fetal: ***bradycardia, late deceleration***

Contraindications: Hypersensitivity, uterine fibrosis, cervical stenosis, pelvic surgery, pelvic inflammatory disease (PID), respiratory disease

Precautions: Hepatic disease, renal disease, cardiac disease, asthma, anemia, jaundice, diabetes mellitus, convulsive disorders, hypertension, hypotension

Pharmacokinetics

Absorption	Rapidly absorbed
Distribution	Unknown
Metabolism	Enzymes
Excretion	Kidneys
Half-life	Unknown

Pharmacodynamics

	GEL	SUPP
Onset	Rapid	10 min
Peak	30-45 min	Unknown
Duration	Unknown	2-3 hr

Interactions

Individual drugs

Oxytocin: ↑ effect

NURSING CONSIDERATIONS
Assessment
- Assess dilatation and effacement of the cervix, uterine contractions, fetal heart tones; watch for contractions lasting over 1 min, hypertonus, fetal distress; drug should be slowed or discontinued
- Assess for fever that occurs approximately 30 min following supp insertion (abortion)
- Monitor for nausea, vomiting, diarrhea; these may require medication
- Assess for hypersensitive reaction: dyspnea, rash, chest discomfort
- Assess respiratory rate, rhythm, depth; notify prescriber of abnormalities, in pulse, B/P
- Check vaginal discharge; itching, irritation indicates vaginal infection

Nursing diagnoses
- ✓ Injury, high risk for (side effects)
- ✓ Knowledge deficit (teaching)

Implementation
Supp route
- Warm suppository by running warm water over package; insert high in vagina, wear gloves to prevent absorption; have patient recumbent for at least 10 min

Gel route
- Do not allow to come in contact with skin; use soap and water to wash after use
- Gel should be at room temp
- Place patient in dorsal or lithotomy position to insert gel into cervical canal; remove catheter; discard all items after use; keep supine 15-30 min

Insert route
- Insert transversely in the posterior fornix of the vagina immediately after removal from foil package; do not insert without retrieval system

Patient/family education
- Teach patient all aspects of treatment including purpose of medication and expected results
- Tell patient that gel may produce warmth in her vagina
- Caution patient that if contractions are longer than 1 min to notify nurse or prescriber
- Advise patient to notify prescriber of cramping, pain, increased bleeding, chills, increased temp, or foul-smelling discharge; these symptoms may indicate uterine infection

Evaluation
Positive therapeutic outcome
- Progression of labor
- Abortion

diphenhydramine ⊶ (OTC, ℞)
(dye-fen-hye'dra-meen)
Allerdryl ✦, AllerMax, Banophen, Belix, Bena-D 10, Bena-D 50, Benadryl, Benadryl 25, Benadryl Kapseals, Benahist 10, Benahist 50, Ben-Allergin-50, Benoject, Benoject-10, Benoject-50, Benylin Cough, Bydramine, Compoz, Dermamycin, Diahist, Diphenacen-50, Diphen Cough, Diphenhist, diphenhydramine HCl, Dormarex 2, Dormin, Dyrexin, Genahist, Hydramine, Hydramyn, Hyrexin-50, Insomnal ✦, Nidryl, Nordryl, Nordryl Cough, Nytol, Phendry, Scot-Tussin Allergy, Silphen Cough, Sleep-Eze 3, Sleepinal, Sominex 2, Sominex Caplets, Tusstat, Twilite, Uni-Bent Cough, Wehdryl

Func. class.: Antihistamine, antitussive

Chem. class.: Ethanolamine derivative, H_1-receptor antagonist

Pregnancy category C

Action: Acts on blood vessels, GI, respiratory system by competing with histamine for H_1-receptor site; decreases allergic response by blocking histamine; causes increased heart rate, vasodilatation, secretions

➔ **Therapeutic Outcome:** Absence of allergy symptoms and rhinitis, decreased dystonic symptoms, absence of motion sickness, absence of cough, ability to sleep

Uses: Allergy symptoms, rhinitis, motion sickness, antiparkinsonism, nighttime sedation, infant colic, nonproductive cough, anaphylaxis, nasal allergies, allergic dermatoses, dystonic reactions

Dosage and routes

Adult: PO 25-50 mg q4-6h, not to exceed 400 mg/day; IM/**IV** 10-50 mg, not to exceed 400 mg/day

P ***Child >12 kg:*** PO/IM/**IV** 5 mg/kg/day in 4 divided doses, not to exceed 300 mg/day

Available forms: Caps 25, 50 mg; tabs 25, 50 mg; elix 12.5 mg/5 ml; syr 12.5 mg/5 ml; inj IM, **IV** 50 mg/ml; cream 1%, 2%; lotion 1%

Adverse effects

CNS: Dizziness, drowsiness, poor coordination, fatigue, anxiety, euphoria, confusion, paresthesia, neuritis

EENT: Blurred vision, dilated pupils, tinnitus, nasal stuffiness, dry nose, throat, mouth

GI: Dry mouth, nausea, anorexia, diarrhea

GU: Retention, dysuria, frequency

HEMA: ***Thrombocytopenia, agranulocytosis, hemolytic anemia***

INTEG: Photosensitivity

RESP: Increased thick secretions, wheezing, chest tightness

Contraindications: Hypersensitivity to H_1-receptor antagonist, acute asthma attack, lower respiratory tract disease

Precautions: Increased intraocular pressure, renal disease, cardiac disease, hypertension, bronchial asthma, seizure disorder, stenosed peptic ulcers, hyperthyroidism, prostatic hypertrophy, bladder neck obstruction, pregnancy **C**

Pharmacokinetics

Absorption	Well absorbed (PO, IM); minimally absorbed (top); completely absorbed (**IV**)
Distribution	Widely distributed; crosses placenta
Metabolism	Liver (95%)
Excretion	Kidneys, breast milk
Half-life	2½-7 hr

Pharmacodynamics

	PO	IM	IV
Onset	15-60 min	30 min	Immediate
Peak	1-4 hr	1-4 hr	Unknown
Duration	4-8 hr	4-8 hr	4-8 hr

Interactions

Individual drugs

Alcohol: ↑ CNS depression
Disopyramide: ↑ anticholinergic response
Quinidine: ↑ anticholinergic response

Drug classifications

Antidepressants, tricyclic: ↑ anticholinergic response
CNS depressants: ↑ CNS depression
MAOI: ↑ anticholinergic effect
Narcotics: ↑ CNS depression
Sedative/hypnotics: ↑ CNS depression

Lab test interferences

False negative: Skin allergy tests (discontinue antihistamines 3 days before testing)

NURSING CONSIDERATIONS

Assessment

- Assess respiratory status: rate, rhythm, increase in bronchial secretions, wheezing, chest tightness; provide fluids to 2 L/day to decrease secretion thickness
- Monitor I&O ratio: be alert for urinary retention, frequency, dysuria, especially **G** elderly; drug should be discontinued if these occur
- Monitor CBC during long-term therapy; blood dyscrasias may occur but are rare
- If giving for dystonic reactions, assess type of involuntary movements and evaluate response to this medication
- Assess cough characteristics including type, frequency, thickness of secretions, and evaluate response to this medication if using for cough

Nursing diagnoses

✓ Injury, risk for (side effects)
✓ Sleep pattern disturbance (uses)
✓ Knowledge deficit (teaching)

Implementation

- Give 20 min before hs if using for sleep aid

PO route

- Give with meals if GI symptoms occur; absorption may be slightly decreased; cap may be opened and drug mixed with food/fluids for patients with swallowing difficulties

IM route

- Give IM injection in large muscle mass; aspirate to avoid **IV** administration; rotate sites

IV **IV route**

- Give **IV** undiluted 25 mg/min; may be diluted with 0.9% NaCl, D_5W, $D_{10}W$, 0.45% NaCl, D_5/0.9% NaCl, D_5/0.45% NaCl, D_5/0.25% NaCl, LR, Ringer's, give 25 mg/min or less

Syringe incompatibilities: Pentobarbital, phenytoin, thiopental

Syringe compatibilities: Atropine, butorphanol, chlorpromazine, cimetidine, dimenhydrinate, droperidol, fentanyl, glycopyrrolate, hydromorphone, hydroxyzine, meperidine, metoclopramide, midazolam, morphine, nalbuphine, pentazocine, perphenazine, prochlorperazine, promazine, promethazine, ranitidine, scopolamine

Y-site compatibilities: Acyclovir, aldesleukin, amifostine, amsacrine, fluconazole, fludarabine, granisetron, heparin, idarubicin, melphalan, meperidine, ondansetron, paclitaxel, sargramostim, thiotepa, vinorelbine

Y-site incompatibility: Foscarnet

Additive compatibilities: Amikacin, aminophylline, bleomycin, cephapirin, erythromycin, methyldopate, nafcillin, netilmicin, methicillin, penicillin G potassium, polymyxin B, tetracycline, vitamin B with C

Additive incompatibilities: Amobarbital, cephalothin, thiopental

Patient/family education

- Tell patient that a false-negative result may occur with skin testing; these procedures should not be scheduled until 3 days after discontinuing use
- Caution patient to avoid hazardous activities and activities requiring alertness, since dizziness may occur; instruct patient to request assistance with ambulation
- Advise patient to avoid alcohol, other depressants; CNS depression may occur
- Teach all aspects of drug uses; to notify prescriber if confusion, sedation, hypotension occur; to avoid driving and other hazardous activity if drowsiness occurs; to avoid alcohol or other CNS depressants that may potentiate effect
- Teach patient hard candy, gum, frequent rinsing of mouth may be used for dryness

Evaluation

Positive therapeutic outcome

- Absence of motion sickness
- Absence of nausea, vomiting
- Ability to sleep
- Absence of cough
- Decrease in involuntary movements

Treatment of overdose:

- Administer ipecac syrup or lavage, diazepam, vasopressors, barbiturates (short acting)

D

diphenoxylate with atropine/difenoxin with atropine (℞)

(dye-fen-ox′i-late)

Diphenatol, Lofene, Logen, Lomanate, Lomotil, Lonox, Lo-Trop, Motofen, Nor-mil

Func. class.: Antidiarrheal

Chem. class.: Phenylpiperidine derivative, opiate agonist

Pregnancy category C

Controlled substance schedule V (diphenoxylate/atropine); IV (difenoxin/atropine)

Action: Inhibits gastric motility by acting on mucosal receptors responsible for peristalsis; related to narcotic analgesics as adjunct

Therapeutic Outcome: Decreased loose stools

Uses: Diarrhea (cause undetermined)

Dosage and routes

Adult: PO 2.5-5 mg qid, titrated to patient response

P ***Child 2-12 yr:*** PO 0.3-0.4 mg/kg/day in divided doses

Available forms: Tab 2.5 mg diphenoxylate/0.025 mg atropine; tab 1 mg difenoxin/0.025 mg atropine; liq 2.5 mg diphenoxylate/0.025 mg atropine/5 ml

Adverse effects

CNS: Drowsiness, headache, sedation, depression, weakness, lethargy, flushing, hyperthermia

CV: Tachycardia

EENT: Blurred vision, nystagmus, mydriasis

GI: Nausea, vomiting, abdominal pain, glossitis, colitis

GU: Urine retention

INTEG: Rash, urticaria, pruritus, ***angioneurotic edema***

Contraindications: Hypersensitivity, severe liver disease, pseudomembranous enterocolitis, glaucoma, P child <2 yr, electrolyte imbalances

Precautions: Hepatic disease, renal disease, ulcerative colitis, G pregnancy **C**, lactation, elderly

Pharmacokinetics	
Absorption	Well absorbed
Distribution	Unknown
Metabolism	Liver, active metabolite
Excretion	Kidneys
Half-life	2½ hr

Pharmacodynamics	
Onset	45-60 min
Peak	2 hr
Duration	3-4 hr

Interactions

Individual drugs

Alcohol: ↑ action of alcohol
Disopyramide: ↑ anticholinergic effect

Drug classifications

Anticholinergics: ↑ anticholinergic effect
Antidepressants, tricyclic: ↑ anticholinergic effect
Antihistamines: ↑ CNS depression
Barbiturates: ↑ action of barbiturates
CNS depressants: ↑ action of CNS depressants
MAOI: Hypertensive crisis; do not use together
Narcotics: ↑ action of narcotics
Sedative/hypnotics: ↑ CNS depression

NURSING CONSIDERATIONS

Assessment

- Monitor electrolytes (potassium, sodium, chloride) if on long-term therapy; fluid status, skin turgor
- Assess bowel pattern before, during treatment; check for rebound constipation after termination of medication; check bowel sounds
- Check response after 48 hr; if no response, drug should be discontinued and other treatment initiated
- Assess for abdominal distention and toxic megacolon, which may occur in ulcerative colitis

Nursing diagnoses

✓ Diarrhea (uses)
✓ Constipation (adverse reactions)
✓ Knowledge deficit (teaching)
✓ Noncompliance (teaching)

Implementation

- Give for 48 hr only; tabs may

be given with food, crushed and mixed with fluids; liq should be measured accurately

Patient/family education

- Advise patient to avoid alcohol and OTC products unless directed by prescriber; may cause increased CNS depression
- Caution patient not to exceed recommended dosage; that drug may be habit forming
- Advise patient that drug may cause drowsiness; to avoid hazardous activities until response to drug is determined
- Teach patient that dry mouth can be decreased by frequent sips of water, hard candy, sugarless gum

Evaluation

Positive therapeutic outcome

- Decreased diarrhea

dipyridamole (℞)

(dye-peer-id'a-mole)

Apo-Dipyridamole ♣, dipyridamole, Persantine, Persantine IV

Func. class.: Coronary vasodilator, antiplatelet agent

Chem. class.: Nonnitrate

Pregnancy category B

Action: Inhibits adenosine uptake, which produces coronary vasodilatation; increases oxygen saturation in coronary tissues, coronary blood flow; acts on small vessels with little effect on vascular resistance; may increase development of collateral circulation; decreased platelet aggregation by the inhibition of phosphodiesterases (enzymes)

➔ **Therapeutic Outcome:** Inhibition of platelet aggregation; absence of ischemic attacks, reinfarction

Uses: Prevention of transient ischemic attacks, inhibition of platelet adhesion to prevent myocardial reinfarction, thromboembolism, with warfarin in prosthetic heart valves, prevention of coronary bypass graft occlusion with aspirin; possibly effective for long-term therapy of chronic angina pectoris

Dosage and routes

Transient ischemic attacks

Adult: PO 50 mg tid, 1 hr ac, not to exceed 400 mg qd

Inhibition of platelet adhesion

Adult: PO 50-75 mg qid in combination with aspirin or warfarin

Available forms: Tabs 25, 50, 75 mg; **IV**

Adverse effects

CNS: Headache, dizziness, weakness, fainting, syncope

CV: Postural hypotension

GI: Nausea, vomiting, anorexia, diarrhea

INTEG: Rash, flushing

Contraindications: Hypersensitivity, hypotension

Precautions: Pregnancy **B**

Pharmacokinetics	
Absorption	30%-50% (PO)
Distribution	Widely distributed; crosses placenta
Metabolism	Liver
Excretion	Bile, undergoes enterohepatic recirculation; enters breast milk
Half-life	10 hr

Pharmacodynamics	PO	IV
Onset	Unknown	Unknown
Peak	2½ hr	6 min
Duration	6 hr	½ hr
Therapeutic effect	Several mo	

Interactions
Individual drugs
Aspirin: ↑ antiplatelet effect
Coumadin: ↑ bleeding
Theophylline: ↓ effects of disopyramide (thallium)
Drug classifications
Anticoagulants: ↑ risk of bleeding
NSAIDs: ↑ risk of bleeding
Thrombolytics: ↑ risk of bleeding

NURSING CONSIDERATIONS
Assessment
- Monitor B/P, pulse baseline and during treatment until stable; take B/P with patient lying, standing; orthostatic hypotension is common
- Assess cardiac status: chest pain, what aggravates or ameliorates condition
- If using by **IV** route, monitor vital signs before, during, and after infusion; monitor for chest pain, bronchospasm; use ECG for identifying dysrhythmias; use aminophylline up to 250 mg **IV** for bronchospasm and chest pain if chest pain is unrelieved with the 250 mg dose of aminophylline; give SL dose of nitroglycerin

Nursing diagnoses
✓ Cardiac output, decreased (uses)
✓ Pain (uses)
✓ Knowledge deficit (teaching)

Implementation
PO route
- Give with 8 oz of water; to improve absorption give on an empty stomach; if GI symptoms occur may give with meals
- Tabs may be crushed, mixed with food or fluids for swallowing difficulty or swallowed whole
- Store at room temp

IV **IV Intermittent inf**
- Give by **IV** after diluting each 5 mg/2 ml or more in D_5W, 0.45% NaCl, or 0.9% NaCl 20-50 ml should be given; give over 4 min; do not give undiluted

Patient/family education
- Teach patient that this medication is not a cure; that drug may have to be taken continuously in evenly spaced doses only as directed; if a dose is missed, take one when remembered up to 4 hr; do not double doses
- Inform patient that it is necessary to quit smoking to prevent excessive vasoconstriction
- Advise patient to rise slowly from sitting or lying down to prevent orthostatic hypotension
- Caution patient not to use alcohol or OTC medication unless approved by prescriber
- Caution patient to avoid hazardous activities until stabilized on medication; dizziness may occur

Evaluation
Positive therapeutic outcome
- Absence of reinfarction, ischemic attacks

Treatment of overdose:
Administer **IV** phenylephrine

dirithromycin (℞)

(die-rith-roe-mie′sin)

Dynabac

Func. class.: Antibacterial

Chem. class.: Macrolide

Pregnancy category C

Action: Binds to 50S ribosomal subunits of susceptible bacteria; suppresses protein synthesis

➔ **Therapeutic Outcome:** Bactericidal action against *Moraxella catarrhalis, Streptococcus pneumoniae, Legionella pneumophilia, Mycoplasma pneumoniae, S. pyogenes, Staphylococcus aureus, S. agalactiae, Streptococcus* sp., *S. viridans, Bordetella pertussis, Propionibacterium acnes*

Uses: Infections of upper and lower respiratory tract

Dosage and routes

Adult: PO 500 mg qd, given for 7-14 days depending on infections

Available forms: Tab, enteric coated 250 mg

Adverse effects

GI: Abdominal pain, nausea, diarrhea, vomiting, dyspepsia, GI disorders, flatulence, abnormal stools, anorexia, constipation, ***pseudomembranous colitis***

CNS: Headache, dizziness, insomnia

HEMA: Increased platelet count, increased eosinophils

RESP: Cough, dyspnea

INTEG: Pruritus, urticaria

Contraindications: Hypersensitivity to this drug or any other macrolide, or erythromycin, bacteremias

G P **Precautions:** Elderly, pregnancy **C**, lactation, children, hepatic, renal disease

Pharmacokinetics

Absorption	Rapidly absorbed
Distribution	Widely distributed
Metabolism	No hepatic metabolism
Excretion	Bile, feces (up to 97%)
Half-life	Plasma half-life 8 hr, terminal 44 hr

Pharmacodynamics

Unknown

Interactions

Drug classifications

Antacids: Slightly enhanced absorption of dirithromycin

H_2 antagonists: Slightly enhanced absorption of dirithromycin

NURSING CONSIDERATIONS

Assessment

- Assess I&O ratio; report hematuria, oliguria in renal disease
- Monitor liver function studies: AST (SGOT), ALT (SGPT)
- Monitor renal studies: Urinalysis, protein, blood
- Monitor C&S before drug therapy; drug may be given as soon as culture is taken; C&S may be repeated after treatment
- Assess bowel pattern before, during treatment; pseudomembranous colitis may occur
- Assess for skin eruptions, itching
- Assess respiratory status: rate, character, wheezing, tightness in chest; discontinue drug
- Identify allergies before treatment, reaction of each

D

medication; place allergies on chart, notify all people giving drugs

Nursing diagnoses

- ✓ Infection, risk for (uses)
- ✓ Diarrhea (side effects)
- ✓ Knowledge deficit (teaching)
- ✓ Noncompliance (teaching)

Implementation

- Give adequate intake of fluids (2 L) during diarrhea episodes
- ⊘ Administer whole; do not cut, crush, chew tablets
- Give with food or within 1 hr of food
- Store at room temperature in tight container

Patient/family education

- Teach patient to take with full glass of water; give with food
- Instruct patient to report sore throat, fever, fatigue; may indicate superinfection
- Teach patient to notify nurse of diarrhea stools, dark urine, pale stools, yellow discoloration of eyes or skin, severe abdominal pain
- Instruct patient to take at evenly spaced intervals; complete dosage regimen

Evaluation

Positive therapeutic outcome

- C&S negative for infection

Treatment of hypersensitivity: Withdraw drug, maintain airway, administer epinephrine, aminophylline, O_2, **IV** corticosteroids

disopyramide (℞)

(dye-soe-peer'a-mide)

disopyramide, Napamide, Norpace, Norpace CR, Rhythmodan

Func. class.: Antidysrhythmic (class IA)

Chem. class.: Nonnitrate

Pregnancy category C

Action: Prolongs action potential duration and effective refractory period; reduces disparity in refractory between normal and infarcted myocardium; prevents increased myocardial excitability and conduction contractility

➔ **Therapeutic Outcome:** Suppression of supraventricular dysrhythmias

Uses: PVCs, ventricular tachycardia, supraventricular tachycardia, atrial flutter, fibrillation

Investigational uses: Supraventricular tachycardia (prevention, treatment)

Dosage and routes

Adult: PO 100-200 mg q6h; in renal dysfunction 100 mg q6h; sus rel cap 200 mg q12h

P ***Child 12-18 yr:*** PO 6-15 mg/kg/day, in divided doses q6h

P ***Child 4-12 yr:*** PO 10-15 mg/kg/day in divided doses q6h

P ***Child 1-4 yr:*** PO 10-20 mg/kg/day in divided doses q6h

P ***Child <1 yr:*** PO 10-30 mg/kg/day, in divided doses q6h

Available forms: Caps 100, 150 mg (as phosphate); sus rel caps 100, 150 mg

Adverse effects

CNS: Headache, dizziness, psychosis, fatigue, depression, paresthesias, anxiety, insomnia
CV: Hypotension, bradycardia, angina, PVCs, tachycardia, increases in QRS and QT segments, ***cardiac arrest,*** edema, weight gain, AV block, *CHF,* syncope, chest pain
GI: Dry mouth, constipation, nausea, anorexia, flatulence, diarrhea, vomiting
GU: Retention, hesitancy, impotence, urinary frequency, urgency
EENT: Blurred vision, dry nose, throat, eyes, narrow-angle glaucoma
HEMA: ***Thrombocytopenia, agranulocytosis,*** anemia (rare), decreased Hgb, Hct
INTEG: Rash, pruritus, urticaria
META: Hypoglycemia
MS: Weakness, pain in extremities

Contraindications: Hypersensitivity, 2nd- or 3rd-degree heart block, cardiogenic shock, CHF (uncompensated), sick sinus syndrome, QT prolongation

Precautions: Pregnancy **C,** lactation, diabetes mellitus, P renal disease, children, hepatic disease, myasthenia gravis, narrow-angle glaucoma, cardiomyopathy, conduction abnormalities

Pharmacokinetics

Absorption	Well absorbed
Distribution	Widely distributed
Metabolism	Liver
Excretion	Kidneys
Half-life	4-10 hr

Pharmacodynamics

	PO	PO–SUS REL
Onset	½-3½ hr	Unknown
Peak	2 hr	Unknown
Duration	1½-8 hr	12 hr

Interactions

Individual drugs

Flecainide: ↑ levels, toxicity
Lidocaine: Bradycardia, arrest
Mexiletine: ↑ levels, toxicity
Phenytoin: ↑ blood levels, toxicity
Procainamide: ↑ levels, toxicity
Quinidine: ↑ levels, toxicity
Rifampin: ↓ disopyramide levels
Warfarin: ↑ level, bleeding

Drug classifications

Anticoagulants: ↓ prothrombin time
Antidysrhythmics: Widening of QRS or QRT
β-Blockers: ↑ dysrhythmias, arrest

Lab test interferences

↑ CPK

NURSING CONSIDERATIONS

Assessment

- Assess respiratory status: auscultate lung fields for bibasilar crackles in patients with advanced CHF
- Monitor I&O ratio and electrolytes: potassium, sodium, chloride; watch for decreasing urinary output, possible retention
- Monitor liver function studies: AST (SGOT), ALT (SGPT), bilirubin, alkaline phosphatase
- Monitor ECG to determine drug effectiveness, measure PR, QRS, QT intervals; check for PVCs, other dysrhythmias; monitor B/P for hypotension; check for prolonged widening

QT intervals, QRS complex; if QT or QRS increase by 50% or more, withhold next dose, notify prescriber
- Monitor for dehydration or hypovolemia
- Monitor for CNS symptoms: psychosis, numbness, depression; if these occur, drug should be discontinued

Nursing diagnoses

✓ Cardiac output, decreased (uses)
✓ Knowledge deficit (teaching)

Implementation

- Do not crush or break sus rel caps
- Give 1 hr ac or 2 hr pc
- If changing from regular release to sus rel cap, give sus rel 6 hr after last dose of regular release

Patient/family education

- Teach patient to report side effects immediately to prescriber; to take exactly as prescribed; if dose is missed take when remembered if within 3-4 hr of next dose; do not double doses
- Teach patient to complete follow-up appointment with prescriber including pulmonary function studies, chest x-ray
- Instruct patient that dry mouth may be relieved by frequent sips of water, hard candy, sugarless gum
- Caution patient to make position changes from lying to standing slowly to prevent orthostatic hypotension

Evaluation

Positive therapeutic outcome
- Decreased PVCs, ventricular tachycardia

Treatment of overdose: Administer O_2, artificial ventilation, ECG; administer dopamine for circulatory depression; administer diazepam or thiopental for convulsions, isoproterenol

disulfiram (℞)
(dye-sul′fi-ram)
Antabuse, disulfiram
Func. class.: Alcohol deterrent
Chem. class.: Aldehyde dehydrogenase inhibitor
Pregnancy category X

Action: Blocks oxidation of alcohol at acetaldehyde stage; accumulation of acetaldehyde produces the disulfiram-alcohol reaction

Therapeutic Outcome: Disulfiram reaction when alcohol is ingested

Uses: Chronic alcoholism (as adjunct)

Dosage and routes

Adult: PO 250-500 mg qd × 1-2 wk, then 125-500 mg qd until fully socially recovered

Available forms: Tabs 250, 500 mg

Adverse effects

CNS: Headache, drowsiness, restlessness, dizziness, fatigue, tremors, psychosis, neuritis, sweating, ***convulsions, death,*** peripheral neuropathy
GI: Nausea, vomiting, anorexia, severe thirst, ***hepatotoxicity,*** metallic, garliclike aftertaste
INTEG: Rash, dermatitis, urticaria
Disulfiram reaction: Alcohol reaction: flushing, throbbing headache, respiratory difficulty, nausea, vomiting, sweating,

thirst, chest pain, palpitations, dyspnea, hyperventilation, tachycardia, confusion, CV collapse, MI, CHF, convulsions, death

Contraindications: Hypersensitivity, alcohol intoxication, psychoses, CV disease, pregnancy **X**

Precautions: Hypothyroidism, hepatic disease, diabetes mellitus, seizure disorders, nephritis, cerebral damage

Pharmacokinetics	
Absorption	Well absorbed
Distribution	Fat
Metabolism	Liver, oxidized
Excretion	Feces (unchanged)
Half-life	4-10 hr

Pharmacodynamics	
Onset	10 min
Peak	Unknown
Duration	Unknown

Interactions

Individual drugs

Alcohol: Disulfiram reaction
Diazepam: ↑ effects of diazepam
Isoniazid: ↑ effects of isoniazid
Metronidazole: Psychosis
Paraldehyde: ↑ effects of paraldehyde
Phenytoin: ↑ effects of phenytoin

Drug classifications

Antidepressants, tricyclic: ↑ effect of antidepressants

Lab test interferences

↑ Cholesterol
↓ ^{131}I uptake, ↓ PBI, ↓ VMA

NURSING CONSIDERATIONS

Assessment

- Monitor liver function studies q2 wk during therapy: AST (SGOT), ALT (SGPT); these may be elevated
- Monitor CBC, SMA q3-6 mo to detect any abnormality, including increased cholesterol q6 months during treatment
- Assess mental status: affect, mood, drug history, ability to follow treatment, abstain from alcohol
- Assess for signs of hepatotoxicity: jaundice, dark urine, clay-colored stools, abdominal pain

Nursing diagnoses

✓ Coping, ineffective individual (uses)
✓ Noncompliance (teaching)
✓ Knowledge deficit (teaching)

Implementation

- Give only with patient's knowledge; do not give to intoxicated individuals; check other medication for alcohol content
- Give once per day in AM or hs if drowsiness occurs
- Give only after patient has not been drinking for >12 hr
- Tab may be crushed and mixed with beverages

Patient/family education

- Teach patient effect of this drug if alcohol is taken; written consent for disulfiram therapy should be obtained
- Caution patient that shaving lotions, creams, lotions, cough preparations, skin products must be checked for alcohol content; even in small amount, alcohol can produce a reaction; tolerance will not develop if treatment is prolonged
- Teach patient that disulfiram reaction may occur for 2 wk after last dose; to carry ID listing disulfiram therapy
- Teach patient that tabs can be crushed, mixed with beverage
- Advise patient to avoid driv-

ing and hazardous tasks if drowsiness occurs
• Caution patient that disulfiram reaction can be fatal; occurs 15 min after drinking and may last several hr
• Give patient written instructions and symptoms of alcohol-antabuse reaction (nausea, vomiting, flushing, dyspnea, sweating, convulsions, weakness, blurred vision, chest pain, confusion, dizziness, pounding heartbeat, loss of consciousness, heart attack, death)

Evaluation

Positive therapeutic outcome
• Prevention of alcohol intake

Treatment of overdose: IV vitamin C, ephedrine sulfate, antihistamines, O_2

dobutamine (℞)

(doe-byoo′ta-meen)
dobutamine, Dobutrex
Func. class.: Adrenergic direct-acting β_1-agonist, inotropic agent
Chem. class.: Catecholamine

Pregnancy category C

Action: Causes increased contractility, increased coronary blood flow and heart rate by acting on β_1-receptors in heart; minor alpha/beta$_2$ effects

Therapeutic Outcome: Cardiac output increased with decreased fatigue and dyspnea

Uses: Cardiac surgery, refractory heart failure, cardiac decompensation

Investigational uses: Cardiogenic shock in children, congenital heart disease in children undergoing cardiac cath

Dosage and routes

Adult: **IV** inf 2.5-10 μg/kg/min; may increase to 40 μg/kg/min if needed

Child: **IV** inf 7.75 μg/kg/min over 10 min for cardiac cath

Available forms: Inj 12.5 mg/ml

Adverse effects

CNS: *Anxiety,* headache, dizziness
CV: Palpitations, tachycardia, hypertension, PVCs, angina
GI: Heartburn, nausea, vomiting
MS: Muscle cramps (leg)

Contraindications: Hypersensitivity, idiopathic hypertrophic subaortic stenosis

Precautions: Pregnancy **C,** lactation, children, hypertension

Pharmacokinetics	
Absorption	Complete
Distribution	Unknown
Metabolism	Liver
Excretion	Kidney
Half-life	2 min

Pharmacodynamics	
Onset	1-5 min
Peak	10 min
Duration	<10 min

Interactions

Individual drugs

Bretylium: ↑ dysrhythmias
Disopyramide: ↑ hypotension
Guanethidine: ↑ pressor response
Oxytocin: ↑ dysrhythmias
Phenytoin: ↑ hypotension, bradycardia

Drug classifications

Anesthetics: ↑ dysrhythmias
Antidepressants, tricyclic: ↑ pressor response

Antihypertensives: ↑ hypotension
β-Blockers: ↑ pressor response
Cardiac glycosides: ↑ inotropic effect
MAOI: ↑ dysrhythmias

NURSING CONSIDERATIONS
Assessment
- Assess for hypovolemia; if present, correct before beginning treatment with dobutamine; avoid use in patients with atrial fibrillation before digitalization
- Monitor ECG for dysrhythmias, ischemia during treatment; some patients may not need continuous ECG monitoring; also monitor PCWP, CVP, CO_2, urinary output; notify prescriber if <30 ml hr
- Assess for heart failure: bibasilar crackles, S_3 gallop, dyspnea, neck vein distention in patients with cardiomyopathy or CHF
- Assess for oxygenation or perfusion deficit: decreased B/P, chest pain, dizziness, loss of consciousness
- Monitor B/P and pulse q5 min during inf; if B/P drops 30 mm Hg, stop inf and call prescriber
- Monitor ALT (SGOT), AST (SGPT), bilirubin daily
- Monitor for sulfite sensitivity, which may be life threatening

Nursing diagnoses
✓ Cardiac output, decreased (uses)
✓ Knowledge deficit (teaching)

Implementation
IV IV route
- Reconstitute 250 mg/10 ml of D_5W or sterile water for inj; may add another 10 ml to dissolve completely if needed, then dilute in 50 ml or more D_5W, 0.9% NaCl, 0.45% NaCl, D_5/0.45% NaCl, D_5/0.9% NaCl, D_5/LR, LR; titrate to patient response; use inf pump for correct dose

Syringe incompatibility: Doxapram

Syringe compatibilities: Heparin, ranitidine

Y-site compatibilities: Amifostine, amrinone, atracurium, bretylium, calcium chloride, calcium gluconate, ciprofloxacin, diazepam, diltiazem, dopamine, enalaprilat, famotidine, fluconazole, haloperidol, regular insulin, labetalol, lidocaine, magnesium sulfate, meperidine, nitroglycerin, pancuronium, potassium chloride, ranitidine, sodium nitroprusside, streptokinase, tacrolimus, theophylline, thiotepa, tolazoline, vecuronium, verapamil, zidovudine

Y-site incompatibilities: Acyclovir, alteplase, aminophylline, foscarnet, phytonadione

Additive compatibilities: Amiodarone, atracurium, atropine, dopamine, enalaprilat, epinephrine, flumazenil, hydralazine, isoproterenol, lidocaine, meperidine, metaraminol, morphine, nitroglycerin, norepinephrine, phentolamine, phenylephrine, procainamide, propranolol, ranitidine, verapamil

Additive incompatibilities: Acyclovir, aminophylline, bumetanide, calcium gluconate, diazepam, digoxin, furosemide, insulin, magnesium sulfate, phenytoin, potassium phosphate, sodium bicarbonate

D

Patient/family education
- Teach patient reason for medication and expected results, reason for all monitoring and procedures
- Advise patient to report all side effects

Evaluation

Positive therapeutic outcome
- Increased cardiac output
- Decreased PCWP, adequate CVP
- Decreased dyspnea, fatigue, edema, ECG
- Increased urine output

Treatment of overdose: Discontinue drug, support circulation

docusate calcium/ docusate potassium/ docusate sodium (OTC)

(dok'yoo-sate)

DC Softgels, docusate calcium, Pro-Cal-Sof, Sulfalax Calcium, Surfak/Dialose, Diocto-K, Kasof/Colace, Correctol Extra Gentle, Diocto, Dioeze, Disonate, docusate sodium, DOK, DOS Softgel, Doxinate, D-S-S, Modane Soft, Regulex SS, Regutol

Func. class.: Laxative, emollient

Chem. class.: Anionic surfactant

Pregnancy category C

Action: Increases water, fat penetration in intestine; allows for easier passage of stool; increases electrolyte, water secretion in colon

Therapeutic Outcome: Passage of softened stool, absence of constipation

Uses: To soften stools, prevent constipation, soften fecal impaction (rec route)

Dosage and routes

Adult: PO 50-300 mg qd (docusate sodium) or 240 mg (docusate calcium or docusate potassium) prn; enema 5 ml (docusate sodium)

P ***Child >12 yr:*** Enema 2 ml (docusate sodium)

P ***Child 6-12 yr:*** PO 40-120 mg qd (docusate sodium)

P ***Child 3-6 yr:*** PO 20-60 mg qd (docusate sodium)

P ***Child <3 yr:*** PO 10-40 mg qd (docusate sodium)

Available forms: Caps 50, 100, 240, 250, 300 mg; tabs 50, 100 mg; oral sol 10, 50 mg/ml, 16.7, 20 mg/ml; enema conc 18 g/100 ml
Docusate calcium: Caps 50, 240 mg
Docusate potassium: Caps 100, 240 mg
Docusate sodium: Caps 50, 100, 240, 250 mg; tabs 100 mg; syr 50, 60 mg/15 ml; liq 150 mg/15 ml; sol 50 ml/ml; enema 283 mg/3.9 g cap

Adverse effects

EENT: Bitter taste, throat irritation
GI: Nausea, anorexia, cramps, diarrhea
INTEG: Rash

Contraindications: Hypersensitivity, obstruction, fecal impaction, nausea/vomiting

Precautions: Pregnancy **C**

Pharmacokinetics	
Absorption	Minimal (PO)
Distribution	Unknown
Metabolism	Not metabolized
Excretion	Bile
Half-life	Unknown

Pharmacodynamics	PO	REC
Onset	24-72 hr	4-6 hr
Peak	Unknown	Unknown
Duration	Unknown	Unknown

Interactions: None

NURSING CONSIDERATIONS

Assessment

- Assess cramping, rectal bleeding, nausea, vomiting; if these symptoms occur, drug should be discontinued; identify cause of constipation; identify whether fluids, bulk, or exercise is missing from lifestyle

Nursing diagnoses

- ✓ Bowel elimination, altered: constipation (uses)
- ✓ Bowel elimination, altered: diarrhea (side effects)
- ✓ Knowledge deficit (teaching)
- ✓ Noncompliance (teaching)

Implementation

PO route

- Dilute oral sol in juice or other fluid to disguise taste
- Give tabs or caps with 8 oz of liq; give on empty stomach for increased absorption, results

Patient/family education

- Discuss with patient that adequate fluid consumption is as necessary as bulk, exercise for adequate bowel function
- Teach patient that normal bowel movements do not always occur daily
- Advise patient not to use in presence of abdominal pain, nausea, vomiting; tell patient to notify prescriber if unrelieved constipation or if symptoms of electrolyte imbalance occur: muscle cramps, pain, weakness, dizziness, excessive thirst
- Caution patients with heart disease to avoid using the Valsalva maneuver to expedite evacuation

Evaluation

Positive therapeutic outcome

- Decreased constipation within 3 days

donepezil (℞)

(don-ep-ee′zill)

Aricept

Func. class.: Reversible cholinesterase

Pregnancy category C

Action: Elevates acetylcholine concentrations (cerebral cortex) by slowing degradation of acetylcholine released in cholinergic neurons; does not alter underlying dementia

➔ Therapeutic Outcome: Decreased symptoms of Alzheimer's disease

Uses: Treatment of mild to moderate dementia in Alzheimer's disease

Dosage and routes

Adult: PO 5-10 qd

Available forms: Tabs 5, 10 mg

Adverse effects

CNS: Dizziness, insomnia, somnolence, headache, fatigue, abnormal dreams

CV: Hypotension or hypertension

GI: Nausea, vomiting, anorexia

GU: Frequency, UTI, incontinence
INTEG: Rash, flushing
MS: Cramps, arthritis
RESP: Rhinitis, URI, cough, pharyngitis

Contraindications: Hypersensitivity to this drug or piperidine derivatives

Precautions: Sick sinus syndrome, history of ulcers, GI bleeding, hepatic disease, bladder obstruction, asthma, pregnancy **C**, lactation, P children, seizures, asthma, COPD

Pharmacokinetics

Absorption	Well
Distribution	Unknown
Metabolism	Liver to metabolites
Excretion	Unknown
Half-life	10 hr

Pharmacodynamics

Unknown

Interactions

Drug classification

Anticholinergics: ↓ activity
Cholinesterase inhibitors: synergistic effects
Cholinergic agonists: synergistic effects
NSAIDs: ↑ gastric acid secretions

NURSING CONSIDERATIONS

Assessment

- Monitor B/P: hypotension, hypertension
- Assess mental status: affect, mood, behavioral changes, depression, complete suicide assessment
- Assess GI status: nausea, vomiting, anorexia, diarrhea
- Assess GU status: urinary frequency, incontinence

Nursing diagnoses

✓ Confusion, chronic (uses)
✓ Memory, impaired (uses)

Implementation

- Give between meals; may be given with meals for GI symptoms
- Administer dosage adjusted to response no more than q6wk
- Provide assistance with ambulation during beginning therapy; dizziness, ataxia may occur

Patient/family education

- Advise to report side effects: twitching, nausea, vomiting, sweating; indicates overdose
- Advise to use drug exactly as prescribed; at regular intervals, preferably between meals; may be taken with meals for GI upset
- Advise to notify prescriber of nausea, vomiting, diarrhea (dose increase or beginning treatment), or rash
- Advise not to increase or abruptly decrease dose, serious consequences may result

Evaluation

Positive therapeutic outcome

- Decrease in confusion; improved mood

Treatment of overdose: Withdraw drug, administer tertiary anticholinergics, provide supportive care

dopamine (℞)
(doe'pa-meen)
Dopastat, dopamine HCl, Intropin, Revimine ♣
Func. class.: Agonist, vasopressor, inotropic agent
Chem. class.: Catecholamine
Pregnancy category C

Action: Causes increased cardiac output; acts on β_1- and α-receptors, causing vasoconstriction in blood vessels; when low doses are administered, causes renal and mesenteric vasodilatation; β_1 stimulation produces inotropic effects with ↑ cardiac output

Therapeutic Outcome: Increased B/P, cardiac output

Uses: Shock; to increase perfusion; hypotension

Investigational uses: COPD, RDS in infants

Dosage and routes
Adult: **IV** inf 2-5 μg/kg/min, not to exceed 50 μg/kg/min; titrate to patient's response

COPD
Adult: **IV** 4 μg/kg/min

CHF
Adult: **IV** 2-5 μg/kg/min

RDS
Infants: **IV** 5 μg/kg/min

Available forms: Inj 0.8, 1.6, 40, 80, 160 mg/ml

Adverse effects
CNS: Headache
CV: Palpitations, tachycardia, hypertension, ectopic beats, angina, wide QRS complex, peripheral vasoconstriction
GI: Nausea, vomiting, diarrhea
INTEG: Necrosis, tissue sloughing with extravasation, ***gangrene***
RESP: Dyspnea

Contraindications: Hypersensitivity, ventricular fibrillation, tachydysrhythmias, pheochromocytoma

Precautions: Pregnancy **C,** lactation, arterial embolism, peripheral vascular disease

Pharmacokinetics	
Absorption	Complete
Distribution	Widely
Metabolism	Liver
Excretion	Kidney, plasma
Half-life	2 min

Pharmacodynamics	
Onset	2-5 min
Peak	Unknown
Duration	<10 min

Interactions
Individual drugs
Phenytoin: ↑ hypotension, bradycardia
Drug classifications
Anesthetics: ↑ dysrhythmias
Antidepressants, tricyclic: ↑ pressor response
β-Blockers: ↓ cardiac response
Cardiac glycosides: ↑ inotropic effect
MAOIs: ↑ hypertension (severe)

NURSING CONSIDERATIONS
Assessment
- Monitor ECG for dysrhythmias, ischemia during treatment; some patients may not need continuous ECG monitoring; also monitor PCWP, CVP, CO_2, urinary output; notify prescriber if <30 ml/hr
- Assess for heart failure: bibasilar crackles, S_3 gallop, dyspnea, neck vein distention

in patients with cardiomyopathy or CHF
- Assess for oxygenation or perfusion deficit: decreased B/P, chest pain, dizziness, loss of consciousness
- Monitor B/P and pulse q5 min during inf; if B/P drops 30 mm Hg, stop inf and call prescriber
- Check for extravasation: change site q48h

Nursing diagnoses

- ✓ Cardiac output, decreased (uses)
- ✓ Tissue perfusion, altered (uses)
- ✓ Fluid volume excess (uses)
- ✓ Knowledge deficit (teaching)

Implementation

- Give by continuous inf; dilute 200-400 mg/250-500 ml D_5W, 0.9% NaCl, D_5/LR, D_5/0.45% NaCl, D_5/0.9% NaCl, LR; do not use discolored sol; sol is stable for 24 hr; give 0.5-5 μg/kg/min; may increase by 1-4 μg/kg/min q15-30 min until desired patient response; use inf pump

Y-site incompatibilities: Acyclovir, alteplase, indomethacin

Y-site compatibilities: Aldesleukin, amifostine, amrinone, atracurium, ciprofloxacin, diltiazem, dobutamine, enalaprilat, esmolol, famotidine, fluconazole, foscarnet, haloperidol, heparin, hydrocortisone, labetalol, lidocaine, meperidine, midazolam, morphine, nitroglycerin, nitroprusside, norepinephrine, pancuronium, potassium chloride, ranitidine, streptokinase, tacrolimus, theophylline, thiotepa, tolazoline, vecuronium, verapamil, vitamin B with C, zidovudine

Addidtive compatibilities: Aminophylline, atracurium, bretylium, calcium chloride, chloramphenicol, dobutamine, enalaprilat, flumazenil, heparin, hydrocortisone, kanamycin, lidocaine, methylprednisolone, nitroglycerin, oxacillin, potassium chloride, ranitidine, verapamil

Patient/family education

- Teach patient reason for medication, expected results, reason for all monitoring, and procedures
- Advise patient to report all side effects

Evaluation

Positive therapeutic outcome

- Increased cardiac output

Treatment of overdose: Discontinue drug, support circulation; give a short-acting α-blocker (phentolamine)

doxacurium (℞)

(dox'a-cure-ee-yum)

Nuromax

Func. class.: Neuromuscular blocker (nondepolarizing)

Pregnancy category C

Action: Inhibits transmission of nerve impulses by binding with cholinergic receptor sites, antagonizing action of acetylcholine; no analgesic response

➔ **Therapeutic Outcome:** Paralysis of all skeletal muscles

Uses: Facilitation of endotracheal intubation, skeletal muscle relaxation during mechanical ventilation, surgery, or general anesthesia

Dosage and routes
Adult: **IV** 0.05 mg/kg; 0.08 mg/kg is used for prolonged neuromuscular blockade; maintenance 0.025 mg/kg
P ***Child 2-12 yr:*** **IV** 0.03-0.05 mg/kg; may increase for maintenance dose

Available forms: Inj 1 mg/ml

Adverse effects
CV: ***Decreased B/P, ventricular fibrillation, MI, cardiovascular accident***
EENT: Diplopia
INTEG: Rash, urticaria
RESP: ***Prolonged apnea, bronchospasm, wheezing, respiratory depression***
MS: *Weakness,* prolonged skeletal muscle relaxation, ***paralysis***

Contraindications: Hypersensitivity

Precautions: Pregnancy **C**, renal hepatic disease, lactation, P children <3 mo, fluid and electrolyte imbalances, neuromuscular disease, respiratory G disease, obesity, elderly, severe burns

Pharmacokinetics	
Absorption	Complete
Distribution	Unknown
Metabolism	Unknown
Excretion	Kidneys, bile, unchanged
Half-life	½-2 hr; increased in renal transplant patient

Pharmacodynamics	
Onset	Up to 5 min
Peak	Unknown
Duration	1½ hr

Interactions
Individual drugs
Clindamycin: ↑ paralysis length and intensity
Colistin: ↑ paralysis length and intensity
Lidocaine: ↑ paralysis length and intensity
Lithium: ↑ paralysis length and intensity
Magnesium: ↑ paralysis length and intensity
Polymyxin B: ↑ paralysis length and intensity
Procainamide: ↑ paralysis length and intensity
Quinidine: ↑ paralysis length and intensity
Succinylcholine: ↑ paralysis length and intensity
Drug classifications
Aminoglycosides: ↑ paralysis length and intensity
β-Blockers: ↑ paralysis length and intensity
Diuretics, potassium-losing: ↑ paralysis length and intensity
General anesthesia: ↑ paralysis length and intensity

NURSING CONSIDERATIONS
Assessment

- Monitor for electrolyte imbalances (potassium, magnesium) before drug is used; electrolyte imbalances may lead to increased action of this drug
- Monitor vital signs (B/P, pulse, respirations, airway) until fully recovered; rate, depth, pattern of respirations, strength of hand grip; patient should be intubated before use
- Monitor recovery: decreased paralysis of face, diaphragm, leg, arm, rest of body; residual weakness and respiratory problems may occur during recovery period
- Monitor allergic reactions: rash, fever, respiratory distress, pruritus; drug should be discontinued

D

Nursing diagnoses

- ✓ Breathing pattern, ineffective (uses)
- ✓ Communication, impaired verbal (adverse reactions)
- ✓ Anxiety (adverse reactions)
- ✓ Knowledge deficit (teaching)

Implementation

- Anesthesiologist uses peripheral nerve stimulator to determine neuromuscular blockade; deep tendon reflexes should be monitored during extended periods
- Give direct **IV** undiluted over 1 min, or diluted in 1050 ml of D_5W, ½ NaCl or NS and give as an infusion at prescribed rate (only by qualified person, usually an anesthesiologist); do not administer IM
- Further dilute in D_5W, 0.9% NaCl, D_5/0.9% NaCl q15-25 min (intermittent inf)
- Maintenance is given q20-45 min after 1st dose (cont inf); titrate to patient response
- Store in light-resistant area

Solution compatibilities: LR, D_5/LR, D_5/0.9% NaCl

Patient/family education

- Provide reassurance if communication is difficult during recovery from neuromuscular blockade
- Provide explanation to patients regarding all procedures or treatments; patient will remain conscious if anesthesia is not given also

Evaluation

Positive therapeutic outcome

- Paralysis of jaw, eyelid, head, neck, rest of body as evaluated by peripheral nerve stimulator

Treatment of overdose: Administer edrophonium or neostigmine, atropine; monitor VS; may require mechanical ventilation

doxapram (℞)

(dox′a-pram)

Dopram

Func. class.: Analeptic (respiratory/cerebral stimulant)

Pregnancy category B

Action: Respiratory stimulation through activation of peripheral carotid chemoreceptor in low dosages; with higher dosages medullary respiratory centers are stimulated, producing general CNS stimulation

Therapeutic Outcome: Ease of breathing, ABGs at normal limits

Uses: COPD, postanesthesia CNS and respiratory stimulation, prevention of acute hypercapnia, drug-induced CNS depression

Dosage and routes

Postanesthesia stimulation

Adult: **IV** inj 0.5-1 mg/kg, not to exceed 1.5 mg/kg total as a single inj; **IV** inf 250 mg in 250 ml sol, not to exceed 4 mg/kg; run at 1-3 mg/min

Drug-induced CNS depression

Adult: **IV** priming **IV** dose of 2 mg/kg, repeated in 5 min; repeat q1-2h until patient awakens; **IV** inf priming dose 2 mg/kg at 1-3 mg/min, not to exceed 3 g/day

COPD (hypercapnia)

Adult: **IV** inf 1-2 mg/min, not to exceed 3 mg/min for no longer than 2 hr

Available forms: Inj **IV** 20 mg/ml

Adverse effects

CNS: ***Convulsions*** (clonus/generalized), *headache,* restlessness, dizziness, confusion, paresthesias, flushing, sweating, bilateral Babinski's sign, rigidity, depression

CV: Chest pain, hypertension, change in heart rate, lowered T waves, tachycardia, arrhythmias

EENT: Pupil dilation, sneezing

GI: Nausea, vomiting, diarrhea, hiccups

GU: Retention, incontinence

INTEG: Pruritus, irritation at inj site

RESP: ***Laryngospasm, bronchospasm,*** rebound hypoventilation, dyspnea, cough, tachypnea, hiccups

Contraindications: Hypersensitivity, seizure disorders, severe hypertension, severe bronchial asthma, severe dyspnea, severe cardiac disorders, pneumothorax, pulmonary embolism, severe respiratory disease, P newborns

Precautions: Bronchial asthma, pheochromocytoma, severe tachycardia, dysrhythmias, pregnancy **B,** hypertension, lactation, P children

Pharmacokinetics	
Absorption	Complete
Distribution	Unknown
Metabolism	Liver
Excretion	Kidneys, metabolites
Half-life	2.5-4 hr

Pharmacodynamics	
Onset	20-40 sec
Peak	1-2 min
Duration	5-10 min

Interactions

Individual drugs

Enflurane: ↑ dysrhythmias

Halothane: ↑ dysrhythmias

Drug classifications

MAOI: ↑ hypertension

Skeletal muscle relaxants: May mask the effects of skeletal muscle relaxants

Sympathomimetics: Synergistic pressor effect

NURSING CONSIDERATIONS

Assessment

- Monitor B/P, heart rate, deep tendon reflexes, level of consciousness, ABGs before administration q30 min; check for Po_2, Pco_2, O_2 saturation during treatment
- Monitor ECG; watch for hypertension, increased pulse, increased pulmonary artery pressures
- Monitor for hypertension; dysrhythmias, tachycardia, dyspnea, skeletal muscle hyperactivity; may indicate overdosage; discontinue if these occur
- Assess for respiratory stimulation: increased respiratory rate, depth, abnormal rhythm; check for patent airway; elevate head of bed to 45 degrees or higher, position patient on side
- Check for extravasation: redness, inflammation, pain; may cause phlebitis; change **IV** site q48h

Nursing diagnoses

✓ Breathing pattern, ineffective (uses)
✓ Impaired gas exchange (uses)
✓ Knowledge deficit (teaching)

Implementation

- May give by **IV** diluted with equal parts of sterile water for inj; may be diluted 250 mg/250 ml (1 mg/ml) of D_5W, $D_{10}W$ (dilute 400 mg/180 ml

D

of compatible IV sol [2 mg/ml]) and run as inf over 2 hr
• Give **IV** undiluted over 5 min; **IV** inf at 1-3 mg/min; adjust for desired respiratory response, using inf pump **IV**; if an inf is used after initial dose, start at 1-3 mg/min; adjust for desired respiratory response, using inf pump **IV**; if an inf is used after initial dose, start at 1-3 mg/min depending on patient response; D/C after 2 hr; wait 1-2 hr and repeat
• Give only after adequate airway is established; ensure O_2, **IV** barbiturates, resuscitative equipment available
• Discontinue inf if side effects occur; narrow margin of safety

Syringe compatibilities: Amikacin, bumetadine, chlorpromazine, cimetidine, cisplatin, cyclophosphamide, dopamine, doxycycline, epinephrine, hydroxyzine, imipramine, isoniazid, lincomycin, methotrexate, netilmicin, phytonadione, pyridoxine, terbutaline, thiamine, tobramycin, vincristine

Syringe incompatibilities: Aminophylline, ascorbic acid, cefoperazone, cefotaxime, cefotetan, cefuroxime, dexamethasone, diazepam, digoxin, dobutamine, folic acid, furosemide, hydrocortisone, ketamine, methylprednisolone, minocycline, thiopental, ticarcillin

Patient/family education
• Teach all aspects of drug, purpose, expected reactions
• Caution patient if difficulty breathing or shortness of breath occurs to notify nurse or prescriber

Evaluation
Positive therapeutic outcome
• Increased breathing capacity
• ABGs WNL for patient

Treatment of overdose: Lavage, activated charcoal; monitor electrolytes, VS; diazepam for seizures; discontinue inf

doxazosin (℞)
(dox-ay'zoe-sin)
Cardura
Func. class.: Peripheral α-adrenergic blocker, antihypertensive
Chem. class.: Quinazoline
Pregnancy category B

Action: Peripheral blood vessels are dilated, peripheral resistance lowered; reduction in B/P results from α-adrenergic receptors being blocked

Therapeutic Outcome: Decreased B/P, decreased symptoms of BPH

Uses: Hypertension alone or as an adjunct, urinary outflow obstruction, symptoms of benign prostatic hyperplasia

Investigational uses: CHF with digoxin and diuretics

Dosage and routes
Adult: PO 1 mg qd, increasing up to 16 mg qd if required; usual range 4-16 mg/day

Available forms: Tabs 1, 2, 4, 8 mg

Adverse effects
CNS: Dizziness, headache, drowsiness, anxiety, depression, vertigo, weakness, fatigue, asthenia

CV: Palpitations, orthostatic hypotension, tachycardia, edema, dysrhythmias, chest pain
EENT: Epistaxis, tinnitus, dry mouth, red sclera, pharyngitis, rhinitis
GI: Nausea, vomiting, diarrhea, constipation, abdominal pain
GU: Incontinence, polyuria

Contraindications: Hypersensitivity to quinazolines

Precautions: Pregnancy **B**, P children, lactation, hepatic disease

Pharmacokinetics

Absorption	Well absorbed
Distribution	Not known; 98% plasma protein bound
Metabolism	Liver, extensively (<63%)
Excretion	Kidneys
Half-life	22 hr

Pharmacodynamics

Onset	2 hr
Peak	2-6 hr
Duration	6-12 hr

Interactions

Individual drugs

Clonidine: ↓ effects of clonidine
Indomethacin: ↓ hypotensive effects
Verapamil: ↑ hypotensive effects

Drug classifications

β-blockers: ↑ postural hypotension

Lab test interferences

False positive: Urine acetone

NURSING CONSIDERATIONS

Assessment

- Monitor B/P, orthostatic hypotension, syncope; check for edema in feet, legs daily; I&O; monitor for weight daily; notify prescriber of changes
- Assess for orthostatic hypotension; tell patient to rise slowly from sitting or lying position

Nursing diagnoses

- ✓ Cardiac output, decreased (uses)
- ✓ Injury, potential for physical (side effects)
- ✓ Knowledge deficit (teaching)
- ✓ Noncompliance (teaching)

Implementation

- Store in tight container at 86° F (30° C) or less
- May be used in combination with other antihypertensives
- May be given with food to prevent GI symptoms

Patient/family education

- Teach patient not to discontinue drug abruptly; emphasize the importance of complying with dosage schedule, even if feeling better; if dose is missed take as soon as remembered; take at same time each day
- Teach patient not to use OTC products (cough, cold, allergy) unless directed by prescriber; also to avoid large amounts of caffeine
- Emphasize the need to rise slowly to sitting or standing position to minimize orthostatic hypotension
- Teach patient to notify prescriber of mouth sores, sore throat, fever, swelling of hands or feet, irregular heartbeat, chest pain
- Caution patient to report excessive perspiration, dehydration, vomiting, diarrhea; may lead to fall in B/P
- Caution patient that drug may cause dizziness, fainting, lightheadedness; may occur

during 1st few days of therapy; to avoid hazardous activities
• Teach patient how to take B/P, and normal readings for age group; to take B/P q7 days

Evaluation

Positive therapeutic outcome
• Decreased B/P in hypertension
• Decreased symptoms in BP

Treatment of overdose: Administer volume expanders or vasopressors; discontinue drug; place in supine position

doxepin (℞)

(dox'e-pin)

doxepin HCl, Sinequan, Sinequan Concentrate, Triadapin ✤

Func. class.: Antidepressant, tricyclic; antianxiety

Chem. class.: Dibenzoxepin, tertiary amine

Pregnancy category C

Action: Blocks reuptake of norepinephrine, serotonin into nerve endings, increasing action of norepinephrine, serotonin in nerve cells; has anticholinergic effects

➔ Therapeutic Outcome: Decreased symptoms of depression after 2-3 wk

Uses: Major depression, anxiety

Investigational uses: Chronic pain management

Dosage and routes

Adult: PO 50-75 mg/day in divided doses; may increase to 300 mg/day or may give daily dose hs

Available forms: Caps 10, 25, 50, 75, 100, 150 mg; oral conc 10 mg/ml

Adverse effects

CNS: Dizziness, drowsiness, confusion, headache, anxiety, tremors, stimulation, weakness, insomnia, nightmares, G extrapyramidal symptoms (elderly), increased psychiatric symptoms, paresthesia

CV: Orthostatic hypotension, ECG changes, tachycardia, ***hypertension,*** palpitations

EENT: Blurred vision, tinnitus, mydriasis, ophthalmoplegia, glossitis

GI: Diarrhea, dry mouth, nausea, vomiting, ***paralytic ileus,*** increased appetite, cramps, epigastric distress, jaundice, ***hepatitis,*** stomatitis, constipation

GU: Retention, ***acute renal failure***

HEMA: ***Agranulocytosis, thrombocytopenia, eosinophilia, leukopenia***

INTEG: Rash, urticaria, sweating, pruritus, photosensitivity

Contraindications: Hypersensitivity to tricyclic antidepressants, urinary retention, narrow-angle glaucoma, prostatic hypertrophy

Precautions: Suicidal patients, G elderly, pregnancy **C**

Pharmacokinetics	
Absorption	Well absorbed
Distribution	Widely distributed; crosses placenta
Metabolism	Liver, extensively
Excretion	Kidneys, breast milk
Half-life	8-21 hr

Pharmacodynamics
Unknown

Interactions

Individual drugs

Alcohol: ↑ CNS depression
Cimetidine: ↑ levels, toxicity
Clonidine: Severe hypotension; avoid use
Disulfiram: Organic brain syndrome
Fluoxetine: ↑ levels, toxicity
Guanethidine: ↓ effects of guanethidine

Drug classifications

Analgesics: ↑ CNS depression
Anticholinergics: ↑ side effects
Antihistamines: ↑ CNS depression
Antihypertensives: May block antihypertensive effect
Barbiturates: ↑ effects
Benzodiazepines: ↑ effects
CNS depressants: ↑ effects
MAOI: Hypertensive crisis, convulsions
Oral contraceptives: ↑ effects, toxicity
Phenothiazines: ↑ toxicity
Sedative/hypnotics: ↑ CNS depression
Sympathomimetics, indirect acting: ↓ effects

Smoking

↑ metabolism, ↓ effects

Lab test interferences

↑ Serum bilirubin, ↑ blood glucose, ↑ alkaline phosphatase
↓ VMA, ↓ 5-HIAA, ↓ blood glucose
False ↑ Urinary catecholamines

NURSING CONSIDERATIONS

Assessment

- Monitor B/P (with patient lying, standing), pulse q4h; if systolic B/P drops 20 mm Hg, hold drug, notify prescriber; take vs q4h in patients with cardiovascular disease
- Monitor blood studies: CBC, leukocytes, differential, cardiac enzymes if patient is receiving long-term therapy
- Monitor hepatic studies: AST (SGOT), ALT (SGPT), bilirubin
- Check weight weekly; appetite may increase with drug
- Assess ECG for flattening of T wave, bundle branch block, AV block, dysrhythmias in cardiac patients
- Assess for extrapyramidal G symptoms primarily in elderly: rigidity, dystonia, akathisia
- Assess mental status: mood, sensorium, affect, suicidal tendencies; increase in psychiatric symptoms: depression, panic
- Monitor urinary retention, constipation; constipation is P more likely to occur in children G or elderly
- Assess for withdrawal symptoms: headache, nausea, vomiting, muscle pain, weakness; do not usually occur unless drug was discontinued abruptly
- Identify alcohol consumption; if alcohol is consumed, hold dose until AM

Nursing diagnoses

✓ Coping, ineffective individual (uses)
✓ Injury, risk for (side effects)
✓ Knowledge deficit (teaching)

Implementation

- Give with food or milk for GI symptoms; dilute concentrate with fruit juice, water, milk to disguise taste
- Give dosage hs if oversedation occurs during day; may G take entire dose hs; elderly may not tolerate once/day dosing
- Store at room temp; do not freeze

Patient/family education

- Tell patient that therapeutic effects may take 2-3 wk; to use caution in driving and other activities requiring alertness because of drowsiness, dizziness, blurred vision
- Advise patient to avoid rising quickly from sitting to standing, especially elderly
- Teach patient to avoid alcohol ingestion, other CNS depressants; not to discontinue medication quickly after long-term use: may cause nausea, headache, malaise
- Teach patient to wear sunscreen or large hat, since photosensitivity occurs
- Teach patient to increase fluids, bulk in diet if constipation, urinary retention occur, especially elderly; to take gum, hard sugarless candy, or frequent sips of water for dry mouth

Evaluation

Positive therapeutic outcome

- Decrease in depression
- Absence of suicidal thoughts

Treatment of overdose: ECG monitoring, induce emesis, lavage, activated charcoal, administer anticonvulsant

doxorubicin (℞)

(dox-oh-roo'bi-sin)

Adriamycin, Adriamycin PFS, Adriamycin RDF, doxorubicin HCl, Rubex

Func. class.: Antineoplastic, antibiotic

Chem. class.: Anthracycline glycoside

Pregnancy category D

Action: Inhibits DNA synthesis primarily; derived from *Streptomyces peucetius;* replication is decreased by binding to DNA, which causes strand splitting; active throughout entire cell cycle; a vesicant

Therapeutic Outcome: Prevention of rapidly growing malignant cells

Uses: Wilms' tumor; bladder, breast, cervical, head, neck, liver, lung, ovarian, prostatic, stomach, testicular, thyroid cancer; Hodgkin's disease; acute lymphoblastic leukemia; myeloblastic leukemia; neuroblastomas; lymphomas; sarcomas

Dosage and routes

Adult: 60-75 mg/m^2 q3 wk, or 30 mg/m^2 on days 1-3 of 4-wk cycle, not to exceed 550 mg/m^2 cumulative dose

Available forms: Inj 10, 20, 50 mg

Adverse effects

CV: Increased B/P, ***sinus tachycardia, PVCs,*** chest pain, ***bradycardia, extrasystole***

GI: Nausea, vomiting, anorexia, mucositis, ***hepatotoxicity***

GU: Impotence, sterility, amenorrhea, gynecomastia, hyperuricemia

HEMA: Thrombocytopenia, leukopenia, anemia
INTEG: Rash, necrosis at inj site, dermatitis, reversible alopecia, cellulitis, thrombophlebitis at inj site

Contraindications: Hypersensitivity, pregnancy (1st trimester) **D,** lactation, systemic infections

Precautions: Renal, hepatic, cardiac disease, gout, bone marrow suppression (severe)

Pharmacokinetics

Absorption	Complete bioavailability
Distribution	Widely distributed; crosses placenta
Metabolism	Liver, extensively
Excretion	Bile (40%-50%)
Half-life	12 min; 3½ hr, 29⅔ hr

Pharmacodynamics

Unknown

Interactions

Individual drugs
Cyclophosphamide: ↑ cardiotoxicity, CHF
Mercaptopurine: ↑ liver disorders, hepatitis
Radiation: ↑ toxicity, bone marrow suppression
Drug classifications
Antineoplastics: ↑ toxicity, bone marrow suppression
Live virus vaccines: ↑ adverse reactions, ↓ antibody response
Lab test interferences
↑ Uric acid

NURSING CONSIDERATIONS

Assessment

- Monitor ECG; watch for ST-T wave changes, low QRS and T; possible dysrhythmias (sinus tachycardia, heart block, PVCs) may occur
- Assess buccal cavity q8h for dryness, sores or ulceration, white patches, pain, bleeding, dysphagia; obtain prescription for viscous lidocaine (Xylocaine)
- Assess symptoms indicating severe allergic reaction: rash, pruritus, urticaria, purpuric skin lesions, itching, flushing; drug should be discontinued
- Assess tachypnea, ECG changes, dyspnea, edema, fatigue
- Monitor CBC, differential, platelet count weekly; withhold drug if WBC count is <4000/mm³ or platelet count is <100,000/mm³; notify prescriber of results if WBC <20,000/mm³, platelets <150,000/mm³
- Assess for increased uric acid levels, swelling, joint pain, primarily extremities; patient should be well hydrated to prevent urate deposits
- Monitor renal function studies: BUN, creatinine, serum uric acid, urine CrCl before and during therapy; I&O ratio; report fall in urine output to <30 ml/hr
- Monitor temp q4h (may indicate beginning of infection)
- Monitor liver function tests before and during therapy (bilirubin, AST [SGOT], ALT [SGPT], LDH) as needed or monthly; note yellowing of skin or sclera, dark urine, clay-colored stools, itchy skin, abdominal pain, fever, diarrhea
- Assess for bleeding: hematuria, stool guaiac, bruising or petechiae, mucosa or orifices q8h; inflammation of mucosa, breaks in skin
- Identify effects of alopecia on body image; discuss feelings about body changes

Nursing diagnoses

- ✓ Injury, risk for (adverse reactions)
- ✓ Body image disturbance (adverse reactions)
- ✓ Infection, risk for (adverse reactions)
- ✓ Knowledge deficit (teaching)

Implementation

- Avoid contact with skin; very irritating; wash completely to remove; give fluids **IV** or PO before chemotherapy to hydrate patient
- Give antiemetic 30-60 min before giving drug to prevent vomiting and prn; give antibiotics for prophylaxis of infection
- Provide liq diet: carbonated beverages; gelatin may be added if patient is not nauseated or vomiting
- Help patient to rinse mouth tid-qid with water or club soda, brush teeth bid-qid with soft brush or cotton-tipped applicators for stomatitis, use unwaxed dental floss
- Drug should be prepared by experienced personnel using proper precautions
- Give **IV** after diluting 10 mg/5 ml of NaCl for inj; another 5 ml of diluent/10 mg is recommended; shake; give over 3-5 min; give through Y-tube or 3-way stopcock through free-flowing D_5 inf or NS
- Use hydrocortisone, dexamethasone, or sodium bicarbonate (1 mEq/1 ml) for extravasation: apply ice compress

Syringe compatibilities: Bleomycin, cisplatin, cyclophosphamide, droperidol, fluorouracil, leucovorin, methotrexate, metoclopramide, mitomycin, vincristine

Syringe compatibilities: Furoscmide, heparin

Y-site compatibilities: Amifostine, aztreonam, bleomycin, cimetidine, cisplatin, cyclophosphamide, droperidol, famotidine, filgrastim, fludarabine, fluorouracil, granisetron, leucovorin calcium, methotrexate, metoclopramide, mitomycin, paclitaxel, teniposide, thiotepa,vinblastine, vincristine

Y-site incompatibilities: Furosemide, heparin

Additive incompatibilities: Aminophylline, cephalothin, dexamethasone, diazepam, fluorouracil, hydrocortisone

Additive compatibilities: Ondansetron

Patient/family education

- Tell patient that urine and other body fluids may be red-orange for 48 hr; contraceptive measures are recommended during therapy; drug is teratogenic to fetus
- Advise patient to avoid use of products containing aspirin or ibuprofen, razors, commercial mouthwash, since bleeding may occur; to report symptoms of bleeding (hematuria, tarry stools)
- Instruct patient to report signs of anemia (fatigue, headache, irritability, faintness, shortness of breath)
- Inform patient that hair may be lost during treatment; a wig or hair piece may make patient feel better; new hair may be different in color, texture
- Caution patient not to have any vaccinations without the advice of the prescriber; serious reactions can occur

Evaluation

Positive therapeutic outcome

- Prevention of rapid division of malignant cells

doxycycline (℞)

(dox-i-sye'kleen)

Apo-Doxy ✱, Doryx, Doxy 100, Doxy 200, Doxy-Caps, Doxychel Hyclate, Doxycin ✱, doxycycline, Monodox, Novodoxyclin ✱, Vibramycin, Vibramycin IV, Vibra-Tabs, Vovox

Func. class.: Broad-spectrum antibiotic/antiinfective

Chem. class.: Tetracycline

Pregnancy category D

Action: Inhibits protein synthesis, phosphorylation in microorganisms by binding to 30S ribosomal subunits, reversibly binding to 50S ribosomal subunits; bacteriostatic

Therapeutic Outcome: Bactericidal action against the following: gram-positive pathogens *Bacillus anthracis, Clostridium perfringens, C. tetani, Listeria monocytogenes, Nocardia, Propionibacterium acnes, Actinomyces israelii;* gram-negative pathogens *Haemophilus influenzae, Legionella pneumophila, Yersinia enterocolitica, V. pestis, Neisseria gonorrhoeae, N. meningitidis, Mycoplasma, Chlamydia, Rickettsia*

Uses: Syphilis, gonorrhea, lymphogranuloma venereum, uncommon gram-negative or positive organisms, malaria prophylaxis

Investigational uses: Traveler's diarrhea, Lyme disease, prevention of chronic bronchitis

Dosage and routes

Adult: PO 100 mg q12h on day 1, then 100 mg/day; **IV** 200 mg in 1-2 inf on day 1, then 100-200 mg/day

P ***Child >8 yr:*** PO/**IV** 4.4 mg/kg/day in divided doses q12h on day 1, then 2.2-4.4 mg/kg/day

Gonorrhea (Patients allergic to penicillin)

Adult: Uncomplicated, PO 200 mg, then 100 mg hs and 100 mg bid × 3 days or 300 mg, then 300 mg in 1 hr; disseminated, 100 mg PO bid × at least 7 days

Chlamydia trachomatis

Adult: PO 100 mg bid × 7days

Syphilis

Adult: PO 300 mg/day in divided doses × 10 days

Available forms: Tabs 50, 100 mg; caps 50, 100 mg; syr 50 mg/ml; powder for inj 100, 200 mg; powder for oral susp 25 mg/5 ml

Adverse effects

CNS: Fever

CV: Pericarditis

EENT: Dysphagia, glossitis, decreased calcification of deciduous teeth, oral candidiasis

GI: Nausea, abdominal pain, vomiting, diarrhea, anorexia, enterocolitis, ***hepatotoxicity,*** flatulence, abdominal cramps, gastric burning, stomatitis

GU: Increased BUN

HEMA: ***Eosinophilia, neutropenia, thrombocytopenia, hemolytic anemia***

INTEG: Rash, urticaria, photosensitivity, increased pigmentation, ***exfoliative dermatitis,*** pruritus, ***angioedema***

Contraindications: Hypersensitivity to tetracyclines, P children <8 yr, pregnancy **D**

Precautions: Hepatic disease, lactation

Pharmacokinetics

Absorption	Well absorbed
Distribution	Widely distributed, crosses placenta
Metabolism	Some hepatic recycling
Excretion	Bile, feces; kidneys unchanged (20%-40%)
Half-life	15-22 hr; increased in severe renal disease

Pharmacodynamics

	PO	IV
Onset	1½-4 hr	Immediate
Peak	1.5-4 hr	Infusion's end

Interactions

Individual drugs

Calcium: Forms chelates, ↓ absorption

Carbamazepine: ↑ effect of carbamazepine

Iron: Forms chelates, ↓ absorption

Magnesium: Forms chelates, ↓ absorption

Phenytoin: ↓ effect of doxycycline

Drug classifications

Anticoagulants, oral: ↑ effect of anticoagulants

Barbiturates: ↓ effect of doxycycline

Contraceptives, oral: ↓ effect of oral contraceptive

Food

↓ absorption with dairy products

Lab test interferences

False ↑ Urinary catecholamines, false ↑ ALT (SGOT), false ↑ AST (SGPT)

False negative: Urine glucose

NURSING CONSIDERATIONS

Assessment

- Assess patient for previous sensitivity reaction
- Assess patient for signs and symptoms of infection including characteristics of wounds, sputum, urine, stool, WBC >10,000, fever; obtain baseline information before and during treatment
- Obtain C&S before beginning drug therapy to identify if correct treatment has been initiated
- Assess for allergic reactions: rash, urticaria, pruritus, chills, fever, joint pain; angioedema may occur a few days after therapy begins
- Assess bowel pattern daily; if severe diarrhea occurs, drug should be discontinued
- Monitor for bleeding: ecchymosis, bleeding gums, hematuria, stool guaiac daily if on long-term therapy; blood dyscrasias may occur
- Assess for overgrowth of infection: perineal itching, fever, malaise, redness, pain, swelling, drainage, rash, diarrhea, change in cough, sputum

Nursing diagnoses

- ✓ Infection, risk for (uses)
- ✓ Diarrhea (side effects)
- ✓ Injury, risk for (side effects)
- ✓ Knowledge deficit (teaching)
- ✓ Noncompliance (teaching)

Implementation

PO route

- ⊘ Do not crush, chew caps
- Give around the clock to maintain proper blood levels; give with food to increase absorption of drug; do not give within 3 hr of other agents; drug reactions may occur

• Give with 8 oz of water, 1 hr before hs to prevent ulceration
• Shake liq preparation well before giving; use calibrated device for proper dosing
• Do not give with iron, calcium, magnesium products or antacids, which decrease absorption and form insoluble chelate

IV **IV route**
• Check for irritation, extravasation, phlebitis daily; change site q72h
• For intermittent inf, dilute each 100 mg/10 ml 0.9% NaCl, sterile water for inj; further dilute in at least 100 ml 0.9% NaCl, D_5W, Ringer's, LR, D_5/LR; protect from direct light; give over 1-4 hr

Y-site incompatibility: Hetastarch

Y-site compatibilities: Acyclovir, amifostine, amiodarone, aztreonam, cyclophosphamide, diltiazem, filgrastim, fludarabine, hydromorphone, magnesium sulfate, melphalan, meperidine, morphine, ondansetron, perphenazine, sargramostim, tacrolimus, teniposide, theophylline, thiotepa, vinorelbine

Additive compatibility: Ranitidine

Syringe compatibility: Doxapram

Patient/family education
• Teach patient to report sore throat, bruising, bleeding, joint pain; may indicate blood dyscrasias (rare)
• Advise patient to contact prescriber if vaginal itching, loose, foul-smelling stools, furry tongue occur; may indicate superinfection; report itching, rash, pruritus, urticaria
• Instruct patient to take all medication prescribed for the length of time ordered; drug must be taken around the clock to maintain blood levels; do not give medication to others
• Advise patient to notify prescriber of diarrhea with blood or pus

Evaluation
Positive therapeutic outcome
• Absence of signs/symptoms of infection (WBC <10,000, temp WNL, absence of red draining wounds)
• Reported improvement in symptoms of infection

droperidol (℞)
(droe-per'i-dole)
Droperidol, Inapsine
Func. class.: Neuroleptic, tranquilizer, antiemetic
Chem. class.: Butyrophenone derivative
Pregnancy category C

Action: Acts on CNS at subcortical levels, producing tranquilization, sleep; antiemetic

➔ **Therapeutic Outcome:** Maintenance of anesthesia

Uses: Premedication for surgery; induction, maintenance in general anesthesia; postoperatively for nausea and vomiting

Dosage and routes
Induction
Adult: **IV**/IM 0.22-0.275 mg/kg given with analgesic or general anesthetic; may give 1.25-2.5 mg additionally

P ***Child 2-12 yr:*** **IV**/IM 88-165

μg/kg, titrated to response needed

Premedication

Adult: IM/**IV** 2.5-10 mg ½-1 hr before surgery

P ***Child 2-12 yr:*** IM/**IV** 88-165 μg/kg

Maintaining general anesthesia

Adult: **IV** 1.25-2.5 mg

Regional anesthesia adjunct

Adult: IM/**IV** 2.5-5 mg

Diagnostic procedures without general anesthesia

Adult: IM 2.5-10 mg ½-1 hr before procedure; 1.25-2.5 mg may be needed additionally

Available forms: Inj 2.5 mg/ml

Adverse effects

CNS: Dystonia, akathisia, flexion of arms, fine tremors, dizziness, anxiety, drowsiness, restlessness, hallucinations, depression
CV: Tachycardia, hypotension
EENT: Upward rotation of eyes, oculogyric crisis
INTEG: Chills, facial sweating, shivering
RESP: Laryngospasm, bronchospasm

Contraindications: Hyper-P sensitivity, child <2 yr, pregnancy **C**

G **Precautions:** Elderly, cardiovascular disease (hypotension, bradydysrhythmias), renal disease, liver disease, Parkinson's disease

Pharmacokinetics

Absorption	Well absorbed (IM)
Distribution	Crosses blood-brain barrier, placenta
Metabolism	Liver
Excretion	Kidneys, unchanged (10%)
Half-life	Unknown

Pharmacodynamics

	IM/IV
Onset	3-10 min
Peak	30 min
Duration	3-6 hr

Interactions

Individual drugs

Alcohol: ↑ CNS depression
Lithium: ↑ side effects of lithium

Drug classifications

Amphetamines: ↓ effects of amphetamines
Anticholinergics: ↓ effects of anticholinergics
Anticoagulants: ↓ effects of anticoagulants
Anticonvulsants: ↓ effects of anticonvulsants
Antiparkinsonian agents: ↓ effects of antiparkinsonian agents
Antipsychotics: ↑ CNS depression
Barbiturates: ↑ CNS depression
CNS depressants: ↑ CNS depression
Narcotics: ↑ CNS depression

NURSING CONSIDERATIONS

Assessment

- Check VS q10 min during **IV** administration, q30 min after IM dose; for increasing heart rate or decreasing B/P, notify prescriber at once; do not place patient in Trendelenburg's position, or sympathetic blockade may occur, causing respiratory arrest
- Assess extrapyramidal reactions: dystonia, akathisia, extended neck, restlessness, tremors; if these occur, an anticholinergic should be given
- If given for nausea or vomiting, monitor for significant loss

of fluids, bowel sounds before and during administration

Nursing diagnoses

✓ Injury, risk for (adverse reactions)

✓ Knowledge deficit (teaching)

Implementation

IM route

- Give deeply in large muscle mass

IV **IV route**

- Give direct **IV** undiluted; give through Y-tube or 3-way stopcock at 10 mg or less/min; titrate to patient response
- Intermittent inf may be given by adding dose to 250 ml LR, D_5W, 0.9% NaCl; give slowly
- Give anticholinergics (benztropine, diphenhydramine) for extrapyramidal reaction
- Give only with crash cart, resuscitative equipment nearby

Syringe compatibilities: Atropine, bleomycin, butorphanol, chlorpromazine, cimetidine, cisplatin, cyclophosphamide, dimenhydrinate, diphenhydramine, doxorubicin, fentanyl, glycopyrrolate, hydroxyzine, meperidine, metoclopramide, midazolam, mitomycin, morphine, nalbuphine, pentazocine, perphenazine, prochlorperazine, promazine, promethazine, scopolamine, vinblastine, vincristine

Syringe incompatibilities: Fluorouracil, furosemide, heparin, leucovorin, methotrexate, pentobarbital

Y-site compatibilities: Amifostine, aztreonam, bleomycin, buprenorphine, cisplatin, cyclophosphamide, cytarabine, doxorubicin, filgrastim, fluconazole, fludarabine, hydrocortisone sodium succinate, idarubicin, melphalen, meperidine, metoclopramide, mitomycin, ondansetron, paclitaxel, potassium chloride, sargramostim, teniposide, thiotepa, vinblastine, vincristine, vitamin B with C

Y-site incompatibilities: Fluorouracil, foscarnet, furosemide, leucovorin, methotrexate, nafcillin

Additive incompatibility: Barbiturates

Patient/family education

- Advise patient that orthostatic hypotension is common; to rise from lying or sitting position slowly
- Caution patient that drowsiness may occur; to call for assistance for ambulation

Evaluation

Positive therapeutic outcome

- Decreased anxiety
- Absence of vomiting during and after surgery

dyphylline (℞)

(dye'fi-lin)

Dilor, Dyflex-200, Dyflex-400, Dylline, dyphylline, Lufyllin, Lufyllin-400, Neothylline, Protophylline ❁

Func. class.: Bronchodilator, phosphodiesterase inhibitor

Chem. class.: Xanthine, ethylenediamide

Pregnancy category C

Action: Relaxes smooth muscle of respiratory system by blocking phosphodiesterase, which increases cyclic AMP;

cyclic AMP results in positive inotropic, chronotropic effects, bronchodilatation, stimulation of CNS

➔ **Therapeutic Outcome:** Bronchodilatation with ease of breathing

Uses: Bronchial asthma, bronchospasm in chronic bronchitis, COPD

Dosage and routes

Adult: PO 200-800 mg q6h; IM 250-500 mg q6h injected slowly

Available forms: Tabs 200, 400 mg; elix 100, 160 mg/15 ml; inj 250 mg/ml

Adverse effects

CNS: Anxiety, restlessness, insomnia, dizziness, ***convulsions,*** headache, lightheadedness, muscle twitching

CV: Palpitations, sinus tachycardia, hypotension, flushing, dysrhythmias

GI: Nausea, vomiting, anorexia, dyspepsia, epigastric pain

INTEG: Flushing, urticaria

OTHER: Fever, dehydration, ***albuminuria,*** hyperglycemia

RESP: Tachypnea

Contraindications: Hypersensitivity to xanthines, tachydysrhythmias

G **Precautions:** Elderly, CHF, cor pulmonale, hepatic disease, active peptic ulcer disease, diabetes mellitus, hyperthy-
P roidism, hypertension, children, renal disease, pregnancy **C**, glaucoma

Pharmacokinetics

Absorption	Well absorbed (PO)
Distribution	Unknown
Metabolism	Liver
Excretion	Kidneys (85%)
Half-life	2 hr; increased in renal disease

Pharmacodynamics

	PO	IM
Onset	Unknown	Unknown
Peak	1 hr	Unknown
Duration	6 hr	Unknown

Interactions

Individual drugs

Cimetidine: ↓ metabolism, ↑ toxicity

Ketamine: Do not use together; seizures may occur

Drug classifications

Barbiturates: ↓ effect of dyphylline

β-Adrenergic blockers: ↓ metabolism, ↑ toxicity

Benzodiazepines: ↓ sedative effect

Sympathomimetics: ↑ CNS, CV adverse reactions

Smoking

↑ metabolism, ↓ effect

Food

Caffeinated foods (cola, coffee, tea, chocolate): ↑ CNS, CV, adverse reactions

NURSING CONSIDERATIONS

Assessment

- Monitor dyphylline blood levels (therapeutic level is <20 μg/ml); toxicity may occur with small increase above 20
G μg/ml, especially elderly; determine whether theophylline was given recently (24 hr)
- Monitor I&O; an increase in diuresis occurs; dehydration
G may result in elderly or
P children
- Assess respiratory rate, rhythm, depth; before and during treatment auscultate

lung fields bilaterally; notify prescriber of abnormalities
• Assess for allergic reactions: rash, urticaria; if these occur, drug should be discontinued

Nursing diagnoses
✓ Injury, high risk for (uses, adverse reactions)
✓ Airway clearance, ineffective (uses)
✓ Activity intolerance (uses)
✓ Knowledge deficit (teaching)

Implementation
PO route
• Give 1 hr ac and 2 hr pc to increase absorption; elix should be measured accurately
IM route
• Inject slowly; do not give by **IV** route; do not administer if cloudy or a precipitate occurs

Patient/family education
• Teach patient to take doses as prescribed, not to skip doses or double dose; patient should check OTC medications and current prescription medications for ephedrine, which increases CNS stimulation; tell patient not to drink alcohol or caffeine products (tea, coffee, chocolate, colas) or cardiovascular effects may occur
• Advise patient to avoid hazardous activities; dizziness may occur
• Caution patient if GI upset occurs, to take drug with 8 oz water; avoid food, since absorption may be decreased
• Teach patient to notify prescriber of change in smoking habit; a change in dosage may be required
• Instruct patient to report nausea, vomiting, insomnia, tachycardia, dysrhythmias, convulsions, or restlessness; can indicate toxicity
• Teach patient to increase fluids to 2 L/day to decrease viscosity of secretions

Evaluation
Positive therapeutic outcome
• Decreased dyspnea
• Clear lung fields bilaterally

edetate calcium disodium (℞)

(ee'de-tate)

calcium disodium versenate, calcium EDTA, edathamil calcium disodium, sodium chloride edetate

Func. class.: Heavy metal antagonist; antidote
Chem. class.: Chelating agent

Pregnancy category C

Action: Binds ions of lead by displacement of calcium to form a water-soluble complex that is removed by kidneys

➔ **Therapeutic Outcome:** Decreased lead levels, absence of toxicity

Uses: Lead poisoning, acute lead encephalopathy

Dosage and routes
Acute lead encephalopathy
P ***Adult and child:*** 1.5 g/m^2/day × 3-5 days, with dimercaprol; may be given again after 4 days off drug

Lead poisoning
Adult: **IV** 1 g/250-500 ml D_5W or 0.9% NaCl over 1-2 hr or q12h × 3-5 days; may repeat after 2 days; not to exceed 50 mg/kg/day; may be given as a continuous inf over 8-24 hr

Adult: IM 35 mg/kg bid

P ***Child:*** IM 35 mg/kg/day in divided doses q8-12h, not to exceed 50 mg/kg/day; may give for 3-5 days, off 4 days before next course

Available forms: Inj 200 mg/ml

Adverse effects

CNS: Headache, paresthesia, numbness

CV: Hypotension, dysrhythmias, thrombophlebitis

EENT: Nasal congestion, sneezing

GI: Vomiting, ***diarrhea, abdominal cramps, anorexia,*** cheilosis, histamine-like reaction with GI distress

GU: Hematuria, renal tubular necrosis, proteinuria

INTEG: Urticaria, erythema, pruritus, pain at injection site, fever, cheilosis

MS: Leg cramps, myalgia, arthralgia, weakness

Contraindications: Hypersensitivity, anuria, poisoning of other metals, severe renal disease, P child <3 yr

Precautions: Hypertension, pregnancy **C,** lactation, gout, active TB

Pharmacokinetics	
Absorption	Well absorbed (IM), complete (**IV**)
Distribution	Extracellular fluid
Metabolism	Not metabolized
Excretion	Kidneys, unchanged; lead complex
Half-life	**IV** 20-60 min, IM 1½ hr

Pharmacodynamics
Unknown

Interactions: None

NURSING CONSIDERATIONS

Assessment

- Assess patient's VS, B/P, pulse, respirations; weigh daily
- Monitor I&O, kidney function studies, BUN, creatinine, CrCl; watch for decreasing urine output
- Assess neuro status: watch for paresthesias, beginning convulsions
- Monitor urine: pH, albumin, casts, blood, coproporphyrins, calcium
- Assess for febrile reactions that may occur 4-8 hr following drug therapy
- Monitor for cardiac abnormalities: dysrhythmias, hypotension, tachycardia
- Assess for allergic reactions (rash, urticaria); if these occur, drug should be discontinued

Nursing diagnoses

- ✓ Poisoning, risk for (uses)
- ✓ Injury, risk for (uses, adverse reactions)
- ✓ Knowledge deficit (teaching)

Implementation

IV route

- Give by intermitent inf after diluting 5 ml EDTA/250-500 ml D_5W or 0.9% NaCl; give over 1 hr in less severe lead toxicity and over 2 hr in severe lead toxicity
- Cont inf may be given over 8-24 hr

Additive incompatibilities: Amphotericin B, hydralazine

Additive compatibility: Netilmicin

IM route

- Give by IM 1 ml procaine HCl 1% per 1 ml of drug; rotate inj sites, administer deeply in large muscle mass

Patient/family education

- Explain reason for medication and expected results
- Provide a referral to health department to assess lead levels in home or work place

Evaluation

Positive therapeutic outcome

- Decreased symptoms of lead intoxication
- Decreased lead level <50 μg/dl

Treatment of overdose: IV calcium salt

edrophonium (℞)

(ed-roe-fone'ee-yum)

Enlon, Reversol, Tensilon

Func. class.: Cholinergics, anticholinesterase

Chem. class.: Quaternary ammonium compound

Pregnancy category C

Action: Inhibits destruction of acetylcholine, which increases concentration at sites where acetylcholine is released; this facilitates transmission of impulses across myoneural junction

➔ **Therapeutic Outcome:** Reversal of nondepolarizing neuromuscular blockers; absence of difficulty with muscular function in myasthenia gravis

Uses: Diagnosis of myasthenia gravis; curare antagonist; differentiation of myasthenic crisis from cholinergic crisis; reversal of nondepolarizing neuromuscular blockers

Dosage and routes

Tensilon test (myasthenia gravis diagnosis)

Adult: **IV** 1-2 mg over 15-30 sec, then 8 mg if no response; IM: 10 mg; if cholinergic reaction occurs, retest after ½ hr with 2 mg IM

P ***Child >34 kg:*** **IV** 2 mg; if no response in 45 sec, then 1 mg q45 sec, not to exceed 10 mg; IM 5 mg

P ***Child <34 kg:*** **IV** 1 mg; if no response in 45 sec, then 1 mg q45 sec, not to exceed 5 mg; IM 2 mg

P ***Infant:*** **IV** 0.5 mg

Reversal of nondepolarizing neuromuscular blockers

Adult: **IV** 10 mg over 30-45 sec, may repeat, not to exceed 40 mg

Differentiation of myasthenic crisis from cholinergic crisis

Adult: **IV** 1 mg, if no response in 1 min, may repeat

Available forms: Inj 10 mg/ml

Adverse effects

CNS: Dizziness, headache, sweating, weakness, ***convulsions***, uncoordination, ***paralysis***, drowsiness, ***loss of consciousness***

CV: Tachycardia, dysrhythmias, bradycardia, hypotension, AV block, ECG changes, ***cardiac arrest***, syncope

EENT: Miosis, blurred vision, lacrimation, visual changes

GI: *Nausea, diarrhea, vomiting, cramps, increased salivary and gastric secretions, dysphagia, increased peristalsis*

GU: Frequency, incontinence, urgency

INTEG: Rash, urticaria

RESP: Respiratory depression, bronchospasm, constriction, laryngospasm, respiratory arrest, dyspnea

Contraindications: Obstruction of intestine, renal system, hypersensitivity

Precautions: Seizure disorders, bronchial asthma, coronary occlusion, hyperthyroidism, dysrhythmias, peptic ulcer, megacolon, poor GI motility, pregnancy **C**, bradycardia, hypotension

Pharmacokinetics

Absorption	Unknown
Distribution	Unknown
Metabolism	Unknown
Excretion	Unknown
Half-life	Unknown

Pharmacodynamics

	IM	IV
Onset	2-10 min	30-60 sec
Peak	Unknown	Unknown
Duration	12-45 min	6-25 min

Interactions

Drug classifications

Anticholinergics: ↓ effect of edrophonium

NURSING CONSIDERATIONS

Assessment

- Assess vital signs, respiration during test
- Monitor diabetic patient carefully—this drug lowers blood glucose

Nursing diagnoses

✓ Breathing pattern, ineffective (uses)

✓ Knowledge deficit (teaching)

Implementation

IV **IV route**

- Administer undiluted 2 mg or less over 15-30 sec, or give as continuous inf in myasthenia crisis
- Give only after ensuring that atropine sulfate is available for cholinergic crisis
- Give only after all other cholinergics have been discontinued
- Store at room temp

Y-site compatibilities: Heparin, hydrocortisone, potassium chloride, vitamin B with C

Patient/family education

- Instruct patient to wear Medic Alert ID specifying myasthenia gravis and drugs taken

Evaluation

Positive therapeutic outcome

- Increased muscle strength, hand grasp; improved gait; absence of labored breathing (if severe)

Treatment of overdose: Respiratory support, atropine 1-4 mg (**IV**)

enalapril/ enalaprilat (℞)

(e-nal'april/e-nal'a-pril-at)

Vasotec, Vasotec IV

Func. class.: Antihypertensive

Chem. class.: Angiotensin-converting enzyme inhibitor

Pregnancy category C

Action: Selectively suppresses renin-angiotensin-aldosterone system; inhibits ACE; prevents conversion of angiotensin I to angiotensin II, resulting in dilatation of arterial and venous vessels

Therapeutic Outcome: Decreased B/P in hypertension; decreased preload, afterload in CHF

Uses: Hypertension, CHF, alone or in combination

Dosage and routes

Adult: PO 5 mg/day, may increase or decrease to desired response; range 10-40 mg/day

Hypertension
Adult: **IV** 1.25 mg q6h over 5 min
Patients on diuretics
Adult: **IV** 0.625 mg over 5 min, may give additional doses of 1.25 mg q6h
Renal impairment
Adult: **IV** 1.25 mg q6h with CrCl <3 mg/dl or 0.625 mg if CrCl >3 mg/dl

Available forms: Tabs 2.5, 5, 10, 20 mg; inj 1.25 mg/ml

Adverse effects
CNS: Insomnia, dizziness, paresthesias, headache, fatigue, anxiety
CV: Hypotension, chest pain, tachycardia, dysrhythmias
EENT: Tinnitus, visual changes, sore throat, double vision, dry burning eyes
GI: Nausea, vomiting, colitis, cramps, diarrhea, constipation, flatulence, dry mouth, loss of taste
GU: ***Proteinuria, renal failure,*** increased frequency of polyuria or oliguria
HEMA: ***Agranulocytosis, neutropenia***
INTEG: Rash, purpura, alopecia, hyperhidrosis
META: Hyperkalemia
RESP: Dyspnea, cough, rales, angioedema

Contraindications: Pregnancy C, lactation

Precautions: Renal disease, hyperkalemia

Pharmacokinetics

Absorption	Well absorbed (PO), complete (IV)
Distribution	Unknown
Metabolism	Liver (active metabolite—enalaprilat)
Excretion	Kidneys (60%—enalaprilat, 20%—enalapril)
Half-life	Enalaprilat 11 hr, increased in renal disease

Pharmacodynamics

	PO	IV
Onset	1 hr	15 min
Peak	4-6 hr	1-4 hr
Duration	24 hr	6 hr

Interactions
Individual drugs
Alcohol: ↑ hypotension (large amounts)
Allopurinol: ↑ hypersensitivity
Digoxin: ↑ serum levels
Hydralazine: ↑ toxicity
Indomethacin: ↓ antihypertensive effect
Lithium: ↑ serum levels
Prazosin: ↑ toxicity
Drug classifications
Adrenergic blockers: ↑ hypotension
Antacids: ↓ absorption
Antihypertensives: ↑ hypotension
Diuretics: ↑ hypotension
Diuretics, potassium-sparing: ↑ toxicity
Ganglionic blockers: ↑ hypotension
Potassium supplements: ↑ toxicity
Sympathomimetics: ↑ toxicity
Lab test interferences
Interferences: Glucose/insulin tolerance tests

NURSING CONSIDERATIONS
Assessment
- Monitor blood studies: neutrophils, decreased platelets
- Monitor B/P, orthostatic

E

hypotension, syncope; if changes occur dosage change may be required

• Monitor renal studies: protein, BUN, creatinine; increased levels may indicate nephrotic syndrome and renal failure

• Monitor renal symptoms: polyuria, oliguria, frequency, dysuria

• Establish baselines in renal, liver function tests before therapy begins

• Check potassium levels throughout treatment, although hyperkalemia rarely occurs

• Check for edema in feet, legs daily

• Assess for allergic reactions: rash, fever, pruritus, urticaria; drug should be discontinued if antihistamines fail to help

Nursing diagnoses

✓ Cardiac output, decreased (uses)

✓ Injury, potential for (adverse reactions)

✓ Knowledge deficit (teaching)

✓ Noncompliance (teaching)

Implementation

PO route

• Store in air-tight container at 86° F (30° C) or less

• Severe hypotension may occur after 1st dose of this medication; decreased hypotension may be prevented by reducing or discontinuing diuretic therapy 3 days before beginning benazepril therapy

• Give by **IV** inf of 0.9% NaCl (as ordered) to expand fluid volume if severe hypotension occurs

IV IV route

• Give **IV** direct over 5 min

• Dilute in 50 ml 0.9% NaCl, D_5W, D_5/0.9% NaCl, D_5/LR; diluted solution may be used for 24 hr

Y-site compatibilities: Allopurinol, amifostine, amikacin, aminophylline, ampicillin, ampicillin/sulbactam, aztreonam, butorphanol, calcium gluconate, cefazolin, cefoperazone, ceftazidime, ceftizoxime, chloramphenicol, cimetidine, clindamycin, dobutamine, dopamine, erythromycin lactobionate, esmolol, famotidine, fentanyl, filgrastim, ganciclovir, gentamicin, heparin, hetastarch, hydrocortisone, labetalol, lidocaine, magnesium sulfate, melphalan, methylprednisolone, metronidazole, morphine, nafcillin, nicardipine, penicillin G, potassium, phenobarbital, piperacillin, potassium chloride, potassium phosphate, ranitidine, teniposide, thiotepa, tobramycin, trimethoprim/sulfamethoxazole, vancomycin, vinorelbine

Y-site incompatibilities: Amphotericin B, phenytoin

Additive compatibilities: Dobutamine, dopamine, heparin, nitroglycerin, nitroprusside, potassium chloride

Patient/family education

• Advise patient not to discontinue drug abruptly; advise patient to tell all persons associated with health care

• Teach patient not to use OTC products (cough, cold, allergy medications) unless directed by physician; serious side effects can occur; xanthines, such as coffee, tea, chocolate, cola can prevent action of drug

• Instruct patient on the importance of complying with

dosage schedule, even if feeling better; to continue with medical regimen to decrease B/P: exercise, cessation of smoking, decreasing stress, diet modifications

- Emphasize the need to rise slowly to sitting or standing position to minimize orthostatic hypotension; not to exercise in hot weather, which can cause increased hypotension
- Advise patient to notify prescriber of mouth sores, sore throat, fever, swelling of hands or feet, irregular heartbeat, chest pain, coughing, shortness of breath
- Caution patient to report excessive perspiration, dehydration, vomiting, diarrhea; may lead to fall in B/P
- Caution patient that drug may cause dizziness, fainting, light-headedness; may occur during 1st few days of therapy; to avoid activities that may be hazardous
- Teach patient how to take B/P, and normal readings for age group

Evaluation

Positive therapeutic outcome

- Decreased B/P in hypertension

Treatment of overdose: Lavage, **IV** atropine for bradycardia; **IV** theophylline for bronchospasm, digitalis, O_2; diuretic for cardiac failure, hemodialysis

enoxacin (℞)

(en-ox'a-sin)

Penetrex

Func. class.: Antiinfective

Chem. class.: Fluoroquinolone

Pregnancy category C

Action: Interferes with conversion of intermediate DNA fragments into high–molecular-weight DNA in bacteria; DNA gyrase inhibitor

➔ Therapeutic Outcome: Bactericidal against the following organisms: staphylococci, *Enterobacter* sp, *Escherichia coli, Klebsiella* sp, *Neisseria gonorrhea, Pseudomonas aeruginosa*

Uses: Uncomplicated urethral or cervical gonorrhea, uncomplicated and complicated urinary tract infections (UTI)

Dosage and routes

Gonorrhea

Adult: PO 400 mg as a single dose

Uncomplicated UTI

Adult: PO 200 mg bid × 7 days

Complicated UTI

Adult: PO 400 mg bid × 14 days

Available forms: Tabs 200, 400 mg

Adverse effects

CNS: Dizziness, headache, fatigue, somnolence, depression, insomnia, anxiety

EENT: Visual disturbances, dizziness

GI: Diarrhea, nausea, vomiting, anorexia, flatulence, heartburn, abdominal pain,

dry mouth, increased AST (SGOT), ALT (SGPT)
INTEG: Rash, pruritus, photosensitivity

Contraindications: Hypersensitivity to quinolones

P G **Precautions:** Pregnancy **C,** lactation, children, elderly, renal disease, seizure disorders

Pharmacokinetics	
Absorption	Well absorbed
Distribution	Widely
Metabolism	Liver 20%
Excretion	Kidneys 50%-80%
Half-life	3-6 hr, increased in renal disease

Pharmacodynamics	
Onset	Unknown
Peak	Unknown

Interactions

Individual drugs

Bismuth subsalicylate: ↓ enoxacin level
Caffeine: ↓ effect of enoxacin
Cyclosporine: ↑ nephrotoxicity
Digoxin: ↑ digoxin levels
Nitrofurantoin: ↓ effectiveness
Probenecid: ↑ blood levels
Sucralfate: ↓ absorption of enoxacin
Theophylline: ↑ toxicity
Warfarin: ↑ warfarin effect
Zinc sulfate: ↓ absorption of enoxacin

NURSING CONSIDERATIONS

Assessment

- Assess patient for previous sensitivity reaction to quinolones
- Assess patient for signs and symptoms of infection including WBC >10,000, hematuria, foul-smelling urine; obtain baseline information before and during treatment
- Complete C&S testing before beginning drug therapy; this will identify if correct treatment has been initiated
- Assess for allergic reactions: rash, urticaria, pruritus
- Identify urine output; also monitor increases in BUN, creatinine
- Monitor blood studies: AST (SGOT), ALT (SGPT)

Nursing diagnoses

✓ Infection, risk for (uses)
✓ Diarrhea (adverse reactions)
✓ Knowledge deficit (teaching)
✓ Noncompliance (teaching)

Implementation

- Give 1 hr ac or 2 hr pc to maintain proper blood levels
- Give with 8 oz of water, 1 hr before hs to prevent ulceration
- Do not give with iron products or antacids, which will decrease absorption; should not be given 4 hr before or 2 hr after medication

Patient/family education

- Instruct patient to increase fluids to 3L/day to prevent crystallization in the kidney
- Instruct patient to report itching, rash, pruritus, urticaria
- Instruct patient to take all medication prescribed for the length of time ordered; drug must be taken as ordered
- Advise patient to limit intake of alkaline foods and drugs: milk, dairy products, peanuts, vegetables, alkaline antacids, sodium bicarbonate

Evaluation

Positive therapeutic outcome

- Reported improvement in symptoms of infection
- Negative C&S test results

enoxaparin (℞)
(ee-nox'a-par-in)
Lovenox
Func. class.: Antithrombotic
Chem. class.: Unfractionated porcine heparin (low-molecular heparin)
Pregnancy category C

Action: Prevents conversion of fibrinogen to fibrin and prothrombin to thrombin by enhancing inhibitory effects of antithrombin III; produces higher ratio of anti-factor Xa to anti-factor IIa

➔ **Therapeutic Outcome:** Prevention of deep vein thrombosis

Uses: Prevention of deep vein thrombosis, pulmonary emboli in hip and knee replacement

Dosage and routes
Hip/knee replacement
Adult: SC 30 mg bid given 12-24 hr post-op for 7-10 day, provided that hemostasis has been established

Abdominal surgery
Adult: SC 40 mg qd x 7-10 days to prevent thromboembolic complications

Available forms: Inj 30 mg/0.3 ml, 40 mg/0.4 ml (prefilled syringes)

Adverse effects
CNS: Fever, confusion
GI: Nausea
GU: Edema, peripheral edema
HEMA: Hypochromic anemia, thrombocytopenia, bleeding
INTEG: Ecchymosis

Contraindications: Hypersensitivity to this drug, heparin, or pork; hemophilia; leukemia with bleeding; peptic ulcer disease; thrombocytopenic purpura, heparin-induced thrombocytoparia

Precautions: Alcoholism, G elderly, pregnancy **C,** hepatic disease (severe), renal disease (severe), blood dyscrasias, severe hypertension, subacute bacterial endocarditis, acute P nephritis, lactation, children

Pharmacokinetics	
Absorption	Well absorbed
Distribution	Unknown
Metabolism	Unknown
Excretion	Unknown
Half-life	4½ hr

Pharmacodynamics	
Onset	Unknown
Peak	3-5 hr
Duration	Unknown

Interactions
Drug classifications
Anticoagulants: ↑ bleeding
Nonsteroidal antiinflammatories: ↑ bleeding
Salicylates: ↑ bleeding
Lab test interferences
↑ T_3 uptake
↓ Uric acid

NURSING CONSIDERATIONS
Assessment
- Monitor blood studies (Hct, occult blood in stools), anti-Xa levels q3mo; platelet count q2-3 days; thrombocytopenia may occur
- Assess patient for bleeding gums, petechiae, ecchymosis, black tarry stools, hematuria, epistaxis, decrease in B/P; indicate bleeding and possible hemorrhage; notify prescriber immediately

Nursing diagnoses

- ✓ Injury, risk for (uses, adverse reactions)
- ✓ Tissue perfusion, altered (uses)
- ✓ Knowledge deficit (teaching)

Implementation

- Give at same time each day to maintain steady blood levels
- Administer SC deeply; do not give IM; sol is clear to yellow; do not use sol with precipitate; rotate sites; apply gentle pressure for 1 min

Patient/family education

- Warn patient to avoid OTC preparations unless directed by prescriber because they could cause serious drug interactions
- Instruct patient to use soft-bristled toothbrush to avoid bleeding gums; to avoid contact sports; to use electric razor; to avoid IM inj
- Advise patient to report any signs of bleeding, bruising: gums, under skin, urine, stools

Evaluation

Positive therapeutic outcome

- Absence of deep vein thrombosis

ephedrine (℞, OTC)

(e-fed'rin)

ephedrine, ephedrine sulfate, Neorespin, Kondon's Nasal Jelly, Pretz-D

Func. class.: Adrenergic, mixed direct and indirect effects; bronchodilator, nasal decongestant, vasopressor

Chem. class.: Phenylisopropylamine

Pregnancy category C

Action: Increases contractility and heart rate by acting on β-receptors in the heart; also acts on α-receptors, causing vasoconstriction in blood vessels

➔ **Therapeutic Outcome:** Decreased nasal congestion, bronchodilatation, stimulation, increased B/P

Uses: Shock; increased perfusion; hypotension, bronchodilatation; nasal congestion; orthostatic hypotension, depression, narcolepsy; vasopressor

Dosage and routes

Adult: IM/SC 25-50 mg, not to exceed 150 mg/24 hr; **IV** 10-25 mg, not to exceed 150 mg/24 hr

P ***Child:*** SC/**IV** 3 mg/kg/day or 100 mg/m^2/day in divided doses q4-6h

Bronchodilator

Adult: PO 25-50 mg bid-qid, not to exceed 400 mg/day; IM/SC 12½-25 mg

P ***Child:*** PO 2-3 mg/kg/day or 100 mg/m^2/day in 4-6 divided doses

Nasal decongestant

P ***Adult and child >6 yr:*** Nasal i-ii sprays in each nostril prn q4hr for <3-4 days

Stimulation

Adult: PO 25-50 mg q3-4 hr prn

P ***Child:*** PO 3 mg/kg/day or 100 mg/m^2/day in 4-6 divided doses

Orthostatic hypotension

Adult: PO 25 mg qd-qid

P ***Child:*** PO 3 mg/kg/day in 4-6 divided doses

Labor

Adult: Administer dose to maintain B/P at or <130/80 mm Hg

Available forms: Inj 25, 50 mg/ml; caps 25, 50 mg; syr 20 mg/5 ml; nasal spray 0.25% nasal drops 0.5%; nasal jelly 1%

Adverse effects

CNS: Tremors, anxiety, insomnia, headache, dizziness, confusion, hallucinations, ***convulsions, CNS depression***

CV: Palpitations, tachycardia, hypertension, chest pain, ***dysrhythmias***

EENT: Rebound congestion (nasal)

GI: Anorexia, nausea, vomiting

GU: Dysuria, urinary retention

*RESP: **Dyspnea***

Contraindications: Hypersensitivity to sympathomimetics, angle-closure glaucoma

Precautions: Pregnancy **C**, cardiac disorders, hyperthyroidism, diabetes mellitus, prostatic hypertrophy

Pharmacokinetics

Absorption	Well absorbed (PO/IM/SC) complete (IV)
Distribution	Unknown
Metabolism	Liver
Excretion	Kidneys—unchanged
Half-life	3-5 hr

Pharmacodynamics

	PO	SC	IM	IV	NASAL
Onset	¼-1 hr	Unkn	15-30 min	5 min	Unkn
Peak	Unkn	Unkn	Unkn	Unkn	Unkn
Duration	2-4 hr	1 hr	1 hr	2 hr	6 hr

Interactions

Drug classifications

Antidepressants, tricyclics: ↓ effect of vasopressor

Anesthetics, halothane: Increased dysrhythmias

β-adrenergic blockers: Blocks therapeutic effect

Bronchodilators, aerosol: ↑ action of bronchodilator

MAOI: ↑ chance of hypertensive crisis

Oxytoxics: ↑ severe hypertension

Sympathomimetics: ↑ adrenergic side effects

NURSING CONSIDERATIONS

Assessment

- Monitor respiratory function: vital capacity, forced expiratory volume, ABGs, lung sounds, heart rate, baseline rhythm (bronchodilator)
- Monitor for evidence of allergic reactions; paradoxical bronchospasm; withhold dose; notify prescriber
- Monitor ECG, B/P, pulse, q5 min when using **IV** route (shock)
- Assess nasal congestion to identify factors contributing to ongoing congestion (nasal use)
- Assess mental status and sleeping patterns; mood, sensorium, ability to stay awake

Nursing diagnoses

✓ Airway clearance, ineffective (uses)
✓ Gas exchange impaired (uses)
✓ Sleep pattern disturbance (uses)
✓ Knowledge deficit (teaching)

Implementation

PO route

- Administer several hr (up to 6 hr) before hs to prevent sleeplessness

IV **IV route**

- Give **IV** directly undiluted using 3-way stopcock or Y-site; give 10 mg/min or less
- Use clear sol without precipitate; unused sol should be discarded

Additive compatibilities: Chloramphenicol, lidocaine,

metaraminol, nafcillin, penicillin G, potassium

Syringe compatibilities:
Pentobarbital

Y-site compatibilities:
Etomidate

Solution compatibilities:
0.9% NaCl, 0.45% NaCl, D5W, D10W, Ringers, LR, ionosol

Patient/family education

• Advise patient to avoid use of OTC medications—extra stimulation may occur, and not to use alcohol

Evaluation

Positive therapeutic outcome

• Increased B/P (vasopressor)
• Ability to stay awake (absence of narcolepsy) or improved mood (absence of depression)
• Absence of bronchospasm
• Decreased nasal congestion

Treatment of overdose:
Administer a β_2-adrenergic blocker

epinephrine (℞, OTC)

(ep-i-nef'rin)

Adrenalin Chloride, Adrenalin Chloride Solution, AsthmaHaler, Asthma Nefrin, Bronitin Mist, Bronkaid Mist, Dysne-Inhal, epinephrine, Epinal, Epitrate, Eppy/N, Glaucon, epinephrine HCl, Epinephrine Pediatric, EpiPen Jr., Medihaler-Epi, micronefrin, Nephron Inhalant, Primatene Mist, S-2 Inhalant, Sus-Phrine, Vaponefrin

Func. class.: Adrenergic, bronchodilator, cardiac stimulant

Chem. class.: Catecholamine

Pregnancy category C

Action: β_1- and β_2-agonist causing increased levels of cyclic AMP producing bronchodilatation, cardiac, and CNS stimulation; large doses cause vasoconstriction; small doses can cause vasodilation via β_2-vascular receptors

Therapeutic Outcome: Vasoconstrictor, cardiac stimulator, bronchodilator, decreased aqueous humor

Uses: Acute asthmatic attacks, hemostasis, bronchospasm, anaphylaxis, allergic reactions, cardiac arrest, adjunct in anesthesia

Dosage and routes

Asthma

P ***Adult and child:*** Inh 1-2 puffs of 1:100 or 2.25% racemic q15 min

Bronchodilator (parenteral epinephrine solution)
Adult: SC 0.2-0.5 mg, q20 min-4 hr max/mg/dose

Anaphylactic shock/vasopressor
Adult: SC/IM 0.5, repeat q5 min if needed, then **IV** 0.1-0.25 mg, repeat q5-15 min or infusion 1 mg/min, increase to 4 mg/min

P ***Child:*** SC/IM/**IV** 10 μg/ kg, repeat q5-15 min, up to 0.3 mg

Anaphylactic reaction
Adult: SC/IM 0.2-0.5 mg, repeat q10-15 min, not to exceed 1 mg/dose

P ***Child:*** SC 0.01 mg/kg, repeat q15min × 2 doses, then q4h as needed, up to 0.5 mg/dose

Bronchodilator
P ***Adult and child:*** Inh 1-2 inh of 1:100 or 2.25% racepineprine - 0.2 mg/dose, may repeat q3h

Adult: Ophth: 1 gtt qd or bid

Cardiac arrest
Adult: IC, **IV**, endotracheal 0.1-1 mg repeat q5 min prn

P ***Child:*** IC, **IV**, endotracheal 5-10 μg q5 min, may use 0.1 μ/kg/min **IV** inf after initial dose

Available forms: Aerosol 0.16 mg/spray, 0.2 mg/spray, 0.25 mg/spray, inj 1:1000 (1 mg/ml), 1:200 (5 mg/ml), 0.01 mg/ml (1:100,000), 0.1 mg/ml (1:10,000), 0.5 mg/ml (1:2,000); IM, **IV**, SC; sol for nebulization 1:100, 1.25% 2.25% (base)

Adverse effects
CNS: Tremors, anxiety, insomnia, headache, dizziness, confusion, hallucinations, ***cerebral hemorrhage***
CV: Palpitations, tachycardia, hypertension, *dysrhythmias,* increased T wave
GI: Anorexia, nausea, vomiting
GU: Urinary retention, hesitancy
RESP: Dyspnea

Contraindications: Hypersensitivity to sympathomimetics, narrow-angle glaucoma

Precautions: Pregnancy **C,** cardiac disorders, hyperthyroidism, diabetes mellitus, G prostatic hypertrophy, elderly, lactation

Pharmacokinetics

Absorption	Well absorbed (PO), complete (IV)
Distribution	Unknown, crosses placenta
Metabolism	Liver
Excretion	Breast milk
Half-life	Unknown

Pharmacodynamics

	SC	IM	IV	INH
Onset	3-5 min	5-10 min	Immediate	1 min hr
Peak	Unknown	Unknown	Unknown	Unknown
Duration	1-4 hr	1-4 hr	Unknown	1-4 hr

Interactions
Drug classifications
α-Adrenergic blockers: ↓ hypertensive effects
Anesthetics, general: ↑ dysrythmias
Antidepressants, tricyclics: ↑ pressor response
Antihistamines: ↑ pressor response
β-adrenergic blockers: Block therapeutic effect
Bronchodilators, aerosol: ↑ action of bronchodilator

Cardiac glycosides: ↑ dysrhythmias
Diuretics: ↓ vascular response
Ergots: ↓ vascular response
Insulin: ↑ need for insulin in diabetics
Lithium: ↓ effect of epinephrine
Methyldopa: ↑ pressor response
MAOI: ↑ chance of hypertensive crisis
Other sympathomimetics: ↑ adrenergic side effects, additive effects
Phenothiazines: ↓ vascular response

NURSING CONSIDERATIONS

Assessment

- Monitor respiratory function: vital capacity, forced expiratory volume, ABGs, lung sounds, heart rate, rhythm (baseline); amount, color of sputum
- Monitor ECG during administration continuously; if B/P increases, drug should be decreased; check B/P, pulse q5min after parenteral route; CVP, PCWP, SVR
- Check inj site for tissue sloughing; if this occurs, administer phentolamine mixed with 0.9% NaCl
- Monitor for evidence of allergic reactions, paradoxical bronchospasm, withhold dose, notify prescriber; sulfite sensitivity, which may be life threatening

Nursing diagnoses

☑ Airway clearance, ineffective (uses)
☑ Gas exchange impaired (uses)
☑ Cardiac output, decreased (uses)
☑ Sensory-perceptual alteration, visual (uses) (ophth)
☑ Knowledge deficit (teaching)

Implementation

IV IV route

- Give after diluting 1 mg of 1:1000 sol/10 ml or more; 0.9% NaCl yields 1:10,000 sol, give l mg/min
- Give by continuous inf after further diluting in 0.9% NaCl, D5W, D10W, D5/LR, LR—give via 3-way stopcock; for Y-site, use inf pump; ↑ dose of insulin in diabetic patients

Y-site incompatibility:
Ampicillin

Y-site compatibilities:
Amrinone, atracurium, calcium chloride, calcium gluconate, diltiazem, famotidine, heparin, hydrocortisone sodium succinate, pancuronium, phytonadione, potassium chloride, vecuronium, vitamin B with C

Syringe compatibilities:
Doxapram, heparin, milrinone

Additive compatibilities:
Amikacin, cimetidine, dobutamine, floxacillin, furosemide, metaraminol, ranitidine, verapamil

Additive incompatibilities:
Aminophylline, mephentermine, sodium bicarbonate, warfarin

SC/IM route

- Rotate inj sites, massage well, do not use gluteal (IM) site
- Shake suspension before using

Inh route

- Use 2.25% sol diluted in nebulizer/respirator
- 10 gtt of a 1% sol should be placed in nebulizer

Endotracheal route

- Only used in intubated patient; use **IV** dose that should be injected by endotracheal tube into bronchi

Patient/family education
• Tell patient not to use OTC medications; extra stimulation may occur; to use this medication before other medications and allow at least 5 min between each, to prevent overstimulation
• Teach patient that paradoxical bronchospasm may occur and to stop drug immediately and notify health care provider; to limit caffeine products such as chocolate, coffee, tea, and colas
• Patient should rinse mouth after inh
• Patient should report blurred vision, irritation with ophth preparations

Evaluation

Positive therapeutic outcome
• Absence of dyspnea, wheezing
• Improved airway exchange, improved ABGs
• Decreased aqueous humor
• Stabilization of heart rate and cardiac output

Treatment of overdose: Administer a B_2-adrenergic blocker, vasodilators, α-blocker

epoetin alfa (℞)
(ee-poe'e-tin al'fa)
Epogen, rHU-EPO, Eprex ✤, Erythropoietin, Procrit
Func. class.: Hormone
Chem. class.: Amino acid polypeptide
Pregnancy category C

Action: Erythropoietin is one factor controlling rate of red cell production; drug is developed by recombinant DNA technology

➔ Therapeutic Outcome: Decreased anemia with increased RBCs

Uses: Anemia caused by reduced endogenous erythropoietin production, primarily end-stage renal disease; to correct hemostatic defect in uremia; anemia caused by AZT (zidovudine) treatment in HIV-positive patients; anemia caused by chemotherapy; reduction of allogeneic blood transfusion in surgery patients

Dosage and routes

Anemia secondary to chemotherapy
Adult: SC 150 U/kg 3×/wk, may increase after 2 mo up to 300 U/kg 3×/wk

Anemia in chronic renal failure
Adult: SC/**IV** 50-100 U/kg 3×/wk, then adjust dose by 25 U/kg/dose to maintain appropriate Hct

Anemia secondary to zidovudine treatment
Adult: SC/**IV** 100 U/kg 3×/wk × 2 mo; may increase by 50-100 U/kg q1-2 mo, up to 300 U/kg 3×/wk

Available forms: Inj 2000, 3000, 4000, 10,000, 20,000 U/ml

Adverse effects
CNS: ***Seizures,*** coldness, sweating, headache
CV: Hypertension, ***hypertensive encephalopathy***
MS: Bone pain

Contraindications: Hypersensitivity to albumin, severe hypertension, erythropoietin levels of >200 mU/ml

Precautions: Pregnancy **C**

Pharmacokinetics

Absorption	Well absorbed (SC), completely absorbed (IV)
Distribution	Unknown
Metabolism	Unknown
Excretion	Unknown
Half-life	5-14 hr

Pharmacodynamics

	SC/IV
Onset	Unknown
Peak	Unknown
Duration	Unknown
Increased RBC count	1-2 wk

Interactions: None

NURSING CONSIDERATIONS

Assessment

- Monitor renal studies: urinalysis, protein, blood, BUN, creatinine; I&O; report drop in output to <50 ml/hr
- Monitor blood studies: reticulocyte count weekly; check for symptoms of anemia: fatigue, pallor, dyspnea
- Assess for CNS symptoms: coldness, sweating
- Assess CV status: B/P before and during treatment; hypertension may occur rapidly leading to hypertension encephalopathy
- Assess patient during hemodialysis for bruits, thrills of shunts; drug prevents severe anemia in chronic renal failure; clotting may need to be treated with increased anticoagulant
- Monitor serum iron levels, ferritin, transferrin levels; iron therapy may be needed to prevent recurring anemia
- Monitor blood studies: BUN, creatinine, uric acid, platelets, WBC, phosphorus, potassium, bleeding time. Hct, Hgb, RBCs, reticulocytes should be checked in chronic renal failure

Nursing diagnoses

- ✓ Fatigue (uses)
- ✓ Activity intolerance (uses)
- ✓ Knowledge deficit (teaching)

Implementation

IV IV route

- Administer by direct route at end of dialysis by venous line, do not shake

Solution compatibilities: NaCl 0.9%, $D_{10}W$, $D_{10}W$/ Albumin, sterile water for inj, TPN

SC route

- Give by SC route in patients not using dialysis

Patient/family education

- Teach patients with renal disease to include high-iron and low-potassium foods in their diets (meat, dark green leafy vegetables, eggs, enriched breads)
- Teach patient the reason for treatment, expected results
- Advise patient to use contraception (pregnancy may occur)

Evaluation

Positive therapeutic outcome

- Increased appetite
- Enhanced sense of well-being
- Increase in reticulocyte count in 1-2 wk

ergonovine (℞)

(er-goe-noe'veen)

Ergometrine, ergotrate maleate

Func. class.: Oxytocic

Chem. class.: Ergot alkaloid

Pregnancy category N/A

Action: Stimulates uterine and vascular smooth muscle contractions, decreases bleeding

Therapeutic Outcome: Uterine contraction, decreases bleeding

Uses: Treatment of postpartum or postabortion hemorrhage

Investigational uses: To induce a coronary artery spasm

Dosage and routes

Oxytoxic

Adult: IM 0.2 mg q2-4h, not to exceed 5 doses; **IV** 0.2 mg given over 1 min

Induced coronary artery spasm

Adult: **IV** 50 mg q5 min up to 400 μg or until chest pain occurs

Available forms: Inj 0.2 mg/ml

Adverse effects

CNS: *Headache, dizziness,* fainting

CV: Hypertension, chest pain

EENT: Tinnitus

GI: *Nausea, vomiting*

GU: Cramping

INTEG: Sweating

RESP: Dyspnea

Contraindications: Hypersensitivity to ergot medication, augmentation of labor, before delivery of placenta, spontaneous abortion (threatened), pelvic inflammatory disease (PID)

Precautions: Hepatic disease, renal disease, cardiac disease, asthma, anemia, convulsive disorders, hypertension, glaucoma, obliterative vascular disease

Pharmacokinetics

Absorption	Well absorbed (IM), completely absorbed (IV)
Distribution	Unknown
Metabolism	Liver
Excretion	Kidneys
Half-life	Unknown

Pharmacodynamics

	IM	IV
Onset	2-5 min	Immediate
Peak	Unknown	Unknown
Duration	3 hr	45 min

Interactions

Drug classifications

Ergots: ↑ hypertension

Sympathomimetics: ↑ hypertension

NURSING CONSIDERATIONS

Assessment

- Monitor B/P, pulse; watch for change that may indicate hemorrhage; check respiratory rate, rhythm, depth; notify prescriber of abnormalities
- Assess fundal tone, nonphasic contractions; check for relaxation or severe cramping
- Assess for ergotism or overdose: nausea, vomiting, weakness, muscular pain, insensitivity to cold, paresthesia of extremities; drug should be decreased or inf discontinued
- Before administering ergonovine, calcium levels should be checked; if hypocalcemia is present, correction should be made to increase effectiveness of this drug
- Monitor prolactin levels and decreased breast milk production

Nursing diagnoses

- ✓ Tissue perfusion, decreased (uses)
- ✓ Injury, risk for (adverse reactions)
- ✓ Knowledge deficit (teaching)

Implementation

IM route

- Contractions begin in 2-5 min, drug is given q2-4h for contractions to continue; give deeply in large muscle mass; rotate inj sites if additional doses are given

IV **IV route**

- Give **IV** directly after dilution with 5 ml of 0.9% NaCl, give over >1 min through Y-site of free-running **IV** of 0.9% NaCl or D_5W

Additive compatibilities: Amikacin, cephapirin, sodium bicarbonate

Patient/family education

- Advise patient to report increased blood loss, increased temp or foul-smelling lochia
- Inform patient that cramping is normal—pad count should be done to determine amount of bleeding
- Tell patient not to smoke during treatment to prevent excessive vasoconstriction

Evaluation

Positive therapeutic outcome

- Absence of severe bleeding

Treatment of overdose: Stop drug; give vasodilators, heparin, dextran

ergotamine (℞)

(er-got'a-meen)

Ergostat, Ergomar ✤, Gynergen ✤, Medihaler Ergotamine ✤

Func. class.: α-Adrenergic blocker, vascular headache suppressant

Chem. class.: Ergot alkaloid-amino acid

Pregnancy category X

Action: Constricts smooth muscle in peripheral, cranial blood vessels, relaxes uterine muscle; blocks serotonin release

➔ **Therapeutic Outcome:** Absence of headache

Uses: Vascular headache (migraine, histamine, cluster)

Dosage and routes

Adult: 2 mg, then 1-2 mg qh or q½h for SL, not to exceed 6 mg/day or 10 mg/wk; inh 1 puff, may repeat in 5 min, not to exceed 6/24 hr

Available forms: SL tab 2 mg; tab 1 mg; oral inh 360 µg/dose

Adverse effects

CNS: Numbness in fingers, toes, headache, weakness

CV: Transient tachycardia, chest pain, bradycardia, edema, claudication, increase or decrease in B/P

GI: Nausea, vomiting

MS: Muscle pain

Contraindications: Hypersensitivity to ergot preparations, occlusion (peripheral, vascular), CAD, hepatic disease, renal disease, peptic ulcer, hypertension, pregnancy **X**

Precautions: Lactation, P children, anemia

Pharmacokinetics

Absorption	Erratic (PO), poor (SL), rapidly (SC, IM)
Distribution	Crosses blood-brain barrier
Metabolism	Liver—extensively
Excretion	Kidneys (metabolites)
Half-life	Biphasic 2.7 hr, 21 hr

Pharmacodynamics

	PO	SL
Onset	1-2 hr	Unknown
Peak	½-3 hr	Unknown
Duration	Unknown	Unknown

Interactions

Individual drugs

Methysergide: ↑ effect
Sumatriptan: ↑ vasoconstriction

Drug classifications

Antiinfectives (macrolide): ↑ vasoconstriction
Ergots: ↑ hypertension
Oral contraceptives: ↑ vasoconstriction
Sympathomimetics: ↑ hypertension

NURSING CONSIDERATIONS

Assessment

- Assess characteristics of pain: duration, intensity, location, frequency, alleviating factors; also identify if halos, nausea, vomiting, blurred vision occur with headache. Assess before and during treatment
- Assess for ergotism or overdose: nausea, vomiting, weakness, muscular pain, insensitivity to cold, paresthesia of extremities; drug should be decreased or infusion discontinued
- Check for hypertension: B/P, pulse, monitor all peripheral pulses; if hypertension occurs, notify prescriber; also check for tachycardia or bradycardia

Nursing diagnoses

- ✓ Pain, acute (uses)
- ✓ Injury, risk for (adverse reactions)
- ✓ Knowledge deficit (teaching)

Implementation

SL route

- Have patient place tab under tongue; patient should not chew, crush, or swallow SL tab
- Patient should not drink, eat, or smoke until tab has dissolved

Inh route

- Teach patient how to use inhaler, protect ampules from heat/light

Patient/family education

- Caution patient not to smoke during treatment to prevent excessive vasoconstriction
- Advise patient to avoid alcohol or OTC medications unless approved by prescriber
- Tell patient to inform prescriber if pregnancy occurs

Treatment of overdose: Stop drug, give vasodilators, heparin, dextran

E

erythromycin base, erythromycin estolate, erythromycin ethylsuccinate, erythromycin gluceptate, erythromycin lactobionate, erythromycin stearate (℞)

(eh-rith-roe-mye'sin)

Apo Erythro-El ♣, Erybid ♣, E-Base, E-Mycin, ERYC, Ery-Tab, erythromycin, erythromycin base, Erythromycin Filmtabs, Novorythro ♣, PCE Dispertab, Robimycin Robitabs/Erythromid ♣, erythromycin estolate, Ilosone, Ilosone Pulvules/ E.E.S. 200, E.E.S. 400, Eryped, Ery Ped Drops, Eryped 200, Eryped 400, erythromycin ethylsuccinate, erythromycin lactobionate, Ilotycin Gluceptate

Func. class.: Antibacterial

Chem. class.: Macrolide antibiotic

Pregnancy category C

Action: Binds to 50S ribosomal subunits of susceptible bacteria and suppresses protein synthesis

Therapeutic Outcome: Bactericidal action against the following organisms: *N. gonorrhoeae, D. pneumoniae, M. pneumoniae, C. diphtheriae, B. pertussis, B. burgdorferi, L. monocytogenes;* syphilis, Legionnaire's disease; *C. trachomatis; H. influenzae,* streptococci, staphylocci; gram-positive bacilli: *Clostridium, Corynebacterium;* gram-negative pathogens: *Neisseria, Haemophilus influenzae,* Legionclla pneumophila, mycoplasma, and chlamydia trachomatis, *Entamoeba histolytica*

Uses: Mild to moderate respiratory tract, skin, soft tissue infections

Dosage and routes

Soft tissue infections

Adult: PO 250-500 mg q6h (base, estolate, stearate); PO 400-800 mg q6h (ethylsuccinate); **IV** inf 15-20 mg/kg/day (lactobionate)

P ***Child:*** PO 30-50 mg/kg/day in divided doses q6h (salts); **IV** 15-20 mg/kg/day in divided doses q4-6h (lactobionate)

N. gonorrhoeae/PID

Adult: **IV** 500 mg q6h × 3 days (gluceptate, lactobionate), then PO 250 mg (base, estolate, stearate) or 400 mg (ethylsuccinate) q6h × 1 wk

Syphilis

Adult: PO 20 g in divided doses over 15 days (base, estolate, stearate)

Chlamydia

Adult: PO 500 mg q6h × 1 wk or 250 mg qid × 2 wk

P ***Infant:*** PO 50 mg/kg/day in 4 divided doses × 3 wk or more

P ***Newborn:*** PO 50 mg/kg/day in 4 divided doses × 2 wk or more

Intestinal amebiasis

Adult: PO 250 mg q6h × 10-14 days (base, estolate, stearate)

P ***Child:*** PO 30-50 mg/kg/day in divided doses q6h × 10-14 days (base, estolate, stearate)

Available forms: Base: tab,

enteric-coated 250, 333, 500 mg; tabs, film-coated 250, 500 mg; caps, enteric-coated 125, 250 mg; estolate: tabs, chewable 125, 250 mg; tab 500 mg; caps 125, 250 mg; drops 100 mg/ml; susp 125, 250 mg/5 ml; stearate: tabs, film-coated 250, 500 mg; ethylsuccinate: tabs, chewable 200, 100 mg/ 2.5 ml, 200, 400 mg/5 ml; susp 200, 400 mg; powder for susp 100 mg/2.5 ml, 200 and 400 mg/ 5 ml powder for inj; 500 mg and 1 g (lactobionate); 250 mg, 500 mg, 1 g (as gluceptate)

Adverse effects

EENT: Hearing loss, tinnitus
GI: Nausea, vomiting, diarrhea, **hepatotoxicity,** abdominal pain, stomatitis, heartburn, anorexia, pruritus ani
GU: Vaginitis, moniliasis
INTEG: Rash, urticaria, pruritus, thrombophlebitis (**IV** site)

Contraindications: Hypersensitivity

Precautions: Pregnancy **C**, hepatic disease, lactation

Pharmacokinetics

Absorption	Well absorbed (PO), minimally absorbed (top, ophth)
Distribution	Widely distributed; minimally distributed (CSF); crosses placenta
Metabolism	Liver, partially
Excretion	Bile, unchanged; kidneys (minimal), unchanged
Half-life	1-3 hr

Pharmacodynamics

	PO	IV
Onset	1 hr	Rapid
Peak	4 hr	Infusion's end

Interactions

Individual drugs

Alfentanil: ↑ toxicity
Bromocriptine: ↑ toxicity
Carbamazepine: ↑ toxicity, from ↑ levels
Cisapride: Life-threatening dysrhythmias
Clindamycin: ↓ action of clindamycin
Cyclosporine: ↑ toxicity
Digoxin: ↑ blood levels of digoxin
Disopyramide: ↑ toxicity
Methylprednisolone: ↑ toxicity
Theophylline: ↑ toxicity from ↑ levels
Triazolam: ↑ effects of triazolam

Drug classifications

Antihistamines: ↑ levels of antihistamine
Ergots: ↑ ergotism
Oral anticoagulants: ↑ effects of oral anticoagulants
Penicillins: ↑ or ↓ action of penicillins

Lab test interferences

False ↑ 17-OHCS/17-KS, false ↑ AST (SGOT)/ALT (SGPT)
↓ Folate assay

NURSING CONSIDERATIONS

Assessment

- Assess patient for previous sensitivity reaction
- Assess patient for signs and symptoms of infection including characteristics of wounds, sputum, urine, stool, WBC >10,000, earache, fever; obtain baseline information before and during treatment
- Obtain C&S test results before beginning drug therapy to identify if correct treatment has been initiated
- Assess for allergic reactions:

rash, urticaria may occur a few days after therapy begins
- Identify urine output; if decreasing, notify prescriber (may indicate nephrotoxicity); also monitor increases in BUN, creatinine
- Monitor blood studies: AST (SGOT), ALT (SGPT), CBC, Hct, bilirubin, LDH, alk phosphatase, Coombs' test monthly if patient is on long-term therapy
- Monitor electrolytes: potassium, sodium, chloride monthly if patient is on long-term therapy
- Assess bowel pattern qd; if severe diarrhea occurs, drug should be discontinued
- Assess for overgrowth of infection: perineal itching, fever, malaise, redness, pain, swelling, drainage, rash, diarrhea, change in cough, sputum

Nursing diagnoses

- ✓ Infection, risk for (uses)
- ✓ Diarrhea (adverse reactions)
- ✓ Knowledge deficit (teaching)
- ✓ Noncompliance (teaching)
- ✓ Injury, risk for (adverse reactions)

Implementation

PO route

- Give around the clock on an empty stomach, at least 1 hr ac or 2 hr pc; may be taken with food if GI upset occurs; do not take with juices; take dose with a full glass of water: use calibrated measuring device for drops or susp; shake well
- Chewable tab may be crushed or chewed, not swallowed whole
- Do not open, crush, or chew time-release cap or tab, enteric-coated tab may be given

IV **IV route**

- Add 10 ml of sterile water for inj without preservatives to 250- or 500-mg vials and 20 ml to 1-g vial; sol is stable for 1 wk after reconstitution if refrigerated
- Intermittent inf: dilute further in 100-250 ml of 0.9% NaCl or D_5W
- Give over 20-60 min to avoid phlebitis; assess for pain along vein; slow inf if pain occurs; apply ice to site and notify prescriber if unable to relieve pain
- Continuous inf: may also be administered as an infusion in a dilution of 1 g/l of 0.9% NaCl, D_5W, over 4 hr

Additive compatibilities:
Calcium gluconate, corticotropin, dimenhydrinate, heparin, hydrocortisone, lidocaine, methicillin, penicillin G potassium, potassium chloride, sodium bicarbonate

Additive incompatibilities:
Aminophylline, cephapirin, pentobarbital, secobarbital, streptomycin, tetracycline

Syringe incompatibility:
Heparin

Erythromycin lactobionate

Additive incompatibilities:
Cephalothin, colistimethate, floxacillin, furosemide, heparin, metaraminol, metoclopramide, tetracycline, vitamin B with C

Additive compatibilities:
Aminophylline, ampicillin, cimetidine, diphenhydramine, hydrocortisone, lidocaine, methicillin, penicillin G potassium, penicillin G sodium, pentobarbital, polymyxin B, potassium chloride, prednisolone, prochlorperazine, promazine, sodium bicarbonate, sodium iodide, verapamil

Syringe incompatibilities: Ampicillin, heparin

Syringe compatibility: Methicillin

Y-site incompatibility: Fluconazole

Y-site compatibilities: Acyclovir, amiodarone, cyclophosphamide, enalaprilat, esmolol, famotidine, foscarnet, hydromorphone, idarubicin, labetol, lorazepam, magnesium sulfate, merperidine, midazolam, morphine, multivitamins, perphenazine, vitamin B with C, zidovudine

Patient/family education

• Teach patient to report sore throat, bruising, bleeding, joint pain—may indicate blood dyscrasias (rare)

• Advise patient to contact prescriber if vaginal itching, loose, foul-smelling stools, furry tongue occur—may indicate superimposed infection

• Instruct patient to take all medication prescribed for the length of time ordered

Evaluation

Positive therapeutic outcome

• Absence of signs/symptoms of infection (WBC <10,000, temp WNL, absence of red, draining wounds, earache)

• Reported improvement in symptoms of infection

Treatment of overdose: Withdraw drug, maintain airway, administer epinephrine, aminophylline, O_2, **IV** corticosteroids

esmolol (℞)

(ez'moe-lole)

Brevibloc

Func. class.: β-Adrenergic blocker (antidysrhythmic II)

Pregnancy category C

E

Action: Competitively blocks stimulation of β_1-adrenergic receptors in the myocardium; produces negative chronotropic, inotropic activity (decreases rate of SA node discharge, increases recovery time), slows conduction of AV node, decreases heart rate, decreases O_2 consumption in myocardium; also decreases renin-aldosterone-angiotensin system at high doses; inhibits β_2-receptors in bronchial system slightly

➔ **Therapeutic Outcome:** Decreased supraventricular tachycardia

Uses: Supraventricular tachycardias, noncompensatory tachycardia, hypertensive crisis

Dosage and routes

Adult: **IV** loading dose— 500 μg/kg/min over 1 min; maintenance—50 μg/kg/min for 4 min; may repeat q5 min, increasing maintenance inf by 50 μg/kg/min (max of 200 μg/kg/min); titrate to patient response

Available forms: Inj 10 mg, 250 mg/ml

Adverse effects

CNS: Confusion, lightheadedness, paresthesia, somnolence, fever, dizziness, fatigue, headache, depression, anxiety

CV: Hypotension, bradycardia,

chest pain, peripheral ischemia, shortness of breath, CHF, conduction disturbances
GI: Nausea, vomiting, anorexia, gastric pain, flatulence, constipation, heartburn, bloating
GU: Urinary retention, impotence, dysuria
INTEG: Induration, inflammation at site, discoloration, edema, erythema, burning pallor, flushing, rash, pruritus, dry skin, alopecia
RESP: ***Bronchospasm,*** dyspnea, cough, wheezing, nasal stuffiness

Contraindications: 2nd- or 3rd-degree heart block, cardiogenic shock, CHF, cardiac failure, hypersensitivity

Precautions: Hypotension, pregnancy **C,** peripheral vascular disease, diabetes, hypoglycemia, thyrotoxicosis, renal disease, lactation

Pharmacokinetics	
Absorption	Complete
Distribution	Unknown
Metabolism	Liver
Excretion	Kidneys
Half-life	9 min

Pharmacodynamics	
Onset	Rapid
Peak	Unknown
Duration	1-2 min

Interactions

Individual drugs

Alcohol: ↑ hypotension (large amounts)
Epinephrine: α-Adrenergic stimulation
Hydralazine: ↑ hypotension, bradycardia
Prazosin: ↑ hypotension, bradycardia
Thyroid: ↓ effect of esmolol
Verapamil: ↑ myocardial depression

Drug classifications

Antihypertensives: ↑ hypertension
β_2-Agonists: ↓ bronchodilatation
Cardiac glycosides: ↑ bradycardia
Nitrates: ↑ hypotension
Theophyllines: ↓ bronchodilatation

Smoking

↑ tachycardia

Lab test interferences

↑ Liver function tests

NURSING CONSIDERATIONS

Assessment

- Monitor B/P during beginning treatment, periodically thereafter; pulse q4hr; note rate, rhythm, quality; apical/radial pulse before administration; notify prescriber of any significant changes (pulse <50 bpm)
- Check for baselines in renal, liver function tests before therapy begins
- Assess for edema in feet, legs daily, monitor I&O, daily weight; check for jugular vein distention, rales bilaterally, dyspnea (CHF)
- Monitor skin turgor, dryness of mucous membranes for hydration status, especially G elderly

Nursing diagnoses

- ✓ Cardiac output, decreased (uses)
- ✓ Injury, risk for (adverse reactions)
- ✓ Knowledge deficit (teaching)
- ✓ Noncompliance (teaching)

Implementation

- Give by intermittent inf after diluting 5 g/500 ml D_5W, 0.9% NaCl, D_5/0.45% NaCl,

D_5/LR, D_5/0.9% NaCl, 0.45% NaCl, LR, (10 mg/ml)
• Give loading dose over 1 min, then maintenance dose over 4 min, may repeat loading dose q5 min with increased maintenance dose; maintenance should not be >200 mcg/kg/min and be administered up to 48 hr; dosage should be tapered at a rate of 25 μg/kg/min
• Store at room temp for 24 hr; sol should be clear

Y-site compatibilities: Amikacin, aminophylline, ampicillin, amiodarone, atracurium, butorphanol, calcium chloride, cefazolin, cefoperazone, ceftazidime, ceftizoxime, chloramphenicol, cimetidine, clindamycin, diltiazem, dopamine, enalaprilat, erythromycin, famotidine, fentanyl, gentamicin, heparin, hydrocortisone, regular insulin, labetalol, magnesium sulfate, methyldopate, metronidazole, midazolam, morphine, nafcillin, nitroglycerin, norepinephrine, nitroprusside, pancuronium, penicillin G potassium, phenytoin, piperacillin, polymyxin B, potassium chloride, potassium phosphate, ranitidine, streptomycin, tacrolimus, tobramycin, vancomycin, vecuronium

Y-site compatibility: Furosemide

Additive compatibilities: Aminophylline, bretylium, heparin

Additive incompatibilities: Diazepam, procainamide, sodium bicarbonate, thiopental

Patient/family education
• Teach patient need for medication and expected results
• Caution patient to rise slowly to prevent orthostatic hypotension

Evaluation

Positive therapeutic outcome
• Absence of dysrhythmias

Treatment of overdose: Defibrillation, vasopressor for hypotension

E

esoprostenol (℞)
(e-soh-proh'sti-nole)
Flolan
Func. class.: Antihypertensive
Pregnancy category B

Action: Produces falls in B/P by direct vasodilation of pulmonary and systemic arterial vascular beds, inhibition of platelet aggregation

➔ **Therapeutic Outcome:** Decreased B/P

Uses: Pulmonary hypertension; long-term **IV** treatment (NYHA Class III, **IV**)

Dosage and routes
Hypertension
Adult: **IV** via central-line catheter; 4 ng/kg/min (continuous chronic infusion) or 8.6 ng/kg/min (acute dose ranging)

Available forms: Powder for reconstitution 0.5 mg, 1.5 mg

Adverse effects
CNS: Dizziness, headache, anxiety, depression, paresthesias
CV: Hypotension, bradycardia, tachycardia, flushing, heart failure, syncope, shock, chest pain

GI: Nausea, vomiting, diarrhea
INTEG: Rash, pruritus
MS: MS pain, back pain, jaw pain, myalgia
RESP: Dyspnea, cough, hypoxia

Contraindications: Hypersensitivity; CHF

P G **Precautions:** Pregnancy **B**, lactation, children, elderly

Pharmacokinetics

Absorption	Complete
Distribution	Unknown
Metabolism	Liver
Excretion	Urine
Half-life	6½ min

Pharmacodynamics

Unknown

Interactions

Drug classifications

Antihypertensives: ↑ hypotension
Antiplatelets: ↑ bleeding
Anticoagulants: ↑ bleeding
Diuretics: ↑ hypotension

NURSING CONSIDERATIONS

Assessment

- Assess I&O, weight daily
- Assess B/P during beginning treatment, periodically thereafter; pulse q4h, note rate, rhythm, quality
- Monitor apical/radial pulse; notify prescriber of any significant changes
- Monitor baseline in renal, liver function tests before therapy begins
- Monitor edema in feet, legs daily
- Monitor skin turgor, dryness of mucous membranes for hydration status

Nursing diagnoses

✓ Cardiac output, decreased (uses)
✓ Tissue perfusion, altered (adverse reactions)
✓ Knowledge deficit (teaching)

Implementation

- Give **IV** in diluent only; for 3,000 ng/ml, dissolve vial of 0.5 mg/5 ml diluent, withdraw 3 ml, add sufficient diluent to make 100 ml
- Use following calculation:

$$\frac{\text{INF rate (ml/hr)} = \text{dose (ng/Kg/min)}}{\times \text{ weight (Kg)} \times 60}$$

- Store in dry area at room temp

Patient/family education

- Advise not to discontinue drug abruptly; taper over 2 wk; may cause precipitate angina
- Advise not to use OTC products unless directed by prescriber
- Teach to report bradycardia, dizziness, depression
- Teach to comply with weight control, dietary adjustment, modified exercise program
- Teach to carry Medic Alert ID to identify drug, allergies
- Teach to report symptoms of CHF: difficult breathing, especially on exertion or when lying down, night cough, swelling of extremities

Evaluation

Positive therapeutic outcome

- Decreased B/P

estazolam (℞)
(ess-taz'oh-lam)
ProSom
Func. class.: Sedative-hypnotic
Chem. class.: Benzodiazepine derivative
Pregnancy category X
Controlled substance schedule IV

Action: Produces CNS depression at the limbic, thalamic, hypothalamic levels of the CNS; may be mediated by neurotransmitter γ-aminobutyric acid (GABA); results are sedation, hypnosis, skeletal muscle activity, anxiolytic action

Therapeutic Outcome: Ability to sleep, relaxation

Uses: Insomnia (short-term)

Dosage and routes
Adult: PO 1-2 mg hs

Available forms: Tabs 1, 2 mg

Adverse effects
CNS: Lethargy, drowsiness, daytime sedation, dizziness, confusion, light-headedness, headache, anxiety, irritability, weakness, tremors, depression, lack of coordination
CV: Chest pain, pulse changes, palpitations, tachycardia
GI: Nausea, vomiting, diarrhea, heartburn, abdominal pain, constipation, anorexia, taste alteration
HEMA: Leukopenia, granulocytopenia (rare)
INTEG: Dermatitis, allergy, sweating, flushing, pruritus
MISC: Joint pain, respiratory congestion, dependency

Contraindications: Hypersensitivity to benzodiazepines, pregnancy **X**, sleep apnea

Precautions: Hepatic disease, renal disease, suicidal individuals, drug abuse, elderly, psychosis, child <18, lactation, depression, **pulmonary insufficiency**

Pharmacokinetics

Absorption	Well absorbed
Distribution	Crosses blood-brain barrier, placenta
Metabolism	Liver
Excretion	Kidneys, feces, breast milk
Half-life	10-24 hr

Pharmacodynamics

Onset	15-45 min
Peak	1½-2 hr
Duration	7-8 hr

Interactions
Individual drugs
Alcohol: ↑ CNS depression
Cimetidine: ↑ action
Disulfiram: ↑ action
Fluoxetine: ↑ action
Isoniazid: ↑ action
Ketoconazole: ↑ action
Levodopa: ↓ action of levodopa
Metoprolol: ↑ action
Propoxyphene: ↑ action
Propranolol: ↑ action
Rifampin: ↓ action of chlordiazepoxide
Theophylline: ↓ sedative effects
Valproic acid: ↑ action
Drug classifications
Analgesics, opioid: ↑ CNS depression
Antidepressants: ↑ CNS depression
Antihistamines: ↑ CNS depression
Barbiturates: ↓ effect of chlordiazepoxide
Contraceptives: ↑ effect
MAOI: ↑ CNS depression

NURSING CONSIDERATIONS

Assessment

- Assess patient's sleep pattern and note physical circumstances that interrupt sleep (sleep apnea, obstructed airway, pain/discomfort, urinary frequency) and psychologic (fear, anxiety); patient's bedtime routine, pre-sleep cues/props
- Identify potential for abuse; this drug may lead to physical and psychologic dependency; amount of drug should be limited
- Monitor blood studies: Hct, Hgb, RBCs, serum folate (if on long-term therapy), protime in patients receiving anticoagulants because action of anticoagulant may be increased
- Assess patient's mental status: mood, sensorium, affect, memory (long-term, short-term); for physical dependency: more frequent requests for medication, shakes, anxiety, pinpoint pupils

Nursing diagnoses

☑ Sleep pattern disturbance
☑ Knowledge deficit (teaching)
☑ Noncompliance (teaching)

Implementation

- Give ½-1 hr before hs for sleeplessness; on empty stomach for fast onset, but may be taken with food if GI symptoms occur
- Store in air-tight container in cool environment

Patient/family education

- Advise patient to avoid driving or other activities requiring alertness; to avoid alcohol ingestion or CNS depressants; serious CNS depression may result plus tachycardia, flushing, headache, hypotension
- Provide patient with alternate measures to improve sleep (reading, exercise several hr before hs, warm bath, warm milk, TV, self-hypnosis, deep breathing)
- G Inform patient that hangover is common in elderly but less common than with barbiturates
- Teach patient symptoms of withdrawal: nausea, vomiting, anxiety, hallucinations, insomnia, tachycardia, fever, cramps, tremors, seizures
- Advise patient to watch for allergic reaction (rash) and to discontinue drug if rash occurs

Evaluation

Positive therapeutic outcome

- Ability to sleep at night
- Decreased amount of early AM awakenings

estradiol/estradiol cypionate/estradiol valerate/estradiol transdermal system (℞)

(ess-tra-dye'ole)

Alora, Cypionate, depGynogen, Depo Estradiol, Depogen, Dura-Estrin, Estra-D, Estradlol Cypionate, Estro-Cyp, Estroject-L.A., Estronol-LA/ Estrace, Esaderm/Deladiol-40, Delestrogen, Dioval 40, Dioval XX, Duragen-10, Duragen-20, Duragen-40, Estradiol Valerate, Estra-L 20, Estra-L 40, FemPatch, Gynogen L.A. "10", Gynogen L.A. "20", Gynogen L.A. "40", L.A.E. 20, Valergen 10, Valergen 20, Valergen 40/ Estrace, Estraderm TTS

Func. class.: Estrogen

Chem. class.: Nonsteroidal synthetic estrogen

Pregnancy category X

Action: Needed for adequate functioning of female reproductive system; affects release of pituitary gonadatropins, inhibits ovulation, promotes adequate calcium use in bone structure

Therapeutic Outcome: Decreased tumor size in prostatic cancer; increased estrogen levels in menopause, female hypogonadism

Uses: Menopause, breast cancer, prostatic cancer, atrophic vaginitis, kraurosis vulvae, hypogonadism, castration, primary ovarian failure, prevention of osteoporosis

Dosage and routes

Menopause/hypogonadism/castration/ovarian failure

Adult: PO 1-2 mg qd 3 wk on, 1 wk off or 5 days on, 2 days off; IM 0.2-1 mg qwk

Prostatic cancer

Adult: PO 1-2 mg qd 3 wk on, 1 wk off or 5 days on, 2 days off; IM 0.2-1 mg qwk

Breast cancer

Adult: PO 10 mg tid × 3 mo or longer

Atropic vaginitis

Adult: Vag cream 2-4 g qd × 1-2 wk, then 1 g 1-3 ×/wk

Kraurosis vulvae

Adult: IM 1-1.5 mg 1-2 ×/wk

Available forms: Extradiol tabs 1, 2 mg; cypionate inj IM 5 mg/ml; valerate inj IM 10, 20, 40 mg/ml; transderm 0.025, 0.05, 0.075, mg/24-hr release rate, 0.1 mg/24-hr release rate; vag cream 100 μg/g

Adverse effects

CNS: Dizziness, headache, migraine, depression

CV: Hypotension, thrombophlebitis, edema, ***thromboembolism, stroke, pulmonary embolism, myocardial infarction***

EENT: Contact lens intolerance, increased myopia, astigmatism

GI: *Nausea*, vomiting, diarrhea, anorexia, pancreatitis, cramps, constipation, increased appetite, increased weight, ***cholestatic jaundice***

GU: Amenorrhea, cervical erosion, breakthrough bleeding, dysmenorrhea, vaginal candidiasis, breast changes, *gynecomastia, testicular atrophy, impotence*

INTEG: Rash, urticaria, acne, hirsutism, alopecia, oily skin, seborrhea, purpura, melasma
META: Folic acid deficiency, hypercalcemia, hyperglycemia

Contraindications: Breast cancer, thromboembolic disorders, reproductive cancer, genital bleeding (abnormal, undiagnosed), pregnancy **X**

Precautions: Hypertension, asthma, blood dyscrasias, gallbladder disease, CHF, diabetes mellitus, bone disease, depression, migraine headache, convulsive disorders, hepatic disease, renal disease, family history of cancer of breast or reproductive tract

Pharmacokinetics

Absorption	Well absorbed
Distribution	Widely distributed, crosses placenta
Metabolism	Unknown
Excretion	Unknown
Half-life	Unknown

Pharmacodynamics

	PO	IM	IV
Onset	Rapid	Slow	Rapid
Peak	Unknown	Unknown	Unknown
Duration	Unknown	Unknown	Unknown

Interactions

Drug classifications

Anticoagulants: ↓ action of anticoagulants
Antidepressants, tricyclics: ↑ toxicity
Barbiturates: ↓ action of chlorotrianisene
Corticosteroids: ↑ action of corticosteroids
Oral hypoglycemics: ↓ action of hypoglycemics

Lab test interferences

↑ BSP retention test; ↑ PBI; ↑ T_4; ↑ serum sodium; ↑ platelet aggregation; ↑ thyroxine-binding globulin (TBS); ↑ prothrombin; ↑ factors VII, VIII, IX, X; ↑ triglycerides
↓ Serum folate, ↓ serum triglyceride, ↓ T_3 resin uptake test, ↓ glucose tolerance test, ↓ antithrombin III, ↓ pregnanediol, ↓ metyrapone test
False positive: LE prep, antinuclear antibodies

NURSING CONSIDERATIONS

Assessment

- Monitor blood glucose in patient with diabetes; increased urine glucose may occur
- Monitor B/P q4h; watch for increase caused by water and sodium retention
- Monitor I&O ratio; be alert for decreasing urinary output and increasing edema; monitor weight daily; notify prescriber if weekly weight gain is >5 lb; if increased, diuretic may be ordered
- Obtain liver function studies, including AST (SGOT), ALT (SGPT), bilirubin, alk phosphatase
- Assess edema, hypertension, cardiac symptoms, jaundice
- Assess mental status: affect, mood, behavioral changes, aggression; depression may occur, drug may need to be discontinued

Nursing diagnoses

☑ Sexual dysfunction (uses)
☑ Injury, risk for (adverse reactions)

Implementation

PO route

- Give titrated dose, use lowest effective dose
- Give with food or milk to decrease GI symptoms

IM route

- Administer deeply in large muscle mass; drug is painful

- Rotate syringe to mix oil and medication

Trans route

- Apply to area free of hair to ensure adhesion
- Start trans dose 7 days before last PO dose if routes are to be changed

Vag route

- Place cream in applicator by attaching tube to applicator; squeeze cream into tube to mark; insert with patient reclining
- Applicator should be washed after each use

Patient/family education

- Tell patient to take exactly as prescribed; do not double doses
- Advise patient that increased weight gain and symptoms of fluid retention should be reported to prescriber: edema of feet, ankles, sacral area; abnormal vaginal bleeding; breast lumps; hepatic disease (dark urine, clay-colored stools, jaundice of skin, sclera, pruritus)
- Caution patient that thromboembolic symptoms should be reported: tenderness in legs, chest pain, dyspnea, headaches, blurred vision
- Inform patient to use sunscreen and protective clothing because sunburns may occur
- Advise patient to stop smoking—smokers have a greater chance of thromboembolic disorder
- Tell patient to use a nonhormonal birth control, and to notify prescriber if pregnancy is suspected

Evaluation

Positive therapeutic outcome

- Reversal of menopausal symptoms
- Decrease in tumor size in prostatic or breast cancer
- Decrease in itching, inflammation of vagina
- Absence of symptoms of osteoporosis

estramustine (℞)

(ess-tra-muss′teen)

Emcyt

Func. class.: Antineoplastic

Chem. class.: Hormone, alkylating agent

Pregnancy category D

Action: Combination drug consisting of nitrogen mustard/estrogen; estrogen is a carrier for the nitrogen mustard into estrogen-dependent tissue; acts like a weak alkylating agent; decreases serum testosterone levels

➔ **Therapeutic Outcome:** Prevention of rapidly growing malignant cells

Uses: Metastatic prostate cancer (palliative treatment only)

Dosage and routes

Adult: PO 10-16 mg/kg in 3-4 divided doses/day; treatment may continue for 3 mo; 600 mg/m^2/day in 3 divided doses

Available forms: Cap 140 mg

Adverse effects

CNS: Headache, anxiety, seizures, insomnia, mood swings

CV: ***Myocardial infarction,*** hypertension, ***CHF, CVA***

GI: Nausea, vomiting, anorexia, ***hepatotoxicity***

GU: ***Renal failure,*** impotence, gynecomastia

HEMA: Anemia, thrombocytopenia, leukopenia
INTEG: *Rash,* urticaria, pruritus, flushing, alopecia
RESP: Dyspnea, ***emboli,*** hoarseness

Contraindications: Hypersensitivity to estradiol, thromboembolic disorders, pregnancy **D**

Precautions: Edema, hepatic disease, CVA, MI, seizures, hypertension, diabetes mellitus

Pharmacokinetics	
Absorption	Well absorbed
Distribution	Prostatic area
Metabolism	Liver
Excretion	Bile, feces
Half-life	20 hr (terminal)

Pharmacodynamics	
Onset	1-2 hr
Peak	1-2 hr
Duration	1-2 hr

Interactions
Drug classifications
Calcium supplements: Blocked absorption
Live virus vaccines: ↑ adverse reactions
Food
Calcium (dairy foods): Blocked absorption
Smoking
↑ cardiotoxicity

NURSING CONSIDERATIONS
Assessment
- Assess symptoms indicating severe allergic reaction: rash, pruritus, urticaria, purpuric skin lesions, itching, flushing
- Monitor temp q4h (may indicate beginning of infection)
- Monitor liver function tests before and during therapy (bilirubin, AST [SGOT], ALT [SGPT], LDH) as needed or monthly; yellowing of skin, sclera, dark urine, clay-colored stools, itchy skin, abdominal pain, fever, diarrhea; renal function studies: BUN, urine CrCl, electrolytes before and during therapy
- Assess patient for bleeding: hematuria, stool guaiac, bruising or petechiae, mucosa or orifices q8h; inflammation of mucosa, breaks in skin

Nursing diagnoses
- ✓ Injury, risk for (adverse reactions)
- ✓ Body image disturbance (adverse reactions)
- ✓ Infection, risk for (adverse reactions)
- ✓ Knowledge deficit (teaching)

Implementation
- Give in divided doses over 1-3 mo; administer with water 1 hr ac or 2 hr pc; give antiemetic if nausea, vomiting, or anorexia become severe; do not give with calcium-rich products or antacids with calcium
- ⊘ Do not crush, chew caps

Patient/family education
- Teach patient to avoid use of products containing aspirin or ibuprofen, razors, commercial mouthwash—bleeding may occur; to report symptoms of bleeding (hematuria, tarry stools)
- Instruct patient to report signs of anemia, (fatigue, headache, irritability, faintness, shortness of breath)
- Caution patient that contraception is needed during treatment and several mo after
- Teach patient to watch for pain, swelling, redness, tenderness, change in vision and chest pain; should be reported

immediately to prescriber (thromboembolic disorders)

Evaluation

Positive therapeutic outcome

- Prevention of rapid division of malignant cells

estrogenic substances, conjugated (℞)

C.E.S ✱, conjugated estrogens, Conjugated Estrogens C.S.D. ✱, Premarin, Premarin Intravenous

Func. class.: Estrogen hormone

Chem. class.: Nonsteroidal synthetic estrogen

Pregnancy category X

Action: Needed for adequate functioning of female reproductive system; affects release of pituitary gonadotropins; inhibits ovulation; promotes adequate calcium use in bone structures

Therapeutic Outcome: Decreased tumor size in prostatic cancer; increased estrogen levels in menopause, female hypogonadism

Uses: Menopause, breast cancer, prostatic cancer, abnormal uterine bleeding, hypogonadism, castration, primary ovarian failure, osteoporosis

Dosage and routes

Menopause

Adult: PO 0.3-1.25 mg qd 3 wk on, 1 wk off

Osteoporosis

Adult: PO 0.625 mg qd or in a cycle

Atrophic vaginitis

Adult: Vag 2-4g cream qd × 21 days, off 7 days, repeat

Prostatic cancer

Adult: PO 1.25-2.5 mg tid

Breast cancer

Adult: PO 10 mg tid × 3 mo or longer

Abnormal uterine bleeding

Adult: **IV**/IM 25 mg, repeat in 6-12 hr

Ovariectomy/primary ovarian failure

Adult: PO 1.25 mg qd 3 wk on, 1 wk off

Hypogonadism

Adult: PO 2.5 mg bid-tid × 20 days/mo

Available forms: Tabs 0.3, 0.625, 0.9, 1.25, 2.5 mg; inj 25 mg/vial; vag cream 0.625 mg/g

Adverse effects

CNS: Dizziness, headache, migraine, depression

CV: Hypotension, thrombophlebitis, edema, ***thromboembolism, stroke, pulmonary embolism, MI***

EENT: Contact lens intolerance, increased myopia, astigmatism

GI: *Nausea,* vomiting, diarrhea, anorexia, pancreatitis, cramps, constipation, increased appetite, increased weight, ***cholestatic jaundice***

GU: Amenorrhea, cervical erosion, breakthrough bleeding, dysmenorrhea, vaginal candidiasis, breast changes, *gynecomastia, testicular atrophy, impotence*

INTEG: Rash, urticaria, acne, hirsutism, alopecia, oily skin, seborrhea, purpura, melasma

META: Folic acid deficiency, hypercalcemia, hyperglycemia

Contraindications: Breast cancer, thromboembolic disorders, reproductive cancer, genital bleeding (abnormal, undiagnosed), pregnancy **X**, lactation

Precautions: Hypertension, asthma, blood dyscrasias, gallbladder disease, CHF, diabetes mellitus, bone disease, depression, migraine headache, convulsive disorders, hepatic disease, renal disease, family history of cancer of breast or reproductive tract

Pharmacokinetics

Absorption	Well absorbed (PO), completely absorbed (IV)
Distribution	Widely distributed, crosses placenta
Metabolism	Liver—exclusively; hepatic recirculation
Excretion	Kidney
Half-life	Unknown

Pharmacodynamics

	PO	IM	IV
Onset	Rapid	Slow	Immediate
Peak	Unknown	Unknown	Unknown
Duration	Unknown	Unknown	Unknown

Interactions
Individual drugs
Phenylbutazone: ↓ action of phenylbutazone
Rifampin: ↓ action of phenylbutazone
Drug classifications
Anticoagulants: ↓ action of anticoagulants
Anticonvulsants: ↓ action of chlorotrianisene
Antidepressants, tricyclics: ↑ toxicity
Barbiturates: ↓ action of chlorotrianisene
Corticosteroids: ↑ action of corticosteroids
Oral hypoglycemics: ↓ action of hypoglycemics
Lab test interferences
↑ BSP retention test; ↑ PBI, ↑ T_4; ↑ serum sodium; ↑ platelet aggressability; ↑ thyroxine-binding globulin (TBG); ↑ prothrombin; ↑ factors VII, VIII, IX, X; ↑ triglycerides
↓ Serum folate, ↓ serum triglyceride, ↓ T_3 resin uptake test, ↓ glucose tolerance test, ↓ antithrombin III, ↓ pregnanediol, ↓ metyrapone test
False positive: LE prep, antinuclear antibodies

NURSING CONSIDERATIONS
Assessment
- Monitor blood glucose in patient with diabetes; increased urine glucose may occur
- Monitor B/P q4h; watch for increase caused by water and sodium retention
- Monitor I&O ratio; be alert for decreasing urinary output and increasing edema; monitor weight daily; notify prescriber if weekly weight gain is >5 lb; if increased, diuretic may be ordered
- Obtain liver function studies, including AST (SGOT), ALT (SGPT), bilirubin, alk phosphatase
- Assess edema, hypertension, cardiac symptoms, jaundice
- Assess mental status: affect, mood, behavioral changes, aggression; depression may occur, drug may need to be discontinued

Nursing diagnoses
✓ Sexual dysfunction (uses)
✓ Injury, risk for (adverse reactions)

Implementation

PO route

• Give titrated dose, use lowest effective dose
• Give in one dose in AM for prostatic cancer, vaginitis, hypogonadism
• Give with food or milk to decrease GI symptoms

IM route

• Reconstitute after withdrawing at least 5 ml of air from container and inject sterile diluent on vial side, rotate to dissolve
• Give IM injection deeply in large muscle

IV **IV route**

• Direct **IV**: Reconstitute as for IM, inject into distal port of running **IV** line of D_5W, 0.9% NaCl, LR, at a rate of 5 mg/min or less

Y-site compatibilities: Potassium chloride, vit B/C

Vag route

• Place cream in applicator by attaching tube to applicator, squeeze cream into tube to mark, insert with patient recumbent
• Applicator should be washed after each use

Patient/family education

• Caution patient to take exactly as prescribed and not to double doses
• Advise patient that increased weight gain and symptoms of fluid retention should be reported to prescriber: edema of feet, ankles, sacral area; abnormal vaginal bleeding; breast lumps; hepatic disease (dark urine, clay-colored stools, jaundice of skin, sclera, pruritus)
• Caution patient that thromboembolic symptoms should be reported: tenderness in legs, chest pain, dyspnea, headaches, blurred vision
• Inform patient that sunburns may occur and to use sunscreen and protective clothing
• Advise patient to stop smoking because smoking increases the chance of developing a thromboembolic disorder
• Tell patient to use a nonhormonal birth control, and to notify prescriber if pregnancy is suspected

Evaluation

Positive therapeutic outcome

• Reversal of menopause symptoms
• Decrease in tumor size in prostatic, breast cancer
• Decrease in itching, inflammation of vagina
• Absence of symptoms of osteoporosis

ethambutol (℞)

(e-tham′byoo tole)

Etibi ✤, Myambutol

Func. class.: Antitubercular

Chem. class.: Diisopropylethylene diamide derivative

Pregnancy category D

Action: Inhibits RNA synthesis, decreases tubercle bacilli replication

Therapeutic Outcome: Resolution of TB infection

Uses: Pulmonary tuberculosis, as an adjunct of other mycobacterial infections

Dosage and routes

P ***Adult and child >13 yr:*** PO 15-25 mg/kg/day as a single dose

Retreatment
P ***Adult and child >13 yr:*** PO 25 mg/kg/day as single dose × 2 mo with at least 1 other drug, then decrease to 15 mg/kg/day as single dose

Available forms: Tabs 100, 400 mg

Adverse effects
CNS: Headache, confusion, fever, malaise, dizziness, disorientation, hallucinations
EENT: Blurred vision, optic neuritis, photophobia, decreased visual acuity
GI: Abdominal distress, anorexia, nausea, vomiting
INTEG: Dermatitis, pruritis
META: Elevated uric acid, acute gout, liver function impairment
MISC: Thrombocytopenia, joint pain, bloody sputum

Contraindications: Hypersensitivity, optic neuritis, **P** child <13 yr; pregnancy **D**

Precautions: Renal disease, diabetic retinopathy, cataracts, ocular defects, hepatic and hematopoietic disorders

Pharmacokinetics	
Absorption	Rapidly absorbed
Distribution	Widely distributed, crosses blood-brain barrier, placenta
Metabolism	Liver
Excretion	Kidneys— unchanged
Half-life	3 hr, increased in liver, kidney disease

Pharmacodynamics	
Onset	Rapid
Peak	2-4 hr

Interactions
Individual drugs
Cisplatin: ↑ renal toxicity
Drug classifications
Antacids, aluminum: ↓ absorption

NURSING CONSIDERATIONS
Assessment
- Obtain C&S tests including sputum tests before initiating treatment; monitor q mo to detect resistance
- Monitor liver studies qwk: ALT (SGPT), AST (SGOT), bilirubin; renal studies: before, qmo: BUN, creatinine, output, specific gravity, urinalysis, uric acid
- Assess patient's mental status often: affect, mood, behavioral changes; psychosis may occur with hallucinations, confusion
- Assess patient's hepatic status: decreased appetite, jaundice, dark urine, fatigue
- Assess patient for visual disturbance that may indicate optic neuritis: blurred vision, change in color perception may lead to blindness

Nursing diagnoses
✓ Infection, risk for (uses)
✓ Diarrhea (adverse reactions)
✓ Sensory-perceptual alterations (adverse reactions)
✓ Knowledge deficit (teaching)
✓ Noncompliance (teaching)

Implementation
- Give with meals to decrease GI symptoms, at same time each day to maintain blood level
- Give antiemetic if vomiting occurs

Patient/family education
- Advise patient that compliance with dosage schedule and duration is necessary to eradicate disease; to keep scheduled appointments including ophthalmic appointments or relapse may occur
- Caution patient to report weakness, fatigue, loss of appetite, nausea, vomiting, yellowing of skin or eyes, tingling/

numbness of hands/feet, weight gain, or decreased urine output
• Caution patient to inform prescriber if pregnancy is suspected

Evaluation

Positive therapeutic outcome
• Decreased symptoms of TB

ethosuximide (℞)

(eth-oh-sux'i-mide)

Zarontin

Func. class.: Anticonvulsant

Chem. class.: Succinimide

Pregnancy category C

Action: Inhibits spike and wave formation in absence seizures (petit mal); decreases amplitude, frequency, duration, spread of discharge in minor motor seizures

Therapeutic Outcome: Decreased seizure activity

Uses: Absence seizures, partial seizures, tonic-clonic seizures

Dosage and routes

P ***Adult and child >6 yr:*** PO 250 mg bid initially; may increase by 250 mg q4-7d, not to exceed 1.5 g/day

P ***Child 3-6 yr:*** PO 250 mg/day or 125 mg bid; may increase by 250 mg q4-7d, not to exceed 1.5 g/day

Available forms: Cap 250 mg; syr 250 mg/5 ml

Adverse effects

CNS: Drowsiness, dizziness, fatigue, euphoria, lethargy, anxiety, aggressiveness, irritability, depression, insomnia, headache

EENT: Myopia, blurred vision

GI: Nausea, vomiting, heartburn, anorexia, diarrhea, abdominal pain, cramps, constipation, hiccups, weight loss, gum hypertrophy, tongue swelling

GU: Vaginal bleeding; pink, brown urine

HEMA: ***Agranulocytosis, aplastic anemia, thrombocytopenia, leukocytosis, eosinophilia, pancytopenia***

INTEG: Urticaria, pruritic erythema, hirsutism, **Stevens-Johnson syndrome**

Contraindications: Hypersensitivity to succinimide derivatives

Precautions: Lactation, pregnancy **C**, hepatic disease, renal disease

Pharmacokinetics	
Absorption	Rapidly, completely absorbed
Distribution	Body water
Metabolism	Liver
Excretion	Kidneys, 10% unchanged
Half-life	Adult—60 hr; child—24-30 hr

Pharmacodynamics	
Onset	Several hr, days
Peak	1-7 days
Duration	Days
Steady state	4-7 days

Interactions

Individual drugs

Alcohol: ↑ CNS depression

Phenytoin: ↑ metabolism, ↓ effectiveness

Drug classification

Antidepressants: ↑ CNS depression, decreased seizure threshold

Antihistamines: ↑ CNS depression

MAOI: ↓ seizure threshold

Narcotics: ↑ CNS depression

Phenothiazines: ↓ seizure threshold
Sedative/hypnotics: ↑ CNS depression

NURSING CONSIDERATIONS
Assessment
- Monitor drug level: therapeutic level 30-50 μg/ml
- Assess blood studies; CBC platelets q2 wk until stabilized, then qmo × 12, then q3 mo
- Assess mental status: mood, sensorium, affect, memory (long, short)
- Assess respiratory depression: rate, depth, character
- Assess blood dyscrasias: fever, sore throat, bruising, rash, jaundice

Nursing diagnoses
✓ Injury, risk for (adverse reactions)
✓ Knowledge deficit (teaching)

Implementation
- Administer on empty stomach for best absorption

Patient/family education
- Teach patient to carry ID card or Medic-Alert bracelet stating patient's name, drugs taken, condition, prescriber's name, phone number
- Caution patient to avoid driving, other activities that require alertness; to avoid alcohol ingestion and CNS depressants because increased sedation may occur
- Advise patient not to discontinue medication abruptly after long-term use; absence seizures may occur
- Inform patient that drug must be taken as prescribed; not to double doses because serious reactions may occur; may take drug within 4 hr if missed
- Advise patient to notify prescriber of hepatic symptoms, blood dyscrasia (fatigue, fever, sore throat, bruises, rash)
- Caution patient to notify prescriber if pregnancy is anticipated or suspected
- Inform patient that urine may become pink or brown
- ⊘ Do not chew, crush caps

Evaluation
Positive therapeutic outcome
- Decreased seizure activity

Treatment of overdose: Lavage, activated charcoal, warming blanket, vital signs; monitor electrolytes

etidronate (℞)
(eh-tih-droe'nate)
Didronel, Didronel IV
Func. class.: Parathyroid agent (calcium regulator)
Chem. class.: Diphosphate
Pregnancy category B

Action: Decreases bone resorption and new bone development (accretion)

→ **Therapeutic Outcome:** Decreased bone reabsorption, calcium levels WNL

Uses: Paget's disease, heterotopic ossification, hypercalcemia of malignancy

Dosage and routes
Paget's disease
Adult: PO 5-10 mg/kg/ day 2 hr ac with water, not to exceed 20 mg/kg/day, max 6 mo or 11-20 mg/kg/day for max of 3 mo

Heterotopic ossification
Adult: PO 20 mg/kg qd × 2 wk, then 10 mg/kg/day for 10 wk, total 12 wk

Hypercalcemia
Adult: **IV** 7.5 mg/kg/day × 3 days, then 20 mg/kg/day (PO)
Heterotopic ossification/hip replacement
Adult: PO 20 mg/kg/day × 4 wk before and 3 mo after surgery

Available forms: Tabs 200, 400 mg; inj 300 mg/6 ml

Adverse effects
GI: Nausea, diarrhea
GU: Nephrotoxicity
MS: Bone pain, hypocalcemia, decreased mineralization of nonaffected bones

Contraindications: Pathologic P fractures, children, colitis, severe renal disease with creatinine >5 mg/dl

Precautions: Pregnancy **B,** renal disease, lactation, restricted vit D/Ca

Pharmacokinetics

Absorption	Poorly absorbed (PO), completely absorbed (IV)
Distribution	50% bond to crystals in osteogenesis
Metabolism	None
Excretion	Feces (unabsorbed), kidney (unchanged)
Half-life	5-7 hr; in bone >3 mo

Pharmacodynamics

	PO	IV
Onset	4 wk	24 hr
Peak	Unknown	3-4 days
Duration	Up to 1 yr	10-12 days

Interactions
Drug classifications
Antacids: ↓ absorption of etidronate
Mineral supplements with magnesium, calcium, or aluminum: ↓ absorption of etidronate
Individual drugs
Didanosine: ↓ absorption of etidronate
Calcitonin: ↑ effect of calcitonin
Food
Dairy products: ↓ absorption of etidronate

NURSING CONSIDERATIONS

E

Assessment
- Assess for GI symptoms, polyuria, flushing, head swelling, tingling, headache—may indicate hypercalcemia; nervousness, irritability, twitching, seizures, spasm, paresthesia indicates hypocalcemia at start of treatment
- Identify nutritional status; evaluate diet for sources of vitamin D (milk, some seafood), calcium (dairy products, dark green vegetables), phosphates
- Monitor BUN, creatinine, uric acid, chloride, electrolytes, urine pH, urinary calcium, magnesium, phosphate, urinalysis (calcium should be kept at 9-10 mg/dl), albumin, alk phosphatase baseline and q3-6 mo; check urine sediment for casts throughout treatment
- Assess for increased drug level—toxic reactions occur rapidly; have calcium chloride or gluconate on hand if calcium level drops too low; check for tetany

Nursing diagnoses
✓ Injury, risk for (adverse reactions)
✓ Pain, chronic (uses)
✓ Knowledge deficit (teaching)

Implementation
PO route
- Administer on empty stomach to improve absorption (2 hr ac)

IV route
- Used in hypercalcemias—give by intermittent inf after diluting 300 mg/250 ml or more 0.9% NaCl; run over 2-3 hr

Patient/family education
- Teach method of inj if patient will be responsible for self-medication
- Caution patient to notify prescriber of hypercalcemic relapse: renal calculi, nausea, vomiting, thirst, lethargy, deep bone or flank pain
- Teach patient that warmth and flushing occur and last 1 hr
- Teach patient to follow a low-calcium diet as prescribed (Paget's disease, hypercalcemia)
- Advise patient to notify prescriber of diarrhea, nausea; dose may be divided to lessen these symptoms
- Inform patient that metallic taste may occur with **IV** dosing

Evaluation

Positive therapeutic outcome
- Calcium levels 9-10 mg/dl
- Decreasing symptoms of Paget's disease including pain
- Decreased bone loss in osteoporosis

etodolac (℞)
(ee-toe-doe'lak)
Lodine, Lodine XL
Func. class.: Nonsteroidal antiinflammatory, nonnarcotic analgesic
Pregnancy category C

Action: Inhibits prostaglandin synthesis by decreasing enzyme needed for biosynthesis; analgesic, antiinflammatory properties

Therapeutic Outcome: Decreased pain, inflammation

Uses: Mild to moderate pain, osteoarthritis

Dosage and routes

Osteoarthritis

Adult: PO 800-1200 mg/day in divided doses to 600-1200 mg/day in divided doses; do not exceed 1200 mg/day; patients <60 kg not to exceed 20 mg/kg

Analgesia

Adult: PO 200-400 mg q6-8h prn for acute pain; do not exceed 1200 mg/day; patients 60 kg, not to exceed 20 mg/kg

Available forms: Caps 200, 300 mg; tabs, ext rel 400 mg

Adverse effects

CNS: Dizziness, headache, drowsiness, fatigue, tremors, confusion, insomnia, anxiety, depression, light-headedness, vertigo
CV: Tachycardia, peripheral edema, fluid retention, palpitations, dysrhythmias, CHF
EENT: Tinnitus, hearing loss, blurred vision
GI: ***Nausea, anorexia,*** vomiting, diarrhea, jaundice, ***cholestatic hepatitis,*** constipation, flatulence, cramps, dry mouth, peptic ulcer, dyspepsia, ***GI bleeding***
GU: ***Nephrotoxicity: dysuria, hematuria, oliguria, azotemia, cystitis, UTI***
HEMA: ***Blood dyscrasias,*** epistaxis, bruising
INTEG: Erythema, urticaria, purpura, rash, pruritus, sweating

Contraindications: Hypersensitivity; patients in whom aspirin, iodides, or other NSAIDs have produced asthma, rhinitis, urticaria, nasal polyps, angioedema, bronchospasm

Precautions: Pregnancy **C**, P lactation, children, bleeding, G GI, cardiac disorders, elderly; renal, hepatic disorders

Pharmacokinetics

Absorption	Well absorbed
Distribution	Highly bound to plasma protein
Metabolism	Unknown
Excretion	Unknown
Half-life	7 hr

Pharmacodynamics

Onset	½ hr
Peak	1-2 hr
Duration	4-12 hr

Interactions

Individual drugs

Acetaminophen (long-term use): ↑ renal reactions
Alcohol: ↑ adverse reactions
Aspirin: ↓ effectiveness, ↑ adverse reactions
Coumadin: ↑ anticoagulant effects
Digoxin: ↑ toxicity, ↑ levels
Insulin: ↓ insulin effect
Lithium: ↑ toxicity
Methotrexate: ↑ toxicity
Phenytoin: ↑ toxicity
Probenecid: ↑ toxicity
Sulfonylurea: ↑ toxicity

Drug classifications

Anticoagulants: ↑ risk of bleeding
Antihypertensives: ↓ effect of antihypertensives
Antineoplastics: ↑ risk of hematologic toxicity
β-blockers: ↑ antihypertension
Cephalosporins: ↑ risk of bleeding
Diuretics: ↓ effectiveness of diuretics
Glucocorticoids: ↑ adverse reactions
Hypoglycemics: ↓ hypoglycemic effect
Nonsteroidal antiinflammatories: ↑ adverse reactions
Potassium supplements: ↑ adverse reactions
Radiation: ↑ risk of hematologic toxicity
Sulfonamides: ↑ toxicity

NURSING CONSIDERATIONS

Assessment

- Monitor blood counts during therapy; watch for decreasing platelets; if low, therapy may need to be discontinued, then restarted after hematologic recovery; watch for blood dyscrasia (thrombocytopenia): bruising, fatigue, bleeding, poor healing

Nursing diagnoses

- ✓ Pain (uses)
- ✓ Mobility, impaired physical mobility (uses)
- ✓ Knowledge deficit (teaching)
- ✓ Injury, risk for (adverse reactions)

Implementation

- Administer with food or milk to decrease gastric symptoms; food will slow absorption slightly, will not decrease absorption.
- Do not crush, chew ext rel tabs

Patient / family education

- Inform patient that drug must be continued for prescribed time to be effective; to avoid aspirin, alcoholic beverages
- Caution patient to report bleeding, bruising, fatigue,

malaise because blood dyscrasias can occur
- Instruct patient to use caution when driving; drowsiness, dizziness may occur
- Teach patient to take with a full glass of water to enhance absorption; do not crush, break, or chew medication

Evaluation
Positive therapeutic outcome
- Decreased pain
- Decreased inflammation
- Increased mobility

etoposide (VP-16) (℞)
(e-toe'poe-side)
Etopophos, VePesid
Func. class.: Antineoplastic
Chem. class.: Semisynthetic podophyllotoxin
Pregnancy category D

Action: Inhibits mitotic activity through metaphase to mitosis; also inhibits cells from entering mitosis, depresses DNA, RNA synthesis

Therapeutic Outcome: Prevention of rapid growth of malignant cells

Uses: Leukemias, lung, testicular cancer, lymphomas, neuroblastoma, melanoma, ovarian cancer; being investigated for use in leukemia, lymphoma

Dosage and routes
Adult: **IV** 45-75 mg/m^2/day × 3-5 days given q3-5 wk or 200-250 mg/m^2/wk, or 125-140 mg/m^2/day 3 × wk, q5 wk
Adult: PO 70 mg/m^2/day × 4 days, repeated q3-4 wk up to 100 mg/m^2/day × 5 days q3-4 wk

Available forms: Inj 20 mg/ml; powder for inj (lyophilized) 119.3 mg/300 mg dextran; caps 50 mg

Adverse effects
CNS: Headache, *fever*
CV: Hypotension
GI: Nausea, vomiting, anorexia, ***hepatotoxicity***
GU: ***Nephrotoxicity***
HEMA: ***Thrombocytopenia, leukopenia, myelosuppression, anemia***
INTEG: Rash, alopecia, phlebitis at **IV** site
RESP: ***Bronchospasm***

Contraindications: Hypersensitivity, bone marrow depression, severe hepatic disease, severe renal disease, bacterial infection, pregnancy **D**

Precautions: Renal disease, hepatic disease, lactation, P children, gout

Pharmacokinetics

Absorption	Variably absorbed
Distribution	Rapidly absorbed, 97% protein binding, crosses placenta
Metabolism	Liver—some
Excretion	Kidneys, unchanged 50%, breast milk
Half-life	3 hr initially, 15 hr terminally

Pharmacodynamics
Unknown

Interactions
Individual drugs
Radiation: ↑ toxicity, bone marrow suppression
Drug classifications
Antineoplastics: ↑ toxicity, bone marrow suppression
Live virus vaccines: ↑ adverse reactions

NURSING CONSIDERATIONS
Assessment
- Monitor B/P, (baseline and

q15 min) during administration

- Monitor CBC, differential, platelet count weekly; withhold drug if WBC is <4000 or platelet count is <75,000; notify prescriber of results—recovery will take 3 wk
- Monitor renal function studies: BUN, urine CrCl before, during therapy; I&O ratio; report fall in urine output of 30 ml/hr; for decreased hyperuricemia
- Monitor for cold, fever, sore throat (may indicate beginning infection); notify prescriber if these occur
- Assess for bleeding: hematuria, guaiac, bruising or petechiae, mucosa or orifices q8h; no rectal temp; avoid IM inj; use pressure to venipuncture sites
- Identify nutritional status: an antiemetic may need to be prescribed
- Assess for symptoms indicating severe allergic reactions: rash, pruritus, urticaria, itching, flushing, bronchospasm, hypotension; epinephrine and crash cart should be nearby

Nursing diagnoses

- ✓ Injury, risk for (adverse reactions)
- ✓ Body image disturbance (adverse reactions)
- ✓ Infection, risk for (adverse reactions)
- ✓ Knowledge deficit (teaching)

Implementation

PO route

- Caps need to be refrigerated

IV IV route

- Give by intermittent inf
- Sol should be prepared by qualified personnel and only under controlled conditions
- Use Luer Loc tubing to prevent leakage; do not let sol come in contact with skin—if contact occurs, wash well with soap and water
- Give after diluting 100 mg/250 ml or more D_5W or NaCl to a concentration of 0.2-0.4 mg/ml; infuse over 30-60 min
- Give hyaluronidase 150 U/ml to 1 ml NaCl to infiltration area; ice compress for treatment of vesicant activity

Y-site compatibilities: Allopurinol, amifostine, aztreonam, fludarabine, granisetron, melphalan, ondansetron, paclitaxel, sargramostim, teniposide, thiotepa, vinorelbine

Y-site incompatibility: Idarubicin

Additive compatibilities: Cisplatin, cytarabine, floxuridine, fluorouracil, hydroxyzine, ifosfamide, ondansetron

Patient/family education

- Teach patient to avoid use of products containing aspirin or ibuprofen, razors, commercial mouthwash because bleeding may occur; to report symptoms of bleeding (hematuria, tarry stools)
- Instruct patient to report signs of anemia (fatigue, headache, irritability, faintness, shortness of breath)
- Teach patient to report any changes in breathing or coughing even several months after treatment
- Advise patient that contraception will be necessary during treatment because teratogenesis may occur
- Caution patient that hair loss may occur during treatment; a wig or hairpiece may make patient feel better; new hair will be different in color, texture

E

• Advise patient to avoid vaccinations during treatment because serious reactions may occur
• Teach patient to report signs/symptoms of infection; fever, chills, sore throat; patient should avoid crowds and persons with known infections

Evaluation
Positive therapeutic outcome
• Decreased spread of malignant, leukemic cells

etretinate (℞)
(e-tret′inate)
Tegison
Func. class.: Systemic antipsoriatic
Chem. class.: Retinol derivative
Pregnancy category X

Action: Unknown; drug is related to retinol

Therapeutic Outcome: Decrease in size and number of lesions

Uses: Severe recalcitrant psoriasis including erythrodermic and generalized pustular types

Dosage and routes
Adult: PO 0.75-1 mg/kg/day in divided doses, not to exceed 1.5 mg/kg/day; maintenance dose 0.5-0.75 mg/kg/day generally beginning after 8-16 wk of therapy

Available forms: Caps 10, 25 mg

Adverse effects
CNS: Fatigue, headache, dizziness, fever, pain, anxiety, amnesia, depression
CV: Edema, ***CV obstruction, atrial fibrillation,*** chest pain, coagulation disorders
EENT: Eye irritation, eye pain, double vision, change in lacrimation; earache, otitis externa, dry nose, eyes, mouth; nosebleed, chelitis, sore tongue
GI: Anorexia, abdominal pain, nausea, ***hepatitis,*** constipation, diarrhea, flatulence, weight loss
GU: WBC in urine, ***proteinuria,*** glycosuria, *increased BUN, creatinine,* ***hematuria,*** *casts,* ***acetonuria, hemoglobinuria, dysuria***
INTEG: Alopecia; peeling of palms, soles, fingertips; itching; rash; dryness; red scaling on face; bruising; sunburn; pyogenic granuloma; paronychia; onycholysis; perspiration change, nail changes
META: Increase or decrease in potassium, calcium, phosphate, sodium, chloride
MS: Hyperostosis, bone pain, cramps, myalgia, gout, hypertonia
RESP: Dyspnea, cough

Contraindications: Pregnancy **X**

Precautions: Lactation, children, hepatic disease, diabetes, obesity

Pharmacokinetics

Absorption	Well absorbed
Distribution	Stored in fatty tissue, crosses placenta, 99% protein binding
Metabolism	Liver (extensively)
Excretion	Kidney (metabolite)
Half-life	Terminal 120 days

Pharmacodynamics

Onset	1-6 wk
Peak	4-9 mo
Duration	Years

Interactions
Individual drugs
Vitamin D: ↑ toxicity
Drug classifications
Abrasives: ↑ irritation
Desquamating agents: ↑ irritation
Tetracyclines: ↑ pseudotumor cerebri
Food
↑ absorption with food (fatty)

NURSING CONSIDERATIONS
Assessment

- Assess patient for pseudotumor cerebri: headache, nausea, vomiting, visual problems, papilledema
- Monitor hepatic studies: AST (SGOT), ALT (SGPT), LDH, q1-2 wk × 3 mo, q1-3 mo thereafter because hepatotoxicity may occur
- Assess patient for visual problems: blurring, decreased night vision, poor visual acuity; drug should be discontinued and ophthalmologist consulted
- Check lipids (cholesterol, triglycerides, HDL) before, q1-2 wk during treatment; after discontinuing treatment, lipids will return to normal
- Monitor blood and renal studies: CBC (Hct, Hgh, platelets, WBC); urinalysis, BUN, creatinine (may be increased); urine may show protein, glucose, acetone, blood; electrolytes may be increased or decreased (sodium, potassium, calcium, phosphate)

Nursing diagnoses

✓ Body image disturbance (uses)
✓ Injury, risk for (adverse reactions)
✓ Knowledge deficit (teaching)

Implementation

- Give with food (fatty) to increase absorption
- Do not chew, crush caps

Patient/family education

- Advise patient to take with food to enhance absorption
- Caution patient not to use during pregnancy; contraception must be used for 1 mo before or after therapy; teratogenic effects are longlasting
- Caution patient not to take vitamin A supplements because increased vitamin A levels may occur and to avoid alcohol and fatty diet or lipid levels will increase
- Inform patient that contact lens intolerance is common; glasses may need to be used
- Advise patient to use gum, hard candy, or frequent sips of water to prevent dry mouth, and to prevent burns by using sunscreen or protective clothing
- Inform patient that blurred vision, change in color perception, joint pain, jaundice, cramping should be reported to prescriber

Evaluation
Positive therapeutic outcome

- Decrease in scaling, itching, amount of psoriasis

factor IX complex (human)/factor IX (human) (℞)

Konyne 80, Proplex T, Proplex SX-T, Profilnine Heat-Treated/Alphanine, Alpha Nine SD, Mononine
Func. class.: Hemostatic
Chem. class.: Factors II, VII, IX, X
Pregnancy category C

Action: Causes an increase in blood levels of clotting factors

II, VII, IX, X; factor IX (human) has IX activity only

Therapeutic Outcome: Replacement of factors II, VII, IX, X

Uses: Hemophilia B (Christmas disease), factor IX deficiency, anticoagulant reversal, control of bleeding in patients with factor VIII inhibitors; reversal of overdose of anticoagulants in emergencies

Dosage and routes

Bleeding in hemophilia A and inhibitors of factor VIII

P ***Adult/child:*** 75 U/kg, repeat in 12 hr

Bleeding in hemophilia B

P ***Adult/child:*** Give to establish 25% of normal Factor IX activity or 60-75 U/kg/day then 10-20 U/kg/day × 1 wk

Prophylaxis of bleeding in hemophilia B

P ***Adult/child:*** 10-20 U/kg/day × 1 wk

Reversal of oral anticoagulant

P ***Adult/child:*** 15 U/kg

Factor VII deficiency (use Proplex T)

P ***Adult/child:*** 0.5 U/kg × body weight (kg) × desired factor IX increase (in % of normal); repeat q4-6h if needed

Factor IX (human)

AlphaNine, AlphaNine SD (minor to moderate hemorrhage)

P ***Adult/child:*** Give amount to increase plasma Factor IX level to 20%-30%

Serious hemorrhage

P ***Adult/child:*** Give amount to increase plasma Factor IX level to 30%-50% given as daily inf

Mononine

Minor hemorrhage

P ***Adult/child:*** Give amount to increase plasma Factor IX level to 15%-25% (20-30 U/kg), may repeat in 24 hr

Major trauma

P ***Adult/child:*** Give amount to increase plasma Factor IX level to 25%-50% (75 U/kg) q1830 h for up to 10 days

Available forms: Inj (number of units noted on label)

Adverse effects

CNS: Headache, dizziness, malaise, paresthesia, *lethargy, chills, fever, flushing*

CV: Hypotension, tachycardia, *MI,* ***venous thrombosis, pulmonary embolism***

EENT: Tinnitus, eyelid swelling

GI: Nausea, vomiting, abdominal cramps, jaundice, ***viral hepatitis***

HEMA: ***Thrombosis, hemolysis, AIDS, DIC***

INTEG: Rash, flushing, *urticaria*

RESP: ***Bronchospasm***

Contraindications: Hypersensitivity, hepatic disease, DIC, elective surgery, mild factor IX deficiency

Precautions: Neonates/ P infants, pregnancy **C**

Pharmacokinetics	
Absorption	40% (PO), complete (IV)
Distribution	Unknown
Metabolism	Rapidly cleared from plasma, liver 30%
Excretion	70% unchanged—kidneys
Half-life	24 hr

Pharmacodynamics

Unknown

Interactions

Individual drugs

Aminocaproic acid: ↑ risk of thrombosis; do not use together

NURSING CONSIDERATIONS

Assesment

- Monitor blood studies (coagulation factor assays by % normal: 5% prevents spontaneous hemorrhage, 30%-50% for surgery, 80%-100% for severe hemorrhage); check for bleeding q15-30 min, immobilize and apply ice to affected joints
- Monitor for increased B/P, pulse
- Monitor I&O; if urine becomes orange or red, notify prescriber
- Assess for allergic or pyrogenic reaction: fever, chills, rash, itching; slow inf rate if not severe
- Assess for DIC: bleeding, ecchymosis, hypersensitivity, changes in coagulation tests

Nursing diagnoses

- Injury, risk for (uses)
- Tissue perfusion, altered (uses)
- Knowledge deficit (teaching)

Implementation

IV route

- Give **IV** after warming to room temp 3 ml/min or less, with plastic syringe only; do not admix
- Give after dilution with provided diluent, 50 U/ml or 25 U/ml; give so as not to exceed 10 ml/min; decrease rate if fever, headache, flushing, tingling occur
- Give after crossmatch is completed if patient has blood type A, B, AB, to determine incompatibility with factor
- Store reconstituted sol for 3 hr at room temp or up to 2 yr if refrigerated (powder); check expiration date

Patient/family education

- Advise patient to report any signs of bleeding: gums, under skin, urine, stools, emesis
- Caution patient about risk of viral hepatitis, AIDS; that immunization for hepatitis B may be given first; to be tested q2-3 mo for HIV
- Tell patient to carry ID identifying disease and treatment; avoid salicylates, to inform other health professionals about condition

Evaluation

Positive therapeutic outcome

- Prevention of hemorrhage

famciclovir (℞)

(fam-sye-klo'vir)

Famvir

Func. class.: Antiviral

Chem. class.: Guanosine nucleoside

Pregnancy category B

Action: Inhibits DNA polymerase and viral DNS synthesis by the conversion of this guanosine nucleoside to penciclovir

Therapeutic Outcome: Decreasing size and number of lesions

Uses: Treatment of acute herpes zoster, genital herpes

Dosage and routes

Adult: PO 500 mg q8h; in renal disease if creatinine clearance is ≥60 ml/min/1.73 m^2 (500 mg q8h); if 40-59 ml/min/1.73 m^2 (500 mg q12h); if 20-39 ml/min/1.73 m^2 (500 mg q24h)

Available forms: Tab 500 mg

Adverse effects

CNS: Headache, fatigue
GI: Nausea, vomiting, diarrhea, constipation, abdominal pain
GU: Decreased sperm count
INTEG: Pruritis
MS: Back pain
RESP: Pharyngitis, sinusitis

Contraindications: Hypersensitivity to this drug or penciclovir

Precautions: Renal disease, pregnancy **B,** hypersensitivity to acyclovir, ganciclovir

Pharmacokinetics

Absorption	Well absorbed
Distribution	Unknown
Metabolism	Intestinal tissue, blood, liver
Excretion	Breast milk, kidney, bile
Half-life	3 hr

Pharmacodynamics

Onset	Unknown
Peak	1 hr
Duration	8 hr

Interactions: None known

NURSING CONSIDERATIONS

Assessment

- Assess amount and distribution of lesions; also burning, itching, or pain (early symptoms of herpes infection)
- Monitor renal function studies: urine CrCl, BUN before and during treatment if patient has decreased renal function; dose may need to be lowered
- Monitor bowel pattern before, during treatment; diarrhea may occur

Nursing diagnoses

☑ Infection, risk for (uses)
☑ Knowledge deficit (teaching)

Implementation

- Give with or without meals; absorption does not appear to be lowered when taken with food

Patient/family education

- Teach patient how to recognize signs of beginning infection
- Teach patient how to prevent the spread of infection to others
- Teach patient reason for medication and expected results

Evaluation

Positive therapeutic outcome

- Decreased size and spread of lesions

famotidine (℞)

(fa-moe′to-deen)

Pepcid AC acid controller, Pepcid, Pepcid IV

Func. class.: H_2-Histamine receptor antagonist, antiulcer agent

Pregnancy category B

Action: Inhibits histamine at H_2-receptor site in gastric parietal cells, which inhibits gastric acid secretion

➔ **Therapeutic Outcome:** Healing of duodenal ulcers or gastric ulcers; prevention of duodenal ulcers; decreases symptoms of GERD or Zollinger-Ellison syndrome, heartburn

Uses: Short-term treatment of active duodenal ulcer, maintenance therapy for duodenal ulcer, Zollinger-Ellison syndrome, multiple endocrine adenomas, gastric ulcers, heartburn

Dosage and routes

Duodenal ulcer

Adult: PO 40 mg qd hs × 4-8 wk, then 20 mg qd hs if needed (maintenance); **IV** 20 mg q12h if unable to take PO

Hypersecretory conditions

Adult: PO 20 mg q6h; may give 160 mg q6h if needed; **IV** 20 mg q12h if unable to take PO

Heartburn relief/prevention

Adult: 10 mg with water or 1 hr before eating

Available forms: Tabs 10, 20, 40 mg; powder for oral susp 10 mg/5 ml; inj 10 mg/ml, 20 mg/50 ml 0.9% NaCl

Adverse effects

CNS: Headache, dizziness, paresthesia, ***seizure,*** depression, anxiety, somnolence, insomnia, fever

EENT: Taste change, tinnitus, orbital edema

GI: Constipation, nausea, vomiting, anorexia, cramps, abnormal liver enzymes

HEMA: Thrombocytopenia

INTEG: Rash

MS: Myalgia, arthralgia

RESP: Bronchospasm

Contraindications: Hypersensitivity

Precautions: Pregnancy **B,** P lactation, children <12 yr, severe renal disease, severe G hepatic function, elderly

Pharmacokinetics

Absorption	50% absorbed (PO)
Distribution	Plasma, protein binding (15%-20%)
Metabolism	Liver (30% active metabolizing)
Excretion	Kidneys (70%)
Half-life	2½-3½ hr

Pharmacodynamics

	PO	IV
Onset	30-60 min	Immediate
Peak	1-3 hr	½-3 hr
Duration	6-12 hr	6-12 hr

Interactions

Individual drugs

Ketoconazole: ↓ absorption of ketoconazole

Drug classifications

Antacids: ↓ absorption of famotidine

NURSING CONSIDERATIONS

Assessment

- Assess patient with ulcers or suspected ulcers: epigastric, abdominal pain, hematemesis, occult blood in stools, blood in gastric, aspirate prior to treatment—throughout treatment, monitor gastric pH (5 should be maintained)
- Monitor I&O ratio, BUN, creatinine, CBC with differential monthly

Nursing diagnoses

✓ Pain (uses)
✓ Knowledge deficit (teaching)

Implementation

PO route

- Give antacids 1 hr before or 2 hr after famotidine; may be given with foods or liq
- Administer oral susp after shaking well; discard unused sol after 1 mo

IV **IV route**

- Give **IV** direct after diluting 2 ml of drug (10 mg/ml) in 0.9% NaCl to total volume of 5-10 ml; inject over 2 min to prevent hypotension
- Administer **IV** intermittent inf after diluting 20 mg of drug in 100 ml of LR, 0.9% NaCl, D_5W, $D_{10}W$; run over 15-30 min
- Store in cool environment

F

(oral); **IV** solution is stable for 48 hr at room temp; do not use discolored sol

Additive compatibilities: Cefazolin, flumazenil

Y-*site compatibilities:* Allopurinol, amifostine, aminophylline, ampicillin, ampicillin/sulbactam, amrinone, atropine, aztreonam, bretylium, calcium gluconate, cefazolin, cefmetazole, cefoperazone, cefotaxime, cefotetan, cefoxitin, ceftazidime, ceftizoxime, cefuroxime, cephalothin, cephapirin, dexamethasone, dextran 40, digoxin, dobutamine, dopamine, doxorubicin, enalaprilat, epinephrine, erythromycin lactobionate, esmolol, folic acid, furosemide, gentamicin, haloperidol, heparin, hydrocortisone, imipenem/cilastatin, regular insulin, isoproterenol, labetalol, lidocaine, magnesium sulfate, melphalan, methylprednisolone, metoclopramide, mezlocillin, nitroglycerin, nitroprusside, norepinephrine, ondansetron, oxacillin, paclitaxel, perphenazine, phenylephrine, phenytoin, phytonadione, piperacillin, potassium chloride, potassium phosphate, procainamide, sodium bicarbonate, theophylline, thiamine, thiotepa, ticarcillin, verapamil

Patient/family education

- Caution patient to avoid driving, other hazardous activities until stabilized on this medication; dizziness may occur
- Advise patient to avoid black pepper, caffeine, alcohol, harsh spices, extremes in temperature of food; tell patient to avoid OTC preparations: aspirin, cough, cold preparations; condition may worsen
- Tell patient that smoking decreases the effectiveness of the drug; that smoking cessation should be considered
- Instruct patient that drug must be continued for prescribed time to be effective and taken exactly as prescribed; doses are not to be doubled; to take missed dose when remembered up to 1 hr before next dose
- Tell patient to report bruising, fatigue, malaise; blood dyscrasias may occur
- Tell patient to report diarrhea, black tarry stools, sore throat, rash, dizziness, confusion, rash, or delirium to prescriber immediately

Evaluation

Positive therapeutic outcome

- Decreased pain in abdomen
- Healing of ulcers

fat emulsions (℞)

(fat ee-mul'shuns)

Intralipid 10%, Intralipid 20%, Liposyn II 10%, Liposyn II 20%, Liposyn III 10%, Liposyn III 20%, Soyacal 20%

Func. class.: Caloric

Chem. class.: Fatty acid, long chain

Pregnancy category C

Action: Needed for energy, heat production; consists of neutral triglycerides, primarily unsaturated fatty acids

Therapeutic Outcome: Increased available calories and fatty acids

Uses: Increase calorie intake, prevent fatty acid deficiency

Dosage and routes

Deficiency

P ***Adult and child:*** **IV** 8%-10% of required calorie intake (intralipid)

Adjunct to TPN

Adult: **IV** 1 ml/min over 15-30 min (10%) or 0.5 ml/min over 15-30 min (20%); may increase to 500 ml over 4-8 hr if no adverse reactions occur; not to exceed 2.5 g/kg

P ***Child:*** **IV** 0.1 ml/min over 10-15 min (10%) or 0.05 ml/min over 10-15 min (20%); may increase to 1 g/kg over 4 hr if no adverse reactions occur; not to exceed 4 g/kg

Prevention of deficiency

Adult: **IV** 500 ml 2 × wk (10%), given 1 ml/min for 30 min, not to exceed 500 ml over 6 hr

P ***Child:*** **IV** 5-10 ml/kg/day (10%), given 0.1 ml/min for 30 min, not to exceed 100 ml/hr

Available forms: 10% (50, 100, 200, 250, 500 ml), 20% (50, 100, 200, 250, 500 ml)

Adverse effects

CNS: Dizziness, headache, drowsiness, focal seizures

CV: ***Shock***

GI: Nausea, vomiting, ***hepatomegaly***

HEMA: ***Hyperlipemia, hypercoagulation, thrombocytopenia, leukopenia, leukocytosis***

RESP: Dyspnea, ***fat in lung tissue***

Contraindications: Hypersensitivity, hyperlipemia, lipid necrosis, acute pancreatitis accompanied by hyperlipemia, hyperbilirubinemia of the

P newborn

Precautions: Severe liver disease, diabetes mellitus, thrombocytopenia, gastric ulcers, premature, term

P newborns, pregnancy **C**, sepsis

Pharmacokinetics	
Absorption	Completely absorbed
Distribution	Intravascular space
Metabolism	Conversion to triglycerides, to free fatty acids
Excretion	Unknown
Half-life	Unknown

Pharmacodynamics

Unknown

Interactions: None

NURSING CONSIDERATIONS

Assessment

- Monitor triglycerides, free fatty acid levels, platelet counts daily to prevent fat overload, thrombocytopenia
- Monitor liver function studies: AST (SGOT), ALT (SGPT), Hct, Hgb—notify prescriber if abnormal
- Assess nutritional status: calorie count by dietician; monitor weight daily

Nursing diagnoses

✓ Nutrition, less than body requirements (uses)

✓ Knowledge deficit (teaching)

Implementation

- Administer using inf pump at prescribed rate; do not use in-line filter sized for lipid emulsion; clogging will occur
- Do not use mixed sol that look oily or are not separated; discard unused sol
- Change **IV** tubing at each inf: infection may occur with old tubing
- Give by intermittent inf at a rate of 10% sol (1 ml/min); 20% sol (0.5 ml/min) initially for 15-30 min; may be in-

F

creased to 10% sol (120 ml/hr) or 20% sol (62.5 ml/hr) if no adverse reactions occur; do not give more than 500 ml during the first day; children should be given 10% (0.1 mg/ml) or 20% (0.05 ml/min) initially for 15-30 min, may be increased 1 g/kg/4hr, do not give more than 10% (100 ml/hr) or 20% (50 ml/hr)

Y-site compatibilities: Ampicillin, cefamandole, cefazolin, cefoxitin, cephapirin, clindamycin, digoxin, dopamine, erythromycin, furosemide, gentamicin, IL-2, isoproterenol, lidocaine, kanamycin, norepinephrine, oxacillin, penicillin G potassium, ticarcillin, tobramycin

Y-site incompatibilities: Amikacin, tetracycline

Additive compatibilities: Cefamandole, chloramphenicol, cimetidine, cyclosporine, diphenhydramine, famotidine, heparin, hydrocortisone, multivitamins, nizatidine, penicillin G potassium

Patient/family education

- Teach patient reason for use of lipids and expected results

Evaluation

Positive therapeutic outcome

- Increased weight
- Fatty acids at adequate levels

felbamate (℞)

(fell-ba'mate)

Felbatol

Func. class.: Anticonvulsant

Chem. class.: Carbamate derivative

Pregnancy category C

Action: Mechanism of action unknown; may increase seizure threshold; has weak inhibitory effects on GABA-receptor and benzodiazepine-receptor binding

Therapeutic Outcome: Absence of seizures

Uses: Partial seizures, with or without generalization in adults; partial and generalized seizures in children with Lennox-Gastaut syndrome

Dosage and routes

Adjunctive therapy

Adult: PO add 1.2 g/day in 3-4 divided doses; reduce other anticonvulsants (valproic acid, phenytoin, carbamazepine, and derivatives) by 20% to control plasma concentrations; may increase felbamate in 1.2 g/day increments qwk, up to 3.6 g/day

Monotherapy

Adult: PO 1.2 g/day in 3-4 divided doses; titrate with close supervision; increase dose in 600-mg increments q2wk to 3.6 g/day if needed

Lennox-Gastaut syndrome

Child (2-14 yr): PO add 15 mg/kg/day in 3-4 divided doses; reduce other anticonvulsants (valproic acid, phenytoin, carbamazepine, and derivatives) by 20% to control plasma concentrations; may increase felbamate 15 mg/kg/day qwk up to 45 mg/day

Available forms: Tabs 400, 600 mg; susp 600 mg/5 ml

Adverse effects

CNS: Dizziness, fatigue, *headache, insomnia,* anxiety, tremor, unsteady gait, depression, paresthesia
CV: Chest pain
EENT: Dry mouth, blurred vision, diplopia, otitis media
GI: Nausea, constipation, diarrhea, anorexia, vomiting, abdominal pain, increased liver enzymes, hiccups, *dyspepsia*
GU: Urinary incontinence, intramenstrual bleeding, *UTI*
HEMA: Purpura, ***leukopenia***
INTEG: Rash, acne
RESP: Upper respiratory tract infection, rhinitis, sinusitis, pharyngitis, coughing

Contraindications: Hypersensitivity to this drug, other carbamates

Precautions: Hepatic disease, renal disease, cardiac disease, P psychosis, pregnancy **C,** lacta- G tion, child <6 yr, elderly

Pharmacokinetics

Absorption	Well absorbed
Distribution	Crosses placenta, plamsa protein binding (22%-25% to albumin)
Metabolism	Liver
Excretion	Kidneys—unchanged (40%-50%)
Half-life	20-23 hr

Pharmacodynamics

Unknown

Interactions

Individual drugs

Carbamazepine: ↓ levels of carbamazepine
Phenytoin: ↑ levels of phenytoin
Valproic acid: ↑ levels of phenytoin

NURSING CONSIDERATIONS

Assessment

- Assess mental status: mood, sensorium, affect, memory (long, short), especially in G elderly
- Assess for blood dyscrasias: fever, sore throat, bruising, rash, jaundice, epistaxis (long-term treatment only)
- Assess seizure activity including type, location, duration, and character; provide seizure precaution

Nursing diagnoses

✓ Injury, risk for (side effects)
✓ Knowledge deficit (teaching)

Implementation

- Give on empty stomach for best absorption

Patient/family education

- Teach patient to carry Medic Alert ID stating name, drugs taken, condition, prescriber's name, phone number
- Advise patient to avoid driving, other activities that require alertness
- Teach patient not to discontinue medication abruptly after long-term use

Evaluation

Positive therapeutic outcome

- Decreased seizure activity

Treatment of overdose: Lavage, vital signs

felodipine (℞)
(fell-oh′di-peen)
Plendil
Func. class.: Calcium-channel blocker, antihypertensive
Chem. class.: Dihydropyridine
Pregnancy category C

Action: Inhibits calcium ion influx across cell membrane, resulting in dilation of peripheral arteries

➡ **Therapeutic Outcome:** Decreased B/P in hypertension

Uses: Essential hypertension, alone or with other antihypertensives

Dosage and routes
Adult: PO 5 mg qd initially, usual range 5-10 mg qd; do not exceed 20 mg qd; do not adjust dosage at intervals of <2 wk

Available forms: Ext rel tabs 5, 10 mg

Adverse effects
CNS: Headache, fatigue, drowsiness, dizziness, anxiety, depression, nervousness, insomnia, light-headedness, paresthesia, tinnitus, psychosis, somnolence
CV: Dysrhythmias, edema, CHF, hypotension, palpitations, ***MI, pulmonary edema,*** tachycardia, syncope, AV block, angina
GI: Nausea, vomiting, diarrhea, gastric upset, constipation, increased liver function studies, dry mouth
HEMA: Anemia
INTEG: Rash, pruritus
MISC: Flushing, sexual difficulties, cough, nasal congestion, shortness of breath, wheezing, epistaxis, respiratory infection, chest pain

Contraindications: Hypersensitivity, sick sinus syndrome, 2nd- or 3rd-degree heart block

Precautions: CHF, hypotension <90 mm Hg systolic, hepatic injury, pregnancy **C,** P lactation, children, renal disease, G elderly

Pharmacokinetics

Absorption	Well absorbed
Distribution	Unknown; protein binding >99%
Metabolism	Liver, extensively
Excretion	Kidneys
Half-life	11-16 hr

Pharmacodynamics

Onset	2-3 hr
Peak	2½-5 hr
Duration	<24 hr

Interactions
Individual drugs
Alcohol: ↑ hypotension
Carbamazepine: ↑ toxicity
Digoxin: ↑ digoxin levels, ↑ bradycardia, CHF
Phenobarbital: ↓ effectiveness
Phenytoin: ↓ effectiveness
Propranolol: ↑ toxicity
Drug classifications
Antihypertensives: ↑ hypotension
β-Adrenergic blockers: ↑ bradycardia, CHF
Nitrates: ↑ nitrates

NURSING CONSIDERATIONS
Assessment
• Assess fluid volume status: I&O ratio and record; weight; skin turgor; adequacy of pulses; moist mucous membranes; bilateral lung sounds; peripheral pitting edema—dehydration symptoms of decreasing output, thirst, hypotension,

dry mouth, and mucous membranes should be reported
- Monitor ALT (SGPT), AST (SGOT), bilirubin daily if these are elevated
- Monitor cardiac status: B/P, pulse, respiration, ECG

Nursing diagnoses

✓ Cardiac output, decreased (uses)
✓ Knowledge deficit (teaching)

Implementation

- Give once a day, with food for GI symptoms
- Do not crush, chew tabs

Patient/family education

- Caution patient to avoid hazardous activities until stabilized on drug, and dizziness is no longer a problem
- Instruct patient to limit caffeine consumption; to avoid alcohol and OTC drugs unless directed by prescriber
- Urge patient to comply in all areas of medical regimen: diet, exercise, stress reduction, drug therapy; to notify prescriber of irregular heart beat, shortness of breath, swelling of feet and hands, pronounced dizziness, constipation, nausea, hypotension
- Teach patient to use as directed even if feeling better; may be taken with other cardiovascular drugs (nitrates, beta blockers)

Evaluation

Positive therapeutic outcome

- Decreased B/P

fenofibrate (℞)
(fen-oh-fee′ brate)
Lipidil

Func. class.: Antilipemic
Chem. class.: Aryloxisobutyric acid derivative

Pregnancy category C

Action: Inhibits biosynthesis of low-density and very low-density lipoproteins, which are responsible for triglyceride development; mobilizes triglycerides from tissue; increases excretion of neutral sterols

Therapeutic Outcome: Decreasing cholesterol levels and low-density lipoproteins, decreased pruritus

Uses: Types IV, V hyperlipidemia

Dosage and routes

Adult: PO 100 mg/day

Available forms: Cap 100 mg

Adverse effects

CNS: Fatigue, weakness, drowsiness, dizziness
CV: Angina, dysrhythmias, thrombophlebitis, ***pulmonary emboli***
GI: Nausea, vomiting, dyspepsia, increased liver enzymes, stomatitis, flatulence, hepatomegaly, gastritis, increased cholethiasis, weight gain
GU: Decreased libido, impotence, dysuria, proteinuria, oliguria, ***hematuria***
HEMA: ***Leukopenia,*** anemia, ***eosinophilia,*** bleeding
INTEG: *Rash,* urticaria, pruritus, dry hair and skin, alopecia
MISC: Polyphagia, weight gain
MS: Myalgias, arthralgias

Contraindications: Severe hepatic disease, severe renal

disease, primary biliary cirrhosis

Precautions: Peptic ulcer, pregnancy **C**, lactation

Pharmacokinetics	
Absorption	Unknown
Distribution	Unknown
Metabolism	Unknown
Excretion	Unknown
Half-life	Unknown

Pharmacodynamics

Unknown

Interactions

Drug classifications

Anticoagulants, oral: ↑ effect of anticoagulants

Diuretics, thiazide: ↓ action of fenofibrate

Estrogens: ↓ action of fenofibrate

Lab test interferences

↑ Liver function studies, ↑ CPK, ↑ BSP, ↑ thymol turbidity, ↑ glucose

↓ Hgb, ↓ Hct, ↓ WBC

NURSING CONSIDERATIONS

Assessment

- Assess nutrition: fat, protein, carbohydrates, nutritional analysis should be completed by dietician
- Assess skin integrity after patient has been receiving drug; itching, pruritus often occur from bile deposits on skin
- Monitor cardiac glycoside level if both drugs are being administered—cardiac glycoside levels will be decreased
- Monitor for signs of vit A, D, K deficiency; serum cholesterol, triglyceride levels, electrolytes if on extended therapy
- Monitor bowel pattern daily; increase bulk, water in diet if constipation develops

Nursing diagnoses

✓ Knowledge deficit (teaching)

✓ Noncompliance (teaching)

Implementation

- Give with evening meal; if dose is increased, take with breakfast and evening meal
- ⊘ Do not chew, crush caps
- Store in cool environment in tight, light-resistant container

Patient/family education

- Inform patient that compliance is needed because toxicity may result if doses are missed
- Teach patient that risk factors—high-fat diet, smoking, alcohol consumption, absence of exercise—should be decreased
- Caution patient to practice birth control while on this drug
- Teach patient to notify prescriber if the GI symptoms of diarrhea, abdominal or epigastric pain, nausea, or vomiting occur
- Instruct patient to report GU symptoms: dysuria, proteinuria, oliguria, decreased libido, impotence

Evaluation

Positive therapeutic outcome

- Decrease in cholesterol to desired level after 8 wk

fenoprofen (℞)

(fen-oh-proe'fen)

fenoprofen, Nalfon

Func. class.: Nonsteroidal antiinflammatory, nonnarcotic analgesic

Chem. class.: Propionic acid derivative

Pregnancy category B

Action: Inhibits prostaglandin synthesis by decreasing enzyme needed for biosynthesis; analgesic, antiinflammatory, antipyretic

Therapeutic Outcome: Decreased pain, inflammation

Uses: Mild to moderate pain, osteoarthritis, rheumatoid arthritis, acute gout, arthritis, ankylosing spondylitis, inflammation, dysmenorrhea

Dosage and routes

Pain

Adult: PO 200 mg q4-6h as needed

Arthritis

Adult: PO 300-600 mg qid, not to exceed 3.2 g/day

Available forms: Caps 200, 300 mg; tab 600 mg

Adverse effects

CNS: Dizziness, headache, drowsiness, fatigue, tremors, confusion, insomnia, anxiety, depression

CV: Tachycardia, peripheral edema, palpitations, dysrhythmias

EENT: Tinnitus, hearing loss, blurred vision

GI: Nausea, anorexia, vomiting, diarrhea, jaundice, ***cholestatic hepatitis,*** constipation, flatulence, cramps, dry mouth, peptic ulcer

GU: ***Nephrotoxicity: dysuria, hematuria, oliguria, azotemia***

HEMA: ***Blood dyscrasias***

INTEG: Purpura, rash, pruritus, sweating

Contraindications: Hypersensitivity, asthma, severe renal disease, severe hepatic disease

Precautions: Pregnancy **B,** 1st and 2nd trimester, lactation, children, bleeding disorders, GI disorders, cardiac disorders, hypersensitivity to other antiinflammatory agents

Pharmacokinetics

Absorption	Well absorbed
Distribution	Does not cross placenta
Metabolism	Extensively—liver
Excretion	Unchanged—kidneys
Half-life	3½ hr

Pharmacodynamics

Onset	15-30 min
Peak	2 hr
Duration	4-6 hr

Interactions

Individual drugs

Cefamandole: ↑ bleeding

Furosemide: ↑ toxic effects

Heparin: ↑ bleeding

Insulin: ↑ effects

Methotrexate: ↑ effects

Phenytoin: ↑ effects

Plicamycin: ↑ bleeding

Probenecid: ↓ effects

Spironolactone: ↓ effects

Sulfinpyrazone: ↓ effects

Valproic acid: ↑ effects, ↑ bleeding

Vancomycin: ↑ ototoxicity

Drug classifications

Antacids: ↓ effects of fenoprofen

Anticoagulants: ↑ effects

Carbonic anhydrase inhibitors: ↑ toxic effects

Nonsteroidal antiinflammatories: ↑ gastric ulcers
Salicylates: ↓ blood sugar levels
Steroids: ↓ effects of fenoprofen, ↑ gastric ulcers
Sulfonylamides: ↓ effects

NURSING CONSIDERATIONS

Assessment

- Monitor liver function; renal function, other blood studies: AST (SGOT), ALT (SGPT), bilirubin, creatinine, BUN, CBC, Hct, Hgb, pro-time if patient is on long-term therapy
- Check I&O ratio; decreasing output may indicate renal failure (long-term therapy)
- Assess for allergic reactions: rash, urticaria; if these occur, drug may have to be discontinued
- Assess for ototoxicity: tinnitus, ringing, roaring in ears; audiometric testing needed before, after long-term therapy
- Assess for visual changes: blurring, halos; corneal, retinal damage
- Check edema in feet, ankles, legs
- Identify prior drug history; there are many drug interactions
- Monitor pain: location, duration, type, intensity, prior to dose and 1 hr after; ROM prior to dose and after

Nursing diagnoses

✓ Pain (uses)
✓ Mobility, impaired (uses)
✓ Knowledge deficit (teaching)
✓ Injury, risk for (adverse reactions)

Implementation

- Administer to patient crushed or whole; chewable tab may be chewed (do not crush enteric product)
- Give with food or milk to decrease gastric symptoms; absorption may be slowed; give 30 min ac or 2 hr pc

Patient/family education

- Teach patient to report any symptoms of renal toxicity, visual changes, ototoxicity, allergic reactions, bleeding (long-term therapy)
- Advise patient to take with 8 oz of water and sit upright for ½ hr after dose to prevent ulceration
- Caution patient not to exceed recommended dosage—acute poisoning may result—and to take as prescribed, do not double dose
- Instruct patient to read label on other OTC drugs; many contain other antiinflammatories
- Inform patient that the therapeutic response takes 2 wk (arthritis)
- Teach patient to report tinnitus, confusion, diarrhea, sweating, hyperventilation, blurred vision, fever, joint aches
- Caution patient to avoid alcohol ingestion; GI bleeding may occur

Evaluation

Positive therapeutic outcome

- Decreased pain
- Decreased inflammation
- Increased mobility

fexofenadine (℞)

(fex-oh-fin'a-deen)

Allegra

Func. class.: H_1 histamine antagonist

Pregnancy category C

Action: Acts on blood vessels, GI, respiratory system by competing with histamine for H_1-receptor site; decreases allergic response by blocking pharmacologic effects of histamine; less sedation rate than with other antihistamines; causes increased heart rate, vasodilation, increased secretions

Therapeutic Outcome: Absence of allergy symptoms and rhinitis

Uses: Rhinitis, allergy symptoms, chronic idiopathic urticaria

Dosage and routes

P ***Adult and child >12 yr:*** 60 mg bid

Renal function impairment 60 mg qd

Available forms: Cap 60 mg

Adverse effects

CNS: Headache, stimulation, drowsiness, sedation, fatigue, confusion, blurred vision, tinnitus, restlessness, tremors, P paradoxical excitation in chil- G dren or elderly

CV: Hypotension, palpitations, bradycardia, tachycardia, dysrhythmias (rare)

GI: Nausea, diarrhea, abdominal pain, vomiting, constipation

GU: Frequency, dysuria, urinary retention, impotence

HEMA: Hemolytic anemia, thrombocytopenia, leukopenia, agranulocytosis, pancytopenia

INTEG: Rash, eczema, photosensitivity, urticaria

RESP: Thickening of bronchial secretions; dry nose, throat

Contraindications: Hypersen- P sitivity, newborn or premature infants, lactation, severe hepatic disease

Precautions: Pregnancy **C,** G elderly, children, respiratory P disease, narrow-angle glaucoma, prostatic hypertrophy, bladder neck obstruction, asthma

Pharmacokinetics

Absorption	Well absorbed
Distribution	Unknown
Metabolism	Liver
Excretion	Kidneys

Pharmacodynamics

Onset	15-30 min
Peak	1-2 hr
Duration	8-12 hr

Interactions

Individual drugs

Alcohol: ↑ CNS depression

Erythromycin: ↑ CV reaction

Itraconazole: ↑ CV reaction

Ketoconazole: ↑ CV reaction

Procarbazine: ↑ CNS depression

Drug classifications

Anticoagulants, oral: ↓ action

CNS depressants: ↑ CNS depression

MAOI: ↑ anticholinergic effect

Narcotics: ↑ CNS depression

Sedative/hypnotics: ↑ CNS depression

Food

↓ absorption

Lab test interferences

False negative: Skin allergy tests (discontinue antihistamine 3 days before testing)

F

NURSING CONSIDERATIONS
Assessment
- Assess respiratory status: rate, rhythm, increase in bronchial secretions, wheezing, chest tightness; provide fluids to 2 L/day to decrease secretion thickness
- Monitor I&O ratio: be alert for urinary retention, frequency, dysuria, especially G elderly; drug should be discontinued if these occur

Nursing diagnoses
- ✓ Airway clearance, ineffective (uses)
- ✓ Injury, risk for (side effects)
- ✓ Knowledge deficit (teaching)
- ✓ Noncompliance (teaching, overuse)

Implementation
- Give on an empty stomach 1 hr before or 2 hr pc to facilitate absorption
- Store in tight, light-resistant container

Patient/family education
- Teach all aspects of drug uses; to notify prescriber if confusion, sedation, hypotension occur; to avoid driving or other hazardous activity if drowsiness occurs; to avoid alcohol or other CNS depressants that may potentiate effect
- Instruct patient to take 1 hr before or 2 hr pc to facilitate absorption
- Instruct patient not to exceed recommended dose; dysrhythmias may occur
- Teach patient that hard candy, gum, frequent rinsing of mouth may be used for dryness

Evaluation
Positive therapeutic outcome
- Absence of running or congested nose, rashes

Treatment of overdose: Administer ipecac syrup or lavage, diazepam, vasopressors, barbiturates (short acting)

fentanyl (℞)
(fen'ta-nill)
fentanyl, Sublimaze
Func. class.: Narcotic analgesic
Chem. class.: Opiate, synthetic phenylpiperidine derivative
Pregnancy category C
Controlled substance schedule II

Action: Inhibits ascending pain pathways in CNS, increases pain threshold, alters pain perception by binding to opiate receptors

➔ **Therapeutic Outcome:** Relief of pain, supplement to anesthesia

Uses: Preoperatively, postoperatively; adjunct to general anesthetic, when combined with droperidol

Dosage and routes
Anesthetic
Adult: **IV** 0.05-0.1 mg q2-3 min prn
Preoperatively
Adult: IM 0.05-0.1 mg q30-60 min before surgery
Postoperatively
Adult: IM 0.05-0.1 mg q1-2hr prn
P ***Child:*** IM 0.02-0.03 mg/9 kg

Available forms: Inj 0.05 mg/ml

Adverse effects
CNS: Dizziness, delirium, euphoria, light-headedness,

sedation, dysphoria, agitation, anxiety
CV: ***Bradycardia, cardiac arrest,*** hypotension or hypertension, facial flushing, chills
EENT: Blurred vision, miosis
GI: Nausea, vomiting, diarrhea, cramps
MS: Muscle rigidity
RESP: ***Respiratory depression, arrest, laryngospasm***

Contraindications: Hypersensitivity to opiates, myasthenia gravis

G **Precautions:** Elderly, respiratory depression, increased intracranial pressure, seizure disorders, severe respiratory disorders, cardiac dysrhythmias, pregnancy C

Pharmacokinetics

Absorption	Well absorbed (IM), completely absorbed (IV)
Distribution	Unknown, crosses placenta
Metabolism	Extensively—liver, 80% bound to plasma proteins
Excretion	Kidneys—up to 25% unchanged, breast milk
Half-life	1½-6 hr

Pharmacodynamics

	IM	IV
Onset	7-8 min	Rapid
Peak	30 min	3-5 min
Duration	1-2 hr	½-1 hr

Interactions

Individual drugs

Alcohol: ↑ respiratory depression, hypotension, ↑ sedation
Cimetidine: ↑ recovery
Erythromycin: ↑ recovery
Nalbuphine: ↓ analgesia
Pentazocine: ↓ analgesia

Drug classifications

Antihistamines: ↑ respiratory depression, hypotension
CNS depressants: ↑ respiratory depression, hypotension
MAOI: Do not use 2 wk before fentanyl
Phenothiazines: ↑ respiratory depression, hypotension
Sedative/hypnotics: ↑ respiratory depression, hypotension

Lab test interferences

↑ Amylase, ↑ lipase

NURSING CONSIDERATIONS

F

Assessment

- Monitor vital signs after parenteral route (B/P, pulse, respiration); note muscle rigidity; take drug history before administering drug; check liver, kidney function tests; assess for respiratory dysfunction: respiratory depression, character, rate, rhythm; notify prescriber if respirations are <10/min
- Monitor CNS changes: dizziness, drowsiness, hallucinations, euphoria, LOC, pupil reaction
- Monitor allergic reactions: rash, urticaria; drug should be discontinued
- Assess for pain: intensity, location, duration, type, before and 15 min after IM route or 3-5 min after **IV** route

Nursing diagnoses

- ✓ Pain (uses)
- ✓ Sensory-perceptual alteration: visual, auditory (adverse reactions)
- ✓ Breathing pattern, ineffective (adverse reactions)
- ✓ Knowledge deficit (teaching)

Implementation

- Give by inj (IM, **IV**), only with resuscitative equipment available; give slowly to prevent rigidity
- Give **IV** undiluted by anesthesiologist or diluted with 5

ml or more sterile water or 0.9% NcCl given through Y-tube or 3-way stopcock given at 0.1 mg or less/ 1.2 min

- Store in light-resistant area at room temp

Syringe compatibilities: Atracurium, atropine, butorphanol, chlorpromazine, cimetidine, dimenhydrinate, diphenhydramine, droperidol, heparin, hydromorphone, hydroxyzine, meperidine, metoclopramide, midazolam, morphine, pentazocine, perphenazine, prochlorperazine, promazine, promethazine, ranitidine, scopolamine

Syringe incompatibility: Pentobarbital

Y-site compatibilities: Atracurium, enalaprilat, esmolol, heparin, hydrocortisone, labetalol, lorazepam, midazolam, nafcillin, pancuronium, potassium chloride, vecuronium, vit B/C

Additive compatibilities: Bupivacaine, sodium bicarbonate

Additive incompatibilities: Methohexital, pentobarbital, thiopental

Solution compatibilities: D_5W, 0.9% NaCl

Patient/family education

- Advise patient to report any symptoms of CNS changes, allergic reactions
- Instruct patient to avoid CNS depressants: alcohol, sedative/hypnotics for at least 24 hr after taking this drug
- Teach patient that dizziness, drowsiness, confusion are common, and to avoid getting up without assistance
- Discuss in detail with patient all aspects of the drug

Evaluation

Positive therapeutic outcome

- Maintenance of anesthesia
- Decreased pain

Treatment of overdose: Narcan 0.2-0.8 **IV**, O_2, **IV** fluids, vasopressors

fentanyl transdermal (℞)

(fen′ta-nill)

Duragesic-25, Duragesic-50, Duragesic-75, Duragesic-100

Func. class.: Narcotic, analgesic

Chem. class.: Opiate, synthetic phenylpiperidine

Pregnancy category C

Controlled substance schedule II

Action: Inhibits ascending pain pathways in CNS, increases pain threshold, alters pain perception by binding to opiate receptors

➔ **Therapeutic Outcome:** Relief of chronic pain

Uses: Management of chronic pain for those requiring opioid analgesia

Dosage and routes

Adult: 25 μg/hr; may increase until pain relief occurs; apply patch to flat surface on upper torso and wear for 72 hr; apply new patch on different site for continued relief

Available forms: Patches 2.5, 5, 7.5, 10 mg

Adverse effects

CNS: Dizziness, delirium, euphoria, light-headedness,

sedation, dysphoria, agitation, anxiety
CV: Bradycardia, ***cardiac arrest***, hypotension or hypertension, facial flushing, chills
EENT: Blurred vision, miosis
GI: Nausea, vomiting, diarrhea, cramps
RESP: Respiratory depression, laryngospasm, bronchospasm; depresses cough; hypoventilation

Contraindications: Hypersensitivity to opiates, myasthenia gravis

G **Precautions:** Elderly, respiratory depression, increased intracranial pressure, seizure disorders, severe respiratory disorders, cardiac dysrhythmias, pregnancy **C**, fever

Pharmacokinetics	
Absorption	92% (skin), continuously for 72 hr
Distribution	Crosses placenta
Metabolism	Extensively—liver
Excretion	Up to 25%—kidneys unchanged
Half-life	17 hr after removal of patch

Pharmacodynamics	
Onset	6 hr
Peak	12-24 hr
Duration	72 hr

Interactions

Individual drugs

Alcohol: ↑ respiratory depression, hypotension, ↑ sedation
Cimetidine: ↑ recovery
Erythromycin: ↑ recovery
Nalbuphine: ↓ analgesia
Pentazocine: ↓ analgesia

Drug classifications

Antihistamines: ↑ respiratory depression, hypotension
CNS depressants: ↑ respiratory depression, hypotension
MAOI: Do not use 2 wk before fentanyl
Phenothiazines: ↑ respiratory depression, hypotension
Sedative/hypnotics: ↑ respiratory depression, hypotension

Lab test interferences

↑ Amylase, ↑ lipase

NURSING CONSIDERATIONS

Assessment

- Assess for respiratory dysfunction: respiratory depression, character, rate, rhythm; notify prescriber if respirations are <10/min
- Monitor CNS changes: dizziness, drowsiness, hallucinations, euphoria, LOC, pupil reaction
- Monitor allergic reactions: rash, urticaria; drug should be discontinued
- Assess for pain: intensity, location, duration, type—before and after administration

Nursing diagnoses

✓ Pain (uses)
✓ Sensory-perceptual alteration: visual, auditory (adverse reactions)
✓ Breathing pattern, ineffective (adverse reactions)
✓ Knowledge deficit (teaching)

Implementation

- Narcotic analgesics should be used to control pain until relief is obtained with transdermal patch; patients may continue to require other narcotics for breakthrough pain; if >100 μg/hr is required, use multiple systems
- Apply patch to chest on a flat area with skin intact; for skin preparation, use clear water with no soap; clip hair, skin should be dry before applying patch; apply immediately after removing from package and press firmly in place with palm of hand; flush old patch down

toilet immediately upon removal

Use pain dosing

• Dosage is titrated based on patient's report of pain; dosage is determined by calculating the previous 24-hr requirement and converting to equianalgesic morphine dose

• To convert to another narcotic analgesic, remove transdermal patch and begin treatment with half the equal pain controlling dose of the new analgesic in 12-18 hr

• Medication should be tapered gradually after longterm use to prevent withdrawal symptoms

Patient/family education

• Advise patient to report any symptoms of CNS changes, allergic reactions

• Instruct patients to avoid CNS depressants: alcohol, sedative/hypnotics for at least 24 hr after this drug

• Discuss with patient that dizziness, drowsiness, and confusion are common and to avoid getting up without assistance

• Discuss all aspects of the drug in detail

Evaluation

Positive therapeutic outcome

• Decreased pain

Treatment of overdose: Narcan 0.2-0.8 **IV**, O_2, **IV** fluids, vasopressors

ferrous fumarate/ ferrous gluconate/ ferrous sulfate (℞, OTC)

(fer'us)

Femiron, Feostat, Ferrets, Ferrous Fumarate, Fumasorb, Fumerin, Hemocyte, Ircon, Nephro-Fer, Span-FF, Fergon, Ferralet, Ferralet S.R., ferrous gluconate, Simron, Feosol, Feratab, Fer-In-Sol, Fer-Iron, Fero-Gradumet, Ferospace, Ferralyn, Ferra-TD, ferrous sulfate, Mol-Iron, Slow-Fe

Func. class.: Hematinic

Chem. class.: Iron preparation

Pregnancy category A

Action: Replaces iron stores needed for red blood cell development, energy and O_2 transport, utilization; fumarate contains 33% elemental iron; gluconate, 12%; sulfate, 20%; iron, 30%; ferrous sulfate exsiccated

Therapeutic Outcome: Prevention and correction of iron deficiency

Uses: Iron deficiency anemia, prophylaxis for iron deficiency in pregnancy

Dosage and routes

Fumarate

Adult: PO 200 mg tid-qid

P ***Child 2-12 yr:*** PO 3 mg/kg/day (elemental iron) tid-qid

P ***Child 6 mo-2 yr:*** PO up to 6 mg/kg/day (elemental iron) tid-qid

P ***Child 6 mo-2 yr:*** PO 6 mg/kg/day in 3-4 divided doses

P ***Infants:*** PO 10-25 mg/day (elemental iron) in 3-4 divided doses

Gluconate
Adult: PO 200-600 mg tid

P ***Child 6-12 yr:*** PO 300-900 mg qd

P ***Child <6 yr:*** PO 100-300 mg-qd

Sulfate
Adult: PO 0.750-1.5 g/day in divided doses tid

P ***Child 6-12 yr:*** 600 mg/day in divided doses

Pregnancy
Adult: PO 300-600 mg/day in divided doses

Available forms:
Fumarate:
Tabs 63, 195, 200, 324, 325 mg; tab, chewable 100 mg; tab, controlled-release 300 mg; oral susp 100 mg/5 ml, 45 mg/0.6 ml

Gluconate:
Tabs 300, 320, 325, mg; caps 86, 325, 435 mg; tab, film-coated 300 mg; elix 300 mg/5 ml

Sulfate:
Tabs 195, 300, 325, mg; tab, enteric-coated 325 mg; tab, extended-release; time-release cap 525 mg

Adverse effects
GI: Nausea, constipation, epigastric pain, black and red tarry stools, vomiting, diarrhea
INTEG: Temporarily discolored tooth enamel and eyes

Contraindications: Hypersensitivity, ulcerative colitis/regional enteritis, hemosiderosis/hemochromatosis, peptic ulcer disease, hemolytic anemia, cirrhosis

Precautions: Anemia (long-term), pregnancy **A**

Pharmacokinetics

Absorption	Up to 30%
Distribution	Bound to transferrin, crosses placenta
Metabolism	Recycled
Excretion	Feces, urine, skin, breast milk
Half-life	Unknown

Pharmacodynamics

Unknown

Interactions
Individual drugs
Chloramphenicol: ↑ absorption of iron products
Levodopa: ↓ absorption of levodopa
Methyldopa: ↓ absorption of methyldopa
Penicillamine: ↓ absorption of penicillamine
Quinolone: ↓ absorption of quinolone
Tetracycline: ↓ absorption of iron products
Vitamin C: ↑ absorption of iron products
Lab test interferences
False positive: Occult blood

NURSING CONSIDERATIONS
Assessment
- Monitor blood studies: Hct, Hgb, reticulocytes, bilirubin before treatment, at least monthly
- Assess for toxicity: nausea, vomiting, diarrhea (green, then tarry stools,) hematemesis, pallor, cyanosis, shock, coma
- Assess bowel elimination; if constipation occurs, increase water, bulk, activity before laxatives are required
- Assess nutrition: amount of iron in diet (meat, dark green leafy vegetables, dried beans,

dried fruits, eggs); provide referral to dietician if indicated
- Identify cause of iron loss or anemia, including salicylates, sulfonamides, antimalarials, quinidine

Nursing diagnoses
- ✓ Nutrition, less than body requirements (uses)
- ✓ Fatigue (uses)
- ✓ Knowledge deficit (teaching)

Implementation
- P Give only with vit E supplements to infants or hemolytic anemia may occur
- Give between meals for best absorption; may give with juice; do not give with antacids or milk, delay at least 1 hr; if GI symptoms occur, give PC even if absorption is decreased; eggs, milk products, chocolate, caffeine interfere with absorption
- ⊘ Do not crush, chew tabs
- Give liq preparations through plastic straw to avoid discoloration of tooth enamel; dilute thoroughly
- Give at least 1 hr before bedtime because corrosion may occur in stomach
- Give for <6 mo for anemia
- Store in air-tight, light-resistant container

Patient/family education
- Advise patient that iron will make stools black or dark green; that iron poisoning may occur if increased beyond recommended level
- Tell patient not to crush; swallow tab whole; to keep out P of reach of children
- Caution patient not to substitute one iron salt for another; elemental iron content differs (e.g., 300 mg ferrous fumarate contains about 100 mg elemental iron, whereas 300 mg ferrous gluconate contains only about 30 mg elemental iron)
- Caution patient to avoid reclining position for 15-30 min after taking drug to avoid esophageal corrosion; to follow diet high in iron

Evaluation

Positive therapeutic outcome
- Decreased fatigue, weakness
- Improvement in Hct, Hgb, reticulocytes

Treatment of overdose: Induce vomiting; give eggs, milk until lavage can be done

fibrinolysin/desoxyribonuclease (℞)

(fye-brin-oe-lye′sin/dez-ox-ee-rye-boe-nuke′lee-ase)

Elase

Func. class.: Enzyme

Chem. class.: Proteolytic-bovine

Pregnancy category C

Action: Dissolves fibrin in clots and fibrinous exudates, attacks DNA in areas of disintegrating cells

➔ **Therapeutic Outcome:** A clean wound

Uses: Debridement of wounds, vaginitis, cervicitis, ulcerative colitis, 2nd-, 3rd-degree burns; irrigating wounds, topically

Dosage and routes

Debridement/intravaginally

Adult: Oint 5 g × 5 applications

Irrigating
Adult: Irrig dilution depends on type of wound

Available forms: Fibrinolysin with desoxyribonuclease 666.6 U/g; powder for reconstitution fibrinolysin 25 U/desoxyribonuclease 15,000 U

Adverse effects
INTEG: Hyperemia

Contraindications: Hypersensitivity to bovine or mercury products, hematoma

Precautions: Pregnancy **C**

Pharmacokinetics	
Absorption	Not absorbed
Distribution	Unknown
Metabolism	Unknown
Excretion	Unknown
Half-life	Unknown

Pharmacodynamics

Unknown

Interactions: None

NURSING CONSIDERATIONS

Assessment
- Assess for signs of irritation and inflammation around wound; drug should be discontinued
- Assess wound for drainage, color, odor, size, depth before and during therapy

Nursing diagnoses
✓ Skin integrity, altered (uses)
✓ Knowledge deficit (teaching)

Implementation

Top route
- Apply after reconstituting top sol with 10-50 ml sterile NaCl sol; use only fresh sol; reconstituted sol is stable for 24 hr; remove necrotic debris, dry eschar
- Saturate gauze with sol; pack area; remove in 6-8 hr and clean; repeat tid-qid
- Apply top oint after flushing wound with saline, water or hydrogen peroxide, let dry or pat dry, then apply a small amount of oint to area and cover with a nonadhesive dressing; change qd or bid

Vag route
- Place 5 ml in applicator, apply with patient recumbent

Patient/family education
- Teach patient reason for treatment and expected results

Evaluation

Positive therapeutic outcome
- Decrease in wound scarring, tissue necrosis

filgrastim (℞)

(fill-gras′stim)

Neupogen

Func. class.: Biologic modifier

Chem. class.: Granulocyte colony-stimulating factor

Pregnancy category C

Action: Stimulates proliferation and differentiation of neutrophils; a glycoprotein

➡ **Therapeutic Outcome:** Absence of infection

Uses: To decrease infection in patients receiving antineoplastics that are myelosuppressive; to increase WBC in patients with drug-induced neutropenia

Dosage and routes
Adult: **IV**/SC 5 μg/kg/day in a single dose; may increase by 5 μg/kg in each chemotherapy cycle; give qd for up to 2 wk until the absolute neutrophil count (ANC) has reached 10,000/mm^3; response to

G-CSF is much greater with SC than **IV** therapy

Available forms: Inj 300 μg/ml

Adverse effects

CNS: Fever

GI: Nausea, vomiting, diarrhea, mucositis, anorexia

HEMA: Thrombocytopenia

INTEG: Alopecia, exacerbation of skin conditions

MS: Osteoporosis, skeletal pain

RESP: Respiratory distress syndrome

Contraindications: Hypersensitivity to proteins of *E. coli*

Precautions: Pregnancy **C,** lactation, cardiac conditions, P children, myeloid malignancies

Pharmacokinetics

Absorption	Well absorbed (SC), completely absorbed (IV)
Distribution	Unknown
Metabolism	Unknown
Excretion	Unknown
Half-life	Unknown

Pharmacodynamics

Unknown

Interactions

Drug classifications

Antineoplastics: ↑ neutrophils, do not use together 24 hr before or after antineoplastics

Lab test interferences

↑ Uric acid, ↑ lactate dehydrogenase, ↑ alk phosphatase

NURSING CONSIDERATIONS

Assessment

• Monitor blood studies: CBC, platelet count before treatment and twice weekly; neutrophil counts (ANC) may be increased for 2 days after therapy, but treatment should continue until ANC >10,000/mm^3

• Assess for bone pain: frequency, intensity, duration; analgesics may be given; opiates should not be used

• Check B/P, heart rate, respiration, baseline and during treatment

Nursing diagnoses

✓ Infection, risk for (uses)
✓ Pain, acute (adverse reaction)
✓ Knowledge deficit (teaching)

Implementation

IV **IV route**

• Give 300 μg/ml or 480 μg/1.6 ml; allow to warm to room temp; give single dose over 1 min or less through Y-tube or medport

• Use single-use vials; after dose is withdrawn, do not reenter vial

• Give for 2 wk or until ANC is 10,000/mm^3 after the expected chemotherapy neutrophil nadir

• Store in refrigerator; do not freeze; may store at room temp for up to 6 hr; avoid shaking

Y-site compatibilities: Acyclovir, allopurinol, amikacin, aminophylline, ampicillin, aztreonam, bleomycin, bumetanide, buprenorphine, butorphanol, calcium gluconate, carboplatin, carmustine, cefazolin, cefotetan, ceftazidime, chlorpromazine, cimetidine, cisplatin, cyclophosphamide, cytarabine, dacarbazine, daunorubicin, dexamethasone, diphenhydramine, doxorubicin, doxycycline, droperidol, enalaprilat, famotidine, floxuridine, fluconazole, fludarabine, ganciclovir, gentamicin, haloperidol, hydrocortisone, hydromorphone, hydroxyzine, idarubicin, ifosfamide, imipenem/cilastatin, leucovorin, lorazepam, mechlorethamine, melphalan, meperidine, mesna, methotrexate, metoclopramide, miconazole, minocycline, mitoxantrone, morphine, nalbuphine, netilmicin, ondansetron, plicamycin, potassium chloride, promethazine, ranitidine, sodium bicarbonate, streptozocin, ticarcillin, tobramycin, trimethoprim-sulfamethoxazole, vancomycin, vinblastine, vincristine, vinorelbine, zidovudine

Patient/family education
- Teach patient technique for self-administration: dose, side effects, disposal of containers and needles, provide instruction sheet

Evaluation
Positive therapeutic outcome
- Absence of infection

finasteride (℞)
(fin-ass'te-ride)
Proscar
Func. class.: Androgen hormone inhibitor
Chem. class.: 5-α-reductase inhibitor
Pregnancy category X

Action: Inhibits 5-α-reductase and reduction in DHT; DHT induces androgenic effects by binding to androgen receptors in the cell nuclei of the prostate gland, liver, skin; produces lower levels of 5-α-reductase, which prevents development of benign prostatic hypertrophy (BPH)

➔ **Therapeutic Outcome:** Reduced prostate size

Uses: Symptomatic benign prostatic hyperplasia

Dosage and routes
Adult: PO 5 mg qd × 6-12 mo

Available forms: Tab 5 mg

Adverse effects
GU: Impotence, decreased libido, decreased volume of ejaculate

Contraindications: Hypersensitivity, pregnancy **X**, P children, women

Precautions: Large residual urinary volume, severely diminished urinary flow, liver function abnormalities

Pharmacokinetics

Absorption	(63%)
Distribution	Plasma protein binding, crosses blood-brain barrier
Metabolism	Liver
Excretion	Kidneys—metabolites (39%), feces (57%)
Half-life	6-15 hr

Pharmacodynamics

Onset	Immediate
Peak	8 hr
Duration	14 days

Interactions
Drug classifications
Anticholinergics: ↓ effect of finasteride
Bronchodilators, adrenergic: ↓ effect of finasteride
Theophylline: ↓ effect of finasteride

NURSING CONSIDERATIONS
Assessment
- Assess urinary patterns, residual urinary volume, severely diminished urinary flow; PSA levels and digital rectal

F

exam before initiating therapy and periodically thereafter
• Monitor liver function studies before initiating treatment; extensively metabolized in liver

Nursing diagnoses
✓ Urinary elimination, altered (uses)
✓ Knowledge deficit (teaching)

Implementation
• Administer without regard to meals
• Store at temp <86° F (30° C); protect from light; keep container tightly closed

Patient/family education
• Advise patient that pregnant women should not touch crushed tab or come into contact with semen of a patient taking this drug; may adversely affect development of male fetus
• Inform patient that volume of ejaculate may be decreased during treatment; impotence and decreased libido may also occur

Evaluation
Positive therapeutic outcome
• Decreased postvoiding dribbling, frequency, nocturia
• Increased urinary flow

flecainide (℞)
(flek′a-nide)
Tambocor
Func. class.: Antidysrhythmic (Class IC)
Pregnancy category C

Action: Decreases conduction in all parts of the heart, with greatest effect on the His-Purkinje system, which stabilizes the cardiac membrane

➔ **Therapeutic Outcome:** Absence of dysrhythmias

Uses: Life-threatening ventricular dysrhythmias, sustained ventricular tachycardia; supraventricular tachydysrhythmias

Dosage and routes
Adult: PO 50-100 mg q12h; may increase every 4 days by 50 mg q12h to desired response, not to exceed 400 mg/day

Available forms: Tabs 50, 100, 150 mg

Adverse effects
CNS: Headache, dizziness, involuntary movement, confusion, psychosis, restlessness, irritability, paresthesias, ataxia, flushing, somnolence, depression, anxiety, malaise
CV: Hypotension, bradycardia, angina, PVCs, ***heart block, cardiovascular collapse, arrest,*** *dysrhythmias,* ***CHF, fatal ventricular tachycardia***
EENT: Tinnitus, *blurred vision,* hearing loss
GI: Nausea, vomiting, anorexia, constipation, abdominal pain, flatulence, change in taste
GU: Impotence, decreased libido, polyuria, urinary retention
HEMA: Leukopenia, thrombocytopenia
INTEG: Rash, urticaria, edema, swelling
RESP: Dyspnea, ***respiratory depression***

Contraindications: Hypersensitivity, severe heart block, cardiogenic shock, nonsustained ventricular dysrhythmias, frequent PVCs, non–life-threatening dysrhythmias

Precautions: Pregnancy **C,** lactation, **P** children, renal disease, liver disease, CHF, respiratory depression, myasthenia gravis

Pharmacokinetics

Absorption	Well absorbed
Distribution	Widely distributed
Metabolism	Liver
Excretion	30% kidneys, unchanged
Half-life	14 hr

Pharmacodynamics

Onset	Unknown
Peak	3 hr
Duration	Unknown

Interactions

Individual drugs

Amiodarone: ↑ blood levels, ↑ toxicity
Digoxin: ↑ blood levels, ↑ toxicity
Disopyramide: ↑ levels, ↑ toxicity
Flecainide: ↑ levels, ↑ toxicity
Lidocaine: Bradycardia, arrest
Mexiletine: ↑ levels, ↑ toxicity
Phenytoin: ↑ blood levels
Procainamide: ↑ levels, ↑ toxicity
Quinidine: ↑ levels, ↑ toxicity
Warfarin: ↑ level, ↑ bleeding

Drug classifications

β-blockers: ↑ dysrhythmias, arrest
Calcium channel blockers: ↑ dysrhythmias, arrest

NURSING CONSIDERATIONS

Assessment

- Monitor ECG continuously to determine drug effectiveness; measure PR, QRS, QT intervals; check for PVCs, other dysrhythmias; monitor B/P continuously for hypotension, hypertension and rebound hypertension (after 1-2 hr); check for dehydration or hypovolemia
- Monitor I&O ratio; electrolytes: [K (potassium), Na (sodium)], Cl (chloride); check weight daily and for signs of CHG or pulmonary toxicity: dyspnea, fatigue, cough, fever, chest pain; if these occur, drug should be discontinued
- Monitor liver function studies: AST (SGOT), ALT (SGPT), bilirubin, alk phosphatase
- Assess patient for CNS symptoms: confusion, psychosis, numbness, depression, involuntary movements; if these occur, drug should be discontinued
- Assess patient for hyperthyroidism: lethargy, dizziness, constipation, enlarged thyroid gland, edema of extremities, cool, pale skin; assess patient for hyperthyroidism: restlessness; tachycardia; eyelid puffiness; weight loss; frequent urination; menstrual irregularities; dyspnea; warm, moist skin
- Monitor cardiac rate, respiration: rate, rhythm, character, chest pain; watch for ventricular tachycardia, supraventricular tachycardia, or fibrillation

Nursing diagnoses

✓ Cardiac output, decreased (uses)
✓ Knowledge deficit (teaching)

Implementation

- Give reduced dosage slowly with ECG monitoring; do not increase dose fewer than 4 days apart
- Give with meals if GI upset occurs

Patient/family education

- Instruct patient to report side effects immediately to health care provider

• Instruct patient to complete follow-up appointment with health care provider including pulmonary function studies, chest x-ray

Evaluation
Positive therapeutic outcome
• Absence of dysrythmias

floxuridine (℞)
(flox-yoor′i-deen)
floxuridine, FUDR
Func. class.: Antineoplastic, antimetabolite
Chem. class.: Pyrimidine antagonist
Pregnancy category D

Action: Inhibits DNA synthesis; interferes with cell replication by competitively inhibiting thymidylate synthesis S phase of cell cycle

Therapeutic Outcome: Prevention of rapidly growing malignant cells

Uses: GI adenocarcinoma metastatic to liver; cancer of breast, head, neck, liver, brain, gallbladder, bile duct

Dosage and routes
Adult: Intraarterial by continuous inf 0.1-0.6 mg/kg/day × 1-6 wk; hepatic artery inj 0.4-0.6 mg/kg/day × 1-6 wk

Available forms: Powder for inj 500 mg/5 ml vial

Adverse effects
CNS: Lethargy, malaise, weakness
EENT: Epistaxis
GI: Anorexia, diarrhea, nausea, vomiting, ***hemorrhage,*** stomatitis
GU: Renal failure
HEMA: Thrombocytopenia, leukopenia, myelosuppression, anemia
INTEG: Rash, fever, alopecia

Contraindications: Hypersensitivity, myelosuppression, pregnancy **D,** poor nutritional status, serious infections

Precautions: Renal disease, hepatic disease, bone marrow depression

Pharmacokinetics	
Absorption	Direct to tumor
Distribution	To tumor, crosses blood-brain barrier
Metabolism	Liver
Excretion	60%-80% lungs, kidneys (small)
Half-life	Initial 10-20 min, 20 hr terminal

Pharmacodynamics	
Onset	1 wk
Peak	1-3 wk
Duration	4 wk

Interactions
Individual drugs
Radiation: ↑ toxicity, bone marrow suppression
Drug classifications
Antineoplastics: ↑ toxicity bone marrow suppression
Live virus vaccine: ↑ adverse reactions
Lab test interferences
↑ Liver function studies

NURSING CONSIDERATIONS
Assessment
• Assess buccal cavity q8h for dryness, sores or ulceration, white patches, oral pain, bleeding, dysphagia; obtain prescription for viscous lidocaine (Xylocaine)
• Monitor CBC, differential, platelet count weekly; withhold drug if WBC count is <4000/

mm^3 or platelet count is <100,000/mm^3; notify prescriber of results if WBC <20,000/mm^3, platelets <50,000/mm^3

- Monitor renal function studies: BUN, creatinine, serum uric acid, urine CrCl before and during therapy; I&O ratio; report fall in urine output to <30 ml/hr
- Monitor temp q4h (may indicate beginning of infection)
- Monitor liver function tests before and during therapy (bilirubin, AST (SGOT), ALT (SGPT), LDH) as needed or monthly
- Assess for bleeding: hematuria, stool guaiac, bruising or petechiae, mucosa or orifices q8h; inflammation of mucosa, breaks in skin
- Identify effects of alopecia on body image; discuss feelings about body changes

Nursing diagnoses

- ✓ Injury, risk for (adverse reactions)
- ✓ Body image disturbance (adverse reactions)
- ✓ Infection, risk for (adverse reactions)
- ✓ Knowledge deficit (teaching)

Implementation

- Avoid contact with skin, very irritating, wash completely to remove
- Give fluids **IV** or PO before chemotherapy to hydrate patient
- Give antiemetic 30-60 min before giving drug to prevent vomiting, and prn; administer antibiotics for prophylaxis of infection
- Give top or syst analgesics for pain
- Give in AM so drug can be eliminated before hs
- Provide liq diet: carbonated beverages; gelatin may be added if patient is not nauseated or vomiting
- Recommend that patient rinse mouth tid-qid with water, club soda; brushing of teeth bid-qid with soft brush or cotton-tipped applicators for stomatitis; use unwaxed dental floss

IA route

- Give by intraarterial inf pump after diluting 5 ml drug/5 ml sterile H_2O for inj; dilute further with D_5W or normal saline to required dilution; stable if refrigerated for 14 days.

Additive compatibilites: Carboplatin, cisplatin, cisplatin with etoposide, cisplatin with leucovorin, etoposide, fluorouracil, fluorouracil with leucovorin, leucovorin

Y-site compatibilities: Amifostine, aztreonam, filgrastim, fludarabine, melphalan, ondansetron, paclitaxel, sargramostim, teniposide, thiotepa, vinorelbine

Patient/family education

- Tell patient that contraceptive measures are recommended during therapy
- Teach patient to avoid use of products containing aspirin or ibuprofen, razors, commercial mouthwash because bleeding may occur; to report symptoms of bleeding (hematuria, tarry stools), irritability, faintness, shortness of breath
- Caution patient that hair loss may occur during treatment; a wig or hairpiece may make patient feel better; new hair

F

may be different in color, texture
• Instruct patient not to have any vaccinations without the advice of the prescriber—serious reactions can occur

Evaluation
Positive therapeutic outcome
• Prevention of rapid division of malignant cells

fluconazole (℞)
(floo-kon′a-zole)
Diflucan
Func. class.: Antifungal
Pregnancy category B

Action: Inhibits ergosterol biosynthesis, causes direct damage to membrane phospholipids in the cell wall of fungi

➡ **Therapeutic Outcome:** Fungistatic fungicidal against the following susceptible organisms: ***Candida, Crytococcus neoforms***

Uses: Oropharyngeal esophageal candidiasis in AIDS patients, chronic mucocutaneous candidiasis, urinary candidiasis, cryptococcal meningitis, peritonitis

Dosage and routes
Vaginal candidiasis
Adult: PO 150 mg as a single dose

Serious fungal infections
Adult: PO/**IV** 50-400 mg initially, then 200 mg once daily for 4 wk

Oropharyngeal candidiasis in AIDS patients
Adult: PO 200 mg initially, then 100 mg daily for at least 2 wk

Available forms: Tabs 50, 100, 150, 200 mg; inj 200, 400 mg

Adverse effects
CNS: Headache
GI: Nausea, vomiting, diarrhea, cramping, flatus, increased AST (SGOT), ALT (SGPT), ***hepatotoxicity***
INTEG: Stevens-Johnson syndrome

Contraindications: Hypersensitivity

Precautions: Renal disease, pregnancy **B**

Pharmacokinetics

Absorption	Well absorbed (PO)
Distribution	Widely distributed (peritoneum, cerebrospinal fluid)
Metabolism	<10%—liver
Excretion	>90% kidneys (unchanged)
Half-life	30 hr, increased in renal disease

Pharmacodynamics

	PO	IV
Onset	Unknown	Immediate
Peak	1-2 hr	Infusion's end
Duration	Unknown	Unknown

Interactions
Individual drugs
Warfarin: ↑ anticoagulation
Drug classification
Cyclosporines: ↑ renal dysfunction

NURSING CONSIDERATIONS
Assessment
• Assess for signs and symptoms of infection
• Obtain cultures for C&S before beginning treatment; therapy may be started after culture is taken
❗• Monitor for renal toxicity: increasing BUN, serum creatinine; if BUN is >40 mg/dl or if serum creatinine is

>3 mg/dl, drug may be discontinued or dosage reduced
• Monitor for hepatotoxicity: increased AST (SGOT), ALT (SGPT), alk phosphatase, bilirubin; drug will be discontinued if hepatotoxicity occurs

Nursing diagnoses

✓ Infection, risk for (uses)
✓ Injury, risk for (adverse reactions)
✓ Knowledge deficit (teaching)

Implementation

IV **IV route**

• Give after diluting according to package directions; run at 200 mg/hr or less; do not use plastic containers in connections
• Do not admix
• Administer **IV** using an in-line filter, using distal veins; check for extravasation and necrosis q2h
• Give drug only after C&S confirms organism, drug needed to treat condition
• Store protected from moisture and light, diluted sol is stable for 24 hr

Y-site compatibilities:
Acyclovir, aldesleukin, allopurinol, amifostine, amikacin, aminophylline, ampicillin/sulbactam, aztreonam, benztropine, cefazolin, cefotetan, cefoxitin, chlorpromazine, cimetidine, dexamethasone, diphenhydramine, droperidol, famotidine, filgrastim, fludarabine, foscarnet, ganciclovir, gentamicin, heparin, hydrocortisone, immune globulin, leucovorin, lorazepam, melphalan, meperidine, metoclopramide, metronidazole, midazolam, morphine, nafcillin, nitroglycerin, ondansetron, oxacillin, paclitaxel, pancuronium, penicillin G, potassium, phenytoin, prochlorperazine, promethazine, ranitidine, sargramostim, sulfamethoxazole, tacrolimus, teniposide, theophylline, thiotepa, ticarcillin/clavulanate, tobramycin, trimethoprim, vancomycin, vecuronium, vinorelbine, zidovudine

Y-site incompatibilities:
Amphotericin B, ampicillin, calcium gluconate, cefotaxime, ceftriaxone, ceftazidime, cefuroxime, chloramphenicol, clindamycin, diazepam, digoxin, erythromycin lactobionate, furosemide, haloperidol, hydroxyzine, imipenem/cilastatin, pentamidine, ticarcillin, trimethoprim/sulfamethoxazole

Patient/family education

• Caution patient that long-term therapy may be needed to clear infection; to take entire course of medication; take in equal intervals (PO)
• Teach patient the signs and symptoms of hepatotoxicity: nausea, vomiting, clay-colored stools, dark urine, anorexia, fatigue, jaundice—health care prescriber should be notified immediately

Evaluation

Positive therapeutic outcome
• Decreasing oral candidiasis, fever, malaise, rash
• Negative C&S for infecting organism

F

flucytosine (℞)

(floo-sye'toe-seen)

Ancobon, Ancotil ✱, 5-FC

Func. class.: Antifungal

Chem. class.: Pyrimidine (fluorinated)

Pregnancy category C

Action: Converted to fluorouracil after entering fungi; inhibits RNA, DNA synthesis; synergism action when used with amphotericin B in some infections

➔ **Therapeutic Outcome:** Fungicidal against the following susceptible organisms: *Candida, Cryptococcus*

Uses: *Candida* infections (septicemia, endocarditis, pulmonary, urinary tract infections), *Cryptococcus* (meningitis, pulmonary, urinary tract infections)

Dosage and routes

P ***Adult and child*** **>*50 kg:*** PO 50-150 mg/kg/day q6h

P ***Adult and child*** **<*50 kg:*** PO 1.5-4.5 g/m^2/day in 4 divided doses

Available forms: Caps 250, 500 mg

Adverse effects

CNS: Headache, confusion, dizziness, sedation, vertigo

GI: Nausea, vomiting, anorexia, diarrhea, abdominal distention, cramps, enterocolitis, increased AST (SGOT), ALT (SGPT), alk phosphatase, ***bowel perforation*** (rare)

GU: Increased BUN, creatinine

HEMA: Thrombocytopenia, agranulocytosis, anemia, leukopenia, pancytopenia

INTEG: Rash

Contraindications: Hypersensitivity

Precautions: Renal disease, impaired hepatic function, bone marrow depression, blood dyscrasias, radiation/chemotherapy, pregnancy **C**

Pharmacokinetics

Absorption	Well absorbed
Distribution	Widely distributed, crosses blood-brain barrier, crosses placenta
Metabolism	Unknown
Excretion	90% kidneys—unchanged
Half-life	3-6 hr, increased in renal disease

Pharmacodynamics

Onset	Rapid
Peak	2½-6 hr
Duration	6 hr

Interactions

Individual drugs

Amphotericin B: ↑ toxicity

Cytarabine: ↓ antifungal action

Drug classifications

Antineoplastics: ↑ bone marrow depression

Radiation: ↑ bone marrow depression

Lab test interferences

False ↑ Creatinine

NURSING CONSIDERATIONS

Assessment

- Assess patient for signs and symptoms of infection before beginning treatment and during therapy
- Obtain cultures for C&S before initiating treatment; therapy may be started after culture is taken
- Monitor renal toxicity: increasing BUN, serum creatinine; if BUN is >40 mg/dl or if serum creatinine is

>3 mg/dl, drug may be discontinued or dosage reduced
• Monitor for hepatotoxicity: increased AST (SGOT), ALT (SGPT), alk phosphatase, bilirubin; drug will be discontinued if hepatotoxicity occurs

Nursing diagnoses
✓ Infection, risk for (uses)
✓ Diarrhea (adverse reactions)
✓ Knowledge deficit (teaching)

Implementation
• Give a few caps at a time to decrease nausea, vomiting over 15 min; store in tight, light-resistant containers at room temp
• Do not crush, chew caps
• Use symptomatic treatment as ordered for adverse reactions: aspirin, antihistamines, antiemetics, antispasmodics

Patient/family education
• Advise patient that medication may cause dizziness, drowsiness, and confusion, to avoid hazardous activities until side effects are determined
• Instruct patient to notify prescriber if rash, fever, sore throat, fatigue, muscle weakness, diarrhea, bruising, bleeding occur
• Caution patient to take medication exactly as prescribed; not to double doses—missed doses should be taken when remembered within 1 hr of next dose

Evaluation
Positive therapeutic outcome
• Decreasing oral candidiasis, fever, malaise, rash
• Negative C&S for infection organism

fludarabine (℞)
(floo-dar'a-been)
Fludara
Func. class.: Antineoplastic, antimetabolite
Chem. class.: Vidarabine derivative
Pregnancy category D

F

Action: Competes with physiologic substrate that inhibits DNA synthesis

Therapeutic Outcome: Prevention of rapid growth of malignant cells

Uses: Chronic lymphocytic leukemia; non-Hodgkin's lymphoma

Dosage and routes
***Adult:* IV** 25 mg/m^2 over 30 min qd × 5 days, may repeat q28 days; reconstitute with 2 ml of sterile water for inj; dissolution should occur in <15 sec

Available forms: Lyophilized powder for reconstitution 50 mg/vial

Adverse effects
CNS: Weakness, confusion, headache, depression, sleep disorder, impaired mentation, ***coma,*** peripheral neuropathy
CV: Edema
EENT: Visual disturbances, sinusitis
GI: Nausea, vomiting, anorexia, diarrhea, ***hepatotoxicity,*** abdominal pain, hematemesis, ***hemorrhage***
GU: Dysuria, infection
HEMA: Bleeding, ***thrombocytopenia, leukopenia, myelosuppression, anemia***
INTEG: Rash
META: Hyperuricemia, hyper-

phosphatemia, hypocalcemia, metabolic acidosis, hyperkalemia
*RESP: **Pneumonia**,* dyspnea, cough, interstitial pulmonary infiltrate
SYST: Fever, chills, malaise, fatigue

Contraindications: Hypersensitivity, pregnancy **D**

Precautions: Renal disease, hepatic disease, infants P

Pharmacokinetics

Absorption	Complete
Distribution	Unknown
Metabolism	To active metabolite
Excretion	23% kidneys— unchanged
Half-life	Of metabolite 10 hr

Pharmacodynamics

Unknown

Interactions

Individual drugs

Radiation: ↑ toxicity, bone marrow suppression

Drug classifications

Antineoplastics: ↑ toxicity, bone marrow suppression
Live virus vaccines: ↑ adverse reactions

Lab test interferences

↑ Liver function studies

NURSING CONSIDERATIONS

Assessment

- Assess buccal cavity q8h for dryness, sores or ulcers, white patches, oral pain, bleeding, dysphagia; obtain prescription for viscous lidocaine (Xylocaine)
- Monitor CBC, differential, platelet count weekly; withhold drug if WBC count is <4000/mm^3 or platelet count is <100,000/mm^3, notify prescriber of results
- Monitor renal function studies: BUN, creatinine, serum uric acid, urine CrCl before and during therapy; I&O ratio; report fall in urine output to <30 ml/hr
- Monitor temp q4h (may indicate beginning of infection)
- Monitor liver function tests before and during therapy [bilirubin, AST (SGOT), ALT (SGPT), LDH] as needed or monthly; yellowing of skin, sclera, dark urine, clay-colored stools, itchy skin, abdominal pain, fever, diarrhea
- Assess for bleeding: hematuria, stool guaiac, bruising or petechiae, mucosa or orifices q8h; inflammation of mucosa, breaks in skin
- Identify patient's food preferences; list likes, dislikes
- Identify effects of alopecia on body image; discuss feelings about body changes
- Identify edema in feet, joint pain, stomach pain, tremors
- Identify inflammation of mucosa, breaks in skin

Nursing diagnoses

- ✓ Injury, risk for (adverse reactions)
- ✓ Body image disturbance (adverse reactions)
- ✓ Infection, risk for (adverse reactions)
- ✓ Knowledge deficit (teaching)

Implementation

- Administer fluids **IV** or PO before chemotherapy to hydrate patient
- Give antacid before oral agent, give drug after evening meal, before bedtime; antiemetic 30-60 min before giving drug to prevent vomiting, and prn; antibiotics for prophylaxis of infection

- Give top or syst analgesics for pain
- Give in AM so drug is eliminated before hs
- Put patient on liq diet: carbonated beverages; gelatin may be added if patient is not nauseated or vomiting
- Recommend that patient rinse mouth tid-qid with water, club soda; brush teeth bid-qid with soft brush or cotton-tipped applicators for stomatitis; use unwaxed dental floss
- Reconstitute with 2 ml of sterile water for injection; dissolve lyophilized powder; sol is stable for 8 hr
- Give by intermittent inf; dilute further in 100-125 ml of 0.9% NaCl or D_5W and give over ½ hr

Y-site compatibilities: Allopurinol, amikacin, aminophylline, ampicillin, amsacrine, aztreonam, bleomycin, butorphanol, carboplatin, carmustine, cefazolin, cefepime, cefoperazone, cefotaxime, cefotetan, ceftazidime, ceftriaxone, cefuroxime, cimetidine, cisplatin, clindamycin, cyclophosphamide, cytarabine, dacarbazine, dactinomycin, dexamethasone, diphenhydramine, doxorubicin, doxycycline, droperidol, etoposide, famotidine, filgrastim, floxuridine, fluconazole, fluorouracil, furosemide, gentamicin, haloperidol, heparin, hydrocortisone, ifosfamide, lorazepam, magnesium sulfate, mannitol, mechlorethamine, melphalan, meperidine, mesna, methotrexate, methylprednisolone, metoclopramide, mezlocillin, minocycline, mitoxantrone, morphine, multivitamins, nalbuphine, netilmicin, ondansetron, pentostatin, piperacillin, potassium chloride, promethazine, ranitidine, sodium bicarbonate, teniposide, ticarcillin, tobramycin, trimethoprim-sulfamethoxazole, vancomycin, vinblastine, vincristine, vinorelbine, zidovudine

Y-site incompatibilities: Acyclovir, amphotericin B chlorpromazine, daunorubicin, ganciclovir, hydroxyzine, melphalan, miconazole, prochlorperazine, vinorelbine

Patient/family education

- Caution patient that contraceptive measures are recommended during therapy
- Teach patient to avoid aspirin- or ibuprofen-containing products, razors, commercial mouthwash (bleeding may occur); to report symptoms of bleeding (hematuria, tarry stools)
- Instruct patient to report signs of anemia (fatigue, headache, faintness, shortness of breath)
- Caution patient that hair loss may occur during treatment; a wig or hairpiece may make patient feel better; new hair may be different in color, texture

Evaluation

Positive therapeutic outcome

- Prevention of rapid division of malignant cells

F

fludrocortisone (℞)

(floo-droe-kor′ti-sone)
Florinef Acetate
Func. class.: Corticosteroid
Chem. class.: Mineralocorticoid
Pregnancy category C

Action: Promotes increased reabsorption of sodium and loss of potassium, water, hydrogen from the distal renal tubules

Therapeutic Outcome: Treatment of adrenal insufficiency symptoms

Uses: Adrenal insufficiency, salt-losing adrenogenital syndrome

Dosage and routes

Adult: PO 0.1-0.2 mg qd

Available forms: Tab 0.1 mg

Adverse effects

CNS: Flushing, sweating, headache

CV: Hypertension, ***circulatory collapse, thrombophlebitis, embolism,*** tachycardia

MS: Fractures, osteoporosis, weakness

Contraindications: Hypersensitivity, acute glomerulonephritis, amebiasis

Precautions: Pregnancy **C**, osteoporosis, CHF

Pharmacokinetics

Absorption	Well absorbed
Distribution	Widely
Metabolism	Liver
Excretion	Kidneys, breast milk
Half-life	3½ hr

Pharmacodynamics

Unknown

Interactions

Individual drugs

Amphotericin B: ↑ hypokalemia
Mezlocillin: ↑ hypokalemia
Phenobarbital: ↓ effect of fludrocortisone
Piperacillin: ↑ hypokalemia
Rifampin: ↓ effect of fludrocortisone

Drug classifications

Diuretics: ↑ hypokalemia
Nondepolarizing neuromuscular blocking agents: ↑ neuromuscular blockade

Food

↑ salt/sodium ingestion: ↑ hypokalemia, ↑ hypernatremia

Lab test interferences

↑ Potassium, ↑ chloride
↓ Hematocrit

NURSING CONSIDERATIONS

Assessment

• Monitor patient for fluid retention: weigh daily, notify prescriber of weekly gain >5 lb; B/P q4h, pulse; notify prescriber if chest pain occurs: I&O ratio; be alert for decreasing urinary output and increasing edema

• Check for potassium depletion: paresthesias, fatigue, nausea, vomiting, depression, polyuria, dysrhythmias, weakness

Nursing diagnoses

✓ Fluid volume deficit (uses)
✓ Fluid volume excess (adverse reactions)
✓ Knowledge deficit (teaching)

Implementation

• Administer titrated dose; use lowest effective dose; scored tab may be broken if lower dose is necessary

• Give with food or milk to decrease GI symptoms

Patient/family education

- Advise patient to carry ID as steroid user at all times during diagnosis and treatment
- Caution patient not to discontinue this medication abruptly—Addisonian crisis may occur
- Counsel patient to follow dietary regimen recommended by prescriber—should include high potassium and, possibly, low sodium
- Advise patient to report weight gain >5 lbs; edema in legs, hands; abdominal cramping; nausea; vomiting; anorexia; dizziness or weakness

Evaluation

Positive therapeutic outcome

- Correction of adrenal insufficiency
- Electrolytes and fluids in normal range

flumazenil (℞)

(flu-maz'e-nil)

Mazicon, Ronazicon

Func. class.: Benzodiazepine receptor antagonist

Chem. class.: Imidazobenzodiazepine derivative

Pregnancy category C

Action: Antagonizes the actions of benzodiazepines on the CNS, competitively inhibits the activity at the benzodiazepine receptor complex

➔ **Therapeutic Outcome:** Reversed benzodiazepine toxic effects

Uses: Reversal of the sedative effects of benzodiazepines

Dosage and routes

Reversal of conscious sedation or in general anesthesia

Adult: **IV** 0.2 mg (2 ml) given over 15 sec; wait 45 sec, then give 0.2 mg (2 ml) if consciousness does not occur; may be repeated at 60-sec intervals as needed, up to 4 additional times (max total dose 1 mg); dose is to be individualized

Management of suspected benzodiazepine overdose

Adult: **IV** 0.2 mg (2 ml) given over 30 sec; wait 30 sec, then give 0.3 mg (3 ml) over 30 sec if consciousness does not occur; further doses of 0.5 mg (5 ml) can be given over 30 sec at intervals of 1 min up to cumulative dose of 3 mg

Available forms: Inj 0.1 mg/ml

Adverse effects

CNS: Dizziness, agitation, emotional lability, confusion, ***convulsions,*** somnolence

CV: Hypertension, palpitations, cutaneous vasodilation, dysrhythmias, bradycardia, tachycardia, chest pain

EENT: Abnormal vision, blurred vision, tinnitus

GI: Nausea, vomiting, hiccups

SYST: Headache, injection site pain, increased sweating, fatigue, rigors

Contraindications: Hypersensitivity to this drug or benzodiazepines, serous tricyclic antidepressant overdose, patients given benzodiazepine for control of life-threatening condition

Precautions: Pregnancy **C**, P lactation, children, elderly, G renal disease, seizures, head injury, labor and delivery, hepatic disease, hypoventilation, panic disorder, drug and alcohol dependency, ambulatory patients

Pharmacokinetics

Absorption	Complete
Distribution	Unknown
Metabolism	Liver
Excretion	Unknown
Half-life	41-79 min

Pharmacodynamics

Onset	1 min
Peak	10 min
Duration	Unknown

Interactions: None

NURSING CONSIDERATIONS

Assessment

- Assess cardiac status using continuous monitoring
- Assess for seizures; protect patient from injury
- Assess for GI symptoms: nausea, vomiting; place in side-lying position to prevent aspiration
- Assess for allergic reactions: flushing, rash, urticaria, pruritus

Nursing diagnoses

✓ Injury, risk for (uses)
✓ Poisoning (uses)

Implementation

- Give directly undiluted or diluted in 0.9% NaCl, D_5W, or LR; give over 15 sec
- Check airway and **IV** access before administration

Additive compatibilities: Aminophylline, cimetidine, dobutamine, dopamine, famotidine, heparin, lidocaine, procainamide, ranitidine

Patient/family education

- Caution patient that amnesia may continue
- Instruct patient to avoid any hazardous activities for 18-24 hr after discharge
- Inform patient not to take any alcohol or nonprescription drugs for 18-24 hr—serious reactions may occur

Evaluation

Positive therapeutic outcome

- Decreased sedation, respiratory depression
- Absence of toxicity

fluorouracil (5-fluorouracil) (℞)

(flure-oh-yoor′a-sil)

Adrucil, 5-FU

Func. class.: Antineoplastic, antimetabolite

Chem. class.: Pyrimidine antagonist

Pregnancy category D

Action: Inhibits DNA synthesis; interferes with cell replication by competitively inhibiting thymidylate synthesis, S phase of cell cycle-specific vesicant

➔ **Therapeutic Outcome:** Prevention of rapidly growing malignant cells

Uses: Cancer of breast, colon, rectum, stomach, pancreas; multiple active keratoses; basal cell carcinoma (top)

Dosage and routes

Adult: **IV** 12 mg/kg/day × 4 days, not to exceed 800 mg/day; may repeat with 6 mg/kg on day 6, 8, 10, 12; maintenance is 10-15 mg/kg/wk as a single dose, not to exceed 1 g/wk

Adult: Top 1, 2% sol apply to lesion on head, neck, or on other areas 5% bid

Available forms: Inj 50 mg/ml; cream 1, 5%; sol 1, 2, 5%

Adverse effects

CNS: Lethargy, malaise, weakness

CV: Myocardial ischemia, angina

EENT: Epistaxis

GI: Anorexia, stomatitis, diarrhea, nausea, vomiting, ***hemorrhage, enteritis glossitis***

GU: Renal failure

HEMA: Thrombocytopenia, leukopenia, myelosuppression, anemia, agranulocytosis

INTEG: Rash, fever

Contraindications: Hypersensitivity, myelosuppression, pregnancy **D,** poor nutritional status, serious infections

Precautions: Renal disease, hepatic disease, bone marrow depression, angina, lactation, P children

Pharmacokinetics

Absorption	Completely bioavailable (**IV**), minimal (Top)
Distribution	Widely distributed, concentration in tumor
Metabolism	Liver—converted to active metabolite
Excretion	Lungs (60%-80%), kidneys (up to 15%)
Half-life	20 hr terminal

Pharmacodynamics

Unknown

Interactions

Individual drugs

Radiation: ↑ toxicity, bone marrow suppression

Drug classifications

Antineoplastics: ↑ toxicity bone marrow suppression

Lab test interferences

↑ Liver function studies, ↑ 6-HIAA

↓ Albumin

NURSING CONSIDERATIONS

Assessment

- Monitor ECG; watch for ST-T wave changes, low QRS and T, possible dysrhythmias (sinus tachycardia, heart block, PVCs)
- Assess buccal cavity q8h for dryness, sores or ulceration, white patches, oral pain, bleeding, dysphagia; obtain prescription for viscous lidocaine (Xylocaine)
- Assess symptoms indicating severe allergic reaction: rash, pruritus, urticaria, purpuric skin lesions, itching, flushing
- Assess tachypnea, ECG changes, dyspnea, edema, fatigue; identify dyspnea, rales, unproductive cough, chest pain, tachypnea
- Monitor CBC, differential, platelet count weekly; withhold drug if WBC count is <4000/mm^3 or platelet count is <100,000/mm^3; notify prescriber of results if WBC <20,000/mm^3, platelets <50,000/mm^3
- Monitor renal function studies: BUN, creatinine, serum uric acid, urine CrCl before and during therapy; I&O ratio; report fall in urine output to <30 ml/hr
- Monitor temp q4h (may indicate beginning of infection)
- Monitor liver function tests before and during therapy (bilirubin, AST [SGOT], ALT [SGPT], LDH) as needed or monthly; yellowing of skin, sclera, dark urine, clay-colored stools, itchy skin, abdominal pain, fever, diarrhea
- Assess for bleeding: hematuria, stool guaiac, bruising or petechiae, mucosa or orifices

F

q8h; inflammation of mucosa, breaks in skin

Nursing diagnoses

- ✓ Injury, risk for (adverse reactions)
- ✓ Body image disturbance (adverse reactions)
- ✓ Infection, risk for (adverse reactions)
- ✓ Knowledge deficit (teaching)

Implementation

- Avoid contact with skin (very irritating); wash completely to remove
- Give fluids **IV** or PO before chemotherapy to hydrate patient
- Give antiemetic 30-60 min before giving drug to prevent vomiting, and prn; antibiotics for prophylaxis of infection
- Provide liq diet: carbonated beverages; gelatin may be added if patient is not nauseated or vomiting
- Provide rinsing of mouth tid-qid with water, club soda; brushing of teeth bid-qid with soft brush or cotton-tipped applicators for stomatitis; use unwaxed dental floss

IV IV route

- **IV** undiluted; may inject through Y-tube or 3-way stopcock; give over 1-3 min
- May be diluted in NS, D_5W, given over 2-8 hr as an **IV** inf

Top route

- Wear gloves when applying; may use with a loose dressing

Syringe incompatibility: Droperidol

Syringe compatibilities: Bleomycin, cisplatin, cyclophosphamide, furosemide, heparin, leucovorin, methotrexate, metoclopramide, mitomycin, vinblastine, vincristine

Y-site incompatibilities: Droperidol, vinorelbine

Y-site compatibilities: Allopurinol, amifostine, aztreonam, bleomycin, cefepime, cisplatin, cyclophosphamide, doxorubicin, fludarabine, furosemide, granisetron, heparin, leucovorin, mannitol, melphalan, methotrexate, metoclopramide, mitomycin, paclitaxel, potassium chloride, sargramostin, thiotepa, thiposide, vinblastine, vincristine

Additive incompatibilities: Carboplatin, cisplatin, cytarabine, diazepam, doxorubicin

Additive compatibilities: Bleomycin, cephalothin, etoposides, floxuridine, ifosfamide, leucovorin, methotrexate, prednisolone, vincristine, cyclophosphamide, mitoxantrone

Solution compatibilities: Amino acids 4.25%/D_{25}, D_5/LR, $D_{3.3}$/0.3 NaCl, D_5W, 0.9% NaCl, TPN #23

Patient/family education

- Caution patient that contraceptive measures are recommended during therapy
- Teach patient to avoid using aspirin- or ibuprofen-containing products, razors, commercial mouthwash because bleeding may occur; to report symptoms of bleeding (hematuria, tarry stools)
- Instruct patient to report signs of anemia (fatigue, headache, irritability, faintness, shortness of breath)

Evaluation

Positive therapeutic outcome

- Prevention of rapid division of malignant cells

fluoxetine (℞)
(floo-ox'uh-teen)
Prozac
Func. class.: Bicyclic antidepressant
Pregnancy category B

Action: Inhibits CNS neuron uptake of serotonin, but not of norepinephrine

Therapeutic Outcome: Decreased symptoms of depression after 2-3 wk

Uses: Major depressive disorder, obsessive-compulsive disorder (OCD), bulimia nervosa

Investigational uses: Alcoholism, anorexia nervosa, ADHD, bipolar II affective disorder, borderline personality disorder, cataplexy, narcolepsy, kleptomania, migraine, obesity, post-traumatic stress disorder, schizophrenia, Tourette's syndrome, trichotillomania, levodopa-induced dyskinesia, social phobia

Dosage and routes
Depression/ocs
Adult: PO 20 mg qd AM; after 4 wk if no clinical improvement is noted, dose may be increased to 20 mg bid in AM, afternoon, not to exceed 80 mg/day
Bulimia Nervosa
Adult: PO 60 mg/day in AM

Available forms: Pulvules 10, 20 mg; caps 10, 20 mg; liq 20 mg/5 ml

Adverse effects
CNS: Headache, nervousness, insomnia, drowsiness, anxiety, tremor, dizziness, fatigue, sedation, poor concentration, abnormal dreams, agitation, ***convulsions***
CV: Hot flashes, palpitations, angina pectoris, ***hemorrhage,*** hypertension, first-degree tachycardia
EENT: Visual changes, ear/eye pain, photophobia, tinnitus
GI: Nausea, diarrhea, dry mouth, anorexia, dyspepsia, constipation, cramps, vomiting, taste changes, flatulence, decreased appetite
GU: Dysmenorrhea, decreased libido, urinary frequency, urinary tract infection, amenorrhea, cystitis, impotence
INTEG: Sweating, rash, pruritus, acne, alopecia, urticaria
MS: Pain, arthritis, twitching
RESP: Infection, pharyngitis, nasal congestion, sinus headache, sinusitis, cough dyspnea, bronchitis, asthma, hyperventilation, pneumonia
SYST: Asthenia, viral infection, fever, allergy, chills

Contraindications: Hypersensitivity

Precautions: Pregnancy **B**, lactation, children, elderly

Pharmacokinetics

Absorption	Well absorbed
Distribution	Crosses blood-brain barrier
Metabolism	Liver, extensively to norfluoxetine
Excretion	Kidneys, unchanged (12%), metabolite (7%) Steady state 28-35 days, protein binding 94%
Half-life	1-3 days metabolite up to 1 wk

Pharmacodynamics

Onset	Unknown
Peak	6-8 hr
Duration	Unknown

Interactions

Individual drugs

Alcohol: ↑ CNS depression
Buspirone: ↑ worsening of OCD
Carbamazepine: ↑ toxicity
Clozapine: ↑ clozapine levels
Dextromethorphan: ↑ hallucinations
Lithium: ↑ toxicity
L-tryptophan: ↑ toxicity
Phenytoin: ↑ hydantoin levels

Drug classifications

Barbiturates: ↑ CNS depression
Benzodiazepines: ↑ CNS depression
CNS depressants: ↑ CNS depression
MAOI: Hypertensive crisis, convulsions
Oral anticoagulants: ↑ effects, toxicity
Sedative/hypnotics: ↑ CNS depression

Lab test interferences

↑ Serum bilirubin, ↑ blood glucose, ↑ alk phosphatase
↓ VMA, ↓ 5-HIAA, ↓ blood glucose
False ↑ Urinary catecholamines

NURSING CONSIDERATIONS

Assessment

- Monitor B/P (lying, standing), pulse q4h; if systolic B/P drops 20 mm hg, hold drug and notify prescriber; take vital signs q4h in patients with cardiovascular disease
- Monitor blood studies: CBC, leukocytes, differential, cardiac enzymes if patient is receiving long-term therapy; check platelets, bleeding can occur
- Monitor hepatic studies: AST (SGOT), ALT (SGPT), bilirubin
- Check weight qwk; appetite may increase with drug
- Assess ECG for flattening of T wave, bundle branch block, AV block, dysrhythmias in cardiac patients
- Assess for EPS primarily in elderly: rigidity, dystonia, akathisia
- Assess mental status: mood, sensorium, affect, suicidal tendencies; increase in psychiatric symptoms: depression, panic
- Monitor urinary retention, constipation; constipation is [P] more likely to occur in children [G] or elderly
- [!] Assess for withdrawal symptoms: headache, nausea, vomiting, muscle pain, weakness; do not usually occur unless drug is discontinued abruptly
- Identify patient's alcohol consumption; if alcohol is consumed, hold dose until AM

Nursing diagnoses

- ✓ Coping, ineffective individual (uses)
- ✓ Injury, risk for (side effects)
- ✓ Knowledge deficit (teaching)
- ✓ Noncompliance (teaching)

Implementation

- Give with food or milk for GI symptoms
- Give dosage hs if oversedation occurs during day; may [G] take entire dose hs; elderly may not tolerate once/day dosing
- Store at room temp; do not freeze

Patient/family education

- Teach patient that therapeutic effects may take 2-3 wk
- Instruct patient to use caution in driving or other activities requiring alertness because of drowsiness, dizziness, blurred vision; to avoid rising

quickly from sitting to standing, especially elderly

- Caution patient to avoid alcohol ingestion, other CNS depressants
- Advise patient not to discontinue medication quickly after long-term use: may cause nausea, headache, malaise
- Instruct patient to increase fluids, bulk in diet if constipation, urinary retention occur, especially elderly
- Advise patient to take gum, hard sugarless candy, or frequent sips of water for dry mouth

Evaluation

Positive therapeutic outcome

- Decrease in depression
- Absence of suicidal thoughts

fluphenazine (℞)
(floo-fen′a-zeen)
Apo-Fluphenazine ✦, **Permitil, Prolixin, fluphenazine decanoate, Prolixin Decanoate, Prolixin Enanthate, fluphenazine HCl**
Func. class.: Antipsychotic/neuroleptic
Chem. class.: Phenothiazine, piperazine

Pregnancy category C

Action: Depresses cerebral cortex, hypothalamus, limbic system, which control activity and aggression; blocks neurotransmission produced by dopamine at synapse; exhibits strong α-adrenergic and anticholinergic blocking action; mechanism for antipsychotic effects is unclear

Therapeutic Outcome: Decreased signs and symptoms of psychosis

Uses: Psychotic disorders, schizophrenia

Dosage and routes

Enanthate, decanoate

Adult and child >12 yr: IM 12.5-25 mg q1-3 wk

HCl

Adult: PO 2.5-10 mg, in divided doses q6-8h, not to exceed 20 mg qd; IM initially 1.25 mg then 2.5-10 mg in divided doses q6-8h

Child: PO 0.25-3.5 mg qd in divided doses q4-6h, max 10 mg/qd

Available forms: HCl tabs 1, 2.5, 5, 10 mg; elix 2.5 mg/5 ml; conc 5 mg/ml; inj 10 mg/ml, enanthate, decanoate, inj 25 mg/ml

Adverse effects

CNS: Extrapyramidal symptoms: pseudoparkinsonism, akathisia, dystonia, tardive dyskinesia, drowsiness, headache, ***seizures, neuroleptic malignant syndrome***
CV: Orthostatic hypotension, hypertension, ***cardiac arrest,*** ECG changes, ***tachycardia***
EENT: Blurred vision, glaucoma, dry eyes
GI: Dry mouth, nausea, vomiting, anorexia, constipation, diarrhea, jaundice, weight gain, ***paralytic ileus, hepatitis***
GU: Urinary retention, urinary frequency, enuresis, impotence, amenorrhea, gynecomastia
HEMA: Anemia, ***leukopenia, leukocytosis, agranulocytosis***
INTEG: Rash, photosensitivity, dermatitis
RESP: ***Laryngospasm,*** dyspnea, ***respiratory depression***

Contraindications: Hypersensitivity, circulatory collapse, liver damage, cerebral arteriosclerosis, coronary disease, severe hypertension/hypotension, blood dyscrasias, P coma, child <12 yr, brain damage, bone marrow depression, alcohol and barbiturate withdrawal

Precautions: Pregnancy **C,** lactation, seizure disorders, hypertension, hepatic disease, cardiac disease

Pharmacokinetics

Absorption	Well absorbed (PO, IM)
Distribution	Widely absorbed, crosses blood-brain barrier, placenta
Metabolism	Liver, extensively
Excretion	Kidneys (metabolites)
Half-life	HCl-4.7-15.3 hr, enanthate 3½-4 days, decanoate 6.8-14.3 days

Pharmacodynamics

	PO/IM	IM	IM
	HCl	Enanthate	Decanoate
Onset	1 hr	1-2 days	1-3 days
Peak	1½-2 hr	2-3 days	1-2 days
Duration	6-8 hr	1-3 wk	>4 wk

Interactions

Individual drugs

Alcohol: ↑ effects of both drugs, oversedation
Aluminum hydroxide: ↓ absorption of fluphenazine
Bromocriptine: ↓ antiparkinson activity
Disopyramide: ↑ anticholinergic effects
Epinephrine: ↑ toxicity
Guanethidine: ↓ antihypertensive response
Levodopa: ↓ antiparkinson activity
Lithium: ↓ fluphenazine levels, ↑ extrapyramidal symptoms, masking of lithium toxicity
Magnesium hydroxide: ↓ absorption of fluphenazine
Norepinephrine: ↓ vasoresponse, ↑ toxicity
Phenobarbital: ↓ effectiveness, ↑ metabolism

Drug classifications

Antacids: ↓ absorption of fluphenazine
Anticholinergics: ↑ anticholinergic effects
Antidepressants: ↑ CNS depression
Antidiarrheals, adsorbent: ↓ absorption
Antihistamines: ↑ CNS depression
Antihypertensives: ↑ hypotension
Antithyroid agents: ↑ agranulocytosis
Barbiturate anesthetics: ↑ CNS depression
β-Adrenergics: ↑ effects of both drugs
General anesthetics: ↑ CNS depression
MAOI: ↑ CNS depression
Narcotics: ↑ CNS depression
Sedative/hypnotics: ↑ CNS depression

Lab test interferences

↑ Liver function tests, ↑ cardiac enzymes, ↑ cholesterol, ↑ blood glucose, ↑ prolactin, ↑ bilirubin, ↑ PBI, ↑ cholinesterase I, ↑ alk phosphatase, ↑ leukocytes, ↑ granulocytes, ↑ platelets
↓ Hormones (blood and urine)
False positive: Pregnancy tests, PKU, urine bilirubin
False negative: Urinary steroids, 17-OHCS

NURSING CONSIDERATIONS

Assessment

- Assess mental status: orienta-

tion, mood, behavior, presence of hallucinations, and type before initial administration and monthly; this drug should significantly reduce psychotic behavior
• Check for swallowing of PO medication; check for hoarding or giving of medication to other patients
• Monitor I&O ratio, palpate bladder if low urinary output occurs, especially in elderly; urinalysis recommended before, during prolonged therapy
• Monitor bilirubin, CBC, liver function studies monthly
• Assess affect, orientation, LOC, reflexes, gait, coordination, sleep pattern disturbances
• Monitor B/P with patient sitting, standing, and lying down; take pulse and respirations q4h during initial treatment; establish baseline before starting treatment; report drops of 30 mm Hg; obtain baseline ECG, Q-wave and T-wave changes
• Check for dizziness, faintness, palpitations, tachycardia on rising; severe orthostatic hypotension is common
• Identify for neuroleptic malignant syndrome: hyperpyrexia, muscle rigidity, increased CPK, altered mental status; drug should be discontinued
• Assess for extrapyramidal symptoms including akathisia (inability to sit still, no pattern to movements), tardive dyskinesia (bizarre movements of the jaw, mouth, tongue, extremities), pseudoparkinsonism (rigidity, tremors, pill rolling, shuffling gate), an antiparkinson drug should be prescribed
• Assess for constipation, urinary retention daily; if these occur, increase bulk, water in diet

Nursing diagnoses

- Thought processes, altered (uses)
- Coping, ineffective individual (uses)
- Knowledge deficit (teaching)
- Noncompliance (teaching)

Implementation

PO route

• Give drug in liq form mixed in glass of juice or cola if hoarding is suspected; do not mix in caffeine drinks, tannics, or pectinates; decrease dose in elderly
• Give PO with full glass of water, milk; or give with food to decrease GI upset
• Store in tight, light-resistant container, oral sol in amber bottle

SC route

• May be given by this route; however, it is painful

IM route

• Inject in deep muscle mass, use a 21-G needle into dorsal gluteal site, keep patient recumbent for ½ hr—prevents orthostatic hypotension

Patient/family education

• Teach patient to use good oral hygiene; frequent rinsing of mouth, sugarless gum for dry mouth
• Caution patient to avoid hazardous activities until drug response is determined; dizziness, blurred vision may occur
• Inform patient that orthostatic hypotension occurs often and to rise from sitting or lying position gradually, to remain lying down after IM inj for at least 30 min; tell patient to avoid hot tubs, hot showers, tub baths because hypotension may occur; tell patient that in

hot weather, heat stroke may occur—extra precautions are necessary to stay cool

- Instruct patient to avoid abrupt withdrawal of this drug, or extrapyramidal symptoms may result; drug should be withdrawn slowly
- Teach patient to avoid OTC preparations (cough, hayfever, cold) unless approved by physician because serious drug interactions may occur; avoid use with alcohol, CNS depressants; increased drowsiness may occur
- Instruct patient to use a sunscreen and sunglasses to prevent burns
- Teach patient about extrapyramidal symptoms and necessity of meticulous oral hygiene beause oral candidiasis may occur
- Instruct patient to take antacids 2 hr before or after this drug
- Advise patient to report sore throat, malaise, fever, bleeding, mouth sores; if these occur, CBC should be drawn and drug discontinued

Evaluation

Positive therapeutic outcome

- Decrease in emotional excitement, hallucinations, delusions, paranoia
- Reorganization of patterns of thought, speech

Treatment of overdose: Lavage if orally ingested; provide airway; *do not induce vomiting or use epinephrine*

flurazepam (℞)

(flure-az′e-pam)

Apo-flurazepam ✤, Dalmane, Durapam, flurazepam, Novoflupam ✤, Somnol ✤, Som-Pam ✤

Func. class.: Sedative-hypnotic

Chem. class.: Benzodiazepine derivative

Pregnancy category D

Controlled substance schedule IV (USA), schedule F (Canada)

Action: Produces CNS depression at the limbic, thalamic, hypothalamic levels of CNS; may be mediated by neurotransmitter γ-aminobutyric acid (GABA); results are sedation, hypnosis, skeletal muscle relaxation, anticonvulsant activity, anxiolytic action

➔ **Therapeutic Outcome:** Ability to sleep, relaxation

Uses: Insomnia

Dosage and routes

Adult: PO 15-30 mg hs; may repeat dose once if needed

G ***Geriatric:*** PO 15 mg hs; may increase if needed

Available forms: Caps 15, 30 mg

Adverse effects

CNS: Lethargy, drowsiness, daytime sedation, dizziness, confusion, light-headedness, headache, anxiety, irritability

CV: Chest pain, pulse changes

GI: Nausea, vomiting, diarrhea, heartburn, abdominal pain, constipation

HEMA: Leukopenia, granulocytopenia (rare)

Contraindications: Hypersensitivity to benzodiazepines, pregnancy **D,** lactation, intermittent porphyria, uncontrolled pain

Precautions: Anemia, hepatic disease, renal disease, suicidal individuals, drug abuse, elderly, psychosis, child <15 yr

Pharmacokinetics	
Absorption	Well absorbed
Distribution	Widely absorbed, crosses blood-brain barrier, crosses placenta
Metabolism	Liver to active, inactive metabolites
Excretion	Kidneys, breast milk
Half-life	2½ hr, 30-200 hr active metabolites

Pharmacodynamics	
Onset	15-30 min
Peak	½-1 hr
Duration	7-8 hr

Interactions

Individual drugs

Alcohol: ↑ CNS depression
Cimetidine: ↑ action of flurazepam
Disulfiram: ↑ action of flurazepam
Fluoxetine: ↑ action of flurazepam
Isoniazid: ↑ action of flurazepam
Ketoconazole: ↑ action of flurazepam
Levodopa: ↓ action of levodopa
Metoprolol: ↑ action of flurazepam
Propoxyphene: ↑ action of flurazepam
Propranolol: ↑ action of flurazepam
Rifampin: ↓ action of flurazepam
Theophylline: ↓ sedative effects
Valproic acid: ↑ action of flurazepam

Drug classifications

Analgesics, opioid: ↑ CNS depression
Antidepressants: ↑ CNS depression
Antihistamines: ↑ CNS depression
Barbiturates: ↓ effect of flurazepam
Contraceptives: ↑ effect

Lab test interferences

↑ AST(SGOT)/ALT(SGPT), ↑ serum bilirubin
False ↑ Urinary 17-OHCS
↓ RAI uptake

NURSING CONSIDERATIONS

Assessment

- Assess anxiety reaction: inability to sleep, apprehension, dread, foreboding, or uneasiness related to unidentified source of danger
- Assess for previous drug dependence or tolerance; if drug dependent or tolerant, amount of medication should be restricted
- Monitor B/P (lying, standing), pulse; if systolic B/P drops 20 mm Hg, hold drug, notify prescriber; I&O, may indicate renal dysfunction
- Monitor blood studies: CBC during long-term therapy; blood dyscrasias have occurred rarely
- Monitor hepatic studies: AST (SGOT), ALT (SGPT), bilirubin, creatinine, LDH, alk phosphatase
- Monitor patient's mental status: mood, sensorium, affect, sleeping patterns, drowsiness, dizziness, suicidal tendencies

Nursing diagnoses

✓ Sleep pattern disturbance (uses)

☑ Knowledge deficit (teaching)
☑ Noncompliance (teaching)

Implementation

• Give ½-1 hr before hs for sleeplessness; give on empty stomach with full glass of water or juice for best absorption and to decrease corrosion (do not chew); give pc to decrease GI symptoms if used for sedation

Patient/family education

• Caution patient that drug may be taken with food; if dose is missed take as soon as remembered; do not double doses

• Advise patient to avoid OTC preparations unless approved by a physician, to avoid alcohol ingestion or other psychotropic medications unless prescribed by a health care provider, that 1-2 wk of therapy may be required before therapeutic effects occur

• Caution patient to avoid driving, activities requiring alertness—drowsiness may occur; until medication response is known, tell patient that drowsiness may worsen at beginning of treatment

• Instruct patient not to discontinue medication abruptly after long-term use

• Caution patient to rise slowly or fainting may occur, especially in elderly

Evaluation

Positive therapeutic outcome

• Increased well-being

• Decreased anxiety, restlessness, sleeplessness, dread

Treatment of overdose: Lavage, activated charcoal; monitor electrolytes, vital signs

flurbiprofen (℞)

(flure-bi'proe-fen)

Ansaid, Froben ✤, Ocufen

Func. class.: Nonsteroidal antiinflammatory

Chem. class.: Phenylalkanoic acid

Pregnancy category C

Action: Inhibits prostaglandin synthesis by decreasing enzyme needed for biosynthesis; analgesic, antiinflammatory, antipyretic; inhibits enzyme system necessary for biosynthesis of prostaglandins; inhibits miosis

Therapeutic Outcome: Decreased pain, inflammation

Uses: Mild-to-moderate pain, osteoarthritis, rheumatoid arthritis, acute gout, arthritis, ankylosing spondylitis, inflammation, dysmenorrhea; inhibition of intraoperative miosis, corneal edema

Dosage and routes

Adult: PO 200-300 mg qd in 2-4 divided doses, max 300 mg/day or 100 mg/dose; ophth 1 gtt q½-2h before surgery (4 gtt total)

Available forms: Sol 0.03%; tabs 50, 100 mg

Adverse effects

CNS: Depression, flushing, sweating, headache, mood changes

CV: Hypertension, ***circulatory collapse***, thrombophlebitis, embolism, tachycardia, edema

EENT: Burning, stinging in the eye, irritation, bleeding or redness; fungal infections, increased intraocular pressure, blurred vision

GI: Diarrhea, nausea, abdomi-

nal distention, ***GI hemorrhage,*** increased appetite, pancreatitis
INTEG: Acne, poor wound healing, ecchymosis, petechiae
MS: Fractures, osteoporosis, weakness

Contraindications: Hypersensitivity, epithelial herpes simplex keratitis

Precautions: Pregnancy **C**, lactation, child, aspirin or NSAID hypersensitivity, allergy, bleeding disorder

P

Pharmacokinetics

Absorption	Well absorbed (PO)
Distribution	Widely distributed (PO)
Metabolism	Liver—extensively
Excretion	Kidneys
Half-life	3-6 hr

Pharmacodynamics

Unknown

Interactions

Individual drugs

Alcohol: ↑ GI upset
Aspirin: ↓ effect of flurbiprofen
Carbachol: ↓ effect when used with other ophthalmics
Epinephrine: ↓ effect of epinephrine
Heparin: ↑ bleeding
Radiation: ↑ effects

Drug classifications

Antihypertensives: ↓ antihypertensive effect
Cephalosporins: ↑ bleeding
Hypoglycemics, oral: ↑ hypoglycemic effect
Nonsteroidal antiinflammatory agents: ↑ GI upset

NURSING CONSIDERATIONS

Assessment

- Assess for pain: joint pain (duration, intensity, ROM); baseline and during treatment

Implementation

Ophth route

- Excess sol must be wiped away promptly to prevent its flow into lacrimal system, producing systemic symptoms
- Protect sol from sun

PO route

- Give ½ hr ac or 2 hr pc

Patient/family education

- Advise patient to report change in vision, blurring, or loss of sight during miosis; rash, tinnitus, black stools, headache, chills, fever (systemic)
- Caution patient not to use for any other condition than prescribed
- Inform patient to avoid use with OTC medications for pain or with alcohol unless approved by prescriber
- Advise patient to avoid hazardous activities because dizziness or drowsiness occurs

Evaluation

Positive therapeutic outcome

- Absence of corneal edema, intraoperative miosis (ophth)
- Decreased pain, inflammation

F

flutamide (℞)

(floo′ta-mide)

Eulexin

Func. class.: Antineoplastic hormone

Chem. class.: Antiandrogen

Pregnancy category D

Action: Interferes with testosterone uptake in the nucleus or testosterone activity in target tissues; arrests tumor growth in androgen-sensitive tumors

➔ **Therapeutic Outcome:** Prevention of rapidly growing malignant cells

Uses: Metastatic prostatic carcinoma, stage D2 in combination with LHRH agonistic analogs (leuprolide)

Dosage and routes

Adult: PO 250 mg q8h tid, for a daily dosage of 750 mg

Available forms: Cap 125 mg

Adverse effects

CNS: Hot flashes, drowsiness, confusion, depression, anxiety
GI: Diarrhea, nausea, vomiting, increased liver function studies, ***hepatitis,*** anorexia
GU: Decreased libido, impotence, gynecomastia
INTEG: Irritation at site, rash photosensitivity
MISC: Edema, hematopoietic symptoms, neuromuscular and pulmonary symptoms, hypertension

Contraindications: Hypersensitivity, pregnancy **D**

Pharmacokinetics

Absorption	Well absorbed
Distribution	Unknown
Metabolism	Liver
Excretion	Unknown
Half-life	6 hr

Pharmacodynamics

Unknown

Interactions

Individual drugs

Leuprolide: ↑ synergistic effect

NURSING CONSIDERATIONS

Assessment

• Monitor bilirubin, creatinine, AST (SGOT), ALT (SGPT), alk phosphatase, which may be elevated
• Identify CNS symptoms: drowsiness, confusion, depression, anxiety

Nursing diagnoses

✓ Injury, risk for (adverse reactions)
✓ Sexual dysfunction (adverse reactions)
✓ Body image disturbance (adverse reactions)
✓ Infection, risk for (adverse reactions)
✓ Knowledge deficit (teaching)

Implementation

• Used in combination with LHRH agonist (leuprolide)
• May be given with food or fluids

Patient/family education

• Tell the patient to report side effects: decreased libido, impotence, breast enlargement, hot flashes, diarrhea, which occur when the two drugs are given together
• Inform patient that this drug is taken with leuprolide

Evaluation

Positive therapeutic outcome

• Prevention of rapid division of malignant cells

Treatment of overdose: Induce vomiting, provide supportive care

fluvastatin (℞)

(flu'vah-stay-tin)

Loecol

Func. class.: Antihyperlipidemic

Chem. class.: Synthetically derived fermentation product

Pregnancy category X

Action: Inhibits HMG-CoA reductase enzyme, which reduces cholesterol synthesis

→ Therapeutic Outcome: Decreased cholsterol levels and LDLs, increased HDLs

Uses: As an adjunct in primary hypercholesterolemia (types Ia, Iib)

Dosage and routes

Adult: PO 20-40 mg qd in PM initially, usual range 20-80, not to exceed 80 mg; should be given in 2 doses (40 mg AM, 40 mg PM); dosage adjustments may be made in 4 wk intervals or more

Available forms: Caps 20, 40 mg

Adverse effects

CNS: Headache, dizziness, insomnia
EENT: Lens opacities
GI: Nausea, constipation, diarrhea, dyspepsia, flatus, liver dysfunction, pancreatitis
INTEG: Rash, pruritus
MISC: Fatigue, influenza
MS: Myalgia, myositis, rhabdomyolysis
RESP: Upper respiratory infection, rhinitis, cough, pharyngitis, sinusitis

Contraindications: Hypersensitivity, pregnancy **X,** lactation, active liver disease

Precautions: Past liver disease, alcoholism, severe acute infections, trauma, hypotension, uncontrolled seizure disorders, severe metabolic disorders, electrolyte imbalance

Pharmacokinetics	
Absorption	Unknown
Distribution	Unknown
Metabolism	Liver
Excretion	Feces, kidneys
Half-life	14 hr

Pharmacodynamics

Unknown

Interactions

Individual drugs

Bile acid sequestrants: ↓ effects of fluvastin
Cholestyramine: ↓ action of fluvastin
Colestipol: ↓ action of fluvastin
Cyclosporine: ↑ risk of myopathy
Digoxin: ↑ action
Erthyromycin: ↑ risk of myopathy
Gemfibrozil: ↑ risk of myopathy
Niacin: ↑ risk of myopathy
Rifampin: ↓ effects of fluvastin
Warfarin: ↑ action

NURSING CONSIDERATIONS

Assessment

- Assess nutrition: fat, protein, carbohydrates; nutritional analysis should be completed by dietician before treatment
- Monitor bowel pattern daily; diarrhea may be a problem
- Monitor triglycerides, cholesterol at baseline and throughout treatment; LDL and VLDL should be watched closely; if increased, drug should be discontinued
- Monitor liver function studies q1-2mo during the first 1½ yr of treatment; AST (SGOT), ALT (SGPT), liver function tests may be increased
- Monitor renal studies in patients with compromised renal system: BUN, I&O ratio, creatinine
- Monitor eyes with slit lamp before, 1 mo after treatment begins, annually; lens opacities may occur

Nursing diagnoses

- ✓ Diarrhea (adverse reactions)
- ✓ Knowledge deficit (teaching)
- ✓ Noncompliance (teaching)

F

Implementation
• Give with evening meal; if dosage is increased, take with breakfast and evening meal
• Store in cool environment in airtight, light-resistant container

Patient/family education
• Inform patient that compliance is needed for positive results to occur, not to double doses
• Teach patient that risk factors should be decreased: high-fat diet, smoking, alcohol consumption, absence of exercise
• Advise patient to notify prescriber if the GI symptoms of diarrhea, abdominal or epigastric pain, nausea, vomiting, or if chills, fever, sore throat occur
• Advise patient that treatment will take several years
• Advise patient that blood work and eye exam will be necessary during treatment

Evaluation
Positive therapeutic outcome
• Decreased cholesterol levels, serum triglyceride
• Improved ratio of HDLs

folic acid (vitamin B_9)
(PO, OTC; IM/IV, ℞)
(foe-lik a'sid)
Apo-Folic ✱, Folate, Folvite, Novofolacid ✱, Vitamin B_9
Func. class.: Vitamin B-complex group
Chem. class.: Supplement
Pregnancy category A

Action: Needed for erythropoiesis; increases RBC, WBC, and platelet formation in megaloblastic anemias

➔ **Therapeutic Outcome:** Absence of macrocytic, megaloblastic anemias

Uses: Megaloblastic or macrocytic anemia caused by folic acid deficiency; liver disease; alcoholism; hemolysis; intestinal obstruction; pregnancy

Dosage and routes
Supplement
Adult: PO/IM/SC/**IV** 0.1 mg qd
P ***Child:*** PO/IM/SC/**IV** 0.05 mg qd

Megaloblastic/macrocytic anemia
P ***Adult and child >4 yr:*** PO/SC/IM/**IV** 1 mg qd × 4-5 days
P ***Child <4 yr:*** PO/SC/IM/**IV** 0.3 mg or less qd
Pregnancy/lactation: PO/SC/IM/**IV** 0.8 mg qd

Prevention of megaloblastic/macrocytic anemia
Pregnancy: PO/SC/IM/**IV** 1 mg qd

Available forms: Tabs 0.1, 0.4, 0.8, 1 mg; inj 5, 10 mg/ml

Adverse effects
INTEG: Flushing
RESP: ***Bronchospasm***

Contraindications: Hypersensitivity, anemias other than megaloblastic/macrocytic anemia, vit B_{12} deficiency anemia, uncorrected pernicious anemia

Precautions: Pregnancy **A**

Pharmacokinetics

Absorption	Well absorbed
Distribution	Liver, crosses placenta
Metabolism	Liver (converted to active metabolite)
Excretion	Kidneys (unchanged)
Half-life	Unknown

Pharmacodynamics

Onset	Unknown
Peak	½-1 hr
Duration	Unknown

Interactions

Individual drugs

Methotrexate: ↓ action of folic acid
Phenytoin: ↑ need for folic acid
Sulfasalazine: ↓ action of folic acid
Triamterene: ↓ action of folic acid

Drug classifications

Estrogens: ↑ need for folic acid
Glucocorticoids: ↑ need for folic acid
Sulfonamides: ↓ action of folic acid

NURSING CONSIDERATIONS

Assessment

- Assess patient for fatigue, dyspnea, weakness, shortness of breath, activity intolerance (signs of megaloblastic anemia)
- Monitor Hgb, Hct, and reticulocyte count; folate levels: 6-15 µg/ml baseline and throughout treatment
- Assess nutritional status: bran, yeast, dried beans, nuts, fruits, fresh vegetables, asparagus; if high folic acid foods are missing from the diet, a referral to a dietician may be indicated
- Identify drugs currently taken: alcohol, oral contraceptives, hydantoins, trimethoprim; these drugs may cause increased folic acid use by the body and contribute to deficiency

Nursing diagnoses

- ✓ Nutrition, less than body requirements (uses)
- ✓ Fatigue (uses)
- ✓ Activity intolerance (uses)
- ✓ Knowledge deficit (teaching)

Implementation

IV IV route

- Give **IV** directly, undiluted 5 mg or less/min—or may be added to most **IV** sol or TPN
- Store in light-resistant container

Syringe incompatibility: Doxapram

Y-site compatibility: Famotidine

Solution compatibility: $D_{20}W$

Solution incompatibilities: $D_{40}W$, $D_{50}W$, calcium gluconate

Patient/family education

- Advise patient to take drug exactly as prescribed; not to double doses, toxicity may occur
- Instruct patient to notify prescriber of side effects—rash or fever may indicate hypersensitivity
- Advise patient that urine may become more yellow
- Instruct patient to increase intake of foods rich in folic acid in diet as recommended by dietician or health care provider

Evaluation

Positive therapeutic outcome

- Absence of fatigue, weakness, dyspnea
- Absence of symptoms of megaloblastic anemia

F

foscarnet (℞)
(foss-kar'net)
Foscavir
Func. class.: Antiviral
Chem. class.: Inorganic pyrophosphate organic analog
Pregnancy category C

Action: Antiviral activity is produced by selective inhibition at the pyrophosphate binding site on virus-specific DNA polymerases and reverse transcriptases at concentrations that do not affect cellular DNA polymerases

➔ **Therapeutic Outcome:** Virostatic agents against CMV retinitis

Uses: Treatment of CMV (cytomegalovirus), retinitis, HSV infections; used with ganciclovir for relapsing patients

Dosage and routes

Adult: **IV** inf 60 mg/kg given over at least 1 hr, q8h × 2-3 wk initially, then 90-120 mg/kg/day over 2 hr, usually give with at least 750-1000 ml 0.9% NaCl qd

In renal abnormalities

Adult: **IV** male:

$$\frac{140\text{–age}}{\text{serum creatinine} \times 72} = \text{creatinine clearance}$$

Female: 0.85 x above value

Dose based on table provided in package insert

Available forms: Inj 24 mg/ml

Adverse effects

CNS: Fever, dizziness, headache, ***seizures,*** fatigue, neuropathy, tremor, ataxia, dementia, stupor, EEG abnormalities, vertigo, ***coma,*** abnormal gait, hypertonia, extrapyramidal disorders, hemiparesis, ***paralysis,*** hyperreflexia, paraplegia, ***tetany,*** hyporeflexia, neuralgia, neuritis, celebral edema, paresthesia, depression, confusion, anxiety, insomnia, somnolence, amnesia, hallucinations, agitation

CV: Hypertension, palpitations, ECG abnormalities, 1st degree AV block, nonspecific ST-T segment changes, hypotension, cerebrovascular disorder, cardiomyopathy, ***cardiac arrest,*** bradycardia, dysrhythmias

EENT: Visual field defects, vocal cord paralysis, speech disorders, taste perversion, eye pain, conjunctivitis, tinnitus, otitis

GI: Nausea, vomiting, anorexia, abdominal pain, constipation, dysphagia, rectal hemorrhage, dry mouth, melena, flatulence, ulcerative stomatitis, pancreatitis, enteritis, enterocolitis, glossitis, proctitis, stomatitis, increased amylases, gastroenteritis, ***pseudomembranous colitis,*** duodenal ulcer, ***paralytic ileus, esophageal ulceration,*** abnormal A-G ratio, increased AST (SGPT), ALT (SGOT), cholecystitis, ***hepatitis,*** dyspepsia, tenesmus, hepatosplenomegaly, jaundice

GU: ***Acute renal failure,*** decreased Ccr and increased serum creatinine, ***glomerulonephritis, toxic nephropathy, nephrosis, renal tubular disorders, pyelonephritis, uremia, hematuria, albuminuria,*** dysuria, polyuria

HEMA: Anemia, ***granulocytopenia, leukopenia, thrombocytopenia,*** platelet abnormalities, ***thrombosis, pulmonary***

embolism, coagulation disorders, decreased prothrombin, hypochromic anemia, pancytopenia, hemolysis, leukocytosis, lymphadenopathy, epistaxis, lymphopenia
INTEG: Rash, sweating, pruritus, skin ulceration, seborrhea, skin discoloration, alopecia, acne, dermatitis, pain/inflammation at injection site, facial edema, dry skin, urticaria
MS: Arthralgia, myalgia
RESP: Coughing, dyspnea, pneumonia, sinusitis, pharyngitis, ***pulmonary infiltration,*** stridor, ***pneumothorax, hemoptysis, bronchospasm,*** bronchitis, ***respiratory depression, pleural effusion, pulmonary hemorrhage,*** rhinitis
SYST: Hypokalemia, hypocalcemia, hypomagnesemia, increased alk phosphatase, LDH, BUN, acidosis, hypophosphatemia, hyperphosphatemia, dehydration, glycosuria, increased creatine phosphokinase, hypervolemia, infection, ***sepsis, death, ascites,*** hyponatremia, hypochloremia, hypercalcemia

Contraindications: Hypersensitivity

Precautions: Pregnancy **C**, P lactation, children, elderly, G renal disease, seizure disorders, electrolyte/mineral imbalances, severe anemia

Pharmacokinetics

Absorption	Complete (IV)
Distribution	14%-17% plasma protein binding
Metabolism	Not metabolized
Excretion	Kidneys (90%) unchanged, breast milk
Half-life	2-8 hr; ↑ in renal disease

Pharmacodynamics

Onset	48 hr
Peak	2 wk
Duration	Unknown

Interactions

Individual drugs

Amphotericin B: ↑ nephrotoxicity
Pentamide: ↑ nephrotoxicity
Zidovudine: ↑ anemia

Drug classification

Aminoglycosides: ↑ nephrotoxicity

NURSING CONSIDERATIONS

Assessment

- Culture should be done before treatment with foscarnet is begun; cultures of blood, urine, and throat may all be taken; CMV is not confirmed by this method; the diagnosis is made by an ophth exam
- Assess kidney and liver function; increased hemopoietic studies: BUN, serum creatinine, creatitinine clearance, AST (SGOT), ALT (SGPT), A-G ratio, baseline and during treatment; blood counts should be done q2wk; watch for decreasing granulocytes, Hgb; if low, therapy may have to be discontinued and restarted after hematologic recovery; blood transfusions may be required
- Assess for GI symptoms: severe nausea, vomiting, diarrhea; severe symptoms may necessitate discontinuing drug
- Monitor electrolytes and minerals: calcium, phosphorous, magnesium, sodium, potassium; watch closely for tetany during first administration
- ! Assess for symptoms of

blood dyscrasias (anemia, granulocytopenia); bruising, fatigue, bleeding, poor healing
• Assess for symptoms of allergic reactions: flushing, rash, urticaria, pruritus

Nursing diagnoses
✓ Infection, risk for (uses)
✓ Injury, risk for (adverse reactions)
✓ Knowledge deficit (teaching)

Implementation
IV route
• Administer increased fluids before and during drug administration to induce diuresis and minimize renal toxicity
• Administer via inf pump, at no more than 1 mg/kg/min; do not give by rapid or bolus **IV**; give by central venous line or peripheral vein; standard 24 mg/ml sol may be used without dilution if using by central line; dilute the 24 mg/ml sol to 12 mg/ml with D_5W or 0.9% NaCl if using peripheral vein
• Monitor patient closely during therapy; if tingling, numbness, paresthesias occur, stop inf and obtain lab sample for electrolytes

Y-site incompatibilities: Acyclovir, amphotericin B, calcium, co-trimoxazole, diazepam, digoxin, gancyclovir, haloperidol, leucovorin, midazolam, pentamidine, phenytoin, prochlorperazine, vancomycin

Y-site compatibilities: Aldesleukin, aminophylline, amikacin, ampicillin, aztreonam, benzquinamide, cephalosporins, dexamethasone, dopamine, erythromycin, fluconazole, flucytosine, furosemide, gentamicin, heparin, hydromorphone, hydroxyzine, metoclopramide, metronidazole, miconazole, morphine, nafcillin, oxacillin, penicillin G potassium, phenytoin, piperacillin, ranitidine, tobramycin

Patient/family education
• Advise patient to notify prescriber if sore throat, swollen lymph nodes, malaise, fever occur—may indicate presence of other infections
• Advise patient to report perioral tingling, numbness in extremities, and paresthesias; inf should be stopped and electrolytes should be requested
• Caution patient that serious drug interactions may occur if OTC products are ingested; check first with prescriber
• Inform patient that drug is not a cure, but will control symptoms
• Advise patient that ophth exams must be continued

Evaluation
Positive therapeutic outcome
• Improvement in CMV retinitis

fosinopril (℞)
(foss-in-o'pril)
Monopril
Func. class.: Antihypertensive
Chem. class.: Angiotensin-converting enzyme (ACE) inhibitor
Pregnancy category D

Action: Selectively suppresses renin-angiotensin-aldosterone system; inhibits ACE; prevents conversion of angiotensin I to angiotensin II; results in dilation of arterial, venous vessels

Therapeutic Outcome: Decreased B/P in hypertension

Uses: Hypertension, alone or in combination with thiazide diuretics

Dosage and routes

Adult: PO 10 mg qd initially, then 20-40 mg/day divided bid or qd

Available forms: Tabs 10, 20 mg

Adverse effects

CNS: Insomnia, paresthesia, headache, dizziness, fatigue, memory disturbance, tremor, mood change

CV: Hypotension, chest pain, palpitations, angina, orthostatic hypotension

GI: Nausea, constipation, vomiting, diarrhea

GU: ***Proteinuria,*** increased BUN, creatinine, decreased libido

HEMA: Decreased Hct, Hgb, ***eosinophilia, leukopenia, neutropenia***

INTEG: ***Angioedema,*** rash, flushing, sweating, photosensitivity, pruritus

META: Hyperkalemia

MS: Arthralgia, myalgia

RESP: Cough, sinusitis, dyspnea, ***bronchospasm***

Contraindications: Hypersensitivity to ACE inhibitors, pregnancy **D,** lactation, P children

Precautions: Impaired liver function, hypovolemia, blood dyscrasias, CHF, COPD, G asthma, elderly

Pharmacokinetics

Absorption	30%
Distribution	Crosses placenta
Metabolism	Liver—converted to fosinoprilate
Excretion	50% kidneys (metabolities), 50% feces
Half-life	12 hr—fosinoprilat

Pharmacodynamics

Onset	1 hr
Peak	2-6 hr
Duration	24 hr

F

Interactions

Individual drugs

Alcohol: ↑ hypotension (large amounts)

Allopurinol: ↑ hypersensitivity

Digoxin: ↑ serum levels

Hydralazine: ↑ toxicity

Indomethacin: ↓ antihypertensive effect

Lithium: ↑ serum levels

Prazosin: ↑ toxicity

Drug classifications

Adrenergic blockers: ↑ hypotension

Antacids: ↓ absorption

Antihypertensives: ↑ hypotension

Diuretics: ↑ hypotension

Diuretics, potassium sparing: ↑ toxicity

Ganglionic blockers: ↑ hypotension

Potassium supplements: ↑ toxicity

Sympathomimetics: ↑ toxicity

Lab test interferences

False positive: Urine acetone

NURSING CONSIDERATIONS

Assessment

- Monitor blood studies: neutrophils, decreased platelets
- Monitor B/P, check for orthostatic hypotension, syncope; if changes occur, dosage change may be required
- Monitor renal studies: protein, BUN, creatinine; watch

for increased levels that may indicate nephrotic syndrome and renal failure; monitor renal symptoms: polyuria, oliguria, frequency, dysuria

- Establish baselines in renal, liver function tests before therapy begins
- Check potassium levels throughout treatment although hyperkalemia rarely occurs
- Check for edema in feet, legs daily, monitor weight daily
- Assess for allergic reactions: rash, fever, pruritus, urticaria; drug should be discontinued if antihistamines fail to help

Nursing diagnoses

- ✓ Cardiac output, decreased (uses)
- ✓ Injury, risk for (side effects)
- ✓ Knowledge deficit (teaching)
- ✓ Noncompliance (teaching)

Implementation

- Store in air-tight container at 86° F (30° C) or less
- Severe hypotension may occur after 1st dose of this medication; ↓ hypotension may be prevented by reducing or discontinuing diuretic therapy 3 days before beginning benzapril therapy

Patient/family education

- Advise patient not to discontinue drug abruptly—warn patient to tell all persons associated with his care
- Teach patient not to use OTC products (cough, cold, allergy) unless directed by prescriber because serious side effects can occur; xanthines such as coffee, tea, chocolate, cola can prevent action of drug
- Teach patient the importance of complying with dosage schedule, even if feeling better; to continue with medical regimen to decrease B/P: exercise, smoking cessation, decreasing stress, diet modifications
- Emphasize the need to rise slowly to sitting or standing position to minimize orthostatic hypotension; not to exercise in hot weather or increased hypotension can occur
- Teach patient to notify prescriber of mouth sores, sore throat, fever, swelling of hands or feet, irregular heartbeat, chest pain, coughing, shortness of breath
- Instruct patient to report excessive perspiration, dehydration, vomiting, diarrhea; may lead to fall in B/P
- Caution patient that drug may cause dizziness, fainting, light-headedness; may occur during 1st few days of therapy; to avoid activities that may be hazardous
- Teach patient how to take B/P, and normal readings for age group

Evaluation

Positive therapeutic outcome

- Decreased B/P in hypertension

Treatment of overdose: 0.9% NaCl **IV** inf, hemodialysis

fosfomycin (℞)

(foss-foe-mye'sin)

Monurol

Func. class.: Urinary anti-infective

Pregnancy category B

Action: Interferes with protein synthesis in bacterial cell by binding to ribosomal subunit, causing misreading of genetic code; inaccurate peptide sequence forms in protein chain, causing bacterial death

➔ **Therapeutic Outcome:** Bactericidal effects for the following organisms *E. faecalis, E. coli*

Uses: Urinary tract infections

Dosage and routes

Adult >18 yr: 1 sachet with or without food, always mix with water before ingesting

Available forms: Single-dose sachet (3 g fosfomycin), orange flavored

Adverse effects

CNS: Headache, dizziness, fever, insomnia, somnolence, migraine, asthenia, nervousness

GI: Nausea, vomiting, anorexia, constipation, dry mouth, flatulence, increased SGPT; diarrhea, dyspepsia

GU: Vaginitis, dysuria, hematuria, menstrual disorder

Contraindications: Hypersensitivity

P **Precautions:** Pregnancy **B,** child <12 yrs, lactation

Pharmacokinetics

Absorption	Well absorbed
Distribution	Unknown
Metabolism	Liver
Excretion	Mostly unchanged in kidneys, feces
Half-life	5-7 hr

Pharmacodynamics

Unknown

Interactions

Individual drugs

Metoclopramide: ↑ urinary excretion of fosfomycin

NURSING CONSIDERATIONS

Assessment

- Assess patient for signs and symptoms of infection including characteristics of urine, WBC >10,000, fever; obtain baseline information and during treatment
- Complete culture and sensitivity before beginning drug therapy; this will ensure that correct treatment has been initiated
- Assess for overgrowth of infection: perineal itching, fever, pain
- Assess urine pH; urine should be kept alkaline

Nursing diagnoses

✓ Infection, risk for (uses)
✓ Diarrhea (side effects)
✓ Knowledge deficit (teaching)
✓ Noncompliance (teaching)
✓ Injury, risk for (side effects)

Implementation

- Pour contents of sachet into 3-4 oz (½ cup) of water, stir to dissolve, use cold water, take immediately
- Only a single dose is necessary
- May be taken with or without food
- Give adequate fluids of 2-3 L/day, unless contraindicated
- Store at 59-86° F

Patient/family education

- Give patient directions to dissolve sachet, caution patient not to take in dry form

Evaluation

Positive therapeutic outcome

- Absence of signs/symptoms of infection (WBC <10,000, temp WNL)
- Reported improvement in symptoms of infection
- Negative C&S

fosphenytoin (℞)

(foss-fen′i-toy-in)

Cerebyx

Func. class.: Anticonvulsant

Chem. class.: Hydantoin

Pregnancy category D

Action: Inhibits spread of seizure activity in motor cortex by altering ion transport; increases AV conduction

➔ Therapeutic Outcome: Decreased seizures, absence of dysrhythmias

Uses: Generalized tonic-clonic seizures, status epilepticus

Dosage and routes

Status epilepticus

Adult: **IV** loading dose 15-20 mg PE/kg given at 100-150 mg PE/min

Nonemergent/maintenance dosing

Adult: IM/**IV** loading dose 10-20 mg PE/kg; maintenance dosing 4-6 mg PE/kg/day given at a rate of <150 mg PE/min

Available forms: Inj 150 mg (100 mg phenytoin), 750 mg (500 mg phenytoin)

Adverse effects

CNS: Drowsiness, dizziness, insomnia, paresthesias, depression, suicidal tendencies, aggression, headache, confusion

CV: Hypotension, ventricular fibrillation

EENT: Nystagmus, diplopia, blurred vision

GI: Nausea, vomiting, constipation, anorexia, weight loss, hepatitis, jaundice, gingival hyperplasia

GU: **Nephritis,** urine discoloration

HEMA: Agranulocytosis, leukopenia, aplastic anemia, thrombocytopenia, megaloblastic anemia

INTEG: Rash, lupus erythematosus, *Stevens-Johnson syndrome,* hirsutism

SYST: Hypocalcemia

Contraindications: Hypersensitivity, psychiatric conditions, pregnancy **D,** bradycardia, SA and AV block, Stokes-Adams syndrome

Precautions: Allergies, hepatic disease, renal disease

Pharmacokinetics	
Absorption	Unknown
Distribution	Unknown
Metabolism	Liver
Excretion	Kidneys
Half-life	Unknown

Pharmacodynamics

Unknown

Interactions

Individual drugs

Alcohol: ↑ CNS depression

Carbamazepine: ↓ effectiveness

Isoniazid: ↓ metabolism, ↑ action

Valproic acid: ↑ seizures

Drug classifications

Anticonvulsants: ↑ CNS depression

Antidepressants: ↑ CNS depression

Antihistamines: ↑ CNS depression

Barbiturates: ↑ CNS depression, ↓ effect of fosphonytoin

Benzodiazepines: ↑ blood levels

General anesthetics: ↑ CNS depression

Hypnotics: ↑ CNS depression

Narcotics: ↑ CNS depression

Sedatives: ↑ CNS depression

Lab test interferences

↓ Dexamethasone, ↓ metyrapone test serum, ↓ PBI, ↓ urinary steroids

↑ Glucose, ↑ alkaline phosphatase, ↑ BSP

NURSING CONSIDERATIONS

Assessment

- Assess drug level: toxic level 30-50 μg/ml
- Assess mental status: mood, sensorium, affect, memory (long, short), especially elderly
- Assess for blood dyscrasias: fever, sore throat, bruising, rash, jaundice, epistaxis (long-term treatment only)
- Assess seizure activity including type, location, duration, and character; provide seizure precaution
- Assess renal studies: urinalysis, BUN, urine creatinine
- Monitor blood studies: RBC, Hct, Hgb, reticulocyte counts weekly for 4 wk then monthly; also check thyroid function tests, serum calcium
- Monitor hepatic studies: ALT (SGPT), AST (SGOT), bilirubin, creatinine
- Assess allergic reaction: red raised rash; if this occurs, drug should be discontinued
- Monitor for toxicity: bone marrow depression, nausea, vomiting, ataxia, diplopia, cardiovascular collapse, slurred speech, confusion

Nursing diagnoses

- ✓ Injury, risk for (uses, adverse reactions)
- ✓ Knowledge deficit (teaching)
- ✓ Noncompliance (teaching)

Implementation

IV route

- Administer by direct **IV** after diluting with D_5 or 0.9% NaCl 1.5-2.5 mg PE/ml

Patient/family education

- Reason for and expected outcome of treatment

Evaluation

Positive therapeutic outcome

- Decreased seizure activity

furosemide (℞)

(fur-oh'se-mide)

Apo-Furosemide ♣, Fumide, Furomide M.D., Furosemide, Furoside, Lasix, Lasix Special ♣, Luramide, Myrosemide, Novosemide ♣, Uritol ♣

Func. class.: Loop diuretic

Chem. class.: Sulfonamide derivative

Pregnancy category C

Action: Acts on the ascending loop of Henle in the kidney, inhibiting the reabsorption of the electrolytes sodium and chloride, causing excretion of sodium, calcium, magnesium, chloride, water, and some potassium; decreases reabsorption of sodium and chloride and increases the excretion of potassium in the distal tubule of the kidney; responsible for slight antihypertensive effect and peripheral vasodilation

Therapeutic Outcome: Decreased edema in lung tissue, peripherally; decreased B/P

Uses: Edema in congestive heart failure, nephrotic syndrome, ascites, caused by hepatic disease, hepatic cirrhosis; may be used alone or as adjunct with antihypertensives such as spironolactone, triamterene; should not be used with ethacrynic acid

Investigational uses: Hypercalcemia in malignancy

Dosage and routes

Adult: PO 20-80 mg/day in AM, may give another dose in 6 hrs, up to 600 mg/day; IM/**IV** 20-40 mg, increased by 20 mg q2h until desired response

P ***Child:*** PO/IM/**IV** 2 mg/kg, may increase by 1-2 mg/kg/ q6-8h up to 6 mg/kg

Pulmonary edema

Adult: **IV** 40 mg given over several min, repeated in 1 hr; increase to 80 mg if needed

Available forms: Tabs 20, 40, 80 mg; oral sol 10 mg/ml, 40 mg/5 ml; inj IM, **IV** 10 mg/ml

Adverse effects

CNS: Headache, fatigue, weakness, vertigo, paresthesias
CV: Orthostatic hypotension, chest pain, ECG changes, ***circulatory collapse***
ELECT: Hypokalemia, hypochloremic alkalosis, hypomagnesemia, hyperuricemia, hypocalcemia, hyponatremia, metabolic alkalosis
*EENT: **Loss of hearing**,* ear pain, tinnitus, blurred vision
GI: Nausea, diarrhea, dry mouth, vomiting, anorexia, cramps, oral or gastric irritations, pancreatitis
*GU: Polyuria, **renal failure**, glycosuria*
*HEMA: **Thrombocytopenia, agranulocytosis, leukopenia neutropenia, anemia***
*INTEG: Rash, pruritus, purpura, **Stevens-Johnson syndrome**,* sweating, photosensitivity, urticaria
MS: Cramps, stiffness

Contraindications: Hypersensitivity to sulfonamides, anuria, P hypovolemia, infants, lactation, electrolyte depletion

Precautions: Diabetes mellitus, dehydration, severe renal disease, pregnancy **C,** cirrhosis, ascites

Pharmacokinetics

	PO
Absorption	GI tract (60%-70%)
	PO/IM/IV
Distribution	Crosses placenta
Metabolism	Liver (30%-40%)
Excretion	Breast milk, urine, feces
Half-life	½-1 hr

Pharmacodynamics

	PO	IM	IV
Onset	1 hr	½ hr	5 mins
Peak	1-2 hrs	Unknown	½ hr
Duration	6-8 hrs	4-8 hrs	2 hrs

Interactions

Individual drugs

Alcohol: ↑ orthostatic hypotension
Cisplatin: ↑ risk of ototoxicity
Ethacrynic acid: Combination with furosemide may cause ↑ chance of dysrhythmias (do not use together)
Indomethacin: ↓ diuretic
Lithium: ↓ renal clearance, causing increased toxicity
Phenytoin: ↓ diuretic effect caused by ↓ absorption
Probenecid: ↓ effects of furosemide
Succinylcholine: Action of succinylcholine is ↑ by low doses and ↓ by high doses of furosemide
Theophylline: May ↑ or ↓ the effect of theophylline
Vancomycin: ↑ risk of ototoxicity

Drug classifications

Adrenergic blockers: ↑ effects
Aminoglycosides: ↑ ototoxicity, nephrotoxicity
Anticoagulants: ↑ anticoagu-

lant effect caused by ↓ plasma protein binding
Antidiabetics: ↓ hypoglycemic effect
Antihypertensives: ↑ antihypertensive effect
Cephalosporins: ↑ nephrotoxicity
Chloral hydrate: ↑ sweating, flushing when given with **IV** furosemide
Clofibrate: ↑ furosemide effects
Corticosteroids: ↑ potassium loss caused by potassium depletion effects of both drugs
Digitalis glycosides: ↑ potassium and magnesium loss with relating dysrhythmias
Narcotics: ↑ orthostatic hypotension
Salicylates: ↓ diuretic effect
Food
↓ diuresis

NURSING CONSIDERATIONS
Assessment

- Assess patient for tinnitus, hearing loss, ear pain; periodic testing of hearing is needed when high doses of this drug are given by **IV** route
- Monitor for renal, cardiac, neurologic, GI, pulmonary manifestations of hypokalemia: acidic urine, reduced urine osmolality, nocturia, polyuria and polydipsia; hypotension, broad T-wave, U-wave, ectopy, tachycardia, weak pulse; muscle weakness, altered LOC, drowsiness, apathy, lethargy, confusion, depression; anorexia, nausea, cramps, constipation, distension, paralyticileus; hypoventilation, respiratory muscle weakness
- Monitor for CNS, GI, cardiovascular, integumentary, neurologic manifestations of hypocalcemia: personality changes, anxiety, disturbances, depression and psychosis; nausea, vomiting, constipation, abdominal pain from muscle spasm; decreased contractility, decreased cardiac output, hypotension, lengthened ST segment, prolonged QT interval; scaling eczema, alopecia, hyperpigmentation; tetany, muscle twitching, cramping grimacing, seizure, altered deep tendon reflexes, spasm
- Monitor for CNS, neuromuscular, GI, cardiac manifestations of hypomagnesemia, agitation; muscle twitching, paresthesias, hyperactive re flexes, positive Babinski reflex, dysphagia, nystagmus seizures, tetnany; nausea, vomiting, diarrhea, anorexia, abdominal distention; ectopy, tachycardia, broad, flat or inverted T-waves, depressed ST segment, prolonged OT, decreased cardiac output, hypotension
- Monitor for CV, GI, neurologic manifestations of hyponatremia: ↑ B/P, cold, clammy skin, hypovolemia or hypervolemia; anorexia, nausea, vomiting, diarrhea, abdominal cramps; lethargy, increased ICP, confusion headache, seizures, coma, fatigue, tremors, hyperreflexia
- Monitor for neurologic, respiratory manifestations of hyperchloremia: weakness, lethargy, coma; deep rapid breathing
- Assess fluid volume status: I&O ratios and record, count or weigh diapers as appropriate, weight, distended red veins, crackles in lung, color, quality and sp gr of urine, skin turgor, adequacy of pulses, moist mucous membranes, bilateral lung sounds, periph-

F

eral pitting edema; dehydration symptoms of decreasing output, thirst, hypotension, dry mouth and mucous membranes should be reported

• Monitor electrolytes: potassium, sodium, calcium, magnesium; also include BUN, blood pH, ABGs, uric acid, CBC, blood sugar

• Assess B/P before and during therapy lying, standing and sitting as appropriate; orthostatic hypotension can occur rapidly

Nursing diagnoses

✓ Fluid volume deficit (side effects)

✓ Fluid volume excess (uses)

✓ Knowledge deficit (teaching)

Implementation

• Give in AM to avoid interference with sleep

• Potassium replacement if potassium level is <3.0 whole, or use oral sol slightly, drug may be crushed if patient is unable to swallow

PO route

• With food, if nausea occurs, absorption may be reduced

IV **IV route**

• Do not use sol that is yellow, or has a precipitate, or crystals

Implementation

IV **Direct IV**

• Give undiluted through Y-tube on 3-way stopcock; give 20 mg or less/min

Int Inf

• May be added to NS, D_5W, $D_{10}W$, $D_{20}W$; invert sugar 10% in electrolyte #1, LR, Sodium lactate y_6m, use within 24 hr to assure compatibility; give through Y-tube or 3-way stopcock; give at 4 mg/min or less, use inf pump

Syringe incompatibilities: Doxapram, doxorubicin, droperidol, metaclopramide, milrinone

Y-site incompatibilities: Amsacrine, bleomycin, doxorubicin, droperidol, esmolol, fluconazole, gentamicin, idarubicin, metoclopramide, milrinone, netilmicin, ondansetron, quinidine, vinblastine, vincristine

Additive incompatibilities: Bleomycin, dobutamine, gentamicin, chlorpromazine, diazepam, erythromycin, isoproterenol, meperidine, metoclopramide, netilmicin, opium alkaloids, prochlorperazine, tetracycline

Y-site compatibilities: Allopurinol, amifostine, amikacin, aztrenom, bleomycin, cefepime, cisplatin, cyclophosphamide, cytarabine, dexamethasone, dobutamine, famotidine, fludarabine, fluorouracil, foscarnet, granisetron, heparin, hydrocortisone, indomethacin, kanamycin, leucovorin, lorazepam, methotrexate, mitomycin, morphine, paclitaxel, potassium chloride, sargramostim, thiotepa, tobramycin, tolazoline, vitamin B complex with C

Additive compatibilities: Amikacin, aminophylline, amiodarone, ampicillin, atropine, bumetanide, buprenorphine, flumetanide, calcium gluconate, cefamandole, cefuroxime, cimetidine, cloxacillin, digoxin, epinephrine, heparin, isosorbide, kanamycin, lidocaine, morphine, nitroglycerin, penicillin G, potassium chloride, tobramycin, verapamil, ranitidine, sodium bicarbonate

Patient/family education

General

- Teach patient to take the medication early in the day to prevent nocturia
- Instruct the patient to take with food or milk if GI symptoms of nausea and anorexia occur
- Teach patient to maintain a record of weight on a weekly basis and notify physician of weight loss of >5 lbs
- Caution the patient that this drug causes a loss of potassium, that food rich in potassium should be added to the diet; refer to a dietician for assistance in planning
- Caution the patient not to exercise in hot weather or stand for prolonged periods of time because orthostatic hypotension will be enhanced
- Advise patient to wear protective clothing and sunscreen to prevent photosensitivity
- Teach patient not to use alcohol or any over-the-counter medications without physician's approval, serious drug reactions may occur
- Emphasize the need to contact physician immediately if muscle cramps, weakness, nausea, dizziness or numbness occurs
- Teach patient to take and record their own B/P and pulse
- Caution the patient that orthostatic hypotension may occur and patient should rise slowly from sitting or reclining positions and lie down if dizziness occurs
- Teach patient to continue taking medication even if feeling better, this drug controls symptoms but does not cure the condition
- Advise the patient with hypertension to continue other medical treatment (exercise, weight loss, relaxation techniques, cessation of smoking)

Evaluation

Positive therapeutic outcome

- Decreased edema
- Decreased B/P
- Lowered calcium level in malignancy
- Increased diuresis

G

gallamine (℞)

(gal'a-meen)

Flaxedil

Func. class.: Neuromuscular blocker (nondepolarizing)

Pregnancy category C

Action: Inhibits transmission of nerve impulses by binding with cholinergic receptor sites, antagonizing action of acetylcholine; no analgesic response

➔ **Therapeutic Outcome:** Paralysis of all skeletal muscles

Uses: Facilitation of endotracheal intubation, skeletal muscle relaxation during mechanical ventilation, surgery, or general anesthesia

Dosage and routes

P ***Adult and child >1 mo:*** **IV** 1 mg/kg, not to exceed 100 mg, then 0.5-1 mg/kg q30-40 min

P ***Child <1 mo, >5 kg:*** **IV** 0.25-0.75 mg/kg, then 0.01-0.05 mg/kg q30-40 min

Available forms: Inj 20 mg/ml

Adverse effects

CNS: Malignant hyperthermia

CV: Bradycardia, tachycardia, increased, decreased B/P

EENT: Increased secretions

GI: Decreased motility

INTEG: Rash, flushing, pruritus, urticaria

RESP: Prolonged apnea, bronchospasm, cyanosis, respiratory depression

Contraindications: Hypersensitivity to iodides

Precautions: Pregnancy **C,** thyroid disease, collagen disease, cardiac disease, lactation, P children <2 yr, electrolyte imbalances, dehydration, neuromuscular disease (myasthenia gravis), respiratory disease, renal disease

Pharmacokinetics

Absorption	Complete bioavailability
Distribution	Extracellular space, crosses placenta
Metabolism	Plasma
Excretion	Kidneys—unchanged
Half-life	2½ hr

Pharmacodynamics

Onset	2 min
Peak	5 min
Duration	30 min

Interactions

Individual drugs

Clindamycin: ↑ paralysis, length, and intensity

Colistin: ↑ paralysis, length, and intensity

Lidocaine: ↑ paralysis, length, and intensity

Lithium: ↑ paralysis, length, and intensity

Magnesium: ↑ paralysis, length, and intensity

Polymyxin B: ↑ paralysis, length, and intensity

Procainamide: ↑ paralysis, length, and intensity

Quinidine: ↑ paralysis, length, and intensity

Succinylcholine: ↑ paralysis, length, and intensity

Drug classifications

Aminoglycosides: ↑ paralysis, length, and intensity

β-blockers: ↑ paralysis, length, and intensity

Diuretics, potassium-losing: ↑ paralysis, length, and intensity

General anesthetics: ↑ paralysis, length, and intensity

NURSING CONSIDERATIONS

Assessment

- Monitor for electrolyte imbalances (potassium, magnesium), before drug is used; electrolyte imbalances may lead to increased action of this drug
- Monitor vital signs (B/P, pulse, respirations, airway) until fully recovered; rate, depth, pattern of respirations, strength of hand grip; patient should be intubated before use
- Monitor recovery: decreased paralysis of face, diaphragm, leg, arm, rest of body; residual weakness and respiratory problems may occur during recovery period
- Monitor allergic reactions: rash, fever, respiratory distress, pruritus; if present, drug should be discontinued

Nursing diagnoses

- ✓ Breathing pattern, ineffective (uses)
- ✓ Communication, impaired verbal (adverse reactions)
- ✓ Fear (adverse reactions)
- ✓ Knowledge deficit (teaching)

Implementation

- Use peripheral nerve stimulator by anesthesiologist to determine neuromuscular blockade; deep tendon reflexes should be monitored during extended use

• Give **IV** undiluted by direct **IV** over 1 min, or diluted in 10-50 ml of D_5W, ½ NaCl or NS and give as an infusion at prescribed rate (only by qualified person, usually an anesthesiologist); do not administer IM

• Further dilute in D_5W, 0.9% NaCl, D_5/0.9% NaCl q15-25 min (intermittent infusion)

• Maintenance dose is given q20-45 min after 1st dose (continuous infusion); titrate to patient response

• Store in light-resistant area

Patient/family education

• Provide reassurance if communication is difficult during recovery from neuromuscular blockade

• Provide explanation regarding all procedures or treatments; patient will remain conscious if anesthetic is not given also

Evaluation

Positive therapeutic outcome

• Paralysis of jaw, eyelid, head, neck, rest of body as evaluated by peripheral nerve stimulator

Treatment of overdose: Administer edrophonium or neostigmine, atropine—monitor VS; may require mechanical ventilation

gallium (℞)

(gal'ee-yum)

Ganite

Func. class.: Electrolyte modifier

Chem. class.: Hypocalcemic drug

Pregnancy category C

Action: Lowers serum calcium levels by inhibiting calcium resorption from bone

➔ **Therapeutic Outcome:** Decrease calcium level to 5-9 mg/dl

Uses: Cancer-related hypercalcemia

Dosage and routes

Adult: IV 100-200 mg/m^2 qd × 5 days; inf over 24 hr

Available forms: Inj 25 mg/ml

Adverse effects

CV: Tachycardia

EENT: Blurred vision, optic neuritis, hearing loss

GU: ***Nephrotoxicity,*** increased BUN, creatinine

HEMA: ***Anemia, leukopenia***

META: *Hypophosphatemia,* hypocalcemia, decreased serum bicarbonate

Contraindications: Hypersensitivity, severe renal disease

Precautions: Pregnancy **C**, P lactation, children, mild renal disease

Pharmacokinetics

Absorption	Completely absorbed
Distribution	Unknown
Metabolism	Unknown
Excretion	Kidneys (unchanged)
Half-life	Unknown

Pharmacodynamics	
Onset	12-24 hr
Peak	Unknown
Duration	Unknown

Interactions

Individual drugs

Amphotericin B: ↑ nephrotoxicity

Drug classifications

Aminoglycosides: ↑ nephrotoxicity

NURSING CONSIDERATIONS

Assessment

- Renal status: BUN, creatinine, urine output; if creatinine level is 2.5 mg/dl or more, drug should be discontinued
- Monitor calcium, phosphate, bicarbonate—all levels may be decreased and supplements of phosphate may be needed; calcium daily, phosphate 2-3 ×/wk
- Assess for hypercalcemia: nausea, vomiting, fatigue, weakness, thirst, dehydration, dysrhythmias, headache, confusion, coma, decreased reflexes
- For hypocalcemia: dysrhythmias, hypotension, paresthesia; twitching, colic, laryngospasm; hypercalcemia: poor coordination, myalgia, hypotonia, shortened ST segment and QT interval, prolonged PR interval, cone-shaped T wave, sinus bradycardia; Trousseau's, Chvostek's sign: tremors, tetany, cramping, grimacing, seizures, altered deep tendon reflexes and spasms, personality changes including irritability, depression, psychosis
- Monitor for indications of hypophosphatemia: weakness, malaise, tremors, memory loss, inattention, confusion, decreased reflexes, aching bone pain, joint stiffness, rapid, shallow respiration, decreased tidal volume, nausea, vomiting, anorexia, portal hypertension

Nursing diagnoses

- ✓ Injury, risk for (uses)
- ✓ Knowledge deficit (teaching)

Implementation

- Provide adequate hydration with **IV** saline, 2 L/day during treatment; saline increases the extracellular calcium
- Give by continuous **IV** inf after dilution of dose/1 L 0.9% NaCl or D_5W, run over 24 hr, use inf pump
- Store solution for 48 hr at room temp or 1 wk in refrigerator

Y- *site compatibilities:*

Acyclovir, allopurinol, aminophylline, amifostine, aztreonam, cefazolin, ceftazidime, ceftriaxone, cimetidine, ciprofloxacin, cyclophosphamide, dexamethasone, diphenhydramine, filgrastim, fluconazole, furosemide, heparin, hydrocortisone, fosfimide, magnesium sulfate, mannitol, melphalan, meperidine, mesna, methotrexate, metoclopramide, ondansetron, piperacillin, potassium chloride, ranitidine, sodium bicarbonate, teniposide, thiotepa, trimethoprim, sulfamethoxazole, vancomycin, vinorelbine

Patient/family education

- Instruct patient to follow dietary guidelines given by prescriber, including adequate calcium (dietary products, broccoli) and vit D (fortified milk, grain products, fish oil)
- Explain purpose of drug and expected results

Evaluation

Positive therapeutic outcome

- Decreased serum calcium levels to 5-9 mg/dl

ganciclovir (DHPG) (℞)

(gan-sye'kloe-vir)

Cytovene

Func. class.: Antiviral

Chem. class.: Synthetic nucleoside analog

Pregnancy category C

Action: Inhibits replication of herpes viruses in vitro, in vivo by selective inhibition of the human CMV DNA polymerase and by direct incorporation into viral DNA

Therapeutic Outcome: Decreased proliferation of virus responsible for CMV retinitis

Uses: Cytomegalovirus (CMV) retinitis in immunocompromised persons, including those with AIDS, after indirect ophthalmoscopy confirms diagnosis

Dosage and routes

Induction treatment

Adult: **IV** 5 mg/kg given over 1 hr q12h × 2-3 wk

Maintenance treatment

Adult: **IV** inf 5 mg/kg given over 1 hr, qd × 7 days/wk; or 6 mg/kg qd × 5 days/wk; dosage must be reduced in renal impairment; Intravenous **IV** 200 µg every week

Prevention of CMV

Adult: **IV** 5 mg/kg q12h × 1-2 wks, then 5 mg/kg/day or 6 mg/kg × 5 day of each week

Available forms: Powder 500 mg/vial ganciclovir

Adverse effects

CNS: Fever, chills, ***coma,*** confusion, abnormal thoughts, dizziness, bizarre dreams, headache, psychosis, tremors, somnolence, paresthesia

CV: Dysrhythmia, hypertension/hypotension

EENT: Retinal detachment in CMV retinitis

GI: Abnormal LFTs, nausea, vomiting, anorexia, diarrhea, abdominal pain, ***hemorrhage***

GU: ***Hematuria,*** increased creatinine, BUN

HEMA: ***Granulocytopenia, thrombocytopenia, irreversible neutropenia, anemia, eosinophilia***

INTEG: Rash, alopecia, pruritus, urticaria, pain at inj site, phlebitis

RESP: Dyspnea

Contraindications: Hypersensitivity to acyclovir or ganciclovir

Precautions: Preexisting cytopenias, renal function impairment, pregnancy **C,** lactation, G children <6 mo, elderly, platelet P count <25,000/mm

Pharmacokinetics	
Absorption	Completely absorbed
Distribution	Crosses blood-brain barrier, CSF
Metabolism	Not metabolized
Excretion	Kidneys (90%) unchanged, breast milk
Half-life	3 hr

Pharmacodynamics

Unknown

Interactions

Individual drugs

Imipenem with cilastatin: ↑ chance of seizures

Probenecid: ↑ toxicity

Zidovudine: ↑ bone marrow depression

Radiation: ↑ bone marrow depression

Drug classifications

Antineoplastics: ↑ bone marrow depression

NURSING CONSIDERATIONS

Assessment

- Culture should be done before treatment with ganciclovir is initiated; cultures of blood, urine, and throat may all be taken; CMV is not confirmed by this method; the diagnosis is made by an ophth exam
- Assess kidney, liver function; increased hemopoietic studies: BUN, serum creatinine, AST creatinine clearance (SGOT), ALT (SGPT), A-G ratio, baseline, and drip treatment; blood counts should be done q2wk; watch for decreasing granulocytes, Hgb; if low, therapy may have to be discontinued and restarted after hematologic recovery; blood transfusions may be required
- Assess for GI symptoms: severe nausea, vomiting, diarrhea; severe symptoms may necessitate discontinuing drug
- Monitor electrolytes and minerals: calcium, phosphorous, magnesium, sodium, potassium; watch closely for tetany during 1st administration
- Assess for symptoms of blood dyscrasias (anemia, granulocytopenia); brusing, fatigue, bleeding, poor healing
- Assess for symptoms of allergic reactions: flushing, rash, urticaria, pruritus
- Monitor for leukopenia/neutropenia/thrombocytopenia: WBCs, platelets q2day during 2 ×/day dosing and q1wk thereafter; check for leukopenia with qd WBC count in patients with prior leukopenia with other nucleoside analogs or for whom leukopenia counts are <1000 cells/mm^3 at start of treatment
- Monitor serum creatinine or creatinine clearance at least q2wk

Nursing diagnoses

- ✓ Infection, risk for (uses)
- ✓ Injury, risk for (uses, adverse reactions)
- ✓ Knowledge deficit (teaching)

Implementation

- Medicine should be mixed under strict aseptic conditions using gloves, gown, and mask, and using precautions for antineoplastics
- Administer **IV** after diluting 500 mg/10 ml sterile water for inj (50 mg/ml); shake; further dilute in 100 ml D_5W, 0.9% NaCl, LR and run over 1 hr; use inf pump
- Give slowly; do not give by bolus **IV**, IM, SC inj
- Use diluted sol within 12 hr, do not refrigerate or freeze; do not use sol with particulate matter or discoloration, fludarabine, sargramostim

Y-site incompatibilities: Amsacrine, fludarabine, foscarnet, ondansetron, sargramostim, vinorelbine

Y-site compatibilities: Allopurinol, cisplatin, cyclophosphamide, enalaprilat, filgrastim, fluconazole, melphalan, paclitaxel, tacrolimus, teniposide, thiotepa

Patient/family education

- Advise patient to notify prescriber if sore throat, swollen lymph nodes, malaise, fever

occur—may indicate other infections
• Advise patient to report perioral tingling, numbness in extremities, and paresthesias
• Caution patient that serious drug interactions may occur if OTC products are ingested; check first with prescriber
• Inform patient that drug is not a cure, but will control symptoms
• Advise patient that regular ophth exams must be continued
• Inform patient that major toxicities may necessitate discontinuing drug
• Instruct patient to use contraception during treatment and that infertility may occur; men should use barrier contraception for 90 days after treatment

Evaluation
Positive therapeutic outcome
• Decreased symptoms of CMV

Treatment of overdose: Discontinue drug, use hemodialysis, and increase hydration

gemcitabine (℞)
(gem-sit'a-been)
Gemzar
Func. class.: Misc. antineoplastic
Chem. class.: Nucleoside analog
Pregnancy category D

Action: Exhibits antitumor activity by killing cells undergoing DNA synthesis (S phase) and blocking GL/S-phase boundary

➔ Therapeutic Outcome: Prevention of growth of tumor

Uses: Adenocarcinoma of the pancreas: nonresectable stage II, III, or metastatic stage IV

Dosage and routes
Adult: **IV** 100 mg/m^2 given over ½ hr qwk × 7 wk, then 1 wk rest period; subsequent cycles should be infused once qwk × 3 wk out of every 4 wk

Available forms: Lyophilized powder 20 mg/ml

Adverse effects
GI: Diarrhea, nausea, vomiting, anorexia, constipation, stomatitis
HEMA: ***Leukopenia, anemia, neutropenia, thrombocytopenia***
INTEG: Irritation at site, rash, alopecia
OTHER: Dyspnea, fever, ***hemorrhage***, infection

Contraindications: Hypersensitivity, pregnancy **D**

P G Precautions: Lactation, children, elderly, myelosuppression, irradiation

Pharmacokinetics

Absorption	Unknown
Distribution	Unknown
Metabolism	Unknown
Excretion	Unknown
Half-life	42-79 min

Pharmacodynamics

Unknown

Interactions
Drug classifications
Antineoplastics: ↑ myelosuppression, diarrhea

NURSING CONSIDERATIONS
Assessment
• Monitor CBC, differential, platelet count weekly; withhold drug if WBC is <3500/mm^3, or platelet count <100,000/

mm³; notify prescriber of these results; drug should be discontinued
• Assess food preferences: list likes, dislikes
• Assess buccal cavity q8h for dryness, sores or ulceration, white patches, oral pain, bleeding, dysphagia
• Assess GI symptoms: frequency of stools; cramping
• Assess signs of dehydration: rapid respirations, poor skin turgor, decreased urine output, dry skin, restlessness, weakness

Nursing diagnoses

✓ Infection, risk for (adverse reactions)
✓ Nutrition, altered: less than body requirements (adverse reaction)

Implementation

• Give increased fluid intake to 2-3 L/day to prevent dehydration, unless contraindicated
• Change **IV** site q48h
• Provide for rinsing of mouth tid-qid with water, club soda; brushing of teeth bid-tid with soft brush or cotton-tipped applicator for stomatitis; use unwaxed dental floss
• Give nutritious diet with iron, vitamin supplement, low fiber, few dairy products

Patient/family education

• Advise to avoid foods with citric acid or hot or rough texture if stomatitis is present; to drink adequate fluids
• Advise to report stomatitis; any bleeding, white spots, ulcerations in mouth; tell patient to examine mouth qd, report symptoms
• Advise to report signs of anemia: fatigue, headache, faintness, shortness of breath, irritability
• Advise to use contraception during therapy

Evaluation

Positive therapeutic outcome

• Decrease in tumor size, decrease in spread of cancer

Treatment of overdose: Induce vomiting, provide supportive care

gemfibrozil (℞)

(gem-fye'broe-zil)

Lopid

Func. class.: Antilipemic

Chem. class.: Aryloxisobutyric acid derivative

Pregnancy category C

Action: Inhibits biosynthesis of VLDL, decreased triglycerides, increased HDLs

➔ **Therapeutic Outcome:** Decreased hepatic triglyceride production, VLDL; accelerates removal of cholesterol from liver

Uses: Type III, IV, V hyperlipidemia as adjunct with diet therapy

Dosage and routes

Adult: PO 1200 mg in divided doses bid 30 min ac

Available forms: Caps 300 mg; tabs 600 mg

Adverse effects

CNS: Dizziness, blurred vision
GI: Nausea, vomiting, dyspepsia, diarrhea, abdominal pain
HEMA: Leukopenia, anemia, eosinophilia
INTEG: Rash, urticaria, pruritus
MISC: Task perversion

Contraindications: Severe hepatic disease, preexisting gallbladder disease, severe renal disease, primary biliary cirrhosis, hypersensitivity

Precautions: Monitor hematologic and hepatic function, pregnancy **C,** lactation

Pharmacokinetics

Absorption	Well absorbed
Distribution	Unknown, plasma protein binding >90%
Metabolism	Liver—minimal
Excretion	Kidney—unchanged (70%), feces (6%)
Half-life	1½ hr

Pharmacodynamics

Onset	1-2 hr
Peak	1-2 hr
Duration	2-4 months

Interactions
Drug classifications

Anticoagulants, oral: ↑ effect of anticoagulants
Lovastatin: ↑ rhabdomyolysis
Simivastatin: ↑ rhabdomyolysis

Lab test interferences

↑ Liver function studies, ↑ CPK, ↑ BSP, ↑ thymol turbidity, ↑ glucose
↓ Hgb, ↓ Hct, ↓ WBC

NURSING CONSIDERATIONS
Assessment
- Assess nutrition: fat, protein, carbohydrates—nutritional analysis should be performed by dietician before treatment is initiated
- Monitor bowel pattern daily; diarrhea may be a problem
- Monitor triglycerides, cholesterol baseline and throughout treatment; LDL and VLDL should be watched closely and if increased, drug should be discontinued

Nursing diagnoses
- ✓ Diarrhea (adverse reactions)
- ✓ Knowledge deficit (teaching)
- ✓ Noncompliance (teaching)

Implementation
- Give 30 min before AM and PM meals
- ⊘ Do not crush, chew caps

Patient/family education
- Inform patient that compliance is needed for positive results to occur; not to double doses
- Caution patient to decrease risk factors: high-fat diet, smoking, alcohol consumption, lack of exercise
- Advise patient to notify health care prescriber if the GI symptoms of diarrhea, abdominal or epigastric pain, nausea, vomiting occur; or if chills, fever, sore throat, occur

Evaluation
Positive therapeutic outcome
- Decreased cholesterol levels, serum triglyceride and improved ratio with high-density lipoproteins (HDLs)

gentamicin (℞)
(jen-ta-mye'sin)
Alcomicin ✦, Apogen, Cidomycin ✦, Garamycin, Garamycin Intrathecal, Garamycin IV Piggyback, Garamycin Pediatric, Gentamicin Sulfate, gentamicin sulfate IV Piggyback, Jenamicin, Pediatric Gentamicin Sulfate

Func. class.: Antibiotic
Chem. class.: Aminoglycoside

Pregnancy category C

Action: Interferes with protein synthesis in bacterial cell by binding to ribosomal subunit, causing misreading of genetic code; inaccurate peptide sequence forms in protein chain, causing bacterial death

➔ **Therapeutic Outcome:** Bactericidal effects for the following organisms *P. aeruginosa, Proteus, Klebsiella, Serratia, E. coli, Enterobacter, Citrobacter, Staphylococcus, Shigella, Salmonella, Acinetobacter*

Uses: Severe systemic infections of CNS; respiratory, GI, and urinary tracts; bone; skin; soft tissues caused by susceptible strains

Dosage and routes

Severe systemic infections

Adult: **IV** inf 3-5 mg/kg/day in 3 divided doses q8h; dilute in 50-200 ml NS or D_5W given over 30 min-2 hr; IM 3 mg/kg/day in divided doses q8h

Adult: Intrathec 4-8 mg qd

P ***Child:*** **IV**/IM 2-2.5 mg/ kg q8h

P ***Neonates and infants:*** **IV**/IM 2.5 mg/kg q8h

P ***Neonates <1 wk:*** 2.5 mg/kg q12h

P ***Infants and child >3 mo:*** Intrathec 1-2 mg qd

Dental/respiratory procedures/GI/GU surgery (prophylaxis endocarditis)

Adult: IM 1.5 mg/kg ½-1 hr before procedure with ampicillin

Top

P ***Adult, child:*** Apply to cleansed area 3-4 times daily

Ophth

P ***Adult, child:*** 1-2 drops of ophth sol q2-4h or ophth oint 2-3 times daily

P ***Child:*** IM 2.5 mg/kg ½-1 hr before procedure with ampicillin

Available forms: Inj 10, 40, 60, 80, 100 mg; intrathec 2 mg/ml; ophth sol 0.3%, ophth oint 0.3%, top oint 0.1%, top cream 0.1%

Adverse effects

CNS: Confusion, depression, numbness, tremors, ***convulsions,*** muscle twitching, ***neurotoxicity,*** dizziness, vertigo
CV: Hypotension, hypertension, palpitations
EENT: ***Ototoxicity, deafness,*** visual disturbances, tinnitus
GI: *Nausea, vomiting, anorexia,* increased ALT (SGPT), AST (SGOT), bilirubin, hepatomegaly, ***hepatic necrosis,*** splenomegaly
GU: ***Oliguria, hematuria, renal damage, azotemia, renal failure, nephrotoxicity***
HEMA: ***Agranulocytosis, thrombocytopenia, leukopenia, eosinophilia,*** anemia
INTEG: *Rash,* burning, urticaria, dermatitis, alopecia

Contraindications: Severe renal disease, hypersensitivity

P **Precautions:** Neonates, mild renal disease, pregnancy **C**, hearing deficits, myasthenia G gravis, lactation, elderly, Parkinson's disease

Pharmacokinetics

Absorption	Well absorbed (IM)
Distribution	Distributed in extracellular fluids, poorly distributed in CSF; crosses placenta
Metabolism	Liver, minimal
Excretion	Mostly unchanged (79%) kidneys
Half-life	1-3 hr, increased in renal disease

Pharmacodynamics

	IM	IV
Onset	Rapid	Rapid
Peak	½-1½ hr	Infusion's end

Interactions

Individual drugs

Amphotericin B: ↑ ototoxicity, neurotoxicity, nephrotoxicity
Cisplatin: ↑ ototoxicity, neurotoxicity, nephrotoxicity
Ethacrynic acid: ↑ ototoxicity, neurotoxicity, nephrotoxicity
Furosemide: ↑ ototoxicity, neurotoxicity, nephrotoxicity
Mannitol: ↑ ototoxicity, neurotoxicity, nephrotoxicity
Methoxyflurane: ↑ ototoxicity, neurotoxicity, nephrotoxicity
Polymyxin: ↑ ototoxicity, neurotoxicity, nephrotoxicity
Succinylcholine: ↑ neuromuscular blockade, respiratory depression
Vancomycin: ↑ ototoxicity, neurotoxicity, nephrotoxicity

Drug classifications

Anesthetics: ↑ neuromuscular blockade, respiratory depression
Aminoglycosides: ↑ otoxicity, neurotoxicity
Nondepolarizing neuromuscular blockers: ↑ neuromuscular blockade, respiratory depression

NURSING CONSIDERATIONS

Assessment

- Assess patient for previous sensitivity reaction
- Assess patient for signs and symptoms of infection including characteristics of wounds, sputum, urine, stool, WBC >10,000, fever; obtain baseline information and during treatment
- Complete culture and sensitivity before beginning drug therapy; this will ensure that correct treatment has been initiated
- Assess for allergic reactions: rash, urticaria, pruritus, chills, fever, joint pain may occur a few days after therapy begins
- Identify urine output; if decreasing, notify prescriber (may indicate nephrotoxicity); also, increased BUN, creatinine, urine CrCl <80 ml/min
- Monitor blood studies: AST (SGOT), ALT (SGPT), CBC, Hct, bilirubin, LDH, alk phosphatase, Coombs' test monthly if patient is on long-term therapy
- Monitor electrolytes: potassium, sodium, chloride, magnesium monthly if patient is on long-term therapy
- Monitor for bleeding: ecchymosis, bleeding gums, hematuria; assess stool guaiac daily if on long-term therapy
- Assess for overgrowth of infection: perineal itching, fever, malaise, redness, pain, swelling, drainage, rash, diarrhea, change in cough, sputum
- Obtain weight before treatment; calculation of dosage is usually based on ideal body weight, but may be calculated on actual body weight
- Monitor I&O ratio; urinalysis daily for proteinuria, cells, casts; report sudden change in urine output
- Monitor VS during inf, watch for hypotension, change in pulse
- Assess **IV** site for thrombophlebitis including pain, redness, swelling q30 min, change site if needed; apply warm compresses to discontinued site
- Obtain serum peak, drawn at 30-60 min after **IV** inf or 60 min after IM inj, trough level drawn just before next dose; blood level should be 2-4 times bacteriostatic level

G

• Assess urine pH if drug is used for UTI; urine should be kept alkaline
• Assess for deafness by audiometric testing, ringing, roaring in ears, vertigo; assess hearing before, during, after treatment
• Assess for dehydration: high sp gr, decrease in skin turgor, dry mucous membranes, dark urine

Nursing diagnoses

✓ Infection, risk for (uses)
✓ Diarrhea (side effects)
✓ Knowledge deficit (teaching)
✓ Noncompliance (teaching)
✓ Injury, risk for (side effects)

Implementation

IM route
• Give deeply in large muscle mass; rotate sites

Top route
• Wash hands, wear gloves, clean skin before applying

IV **IV route**
• Give in even doses around the clock; drug must be given for 10-14 days to ensure organism death and prevent superimposed infection
• Give by INT inf over ½-1 hr, flush with 0.9% NaCl or D_5W after inf
• Separate aminoglycosides and penicillins by ≥ 1 hr
• Store in tight container

Y-site incompatibilities: Idarubicin, indomethacin, zidovudine

Y-site compatibilities: Acyclovir, amifostine, atracurium, aztreonam, cyclophosphamide, enalaprilat, esmolol, famotidine, fluconazole, fludarabine, foscarnet, granisetron, hydromorphone, IL-2, insulin, labetalol, lorazepam, magnesium sulfate, meperidine, midazolam, morphine, multivitamins, ondansetron, paclitaxel, pancuronium, thiotepa, vecuronium, vitamin B with C, zidovudine

Additive compatibilities: Atracurium, aztreonam, bleomycin, cefoxitin, cimetidine, ciprofloxacin, methicillin, metronidazole, ofloxacin, penicillin G sodium, ranitidine, verapamil

Patient/family education
• Teach patient to report sore throat, bruising, bleeding, joint pain—may indicate blood dyscrasias (rare)
• Advise patient to contact prescriber if vaginal itching, loose, foul-smelling stools, furry tongue occur—may indicate superimposed infection

Evaluation

Positive therapeutic outcome
• Absence of signs/symptoms of infection (WBC <10,000, temp WNL, absence of red, draining wounds)
• Reported improvement in symptoms of infection

Treatment of overdose: Withdraw drug, hemodialysis

glatiramer (℞)
(glah-teer′a-meer)
Copaxone
Func. class.: Multiple sclerosis agent
Pregnancy category B

Action: Unknown, may modify the immune responses responsible for multiple sclerosis

➔ **Therapeutic outcome:** Decreased symptoms of multiple sclerosis

Uses: Reduction of the frequency of relapses in patients with relapsing-remitting multiple sclerosis

Dosage and routes
Adult: SC 20 mg/day

Available forms: Inj 20 mg/ml

Adverse effects
CNS: Anxiety, hypertonia, tremor, vertigo, speech disorder, agitation, confusion
CV: Migraine, palpitations, syncope, tachycardia, vasodilation
EENT: Eye pain
GI: Nausea, vomiting, diarrhea, anorexia, gastroenteritis
GU: Urgency, dysmenorrhea, vaginal moniliasis
HEMA: Ecchymosis, lymphadenopathy
INTEG: Pruritus, rash, sweating, urticaria, erythema
META: Edema, weight gain
MS: Arthralgia
RESP: Bronchitis, dyspnea

Contraindications: Hypersensitivity to this drug or mannitol

Precautions: Immune disorders, renal disease, pregnancy **B**, lactation

Pharmacokinetics	
Absorption	Unknown
Distribution	Unknown
Metabolism	Unknown
Excretion	Unknown
Half-life	Unknown

Pharmacodynamics

Unknown

NURSING CONSIDERATIONS
Assessment
- Monitor blood, renal, hepatic studies; prior to treatment
- Assess for CNS symptoms: anxiety, confusion, vertigo
- Assess GI status: diarrhea, vomiting, abdominal pain, gastroenteritis
- Assess cardiac status: tachycardia, palpitations, vasodilation

Nursing diagnoses
✓ Knowledge deficit (teaching)
✓ Noncompliance (teaching)

Implementation
- Use a sterile syringe/needle to transfer the supplied diluent into the vial, rotate vial gently, do not shake; withdraw medication using a syringe with 27G needle; administer SC into hip, thigh, arm; discard unused portion
- Use SC route only; do not give IM or **IV**
- Do not use sol that contains precipitate or is discolored

Patient/family education
- Give written, detailed instructions about the drug; provide initial and return demonstrations on inj procedure; give information on use and disposal of drug
- Advise that blurred vision, sweating may occur
- Advise that irregular menses, dysmenorrhea, or metorrhagia as well as breast pain may occur; use contraception during treatment
- Advise that if pregnancy is suspected or if nursing notify prescriber
- Advise not to change dosing or to stop taking drug without advice of prescriber

Evaluation
Positive therapeutic outcome
- Decreased symptoms of multiple sclerosis

G

glipizide (℞)
(glip-i′zide)
Glucotrol
Func. class.: Antidiabetic
Chem. class.: Sulfonylurea (2nd generation)
Pregnancy category C

Action: Causes functioning β-cells in pancreas to release insulin, leading to drop in blood glucose levels; may improve insulin binding to insulin receptors or increase the number of insulin receptors with prolonged administration; may also reduce basal hepatic glucose secretion; not effective if patient lacks functioning β-cells

➡ **Therapeutic Outcome:** Decrease in polyuria, polydipsia, polyphagia, clear sensorium, absence of dizziness, stable gait

Uses: Stable adult-onset diabetes mellitus (type II) NIDDM

Dosage and routes
Adult: PO 5 mg initially, then increase to desired response; max 40 mg/day in divided doses or 15 mg/dose

G ***Elderly hepatic disease:*** PO 2.5 mg initially, then increase to desired response; max 40 mg/day in divided doses or 15 mg/dose

Available forms: Tabs 5, 10 mg scored

Adverse effects
CNS: Headache, weakness, dizziness, drowsiness, tinnitus, fatigue, vertigo
ENDO: ***Hypoglycemia***
GI: ***Hepatotoxicity, cholestatic jaundice,*** nausea, vomiting, diarrhea, heartburn
HEMA: ***Leukopenia, thrombocytopenia, agranulocytosis, aplastic anemia,*** increased AST, ALT, alk phosphatase, ***pancytopenia, hemolytic anemia***
INTEG: Rash, allergic reactions, pruritus, urticaria, eczema, photosensitivity, erythema

Contraindications: Hypersensitivity to sulfonylureas, juvenile or brittle diabetes

Precautions: Pregnancy **C**, G elderly, cardiac disease, severe renal disease, severe hepatic disease, thyroid disease

Pharmacokinetics	
Absorption	Completely absorbed GI tract
Distribution	Unknown
Metabolism	Liver
Excretion	Via kidneys
Half-life	2-4 hr

Pharmacodynamics	
Onset	1-1½ hr
Peak	1-3 hr
Duration	10-24 hr

Interactions
Individual drugs
Diazoxide: Both drugs may have action decreased
Alcohol: Disulfiram-like reaction
Cimetidine: ↑ hypoglycemia
Chloramphenicol: ↑ hypoglycemia
Guanethidine: ↑ hypoglycemia
Methyldopa: ↑ hypoglycemia
Probenecid: ↑ hypoglycemia
Phenytoin: ↓ action of glipizide
Digoxin: ↓ action of glipizide
Isoniazid: ↓ action of glipizide
Insulin: ↑ hypoglycemia
Phenobarbital: ↓ action of glipizide
Rifampin: ↓ action of glipizide

Drug classifications
Anticoagulants: ↑ hypoglycemia
Antiinflammatories, nonsteroidal: ↑ hypoglycemia
Calcium channel blockers: ↓ action of glipizide
Corticosteroids: ↓ action of glipizide
Contraceptives, oral: ↓ action of glipizide
Diuretics, thiazide: ↓ action of glipizide
Estrogens: ↓ action of glipizide
Thyroid preparations: ↓ action of glipizide
Phenothiazine: ↓ action of glipizide
Sympathomimetics: ↓ action of glipizide
Salicylates: ↑ hypoglycemia
MAOIs: ↑ hypoglycemia

NURSING CONSIDERATIONS

Assessment

- Assess for hypoglycemic/hyperglycemic reactions that can occur soon pc; hypoglycemic reactions (sweating, weakness, dizziness, anxiety, tremors, hunger); hyperglycemic reactions
- Monitor CBC (baseline, q3mo) during treatment; check liver function tests periodically AST (SGOT), LDH, and renal studies: BUN, creatinine during treatment

Nursing diagnoses

- ✓ Nutrition, altered: more than body requirements (uses)
- ✓ Nutrition altered: less than body requirements (adverse reactions)
- ✓ Injury, risk for (adverse reactions)
- ✓ Knowledge deficit (teaching)
- ✓ Noncompliance (teaching)

Implementation

- Convert from other oral hypoglycemic agents or insulin dosage of <40 U/day; change may be made without gradual dosage change.
- Convert patients taking >40 U/day of insulin gradually by receiving oral hypoglycemic and 50% of previous insulin dosage for 3-5 days
- Monitor serum or urine glucose and ketones 3 times/day during conversion
- Give drug 30 min before breakfast—if large dose is required, may be divided into two; give with meals to decrease GI upset and provide best absorption
- Give tab crushed and mixed with meal or fluids for patients with difficulty swallowing
- Store in tight container in cool environment

Patient/family education

- Teach patient to check for symptoms of cholestatic jaundice: dark urine, pruritus, yellow sclera; if these occur, prescriber should be notified
- Teach patient to use capillary blood glucose test or Chemstrip 3 ×/day
- Teach patient symptoms of hypo/hyperglycemia, what to do about each
- Instruct patient that drug must be continued on daily basis; explain consequence of discontinuing drug abruptly
- Teach patient to take drug in AM to prevent hypoglycemic reactions at night
- Caution patient to avoid OTC medications unless prescribed by a prescriber
- Teach patient that diabetes is lifelong illness; that this drug is not a cure

• Instruct patient that all food included in diet plan must be eaten to prevent hypoglycemia
• Advise patient to carry Medic-Alert ID and a glucagon emergency kit for emergency purposes

Evaluation

Positive therapeutic outcome
• Decrease in polyuria, polydipsia, polyphagia, clear sensorium, absence of dizziness, stable gait

glyburide (℞)

(glye′byoor-ide)

DiaBeta ✱, Glynase Prestab, Micronase

Func. class.: Antidiabetic
Chem. class.: Sulfonylurea (2nd generation)

Pregnancy category B

Action: Causes functioning β-cells in pancreas to release insulin, leading to drop in blood glucose levels; may improve insulin binding to insulin receptors and increase number of insulin receptors with prolonged administration; may also reduce basal hepatic glucose secretion; not effective if patient lacks functioning β-cells

➔ **Therapeutic Outcome:** Decrease in polyuria, polydipsia, polyphagia, clear sensorium, absence of dizziness, stable gait

Uses: Stable adult-onset diabetes mellitus (type II) NIDDM

Dosage and routes

Adult: PO 2.5-5 mg initially, then increased to desired response

G ***Elderly:*** PO 1.25 mg initially, then increased to desired response; max 20 mg/day, maintenance 1.25-20 mg/qd

Available forms: Tabs 1.25, 2.5, 5 mg

Adverse effects

CNS: Headache, weakness, paresthesia, tinnitus, fatigue, vertigo
ENDO: Hypoglycemia
GI: Nausea, fullness, heartburn, ***hepatoxicity, cholestatic jaundice,*** vomiting, diarrhea
HEMA: Leukopenia, thrombocytopenia, agranulocytosis, aplastic anemia, increased AST, ALT, alk phosphatase
INTEG: Rash, allergic reactions, pruritus, urticaria, eczema, photosensitivity, erythema
MS: Joint pains

Contraindications: Hypersensitivity to sulfonylureas, juvenile or brittle diabetes

Precautions: Pregnancy **B,** G elderly, cardiac disease, severe renal disease, severe hepatic disease, thyroid disease, severe hypoglycemic reactions

Pharmacokinetics	
Absorption	Completely absorbed GI tract
Distribution	90-95% plasma protein binding
Metabolism	Liver
Excretion	Urine, feces (metabolites), crosses placenta
Half-life	10 hr

Pharmacodynamics	
Onset	2-4 hr
Peak	2-8 hr
Duration	24 hr

Interactions

Individual drugs

Diazoxide: Both drugs may have action decreased

Alcohol: Disulfiram-like reaction
Cimetidine: ↑ hypoglycemia
Chloramphenicol:↑ hypoglycemia
Guanethidine: ↑ hypoglycemia
Methyldopa: ↑ hypoglycemia
Probenecid: ↑ hypoglycemia
Phenytoin: ↓ action of glyburide
Digoxin: ↓ digoxin level
Isoniazid: ↓ action of glyburide
Insulin: ↑ hypoglycemia
Phenobarbital: ↓ action of glyburide
Rifampin: ↓ action of glyburide

Drug classifications

Anticoagulants: ↑ hypoglycemia
Antiinflammatories, nonsteroidal: ↑ hypoglycemia
Calcium channel blockers: ↓ action of glyburide
Corticosteroids: ↓ action of glyburide
Contraceptives, oral: ↓ action of glyburide
Diuretics, thiazide: ↓ action of glyburide
Estrogens: ↓ action of glyburide
Thyroid preparations: ↓ action of glyburide
Phenothiazines: ↓ action of glyburide
Sympathomimetics: ↓ action of glyburide
Salicylates: ↑ hypoglycemia
MAOIs: ↑ hypoglycemia

NURSING CONSIDERATIONS

Assessment

- Assess for hypoglycemic/hyperglycemic reactions that can occur soon pc; hypoglycemic reactions (sweating, weakness, dizziness, anxiety, tremors, hunger); hyperglycemic reactions
- Monitor CBC (baseline, q3mo) during treatment; check liver function tests periodically AST (SGOT), LDH and renal studies: BUN, creatinine during treatment

Nursing diagnoses

- ✓ Nutrition, altered: more than body requirements (uses)
- ✓ Nutrition altered: less than body requirements (adverse reactions)
- ✓ Injury, risk for (adverse reactions)
- ✓ Knowledge deficit (teaching)
- ✓ Noncompliance (teaching)

Implementation

- Conversion from other oral hypoglycemic agents or insulin dosage of <40 U/day; change may be made without gradual dosage change
- Patients taking >40 U/day of insulin convert gradually by receiving oral hypoglycemic and 50% of previous insulin dosage for 3-5 days
- Monitor serum or urine glucose and ketones 3 times/day during conversion
- Give drug 30 min before breakfast—if large dose is required, may be divided into two; give with meals to decrease GI upset and provide best absorption
- Give tab crushed and mixed with meal or fluids for patients with difficulty swallowing
- Store in tight container in cool environment

Patient/family education

- Teach patient to check for symptoms of cholestatic jaundice: dark urine, pruritus, yellow sclera; if these occur, prescriber should be notified
- Teach patient to use capillary

G

blood glucose test or Chemstrip 3 ×/day
• Teach patient symptoms of hypo/hyperglycemia, what to do about each
• Instruct patient that drug must be continued on daily basis; explain consequence of discontinuing drug abruptly
• Teach patient to take drug in AM to prevent hypoglycemic reactions at night
• Caution patient to avoid OTC medications unless prescribed by a prescriber
• Teach patient that diabetes is lifelong illness; that this drug is not a cure
• Instruct patient that all food included in diet plan must be eaten to prevent hypoglycemia
• Advise patient to carry Medic Alert ID and a glucagon emergency kit for emergency purposes

Evaluation

Positive therapeutic outcome
• Decrease in polyuria, polydipsia, polyphagia, clear sensorium, absence of dizziness, stable gait

glycerin (OTC)

(gli'ser-in)

Fleet Babylax, glycerin USP, Glycerol, Ophthalgan, Osmoglyn, Sani-Supp

Func. class.: Laxative, hyperosmotic, antiglaucoma agent

Chem. class.: Trihydric alcohol

Pregnancy category C

Action: Increases osmotic pressure by drawing fluid into colon lumen from extravascular spaces to intravascular

➔ **Therapeutic Outcome:** Absence of constipation, intraocular pressure, intracranial pressure, absence of edema in the cornea

Uses: Constipation, intraocular pressure in glaucoma; intracranial pressure, edema in the superficial layers of the cornea

Dosage and routes

P ***Adult and child >6 yr:*** Rec supp 3 g; enema 5-15 ml

P ***Child <6 yr:*** Rec supp 1-1.5 g; enema 2-5 ml

Corneal edema

Adult: Ophth 1-2 gtt q3-4 h

Intraocular pressure reduction

Adult: PO 1-1.5 g/kg once, then 500 mg/kg q6h

P ***Child:*** PO 1-1.5 g/kg qd once, then 500 mg/kg 4-8 hr after first dose

Available forms: Rec sol 4 ml/applicator; supp; oral sol 0.6/ml; ophth sol 7.5 ml/container

Adverse effects

CNS: Headache, confusion, ***convulsions***

GI: Nausea, vomiting, diarrhea

META: Dehydration

Contraindications: Hypersensitivity

Precautions: Pregnancy **C**

Pharmacokinetics	
Absorption	Well absorbed (PO), not absorbed (rectal)
Distribution	To intravascular space
Metabolism	Liver—80%, kidneys—20%
Excretion	Kidneys
Half-life	30 min

Pharmacodynamics

	PO	REC	OPHTH
Onset	10-30 min	Unknown	Unknown
Peak	30-120 min	30 min	Unknown
Duration	6-8 hr	Unknown	Up to 4 hr

Interactions
Drug classifications

Diuretics: ↓ effect of glycerin (ophth)

NURSING CONSIDERATIONS
Assessment
- Assess patient for cause of constipation; identify whether fluids, bulk, or exercise is missing from lifestyle; check for distention, bowel sounds
- After administration, check for cramping, rec bleeding, nausea, vomiting; if these symptoms occur, drug should be discontinued
- Identify stool characteristics: consistency, color, amount, shape, volume

Nursing diagnoses
✓ Constipation (uses)
✓ Knowledge deficit (teaching)

Implementation
Rec route
- Insert glycerin supp after removing wrapper; may cause evacuation in ½ hr
- For evening use 4-ml applications of fluid, have patient in side-lying position, have patient retain for a few min

Ophth route
- Instill 1-2 gtt in one or both eyes by pulling down on conjunctival sac
- Do not use ophth sol that is discolored, has a precipitate, or is cloudy

PO route
- Pour over cracked ice and sip through a straw
- To prevent severe cerebral dehydration headache have patient recumbent during and after administration
- Give by mixing 50% glycerin sol with 0.9% NaCl with flavoring, or use oral sol that is already flavored—flavoring improves taste and prevents GI symptoms
- Storage in cool environment; do not freeze

Patient/family education
- Caution patient not to use laxatives for long-term therapy; normal bowel tone will be lost; that normal bowel movements do not always occur daily
- Advise patient not to use in presence of abdominal pain, nausea, vomiting
- Instruct patient to notify prescriber if constipation is unrelieved or if weakness, dizziness, excessive thirst occur

Evaluation
Positive therapeutic outcome
- Decreased constipation
- Decreased intraocular pressure

glycopyrrolate (℞)
(glye-koe-pye′roe-late)

glycopyrrolate, Robinul, Robinul Forte

Func. class.: Cholinergic blocker

Chem. class.: Quaternary ammonium compound

Pregnancy category C

Action: Inhibits action of acetylcholine at receptor sites in autonomic nervous system, which controls secretions, free acids in stomach

Therapeutic Outcome: Decreased secretions in the respiratory tract, GI system

Uses: Decreased secretions before surgery, reversal of neuromuscular blockade, peptic ulcer disease, irritable bowel syndrome

Dosage and routes

Preoperatively

Adult: IM 0.002 mg/lb ½-1 hr before surgery

P ***Child 2-12 yr:*** IM 0.002-0.004 mg/lb

P ***Child <2 yr:*** IM 0.004 mg/lb

Reversal of neuromuscular blockage

Adult: **IV** 0.2 mg for each mg of neostigmine or 5 mg **IV** of pyridostigmine simultaneously

GI disorders

Adult: PO 1-2 mg bid-tid; IM/**IV** 0.1-0.2 mg tid-qid, titrated to patient response

Available forms: Tabs 1, 2 mg; inj 0.2 mg/ml

Adverse effects

CNS: Confusion, anxiety, restlessness, irritability, delusions, hallucinations, headache, sedation, depression, incoherence, dizziness, lethargy, flushing, weakness

CV: Palpitations, tachycardia, postural hypotension, paradoxical bradycardia

EENT: Blurred vision, photophobia, dilated pupils, difficulty swallowing, increased intraocular pressure, mydriasis, cycloplegia

GI: Dryness of mouth, constipation, nausea, vomiting, abdominal distress, paralytic ileus, altered taste perception

GU: Hesitancy, retention, impotence

INTEG: Urticaria, allergic reactions

MISC: Suppression of lactation, nasal congestion, decreased sweating

Contraindications: Hypersensitivity, narrow-angle glaucoma, myasthenia gravis, P GI/GU obstruction, child <3 yr, tachycardia, myocardial ischemia, hepatic disease, ulcerative colitis, toxic megacolon

Precautions: Pregnancy **C,** G elderly, lactation, prostatic hypertrophy, renal disease, CHF, pulmonary disease, hyperthyroidism

Pharmacokinetics

Absorption	Well absorbed (PO, SC, IM)
Distribution	Unknown
Metabolism	Not metabolized
Excretion	Unchanged feces
Half-life	2 hr

Pharmacodynamics

	PO	IM	IV
Onset	Unknown	15-30 min	Immediate
Peak	1 hr	30-45 min	10-15 min
Duration	8-12 hr	2-7 hr	2-7 hr

Interactions

Individual drugs

Amantadine: ↑ anticholinergic effect

Disopyramide: ↑ anticholinergic effect

Potassium chloride, oral: ↑ GI lesions

Quinidine: ↑ anticholinergic effect

Drug classifications

Antacids: ↓ absorption of glycopyrrolate

Antidiarrheals: ↓ absorption of glycopyrrolate

Anticholinergics: ↑ anticholinergic effect
Antidepressants, tricyclic: ↑ anticholinergic effect
Antihistamines: ↑ anticholinergic effect

NURSING CONSIDERATIONS

Assessment

- Monitor I&O ratio; retention commonly causes decreased urinary output; check for urinary hesitation; palpate bladder if retention occurs
- Monitor ECG for ectopic ventricular beats, PVC, tachycardia
- Monitor for bowel sounds; check for constipation; increase fluids, bulk, exercise if constipation occurs
- Assess for tolerance over long-term therapy; dose may have to be increased or changed
- Assess mental status: affect, mood, CNS depression, worsening of psychiatric symptoms during early therapy

Nursing diagnoses

✓ Knowledge deficit (teaching)

Implementation

IV **IV route**

- Administer **IV** undiluted, give at a rate of 0.2 mg or less over 1-2 min through Y-tube or 3-way stopcock; do not add to **IV** sol
- Administer parenteral dose with patient recumbent to prevent postural hypotension

Syringe compatibilities: Atropine, benzquinamide, butorphanol, chlorpromazine, cimetidine, codeine, dimenhydrinate, diphenhydramine, droperidol, fentanyl, glycopyrrolate, heparin, hydromorphone, hydroxyzine, levorphanol, lidocaine, meperidine, midazolam, morphine, nalbuphine, pentazocine, prochlorperazine, promazine, promethazine, ranitidine, scopolamine

PO route

- Give PO with or after meals to prevent GI upset; may give with fluids other than water

IM route

- Give IM deeply in large muscle mass

Patient/family education

- Caution patient not to operate machinery or engage in hazardous activities if drowsiness occurs
- Advise patient not to take OTC products, cough, cold preparations with alcohol, antihistamines without approval of prescriber
- Caution patient not to discontinue this drug abruptly—tapering should be done over 1 wk

Evaluation

Positive therapeutic outcome

- Decreased secretions, bronchial, GI

gonadorelin HCl (℞)

(goe-nad-oh-rell'in hye-droe-klor'ide)

Factrel

Func. class.: Gonadotropin hormone

Chem. class.: Synthetic luteinizing–hormone-releasing hormone

Pregnancy category B

Action: Combination luteinizing–hormone-releasing hormone that acts on anterior pituitary

Therapeutic Outcome: Elevated luteinizing hormone (LH) levels released by the anterior pituitary

Uses: Evaluation of response of gonadotropic hormone

Dosage and routes

Women: SC/**IV** 100 μg usually given between day 1-7 of menstrual cycle

Available forms: Powder for inj 100, 500 μg/vial

Adverse effects

CNS: Dizziness, headache, flushing

GI: Nausea

INTEG: Inflammation at injection site

SYST: Anaphylaxis, antibody formation (large doses, extended time period)

Contraindications: Hypersensitivity

Precautions: Pregnancy **B**

Pharmacokinetics

Absorption	Completely absorbed (**IV**)
Distribution	Unknown
Metabolism	Liver—inactive compound
Excretion	Kidneys
Half-life	Up to 40 min

Pharmacodynamics

	FEMALES (SC/IV)	MALES (SC)	MALES (IV)
Onset	5 min	5 min	5 min
Peak	½ hr	1 hr	15 min
Duration	2-4 hr	2-4 hr	2-4 hr

Interactions

Individual drugs

Digoxin: ↓ level of gonadorelin

Levodopa: ↑ level of gonadorelin

Spironolactone: ↑ level of gonadorelin

Drug classifications

Dopamine antagonists: ↓ level of gonadorelin

Oral contraceptives: ↓ level of gonadorelin

Phenothiazines: ↓ level of gonadorelin

Lab test interferences

False test results: Androgus, glucocorticoids, estrogens, progestins

NURSING CONSIDERATIONS

Assessment

- Assess test results: pituitary/hypothalamus dysfunction (decreased LH); postmenopausal (increased LH)
- Assess menstrual cycle in females; test should be done during the first wk of menstrual cycle
- Monitor levels by having lab personnel draw blood samples at intervals; baseline levels are drawn 15 min before and just before administration

Nursing diagnoses

✓ Knowledge deficit (teaching)

Implementation

IV IV route

- Administer rapidly by direct **IV** after diluting 100 μg/1 ml or 500 μg/2 ml of provided diluent
- Repeated doses may be necessary to elevate pituitary gonadotropin reserve
- Discard unused portions

Patient/family education

- Teach patient purpose for medication and expected results
- Advise patient to report rash, hives, difficulty breathing, flushing; these should be reported immediately

Evaluation
Positive therapeutic outcome
- Completed test results for gonadotropin-releasing hormone

goserelin (℞)
(goe'se-rel-lin)
Zoladex
Func. class.: Gonadotropin-releasing hormone, antineoplastic
Chem. class.: Synthetic decapeptide analog of LHRH
Pregnancy category X

Action: Inhibitor of pituitary gonadotropin secretion; initially increases LH and FSH, with increases in testosterone, reduction in sex steroid levels

Therapeutic Outcome: Decrease in tumor size and spread of malignant cells

Uses: Advanced prostate cancer

Dosage and routes
Adult: SC 3.6 mg q28 days (implant)

Available forms: Depot inj 3.6 mg

Adverse effects
CNS: Headaches, ***spinal cord compression***, anxiety, depression
CV: ***Dysrhythmia, cerebrovascular accident***, hypertension, ***MI***, chest pain
ENDO: Gynecomastia, breast tenderness, hot flashes
GI: Nausea, vomiting, constipation, diarrhea, ulcer
GU: Spotting, breakthrough bleeding, decreased libido, renal insufficiency, urinary obstruction, urinary tract infection
INTEG: Rash, pain on inj
MS: Osteoneuralgia

Contraindications: Hypersensitivity, pregnancy **X**

Precautions: Children, lactation

Pharmacokinetics	
Absorption	Well absorbed
Distribution	Unknown
Metabolism	Unknown
Excretion	Unknown
Half-life	4½ hr

Pharmacodynamics	
Onset	Unknown
Peak	14-28 days
Duration	Treatment length

Interactions: None
Lab test interferences
↑ Alk phosphatase, ↑ estradiol, ↑ FSH, ↑ LH, ↑ testosterone levels
↓ Testosterone levels, ↓ progesterone

NURSING CONSIDERATIONS
Assessment
- Assess for relief of bone pain (back pain)
- Monitor I&O ratios, palpate bladder for distention (urinary obstruction) at beginning of treatment—renal insufficiency and obstruction may occur

Nursing diagnoses
- ✓ Sexual dysfunction (uses)
- ✓ Knowledge deficit (teaching)

Implementation
- Administer via implant inserted by qualified persons into upper subcutaneous tissue in abdominal wall q28 days

Patient/family education
- Caution patient that gynecomastia and postmenopausal symptoms may occur but will decrease after treatment is discontinued

• Teach patient to contact prescriber if difficulty urinating occurs during treatment

Evaluation

Positive therapeutic outcome

• More normal levels of prostate-specific antigen, acid phosphatase, alk phosphatase; testosterone level of <25 mg/dl

granisetron (℞)

(grane-iss′e-tron)

Kytril

Func. class.: Antiemetic

Chem. class.: 5-HT_3 receptor antagonist

Pregnancy category C

Action: Prevents nausea, vomiting by blocking serotinin peripherally, centrally, and in the small intestine

➔ **Therapeutic Outcome:** Absence of nausea and vomiting

Uses: Prevention of nausea, vomiting associated with cancer chemotherapy including high-dose cisplatin

Dosage and routes

Adult: **IV** 10 μg/kg over 5 min, 30 min before the start of cancer chemotherapy; PO 1 mg bid, give 1st dose 1 hr before chemotherapy and next dose 12 hr after 1st

Available forms: Inj 1 mg/ml; tab 1 mg

Adverse effects

CNS: Headache

GI: Diarrhea, constipation, increased AST (SGOT), ALT (SGPT)

MISC: Rash, ***bronchospasm***

Contraindications: Hypersensitivity

P G **Precautions:** Pregnancy **C**, lactation, children, elderly

Pharmacokinetics

Absorption	Unknown
Distribution	Unknown
Metabolism	Unknown
Excretion	Unknown
Half-life	Unknown

Pharmacodynamics

Unknown

Interactions: None

NURSING CONSIDERATIONS

Assessment

• Assess patient for absence of nausea, vomiting during chemotherapy

• Assess patient for hypersensitive reaction: rash, bronchospasm

Nursing diagnoses

✓ Fluid deficit (uses)

✓ Knowledge deficit (teaching)

Implementation

• Administer **IV** directly over 5 min

• Store at room temp for 48-hr dilution

Y-site incompatibilities: Fluorouracil, furosemide, sodium bicarbonate

Y-site compatibilities: Carboplatin, ceftazidime, cimetidine, cisplatin, cyclophosphamide, cytarabine, dacarbazine, dexamethasone, diphenhydramine, doxorubicin, etoposide, fluorouracil, furosemide, gentamicin, hydromorphone, ifosfamide, lorazepam, magnesium sulfate mechlorethamine, mesna, methotrexate, methylprednisolone, mezlocillin, morphine, paclitaxel, KCl, streptozocin, thiotepa, vincristine

Patient/family education
• Advise patient to report diarrhea, constipation, rash, or changes in respirations

Evaluation
Positive therapeutic outcome
• Absence of nausea, vomiting during cancer chemotherapy

griseofulvin microsize/ griseofulvin ultramicrosize (℞)

(gris-ee-oh-ful'vin)

Fulvicin P/G, Fulvicin-U/F, Grifulvin V, Grisactin, Grisactin 500, Grisactin-Ultra, Grisoven-FP ✦, Gris-PEG

Func. class.: Antifungal
Chem. class.: Penicillium griseofulvum derivative

Pregnancy category C

Action: Arrests fungal cell division at metaphase (mitosis); binds to human keratin, making it resistant to disease

➔ **Therapeutic Outcome:** Absence of fungicidal infection

Uses: Mycotic infections: *Tinea corporis, Tinea pedis, Tinea cruris, Tinea barbae, Tinea capitis, Tinea unguium* if caused by *Epidermophyton, Microsporum, Trichophyton*

Dosage and routes
Adult: PO 500-1000 mg qd in single or divided doses (microsize), 125-165 mg bid (ultramicrosize) or 250-330 mg qd; may need 500-660 mg in divided doses for severe infections

P ***Child:*** PO 10 mg/kg/day or 30 mg/m^2/day (microsize) or 5 mg/kg/day (ultramicrosize)

Available forms: Microcaps 125, 250 mg; tabs 250, 500 mg; oral susp 125 mg/5 ml; ultratabs 125, 165, 250, 330 mg

Adverse effects
CNS: Headache, peripheral neuritis, paresthesias, confusion, dizziness, fatigue
EENT: Transient hearing loss
GU: Proteinuria, cylinduria, precipitate porphyria, increased thirst
GI: Nausea, vomiting, anorexia, diarrhea, cramps, dry mouth, flatulence
HEMA: ***Leukopenia, granulocytopenia, neutropenia, monocytosis***
INTEG: Rash, urticaria, photosensitivity, lichen planus

Contraindications: Hypersensitivity, porphyria, hepatic disease, lupus erythematosus

Precautions: Penicillin sensitivity, pregnancy **C**

Pharmacokinetics

Absorption	Ultra products (completely absorbed), others (variably absorbed)
Distribution	Keratin in skin; liver, muscle, fat
Metabolism	Liver
Excretion	Feces
Half-life	10-24 hr

Pharmacodynamics

Onset	4 hr
Peak	1 day
Duration	2 day

Interactions
Individual drugs
Alcohol: ↑ CNS depression, tachycardia

G

Phenobarbital: ↓ action of griseofulvin

Drug classifications

Anticoagulants, oral: ↓ action of anticoagulant

Contraceptives, oral: ↓ effect of contraceptive

Food

Fat (meat, dairy products): ↑ absorption

NURSING CONSIDERATIONS

Assessment

- Assess patient's skin for fungal infections: peeling, dryness, itching before and throughout treatment
- Monitor blood studies: leukocytes, CBC, platelets, although blood dyscrasias are rare
- ❗ Monitor for renal toxicity: increased BUN, serum creatinine—if serum creatinine >1.7 mg/100 dl, dosage may be reduced (rare)
- Monitor for hepatotoxicity: increasing AST (SGOT), ALT (SGPT), alk phosphatase
- Monitor for allergic reaction: dermatitis, rash; drug should be discontinued, give antihistamines for mild reaction or epinephrine for severe reaction; if patient is allergic to penicillin a cross-sensitivity may exist with this medication

Nursing diagnoses

✓ Skin integrity, impaired (uses)
✓ Infection, risk for (uses)
✓ Knowledge deficit (teaching)

Implementation

- Give with meals (fatty) to prevent GI upset
- Administer drug carefully, making sure there is no confusion with dosage form (microsize vs ultrasize); with meals to decrease GI symptoms; store in tight, light-resistant container at room temp
- Administer drug until three separate cultures are negative for infective organism

Patient/family education

- Teach patient that long-term therapy may be needed to clear infection (2 wk-6 mo depending on organism); compliance is needed even after feeling better
- Instruct patient in proper hygiene: hand-washing technique, nail care, use of concomitant top agents if prescribed to clear infection
- Advise patient to avoid alcohol because nausea, vomiting, hypertension may occur
- Advise patient to use sunscreen or avoid direct sunlight to prevent photosensitivity
- Caution patient to notify prescriber of sore throat, fever, skin rash, which may indicate overgrowth of organisms
- Advise patient to use a nonhormonal form of contraception during treatment and to notify prescriber if pregnancy is anticipated

Evaluation

Positive therapeutic outcome

- Decrease in itching, peeling, dryness

guaifenesin (℞, OTC)
(gwye-fen'e-sin)
Amonidrin, Anti-tuss, Balminil ✤, Breonesin, Fenesin, Gee-Gee, Genatuss, GG-Cen, Glyate, Glycotuss, Glytuss, Guaifenesin, Guiatuss, Halotussin, Humibid, Humibid L.A., Hytuss, Hytuss 2X, Malotuss, Monafed, Mytussin, Naldecon Senior EX, Resyl ✤, Robitussin, Scot-Tussin Expectorant, Sinumist-SR, Uni-Tussin
Func. class.: Expectorant
Pregnancy category C

Action: Acts as an expectorant by stimulating a gastric mucosal reflex to increase the production of lung mucus

➔ **Therapeutic Outcome:** Decreased cough

Uses: Dry, nonproductive cough

Dosage and routes
Adult: PO 100-400 mg q4-6h, or 600-1200 mg q12h (sus-rel) not to exceed 2.4 g/day

P ***Child 6-12 yr:*** PO 100-200 mg q4h or 600 mg q12h (sus-rel); not to exceed 1.2 g/day

P ***Child 2-6 yr:*** PO: 50-100 mg q4h; not to exceed 600 mg/day

Available forms: Tabs 100, 200 mg; tab, sus rel 600 mg; cap 200 mg; syr 100mg/5 ml; liq 200 mg/5 ml; sus-rel cap 300 mg

Adverse effects
CNS: Drowsiness
GI: Nausea, anorexia, vomiting

Contraindications: Hypersensitivity, persistent cough

Precautions: Pregnancy **C**

Pharmacokinetics

Absorption	Well absorbed
Distribution	Unknown
Metabolism	Unknown
Excretion	Unknown
Half-life	Unknown

Pharmacodynamics

	PO	PO SR
Onset	½ hr	Unknown
Peak	Unknown	Unknown
Duration	4-6 hr	12 hr

Interactions: None

NURSING CONSIDERATIONS

Assessment
- Assess cough: type, frequency, character, including characteristics of sputum; lung sounds bilaterally; fluids should be increased to 2 L/day to decrease secretion viscosity (thickness)

Nursing diagnoses
✓ Airway clearance, ineffective (uses)
✓ Knowledge deficit (teaching)

Implementation
- Store at room temp; provide room humidification to assist with liquefying secretions
- Avoid fluids for ½ hr after administration

Patient/family education
- Caution patient to avoid driving, other hazardous activities if drowsiness occurs (rare)
- Advise patient to avoid smoking, smoke-filled rooms, perfumes, dust, environmental pollutants, cleansers
- Instruct patient to notify prescriber if dry, nonproductive cough lasts over 7 days

G

Evaluation

Positive therapeutic outcome
- Absence of dry cough
- Thinner, more productive cough that raises secretions

guanabenz (℞)

(gwan'a-benz)

Wytensin

Func. class.: Antihypertensive

Chem. class.: Central α_2-adrenergic agonist

Pregnancy category C

Action: Stimulates central α_2-adrenergic receptors in the CNS, resulting in decreased sympathetic outflow from brain with decreased peripheral resistance

Therapeutic Outcome: Decreased B/P in hypertension

Uses: Hypertension

Dosage and routes

Adult: PO 4 mg bid, increasing in increments of 4-8 mg/day q1-2 wk, not to exceed 32 mg bid

Available forms: Tabs 4, 8 mg

Adverse effects

CNS: Drowsiness, dizziness, sedation, headache, depression, weakness

CV: ***Severe rebound hypertension,*** chest pain, dysrhythmias, palpitations, hypotension

EENT: Nasal congestion, blurred vision, miosis

GI: Nausea, diarrhea, constipation, dry mouth, anorexia, abnormal taste

GU: Impotence, frequency, gynecomastia

MS: Backache, extremity pain

RESP: Dyspnea

Contraindications: Hypersensitivity to guanabenz

Precautions: Pregnancy **C,** P lactation, children <12 yr, severe coronary insufficiency, recent MI, cerebrovascular disease, severe hepatic or renal failure

Pharmacokinetics

Absorption	70%-80%
Distribution	Widely distributed
Metabolism	Liver, extensively
Excretion	Kidneys
Half-life	6 hr

Pharmacodynamics

Onset	1 hr
Peak	2-4 hr
Duration	12 hr

Interactions

Individual drugs

Alcohol: ↑ hypotension, ↑ sedation

Drug classifications

Analgesics, narcotic: ↑ sedation

Antihypertensives: ↑ hypotension

β-Adrenergic blockers: ↑ bradycardia, CHF

MAOI: ↓ effectiveness of guanabenz

Nitrates: ↑ nitrates

Sedatives/hypnotics: ↑ sedation

NURSING CONSIDERATIONS

Assessment
- Monitor blood studies: neutrophils, decreased platelets
- Monitor renal studies: protein, BUN, creatinine; watch for increased levels that may indicate nephrotic syndrome; polyuria, oliguria, frequency
- Obtain baselines in renal,

liver function tests before therapy begins; potassium levels, although hyperkalemia rarely occurs
• Monitor B/P, pulse if the drug is being used for hypertension; notify prescriber of change
• Watch for allergic reaction: rash, fever, pruritus, urticaria; drug should be discontinued if antihistamines fail to help
• Watch for symptoms of CHF: edema, dyspnea, wet rales, B/P, weight gain

Nursing diagnoses

✓ Cardiac output, decreased (uses)
✓ Injury, risk for (side effects)
✓ Knowledge deficit (teaching)
✓ Noncompliance (teaching)

Implementation

• Give in AM and at bedtime
• Store in air-tight container at room temp

Patient/family education

• Instruct patient not to discontinue drug abruptly—withdrawal symptoms may occur: anxiety, increased B/P, headache, insomnia, increased pulse, tremors, nausea, sweating
• Advise patient not to use OTC cough, cold, or allergy products unless directed by prescriber
• Teach patient to comply with dosage schedule even if feeling better; drug controls symptoms, does not cure
• Caution patient to rise slowly to sitting or standing position to minimize orthostatic hypotension, especially in the G elderly
• Teach patient that excessive perspiration, dehydration, vomiting may occur; diarrhea may lead to fall in blood pressure; consult prescriber if these occur
• Inform patient that drug may cause dizziness, fainting; light-headedness may occur during first few days of therapy; drug may cause dry mouth—use hard candy, saliva product, or frequent rinsing of mouth; that compliance is necessary; not to skip or stop drug unless directed by prescriber; that drug may cause skin rash or impaired perspiration
• Teach patient to avoid hazardous activities because drug may cause drowsiness, dizziness

Evaluation

Positive therapeutic outcome

• Decreased B/P

Treatment of overdose: Vasopressor for hypotension, discontinue drug

guanadrel (℞)

(gwahn'a-drel)
Hylorel
Func. class.: Antihypertensive
Chem. class.: Adrenergic blocker, (peripheral guanethidine derivative)
Pregnancy category B

Action: Inhibits sympathetic vasoconstriction by inhibiting release of norepinephrine; depletes norepinephrine stores in adrenergic nerve endings and the adrenal medulla

➔ **Therapeutic Outcome:** Decreased B/P in hypertension

Uses: Hypertension (moderate to severe) as an adjunct

Dosage and routes
Adult: PO 5 mg bid, adjusted to desired response weekly or monthly; may need 20-75 mg/day in divided doses, higher doses are given tid or qid

Available forms: Tabs 10, 25 mg

Adverse effects
CNS: Drowsiness, fatigue, weakness, feeling of faintness, insomnia, dizziness, mental changes, memory loss, hallucinations, *depression,* anxiety, *confusion, paresthesia, headache*
CV: Orthostatic hypotension, bradycardia, ***CHF,*** palpitations, chest pain, tachycardia, dysrhythmias
EENT: Nasal stuffiness, tinnitus, visual changes, sore throat, double vision, dry burning eyes
GI: Nausea, cramps, diarrhea, constipation, dry mouth, anorexia, indigestion
GU: Ejaculation failure, impotence, dysuria, nocturia, urinary frequency
INTEG: Rash, purpura, alopecia
MS: Leg cramps, aching, pain, inflammation
RESP: Bronchospasm, dyspnea, cough, rales, SOB

Contraindications: Hypersensitivity, pregnancy **B,** pheochromocytoma, lactation, P CHF, child <18 yr

G **Precautions:** Elderly, bronchial asthma, peptic ulcer, electrolyte imbalances, vascular disease

Pharmacokinetics

Absorption	Well absorbed
Distribution	Widely distributed, minimally distributed in the CNS
Metabolism	Liver (50%)
Excretion	Kidneys, unchanged (50%)
Half-life	10-12 hr

Pharmacodynamics

Onset	½-2 hr
Peak	4-6 hr
Duration	4-14 hr

Interactions
Individual drugs
Alcohol: ↑ hypotension
Ephedrine: Blocked antihypertensive effect
Levodopa: ↑ hypotension
Norepinephrine: ↑ pressor, mydriatic effects
Phenylephrine: ↑ pressor, mydriatic effects
Drug classifications
Antidepressants, tricyclic: Blocked effect of guanadrel
Antihypertensive: ↑ hypotension
Amphetamines: ↑ pressor, mydriatic effect
MAOI: Blocked antihypertensive effect
Nitrates: ↑ hypotension
Lab test interferences
False positive: Urine acetone

NURSING CONSIDERATIONS
Assessment
- Monitor blood studies: neutrophils, decreased platelets
- Monitor renal studies: protein, BUN, creatinine; watch for increased levels that may indicate nephrotic syndrome; polyuria, oliguria, urinary frequency
- Obtain baselines in renal, liver function tests before therapy begins; potassium

levels, although hyperkalemia rarely occurs
- Monitor B/P, pulse if the drug is being used for hypertension; notify prescriber of changes
- Assess for allergic reaction: rash, fever, pruritus, urticaria; drug should be discontinued if antihistamines fail to help
- Symptoms of CHF: edema, dyspnea, wet rales, increased B/P, weight gain

Nursing diagnoses

✓ Cardiac output, decreased (uses)
✓ Injury, risk of physical (side effects)
✓ Knowledge deficit (teaching)
✓ Noncompliance (teaching)

Implementation
- Usually given as adjunct with other cardiovascular drugs (diuretics) to decrease edema
- Store in air-tight container at 86° F (30° C) or less

Patient/family education
- Instruct patient not to discontinue drug abruptly, or withdrawal symptoms may occur: anxiety, increased B/P, headache, insomnia, increased pulse, tremors, nausea, sweating
- Advise patient not to use OTC (cough, cold, or allergy) products unless directed by prescriber
- Teach patient to comply with dosage schedule even if feeling better; drug controls symptoms, does not cure
- Caution patient to change position slowly, to rise slowly to sitting or standing position to minimize orthostatic hypotension, especially in the G elderly
- Caution patient that drug may cause dizziness, fainting; light-headedness may occur during first few days of therapy; that drug may cause dry mouth—use hard candy, saliva product, or frequent rinsing of mouth
- Instruct patient that compliance is necessary; not to skip or stop drug unless directed by prescriber
- Inform patient that drug may cause skin rash
- Teach patient to avoid hazardous activities because drug may cause drowsiness, dizziness

Evaluation

Positive therapeutic outcome
- Decreased B/P

guanethidine (℞)
(gwahn-eth-i'deen)

Apo-Guanethidine ✱, guanethidine sulfate, Ismelin

Func. class.: Antihypertensive

Chem. class.: Adrenergic blocker, (peripheral guanethidine derivative)

Pregnancy category B

Action: Inhibits sympathetic vasoconstriction by inhibiting release of norepinephrine, depletes norepinephrine stores in adrenergic nerve endings and the adrenal medulla

➔ **Therapeutic Outcome:** Decreased B/P

Uses: Moderate to severe hypertension

Dosage and routes

Adult: PO 10 mg qd, increase by 10-12.5 mg qwk; may require 25-50 mg qd

Adult: (hospitalized) 25-50 mg; may increase by 25-50 mg/day or qod

P ***Child:*** PO 0.2 mg/kg/day (6 mg/m²/day); increase q 7-10 day 0.2 mg/kg or 6 mg/m²/day

Available forms: Tabs 10, 25 mg

Adverse effects

CNS: Depression, anxiety, drowsiness, fatigue, confusion, headache, sleeping problems
CV: Orthostatic hypotension, dizziness, chest pain, weakness, edema
EENT: Nasal congestion, ptosis, blurred vision
GI: Nausea, vomiting, *diarrhea, constipation, dry mouth,* weight gain, *anorexia,* abdominal pain
GU: Ejaculation failure, impotence, nocturia, edema, *retention,* increased BUN, *frequency*
INTEG: Dermatitis, loss of scalp hair
MS: Aches, leg cramps
RESP: Dyspnea, cough, shortness of breath

Contraindications: Hypersensitivity, pheochromocytoma, recent MI, CHF, cardiac failure, sinus bradycardia

Precautions: Pregnancy **B,** lactation, peptic ulcer, asthma

Pharmacokinetics	
Absorption	Incompletely absorbed (up to 50%)
Distribution	Widely distributed, does not cross blood-brain barrier
Metabolism	Liver—partially
Excretion	Kidneys, breast milk (minimal)
Half-life	5 days

Pharmacodynamics	
Onset	4 wk
Peak	4 wk
Duration	4 wk

Interactions

Individual drugs

Alcohol: ↑ hypotension
Ephedrine: Blocks antihypertensive effect
Levodopa: ↑ hypotension
Metharaminol: ↑ pressor, mydriatic effects
Norepinephrine: ↑ pressor, mydriatic effects
Phenylephrine: ↑ pressor, mydriatic effects

Drug classifications

Antidepressants, tricyclics: ↑ hypotension
Antihypertensives: ↑ hypotension
Amphetamines: ↑ pressor, mydriatic effects
Contraceptives, oral: Blocks antihypertensive effect, ↑ hypertension
MAOI: ↑ hypertension
Nitrates: ↑ hypotension
Phenothiazines: Blocks antihypertensive effect, ↑ hypertension

Lab test interferences

↑ BUN
↓ Blood glucose, ↓ VMA excretion, ↓ urinary norepinephrine

NURSING CONSIDERATIONS

Assessment

- Monitor blood studies: neutrophils, decreased platelets
- Monitor B/P, orthostatic hypotension, syncope
- Monitor renal studies: protein, BUN, creatinine; watch for increased levels that may indicate nephrotic syndrome; polyuria, oliguria, urinary frequency

- Obtain baselines of renal, liver function tests before therapy begins
- Obtain potassium levels, although hyperkalemia rarely occurs
- Check for edema in feet, legs daily; monitor I&O; check for decreasing output
- Assess for allergic reaction: rash, fever, pruritus, urticaria; drug should be discontinued if antihistamines fail to help
- Assess for symptoms of CHF: edema, dyspnea, wet rales, B/P, weight gain

Nursing diagnoses

✓ Cardiac output, decreased (uses)
✓ Injury, risk for (adverse reactions)
✓ Knowledge deficit (teaching)

Implementation

- Usually given as adjunct with other cardiovascular drugs (diuretics) to decrease edema
- Store in air-tight container at 86° F (30° C) or less

Patient/family education

- Instruct patient not to discontinue drug abruptly because withdrawal symptoms may occur: anxiety, increased B/P, headache, insomnia, increased pulse, tremors, nausea, sweating
- Teach patient to comply with dosage schedule even if feeling better; drug controls symptoms, does not cure
- Caution patient to rise slowly to sitting or standing position to minimize orthostatic hypotension, especially in the G elderly
- Instruct patient to notify prescriber of sore throat, fever, swelling of hands or feet, irregular heartbeat, chest pain
- Caution patient that drug may cause dizziness, fainting, light-headedness may occur during first few days of therapy; that drug may cause dry mouth—use hard candy, saliva product, or frequent rinsing of mouth; that compliance is necessary—not to skip or stop drug unless directed by physician; that drug may cause skin rash or impaired perspiration
- Teach patient to avoid hazardous activities—drug may cause drowsiness, dizziness

G

Evaluation

Positive therapeutic outcome

- Decreased B/P in hypertension

Treatment of overdose: Administer vasopressors; discontinue drug

guanfacine (℞)

(gwahn'fa-seen)

Tenex

Func. class.: Antihypertensive

Chem. class.: Central α_2-adrenergic agonist

Pregnancy category B

Action: Stimulates central α_2-adrenergic receptors in the CNS resulting in decreased sympathetic outflow from brain with decreased peripheral resistance

➔ **Therapeutic Outcome:** Decreased B/P in hypertension

Uses: Hypertension in individual using a thaizide diuretic

Dosage and routes

Adult: PO 1 mg/day hs; may increase dose in 2-3 wk to 2-3 mg/day

Available forms: Tab 1 mg

Adverse effects

CNS: Somnolence, dizziness, headache, fatigue
CV: Bradycardia, chest pain
EENT: Taste change, tinnitus, vision change, rhinitis, nasal congestion
GI: Dry mouth, constipation, cramps, nausea, diarrhea
GU: Impotence, urinary incontinence
INTEG: Dermatitis, pruritus, purpura
MS: Leg cramps
RESP: Dyspnea

Contraindications: Hypersensitivity

Precautions: Pregnancy **B**, P lactation, children <12 yr, severe coronary insufficiency, recent MI, renal or hepatic disease, CVA

Pharmacokinetics

Absorption	Well absorbed (80%)
Distribution	Widely distributed
Metabolism	Liver (50%)
Excretion	Kidneys—unchanged (50%)
Half-life	17 hr

Pharmacodynamics

Onset	Unknown
Peak	1-4 hr
Duration	Unknown

Interactions

Individual drugs

Alcohol: ↑ hypotension, ↑ sedation

Drug classifications

Analgesics, narcotic: ↑ sedation
Antidepressants, tricyclic:↓ effectiveness of guanabenz
Antihypertensives: ↑ hypotension
β-Adrenergic blockers: ↑ bradycardia, CHF
MAOI: ↓ effectiveness of guanabenz
Nitrates: ↑ nitrates
Sedatives/hypnotics: ↑ sedation

NURSING CONSIDERATIONS

Assessment

- Monitor blood studies: neutrophils, decreased platelets
- Monitor renal studies: Protein, BUN, creatinine; watch for increased levels that may indicate nephrotic syndrome; polyuria, oliguria, frequency
- Obtain baselines in renal, liver function tests before therapy begins; potassium levels, although hyperkalemia rarely occurs
- Monitor B/P, pulse if the drug is being used for hypertension; notify prescriber of changes
- Assess for edema in feet, legs daily; monitor I&O; check weight for decreasing output
- Assess for allergic reaction: rash, fever, pruritus, urticaria; drug should be discontinued if antihistamines fail to help
- Assess for symptoms of CHF: edema, dyspnea, wet rales, BP, weight gain

Nursing diagnoses

- ✓ Cardiac output, decreased (uses)
- ✓ Injury, risk for (adverse reactions)
- ✓ Knowledge deficit (teaching)
- ✓ Noncompliance (teaching)

Implementation

- Give hs
- Store in air-tight container at room temp

Patient/family education

- Instruct patient not to discontinue drug abruptly, or

withdrawal symptoms may occur: anxiety, increased B/P, headache, insomnia, increased pulse, tremors, nausea, sweating

- Caution patient not to use OTC (cough, cold, or allergy) products unless directed by prescriber
- Teach patient to comply with dosage schedule even if feeling better; drug controls symptoms, does not cure
- Caution patient (especially G the elderly) to change position slowly, to rise slowly to sitting or standing position to minimize orthostatic hypotension
- Instruct patient to notify prescriber of sore throat, fever, swelling of hands or feet, irregular heartbeat, chest pain, increased weight
- Inform patient that drug may cause dizziness, fainting; light-headedness may occur during 1st few days of therapy; drug may cause dry mouth—use hard candy or saliva product, or rinse mouth frequently
- Teach patient that compliance is necessary; not to skip or stop drug unless directed by prescriber
- Caution patient that drug may cause skin rash
- Teach patient to avoid hazardous activities—drug may cause drowsiness; dizziness

Evaluation

Positive therapeutic outcome

- Decreased B/P

halazepam (℞)

(hal-az'e-pam)

Paxipam

Func. class.: Sedative/hypnotic

Chem. class.: Benzodiazepine

Pregnancy category D

Controlled substance schedule IV

Action: Depresses subcortical levels of CNS, including limbic system, reticular formation; potentiates GABA

➡ **Therapeutic Outcome:** Decreased anxiety

Uses: Adjunct in anxiety

Dosage and routes

Adult: PO 20-40 mg tid-qid

G ***Geriatric:*** PO 20 mg qd-bid

Available forms: Tabs 20, 40 mg

Adverse effects

CNS: Dizziness, drowsiness, confusion, headache, anxiety, tremors, stimulation, fatigue, depression, insomnia, hallucinations

CV: Orthostatic hypotension, ***ECG changes, tachycardia,*** hypotension

EENT: Blurred vision, tinnitus, mydriasis

GI: Constipation, dry mouth, nausea, vomiting, anorexia, diarrhea

INTEG: Rash, dermatitis, itching

Contraindications: Hypersensitivity to benzodiazepines, narrow-angle glaucoma, psy- P chosis, pregnancy **D,** child <18 yr

G **Precautions:** Elderly, debilitated, hepatic disease, renal disease

Pharmacokinetics	
Absorption	Well absorbed
Distribution	Widely distributed; crosses placenta
Metabolism	Liver, extensively
Excretion	Kidneys, breast milk
Half-life	2 hr, 30-100 hr active metabolite

Pharmacodynamics	
Onset	Unknown
Peak	1-3 hr
Duration	3-6 hr

Interactions
Individual drugs
Alcohol: ↑ CNS depression
Cimetidine: ↑ action
Digoxin: ↑ risk of digoxin toxicity
Disulfiram: ↑ action
Fluoxetine: ↑ action
Isoniazid: ↑ action
Ketoconazole: ↑ action
Levodopa: ↓ action of levodopa
Metoprolol: ↑ action
Propoxyphene: ↑ action
Propranolol: ↑ action
Rifampin: ↓ action of halazepam
Theophylline: ↓ sedative effects
Valproic acid: ↑ action
Drug classifications
Analgesics, opioid: ↑ CNS depression
Antidepressants: ↑ CNS depression
Antihistamines: ↑ CNS depression
Barbiturates: ↓ effect of halazepam
Contraceptives: ↑ effect
Lab test interferences
↑ AST (SGOT)/ALT (SGPT), ↑ serum bilirubin
False ↑ 17-OHCS
↓ RAIU

NURSING CONSIDERATIONS
Assessment
- Assess mental status: mood, sensorium, anxiety, affect, sleeping pattern, drowsiness, G dizziness, especially elderly; physical dependency, withdrawal symptoms: anxiety, panic attacks, agitation, convulsions, headache, nausea, vomiting, muscle pain, weakness; suicidal tendencies; for indications of increasing tolerance and abuse
- Monitor B/P (with patient lying, standing), pulse; if systolic B/P drops 20 mm Hg, hold drug, notify prescriber
- Monitor hepatic studies: AST (SGOT), ALT (SGPT), bilirubin, creatinine, LDH, alkaline phosphatase

Nursing diagnoses
✓ Anxiety (uses)
✓ Injury, risk for (adverse reactions)
✓ Knowledge deficit (teaching)

Implementation
- Give with food or milk for GI symptoms; tab may be crushed, if patient is unable to swallow medication whole, and mixed with foods or fluids
- Give sugarless gum, hard candy, frequent sips of water for dry mouth

Patient/family education
- Advise patient that drug may be taken with food, or fluids and tab may be crushed or swallowed whole
- Caution patient not to use for everyday stress or longer than 3 mo unless directed by prescriber; not to take more than prescribed amount; may

be habit forming; not to double doses or skip doses
• Advise patient to avoid OTC preparations unless approved by prescriber
• Instruct patient to avoid driving and activities that require alertness, since drowsiness may occur; to avoid alcohol and psychotropic medications; to rise slowly to prevent fainting, especially G elderly; that drowsiness may worsen at beginning of treatment
• Instruct patient not to discontinue medication abruptly after long-term use; withdrawal symptoms include vomiting, cramping, tremors, seizures

Evaluation

Positive therapeutic outcome
• Decreased anxiety, restlessness, sleeplessness (short-term treatment only)

Treatment of overdose: Lavage, VS, supportive care, give flumazenil

haloperidol 🔑 (℞)

(ha-loe-per'i-dole)

Apo-Haloperidol ✱, Haldol, Haloperidol, Haloperidol Decanoate 50, Haloperidol 100, Haldol L.A. ✱, Novoperidol ✱, Peridol ✱

Func. class.: Antipsychotic/neuroleptic

Chem. class.: Butyrophenone

Pregnancy category C

Action: Depresses cerebral cortex, hypothalamus, limbic system, which control activity and aggression; blocks neurotransmission produced by dopamine at synapse; exhibits strong α-adrenergic, anticholinergic blocking action; mechanism for antipsychotic effects unclear

➔ **Therapeutic Outcome:** Decreased signs and symptoms of psychosis

Uses: Psychotic disorders, control of tics, vocal utterances in Gilles de la Tourette syndrome, short-term treatment of hyperactive children showing excessive motor activity, prolonged parenteral therapy in chronic schizophrenia

Dosage and routes

Psychosis

Adult: PO 0.5-5 mg bid or tid initially depending on severity of condition; increase to desired dosage, max 100 mg/day; IM 2-5 mg q1-8h

P ***Child 3-12 yr:*** PO/IM 0.05-0.15 mg/kg/day

Chronic schizophrenia

Adult: IM 10-15 times the PO dosage q4 wk (decanoate)

P ***Child 3-12 yr:*** PO/IM 0.05-0.15 mg/kg/day

Tics/vocal utterances

Adult: PO 0.5-5 mg bid or tid, increased until desired response occurs

P ***Child 3-12 yr:*** PO 0.05-0.075 mg/kg/day

Hyperactive children

P ***Child 3-12 yr:*** PO 0.05-0.075 mg/kg/day

Available forms: Tabs 0.5, 1, 2, 5, 10, 20 mg; conc 2 mg/ml; inj IM 5 mg/ml

Adverse effects

CNS: Extrapyramidal symptoms: pseudoparkinsonism, akathisia, dystonia, tardive

H

dyskinesia, drowsiness, headache, ***seizures neuroleptic malignant syndrome,*** confusion
CV: Orthostatic hypotension, hypertension, ***cardiac arrest,*** ECG changes, ***tachycardia***
EENT: Blurred vision, glaucoma, dry eyes
GI: Dry mouth, nausea, vomiting, anorexia, constipation, diarrhea, jaundice, weight gain, ***ileus, hepatitis***
GU: Urinary retention, urinary frequency, enuresis, impotence, amenorrhea, gynecomastia
INTEG: Rash, photosensitivity, dermatitis
RESP: ***Laryngospasm,*** dyspnea, ***respiratory depression***

Contraindications: Hypersensitivity, blood dyscrasias, coma, P child <3 yr, brain damage, bone marrow depression, alcohol and barbiturate withdrawal states, Parkinson's disease, angina, epilepsy, urinary retention, narrow-angle glaucoma

Precautions: Pregnancy **C**, lactation, seizure disorders, hypertension, hepatic disease, cardiac disease

Pharmacokinetics

Absorption	Well absorbed (PO, IM); decanoate (IM) absorbed slowly
Distribution	High concentrations in liver, crosses placenta
Metabolism	Liver, extensively
Excretion	Kidneys, breast milk
Half-life	21-24 hr

Pharmacodynamics

	PO	IM	IM (decanoate)
Onset	Erratic	½ hr	3-9 days
Peak	2-6 hr	30-45 min	4-11 days
Duration	8-12 hr	4-8 hr	3 wk

Interactions

Individual drugs

Alcohol: ↑ effects of both drugs, oversedation
Aluminum hydroxide: ↓ absorption
Bromocriptine: ↓ antiparkinson activity
Disopyramide: ↑ anticholinergic effects
Epinephrine: ↑ toxicity
Guanethidine: ↓ antihypertensive response
Levodopa: ↓ antiparkinsonian activity
Lithium: ↓ haloperidol levels, ↑ extrapyramidal symptoms, masking of lithium toxicity
Magnesium hydroxide: ↓ absorption
Norepinephrine: ↓ vasoresponse, ↑ toxicity
Phenobarbital: ↓ effectiveness, ↑ metabolism

Drug classifications

Antacids: ↓ absorption
Anticholinergics: ↑ anticholinergic effects
Antidepressants: ↑ CNS depression
Antidiarrheals, adsorbent: ↓ absorption
Antihistamines: ↑ CNS depression
Antihypertensives: ↑ hypotension
Antithyroid agents: ↑ agranulocytosis
Barbiturate anesthetics: ↑ CNS depression

β-Adrenergics: ↑ effects of both drugs
General anesthetics: ↑ CNS depression
MAOI: ↑ CNS depression
Narcotics: ↑ CNS depression
Sedative/hypnotics: ↑ CNS depression

Lab test interferences
↑ Liver function tests, ↑ cardiac enzymes, ↑ cholesterol, ↑ blood glucose, ↑ prolactin, ↑ bilirubin, ↑ PBI, ↑ cholinesterase
↓ Hormones (blood and urine)
False positive: Pregnancy tests, PKU, urine bilirubin
False negative: Urinary steroids, 17-OHCS

NURSING CONSIDERATIONS

Assessment

- Assess mental status: orientation, mood, behavior, presence and type of hallucinations before initial administration and monthly; this drug should significantly reduce psychotic behavior
- Check for swallowing of PO medication; check for hoarding or giving of medication to other patients
- Monitor I&O ratio; palpate bladder if low urinary output G occurs, especially in elderly; urinalysis is recommended before, during prolonged therapy
- Monitor bilirubin, CBC, liver function studies monthly
- Assess affect, orientation, LOC, reflexes, gait, coordination, sleep pattern disturbances
- Monitor B/P with patient sitting, standing, and lying; take pulse and respirations q4h during initial treatment; establish baseline before starting treatment; report drops of 30 mm Hg; obtain baseline ECG, Q wave and T wave changes
- Check for dizziness, faintness, palpitations, tachycardia on rising; severe orthostatic hypotension is common
- Identify for neuroleptic malignant syndrome: hyperpyrexia, muscle rigidity, increased CPK, altered mental status; drug should be discontinued immediately
- Assess for extrapyramidal symptoms including akathisia (inability to sit still, no pattern to movements), tardive dyskinesia (bizarre movements of the jaw, mouth, tongue, extremities), pseudoparkinsonism (ragged tremors, pill rolling, shuffling gate); an antiparkinsonian drug should be prescribed
- Assess for constipation and urinary retention daily; if these occur, increase bulk, water in diet

Nursing diagnoses

- ✓ Thought processes, altered (uses)
- ✓ Coping, ineffective individual (uses)
- ✓ Knowledge deficit (teaching)
- ✓ Noncompliance (teaching)

Implementation

PO route

- Give drug in liquid form mixed in glass of juice or cola if hoarding is suspected; do not mix in caffeine drinks, tannics, pectins
- Give decreased dosage in G elderly because of slower metabolism
- Give PO with full glass of water, milk; or give with food to decrease GI upset
- Store in tight, light-resistant container, oral sol in amber bottle

H

IM route
• Inject in deep muscle mass, do not give SC; use 21 G 2-inch needle; do not administer sol with a precipitate; give <3 ml per inj site; give slowly, may be painful

Syringe incompatibilities: Hydromorphone, sufentanil

Y-site compatibilities: Allopurinol, amifostine, amsacrine, cimetidine, dobutamine, dopamine, famotidine, filgrastim, fludarabine, lidocaine, lorazepam, melphalan, midazolam, nitroglycerin, norepinephrine, ondansetron, paclitaxel, phenylephrine, sufentanil, tacrolimus, teniposide, theophylline, thiotepa, vinorelbine

Y-site incompatibilities: Fluconazole, foscarnet, heparin, sargramostim

Patient/family education
• Teach patient to use good oral hygiene; use frequent rinsing of mouth, sugarless gum for dry mouth
• Advise patient to avoid hazardous activities until drug response is determined; dizziness, blurred vision are common
• Inform patient that orthostatic hypotension occurs often and to rise from sitting or lying position gradually; to remain lying down after IM inj for at least 30 min; tell patient to avoid hot tubs, hot showers, tub baths, since hypotension may occur; tell patient that in hot weather heat stroke may occur; take extra precautions to stay cool
• Instruct patient to avoid abrupt withdrawal of this drug, or extrapyramidal symptoms may result; drug should be withdrawn slowly
• Caution patient to avoid OTC preparations (cough, hay fever, cold) unless approved by prescriber, since serious drug interactions may occur; avoid use with alcohol, CNS depressants since increased drowsiness may occur
• Advise patient to use a sunscreen and sunglasses to prevent burns
• Teach patient about extrapyramidal symptoms and necessity of meticulous oral hygiene, since oral candidiasis may occur
• Instruct patient to take antacids 2 hr before or after this drug
• Tell patient to report sore throat, malaise, fever, bleeding, mouth sores; if these occur, CBC should be completed and drug discontinued

Evaluation

Positive therapeutic outcome
• Decrease in emotional excitement, hallucinations, delusions, paranoia
• Reorganization of patterns of thought, speech

Treatment of overdose: Lavage if orally ingested; provide airway; *do not induce vomiting*

heparin calcium/ heparin sodium

(℞)

(hep'a-rin)

Calcilean ✦, Calciparine, Hepalean ✦, Heparin Sodium and 0.45% Sodium Chloride, Heparin Sodium and 0.9% Sodium Chloride, Heparin Leo ✦, Heparin Lock Flush, Heparin Sodium, Hep-Lock, Hep-Lock U/P, Liquaemin Sodium

Func. class.: Anticoagulant

Pregnancy category C

Action: Prevents conversion of fibrinogen to fibrin and prothrombin to thrombin by enhancing inhibitory effects of antithrombin III

Therapeutic Outcome: Prevention of thrombi

Uses: Deep vein thrombosis and pulmonary emboli (treatment and prevention), MI, open heart surgery, disseminated intravascular clotting syndrome, atrial fibrillation with embolization, as an anticoagulant in transfusion and dialysis procedures

Dosage and routes

Deep vein thrombosis/MI

Adult: **IV** push 5000-7000 U q4h then titrated to PTT or ACT level; **IV** bol 5000-7500 U, then **IV** inf; **IV** inf after bolus dose, then 1000 U/hr titrated to PTT or ACT level

P ***Child:*** **IV** inf 50 U/kg, maintenance 100 U/kg q4h or 20,000 U/m² qd

Anticoagulation

Adult: SC 5000 UIV then 10,000-20,000 U, then 8,000-10,000 U q8hr or 15,000-20,000 U q12hr

Pulmonary embolism

Adult: **IV** push 7500-10,000 q4h then titrated to PTT or ACT level; **IV** bol 7500-10,000, then **IV** inf; **IV** inf after bol dose, then 1000 U/hr titrated to PTT or ACT level

P ***Child:*** **IV** inf 50 U/kg; maintenance 100 U/kg q4h or 20,000 U/m² qd

Open heart surgery

Adult: **IV** inf 150-300 U/kg, prophylaxis for DVT/PE; SC 5,000 U q8-12h

Heparin flush

P ***Adult/child:*** **IV** 10-100 U

Available forms: Heparin sodium inj 10, 1000, 5000, 10,000, 20,000, 40,000 U/ml; heparin calcium inj 5000, 12,500, 20,000 U/dose, 5000 U/0.2 ml

Adverse effects

CNS: Fever, chills

GI: Diarrhea, nausea, vomiting, anorexia, stomatitis, abdominal cramps, ***hepatitis***

GU: ***Hematuria***

HEMA: ***Hemorrhage, thrombocytopenia***

INTEG: Rash, dermatitis, urticaria, alopecia, pruritus

Contraindications: Hypersensitivity, hemophilia, leukemia with bleeding, peptic ulcer disease, thrombocytopenic purpura, hepatic disease (severe), renal disease (severe), blood dyscrasias, severe hypertension, subacute bacterial endocarditis, acute nephritis

Precautions: Alcoholism, G elderly, pregnancy **C**

Pharmacokinetics

Absorption	Well absorbed (SC)
Distribution	Unknown
Metabolism	Unknown
Excretion	Lymph, spleen
Half-life	1½ hr

Pharmacodynamics

	SC	IV
Onset	½-1 hr	5 min
Peak	2 hr	10 min
Duration	8-12 hr	2-6 hr

Lab test interferences

False ↑ T_3 uptake, ↑ serum thyroxine, ↑ BSP
↓ Uric acid
False negative: ^{125}I fibrinogen uptake

NURSING CONSIDERATIONS

Assessment

- Assess for blood studies (Hct, occult blood in stools) q3 mo if patient is on long-term therapy
- Monitor PPT, which should be 1½-2 times control, PTT; often done qd, APTT, ACT
- Monitor platelet count q2-3 days; thrombocytopenia may occur on 4th day of treatment and resolve, or continued thrombocytopenia on 8th day
- Assess for bleeding gums, petechiae, ecchymosis, black tarry stools, hematuria, epistaxis, decrease in Hct, B/P; may indicate bleeding and possible hemorrhage; notify prescriber immediately
- Monitor for hypersensitivity: fever, skin rash, urticaria; notify prescriber immediately

Nursing diagnoses

- ✓ Injury, risk for (uses, adverse reactions)
- ✓ Tissue perfusion, altered (uses)
- ✓ Knowledge deficit (teaching)

Implementation

IV IV route

- Give directly; **IV** loading dose over 1 min
- Give **IV** diluted in 0.9% NaCl, dextrose, Ringer's sol and by intermittent or cont inf; inf may run from 4-24 hr; use inf pump

Y-site compatibilities:
Acyclovir, aldesleukin, allopurinol, amifostine, aminophylline, ampicillin, atracurium, atropine, betamethasone, bleomycin, calcium gluconate, cephalothin, cephapirin, chlordiazepoxide, chlorpromazine, cimetidine, cisplatin, conjugated estrogens, cyanocobalamin, cyclophosphamide, dexamethasone, digoxin, diphenhydramine, dopamine, edrophonium, enalaprilat, epinephrine, esmolol, ethacrynate, famotidine, fentanyl, fluconazole, fludarabine, fluorouracil, foscarnet, furosemide, hydralazine, regular insulin, isoproterenol, kanamycin, labetalol, leucovorin, lidocaine, lorazepam, magnesium sulfate, melphalan, menadiol sodium, meperidine, methicillin, methotrexate, methoxamine, methylergonovine, metoclopramide, midazolam, minocycline, mitomycin, morphine, neostigmine, nitroglycerin, nitroprusside, norepinephrine, ondansetron, oxacillin, oxytocin, paclitaxel, pancuronium, penicillin G potassium, pentazocine, phytonadione, potassium chloride, prednisolone, procainamide, prochlorperazine, propranolol, pyridostigmine, ranitidine, sargramostim, scopolamine, sodium bicarbonate, streptokinase, succinylcholine, tacrolimus, teniposide, thiotepa,

trimethobenzamide, vecuronium, vinblastine, vincristine, vinorelbine, zidovudine

Y-site incompatibilities: Alteplase, ciprofloxacin, dacarbazine, diazepam, dobutamine, doxorubicin, ergotamine, gentamicin, haloperidol, idarubicin, methotrimeprazine, phenytoin, promethazine, tobramycin, triflupromazine

Additive compatibilities: Aminophylline, amphotericin, ampicillin, bleomycin, calcium gluconate, cephalothin, cephapirin, chloramphenicol, clindamycin, colistimethate, dimenhydrinate, doxacillin, dopamine, enalaprilat, erythromycin, esmolol, floxacillin, fluconazole, flumazenil, furosemide, hydrocortisone, isoproterenol, lidocaine, methyldopate methylprednisolone, nafcillin, octreotide, potassium chloride, prednisolone, promazine, ranitidine, sodium bicarbonate, verapamil, vitamin B complex, vitamin B complex with C

Additive incompatibilities: Amikacin, erythromycin lactobionate, gentamicin, kanamycin, meperidine, methadone, morphine, polymyxin B, streptomycin

Heparin lock route
- Inject 10-100 U/0.5-1 ml after each inf or q8-12h

SC route
- Give SC with at least 25 G ⅜-in needle; do not massage area or aspirate fluid when giving SC inj; give in abdomen between pelvic bones, rotate sites; do not pull back on plunger, leave in for 10 sec; apply gentle pressure for 1 min
- Give at same time each day to maintain steady blood levels
- Changing needles is not recommended

Patient/family education
- Advise patient to avoid OTC preparations that may cause serious drug interactions unless directed by prescriber; may contain aspirin or other anticoagulants
- Tell patient that drug may be held during active bleeding (menstruation), depending on condition
- Caution patient to use soft-bristle toothbrush to avoid bleeding gums; avoid contact sports; use electric razor; avoid IM inj
- Instruct patient to carry a Medic Alert ID or other identification identifying drug taken and condition treated
- Advise patient to report any signs of bleeding: gums, under skin, urine, stools; or unusual bruising

Evaluation

Positive therapeutic outcome
- Decrease of deep vein thrombosis
- PTT of 1.5-2.5 times control
- Free-flowing IV

Treatment of overdose: Withdraw drug, give protamine sulfate

hepatitis B immune globulin (℞)

(hep-a-tite'iss)

H-BIG, Hep-B-Gammagee, Hyper Hep

Func. class.: Immune globulin

Pregnancy category C

Action: Provides active immunity to hepatitis B

➔ **Therapeutic Outcome:** Passive immunity to hepatitis B

Uses: Prevention of hepatitis B virus in exposed patients, including passive immunity in **P** neonates born to HBsAg-positive mother

Dosage and routes

P ***Adult and child >10 yr:*** IM 1 ml, then 1 ml after 1 mo, then 1 ml 6 mo after initial dose

P ***Child 3 mo-10 yr:*** IM 0.5 ml, then 0.5 ml after 1 mo, then 0.5 ml 6 mo after initial dose

Patients with decreased immunity: IM 2 ml, then 2 ml after 1 mo, then 2 ml 6 mo after initial dose

Available forms: Inj 10 mg/0.5 ml, 20 μg/ml

Adverse effects

CNS: Headache, dizziness, fever, faintness, weakness
INTEG: Soreness at inj site, urticaria, erythema, swelling, pruritus
MS: Joint pain
SYST: ***Anaphylaxis, angioedema***

Contraindications: Hypersensitivity to immune globulins, thimerosal, glycine

Precautions: Pregnancy, **G** elderly, lactation, children, **P** active infection, IgA deficiency

Pharmacokinetics	
Absorption	Slowly absorbed
Distribution	Unknown
Metabolism	Unknown
Excretion	Unknown
Half-life	3 wk

Pharmacodynamics	
Onset	1-7 days
Peak	3-10 days
Duration	2-6 mo

Interactions

Drug classifications

Live vaccines: ↓ or ↑ immune response

NURSING CONSIDERATIONS

Assessment

- Assess for history of allergies, skin conditions (eczema, psoriasis, dermatitis), reactions to vaccinations
- Assess for skin reactions: rash, induration, urticaria
- Assess for sneezing, pruritus, angioedema, dysphagia, vomiting, abdominal pain
- ❗ Assess for anaphylaxis: inability to breathe, bronchospasm, hypotension, wheezing, diaphoresis, fever, flushing; epinephrine and emergency equipment should be available

Nursing diagnoses

✓ Infection, risk for (uses)
✓ Knowledge deficit (teaching)

Implementation

- Give after rotating vial; do not shake
- Give in deltoid or anterolateral thigh for better protection; give 2-ml dose in two different sites; do not give **IV**
- Refrigerate unused portion; sol should be clear, light amber, and thick

Patient/family education

- Teach patient purpose of medication and expected results
- Give patient a list of adverse reactions that need to be reported immediately: wheezing, vomiting, sneezing, abdominal pain, sweating, tightness in chest
- Advise patient that pain, rash, swelling at inj site can be expected
- Give patient written record of immunization

Evaluation
Positive therapeutic outcome
- Prevention of hepatitis B

hetastarch (℞)
(het'a-starch)
Hespan
Func. class.: Plasma expander
Chem. class.: Synthetic polymer
Pregnancy category C

Action: Similar to human albumin, which expands plasma volume by colloidal osmotic pressure

➡ **Therapeutic Outcome:** Increased plasma volume

Uses: Plasma volume expander for sepsis, trauma, burns, leukopheresis

Dosage and routes
Adult: **IV** inf 500-1000 ml (30-60 g); total dose not to exceed 1500 ml/day, not to exceed 20 ml/kg/hr (hemorrhagic shock)

Leukapheresis
Adult: **IV** inf 250-700 ml infused at 1:8 ratio with whole blood; may be repeated twice weekly up to 10 treatments

Available forms: 6% hetastarch/0.9% NaCl (6 g/100 ml)

Adverse effects
CNS: Headache
GI: Nausea, vomiting
HEMA: Decreased hematocrit, platelet function, increased bleeding/coagulation times, increased erythrosedimentation rate
INTEG: Rash, urticaria, pruritus, angioedema, chills, fever, flushing, peripheral edema
RESP: Wheezing, dyspnea, ***bronchospasm, pulmonary edema***
SYST: ***Anaphylaxis***

Contraindications: Hypersensitivity, severe bleeding disorders, renal failure, CHF (severe)

Precautions: Pregnancy **C**, liver disease, pulmonary edema

Pharmacokinetics	
Absorption	Completely absorbed
Distribution	Unknown
Metabolism	Degraded
Excretion	Kidneys, unchanged
Half-life	17 days (90%); 48 days (10%)

Pharmacodynamics	
Onset	Immediate
Peak	Infusion's end
Duration	Over 24 hr

Interactions: None
Lab test interferences
False ↑ Bilirubin

NURSING CONSIDERATIONS
Assessment
- Monitor VS q5 min for 30 min; CVP during inf (5-10 cm H_2O normal range); PCWP; urine output q1h: watch for increase which is common; if output does not increase, inf should be decreased or discontinued
- Monitor CBC with differential, Hgb, Hct, pro-time, PTT, platelet count, clotting time during treatment; treatment may increase clotting time, PTT, pro-time, sedimentary rates, Hct may drop due to increase volume and hemodilution; do not allow Hct to be <30% by volume
- Monitor I&O ratio and sp

gr, urine osmolarity; if sp gr is very low, renal clearance is low; drug should be discontinued

• Assess for allergy: rash, urticaria, pruritus, wheezing, dyspnea, bronchospasm; drug should be discontinued immediately

• Assess for circulatory overload: increased pulse, respirations, SOB, wheezing, chest tightness, chest pain, increased CVP, jugular vein distention

• Assess for dehydration after inf; decreased output, increased temp, poor skin turgor, increased sp gr, dry skin

Nursing diagnoses

✓ Fluid volume deficit (uses)
✓ Tissue perfusion, altered (uses)
✓ Fluid volume excess (adverse reactions)
✓ Knowledge deficit (teaching)

Implementation

• Give by **IV** cont inf, undiluted, run at 20 ml/kg/hr; reduced rate in septic shock, burns; rate is calculated by blood volume and response of patient

• Give up to 20 ml kg (1.2 g/kg)/hr

• Store at room temp; discard unused portions; do not freeze; do not use if turbid or deep brown or precipitate forms

Y-site incompatibilities: Amikacin, cefamandole, cefoperazone, cefotaxime, cefoxitin, gentamicin, theophylline, tobramycin

Y-site compatibilities: Cimetidine, diltiazem, doxycycline, enalaprilat

Additive compatibility: Cloxacillin

Patient/family education

• Teach patient the reason for administration and expected results

• Advise patient to notify prescriber if flulike symptoms or allergic symptoms occur

Evaluation

Positive therapeutic outcome

• Increased plasma volume as evidenced by higher B/P, blood volume, output

hydralazine (℞)

(hye-dral'a-zeen)

Alazine, Apresoline, Dralzine, Novo-Hylazin ✤, hydralazine HCl, Rolzine

Func. class.: Antihypertensive, direct-acting peripheral vasodilator

Chem. class.: Phthalazine

Pregnancy category C

Action: Vasodilates arterioles in smooth muscle by direct relaxation; reduces B/P with reflex increases in cardiac function

Therapeutic Outcome: Decreased B/P in hypertension, decreased afterload in CHF

Uses: Essential hypertension; *parenteral:* severe essential hypertension, CHF

Dosage and routes

Adult: PO 10 mg qid 2-4 days, then 25 mg for rest of 1st wk, then 50 mg qid individualized to desired response, not to exceed 300 mg qd; **IV**/IM bol 20-40 mg q4-6h; administer PO as soon as possible; IM 20-40 mg q4-6h

P ***Child:*** PO 0.75-3 mg/kg/day in 4 divided doses; max

7.5 mg/kg/24 hr; **IV** bol 0.10.2 mg/kg q4-6h; IM 0.1-0.2 mg/kg q4-6h

Available forms: Inj 20 mg/ml; tabs 10, 25, 50, 100 mg

Adverse effects

CNS: Headache, tremors, dizziness, anxiety, peripheral neuritis, depression
*CV: Palpitations, reflex tachycardia, **angina, shock,*** edema, rebound hypertension
GI: Nausea, vomiting, anorexia, diarrhea, constipation
GU: Impotence, urinary retention, Na^+, H_2O retention
*HEMA: **Leukopenia, agranulocytosis,*** anemia
INTEG: Rash, pruritus
MISC: Nasal congestion, muscle cramps, *lupuslike symptoms*

Contraindications: Hypersensitivity to hydralazines, coronary artery disease, mitral valvular rheumatic heart disease, rheumatic heart disease

Precautions: Pregnancy **C,** CVA, advanced renal disease

Pharmacokinetics

Absorption	Rapidly absorbed (PO); well absorbed (IM); completely absorbed (**IV**)
Distribution	Widely distributed; crosses placenta
Metabolism	GI mucosa, liver extensively
Excretion	Kidneys
Half-life	2-8 hr

Pharmacodynamics

	PO	IM	IV
Onset	½ hr	10-30 min	5-20 min
Peak	1 hr	1 hr	10-80 min
Duration	2-4 hr	4-6 hr	4-6 hr

Interactions
Individual drugs
Alcohol: ↑ hypotension
Drug classifications
Antihypertensives: ↑ hypotension
β-Adrenergic blockers: ↑ bradycardia, CHF
MAOI: ↑ hypotension
Nitrates: ↑ action of nitrates
NSAIDs: ↓ antihypertensive effect

NURSING CONSIDERATIONS

Assessment

- Assess B/P q5 min for 2 hr, then q1h for 2 hr, then q4h; pulse, jugular venous distention q4h
- Monitor electrolytes, blood studies: potassium, sodium, chloride, carbon dioxide, CBC, serum glucose
- Monitor weight daily, I&O; edema in feet, legs daily; check skin turgor, dryness of mucous membranes for hydration status
- Assess for rales, dyspnea, orthopnea; peripheral edema, fatigue, weight gain, jugular vein distention (CHF)

Nursing diagnoses

✓ Cardiac output, decreased (adverse reactions)
✓ Injury, risk for physical (side effects)
✓ Knowledge deficit (teaching)

Implementation

PO route

- Give with meals to enhance absorption
- Store protected from light and heat

IV route

- Give by **IV** undiluted through Y-tube or 3-way stopcock each 10 mg or less/min
- Administer with patient in recumbent position; keep in

H

that position for 1 hr after administration

Y-site incompatibilities: Aminophylline, ampicillin, diazoxide, furosemide, paclitaxel

Y-site compatibilities: Heparin, hydrocortisone, potassium chloride, verapamil, vitamin B with C

Additive incompatibilities: Aminophylline, ampicillin, chlorothiazide, edetate calcium disodium, ethacrynate, hydrocortisone, melphalan, mephentermine, methohexital, nitroglycerin, phenobarbital, verapamil, vinorelbine

Additive compatibility: Dobutamine

Patient/family education

- Teach patient to take with food to increase bioavailability
- Teach patient to avoid OTC preparations unless directed by prescriber
- Advise patient to notify prescriber if chest pain, severe fatigue, fever, muscle or joint pain occur

Evaluation

Positive therapeutic outcome

- Decreased B/P in hypertension

Treatment of overdose: Administer vasopressors, volume expanders for shock; if PO, lavage or give activated charcoal, digitalization

hydrochlorothiazide 🔑 (℞)

(hye-droe-klor-oh-thye′a-zide)

Diaqua, Diachlor H ✤, Esidrix, Hydro-Chlor, hydrochlorothiazide, HydroDiuril, Hydromal, Hydro-T, Hydrozide ✤, Microzide, Neo-Codema ✤, Novohydrazide ✤, Oretic, Thiuretic, Urozide ✤

Func. class: Diuretic, antihypertensive

Chem. class: Thiazide, sulfonamide derivative

Pregnancy category B

Action: Acts on the distal tubule in the kidney, increasing excretion of sodium, water, chloride, magnesium, potassium, and bicarbonate

➔ **Therapeutic Outcome:** Decreased B/P, decreased edema in lung tissues peripherally

Uses: Edema in CHF, nephrotic syndrome; may be used alone or as adjunct with antihypertensives

Dosage and routes

Adult: PO 25-200 mg/day

P ***Child >6 mo:*** PO 2.2 mg/kg/day

P ***Child <6 mo:*** PO up to 3.3 mg/kg/day in divided doses

Available forms: Tabs 25, 50, 100 mg; cap 12.5 mg; sol 50 mg/5 ml, 100 mg/ml

Adverse effects

CNS: Drowsiness, paresthesia, anxiety, depression, headache, *dizziness, fatigue, weakness*

CV: Irregular pulse, orthostatic hypotension, palpitations,

volume depletion, allergic myocarditis
EENT: Blurred vision
ELECT: *Hypokalemia*, hypercalcemia, hyponatremia, hypochloremia, hypomagnesemia
GI: *Nausea, vomiting, anorexia*, constipation, diarrhea, cramps, pancreatitis, GI irritation, ***hepatitis***
GU: *Frequency*, polyuria, ***uremia***, glucosuria
HEMA: ***Aplastic anemia, hemolytic anemia, leukopenia, agranulocytosis, thrombocytopenia, neutropenia***
INTEG: *Rash*, urticaria, purpura, photosensitivity, fever, alopecia, erythema multiform
META: *Hyperglycemia, hyperuricemia*, increased creatinine, BUN

Contraindications: Hypersensitivity to thiazides or sulfonamides, anuria, renal decompensation, pregnancy **B**, lactation

Precautions: Hypokalemia, renal disease, hepatic disease, gout, COPD, lupus erythematosus, diabetes mellitus, G elderly

Pharmacokinetics

Absorption	Variable
	PO/IV
Distribution	Extracellular spaces; crosses placenta
Metabolism	Excreted unchanged in urine
Excretion	Breast milk
Half-life	6-15 hr

Pharmacodynamics

Onset	2 hr
Peak	4 hr
Duration	6-12 hr

Interactions
Individual drugs
Cholestyramine: ↓ absorption of hydrochlorothiazide
Colestipol: ↓ absorption of hydrochlorothiazide
Diazoxide: ↑ hyperglycemia, hyperuricemia, hypotension
Digitalis: ↑ toxicity
Indomethacin: ↓ hypotensive response
Lithium: ↑ toxicity
Mezlocillin: ↑ hypokalemia
Piperacillin: ↑ hypokalemia
Ticarcillin: ↑ hypokalemia
Drug classifications
Anticoagulants: ↓ effects of
Antidiabetics: ↓ effect of antidiabetic agent
Antihypertensives: ↑ antihypertensive effect
Diuretics, loop: ↑ effects of diuretic
Nondepolarizing skeletal muscle relaxants: ↑ toxicity
Glucocorticoids: ↑ hypokalemia
Sulfonylureas: ↓ effect of sulfonylurea
Food
↑ absorption
Lab test interferences
↑ BSP retention, ↑ calcium, ↑ amylase, ↑ parathyroid test
↓ PBI, ↓ PSP

NURSING CONSIDERATIONS
Assessment
- Monitor glucose in urine if patient is diabetic
- Assess improvement in CVP q8h
- Check for rashes, temp elevation qd
- Assess for confusion, especially in elderly; take safety precautions if needed
- Monitor manifestations of hypokalemia: acidic urine, reduced urine, osmolality, nocturia; hypotension, broad

H

T wave, U wave, ectopy, tachycardia, weak pulse; muscle weakness, altered LOC, drowsiness, apathy, lethargy, confusion, depression; anorexia, nausea, cramps, constipation, distention, paralytic ileus; hypoventilation, respiratory muscle weakness

• Monitor for manifestations of hypomagnesemia: agitation, muscle twitching, paresthesias, hyperactive reflexes, positive Babinski reflex, dysphagia, nystagmus seizures, tetany; nausea, vomiting, diarrhea, anorexia, abdominal distention; ectopy, tachycardia, broad, flat, or inverted T waves, depressed ST segment, prolonged QT, decreased cardiac output, hypotension

• Monitor for manifestations of hyponatremia: increased B/P, cold, clammy skin, hypovolemia or hypervolemia; anorexia, nausea, vomiting, diarrhea, abdominal cramps; lethargy, increased ICP, confusion, headache, seizures, coma, fatigue, tremors, hyperreflexia

• Monitor for manifestations of hyperchloremia: weakness, lethargy, coma, deep rapid breathing

• Assess fluid volume status: I&O ratios, record, count, or weigh diapers as appropriate, weight, distended red veins, crackles in lungs, color, quality and sp gr of urine, skin turgor, adequacy of pulses, moist mucous membranes, bilateral lung sounds, peripheral pitting edema; assess for dehydration symptoms of decreasing output, thirst, hypotension; dry mouth and mucous membranes should be reported

• Monitor electrolytes: potassium, sodium, calcium, magnesium; also include BUN, blood pH, ABGs, uric acid, CBC, blood sugar

• Assess B/P before and during therapy with patient lying, standing and sitting as appropriate; orthostatic hypotension can occur rapidly

Nursing diagnoses

- ✓ Altered urinary elimination (side effect)
- ✓ Fluid volume deficit (side effects)
- ✓ Fluid volume excess (uses)
- ✓ Knowledge deficit (teaching)

Implementation

• Give in AM to avoid interference with sleep

• Provide potassium replacement if potassium level is 3.0; give whole tab or use oral sol lightly; drug may be crushed if patient is unable to swallow

• Administer with food; if nausea occurs, absorption may be increased

Patient/family education

• Teach patient to take the medication early in the day to prevent nocturia

• Instruct the patient to take with food or milk if GI symptoms of nausea and anorexia occur

• Teach patient to maintain a weekly record of weight and notify prescriber of weight loss >5 lb

• Caution the patient that this drug causes a loss of potassium and that food rich in potassium should be added to the diet; refer to a dietician for assistance in planning

• Caution the patient not to exercise in hot weather or stand for prolonged periods since orthostatic hypotension will be enhanced

• Teach patient not to use

alcohol or any OTC medications without prescriber's approval; serious drug reactions may occur

- Emphasize the need to contact prescriber immediately if muscle cramps, weakness, nausea, dizziness or numbness occurs
- Teach patient to take own B/P and pulse and record findings
- Caution the patient that orthostatic hypotension may occur; patient should rise slowly from sitting or reclining positions and lie down if dizziness occurs
- Teach patient to continue taking medication even if feeling better; this drug controls symptoms but does not cure the condition
- Advise the patient with hypertension to continue other medical treatment (exercise, weight loss, relaxation techniques, cessation of smoking)

Evaluation

Positive therapeutic outcome

- Decreased edema
- Decreased B/P
- Increased diuresis

Treatment of overdose: Lavage if taken orally, monitor electrolytes, administer dextrose in saline, monitor hydration, CV, renal status

hydrocodone (℞)

(hye-droe-koe'done)

Hycodan ♣, Robidone ♣

Func. class.: Narcotic analgesic

Chem. class.: Opiate

Pregnancy category C

Controlled substance schedule III

Action: Depresses pain impulse transmission at the spinal cord level by interacting with opioid receptors

➔ Therapeutic Outcome: Pain relief, decreased cough, decreased diarrhea

Uses: Hyperactive and nonproductive cough, mild pain

Dosages and routes

Adult: PO 5 mg q4h prn or 10 mg q12h (long acting)

P ***Child:*** PO 2-12 mg 1.25-5 mg q4h prn

Available forms: Cap 5 mg; susp 5 mg/ml; tabs 5 mg, 10 mg (long acting)

Adverse effects

CNS: Drowsiness, dizziness, lightheadedness, confusion, headache, sedation, euphoria, dysphoria, weakness, hallucinations, disorientation, mood changes, dependence, ***convulsions***

CV: Palpitations, tachycardia, bradycardia, change in B/P, ***circulatory depression,*** syncope

EENT: Tinnitus, blurred vision, miosis, diplopia

GI: Nausea, vomiting, anorexia, constipation, cramps, dry mouth

GU: Increased urinary output, dysuria, urinary retention

INTEG: Rash, urticaria, flushing, pruritus
RESP: Respiratory depression

Contraindications: Hypersensitivity, addiction (narcotic)

Precautions: Addictive personality, pregnancy **C,** lactation, increased intracranial pressure, MI (acute), severe heart disease, respiratory depression, hepatic disease, renal **P** disease, child <18 yr

Pharmacokinetics

Absorption	Well absorbed
Distribution	Unknown; crosses placenta
Metabolism	Liver, extensively
Excretion	Kidneys
Half-life	3½-4½ hr

Pharmacodynamics

	PO (analgesic)	PO (antitussive)
Onset	10-20 min	Unknown
Peak	30-60 min	Unknown
Duration	4-6 hr	4-6 hr

Interactions

Individual drugs

Alcohol: ↑ respiratory depression, hypotension, sedation
Cimetidine: ↑ recovery
Erythromycin: ↑ recovery
Nalbuphine: ↓ analgesia
Pentazocine: ↓ analgesia

Drug classifications

Antihistamines: ↑ respiratory depression, hypotension
CNS depressants: ↑ respiratory depression, hypotension
MAOI: Do not use for 2 wk before taking hydrocodone
Phenothiazines: ↑ respiratory depression, hypotension
Sedative/hypnotics: ↑ respiratory depression, hypotension

Lab test interferences

↑ Amylase, ↑ lipase

NURSING CONSIDERATIONS

Assessment

- Monitor VS after parenteral route; note muscle rigidity, drug history, liver, kidney function tests, respiratory dysfunction: respiratory depression, character, rate, rhythm; notify prescriber if respirations are <10/min
- Monitor CNS changes: dizziness, drowsiness, hallucinations, euphoria, LOC, pupil reaction
- Monitor allergic reactions: rash, urticaria

Nursing diagnoses

✓ Pain (uses)
✓ Sensory-perceptual alteration: visual, auditory (adverse reactions)
✓ Breathing pattern, ineffective (adverse reactions)
✓ Knowledge deficit (teaching)

Implementation

- Give with antiemetic if nausea, vomiting occur
- Give when pain is beginning to return; determine dosage interval by patient response; continuous dosing of medication is more effective given prn
- Medication should be slowly withdrawn after long-term use to prevent withdrawal symptoms
- Store in light-resistant container at room temp
- May be given with food or milk to lessen GI upset
- ⊘ Do not crush, chew caps

Patient/family education

- Instruct patient to report any symptoms of CNS changes, allergic reactions; to avoid CNS depressants: alcohol, sedative/hypnotics for at least 24 hr after taking this drug
- Teach patient that dizziness, drowsiness, and confusion are

common and to avoid getting up without assistance
• Discuss in detail all aspects of the drug

Evaluation

Positive therapeutic outcome
• Decreased pain
• Decreased cough

Treatment of overdose: Naloxone HCl (Narcan) 0.2-0.8 **IV**, O_2, **IV** fluids, vasopressors

hydrocortisone/ hydrocortisone acetate/hydrocortisone valerate (℞)

(hye-droe-kor′ti-sone)

Aeroseb-HC, A-Hydrocort, Ala-Cort, Ala-Scalp, Alphaderm, Bactine Hydrocortisone, Caldecort Anti-Itch, Cetacort, Cortaid, Cortaid Maximum Strength, Cort-Dome, Cortef, Cortef Acetate, Cortef Feminine Itch, Cortenema Acticort 100, Cortizone-5, Cortizone-10, Cortril, Delacort, Delcort, Dermacort, Dermicort, Dermolate Anti-Itch, Dermtex HC, HI-COR-1.0, HI-COR-2.5, Hycort, Hydrocortone, Hydrocortone Acetate, Hydrocortone Phosphate, HydroTex, Hytone, Lacticare-HC, Nutracort, Penecort 1% HC, Solu-Cortef, S-T Cort, Synacort, Tega-Cort, Tega-Cort Forte, Texacort, Westcort

Func. class.: Short-acting glucocorticoid

Chem. class.: Natural nonfluorinated, group IV potency (valerate), group VI potency (acetate and plain)

Pregnancy category C

Action: Decreases inflammation by suppressing migration of polymorphonuclear leukocytes and fibroblasts and reversing increased capillary permeability and lysosomal stabilization (systemic); antipruritic, antiinflammatory (top)

H

Therapeutic Outcome: Decreased inflammation

Uses: Severe inflammation, septic shock, adrenal insufficiency, ulcerative colitis, collagen disorders (systemic), psoriasis, eczema, contact dermatitis, pruritus (top)

Dosage and routes

Adrenal insufficiency/inflammation

Adult: PO 5-30 mg bid-qid; IM/**IV** 100-250 mg (succinate), then 50-100 mg IM as needed; IM/**IV** 15-240 mg q12h (phosphate)

Shock

Adult: 500 mg-2 g q2-6h (succinate)

P ***Child:*** IM/**IV** 0.16-1 mg/kg bid-tid (succinate)

Colitis

Adult: Enema 100 mg nightly for 21 days

Top

P ***Adult and child >2 yr:*** Apply to affected area qd-qid

Available forms: Oint 0.5%, 1%, 2.5%; cream 0.25%, 0.5%, 1%, 2.5%; lotion 0.25%, 0.5%, 1%, 2%, 2.5%; gel 1%; sol 1%; aerosol/pump spray 0.5%; *acetate:* oint 0.5%, 1%, 2.5%; cream 0.5%; lotion 0.05%; aerosol 1%; *valerate:* oint 0.2%; cream 0.2% (many others)

Adverse effects

CNS: Depression, flushing, sweating, headache, mood changes

CV: Hypertension, circulatory collapse, thrombophlebitis, embolism, tachycardia, edema

EENT: Fungal infections, increased intraocular pressure, blurred vision

GI: Diarrhea, nausea, abdominal distention, *GI hemorrhage,* increased appetite, pancreatitis

HEMA: Thrombocytopenia

INTEG: Acne, poor wound healing, ecchymosis, petechiae (top) burning, dryness, itching, irritation, acne, folliculitis, hypertrichosis, perioral dermatitis, hypopigmentation, atrophy, striae, miliaria, allergic contact dermatitis, secondary infection

MS: Fractures, osteoporosis, weakness

Contraindications: Psychosis, hypersensitivity, idiopathic thrombocytopenia, acute glomerulonephritis, amebiasis, fungal infections, nonasthmatic
P bronchial disease, child <2 yr, AIDS, TB, fungal infections (top)

Precautions: Pregnancy **C,** diabetes mellitus, glaucoma, osteoporosis, seizure disorders, ulcerative colitis, CHF, myasthenia gravis, renal disease, esophagitis, peptic ulcer, lactation, (top) viral infections, bacterial infections

Pharmacokinetics

Absorption	Well absorbed (PO); systemic (top)
Distribution	Crosses placenta
Metabolism	Liver, extensively
Excretion	Kidney
Half-life	3-5 hr, adrenal suppression 3-4 days

Pharmacodynamics

	PO	IM	IV	TOP
Onset	1-2 hr	20 min	Rapid	Min to hr
Peak	1 hr	4-8 hr	Unkn	Hr to days
Duration	1½ days	1½ days	1½ days	Hr to days

Interactions

Individual drugs

Amphotericin B: ↑ hypokalemia

Cholestyramine: ↓ action of hydrocortisone
Colestipol: ↓ action of hydrocortisone
Ephedrine: ↓ action of hydrocortisone
Insulin: ↑ need for insulin
Mezlocillin: ↑ hypokalemia
Phenytoin: ↓ action, ↑ metabolism
Rifampin: ↓ action, ↑ metabolism
Ticarcillin: ↑ hypokalemia
Theophylline: ↓ action of hydrocortisone

Drug classifications
Anticoagulants: ↓ action of anticoagulant
Barbiturates: ↓ action, ↑ metabolism
Diuretics: ↑ hypokalemia
Hypoglycemic agents: ↑ need for hypoglycemic agents

Lab test interferences
↑ Cholesterol, ↑ sodium, ↑ blood glucose, ↑ uric acid, ↑ calcium, ↑ urine glucose
↓ Calcium, ↓ potassium, ↓ T_4, ↓ T_3, ↓ thyroid ^{131}I uptake test, ↓ urine 17-OHCS, ↓ 17KS, ↓ PBI
False negative: Skin allergy tests

NURSING CONSIDERATIONS

Assessment

- Monitor potassium, blood sugar, urine glucose while patient on long-term therapy; hypokalemia and hyperglycemia may occur
- Monitor I&O ratio; be alert for decreasing urinary output and increasing edema; weigh daily; notify prescriber of weekly gain >5 lb or edema, hypertension, cardiac symptoms
- Monitor plasma cortisol levels during long-term therapy (normal level is 138-635 nmol/L when drawn at 8 AM); check adrenal function periodically for HPA axis suppression
- Assess for infection: increased temp, WBC even after withdrawal of medication; drug masks infection symptoms; if fever develops, drug should be discontinued
- Check for potassium depletion: paresthesias, fatigue, nausea, vomiting, depression, polyuria, dysrhythmias, weakness
- Assess mental status: affect, mood, behavioral changes, aggression
- Check nasal passages during long-term treatment for changes in mucus (nasal)
- Assess for systemic absorption: increased temp, inflammation, irritation (top)

Nursing diagnoses

✓ Infection, risk for (adverse reactions)
✓ Knowledge deficit (teaching)
✓ Noncompliance (teaching) (top/nasal preparation)

Implementation

PO route

- Give with food or milk to decrease GI symptoms

IV **IV route**

- Give only sodium phosphate product **IV**; reconstitute with sol provided; give 100 mg over >1 min
- May be given by intermittent inf in compatible sol
- Give titrated dose; use lowest effective dosage

Sodium phosphate preparations
Syringe compatibilities: Fluconazole, fludarabine, metoclopramide

H

Additive compatibilities: Amphotericin B, bleomycin, dacarbazine

Y-*site compatibilities:* Amifostine, thiotepa

Sodium succinate preparations

Syringe compatibilities: Metoclopramide, thiopental

Y-*site compatibilities:* Acyclovir, amifostine, aminophylline, ampicillin, amrinone, atracurium, atropine, betamethasone, calcium gluconate, cephalothin, cephapirin, chlordiazepoxide, chlorpromazine, cyanocobalamin, dexamethasone, digoxin, diphenhydramine, dopamine, droperidol, edrophonium, enalaprilat, epinephrine, esmolol, conjugated estrogens, ethacrynate, famotidine, fentanyl, fentanyl/droperidol, filgrastim, fludarabine, fluorouracil, foscarnet, furosemide, hydralazine, regular insulin, isoproterenol, kanamycin, lidocaine, lorazepam, magnesium sulfate, melphalan, menadiol, meperidine, methicillin, methoxamine, methylergonovine, minocycline, morphine, neostigmine, norepinephrine, ondansetron, oxacillin, oxytocin, paclitaxel, pancuronium, penicillin G potassium, pentazocine, phytonadione, prednisolone, procainamide, prochlorperazine, propranolol, pyridostigmine, scopolamine, sodium bicarbonate, succinylcholine, tacrolimus, teniposide, thiotepa, trimethobenzamide, vecuronium, vinorelbine

Y-*site incompatibilities:* Diazepam, ergotamine tartrate, idarubicin, phenytoin, sargramostim

Additive compatibilities: Aminophylline, amphotericin, daunorubicin, mitomycin, mitoxantrone, potassium chloride

Additive incompatibilities: Bleomycin, doxorubicin

Rec route

- Use applicator provided
- Clean applicator after each use

Top route

- Apply only to affected areas; do not get in eyes
- Cleanse and dry area before applying medication, then cover with occlusive dressing (only if prescribed); seal to normal skin; change q12h; syst absorption may occur; use only on dermatoses; do not use on weeping, denuded, or infected area
- Use for a few days after area has cleared
- Store at room temp

Nasal route

- Patient should clear nasal passages before administration; use decongestant if needed; shake inhaler, invert, tilt head backward, insert nozzle into nostril, away from septum; hold other nostril closed and depress activator, inhale through nose, exhale through mouth

Patient/family education

- Teach patient all aspects of drug usage, including cushingoid symptoms
- Advise patient that ID as steroid user should be carried; not to discontinue abruptly; adrenal crisis can result
- Instruct patient to notify prescriber if therapeutic response decreases; dosage adjustment may be needed
- Caution patient to avoid

OTC products unless directed by perscriber: salicylates, alcohol in cough products, cold preparations

- Teach patient symptoms of adrenal insufficiency: nausea, anorexia, fatigue, dizziness, dyspnea, weakness, joint pain, and when to notify prescriber
- Advise patient that long-term therapy may be needed to clear infection (1-2 mo depending on type of infection)

Nasal route

- Instruct patient to clear nasal passages if sneezing attack occurs, then repeat dose; to continue using product even if mild nasal bleeding occurs; bleeding is usually transient
- Teach method of instillation after providing written instruction from manufacturer on instillation

Evaluation

Positive therapeutic outcome

- Decrease in runny nose (nasal)
- Ease of respirations, decreased inflammation
- Absence of severe itching, patches on skin, flaking (top)

hydromorphone (℞)
(hye-droe-mor'fone)
Dihydromorphinone, Dilaudid, Dilaudid-HP, Dilaudid Cough Syrup (combination with guaifenesin/alcohol)
Func. class.: Antitussive, narcotic; opioid analgesic agonist
Chem. class.: Phenanthrene derivative, guaifenesin
Pregnancy category C
Controlled substance schedule II

H

Action: Depresses pain impulse transmission at the spinal cord level by interacting with opioid receptors; increases respiratory tract fluid by decreasing surface tension and adhesiveness, which increases removal of mucus; analgesic, antitussive

Therapeutic Outcome: Decreased cough, decreased pain

Uses: As an antitussive to suppress cough; moderate to severe pain

Dosage and routes

Antitussive

Adult: PO 1 mg q3-4h prn

P ***Child 6-12 yr:*** PO 0.5 mg q3-4h prn

Analgesic

Adult: PO 2 mg q3-6h prn; may increase to 4 mg q4-6h; SC/IM 1-2 mg q3-6h prn; may increase to 3-4 mg q4-6h; **IV** 0.5-1 mg q3h prn; rec 3 mg q4-8h prn

Available forms: Syr 1 mg/5 ml; tabs 1, 2, 3, 4 mg; inj 2, 3, 4, 10 mg/ml; supp 3 mg

Adverse effects

CNS: Dizziness, drowsiness, *sedation, confusion,* headache, euphoria, dreaming, hallucinations
CV: Hypotension, bradycardia
EENT: Miosis, diplopia, blurred vision
GI: Nausea, constipation, vomiting, anorexia
GU: Retention
INTEG: Urticaria, rash, sweating, flushing
RESP: Respiratory depression

Contraindications: Hypersensitivity, increased intracranial pressure, status asthmaticus

Precautions: Hypothyroidism, Addison's disease, CNS depression, brain tumor, asthma, hepatic disease, renal disease, COPD, psychosis, alcoholism, convulsive disorders, pregnancy **C**

Pharmacokinetics

Absorption	Well absorbed (PO), complete (IV)
Distribution	Unknown; crosses placenta
Metabolism	Liver, extensively
Excretion	Kidneys
Half-life	2-3 hr

Pharmacodynamics

	PO/IM/SC	IV	REC
Onset	15-30 min	10-15 min	15-30 min
Peak	30-60 min	15-30 min	30-90 min
Duration	4-5 hr	2-3 hr	4-5 hr

Interactions

Individual drugs

Alcohol: ↑ respiratory depression, hypotension, sedation
Nalbuphine: ↓ analgesia
Pentazocine: ↓ analgesia

Drug classifications

Antihistamines: ↑ respiratory depression, hypotension
Antidepressants: ↑ respiratory depression, hypotension
CNS depressants: ↑ respiratory depression, hypotension
MAOI: Serious reactions; dosage should be reduced
Phenothiazines: ↑ respiratory depression, hypotension
Sedative/hypnotics: ↑ respiratory depression, hypotension

Lab test interferences

↑ Amylase, ↑ lipase

NURSING CONSIDERATIONS

Assessment

- Monitor VS after parenteral route; note muscle rigidity, drug history, liver, kidney function tests, respiratory dysfunction: respiratory depression, character, rate, rhythm; notify prescriber if respirations are <10/min
- Monitor CNS changes: dizziness, drowsiness, hallucinations, euphoria, LOC, pupil reaction
- Monitor allergic reactions: rash, urticaria

Nursing diagnoses

- ✓ Pain (uses)
- ✓ Sensory-perceptual alteration: visual, auditory (adverse reactions)
- ✓ Breathing pattern, ineffective (adverse reactions)
- ✓ Knowledge deficit (teaching)

Implementation

- Give with antiemetic if nausea, vomiting occur
- Give when pain is beginning to return; determine dosage interval by patient response; continuous dosing of medication is more effective given prn; explain analgesic effect
- Withdraw medication slowly

after long-term use to prevent withdrawal symptoms

• Store in light-resistant container at room temp

PO route

• May be given with food or milk to lessen GI upset

IM/SC route

• Do not give if sol is cloudy or a precipitate has formed

IV **IV route**

• Give by direct **IV** after diluting with 5 ml or more sterile water or 0.9% NaCl for inj

• Give slowly at 2 mg over 3-5 min or less

Syringe compatibilities: Atropine, chlorpromazine, cimetidine, diphenhydramine, fentanyl, glycopyrrolate, haloperidol, hydroxyzine, midazolam, pentazocine, pentobarbital, promethazine, ranitidine, scopolamine, tetracaine, thiethylperazine, trimethobenzamide

Y-site compatibilities: Acyclovir, amifostine, amikacin, ampicillin, aztreonam, cefamandole, cefazolin, cefoperazone, ceforanide, cefotaxime, ceftazidime, cefoxitin, ceftizoxime, cefuroxime, cephalothin, cephapirin, chloramphenicol, cisplatin, clindamycin, doxycycline, erythromycin, fludarabine, foscarnet, gentamicin, granisetron, kanamycin, magnesium sulfate, melphalan, metronidazole, mezlocillin, moxalactam, nafcillin, ondansetron, oxacillin, paclitaxel, penicillin G potassium, piperacillin, teniposide, thiotepa, ticarcillin, tobramycin, trimethoprim/sulfamethoxazole, vancomycin, vinorelbine

Y-site incompatibilities: Ampicillin, diazepam, minocycline, phenobarbital, phenytoin, sargramostim

Solution compatibilities: D_5W, D_5/0.45% NaCl, D_5/0.9% NaCl, D_5/LR, D_5/Ringer's sol, 0.45% NaCl, 0.9% NaCl, Ringer's and lactated Ringer's sol

Additive incompatibilities: Sodium bicarbonate, thiopental

Patient/family education

• Instruct patient to report any symptoms of CNS changes, allergic reactions; to avoid CNS depressants: alcohol, sedative/hypnotics for at least 24 hr after taking this drug

• Advise patient that dizziness, drowsiness, and confusion are common and to avoid getting up without assistance

• Discuss in detail all aspects of the drug

Evaluation

Positive therapeutic outcome

• Decreased pain

• Decreased cough

Treatment of overdose: Naloxone HCl (Narcan) 0.2-0.8 IV, O_2, **IV** fluids, vasopressors

hydroxyurea (℞)

(hye-drox-ee-yoo-ree'ah)

Hydrea

Func. class.: Antineoplastic, antimetabolite

Chem. class.: Synthetic urea analog

Pregnancy category D

Action: Acts by inhibiting DNA synthesis without interfering with RNA or protein synthesis; incorporates thymidine into DNA, causing direct damage to DNA strands; S phase specific of cell cycle

➔ **Therapeutic Outcome:** Prevention of rapidly growing malignant cells

Uses: Melanoma, chronic myelocytic leukemia, recurrent or metastatic ovarian cancer, squamous cell carcinoma of the head and neck

Dosage and routes
Solid tumors
Adult: PO 80 mg/kg as a single dose q 3 days or 20-30 mg/kg as a single dose qd

In combination with radiation
Adult: PO 80 mg/kg as a single dose q 3 days; should be started 7 days before irradiation

Resistant chronic myelocytic leukemia
Adult: PO 20-30 mg/kg/day as a single daily dose

Available forms: Cap 500 mg

Adverse effects
CNS: Headache, confusion, hallucinations, dizziness, ***convulsions***
CV: Angina, ischemia
GI: Nausea, vomiting, anorexia, diarrhea, stomatitis, constipation
GU: Increased BUN, uric acid, creatinine, temporary renal function impairment
HEMA: Leukopenia, anemia, thrombocytopenia
INTEG: *Rash*, urticaria, pruritus, dry skin

Contraindications: Hypersensitivity, leukopenia (<2500/mm^3), thrombocytopenia (<100,000/mm^3), anemia (severe), pregnancy **D**

Precautions: Renal disease (severe)

Pharmacokinetics	
Absorption	Well absorbed
Distribution	Crosses blood-brain barrier
Metabolism	Liver (50%)
Excretion	Kidneys, unchanged (50%)
Half-life	4 hr

Pharmacodynamics	
Onset	Unknown
Peak	2 hr
Duration	Unknown

Interactions
Individual drugs
Cyclophosphamide: ↑ cardiotoxicity, CHF
Radiation: ↑ toxicity, bone marrow suppression
Drug classifications
Antineoplastics: ↑ toxicity, bone marrow suppression
Lab test interferences
↑ Renal function studies

NURSING CONSIDERATIONS
Assessment
- Assess buccal cavity q8h for dryness, sores or ulceration, white patches, oral pain, bleeding, dysphagia; obtain prescription for viscous lidocaine (Xylocaine)
- Assess symptoms indicating severe allergic reaction: rash, pruritus, urticaria, purpuric skin lesions, itching, flushing
- Monitor CBC, differential, platelet count weekly; withhold drug if WBC count is <4000/mm^3 or platelet count is <100,000/mm^3; notify prescriber of results if WBC <20,000/mm^3, platelets <150,000/mm^3
- Assess for increased uric acid levels, swelling, joint pain primarily in extremities; patient

should be well hydrated to prevent urate deposits

- Monitor renal function studies: BUN, creatinine, serum uric acid, urine CrCl before and during therapy; I&O ratio; report fall in urine output to <30 ml/hr
- Monitor temp q4h (may indicate beginning of infection)
- Monitor liver function tests before and during therapy (bilirubin, AST [SGOT], ALT [SGPT], LDH) as needed or monthly
- Assess for bleeding: hematuria, stool guaiac, bruising or petechiae, mucosa or orifices q8h; check for inflammation of mucosa, breaks in skin

Nursing diagnoses

- ✓ Injury, risk for (adverse reactions)
- ✓ Body image disturbance (adverse reactions)
- ✓ Infection, risk for (adverse reactions)
- ✓ Knowledge deficit (teaching)

Implementation

- Avoid contact with skin, very irritating; wash completely to remove
- Give fluids **IV** or PO before chemotherapy to hydrate patient
- Give antiemetic 30-60 min before giving drug and prn to prevent vomiting; antibiotics for prophylaxis of infection
- Provide liq diet: carbonated beverages; gelatin may be added if patient is not nauseated or vomiting
- Provide rinsing of mouth tid-qid with water, club soda; brushing of teeth bid-qid with soft brush or cotton-tipped applicators for stomatitis; use unwaxed dental floss
- For difficulty swallowing, cap contents may be mixed with water
- ⊘ Do not crush or chew caps

Patient/family education

- Advise patient that contraceptive measures are recommended during therapy
- Teach patient to avoid use of products containing aspirin or ibuprofen, razors, commercial mouthwash, since bleeding may occur; instruct patient to report symptoms of bleeding (hematuria, tarry stools)
- Instruct patient to report signs of anemia (fatigue, headache, irritability, faintness, shortness of breath)
- Advise patient to report any changes in breathing or coughing even several mo after treatment; to avoid crowds and persons with respiratory tract or other infections
- Caution patient not to have any vaccinations without the advice of the prescriber, serious reactions can occur

Evaluation

Positive therapeutic outcome

- Prevention of rapid division of malignant cells

hydroxyzine (℞)
(hye-drox'i-zeen)
Anxanil, Apo-hydroxyzine ✤, Atarax, Atarax 100, Durrex, E-Vista, Hydroxacen, Hydroxyzine HCl, hydroxyzine pamoate, Hyzine-50, Multipax ✤, Novohydroxyzine ✤, Quiess, Vistaject-25, Vistaject-50, Vistaquel 50, Vistaril, Vistazine 50
Func. class.: Sedative/hypnotic, antihistamine
Chem. class.: Piperazine derivative
Pregnancy category C

Action: Depresses subcortical levels of CNS, including limbic system, reticular formation; anticholinergic, antiemetic, antihistaminic responses

➡ **Therapeutic Outcome:** Absence of allergy symptoms, rhinitis, pruritus, absence of nausea/vomiting, sedation, absence of anxiety

Uses: Anxiety preoperatively, postoperatively to prevent nausea, vomiting; to potentiate narcotic analgesics; sedation; pruritus; prevention of alcohol, drug withdrawal

Dosage and routes
Adult: PO 25-100 mg tid-qid
P ***Child >6 yr:*** PO 50-100 mg/day in divided doses
P ***Child <6 yr:*** PO 50 mg/day in divided doses
Preoperatively/postoperatively
Adult: IM 25-100 mg q4-6h
P ***Child:*** IM 1.1 mg/kg q4-6h

Available forms: Tabs 10, 25, 50, 100 mg; caps 25, 50, 100 mg; syrup 100 mg/5 ml; oral susp 25 mg/5 ml; inj 25, 50 mg/ml

Adverse effects
CNS: Dizziness, drowsiness, confusion, headache, tremors, fatigue, depression, ***convulsions***
GI: Dry mouth

Contraindications: Hypersensitivity, pregnancy **C**

G **Precautions:** Elderly, debilitated patients, hepatic disease, renal disease

Pharmacokinetics

Absorption	Well absorbed
Distribution	Not known
Metabolism	Liver, completely
Excretion	Feces, bile
Half-life	3 hr

Pharmacodynamics

	PO/IM
Onset	15-30 min
Peak	2-4 hr
Duration	4-6 hr

Interactions
Individual drugs
Alcohol: ↑ CNS depression
Atropine: ↑ anticholinergic reactions
Disopyramide: ↑ anticholinergic reactions
Haloperidol: ↑ anticholinergic reactions
Quinidine: ↑ anticholinergic reactions
Drug classifications
Antidepressants: ↑ anticholinergic reactions
Antihistamines: ↑ anticholinergic reactions
CNS depressants: ↑ CNS depression
Narcotics: ↑ CNS depression
Phenothiazines: ↑ anticholinergic reactions
Sedative/hypnotics: ↑ CNS depression

Lab test interferences
False ↑ 17-OHCS

NURSING CONSIDERATIONS
Assessment
- Assess respiratory status: rate, rhythm, increase in bronchial secretions, wheezing, chest tightness; provide fluids to 2 L/day to decrease secretion thickness
- Monitor I&O ratio: be alert for urinary retention, frequency, dysuria, especially in G the elderly; drug should be discontinued if these occur
- Observe for drowsiness, dizziness
- Assess cough characteristics including type, frequency, thickness of secretions; evaluate response to this medication if using for cough

Nursing diagnoses
✓ Injury, risk for (side effects)
✓ Anxiety (uses)
✓ Knowledge deficit (teaching)

Implementation
PO route
- Give with meals if GI symptoms occur; absorption may be slightly decreased; cap may be opened and drug mixed with food/fluids for patients with swallowing difficulties

IM route
- Give IM inj in large muscle mass; aspirate to avoid **IV** administration; use Z-track method; severe necrosis can result with improper technique

Y-site compatibilities:
Aztreonam, ciprofloxacin, filgrastim, foscarnet, melphalan, sufentanil, teniposide, thiotepa, vinorelbine

Y-site incompatibility:
Paclitaxel

Syringe incompatibilities:
Aminophylline, chloramphenicol, dimenhydrinate, heparin, penicillin G potassium, pentobarbital, phenobarbital, phenytoin

Syringe compatibilities:
Atropine, benzquinamide, butorphanol, chlorpromazine, cimetidine, codeine, diphenhydramine, doxapram, droperidol, fentanyl, glycopyrrolate, hydromorphone, lidocaine, meperidine, metoclopramide, morphine, nalbuphine, oxymorphone, pentazocine, procaine, prochlorperazine, promazine, scopolamine

H

Patient/family education
- Caution patient to avoid hazardous activities and activities requiring alertness, since dizziness may occur; instruct patient to request assistance with ambulation
- Advise patient to avoid alcohol, other CNS depressants including cough, cold preparations; CNS depression may occur
- Teach all aspects of drug use; to notify prescriber if confusion, sedation, hypotension occur; to avoid driving and other hazardous activity if drowsiness occurs; to avoid alcohol and other CNS depressants that may potentiate effect
- Instruct patient to take 1 hr pc or 2 hr ac to facilitate absorption
- May crush if patient unable to swallow whole
- Caution patient not to exceed recommended dosage; dysrhythmias may occur
- Tell patient hard candy, gum, frequent rinsing of mouth may be used for dryness

Evaluation

Positive therapeutic outcome

- Absence of nausea, vomiting
- Decreased anxiety

Treatment of overdose: Lavage if orally ingested, VS, supportive care, **IV** norepinephrine for hypotension

ibuprofen 🔑 (OTC)

(eye-byoo-proe'fen)

Aches-N-Pain, Actiprofen ✤, Advil, Amersol ✤, Apo-Ibuprofen ✤, Children's Advil, Excedrin IB, Genpril, Haltran, Ibuprin, ibuprofen, Ibuprohm, I-Tab, Medipren, Menadol, Midol-200, Motrin, Motrin IB, Motrin Junior Strength, Novoprosen ✤, Nuprin, Pamprin-IB, Rufen, Saleto-200, Saleto-400, Saleto-600, Saleto-800, Trendar

Func. class.: Nonsteroidal antiinflammatory; nonnarcotic analgesic

Chem. class.: Propionic acid derivative

Pregnancy category B

Action: Inhibits prostaglandin synthesis by decreasing enzyme needed for biosynthesis; analgesic, antiinflammatory, antipyretic

➔ **Therapeutic Outcome:** Decreased pain, inflammation, fever

Uses: Rheumatoid arthritis, osteoarthritis, primary dysmenorrhea, gout, dental pain, musculoskeletal disorders, fever

Dosage and routes

Analgesia

Adult: PO 200-400 mg q4-6h, not to exceed 3.2 g/day

Antipyretic

P ***Child 6 mo-12yr:*** PO 5 mg/kg (temp <102.5° F), 10 mg/kg (temp >102.5° F), may repeat q4-6h; max 40 mg/kg/day

Anti-inflammatory

Adult: PO 300-800 mg tid-qid; max 3.2 g/day

P ***Child:*** PO 30-40 mg/kg/day in 3-4 divided doses; max 50 mg/kg/day

Available forms: Tabs 200, 300, 400, 600, 800 mg; oral susp 100 mg/5 ml, tab, chew 100 mg

Adverse effects

CNS: Dizziness, drowsiness, fatigue, tremors, confusion, insomnia, anxiety, depression

CV: Tachycardia, peripheral edema, palpitations, dysrhythmias, hypertension

EENT: Tinnitus, hearing loss, blurred vision

GI: Nausea, anorexia, vomiting, diarrhea, jaundice, ***cholestatic hepatitis,*** constipation, flatulence, cramps, dry mouth, peptic ulcer

GU: ***Nephrotoxicity;*** dysuria, hematuria, oliguria, azotemia

HEMA: ***Blood dyscrasias***

INTEG: Purpura, rash, pruritus, sweating

Contraindications: Hypersensitivity, asthma, severe renal disease, severe hepatic disease

Precautions: Pregnancy **B** 1st and 2nd trimesters, lactation, P children, bleeding disorders, GI disorders, cardiac disorders, hypersensitivity to other antiinflammatory agents

Pharmacokinetics

Absorption	Well absorbed
Distribution	Not known; crosses placenta
Metabolism	Liver, extensively
Excretion	Kidneys, unchanged (10%)
Half-life	3½ hr

Pharmacodynamics

Onset	½ hr
Peak	1-2 hr
Duration	4-6 hr

Interactions
Individual drugs
Acetaminophen (long-term use): ↑ renal reactions
Alcohol: ↑ adverse reactions
Aspirin: ↓ effectiveness, ↑ adverse reactions
Coumadin: ↑ anticoagulant effects
Digoxin: ↑ toxicity, levels
Insulin: ↓ insulin effect
Lithium: ↑ toxicity
Methotrexate: ↑ toxicity
Phenytoin: ↑ toxicity
Probenecid: ↑ toxicity
Sulfonylurea: ↑ toxicity
Drug classifications
Anticoagulants: ↑ risk of bleeding
Antihypertensives: ↓ effect of antihypertensives
Antineoplastics: ↑ risk of hematologic toxicity
β-Blockers: ↑ antihypertension
Cephalosporins: ↑ risk of bleeding
Diuretics: ↓ effectiveness of diuretics
Glucocorticoids: ↑ adverse reactions
Hypoglycemics: ↓ hypoglycemic effect
NSAIDs: ↑ adverse reactions
Potassium supplements: ↑ adverse reactions
Radiation: ↑ risk of hematologic toxicity
Sulfonamides: ↑ toxicity
Lab test interferences
↑ Bleeding time

NURSING CONSIDERATIONS
Assessment
- Monitor liver function studies: AST (SGOT), ALT (SGPT), bilirubin, creatinine if patient is on long-term therapy
- Monitor renal function studies: BUN, urine creatinine if patient is on long-term therapy
- Monitor blood studies: CBC, Hct, Hgb, pro-time if patient is on long-term therapy
- Check I&O ratio; decreasing output may indicate renal failure if patient is on long-term therapy
- Assess hepatotoxicity: dark urine, clay-colored stools, yellowing of skin and sclera, itching, abdominal pain, fever, diarrhea if patient is on long-term therapy
- Assess for allergic reactions: rash, urticaria; if these occur, drug may have to be discontinued
- Assess for ototoxicity: tinnitus, ringing, roaring in ears; audiometric testing needed before, after long-term therapy
- Assess for visual changes: blurring, halos; may indicate corneal, retinal damage
- Identify prior drug history; there are many drug interactions
- Monitor pain: location, duration, type, intensity before dose and 1 hr after
- Monitor musculoskeletal status: ROM before dose and 1 hr after
- Identify fever: length of time

in evidence and related symptoms

Nursing diagnoses

- ✓ Pain (uses)
- ✓ Mobility, impaired (uses)
- ✓ Injury, risk for (side effects)
- ✓ Knowledge deficit (teaching)

Implementation

- Administer to patient crushed or whole; 800-mg tab may be dissolved in water
- Give with food or milk to decrease gastric symptoms; give 30 min pc or 2 hr ac; absorption may be slowed

Patient/family education

- Teach patient to report any symptoms of hepatotoxicity, renal toxicity, visual changes, ototoxicity, allergic reactions, bleeding if patient is on long-term therapy
- Caution patient not to exceed recommended dosage; acute poisoning may result
- Advise patient to read label on other OTC drugs
- Inform patient that the therapeutic response takes 1 mo (arthritis)
- Caution patient to avoid alcohol ingestion; GI bleeding may occur
- Advise patient with allergies that allergic reactions may develop

Evaluation

Positive therapeutic outcome

- Decreased pain
- Decreased inflammation
- Decreased fever
- Increased mobility

ibutilide (℞)

(eye-byoo′te-lide)

Covert

Func. class.: Antidysrhythmic (Class III)

Pregnancy category C

Action: Prolongs duration of action potential and effective refractory period; noncompetitive α- and β-adrenergic inhibition

→ **Therapeutic Outcome:** Decreased amount and severity of atrial fibrillation/flutter

Uses: Atrial fibrillation/flutter

Dosage and routes

Adult: **IV** inf (≥60 kg) 1 vial (1 mg) given over 10 min; **IV** inf (<60 kg) 0.1 mg/kg (0.01 mg/kg) given over 10 min

Available forms: Sol 0.1 mg/ml

Adverse effects

CNS: Headache

CV: Hypotension, bradycardia, ***sinus arrest***, CHF, dysrhythmias, hypertension, extrasystoles, ventricular tachycardia, bundle branch block, AV block

GI: Nausea

Contraindications: Hypersensitivity

Precautions: SN dysfunction, 2nd- or 3rd-degree AV block, electrolyte imbalances, pregnancy **C,** bradycardia, lactation, P children <18 yr, renal/hepatic, disease, G elderly

Pharmacokinetics

Absorption	Slow, variable
Distribution	Body tissues; crosses placenta
Metabolism	Liver
Excretion	Kidney
Half-life	15-100 days

Pharmacodynamics	
Onset	1-3 wk
Peak	2-10 hr
Duration	Up to months

Interactions

Individual drugs

Digoxin: ↑ blood levels, ↑ toxicity

Disopyramide: ↑ levels, ↑ toxicity

Flecainide: ↑ levels, ↑ toxicity

Phenytoin: ↑ blood levels

Procainamide: ↑ levels, ↑ toxicity

Quinidine: ↑ levels, ↑ toxicity

Drug classifications

Antidepressants, tricyclic/tetracyclic: prodysrhythmia

H_1-Receptor antagonists: ↑ prodysrhythmia

Phenothiazines: ↑ prodysrhythmia

NURSING CONSIDERATIONS

Assessment

- Monitor I&O ratio; monitor electrolytes: potassium, sodium, chloride
- Monitor liver function studies: AST (SGOT), ALT (SGPT), bilirubin, alkaline phosphatase
- Monitor ECG continuously to determine drug effectiveness; measure PR, QRS, QT intervals; check for PVCs, other dysrhythmias; monitor B/P continuously for hypotension, hypertension; check for rebound hypertension after 1-2 hr
- Monitor for dehydration or hypovolemia
- Assess for CNS symptoms: confusion, psychosis, numbness, depression, involuntary movements; if these occur drug should be discontinued
- Monitor cardiac rate, respiration; rate, rhythm, character, chest pain, ventricular tachycardia, supraventricular tachycardia or fibrillation

Nursing diagnoses

- ✓ Cardiac output, decreased (uses)
- ✓ Gas exchange, impaired (adverse reactions)
- ✓ Knowledge deficit (teaching)

Implementation

PO route

- Give reduced dosage slowly with ECG monitoring only
- Give with meals for GI upset

Patient/family education

- Instruct patient to report side effects immediately to prescriber
- Instruct patient to take medication as prescribed, not to double doses
- Instruct patient to complete follow-up appointment with health care provider, including pulmonary function studies, chest x-ray, ophthalmic examinations

Evaluation

Positive therapeutic outcome

- Decrease in atrial fibrillation/flutter

idarubicin (℞)

(eye-da-roo'bi-sin)

Idamycin

Func. class.: Antineoplastic, antibiotic

Chem. class.: Anthracycline glycoside

Pregnancy category D

Action: Inhibits DNS synthesis derived from daunorubicin by binding to DNA, which causes strand splitting; cell cycle specific (S phase); a vesicant

Therapeutic Outcome: Prevention of rapidly growing malignant cells

Uses: Used in combination with other antineoplastics for acute myelocytic leukemia in adults

Dosage and routes

Adult: **IV** 12 mg/m^2/day × 3 days in combination with cytosine arabinoside, or 25 mg/m^2 **IV** bolus followed by 200 mg/m^2/day × 5 days by cont inf

Available forms: Inj 5, 10 mg vials

Adverse effects

CNS: Fever, chills, headache
CV: ***Dysrhythmias, CHF, pericarditis, myocarditis,*** peripheral edema
GI: Nausea, vomiting, abdominal pain, mucositis, diarrhea, ***hepatotoxicity***
HEMA: ***Thrombocytopenia, leukopenia, anemia***
INTEG: Rash, extravasation, dermatitis, reversible alopecia, urticaria, thrombophlebitis at inj site

Contraindications: Hypersensitivity, pregnancy **D**

Precautions: Renal and hepatic disease, gout, bone marrow depression, children **P**

Pharmacokinetics	
Absorption	Complete bioavailability
Distribution	Rapidly distributed; high tissue binding
Metabolism	Liver, extensively
Excretion	Bile
Half-life	22 hr

Pharmacodynamics

Unknown

Interactions

Individual drugs

Radiation: ↑ toxicity, bone marrow suppression

Drug classifications

Antineoplastics: ↑ toxicity, bone marrow suppression

Lab test interferences

↑ Uric acid

NURSING CONSIDERATIONS

Assessment

- Assess symptoms indicating severe allergic reaction: rash, pruritus, urticaria, purpuric skin lesions, itching, flushing; drug should be discontinued
- Assess for tachypnea, ECG changes, dyspnea, edema, fatigue
- Monitor CBC, differential, platelet count weekly; withhold drug if WBC count is <4000/mm^3 or platelet count is <100,000/mm^3; notify prescriber of results if WBC <20,000/mm^3, platelets <150,000/mm^3
- Monitor temp q4h (may indicate beginning of infection)
- Monitor liver function tests before and during therapy (bilirubin, AST [SGOT], ALT [SGPT], LDH) as needed or monthly; note yellowing of skin and sclera, dark urine, clay-colored stools, itchy skin, abdominal pain, fever, diarrhea; hepatotoxicity can be severe
- Assess for bleeding: hematuria, stool guaiac, bruising or petechiae, mucosa or orifices q8h; assess for inflammation of mucosa, breaks in skin
- Identify effects of alopecia on body image; discuss feelings about body changes

Nursing diagnoses

- ✓ Injury, risk for (adverse reactions)
- ✓ Cardiac output, decreased (adverse reactions)
- ✓ Body image disturbance (adverse reactions)
- ✓ Infection, risk for (adverse reactions)
- ✓ Knowledge deficit (teaching)

Implementation

- Avoid contact with skin; very irritating; wash completely to remove
- Give fluids **IV** or PO before chemotherapy to hydrate patient
- Administer antiemetic 30-60 min before giving drug and prn to prevent vomiting; administer antibiotics for prophylaxis of infection
- Give a liq diet: carbonated beverages; gelatin may be added if patient is not nauseated or vomiting
- Provide rinsing of mouth tid-qid with water, club soda; brushing of teeth bid-qid with soft brush or cotton-tipped applicators for stomatitis; use unwaxed dental floss
- Drug should be prepared by experienced personnel using proper precautions (biologic cabinet, wearing gown, gloves, mask)
- Give after reconstituting 5-mg vial with 5 ml 0.9% NaCl (1 mg/1 ml); give over 10-15 min through Y-tube or 3-way stopcock of inf of D_5 or normal saline; discard unused portion
- Inject hydrocortisone for extravasation; apply ice compress after stopping inf
- Store at room temp for 3 days after reconstituting or 7 days refrigerated

Y-site compatibilities: Amifostine, amikacin, aztreonam, cimetidine, cyclophosphamide, cytarabine, diphenhydramine, droperidol, erythromycin, filgrastim, heparin, magnesium sulfate, mannitol, melphalan, metoclopramide, potassium chloride, ranitidine, sargramostim, thiotepa, vinorelbine

Y-site incompatibilities: Acyclovir, ampicillin/sulbactam, cefazolin, ceftazidine, clindamycin, dexamethasone, etoposide, furosemide, gentamicin, hydrocortisone, lorazepam, meperidine, methotrexate, mezlocillin, sargramostim, sodium bicarbonate, vancomycin, vincristine

Solution compatibilities: $D_{3.3}$/0.3% NaCl, D_5/0.9% NaCl, D_5W, Ringer's, 0.9% NaCl, LR

Patient/family education

- Teach patient to avoid use of products containing aspirin or ibuprofen, razors, commercial mouthwash, since bleeding may occur; to report symptoms of bleeding (hematuria, tarry stools)
- Instruct patient to report signs of anemia (fatigue, headache, irritability, faintness, shortness of breath)
- Advise patient that hair may be lost during treatment; a wig or hair piece may make patient feel better; new hair may be different in color, texture
- Tell patient not to have any vaccinations without the advice of the prescriber; serious reactions can occur
- Advise patient that contraception is needed during treatment and for several mo after the completion of therapy

I

Evaluation

Positive therapeutic outcome
- Prevention of rapid division of malignant cells

ifosfamide (℞)

(i-foss'fa-mide)

Ifex

Func. class.: Antineoplastic alkylating agent

Chem. class.: Nitrogen mustard

Pregnancy category D

Action: Alkylates DNA, RNA; inhibits enzymes that allow synthesis of amino acids in proteins; also responsible for cross-linking DNA strands; activity is not cell cycle stage specific

Therapeutic Outcome: Prevention of rapidly growing malignant cells

Uses: Testicular cancer

Dosage and routes

***Adult:* IV** 1.2 g/m^2/day × 5 days; repeat course q3 wk; give with mesna

Available forms: Inj 1, 3 g

Adverse effects

CNS: Facial paresthesia, fever, malaise, somnolence, confusion, depression, hallucinations, dizziness, disorientation, ***seizures, coma***

GI: Nausea, vomiting, anorexia, ***hepatotoxicity,*** stomatitis, constipation

GU: Hematuria, nephrotoxicity, hemorrhagic cystitis, dysuria, urinary frequency

HEMA: Thrombocytopenia, leukopenia, anemia

INTEG: Dermatitis, alopecia, pain at inj site

Contraindications: Hypersensitivity, bone marrow suppression, pregnancy **D**

Precautions: Renal disease, lactation, children

Pharmacokinetics

Absorption	Complete bioavailability
Distribution	Saturation at high dosages
Metabolism	Liver
Excretion	Breast milk
Half-life	15 hr

Pharmacodynamics

Unknown

Interactions

Individual drugs

Radiation: ↑ toxicity, bone marrow suppression

Drug classifications

Antineoplastics: ↑ toxicity, bone marrow suppression

NURSING CONSIDERATIONS

Assessment

- Monitor CBC, differential, platelet count weekly; withhold drug if WBC is <4000 or platelet count is <75,000; notify prescriber of results if WBC <20,000/mm^3, platelets <150,000/mm^3
- Monitor renal function studies: BUN, serum uric acid, urine CrCl before, during therapy; I&O ratio; report fall in urine output of 30 ml/hr
- Monitor for cold, fever, sore throat (may indicate beginning infection); identify edema in feet and joints, stomach pain, shaking; prescriber should be notified
- Assess for bleeding: hematuria, guaiac, bruising or pete chiae, mucosa or orifices q8h; no rec temp

Nursing diagnoses

✓ Injury, risk for (adverse reactions)

✓ Body image disturbance (adverse reactions)
✓ Infection, risk for (adverse reactions)
✓ Knowledge deficit (teaching)

Implementation

• Give fluids **IV** or PO before chemotherapy to hydrate patient
• Give antiemetic 30-60 min before giving drug and prn to prevent vomiting
• Provide liq diet: carbonated beverages; gelatin may be added if patient is not nauseated or vomiting
• Give **IV** after diluting 1 g/20 ml sterile or bacteriostatic water for inj with parabens or benzyl only; shake
• Give by intermittent inf after further diluting with D_5W, LR, 0.9% NaCl, sterile water for inj (1 g/20 ml = 50 mg/ml); (1 g/50 ml = 20 mg/ml; 1 g/200 ml = 5 mg/ml); give over 30 min
• Store powder at room temp; always give with mesna to prevent ifosfamide-induced hemorrhagic cystitis

Syringe compatibility:
Mesna

Y-site compatibilities:
Allopurinol, amifostine, aztreonam, filgrastim, fludarabine, granisetron, melphalan, paclitaxel, ondansetron, sargramostim, teniposide, thiotepa, vinorelbine

Additive compatibilities:
Carboplatin, cisplatin, epirubicin, etoposide, fluorouracil, mesna

Patient/family education

• Teach patient to avoid use of products containing aspirin or ibuprofen, razors, commercial mouthwash, since bleeding may occur; to report symptoms of bleeding (hematuria, tarry stools)
• Instruct patient to report signs of anemia (fatigue, headache, irritability, faintness, shortness of breath)
• Advise patient to report any changes in breathing or coughing even several mo after treatment; to avoid crowds and persons with respiratory tract or other infections
• Teach patient that hair loss is common; discuss the use of wigs or hair pieces
• Caution patient not to have any vaccinations without the advice of the prescriber; serious reactions can occur
• Advise patient contraception is needed during treatment and for several mo after the completion of therapy

Evaluation

Positive therapeutic outcome
• Prevention of rapid division of malignant cells
• Absence of swelling at night
• Increased appetite, increased weight

imipenem/cilastatin (℞)

(i-me-pen′em sye-la-stat′in)
Primaxin IM, Primaxin IV
Func. class.: Antiinfective; miscellaneous penicillin
Pregnancy category C

Action: Interferes with cell wall replication of susceptible organisms; osmotically unstable cell wall swells and bursts from osmotic pressure; addition of cilastatin prevents renal inactivation that occurs with high urinary concentrations of imipenem

➔ **Therapeutic Outcome:** Bactericidal action against the following: *Streptococcus pneumoniae*, group A β-hemolytic streptococci, *Staphylococcus aureus*, enterococcus; gram-negative organisms: *Klebsiella*, *Proteus*, *Escherichia coli*, *Acinetobacter*, *Serratia*, *Pseudomonas aeruginosa*; *Salmonella*, *Shigella*

Uses: Serious infections caused by gram-positive or gram-negative organisms

Dosage and routes

Adult: **IV** 250-500 mg q6h; severe infections may require 1 g q6h; may give IM q12h (total daily IM dose >1500 mg not recommended)

Available forms: **IV** inj 250, 500; IM inj 500, 750 mg

Adverse effects

CNS: Fever, somnolence, ***seizures***, dizziness, weakness
CV: Hypotension, palpitations
GI: Diarrhea, nausea, vomiting, ***pseudomembranous colitis***, ***hepatitis***, glossitis
HEMA: Eosinophilia, ***neutropenia***, decreased HGb, Hct
INTEG: Rash, urticaria, pruritus, pain at inj site, phlebitis, erythema at inj site
RESP: Chest discomfort, dyspnea, hyperventilation
SYST: ***Anaphylaxis***

Contraindications: Hypersensitivity, IM hypersensitivity to local anesthetics of the amide type

Precautions: Pregnancy **C**, G lactation, elderly, hypersensitivity to penicillins, seizure disor- P ders, renal disease, children

Pharmacokinetics

Absorption	Complete bioavailability (IV)
Distribution	Widely distributed; crosses placenta
Metabolism	Liver
Excretion	Kidneys, unchanged (70%); breast milk
Half-life	1 hr; increased in renal disease

Pharmacodynamics

	IV	IM
Onset	Rapid	Unknown
Peak	½-1 hr	Unknown

Interactions

Individual drugs

Ganciclovir: ↑ seizures
Probenecid: ↓ renal excretion, ↑ blood level

Drug classifications

Cephalosporins: ↓ action
Penicillins: ↓ action

Lab test interferences

False ↑ Creatinine (serum urine), ↑ urinary 17-KS
False positive: Urinary protein, direct Coombs' test, urine glucose
Interference: Cross-matching

NURSING CONSIDERATIONS

Assessment

- Assess patient for previous sensitivity reaction
- Assess patient for signs and symptoms of infection, including characteristics of wounds, sputum, urine, stool, WBC >10,000, fever; obtain baseline information before and during treatment
- Complete C&S tests before beginning drug therapy to identify if correct treatment has been initiated
- Assess for allergic reactions: rash, urticaria, pruritus, chills, fever, joint pain; angioedema may occur a few days after therapy begins; epinephrine,

resuscitation equipment should be available for anaphylactic reaction

- Identify urine output; if decreasing, notify prescriber (may indicate nephrotoxicity); also check for increased BUN, creatinine
- Monitor blood studies: AST (SGOT), ALT (SGPT), CBC, Hct, bilirubin, LDH, alkaline phosphatase, Coombs' test monthly if patient is on long-term therapy
- Monitor electrolytes: potassium, sodium, chloride monthly if patient is on long-term therapy
- Assess bowel pattern qd; if severe diarrhea occurs, drug should be discontinued; may indicate pseudomembranous colitis
- Monitor for bleeding: ecchymosis, bleeding gums, hematuria, stool guaiac daily if on long-term therapy
- Assess for overgrowth of infection: perineal itching, fever, malaise, redness, pain, swelling, drainage, rash, diarrhea, change in cough, sputum

Nursing diagnoses

- ✓ Infection, risk for (uses)
- ✓ Diarrhea (adverse reactions)
- ✓ Injury, risk for (adverse reactions)
- ✓ Knowledge deficit (teaching)
- ✓ Noncompliance (teaching)

Implementation

IM route

- Reconstitute 500 mg/2 ml or 750 mg/3 ml lidocaine without epinephrine; shake well, withdraw and administer entire vial; give deep in large muscle mass, massage

IV **IV route**

- Reconstitute each 250 or 500 mg/10 ml of compatible diluent; shake well; transfer the resulting susp to not less than 100 ml of compatible diluent; add 10 ml to each previously reconstituted vial and shake to ensure all medication is used; transfer the remaining contents of the vial to the inf container; do not administer susp by direct inj; reconstitute 120-ml inf bottles/100 ml of a compatible diluent; shake until clear; may use 0.9% NaCl, D_5W, $D_{10}W$, D_5/0.2% sodium bicarbonate, D_5/0.9% NaCl, D_5/0.45% NaCl, D_5/0.225% NaCl, mannitol 2.5%, 5%, or 10%
- Give by intermittent inf: each 250- or 500-mg dose over 20-30 min, and each 1-g dose over 40-60 min; administer over 15-20 min for P pediatric patients; do not administer direct **IV**; do not admix with other antibiotics

Y-site compatibilities: Acyclovir, amifostine, aztreonam, cefepime, diltiazem, famotidine, filgrastim, fludarabine, foscarnet, idarubicin, regular insulin, melphalan, methotrexate, ondansetron, tacrolimus, teniposide, thiotepa, vinorelbine, zidovudine

Y-site incompatibilities: Fluconazole, meperidine, sargramostim

Additive incompatibilities: Fluconazole, meperidine, sargramostim

Patient/family education

- Teach patient to report sore throat, bruising, bleeding, joint pain; may indicate blood dyscrasias (rare)
- Advise patient to contact prescriber if vaginal itching,

loose, foul-smelling stools, furry tongue occur; may indicate superinfection
• Advise patient to notify prescriber of diarrhea with blood or pus, which may indicate pseudomembranous colitis

Evaluation

Positive therapeutic outcome
• Absence of signs/symptoms of infection (WBC <10,000, temp WNL, absence of red, draining wounds)
• Reported improvement in symptoms of infection

Treatment of anaphylaxis: Epinephrine, antihistamines, resuscitate if needed

imipramine ⊶ (℞)

(im-ip'ra-meen)
Apo-Imipramine ♣, Imipramine HCl, Impril ♣, Janimine, Novo-Pramine ♣, SK-Pramine, Tipramine, Tofranil, Tofranil PM
Func. class.: Antidepressant, tricyclic
Chem. class.: Dibenzazepine, tertiary amine
Pregnancy category C

Action: Blocks reuptake of norepinephrine and serotonin into nerve endings, increasing action of norepinephrine and serotonin in nerve cells; has anticholinergic effects

➔ **Therapeutic Outcome:** Decreased symptoms of depression after 2-3 wk; decreased P bedwetting in children

Uses: Depression, enuresis in P children

Investigational uses: Chronic pain, migraine headaches, cluster headaches as adjunct

Dosage and routes

Adult: PO/IM 75-100 mg/day in divided doses; may increase by 25-50 mg up to 200 mg, not to exceed 300 mg/day; may give daily dose hs

P ***Child:*** PO 25-75 mg/day

Available forms: Tabs 10, 25, 50 mg; inj 25 mg/2 ml; caps 75, 100, 125, 150 mg

Adverse effects

CV: Orthostatic hypotension, ECG changes, tachycardia, ***hypertension,*** palpitations
CNS: Dizziness, drowsiness, confusion, headache, anxiety, tremors, stimulation, weakness, insomnia, nightmares, G extrapyramidal symptoms (elderly), increased psychiatric symptoms, paresthesia
EENT: Blurred vision, tinnitus, mydriasis
GI: Diarrhea, dry mouth, nausea, vomiting, ***paralytic ileus,*** increased appetite, cramps, epigastric distress, jaundice, ***hepatitis,*** stomatitis
GU: Retention, ***acute renal failure***
HEMA: ***Agranulocytosis, thrombocytopenia, eosinophilia, leukopenia***
INTEG: Rash, urticaria, sweating, pruritus, photosensitivity

Contraindications: Hypersensitivity to tricyclic antidepressants, recovery phase of MI, convulsive disorders, prostatic hypertrophy

Precautions: Suicidal patients, severe depression, increased intraocular pressure, narrow-angle glaucoma, urinary retention, cardiac disease, hepatic disease, hyperthyroidism, electroshock therapy, elective **G** surgery, elderly, pregnancy **C**

Pharmacokinetics

Absorption	Well absorbed
Distribution	Widely distributed; crosses placenta
Metabolism	Liver, extensively
Excretion	Kidneys, breast milk
Half-life	6-20 hr

Pharmacodynamics

	PO	IM
Onset	1 hr	1 hr
Peak	Unknown	Unknown
Duration	Unknown	Unknown

Interactions

Individual drugs

Alcohol: ↑ CNS depression
Cimetidine: ↑ levels, toxicity
Clonidine: Severe hypotension; avoid use
Disulfiram: Organic brain syndrome
Fluoxetine: ↑ levels, toxicity
Guanethidine: ↓ effects

Drug classifications

Analgesics: ↑ CNS depression
Anticholinergics: ↑ side effects
Antihistamines: ↑ CNS depression
Antihypertensives: May block antihypertensive effect
Barbiturates: ↑ effects
Benzodiazepines: ↑ effects
CNS depressants: ↑ effects
MAOI: Hypertensive crisis, convulsions
Oral contraceptives: ↑ effects, toxicity
Phenothiazines: ↑ toxicity
Sedative/hypnotics: ↑ CNS depression
Sympathomimetics, indirect acting: ↓ effects

Smoking

↑ metabolism, ↓ effects

Lab test interferences

↑ Serum bilirubin, ↑ blood glucose, ↑ alkaline phosphatase
↓ VMA, ↓ 5-HIAA, ↓ blood glucose
False ↑ Urinary catecholamines

NURSING CONSIDERATIONS

Assessment

- Monitor B/P (with patient lying, standing), pulse q4h; if systolic B/P drops 20 mm Hg, hold drug, notify prescriber; take vital signs q4h in patients with cardiovascular disease
- Monitor blood studies: CBC, leukocytes, differential, cardiac enzymes if patient is receiving long-term therapy
- Monitor hepatic studies: AST (SGOT), ALT (SGPT), bilirubin
- Check weight weekly; appetite may increase with drug
- Assess ECG for flattening of T wave, bundle branch block, AV block, dysrhythmias in cardiac patients
- Assess for extrapyramidal **G** symptoms primarily in elderly: rigidity, dystonia, akathisia
- Assess mental status: mood, sensorium, affect, suicidal tendencies; increase in psychiatric symptoms: depression, panic
- Monitor urinary retention, constipation; constipation is **P** more likely to occur in children **G** or elderly
- **!** Assess for withdrawal symptoms: headache, nausea, vomiting, muscle pain, weakness; do not usually occur unless drug was discontinued abruptly
- Identify alcohol consumption; if alcohol is consumed, hold dose until AM

Nursing diagnoses

✓ Coping, ineffective individual (uses)

✓ Injury, risk for physical (side effects)
✓ Knowledge deficit (teaching)
✓ Noncompliance (teaching)

Implementation

PO route

- Give with food or milk
- ⊘ Do not crush, chew caps
- Store at room temp; do not freeze

IM route

- Put ampule under warm running water for 1 min to dissolve crystals; sol may be yellow or red

Patient/family education

- Teach patient that therapeutic effects may take 2-3 wk
- Teach patient to use caution in driving and other activities requiring alertness because of drowsiness, dizziness, blurred vision; to avoid rising quickly from sitting position, especially G elderly
- Teach patient to avoid alcohol ingestion, other CNS depressants
- Teach patient not to discontinue medication quickly after long-term use: may cause nausea, headache, malaise
- Teach patient to wear sunscreen or large hat, since photosensitivity occurs
- Teach patient to increase fluids, bulk in diet if constipation, urinary retention occur, G especially elderly
- Teach patient to take gum, hard sugarless candy, or frequent sips of water for dry mouth

Evaluation

Positive therapeutic outcome

- Decreased depression
- Absence of suicidal thoughts
- Decreased enuresis in children

Treatment of overdose: ECG monitoring, induce emesis, lavage, activated charcoal, administer anticonvulsant

immune globulin (℞)

gamma globulin, Gamimune N, Gammagard S/D, Gammar-P I.V., Iveegam, polygam, polygam S/D, Sandoglobulin, Venoglobulin-I, immune serum globulin

Func. class.: Immune serum

Chem. class.: IgG

Pregnancy category C

Action: Provides passive immunity to hepatitis A, measles, varicella, rubella, immune globulin deficiency; contains γ-globulin antibodies (IgG)

➔ **Therapeutic Outcome:** Absence of infection

Uses: Immunodeficiency syndrome, B-cell chronic lymphocytic leukemia, kawasaki syndrome, bone marrow transplantation, pediatric HIV infection, agammaglobulinemia, hepatitis A exposure, measles exposure, measles vaccine complications, purpura, rubella exposure, chickenpox exposure

Dosage and routes

Adult: IM 30-50 ml q mo; **IV** 100 mg/kg q mo, 0.01-0.02 ml/kg/min over 30 min (Gamimune); **IV** 200 mg/kg qmo, 0.05-1 ml/min over 15-30 min, then increase to 1.5-2.5 ml/min (Sandoglobulin)

P ***Child:*** IM 20-40 ml q mo

Hepatitis A exposure
P ***Adult and child:*** IM 0.02-0.04 ml/kg or 0.1 mg/kg if treatment is delayed

Hepatitis B exposure
P ***Adult and child:*** IM 0.06 ml/kg within 1 wk, q mo

Measles (postexposure)
P ***Child:*** IM 0.25 ml/kg within 6 days

Immunoglobulin deficiency
P ***Adult and child:*** IM 1.3 ml/kg, then 0.66 ml/kg after 2-4 wk and q2-4 wk thereafter

Idiopathic thrombocytopenic purpura
P ***Adult and child:*** **IV** 0.4 g/kg/day × 5 days or 1g/kg/day × 1-2 days

Available forms: IM inj 2, 10 ml/vial; **IV** inj 5% sol, 0.5, 1, 2.5, 3, 6, 10 g vials

Adverse effects

CNS: Headache, fatigue, malaise

GI: Abdominal pain

INTEG: Pain at inj site, rash, pruritus, chills, chest pain

MS: Arthralgia

SYST: Lymphadenopathy, ***anaphylaxis***

Contraindications: Hypersensitivity

Precautions: Pregnancy **C**

Pharmacokinetics

Absorption	Well absorbed (IM); completely absorbed (IV)
Distribution	Rapidly
Metabolism	Liver, catabolism
Excretion	Kidneys
Half-life	3-4 wk

Pharmacodynamics

	IM	IV
Onset	Unknown	Rapid
Peak	Unknown	Unknown
Duration	Unknown	Unknown

Interactions

Live virus vaccines: Do not give within 3 mo

NURSING CONSIDERATIONS

Assessment

- Assess for exposure date: this drug should be given within 6 days of measles, 1 wk of hepatitis B, 14 days of hepatitis A; if the date of exposure is outside these limits, immune globulin will not be effective
- Monitor blood studies in leukemia, idiopathic thrombocytopenic purpura: WBCs (leukemia), platelets
- Identify the number of inj of this drug the patient has received; multiple inj may lead to sensitization (diaphoresis, fever, chills, malaise)
- Assess for anaphylaxis in patient receiving **IV** immune globulin: diaphoresis, flushing, nausea, vomiting, wheezing, difficulty breathing, hypotension, chest tightness, fever, weakness, sneezing, abdominal pain; VS should be monitored during inf and 1 hr after beginning inf; emergency equipment should be available with epinephrine and antihistamines to treat anaphylaxis

Nursing diagnoses

✓ Infection, risk for (uses)
✓ Knowledge deficit (teaching)

Implementation

IM route

- Give IM (IGIM) in deltoid or anterolateral thigh in adults or anterolateral thigh in young P children; if large amounts are given, several inj may be needed
- Do not give the IM preparation **IV**, SC, or intradermally
- Sol should be transparent and clear or slightly colored

IV route
- Warm to room temp before administration (diluent, powder for inj)
- A transfer device is provided by manufacturer; this drug should not be agitated or shaken
- Do not give the **IV** preparation SC, IM, or intradermally
- Check for adverse reaction during inf; stop inf if adverse reactions are present

Y-site compatibilities: Fluconazole, sargramostim

Gamimune N: Dilute **IV** with D_5; give 0.01 ml/kg/min; may increase to 0.02-0.04 ml/kg/min if no adverse reactions are present; may increase to 0.08 ml/kg/hr; sol should be refrigerated; do not freeze

Gammagard: Reconstitute with sterile water for inj (50 mg protein/ml); give within 2 hr of reconstitution; give 0.5 ml/kg/hr; may increase to 4 ml/kg/hr if no adverse reactions occur; use inf set provided

Gammar-IV: Give 0.01 ml/kg/min (50 mg/ml sol) over 15-30 min; may increase to 0.02 ml/kg/min; if adverse reactions are not present, may increase to 0.03-0.06 ml/kg/min; do not freeze; store at room temp

Iveegam (5%): Give 1-2 ml/min; refrigerate, do not freeze

Sandoglobulin: **IV** diluted with provided diluent; give 0.5-1 ml/min over 15-30 min; may increase to 1.5-2.5 ml/min; other inf may be given 2-2.5 ml/min; store at room temp

Venoglobulin-I: Give 50 mg/ml sol 0.01-0.02 ml/kg/min over 30 min if no adverse reactions; increase 0.04 ml/kg/min; store at room temp

Patient/family education
- Advise patient that passive immunity is temporary; explain reason for and expected results of this drug
- Advise patient that pain and tenderness may occur at inj site

Evaluation

Positive therapeutic outcome
- Prevention of infection
- Increased platelets

Treatment of anaphylaxis: Epinephrine, diphenhydramine, O_2, vasopressors, corticosteroids

indapamide (℞)
(in-dap'a-mide)

Lozol

Func. class.: Diuretic, antihypertensive

Chem. class.: Thiazide-like sulfonamide derivative

Pregnancy category B

Action: Acts on the distal tubule and thick ascending loop of Henle in the kidney, increasing excretion of sodium, water, chloride, magnesium, potassium, and bicarbonate

Therapeutic Outcome: Decreased B/P, decreased edema in lung tissues, peripherally

Uses: May be used alone or as adjunct with antihypertensives (mild to moderate)

Dosage and routes

Edema

Adult: PO 2.5 mg qd in AM,

may be increased to 5 mg qd if needed

Antihypertensive
Adult: PO 1.25-5 mg qd; may increase to 5 mg/day over 8 wks

Available forms: Tabs 1.25, 2.5 mg

Adverse effects

CNS: Depression, *headache, dizziness, fatigue, weakness, nervousness, agitation*
CV: Orthostatic hypotension, palpitations, volume depletion, PVCs
EENT: Blurred vision, nasal congestion, increased intraocular pressure
ELECT: Hypokalemia, hypercalcemia, hyponatremia, hypochloremia, hypomagnesemia
GI: Nausea, vomiting, anorexia, constipation, diarrhea, cramps, GI irritation, abdominal pain
GU: Frequency, polyuria, nocturia
INTEG: Rash, *pruritus,*
META: Hyperglycemia, *hyperuricemia,* increased creatinine, BUN
MS: Cramps

Contraindications: Hypersensitivity to thiazides or sulfonamides, anuria, lactation, hepatic coma

Precautions: Hypokalemia, renal disease, hepatic disease, gout, diabetes mellitus, elderly, ascites, dehydration, pregnancy **B**

Pharmacokinetics

Absorption	Well absorbed
Distribution	Widely distributed
Metabolism	Liver; 7%
Excretion	Unchanged (urine)
Half-life	14-18 hr

Pharmacodynamics

Onset	1-2 hr
Peak	2 hr
Duration	Up to 36 hr

Interactions

Individual drugs
Alcohol: ↑ hypotension
Amphotericin B: ↓ effects
Lithium: ↑ toxicity
Mezlocillin: ↑ hypokalemia
Piperacillin: ↑ hypokalemia
Ticarcillin: ↑ hypokalemia

Drug classifications
Anticoagulants: ↓ effects
Antigout agents: ↓ effects
Antihypertensives: ↑ antihypertensive effect
Cardiac glycosides: ↑ hypokalemia, ↑ toxicity
Glucocorticoids: ↑ hypokalemia

Lab test interferences
↑ Calcium, ↑ parathyroid test

NURSING CONSIDERATIONS

Assessment

- Check for rashes, temp elevation qd
- Monitor patients that receive cardiac glycosides for increased hypokalemia, toxicity
- Monitor manifestations of hypokalemia: acidic or reduced urine, osmolality, nocturia; hypotension, broad T wave, U wave, ectopy, tachycardia, weak pulse; muscle weakness, altered LOC, drowsiness, apathy, lethargy, confusion, depression; anorexia, nausea, cramps, constipation, distention, paralytic ileus; hypoventilation, respiratory muscle weakness
- Monitor for manifestations of hypomagnesemia: agitation, muscle twitching, paresthesias, hyperactive reflexes, positive Babinski reflex, dysphagia, nystagmus seizures, tetany; nausea, vomiting, diarrhea,

anorexia, abdominal distention; ectopy, tachycardia, broad, flat or inverted T waves, depressed ST segment, prolonged QT, decreased cardiac output, hypotension
- Monitor for manifestations of hyponatremia: increased B/P, cold, clammy skin, hypovolemia or hypervolemia; anorexia, nausea, vomiting, diarrhea, abdominal cramps; lethargy, increased ICP, confusion, headache, seizures, coma, fatigue, tremors, hyperreflexia
- Monitor for manifestations of hyperchloremia: weakness, lethargy, coma, deep rapid breathing
- Assess fluid volume status: I&O ratios and record, weight, distended red veins, crackles in lung, color, quality and sp gr of urine, skin turgor, adequacy of pulses, moist mucous membranes, bilateral lung sounds, peripheral pitting edema; dehydration symptoms of decreasing output, thirst, hypotension, dry mouth and mucous membranes should be reported
- Monitor electrolytes: potassium, sodium, calcium, magnesium; also include BUN, blood pH, ABGs, uric acid, CBC, blood sugar
- Assess B/P before and during therapy with patient lying, standing and sitting as appropriate; orthostatic hypotension can occur rapidly

Nursing diagnoses

✓ Altered urinary elimination (side effect)
✓ Fluid volume deficit (side effects)
✓ Fluid volume excess (uses)
✓ Knowledge deficit (teaching)

Implementation

- Give in AM to avoid interference with sleep
- Provide potassium replacement if potassium level is <3.0; give whole
- Give with food; if nausea occurs, absorption may be increased

Patient/family education

- Teach patient to take the medication early in the day to prevent nocturia
- Instruct the patient to take with food or milk if GI symptoms of nausea and anorexia occur
- Teach patient to maintain weekly record of weight and notify prescriber of weight loss >5 lb
- Caution the patient that this drug causes a loss of potassium, so food rich in potassium should be added to the diet; refer to a dietician for assistance in planning
- Caution the patient not to exercise in hot weather or stand for prolonged periods, since orthostatic hypotension will be enhanced
- Teach patient not to use alcohol or any OTC medications without prescriber's approval; serious drug reactions may occur
- Emphasize the need to contact prescriber immediately if muscle cramps, weakness, nausea, dizziness, or numbness occurs
- Teach patient to take own B/P and pulse and record findings
- Caution the patient that orthostatic hypotension may occur and to rise slowly from sitting or reclining positions and lie down if dizziness occurs

- Teach patient to continue taking medication even if feeling better; this drug controls symptoms but does not cure the condition
- Advise the patient with hypertension to continue other medical treatment (exercise, weight loss, relaxation techniques, cessation of smoking)

Evaluation

Positive therapeutic outcome

- Decreased edema
- Decreased B/P
- Increased diuresis

Treatment of overdose: Lavage, monitor electrolytes, administer IV fluids, monitor hydration, CV, renal status

indinavir (℞)

(en-den′a-veer)

Crixivan

Func. class.: Antiviral

Chem. class.: Synthetic peptide-like substrate analog

Pregnancy category C

Action: Inhibits human immunodeficiency virus (HIV) protease, this prevents maturation of the infectious virus

Therapeutic Outcome: Decreased signs/symptoms of HIV infection

Uses: HIV alone or in combination

Dosage and routes

Adult: PO 800 mg q8hr; if given with ddc, given 1 hr apart on empty stomach

Available forms: Caps 200, 400 mg

Adverse effects

CNS: Headache, insomnia, dizziness, somnolence

GI: Diarrhea, abdominal pain, nausea, vomiting, anorexia, dry mouth

INTEG: Rash

MS: Pain

OTHER: Asthenia

Contraindications: Hypersensitivity

Precautions: Liver disease, pregnancy **C**, lactation, children, renal disease

Pharmacokinetics	
Absorption	Unknown
Distribution	Unknown
Metabolism	Unknown
Excretion	Unknown
Half-life	Unknown

Pharmacodynamics

Unknown

Interactions

Individual drugs

Clarithromycin: ↑ levels of both drugs

ddc: ↑ levels of both drugs

Ketoconazole: ↑ levels of both drugs

Astemizole: ↑ level of astemizole

Cisapride: ↑ level of cisapride

Midazolam: ↑ level of midazolam

Triazolam: ↑ level of triazolam

Isoniazid: ↑ level of isoniazid

Drug classifications

Rifamycins: ↓ indinavir levels

NURSING CONSIDERATIONS

Assessment

- Monitor signs of infection, anemia
- Monitor liver studies: ALT, AST
- Obtain C&S before drug therapy; drug may be taken as soon as culture is taken; repeat

C&S after treatment; determine the presence of other sexually transmitted diseases
• Assess bowel pattern before, during treatment; if severe abdominal pain with bleeding occurs, drug should be discontinued, monitor hydration
• Assess skin eruptions; rash, urticaria, itching
• Assess allergies before treatment, reaction of each medication; place allergies on chart

Nursing diagnoses
✓ Infection, risk for (uses)
✓ Knowledge deficit (teaching)

Patient/family education
• Advise to take as prescribed; if dose is missed, take as soon as remembered up to 1 hr before next dose; do not double dose
⊘ • Do not crush, chew caps
• Advise that drug must be taken in equal intervals around the clock to maintain blood levels for duration of therapy

Evaluation
Positive therapeutic outcome
• Decreased signs/symptoms of infection

indomethacin (℞)
(in-doe-meth'a-sin)
Apo-Indomethacin ♣, Indameth ♣, Indocid ♣, Indocin PDA ♣, Novomethacin ♣, indomethacin, Indocin, Indocin SR, Indocin IV
Func. class.: NSAID
Chem. class.: Propionic acid derivative

Pregnancy category B

Action: Inhibits prostaglandin synthesis by decreasing enzyme needed for biosynthesis; analgesic, antiinflammatory, antipyretic

Therapeutic Outcome: Decreased pain, inflammation; or closure of patent ductus
P arteriosus (premature infants)

Uses: Rheumatoid arthritis, ankylosing rheumatoid spondylitis, acute gouty arthritis, closure of patent ductus
P arteriosus in premature infants

Dosage and routes
Arthritis/antiinflammatory
Adult: PO/rec 25 mg bid-tid; may increase by 25 mg/day q wk, not to exceed 200 mg/day; sus rel 75 mg qd; may increase to 75 mg bid

Acute arthritis
Adult: PO/rec 50 mg tid; use only for acute attack, then reduce dosage

Patent ductus arteriosus
P ***Infant <2 days:*** **IV** 0.2 mg/kg, then 0.1 mg/kg q12-24h

P ***Infant 2-7 days:*** **IV** 0.2 mg/kg, then 0.2 mg × 2 doses after 12, 24 hr

P ***Infant >7 days:*** **IV** 0.2 mg/kg, then 0.25 mg/kg × 2 doses after 12, 24 hr

Available forms: Caps 25, 50 mg; sus rel cap 75 mg; oral susp 25 mg/5 ml; rec supp 50 mg; inj 1 mg vials

Adverse effects
CNS: Dizziness, drowsiness, fatigue, tremors, confusion, insomnia, anxiety, depression
CV: Tachycardia, peripheral edema, palpitations, dysrhythmias, hypertension
EENT: Tinnitus, hearing loss, blurred vision
GI: Nausea, anorexia, vomiting, diarrhea, jaundice, ***cholestatic hepatitis,*** constipation,

flatulence, cramps, dry mouth, peptic ulcer, ***ulceration, perforation***
GU: Nephrotoxicity (dysuria, hematuria, oliguria, azotemia)
HEMA: Blood dyscrasias
INTEG: Purpura, rash, pruritus, sweating

Contraindications: Hypersensitivity, asthma, severe renal disease, severe hepatic disease, ulcer disease

Precautions: Pregnancy, lactation, children, bleeding disorders, GI disorders, cardiac disorders, hypersensitivity to other antiinflammatory agents, pregnancy **B** 1st and 2nd trimesters, depression

Pharmacokinetics

Absorption	Well absorbed (PO); erratic (rec); complete (**IV**)
Distribution	Crosses blood-brain barrier; placenta, 99% plasma protein binding
Metabolism	Liver, extensively
Excretion	Breast milk
Half-life	2.6-11 hr

Pharmacodynamics

	IV	PO	PO–EXT REL
Onset	2 day	1-2 hr	½ hr
Peak	Unknown	3 hr	Unknown
Duration	Unknown	4-6 hr	4-6 hr

Interactions

Individual drugs

Acetaminophen (long-term use): ↑ renal reactions
Alcohol: ↑ adverse reactions
Aspirin: ↓ effectiveness, ↑ adverse reactions
Coumadin: ↑ anticoagulant effects
Cyclosporine: ↑ nephrotoxicity
Digoxin: ↑ toxicity, levels
Insulin: ↓ insulin effect
Lithium: ↑ toxicity, levels
Methotrexate: ↑ toxicity
Phenytoin: ↑ toxicity
Probenecid: ↑ toxicity
Zidovudine: ↑ toxicity, levels

Drug classifications

Anticoagulants: ↑ risk of bleeding
Antihypertensives: ↓ effect of antihypertensives
Antineoplastics: ↑ risk of hematologic toxicity
β-Blockers: ↑ antihypertension
Cephalosporins: ↑ risk of bleeding
Glucocorticoids: ↑ adverse reactions
Hypoglycemics: ↓ hypoglycemic effect
Diuretics: ↓ effectiveness of diuretics
NSAIDs: ↑ adverse reactions
Potassium supplements: ↑ adverse reactions
Radiation: ↑ risk of hematologic toxicity
Sulfonamides: ↑ toxicity
Sulfonylureas: ↑ toxicity

NURSING CONSIDERATIONS

Assessment

- Assess for joint pain (duration, intensity, ROM), baseline and during treatment

Nursing diagnoses

✓ Pain (uses)
✓ Chronic pain (uses)
✓ Impaired mobility (uses)
✓ Knowledge deficit (teaching)

Implementation

PO route

- Administer to patient whole; do not crush, chew, or break sus rel cap
- Give with food or milk to decrease gastric symptoms, and prevent ulceration

IV **IV route**

- Give after diluting 1 mg/ml or more normal saline or sterile water for inj without preservative; give over 5-10 sec; avoid extravasation

Rec route

- Have patient retain rec supp for 1 hr after insertion

Patient/family education

- Advise patient to report change in vision, blurring, rash, tinnitus, black stools
- Tell patient not to use for any other condition than prescribed
- Advise patient to avoid use with OTC medications for pain unless approved by prescriber
- Advise patient to avoid hazardous activities, since dizziness or drowsiness can occur

Evaluation

Positive therapeutic outcome

- Decreased stiffness
- Increased joint mobility
- Decreased pain

insulin lispro (℞)

Humalog

Func. class.: Pancreatic hormone

Chem. class.: Exogenous, unmodified insulin analog

Pregnancy category B

Action: Decreases blood sugar; by transport of insulin into cells and the conversion of glucose to glycogen indirectly increases blood pyruvate and lactate, decreases phosphate and potassium, rapid onset, shorter duration than regular insulin

➔ **Therapeutic Outcome:** Decreased blood glucose levels in diabetes mellituus

Uses: Adult-onset diabetes, juvenile diabetes, ketoacidosis types I and II, type II (non-insulin-dependent) diabetes mellitus, type I (insulin-dependent) diabetes mellitus

Dosage and routes

Adult: SC dosage individualized by blood, urine glucose levels

Available forms: Inj U 100/ml, 5 1.5 ml cartridge

Adverse effects

EENT: Blurred vision, dry mouth

INTEG: Flushing, rash, urticaria, warmth, lipodystrophy, lipohypertrophy, swelling, redness

META: Hypoglycemia, rebound hyperglycemia (Somogyi effect 12-72 hr or longer)

SYST: Anaphylaxis

Contraindications: Hypersensitivity to protamine

Precautions: Pregnancy **B**

Pharmacokinetics	
Absorption	Rapidly absorbed
Distribution	Widely distributed
Metabolism	Liver, muscle, kidney
Excretion	Kidneys
Half-life	46 min

Pharmacodynamics	
Onset	15 min
Peak	40-60 min
Duration	Unknown

Interactions

Individual drugs

Alcohol: ↑ hypoglycemia
Diltiazem: ↑ insulin need
Dobutamine: ↑ insulin need
Fenfluramine: ↓ insulin need
Guanethidine: ↓ insulin need

Phenylbutazone: ↓ insulin need
Rifampin: ↑ insulin need
Sulfinpyrazone: ↓ insulin need
Tetracycline: ↓ insulin need

Drug classifications

Anabolic steroids: ↓ insulin need
β-Blockers: Signs/symptoms of hypoglycemia may be masked
Glucocorticoid steroids: ↑ insulin need
Estrogens: ↑ insulin need
MAOI: ↓ insulin need
Oral anticoagulants: ↓ insulin need
Oral hypoglycemics: hypoglycemia
Thiazide diuretics: ↑ insulin need
Thyroid hormones: ↑ insulin need

Smoking

↑ insulin need

Lab test interferences

↑ VMA
↓ Potassium, ↓ magnesium, ↓ inorganic phosphate
Interference: Liver function studies, thyroid function studies

NURSING CONSIDERATIONS

Assessment

- Monitor fasting blood glucose, 2 hr PP (80-150 mg/dl, normal fasting level; 70-130 mg/dl, normal 2-hr level); also glycosylated Hgb may be drawn to identify treatment effectiveness
- Monitor urine ketones during illness; insulin requirements may increase during stress, illness, surgery
- Assess for hypoglycemic reaction that can occur during peak time (sweating, weakness, dizziness, chills, confusion, headache, nausea, rapid weak pulse, fatigue, tachycardia, memory lapses, slurred speech, staggering gait, anxiety, tremors, hunger)
- Assess for hyperglycemia: acetone breath, polyuria, fatigue, polydipsia, flushed dry skin, lethargy

Nursing diagnoses

✓ Injury, risk for (adverse reactions)
✓ Knowledge deficit (teaching)
✓ Noncompliance (teaching)

Implementation

- Give after warming to room temp by rotating in palms to prevent injecting cold insulin; use only insulin syringes with markings or syringe matching U/ml; rotate inj sites within one area; abdomen, upper back, thighs, upper arm, buttocks; keep record of sites
- Give increased dosages if tolerance occurs; give human insulin to those allergic to beef or pork
- Store at room temp for <1 mo; keep away from heat and sunlight; refrigerate all other supply; do not use if discolored; do not freeze

Patient/family education

- Advise patient that blurred vision occurs; not to change corrective lenses until vision is stabilized after 1-2 mo of therapy
- Advise patient to keep insulin and equipment available at all times
- Advise patient to carry Medic Alert ID as diabetic
- Teach patient dosage, route, disease process, and to rotate inj sites
- Instruct patient to carry candy or lump of sugar to treat hypoglycemia; have glucagon

emergency kit available; teach how to use kit
- Teach patient symptoms of ketoacidosis: nausea, thirst, polyuria, dry mouth, decreased B/P, dry flushed skin, acetone breath, drowsiness, Kussmaul respirations; to have insulin available at all times
- Advise patient that a plan is necessary for diet, exercise; all food on diet should be eaten, exercise routine should not vary
- Teach patient to avoid OTC drugs and alcohol unless approved by a prescriber
- Instruct patient to notify prescriber if pregnancy is planned
- Caution patient that treatment is life long; insulin does not cure condition

Evaluation

Positive therapeutic outcome
- Decrease in polyuria, polydipsia, polyphagia; clear sensorium, absence of dizziness, stable gait
- Blood glucose level under control

Treatment of overdose: Glucose 25 g **IV**, via dextrose 50% sol, 50 ml or 1 mg glucagon

insulin, isophane suspension (NPH) 🗝 (℞)
Humulin N, Iletin NPH, Illetin II NPH ♣, Novolin ge NPH ♣, Novolin N, Novolin N PenFill, Novolin N Prefilled, NPH Iletin I, NPH Iletin II, NPH-N

insulin, isophane suspension and regular insulin (℞)
Humulin 70/30, Humalin 30/70 ♣, Novolin 70/30, Novolin 70/30 PenFill, Novolin 7/30 Prefilled, Novolin ge 30/70 ♣

insulin, regular 🗝 (℞)
Humulin R, Iletin I, Illetin II ♣, Novolin ge Toronto ♣, Novolin R, Novolin R PenFill, Novolin R Prefilled, Novolin R Velosulin, Regular Illetin I, Regular Illetin II, regular purified pork insulin, Velosulin Human BR

insulin, zinc suspension (Lente) (℞)
Humulin L, Iletin ♣, Illetin II ♣, Lente Iletin I, Lente Iletin II, Lente L, Novolin ge Lente ♣, Novolin L

insulin, zinc suspension extended (Ultralente) (℞)
Humulin U ♣, Humulin U Ultralente, Novolin ge Ultralente

isophane insulin suspension and insulin injection (℞)
Humalin 50/50, Novolin ge 50/50 ♣,

insulin analog injection
Humalog

Func. class.: Pancreatic hormone

Chem. class.: Exogenous unmodified insulin

Pregnancy category B

Action: Decreases blood sugar; by transport of insulin into cells and the conversion of glucose to glycogen indirectly increases blood pyruvate and lactate, decreases phosphate and potassium; insulin may be beef, pork, human (processed by recombinant DNA technologies)

Therapeutic Outcome: Decreased blood glucose levels in diabetes mellitus

Uses: Adult-onset diabetes, juvenile diabetes, ketoacidosis types I and II, type II (non–insulin-dependent) diabetes mellitus, type I (insulin-dependent) diabetes mellitus

Dosage and routes

Insulin lispro

Adult: SC Give 15 min AC

Human reg

Adults: SC Give ½-1 AC

Insulin, isophane suspension

Adult: SC dosage individualized by blood, urine glucose; usual dose 7-26 U; may increase by 2-10 U/day if needed

Regular insulin

Ketoacidosis

Adult: **IV** 5-10 R, then 5-10 U/hr until desired response, then switch to SC dose; **IV**/inf 2-12 U (50 U/500 ml of normal saline)

P ***Child:*** **IV** 0.1 U/kg

Replacement

P ***Adult and child:*** SC 0.5-1 U/kg/day qid given 30 min pc

Adolescents: SC 0.8-1.2 mg/kg/day; this dosage is used during rapid growth

Available forms: NPH inj 100 U/ml; regular **IV**/IM/SC inj 100 U/ml; insulin analog inj 100 U/ml; insulin zinc susp, ext (ultralente) 100 U/ml; isophane insulin/insulin inj 100 U/ml; zinc susp 100 U/ml

Adverse effects

EENT: Blurred vision, dry mouth

INTEG: Flushing, rash, urticaria, warmth, *lipodystrophy,* lipohypertrophy, swelling, redness

META: Hypoglycemia, rebound hyperglycemia (Somogyi effect 12-72 hr or longer)

SYST: ***Anaphylaxis***

Contraindications: Hypersensitivity to protamine

Precautions: Pregnancy **B**

Pharmacokinetics

Absorption	Rapidly absorbed (SC)
Distribution	Widely distributed
Metabolism	Liver, muscle, kidney
Excretion	Kidneys
Half-life	Regular 3-5 min; NPH 10 min

Pharmacodynamics

	NPH	MIXTARD	INSULIN, REGULAR		INSULIN, REGULAR CONC	ZINC SUSP	ZINC SUSP CONC	ZINC SUSP PROMPT
			SC	IV				SC
Onset	1-2 hr	½ hr	½-1 hr'	10-30 min	½-1 hr	1-2½ hr	4-8 hr	1-1½ hr
Peak	4-12 hr	4-8 hr	2-4 hr	30-60 min	2-5 hr	7-15 hr	10-30 hr	5-10 hr
Duration	18-24 hr	12-24 hr	5-7 hr	½-1 hr	5-7 hr	12-24 hr	7-36 hr	12-16 hr

Interactions
Individual drugs
Alcohol: ↑ hypoglycemia
Diltiazem: ↑ insulin need
Dobutamine: ↑ insulin need
Fenfluramine: ↓ insulin need
Guanethidine: ↓ insulin need
Phenylbutazone: ↓ insulin need
Rifampin: ↑ insulin need
Sulfinpyrazone: ↓ insulin need
Tetracycline: ↓ insulin need
Drug classifications
Anabolic steroids: ↓ insulin need
β-Blockers: Signs/symptoms of hypoglycemia may be masked
Glucocorticoid steroids: ↑ insulin need
Estrogens: ↑ insulin need
MAOI: ↓ insulin need
Oral anticoagulants: ↓ insulin need
Oral hypoglycemics: ↑ hypoglycemia
Thiazide diuretics: ↑ insulin need
Thyroid hormones: ↑ insulin need
Smoking
↑ insulin need
Lab test interferences
↑ VMA
↓ Potassium, ↓ magnesium, ↓ inorganic phosphate
Interference: Liver function studies, thyroid function studies

NURSING CONSIDERATIONS
Assessment
• Monitor fasting blood glucose, 2 hr PP (80-150 mg/dl, normal fasting level; 70-130 mg/dl, normal 2-hr level); also glycosylated Hgb may be drawn to identify treatment effectiveness
• Monitor urine ketones during illness; insulin requirements may increase during stress, illness, surgery
• Assess for hypoglycemic reaction that can occur during peak time (sweating, weakness, dizziness, chills, confusion, headache, nausea, rapid weak pulse, fatigue, tachycardia, memory lapses, slurred speech, staggering gait, anxiety, tremors, hunger)
• Assess for hyperglycemia: acetone breath, polyuria, fatigue, polydipsia, flushed, dry skin, lethargy

Nursing diagnoses
✓ Injury, risk for (adverse reactions)
✓ Knowledge deficit (teaching)
✓ Noncompliance (teaching)

Implementation
SC route
• Give after warming to room temp by rotating in palms to prevent injecting cold insulin; use only insulin syringes with markings or syringe matching U/ml; rotate inj sites within one area: abdomen, upper back, thighs, upper arm, buttocks; keep record of sites
• Give increased dosages if tolerance occurs; give human insulin to those allergic to beef or pork
• Store at room temp for <1 mo; keep away from heat and sunlight; refrigerate all other supply; do not use if discolored; do not freeze

IV **IV route, regular only**
• Do not use if cloudy, thick, or discolored
• Give **IV** direct, undiluted via vein, Y-site, 3-way stopcock; give at 50 U/min or less
• Give by cont inf after diluting with **IV** sol and run at prescribed rate; use **IV** inf pump for correct dosing; give

reduced dose at serum glucose level of 250 mg/100 ml

Syringe compatibility: Metoclopramide

Y-site incompatibility: Nafcillin

Y-site compatibilities: Amiodarone, ampicillin, ampicillin/sulbactam, aztreonam, cefazolin, cefotetan, dobutamine, esmolol, famotidine, gentamicin, heparin, imipenen/cilastatin, indomethacin sodium trihydrate, magnesium sulfate, meperidine, midazolam, morphine, nitroglycerin, nitroprusside, oxytocin, pentobarbital, potassium chloride, regular insulin, ritodrine, sodium bicarbonate, terbutalin, ticarcillin, ticarcillin/clavulanate, tobramycin, vancomycin, vitamin B with C

Additive incompatibilities: Aminophylline, amobarbital, chlorothiazide, cytarabine, dobutamine, pentobarbital, phenobarbital, phenytoin, secobarbital, sodium bicarbonate, thiopental

Additive compatibilities: Bretylium, cimetidine, lidocaine, verapamil

Patient/family education

• Advise patient that blurred vision occurs; not to change corrective lenses until vision is stabilized after 1-2 mo of therapy
• Advise patient to keep insulin and equipment available at all times
• Advise patient to carry Medic Alert ID as diabetic
• Teach patient dosage, route, mixing instructions, disease process; tell patient to continue to use the same brand of insulin and to rotate inj sites
• Instruct patient to carry candy or lump of sugar to treat hypoglycemia; have glucagon emergency kit available; teach how to use these
• Teach patient symptoms of ketoacidosis: nausea, thirst, polyuria, dry mouth, decreased B/P, dry, flushed skin, acetone breath, drowsiness, Kussmaul respirations; to have insulin available at all times
• Advise patient that a plan is necessary for diet, exercise; all food on diet should be eaten, exercise routine should not vary
• Teach patient to avoid OTC drugs and alcohol unless approved by a prescriber
• Instruct patient to notify prescriber if pregnancy is planned
• Caution patient that treatment is lifelong; insulin does not cure condition

Evaluation

Positive therapeutic outcome

• Decrease in polyuria, polydipsia, polyphagia; clear sensorium, absence of dizziness, stable gait
• Blood glucose level under control

Treatment of overdose: Glucose 25 g **IV**, via dextrose 50% sol, 50 ml or 1 mg glucagon

I

interferon alfa-2a/ interferon alfa-2b (℞)

(in-ter-feer'on)

Roferon-A/Intron-A

Func. class.: Miscellaneous antineoplastic

Chem. class.: Protein product

Pregnancy category C

Action: Antiviral action inhibits viral replication by reprogramming virus; antitumor action suppresses cell proliferation; immunomodulating action phagocytizes target cells; may also inhibit virus replication

➔ **Therapeutic Outcome:** Prevention of rapid growth of malignant cells; treatment of hepatitis non-A, non-B (liver function improvement)

Uses: Hairy cell leukemia in persons >18 yr, condylomata acuminata (alfa 2b), malignant melanoma, AIDS-related Kaposi's sarcoma, chronic hepatitis non-A, non-B (alfa 2b), chronic hepatitis B, C (alfa 2b)

Investigational uses: Bladder tumors, carcinoid tumors, non-Hodgkin's lymphoma, essential thrombocytopenia, Cytomegaloviruses, herpes simplex

Dosage and routes

Hairy cell leukemia (2a)

Adult: SC/IM 3 million IU/day × 16-24 wk, then 3 million IU 3 times a wk maintenance

Hairy cell leukemia (2b)

2 million IU/m^2 3 times a wk; if severe adverse reactions occur, dose should be skipped or reduced by one half

Kaposi's sarcoma (2a)

Adult: SC/IM 36 million IU/day × 10-12 wk or 3 million IU/day × 3 days, then 9 million IU/day × 3 days, then 18 million IU/day × 3 days, then 36 million IU/day for the rest of the course; if severe reaction occurs reduce dose by one half

Condylomata acuminata (2b)

1 million IU/lesion 3 times a wk × 3 wk

Chronic hepatitis B (2b)

Adult: SC/IM 30-35 million IU/wk or 5 million IU/day or 10 million IU/3x/wk x 16 wk

Chronic hepatitis C

Adult: SC/IM 36 million IU 3 times a wk

Available forms: Alfa-2a inj 3, 6, 36 million IU/ml; alfa-2b inj 3, 5, 10, 18, 25, 50 million U/vial

Adverse effects

CNS: Dizziness, confusion, numbness, paresthesias, hallucinations, ***convulsions, coma,*** amnesia, anxiety, mood changes

CV: Edema, hypotension, hypertension, chest pain, palpitations, dysrhythmias, **CHF, MI, CVA**

GI: Weight loss, taste changes

GU: Impotence

INTEG: Rash, dry skin, itching, alopecia, flushing, photosensitivity

MISC: Flulike syndrome: fever, fatigue, myalgias, headache, chills

Contraindications: Hypersensitivity

Precautions: Severe hypotension, dysrhythmia, tachycardia, P pregnancy **C,** lactation, children, severe renal or hepatic disease, convulsion disorder

Pharmacokinetics

Absorption	80%-90% (SC/IM)
Distribution	Unknown
Metabolism	Renal tubular (degraded)
Excretion	Kidneys
Half-life	3.7-8.5 hr (2a); 2-7 hr (2b)

Pharmacodynamics

Onset	Unknown
Peak	3-8 hr
Duration	Unknown

Interactions

Individual drugs

Aminophylline: ↑ toxicity, blood levels

Radiation: ↑ toxicity, bone marrow suppression

Zidovudine: ↑ neutropenia

Drug classifications

Antineoplastics: ↑ toxicity, bone marrow suppression

Lab test interferences

Interference: AST (SGOT), ALT (SGPT), LDH, alkaline phosphatase, WBC, platelets, granulocytes, creatinine

NURSING CONSIDERATIONS

Assessment

- Assess for symptoms of infection; may be masked by drug fever; fever, chills, headache, sore throat may occur 6 hr after dose; give acetaminophen for symptoms
- In AIDS patients with Kaposi's sarcoma, assess characteristics of lesions during therapy; symptoms should decrease
- Assess for bleeding: hematuria, stool guaiac, bruising or petechiae, mucosa or orifices q8h; check for inflammation of mucosa, breaks in skin; avoid IM injection, rectal temp, or any other procedures that break the skin
- Assess for CNS reaction: LOC, mental status, dizziness, confusion, poor coordination, difficulty speaking, behavior changes; notify prescriber

Nursing diagnoses

- ✓ Injury, risk for (adverse reactions)
- ✓ Body image disturbance (adverse reactions)
- ✓ Infection, risk for (adverse reactions)
- ✓ Knowledge deficit (teaching)

Implementation

- Sol should be prepared by qualified personnel only under controlled conditions in biologic cabinet using gown, gloves, and mask
- Use Luer-Lok tubing to prevent leakage; do not let sol come in contact with skin; if contact occurs, wash well with soap and water
- Give at hs to minimize side effects
- Give acetaminophen as ordered to alleviate fever and headache
- Give by IM/SC after reconstituting 3-5 million IU/1 ml, 10 million IU/2 ml, 25 million IU/5 ml, of diluent provided; mix gently
- Store reconstituted sol for 1 mo in refrigerator

Intralesional route (2b)

- Give by intralesional route after reconstituting 10 million IU/1 ml bacteriostatic water for inj; no more than 5 lesions can safely be treated at a time; using a 25 G needle inject 0.1 ml into base at center

Patient/family education

- Caution patient to avoid hazardous tasks, since confusion, dizziness may occur;

fatigue is common; activity may have to be altered; to take hs to minimize flu-like symptoms; to take acetaminophen for fever; avoid prolonged sunlight
• Advise patient that brands of this drug should not be changed; each form is different, with different dosages
• Caution patient not to become pregnant while taking drug; possible mutagenic effects; impotence may occur during treatment but is temporary
• Advise patient to report signs of infection: sore throat, fever, diarrhea, vomiting
• Advise patient that emotional lability is common; notify prescriber if severe or incapacitating

Evaluation

Positive therapeutic outcome
• Leukocytes, Hgb, platelets, WNL
• Decreased amount of lesions in AIDS patients with Kaposi's sarcoma
• Decreased amount of genital warts

interferon β-1b (℞)

(in-ter-feer′on)

Betaseron

Func. class.: Multiple sclerosis agent, immune modifier

Chem. class.: Escherichia coli derivative

Pregnancy category C

Action: Antiviral, immunoregulatory; action not clearly understood; biologic response-modifying properties mediated through specific receptors on cells, inducing expression of interferon-induced gene products

➲ **Therapeutic Outcome:** Correcting symptoms of multiple sclerosis

Uses: Ambulatory patients with relapsing or remitting multiple sclerosis

Investigational uses: May be useful in treatment of AIDS, AIDS-related Kaposi's sarcoma, malignant melanoma, metastatic renal cell carcinoma, cutaneous T cell lymphoma, acute non-A, non-B hepatitis

Dosage and routes

Relapsing/remitting multiple sclerosis

Adult: SC 0.25 mg (8 IU) qod

Available forms: Powder for inj lyophilized 0.3 mg (9.6 mIU)

Adverse effects

CNS: Headache, fever, pain, chills, mental changes, hypertonia, ***suicide attempts,*** gait disturbances, depression
CV: Migraine, palpitations, hypertension, tachycardia, peripheral vascular disorders
EENT: Conjunctivitis, blurred vision, laryngitis
GI: Diarrhea, constipation, vomiting, abdominal pain
GU: Dysmenorrhea, irregular menses, metrorrhagia, cystitis, breast pain, spontaneous abortion
HEMA: ***Decreased lymphocytes, WBC;*** *lymphadenopathy*
INTEG: Sweating, inj site reaction, necrosis
MS: Myalgia, ***myasthenia,*** back pain
RESP: Sinusitis, dyspnea

Contraindications: Hypersensitivity to natural or recombinant interferon-β or human albumin

Precautions: Pregnancy **C**, P lactation, child <18 yr, chronic progressive MS, depression, mental disorders

Pharmacokinetics

Absorption	50% is absorbed
Distribution	Unknown
Metabolism	Unknown
Excretion	Unknown
Half-life	8 min-4½ hr

Pharmacodynamics

Onset	Rapid
Peak	Up to 8 hr
Duration	Unknown

Interactions: None

NURSING CONSIDERATIONS

Assessment

- Monitor blood, renal, hepatic studies: CBC, differential, platelet counts, BUN, creatinine, ALT (SGPT), urinalysis; if neutrophil count is <750/mm^3, or if AST (SGOT), ALT (SGPT), is 10 times greater than upper normal limit, or if bilirubin is 5 times greater than upper normal limit; when neutrophil count exceeds 750/mm^3 and liver function or renal studies return to normal, treatment may resume at 50% original dosage
- Assess for CNS symptoms: headache, fatigue, depression; if depression occurs and is severe, drug should be discontinued
- Monitor GI status: diarrhea or constipation, vomiting, abdominal pain
- Monitor cardiac status: increased B/P, tachycardia

Nursing diagnoses

✓ Physical mobility, impaired (uses)
✓ Knowledge deficit (teaching)

Implementation

- Reconstitute 0.3 mg (9.6 million IU)/1.2 ml of supplied diluent (0.2 mg or 8 million IU concentration); rotate vial gently, do not shake; withdraw 1 ml using a syringe with 27 G needle; administer SC into hip, thigh, arm; discard unused portion
- Give acetaminophen for fever, headache; use SC route only; do not give IM or **IV**
- Store reconstituted sol in refrigerator; do not freeze; do not use sol that contains precipitate or is discolored

Patient/family education

- Provide patient or family member with written, detailed instructions about the drug; provide initial and return demonstrations on inj procedure; give information on use and disposal of drug
- Inform patient that blurred vision, sweating may occur
- Advise women patients that irregular menses, dysmenorrhea, or metrorrhagia as well as breast pain may occur; use contraception during treatment; drug may cause spontaneous abortion

Evaluation

Positive therapeutic outcome

- Decreased symptoms of multiple sclerosis

I

interferon gamma-1b (℞)

(in-ter-feer′on)

Actimmune

Func. class.: Biologic response modifier

Chem. class.: Lymphokine, interleukin type

Pregnancy category C

Action: Species-specific protein synthesized in response to viruses; potent phagocyte-activating effects; capable of mediating the killing of *Staphylococcus aureus, Toxoplasma gondii, Leishmania donovani, Listeria monocytogenes, Mycobacterium avium-intracellulare;* enhances oxidative metabolism of macrophages; enhances antibody-dependent cellular cytotoxicity

➔ **Therapeutic Outcome:** Decreased signs/symptoms of infection (serious) in chronic granulomatous disease

Uses: Serious infections associated with chronic granulomatous disease

Dosage and routes

Adult: SC 50 μg/m² (1.5 million U/m²) for patients with a surface area of >0.5 m²; 1.5 μg/kg/dose for patient with a surface area of <0.5/m²; give on Monday, Wednesday, Friday for 3 times a wk dosing

Available forms: Inj 100 μg (3 million U)/single-dose vial

Adverse effects

CNS: Headache, fatigue, depression, fever, chills

GI: Nausea, anorexia, abdominal pain, weight loss, diarrhea, vomiting

INTEG: Rash, pain at inj site

MS: Myalgia, arthralgia

Contraindications: Hypersensitivity to interferon gamma, *E. coli*–derived products

Precautions: Pregnancy **C**, cardiac disease, seizure disorders, CNS disorders, myelosuppression, lactation, children [P]

Pharmacokinetics

Absorption	Slowly absorbed; 89%
Distribution	Unknown
Metabolism	Unknown
Excretion	Unknown
Half-life	5.9 hr

Pharmacodynamics

Onset	Unknown
Peak	7 hr
Duration	Unknown

Interactions

Individual drugs

Radiation: ↑ toxicity, bone marrow suppression

Drug classifications

Antineoplastics: ↑ toxicity, bone marrow suppression

NURSING CONSIDERATIONS

Assessment

- Monitor blood, renal, hepatic studies: CBC with differential, platelet count, BUN, creatinine, ALT (SGPT), urinalysis before and q3 mo during treatment
- Assess for infection: headache, fever, chills, fatigue; these are common adverse reactions
- Monitor CNS symptoms: headache, fatigue, depression

Nursing diagnoses

✓ Infection, risk for (uses)

✓ Knowledge deficit (teaching)

Implementation

- Give at hs to minimize adverse reactions; administer acetaminophen for fever, headache; use 50% of the dosage prescribed if severe reactions occur or discontinue treatment until reactions subside

- Administer using sterilized glass or plastic disposable syringes; give in right or left deltoid and anterior thigh; warm to room temp before use; do not leave at room temp over 12 hr (unopened vial); does not contain preservatives
- Store in refrigerator upon receipt; do not freeze; do not shake

Patient/family education

- Provide patient or family member with written, detailed instructions about the drug; provide initial and return demonstrations on inj procedure; give information on use and disposal of drug
- Caution patient to use contraception during treatment

Evaluation

Positive therapeutic outcome

- Decreased serious infections
- Improvement in existing infections and inflammatory conditions

ipecac syrup (OTC)

(ip′e-kak)

Func. class.: Emetic

Chem. class.: Cephaelis ipecacuanha derivative

Pregnancy category C

Action: Acts on chemoreceptor trigger zone to induce vomiting; irritates gastric mucosa

Therapeutic Outcome: Emesis

Uses: In poisoning from noncaustic substances to induce vomiting

Dosage and routes

Adult: PO 15-30 ml, then 200-300 ml water; may repeat in 30 min

Child >1 yr: PO 15 ml, then 200-300 ml water; may repeat in 30 min

Child <1 yr: PO 5-10 ml, then 100-200 ml water; may repeat dose if needed

Available forms: Liq

Adverse effects

CNS: ***Depression, convulsions, coma***

CV: ***Circulatory failure, atrial fibrillation, fatal myocarditis, dysrhythmias***

GI: Nausea, vomiting, bloody diarrhea

Contraindications: Hypersensitivity, unconscious/semiconscious, depressed gag reflex, poisoning with petroleum products or caustic substances, convulsions, shock, alcohol intolerance

Precautions: Lactation, pregnancy **C,** child <6 mo

Pharmacokinetics	
Absorption	Not absorbed
Distribution	Unknown
Metabolism	Unknown
Excretion	Unknown
Half-life	Unknown

Pharmacodynamics	
Onset	15-30 min
Peak	Unknown
Duration	½ hr

Interactions

Individual drugs

Activated charcoal: ↓ effect; do not use together

Drug classifications

Antiemetics: ↓ effect, do not use together

Food

Milk: ↓ effect

Carbonated drinks: ↑ abdominal distention

NURSING CONSIDERATIONS

Assessment

- Assess type of poisoning; do not administer if petroleum products or caustic substances have been ingested: kerosene, gasoline, lye, Drano
- Assess respiratory status before, during, after administration of emetic; check rate, rhythm, character; respiratory depression can occur rapidly G with elderly or debilitated patients
- Monitor LOC; do not give to patients who are semiconscious or unconscious or if gag reflex is not present

Nursing diagnoses

✓ Injury, risk for (uses)

✓ Poisoning (uses)

✓ Knowledge deficit (teaching)

Implementation

PO route

- Give **ipecac *syrup*, not ipecac,** which is 14 times stronger or death may occur
- Give activated charcoal after the patient has finished vomiting; may begin lavage after 10-15 min after 2 doses of ipecac syrup without results
- Give with the patient upright; give water immediately after the ipecac syrup (200-300 ml for adults; 100-P 200 ml child <1 yr; 200-300 ml for a child >1 yr)

Patient family education

- Give patient phone number for poison control
- Give patient written guidelines on poisoning and when to induce vomiting; suggest patient keep ipecac syrup in P house if young children are present

Evaluation

Positive therapeutic outcome

- Vomiting within 30 min

ipratropium (℞)

(i-pra-troe'pee-um)

Atrovent

Func. class.: Anticholinergic, bronchodilator

Chem. class.: Synthetic quaternary ammonium compound

Pregnancy category B

Action: Inhibits interaction of acetylcholine at receptor sites on the bronchial smooth muscle, resulting in decreased cyclic guanosine monophosphate (cGMP) and bronchodilatation

→ **Therapeutic Outcome:** Bronchodilatation

Uses: Bronchodilatation during bronchospasm for patients with COPD

Dosage and routes

Adult: 2 Inh qid, not to exceed 12 inh/24 hr

Available forms: Aerosol 18 µg/actuation

Adverse effects

CNS: Anxiety, dizziness, headache, nervousness

CV: Palpitations

EENT: Dry mouth, blurred vision

GI: Nausea, vomiting, cramps

INTEG: Rash

*RESP: Cough, worsening of symptoms, **bronchospasms***

Contraindications: Hypersensitivity to this drug, atropine, soya lecithin

Precautions: Pregnancy **B**, P lactation, children <12 yr, narrow-angle glaucoma, prostatic hypertrophy, bladder neck obstruction

Pharmacokinetics

Absorption	Minimal
Distribution	Does not cross blood-brain barrier
Metabolism	Liver, minimal
Excretion	Unknown
Half-life	2 hr

Pharmacodynamics

Onset	5-15 min
Peak	1-1½ hr
Duration	3-6 hr

Interactions

Drug classifications

Bronchodilators, aerosol: ↑ action of bronchodilator

NURSING CONSIDERATIONS

Assessment

- Monitor respiratory function: vital capacity, FEV, ABGs, lung sounds, heart rate, rhythm (baseline and during treatment); if severe bronchospasm is present, a more rapid medication is required
- Monitor for evidence of allergic reactions, paradoxic bronchospasm; withhold dose and notify prescriber; identify if patient is allergic to belladonna products or atropine; allergy to this drug may occur

Nursing diagnoses

- ✓ Airway clearance, ineffective (uses)
- ✓ Gas exchange, impaired (uses)
- ✓ Knowledge deficit (teaching)

Implementation

- Give after shaking container; have patient exhale, place mouthpiece in mouth, inhale slowly, hold breath, remove, exhale slowly; allow at least 1 min between inhalations
- Store in light-resistant container; do not expose to temp over 86° F (30° C)

Patient/family education

- Advise patient not to use OTC medications unless approved by prescriber; extra stimulation may occur; to use this medication before other medications and allow at least 5 min between each to prevent overstimulation
- Teach patient the proper use of the inhaler; review package insert with patient; to avoid getting aerosol in eyes; blurring may result; to wash inhaler in warm water qd and dry; to avoid smoking, smoke-filled rooms, persons with respiratory tract infections
- Teach patient if paradoxic bronchospasm occurs to stop drug immediately and notify prescriber; to limit caffeine products such as chocolate, coffee, tea, and colas
- Instruct patient on administration of dose, not to use more than prescribed; serious side effects may occur; if dose is missed, take when remembered; space other doses on new time schedule; do not double doses

Evaluation

Positive therapeutic outcome

- Absence of dyspnea, wheezing after 1 hr
- Improved airway exchange
- Improved ABGs

irinotecan (℞)
(ear-een-oh-tee'kan)
Camptosar
Func. class.: Antineoplastic hormone
Chem. class.: Topoisomerase inhibitor
Pregnancy category D

Action: Cytotoxic by producing damage to double-strand DNA during DNA synthesis

➔ **Therapeutic Outcome:** Prevention in growth of tumor size

Uses: Metastatic carcinoma of the colon or rectum

Dosage and routes
Adult: **IV** 125 mg/m^2 given over 1½ hr given qwk × 4 wk, then 2 wk rest period, may be repeated; 4 wk or 2 wk off, dosage adjustments may be made to 150 mg/m^2 (high) or 50 mg/m^2 (low); adjustments should be made in increments of 25-50 mg/m^2 depending on patient's tolerance

Available forms: Inj 20 mg/ml

Adverse effects
CNS: Fever, headache, chills, dizziness
CV: Vasodilation
GI: Diarrhea, nausea, vomiting, anorexia, constipation, cramps, flatus, stomatitis, dyspepsia
HEMA: Leukopenia, anemia, neutropenia
INTEG: Irritation at site, rash, sweating
RESP: Dyspnea, increased cough, rhinitis
MISC: Edema, asthenia, weight loss

Contraindications: Hypersensitivity, pregnancy **D**

P G **Precautions:** Lactation, children, elderly, myelosuppression, irradiation

Pharmacokinetics

Absorption	Complete
Distribution	Widely, 30%-68% bond to plasma proteins
Metabolism	Unknown
Excretion	Urine/bile
Half-life	Unknown

Pharmacodynamics

Unknown

Interactions
Individual drugs
Dexamethensone: ↑ lymphocytopenia
Prochlorperazine: ↑ akathisia
Drug classifications
Diuretics: ↑ dehydration
Antineoplastics: ↑ myelosuppression, diarrhea

NURSING CONSIDERATIONS
Assessment
- Assess for CNS symptoms: fever, headache, chills, dizziness
- Assess CBC, differential, platelet count weekly; withhold drug if WBC is <3500/mm^3, or platelet count <100,000/mm^3; notify prescriber of these results, drug should be discontinued
- Assess food preferences: list likes, dislikes
- Assess buccal cavity q8h for dryness, sores or ulceration, white patches, oral pain, bleeding, dysphagia
- Assess GI symptoms: frequency of stools; cramping
- Assess signs of dehydration: rapid respirations, poor skin turgor, decreased urine output; dry skin, restlessness, weakness

Nursing diagnoses

- ✓ Infection, risk for (adverse reactions)
- ✓ Knowledge deficit (teaching)

Implementation

- Provide increased fluid intake to 2-3 L/day to prevent dehydration, unless contraindicated
- Change **IV** site q48h
- Provide rinsing of mouth tid-qid with water, club soda; brushing of teeth bid-tid with soft brush or cotton-tipped applicator for stomatitis; use unwaxed dental floss
- Provide nutritious diet with iron, vitamin supplement, low fiber, few dairy products

Patient/family education

- Advise to avoid foods with citric acid or hot or rough texture if stomatitis is present; to drink adequate fluids
- Advise to report stomatitis; any bleeding, white spots, ulcerations in mouth; tell patient to examine mouth qd, report symptoms
- Advise to report signs of anemia: fatigue, headache, faintness, shortness of breath, irritability
- Advise to use contraception during therapy

Evaluation

Positive therapeutic outcome

- Decrease in tumor size, decrease in spread of cancer

Treatment of overdose: Induce vomiting, provide supportive care

iron dextran (℞)

Imferon ✤, InFed

Func. class.: Hematinic

Chem. class.: Ferric hydroxide complex with dextran

Pregnancy category C

Action: Iron is carried by transferrin to the bone marrow, where it is incorporated into hemoglobin

➔ **Therapeutic Outcome:** Prevention and resolution of iron-deficiency anemia

Uses: Iron-deficiency anemia in patients who cannot take oral preparations

Dosage and routes

P ***Adult and child:*** IM 0.5 ml as a test dose by Z-track, then no more than the following per day:

Adult <50 kg: IM 100 mg

Adult >50 kg: IM 250 mg

P ***Infant <5 kg:*** IM 25 mg

P ***Child <9 kg:*** IM 50 mg

Adult: **IV** 0.5 ml test dose, then 100 mg qd after 2-3 days; **IV** 250/1000 ml of NaCl; give 25 mg test dose, wait 5 min, then inf over 6-12 hr or follow equation:

$$\frac{0.3 \times \text{weight (lb)} \times 100\text{-Hgb (g/dl)} \times 100}{14.8}$$

Patients <30 lb (66 kg) should be given 80% of above formula dose

Available forms: Inj IM/**IV** 50 mg/ml; inj IM only 50 mg/ml

Adverse effects

CNS: Headache, paresthesia,

dizziness, shivering, weakness, ***seizures***
CV: Chest pain, ***shock,*** hypotension, tachycardia
GI: *Nausea,* vomiting, metallic taste, abdominal pain
HEMA: *Leukocytosis*
INTEG: Rash, pruritus, urticaria, fever, sweating, chills, brown skin discoloration, pain at inj site, necrosis, sterile abscesses, phlebitis
MISC: ***Anaphylaxis***
RESP: Dyspnea

Contraindications: Hypersensitivity, all anemias excluding iron-deficiency anemia, hepatic disease

Precautions: Acute renal
P disease, children, asthma, lactation, rheumatoid arthritis
P (**IV**), infants <4 mo, pregnancy **C**

Pharmacokinetics

Absorption	Well absorbed; lymphatics over wk or mo
Distribution	Crosses placenta
Metabolism	Slow; blood loss, desquamation
Excretion	Breast milk, feces, urine, bile
Half-life	6 hr

Pharmacodynamics

Unknown

Interactions

Individual drugs

Chloramphenicol: ↓ reticulocyte response
Oral iron: Do not use together
Vitamin E: ↓ reticulocyte response

Lab test interferences

False ↑ Serum bilirubin
False ↓ Serum calcium
False positive: ^{99m}Tc diphosphate bone scan, iron test (large doses >2 ml)

NURSING CONSIDERATIONS

Assessment

- Monitor blood studies: Hct, Hgb, reticulocytes, bilirubin before treatment, at least monthly
- Assess for allergic reaction and ***anaphylaxis;*** rash, pruritus, fever, chills, wheezing, notify prescriber immediately
- Assess cardiac status: anginal pain, hypotension, tachycardia
- Assess for nutrition: amount of iron in diet (meat, dark green leafy vegetables, dried fruits, eggs); cause of iron loss or anemia, including salicylates, sulfonamides
- Monitor pulse, B/P during **IV** administration

Nursing diagnoses

✓ Fatigue (uses)
✓ Activity intolerance (uses)
✓ Knowledge deficit (teaching)

Implementation

IM route

- D/C oral iron before parenteral; give only after test dose of 25 mg by preferred route; wait at least 1 hr before giving remaining portion
- Give IM deep in large muscle mass; use Z-track method and 19-20 G 2-, 3-inch needle; ensure needle is long enough to place drug deep in muscle; change needles after withdrawing medication and injecting to prevent skin and tissue staining

IV **IV route**

- Give **IV** after flushing tubing with 10 ml of 0.9% NaCl; give undiluted; give 1 ml (50 mg) or less over 1 min or more; flush line after use with 10 ml of 0.9% NaCl; patient should remain recumbent for 30-60 min to prevent orthostatic hypotension

• **IV** inj requires single-dose vial without preservative; verify on label **IV** use is approved
• Give by cont inf after diluting in 50-250 normal saline for inf; administer over 4-5 hr
• Give only with epinephrine available in case of anaphylactic reaction during dose
• Store at room temp in cool environment

Patient/family education

• Caution patient that iron poisoning may occur if increased beyond recommended level; to not take oral iron preparation unless approved by prescriber
• Advise patient that delayed reaction may occur 1-2 days after administration and last 3-4 days (**IV**) or 3-7 days (IM); report fever, chills, malaise, muscle, joint aches, nausea, vomiting, backache

Evaluation

Positive therapeutic outcome

• Increased serum iron levels, Hct, Hgb

Treatment of overdose:

• Discontinue drug, treat allergic reaction, give diphenhydramine or epinephrine as needed for anaphylaxis; give iron-chelating drug in acute poisoning

isoniazid (℞)

(eye-soe-nye'a-zid)

INH, isoniazid, Isotamine ✱, Laniazid, Laniazid C.T., Nydrazid, PMS-Isoniazid ✱, Tubizid

Func. class.: Antitubercular
Chem. class.: Isonicotinic acid hydrazide

Pregnancy category C

Action: Inhibits RNA synthesis, decreases tubercle bacilli replication

Therapeutic Outcome: Resolution of TB infection

Uses: Pulmonary TB as an adjunct; other infections caused by mycobacteria

Dosage and routes

Treatment

Adult: PO/IM 5 mg/kg qd as single dose for 9-24 mo, not to exceed 300 mg/day

P ***Child and infant:*** PO/IM 10-20 mg/kg qd as single dose for 18-24 mo, not to exceed 300 mg/day

Prevention

Adult: PO 300 mg qd as single dose × 12 mo

P ***Child and infant:*** PO/IM 10 mg/kg qd as single dose for 12 mo, not to exceed 300 mg/day

Available forms: Tabs 100, 300 mg; inj 100 mg/ml; powder 50 mg/5 ml; syrup 50 mg/5 ml

Adverse effects

Hypersensitivity: fever, skin eruptions, lymphadenopathy, vasculitis

CNS: Peripheral neuropathy, memory impairment, ***toxic***

encephalopathy, convulsions, psychosis
EENT: Blurred vision, optic neuritis, visual disturbance
GI: Nausea, vomiting, epigastric distress, ***jaundice, fatal hepatitis***
HEMA: ***Agranulocytosis, hemolytic anemia, aplastic anemia, thrombocytopenia, eosinophilia, methemoglobinemia***
MISC: Dyspnea, vitamin B_6 deficiency, pellagra, hyperglycemia, metabolic acidosis, gynecomastia, rheumatic syndrome, SLE-like syndrome

Contraindications: Hypersensitivity, optic neuritis

Precautions: Pregnancy **C,** renal disease, diabetic retinopathy, cataracts, ocular defects, hepatic disease, P child <13 yr

Pharmacokinetics

Absorption	Well
Distribution	Widely
Metabolism	Liver
Excretion	Kidneys
Half-life	1-4 hr

Pharmacodynamics

	PO	IM
Onset	Rapid	Rapid
Peak	1-2 hr	45-60 min
Duration	6-8 hr	6-8 hr

Interactions

Individual drugs
Alcohol: ↑ toxicity
BCG vaccine: ↓ effectiveness of BCG vaccine
Carbamazepine: ↑ toxicity
Cycloserine: ↑ toxicity
Ethionamide: ↑ toxicity
Phenytoin: ↓ metabolism of phenytoin
Rifampin: ↑ toxicity
Drug classifications
Antacids, aluminum: ↓ absorption
Food
Tyramine foods: ↑ toxicity

NURSING CONSIDERATIONS

Assessment

- Obtain C&S tests, including sputum tests, before treatment; monitor every mo to detect resistance
- Monitor liver studies weekly: ALT (SGPT), AST (SGOT), bilirubin; renal studies during treatment and monthly before: BUN, creatinine, output, sp gr, urinalysis, uric acid
- Assess mental status often: affect, mood, behavioral changes; psychosis may occur with hallucinations, confusion
- Assess hepatic status: decreased appetite, jaundice, dark urine, fatigue
- Assess for visual disturbance that may indicate optic neuritis: blurred vision, change in color perception; may lead to blindness

Nursing diagnoses

✓ Infection, risk for (uses)
✓ Diarrhea (adverse reactions)
✓ Injury, risk for (adverse reactions)
✓ Knowledge deficit (teaching)
✓ Noncompliance (teaching)

Implementation

- Give antiemetic for vomiting

PO route

- Give with meals to decrease GI symptoms; it is better to take on empty stomach for better absorption, 1 hr ac or 2 hr pc

IM route

- Give deep in large muscle mass, massage; rotate inj sites

Patient/family education

- Instruct patient that compliance with dosage schedule for duration is necessary; not to skip or double doses; that

scheduled appointments must be kept or relapse may occur
- Caution patient to avoid alcohol while taking drug or hepatoxicity may result; to avoid ingestion of aged cheeses, fish or hypertensive crisis may result; give patient written directions on which foods to avoid while taking this medication
- Tell patient to report peripheral neuritis: weakness, tingling/numbness of hands/feet, fatigue, hepatoxicity: loss of appetite, nausea, vomiting, yellowing of skin or eyes

Evaluation

Positive therapeutic outcome
- Decreased symptoms of TB
- Culture negative for TB

isoproterenol (℞)

(eye-soe proe-ter'e-nole)

Aerolone, Dispos-a-Med, Isoproterenol HCl, Isuprel, Isuprel Glossets, Isuprel Mistometer, Medihaler-Iso, Vapo-Iso

Func. class.: β-Adrenergic-agonist, antidysrhythmic, inotropic

Chem. class.: Catecholamine

Pregnancy category C

Action: Has β_1- and β_2-adrenergic action; relaxes bronchial smooth muscle and dilates the trachea and main bronchi by increasing levels of cAMP, which relaxes smooth muscles; causes increased contractility and heart rate by acting on β-receptors in heart

➔ **Therapeutic Outcome:** Bronchodilatation, increased heart rate and cardiac output from action on β-receptors in the heart

Uses: Bronchospasm, asthma, heart block, ventricular dysrhythmias, shock

Dosage and routes

Asthma, bronchospasm

Adult: SL tab 10-20 mg q6-8h; inh 1 puff; may repeat in 2-5 min; maintenance 1-2 puffs 4-6 times/day; **IV** 1020 mg during anesthesia

P ***Child:*** SL tab 5-10 mg q6-8h; inh 1 puff; may repeat in 2-5 min; maintenance 1-2 puffs 4-6 times/day

Heart block/ventricular dysrhythmias

Adult: **IV** 0.02-0.06 mg, then 0.01-0.2 mg or 5 μg/min HCl; 0.2 mg, then 0.02-1 mg as needed

P ***Child:*** **IV** ½ of beginning adult dosage

Shock

Adult: **IV** inf 0.5-5 μg/min (1 mg/500 ml D_5W) titrate to B/P, CVP, hourly urine output

Available forms: Sol for nebulization 1:400 (0.25%), 1:200 (0.5%), 1:100 (1%); aerosol 0.25%, 0.2%; powder for inh 0.1 mg/cartridge; inj 1:5000 (0.2 mg/ml) **IV**; glossets (SL) 10, 15 mg

Adverse effects

CNS: Tremors, anxiety, insomnia, headache, dizziness, stimulation

CV: Palpitations, tachycardia, hypertension, ***cardiac arrest***

GI: Nausea, vomiting

META: Hyperglycemia

RESP: Bronchial irritation, edema, dryness of oropharynx, ***bronchospasms*** (overuse)

Contraindications: Hypersensitivity to sympathomimetics, narrow-angle glaucoma

Precautions: Pregnancy **C**, cardiac disorders, hyperthyroidism, diabetes mellitus, prostatic hypertrophy

Pharmacokinetics

Absorption	Erratic (SL, rec), rapid (inh, IV)
Distribution	Unknown
Metabolism	Lungs, liver, GI tract
Excretion	Kidneys, unchanged (50%)
Half-life	Unknown

Pharmacodynamics

	SL	INH	IV	REC
Onset	1-2 hr	Rapid	Rapid	2-4 hr
Peak	Unknown	Unknown	Unknown	Unknown
Duration	2 hr	1 hr	10 min	3-4 hr

Interactions

Drug classifications

β-Adrenergic blockers: Block therapeutic effect

Bronchodilators, aerosol: ↑ action of bronchodilator

MAOI: ↑ chance of hypertensive crisis

Sympathomimetics: ↑ adrenergic side effects

NURSING CONSIDERATIONS

Assessment

• Assess respiratory function: vital capacity, FEV, ABGs, lung sounds, heart rate, rhythm (baseline and during therapy)

• Monitor for evidence of allergic reactions, paradoxic bronchospasm; withhold dose; notify prescriber

Nursing diagnoses

✓ Airway clearance, ineffective (uses)

✓ Impaired gas exchange (uses)

✓ Knowledge deficit (teaching)

Implementation

Inh

• Give after diluting dose in sterile water or 0.9% NaCl, 0.45% NaCl; give over 15-20 min

• Store in light-resistant container; do not expose to temp over 86° F (30° C)

IV route

• Give by direct **IV** after diluting 0.2 mg or 1 ml (1:5000 sol)/10 ml 0.9% NaCl for inj or D_5W (1:50,000 sol); give 1:50,000 sol over 1 min

• Give by cont inf by diluting 2 mg or 10 ml (1:5000 sol)/ 500 ml 0.9% NaCl, D_5W, $D_{10}W$, 0.45% NaCl, Ringer's, LR (1:250,000 sol); give at a rate of 1 ml/min by inf pump; ratio is adjusted according to patient response

Y-site compatibilities: Amiodarone, amrinone, atracurium, bretylium, famotidine, heparin, hydrocortisone, pancuronium, potassium chloride, vecuronium, vitamin B with C

Syringe compatibility: Ranitidine

Additive compatibilities: Atracurium, calcium chloride, calcium gluceptate, cephalothin, cimetidine, dobutamine, floxacillin, heparin, magnesium sulfate, multivitamins, netilmicin, potassium chloride, ranitidine, succinylchloride, verapamil, vitamin B with C

Patient/family education

• Caution patient not to use OTC medications before consulting prescriber; extra stimulation may occur

• Instruct patient to use this medication before other medications and allow at least 5 min between each; to prevent overstimulation by limiting caffeine products such as chocolate, coffee, tea, and colas

- Teach patient use of inhaler; review package insert with patient; to avoid getting aerosol in eyes; blurring may result; to wash inhaler in warm water qd and dry; rinse mouth after using; to avoid smoking, smoke-filled rooms, persons with respiratory tract infections
- Instruct patient if paradoxic bronchospasm occurs to stop drug immediately and notify prescriber; to limit caffeine products such as chocolate, coffee, tea, and colas
- Instruct patient on administration of dose; not to use more than prescribed; serious side effects may occur; if taking PO regularly and dose is missed, take when remembered; space other doses on new time schedule; do not double doses

Evaluation

Positive therapeutic outcome

- Absence of dyspnea, wheezing
- Improved airway exchange
- Improved ABGs

Treatment of overdose: Administer a β_2-adrenergic blocker

isosorbide (℞)

(eye-soe-sor'bide)

Apo-ISDN ✦, Cedocard-SR ✦, Coronex ✦, Dilatrate-SR, Imdur, ISDN, Iso-Bid, Isonate, Isorbid, Isordil, Isordil Tembids, Isordil Titradose, Isosorbide Dinitrate, Isotrate Timecelles, Monoket, Novasorbide ✦, Sorbitrate, Sorbitrate SA, Sorbitrate/ISMO

Func. class.: Antianginal, Vasodilator

Chem. class.: Nitrate

Pregnancy category C

Action: Decreases preload, afterload, thus decreasing LVEDP, systemic vascular resistance, and reducing cardiac O_2 demand

➔ **Therapeutic Outcome:** Relief and prevention of angina pectoris

Uses: Chronic stable angina pectoris, prophylaxis of angina pain

Dosage and routes

Adult: PO 5-40 mg qid; SL tab 2.5-10 mg; may repeat q2-3h; chew tab 5-10 mg prn or q2-3h as prophylaxis; sus rel cap 40-80 mg q8-12h

Available forms: Sus rel caps 40 mg; ext rel tabs 40, 60 mg; tabs 5, 10, 20, 30, 40 mg; chew tabs 5, 10 mg; SL tabs 2.5, 5, 10 mg

Adverse effects

CNS: Vascular headache, flushing, dizziness, weakness, faintness

CV: Postural hypotension, tachycardia, ***collapse,*** syncope

GI: Nausea, vomiting

INTEG: Pallor, sweating, rash
MISC: Twitching, hemolytic anemia, ***methemoglobinemia***

Contraindications: Hypersensitivity to this drug or nitrates, severe anemia, increased intracranial pressure, cerebral hemorrhage, acute MI

Precautions: Postural hypotension, pregnancy **C,** lactation, children [P]

Pharmacokinetics

Absorption	Well
Distribution	Unknown
Metabolism	Liver
Excretion	Urine, metabolites
Half-life	Dinitrate 1 hr, mononitrate 5 hr

Pharmacodynamics

	SUS REL	SL	PO
Onset	20-45 min	2-5 min	15-30 min
Peak	Unknown	Unknown	Unknown
Duration	8-12 hr	1-4 hr	4-6 hr

Interactions
Individual drugs
Alcohol: ↑ hypotension
Drug classifications
Antihypertensives: ↑ hypotension
β-Blockers: ↑ hypotension
Calcium channel blockers: ↑ hypotension
Phenothiazines: ↑ hypotension

NURSING CONSIDERATIONS
Assessment
- Monitor for orthostatic B/P, pulse at baseline and during treatment
- Assess for pain: duration, time started, activity being performed, character, intensity

Nursing diagnoses
✓ Cardiac output, decreased (uses)
✓ Tissue perfusion, decreased (uses)
✓ Knowledge deficit (teaching)

Implementation
SL route
- Hold SL tab under tongue until dissolved (a few min); do not take anything PO when SL tab is in place

PO route
- Give 1 hr ac or 2 hr pc with 8 oz of water
- ⊘ Sus rel tab should not be chewed, broken, or crushed; chew tab should be chewed thoroughly

Patient/family education
- Instruct patient to swallow sus rel tab whole, do not chew; SL tab should be dissolved under tongue, do not swallow; chew tab should be chewed thoroughly; do not skip or double doses; if dose is missed take when remembered if 2 hr before next dose (dinitrate), 6 hr before next dose (sus rel), or 8 hr before next dose (mononitrate)
- Caution patient to avoid alcohol and OTC medications unless approved by prescriber
- Inform patient that drug may be taken before stressful activity: exercise, sexual activity
- Advise patient that SL tab may sting mucous membranes
- Caution patient to avoid driving and hazardous activities if dizziness occurs
- Advise patient to comply with complete medical regimen
- Caution patient to make position changes slowly to prevent orthostatic hypotension

Evaluation
Positive therapeutic outcome
- Decrease in, prevention of anginal pain

isradipine (℞)
(is-ra′di-peen)
DynaCirc
Func. class.: Calcium channel blocker, antihypertensive
Chem. class.: Dihydropyridine
Pregnancy category C

Action: Inhibits calcium ion influx across cell membrane during cardiac depolarization; produces relaxation of coronary vascular smooth muscle and peripheral vascular smooth muscle; dilates coronary vascular arteries; increases myocardial oxygen delivery in patients with vasospastic angina

➔ **Therapeutic Outcome:** Decreased B/P

Uses: Hypertension

Dosage and routes
Adult: PO 2.5 mg bid; increase at 3-4 wk intervals up to 10 mg bid

Available forms: Caps 2.5, 5 mg

Adverse effects
CNS: Headache, fatigue, dizziness, fainting, sleep disturbances
CV: Peripheral edema, tachycardia, hypotension, chest pain
GI: Nausea, vomiting, diarrhea, gastric upset, constipation, hepatitis
GU: Nocturia, polyuria, ***acute renal failure***
HEMA: Thrombocytopenia, leukopenia, anemia
INTEG: Rash, pruritus, urticaria, photosensitivity, hair loss
MISC: Flushing

Contraindications: Sick sinus syndrome, 2nd- or 3rd-degree heart block, hypotension less than 90 mm Hg systolic, hypersensitivity

Precautions: CHF, hypotension, hepatic disease, pregnancy **C**, lactation, children, renal disease, elderly

Pharmacokinetics	
Absorption	Well absorbed
Distribution	High plasma protein binding (95%)
Metabolism	Liver, extensively and rapidly
Excretion	Kidney
Half-life	8 hr

Pharmacodynamics	
Onset	1-2 hr
Peak	2-3 hr
Duration	12 hr

Interactions
Individual drugs
Alcohol: ↑ hypotension
Fentanyl: ↑ hypotension
Drug classifications
Antihypertensives: ↑ hypotension
Nitrates: ↑ hypotension

NURSING CONSIDERATIONS
Assessment
- Assess fluid volume status: I&O ratio and record, weight, distended red veins, crackles in lung, color, quality and sp gr of urine, skin turgor, adequacy of pulses, moist mucous membranes, bilateral lung sounds, peripheral pitting edema; dehydration symptoms of decreasing output, thirst, hypotension, dry mouth and mucous membranes should be reported
- Monitor ALT (SGPT), AST (SGOT), bilirubin; if these are elevated, hepatotoxicity is suspected
- Monitor cardiac status: B/P, pulse, respiration, ECG

Nursing diagnoses

- ✓ Cardiac output, decreased (uses)
- ✓ Knowledge deficit (teaching)

Implementation

- Give once a day, with food for GI symptoms
- Do not crush, chew caps

Patient/family education

- Instruct patient to avoid hazardous activities until stabilized on drug and dizziness is no longer a problem
- Instruct patient to limit caffeine consumption; to avoid alcohol and OTC drugs unless directed by prescriber
- Advise patient to comply in all areas of medical regimen: diet, exercise, stress reduction, drug therapy; to notify prescriber of irregular heart beat, shortness of breath, swelling of feet and hands, pronounced dizziness, constipation, nausea, hypotension
- Teach patient to use as directed even if feeling better
- Teach patient to take with a full glass of water

Evaluation

Positive therapeutic outcome

- Decreased B/P

Treatment of overdose: Defibrillation, atropine for AV block, vasopressor for hypotension

itraconazole (℞)

(it-tra-kon′a-zol)

Sporanox

Func. class.: Antifungal (systemic)

Chem. class.: Triazole derivative

Pregnancy category C

Action: Increases cell membrane permeability in susceptible organisms by binding sterols in fungal cell membrane; decreases potassium, sodium, and nutrients in cell

➔ **Therapeutic Outcome:** Fungistatic against *Histoplasma capsulatum, Blastomyces dermatitis, Cryptococcus neoformans, Aspergillus fumigatus, Candida*

Uses: Systemic candidiasis, chronic mucocandidiasis, oral thrush, candiduria, coccidioidomycosis, histoplasmosis, chromomycosis, paracoccidioidomycosis, blastomycosis (pulmonary and extrapulmonary)

Dosage and routes

Adult: PO 200 mg tid × 3 days with food; may increase to 400 mg qd if needed; divide doses over 200 mg in 2 doses/day

Available forms: Cap 100 mg

Adverse effects

CNS: Headache, dizziness, insomnia, somnolence, depression

GI: Nausea, vomiting, anorexia, diarrhea, cramps, abdominal pain, flatulence, ***GI bleeding, hepatotoxicity***

GU: Gynecomastia, impotence, decreased libido

INTEG: Pruritus, fever, rash

MISC: Edema, fatigue, malaise, hypertension, hypokalemia, tinnitus

Contraindications: Hypersensitivity, lactation, fungal meningitis, coadministration with terfenadine

Precautions: Hepatic disease, achlorhydria or hypochlorhydria (drug-induced), children, pregnancy **C**

Pharmacokinetics

Absorption	Variable
Distribution	Tissue, plasma, CSF
Metabolism	Liver, extensively
Excretion	Feces, breast milk
Half-life	20-21 hr

Pharmacodynamics

Onset	Unknown
Peak	4 hr
Duration	Unknown

Interactions

Individual drugs

Astemizole: ↑ dysrhythmias
Carbamazepine: ↑ metabolism, ↓ effect of itraconazole
Cyclosporine: ↑ effects of cyclosporine
Digoxin: ↑ effects of digoxin
Isoniazid: ↑ metabolism, ↓ effect of itraconazole
Phenytoin: ↑ metabolism, ↓ effect of itraconazole
Phenobarbital: ↑ metabolism, ↓ effect of itraconazole
Rifampin: ↑ metabolism, ↓ effect of itraconazole
Terfenadine: ↑ dysrhythmias
Warfarin: ↑ effects of warfarin

Drug classifications

Cardiac glycosides: ↑ effects of cardiac glycosides
Oral hypoglycemics: ↑ effects of oral hypoglycemics

Food

↑ absorption

NURSING CONSIDERATIONS

Assessment

- Monitor for hepatotoxicity: increasing AST (SGOT), ALT (SGPT), alkaline phosphatase, bilirubin
- Monitor for allergic reaction: dermatitis, rash; drug should be discontinued, antihistamines (mild reaction) or epinephrine (severe reaction) administered; check inj site for thrombophlebitis
- Monitor for hypokalemia: anorexia, drowsiness, weakness, decreased reflexes, dizziness, increased urinary output, increased thirst, paresthesias; if these occur, drug should be decreased or discontinued and potassium administered

Nursing diagnoses

- ✓ Infection, risk for (uses)
- ✓ Injury, risk for physical (adverse reaction)
- ✓ Knowledge deficit (teaching)

Implementation

- Give with food or milk to prevent nausea and vomiting
- Do not crush, chew caps
- Store in tight container at room temp

Patient/family education

- Advise patient that long-term therapy may be needed to clear infection (2 wk-3 mo depending on type of infection)
- Teach patient side effects and when to notify prescriber

Evaluation

Positive therapeutic outcome

- Decreased fever, malaise, rash
- Negative C&S for infectious organism

kanamycin (℞)
(kan-a-mye'sin)
kanamycin sulfate, Kantrex
Func. class.: Antiinfective
Chem. class.: Aminoglycoside
Pregnancy category D

Action: Interferes with protein synthesis in bacterial cell by binding to the 30S ribosomal subunit, causing inaccurate peptide sequence to form in protein chain, resulting in bacterial death

Therapeutic Outcome: Bactericidal effects for *Escherichia coli, Acinetobacter, Proteus, Serratia, Pseudomonas aeruginosa*

Uses: Severe systemic infections of CNS, respiratory tract, GI tract, urinary tract, bone, skin, soft tissues; also used as adjunct in hepatic coma, peritonitis, preoperatively to sterilize bowel; decreases ammonia-producing bacteria in bowel and intraperitoneally after fecal spill during surgery

Dosage and routes
Severe systemic infections
P ***Adult and child:*** **IV** inf 15 mg/kg/day in divided doses q8-12h; diluted 500 mg/200 ml of NS or D_5W given over 30-60 min, not to exceed 1.5 g/day; IM 15 mg/kg/day in divided doses q8-12h, not to exceed 1.5 g/day; irrigation not to exceed 1.5 g/day

Hepatic coma
Adult: PO 8-12 g/day in divided doses

Preoperative bowel sterilization
Adult: PO 1 g qh × 4 doses, then q6h × 36-72 hr

Available forms: Inj 75, 500 mg/2 ml, 1 g/3 ml; cap 500 mg

Adverse effects
CNS: Confusion, depression, numbness, tremors, ***convulsions,*** muscle twitching, ***neurotoxicity***
CV: Hypotension
EENT: ***Ototoxicity,*** deafness, visual disturbances, dizziness, vertigo, tinnitus
GI: Nausea, vomiting, anorexia, increased ALT (SGPT), AST (SGOT), bilirubin, hepatomegaly, ***hepatic necrosis,*** splenomegaly
GU: ***Oliguria, hematuria, renal damage, azotemia, renal failure, nephrotoxicity***
HEMA: ***Agranulocytosis, thrombocytopenia, leukopenia, eosinophilia, anemia***
INTEG: Rash, burning, urticaria, dermatitis, alopecia
RESP: Respiratory depression

Contraindications: Bowel obstruction, severe renal disease, hypersensitivity, pregnancy **D**

P **Precautions:** Neonates, myasthenia gravis, hearing deficits, mild renal disease, lactation, Parkinson's disease

Pharmacokinetics	
Absorption	Well absorbed (IM)
Distribution	Widely distributed in extracellular fluids; crosses placenta
Metabolism	Liver, minimally
Excretion	Kidneys, mostly unchanged (79%)
Half-life	2-3 hr; increased in renal disease

Pharmacodynamics

	IM	IV
Onset	Rapid	Rapid
Peak	1-2 hr	1-2 hr

Interactions

Individual drugs

Amphotericin B: ↑ ototoxicity, neurotoxicity, nephrotoxicity
Cisplatin: ↑ ototoxicity, neurotoxicity, nephrotoxicity
Ethacrynic acid: ↑ ototoxicity, neurotoxicity, nephrotoxicity
Furosemide: ↑ ototoxicity, neurotoxicity, nephrotoxicity
Mannitol: ↑ ototoxicity, neurotoxicity, nephrotoxicity
Methoxyflurane: ↑ ototoxicity, neurotoxicity, nephrotoxicity
Polymyxin: ↑ ototoxicity, neurotoxicity, nephrotoxicity
Succinylcholine: ↑ neuromuscular blockade, respiratory depression
Vancomycin: ↑ ototoxicity, neurotoxicity, nephrotoxicity

Drug classifications

Anesthetics: ↑ neuromuscular blockade, respiratory depression
Aminoglycosides: ↑ otoxicity, nephrotoxicity, neurotoxicity
Nondepolarizing neuromuscular blockers: ↑ neuromuscular blockade, respiratory depression

NURSING CONSIDERATIONS

Assessment

- Assess patient for previous sensitivity reaction
- Assess patient for signs and symptoms of infection including characteristics of wounds, sputum, urine, stool, WBC >10,000, fever; obtain baseline information and during treatment
- Obtain C&S tests before beginning drug therapy to identify if correct treatment has been initiated
- Assess for allergic reactions: rash, urticaria, pruritus, chills, fever, joint pain; angioedema may occur a few days after therapy begins
- Identify urine output; if decreasing, notify prescriber (may indicate nephrotoxicity); also check for increased BUN, creatinine, urine CrCl <80 ml/min
- Monitor blood studies: AST (SGOT), ALT (SGPT), CBC, Hct, bilirubin, LDH, alkaline phosphatase, Coombs' test monthly if patient is on long-term therapy
- Monitor electrolytes: potassium, sodium, chloride, calcium, magnesium monthly if patient is on long-term therapy
- Assess bowel pattern qd; if severe diarrhea occurs, drug should be discontinued; may indicate pseudomembranous colitis
- Monitor for bleeding: ecchymosis, bleeding gums, hematuria, stool guaiac daily if on long-term therapy
- Assess for overgrowth of infection: perineal itching, fever, malaise, redness, pain, swelling, drainage, rash, diarrhea, change in cough, sputum
- Obtain weight before treatment; calculation of dosage is usually based on ideal body weight, but may be calculated on actual body weight
- Monitor I&O ratio; perform urinalysis daily for proteinuria, cells, casts; report sudden change in urine output
- Monitor VS during inf; watch for hypotension, change in pulse

K

• Assess **IV** site for thrombophlebitis including pain, redness, swelling q30 min; change site if needed; apply warm compresses to discontinued site
• Obtain serum peak, drawn at 30-60 min after **IV** inf or 60 min after IM inj; draw trough level just before next dose; blood level should be 2-4 times bacteriostatic level
• Assess hearing by audiometric testing, ringing, roaring in ears, vertigo before, during, after treatment
• Assess for dehydration: high sp gr, decrease in skin turgor, dry mucous membranes, dark urine
• Assess vestibular dysfunction: nausea, vomiting, dizziness, headache; drug should be discontinued if severe

Nursing diagnoses

✓ Infection, risk for (uses)
✓ Diarrhea (adverse reactions)
✓ Injury, risk for (adverse reactions)
✓ Knowledge deficit (teaching)

Implementation

PO route

• Give in even doses around the clock; if GI upset occurs, give with food; drug must be given for 10-14 days to ensure organism death and prevent superinfection; store in tight container.

IM route

• Inject deep in large muscle mass

IV **IV route**

• Dilute 500 mg/100-200 ml; or 1 g/200-400 ml D_5W, $D_{10}W$, D_5/0.9% NaCl, 0.9% NaCl, LR
• Do not admix; give aminoglycosides and penicillin at least 1 hr apart
• Give by intermittent inf over 30-60 min; flush with 0.9% NaCl or D_5W after inf is complete

Syringe incompatibilities: Ampicillin, carbanicillin, heparin

Additive incompatibilities: Amphotericin B, cephalothin, cephapirin, chlorpheniramine, heparin, methohexital

Additive compatibilities: Ascorbic acid, cefoxitin, chloramphenicol, clindamycin, dopamine, furosemide, polymyxin B, sodium bicarbonate, tetracycline; admixing is not recommended

Y-site compatibilities: Cyclophosphamide, furosemide, heparin with hydrocortisone, hydromorphone, magnesium sulfate, meperidine, morphine, perphenazine, potassium chloride

Patient/family education

• Teach patient to report sore throat, bruising, bleeding, joint pain, may indicate blood dyscrasias (rare)
• Advise patient to contact prescriber if vaginal itching, loose, foul-smelling stools, furry tongue occur; may indicate superinfection

Evaluation

Positive therapeutic outcome

• Absence of signs/symptoms of infection (WBC <10,000, temp WNL, absence of red, draining wounds)
• Reported improvement in symptoms of infection

Treatment of overdose: Withdraw drug, hemodialysis, monitor serum levels of drug

kaolin/pectin (OTC)

(kay′-oh-lin pek′tin)

Func. class.: Antidiarrheal

Chem. class.: Hydrous magnesium aluminum silicate

Pregnancy category C

Action: Decreases gastric motility, water content of stool; adsorbent, demulcent

➔ **Therapeutic Outcome:** Absence of diarrhea

Uses: Diarrhea (cause undetermined)

Dosage and routes

Adult: PO 60-120 ml (45-90 ml conc) after each loose bowel movement

P ***Child >12 yrs:*** PO 60 ml after each loose bowel movement

P ***Child 6-12 yrs:*** PO 30-60 ml (15 ml conc) after each loose bowel movement

P ***Child 3-6 yrs:*** PO 15-30 ml (7.5 ml conc) after each loose bowel movement

Available forms: Susp kaolin 0.87 g/5 ml, pectin 43 mg/5 ml; kaolin 0.98 g/5 ml, pectin 21.7 mg/5 ml

Adverse effects

GI: Constipation (chronic use)

P **Contraindications:** Child <3 yr, severe abdominal pain

Precautions: Pregnancy **C**

Pharmacokinetics

Absorption	Not absorbed
Distribution	Unknown
Metabolism	Unknown
Excretion	Unknown
Half-life	Unknown

Pharmacodynamics

Onset	½ hr
Peak	Unknown
Duration	6 hr

Interactions

All drugs: ↓ action of all other drugs

NURSING CONSIDERATIONS

Assessment

- Assess bowel pattern before, during treatment; for rebound constipation after termination of medication; check bowel sounds
- Check response after 48 hr; if no response, drug should be discontinued and other treatment initiated

Nursing diagnoses

✓ Diarrhea (uses)
✓ Constipation (adverse reactions)
✓ Knowledge deficit (teaching)
✓ Noncompliance (teaching)

Implementation

- Shake susp before use
- Administer for 48 hr only

Patient/family education

- Advise patient not to exceed recommended dosage

Evaluation

Positive therapeutic outcome

- Decreased diarrhea

K

ketamine (℞)

(ket'a-meen)

Ketalar

Func. class.: General anesthetic

Chem. class.: Phencyclidine derivative

Pregnancy category C

Action: Acts on limbic system, cortex by blocking pain impulses to provide anesthesia

Therapeutic Outcome: Anesthesia

Uses: Short anesthesia for diagnostic/surgical procedures; as an adjunct with other anesthetics

Dosage and routes

P ***Adult and child:*** **IV** 1-4.5 mg/kg over 1 min

P ***Adult and child:*** IM 6.5-13 mg/kg

Maintenance: ½ to full induction dose may be repeated

Available forms: Inj IM, **IV** 10, 50, 100 mg/ml

Adverse effects

CNS: Hallucinations, confusion, delirium, tremors, polyneuropathy, fasciculations, pseudoconvulsions

CV: Increased B/P, hypotension, bradycardia

EENT: Diplopia, salivation, small increase in intraocular pressure

INTEG: Rash, pain at inj site

Contraindications: Hypersensitivity, CVA, increased intracranial pressure, severe hypertension, cardiac decompensation, child <2 yr P

Precautions: Pregnancy **C**, seizure disorders, elderly, psychiatric disorders G

Pharmacokinetics

Absorption	Rapidly absorbed (IM); completely absorbed (IV)
Distribution	Rapidly distributed; crosses placenta
Metabolism	Liver
Excretion	Kidneys
Half-life	2½ hr

Pharmacodynamics

	IV	IM
Onset	Unknown	Unknown
Peak	40 sec	3-8 min
Duration	10 min	25 min

Interactions

Individual drugs

Thiopental: ↓ hypnotic effect

Tubocurarine: ↑ action of tubocurarine

Drug classifications

Antihypertensive with CNS depressant effect: ↑ respiratory depression

Barbiturates: ↑ recovery time

Halothane anesthetics: ↓ cardiac output, B/P

Narcotics: ↑ action of ketamine

Nondepolaring muscle relaxants: ↑ respiratory depression

Thyroid hormone: ↑ tachycardia, hypertension

NURSING CONSIDERATIONS

Assessment

- Monitor VS q10 min during **IV** administration, q30 min after IM dose
- Assess for hallucinations, delusions, separation from environment
- Assess for extrapyramidal reactions: dystonia, akathisia
- Monitor for increasing heart rate or decreasing B/P; notify prescriber at once

Nursing diagnoses
✓ Sensory-perceptual alterations (adverse reactions)
✓ Knowledge deficit (teaching)

Implementation

IV **IV route**
- Administer **IV** after diluting 100 mg/ml with equal parts of D_5W, 0.9% NaCl, sterile water for inj; give over 1 min; may be diluted 10 ml (50 mg/ml)/ 500 ml of normal saline or D_5W = 1 mg/ml; run at 1-2 mg/min; titrate to patient response
- Administer anticholinergic preoperatively to decrease secretions
- Give only with resuscitative equipment nearby
- Give narcotic or diazepam to control recovery symptoms

Syringe incompatibilities: Barbiturates, diazepam, doxapram

Syringe compatibility: Benzquinamide

Patient/family education
- Teach patient reason for medication and expected results

Evaluation

Positive therapeutic outcome
- Maintenance of anesthesia

ketoconazole (℞)
(kee-toe-koe'na-zole)
Nizoral
Func. class.: Antifungal
Chem. class.: Imidazole derivative
Pregnancy category C

Action: Alters cell membrane and inhibits several fungal enzymes; prevents production of adrenal sterols; prevents fungal metabolism

➔ **Therapeutic Outcome:** Fungistatic/fungicidal against susceptible organisms: *Blastomycoses, Candida, Coccidioides, Cryptococcus, Histoplasma;* top route: *tinea cruris, tinea corporis, tinea versicolor, pityrosporum ovale*

Uses: Systemic candidiasis, chronic mucocandidiasis, oral thrush, candiduria, coccidioidomycosis, histoplasmosis, chromomycosis, paracoccidioidomycosis, blastomycosis

Investigational uses: Cushing's syndrome, advanced prostatic cancer

Dosage and routes

Adult: PO 200-400 mg once daily

P ***Children >2 yr:*** 3.3-6.6 mg/kg/day as single daily dose; <2 yr daily dose not established

P ***Adult and child >2 yr:*** Top 2% cream applied qd or bid

Adult: Massage shampoo into scalp 1 min, reapply × 3 min, rinse; continue treatment twice/wk × 1 mo, no more than once q3 days

Available forms: Tab 200 mg; cream 2%; shampoo 2%

Adverse effects

CNS: Headache, dizziness, somnolence
GI: Nausea, vomiting, anorexia, diarrhea, abdominal pain, *hepatotoxicity*
GU: Gynecomastia, impotence
HEMA: Thrombocytopenia, leukopenia, hemolytic anemia
INTEG: Pruritus, fever, chills, photophobia, rash, dermatitis, purpura, urticaria
SYST: Anaphylaxis

K

Contraindications: Hypersensitivity, lactation, fungal meningitis; coadministration with terfenadine

Precautions: Renal disease, hepatic disease, achlorhydria (drug induced), pregnancy **C**, P children <2 yr, other hepatotoxic agents including terfenadine

Pharmacokinetics

Absorption	pH dependent; ↓ pH ↑ absorption
Distribution	Widely distributed; crosses placenta
Metabolism	Liver, partially
Excretion	Feces, bile, breast milk
Half-life	Biphasic: 2 hr, 8 hr

Pharmacodynamics

Onset	Unknown
Peak	1-3 hr
Duration	Unknown

Interactions

Individual drugs

Alcohol: ↑ hepatotoxicity
Astemizole: ↑ dysrhythmias
Carbamazepine: ↑ metabolism, ↓ effect of itraconazole
Cimetidine: ↓ absorption
Cyclosporine: ↑ effects of cyclosporine
Digoxin: ↑ effects of digoxin
Famotidine: ↓ absorption
Isoniazid: ↑ metabolism, ↓ effect of itraconazole
Nizatidine: ↓ absorption
Omeprazole: ↓ absorption
Phenobarbital: ↑ metabolism, ↓ effect of itraconazole
Phenytoin: ↑ metabolism, ↓ effect of itraconazole
Ranitidine: ↓ absorption
Rifampin: ↑ metabolism, ↓ effect of itraconazole
Terfenadine: ↑ dysrhythmias
Theophylline: ↓ effectiveness
Warfarin: ↑ effects of warfarin

Drug classifications

Cardiac glycosides: ↑ effects of cardiac glycosides
Oral anticoagulants: ↑ effects of oral anticoagulants
Oral hypoglycemics: ↑ effects of oral hypoglycemics

Food

↑ absorption

NURSING CONSIDERATIONS

Assessment

- Assess for signs and symptoms of infection: drainage, sore throat, urinary pain, hematuria, fever
- Obtain cultures for C&S before beginning treatment; therapy may be started after culture is taken
- ! Monitor for hepatotoxicity: increased AST (SGOT), ALT (SGPT), alkaline phosphatase, bilirubin; drug is discontinued if hepatotoxicity occurs

Nursing diagnoses

- ✓ Infection, risk for (uses)
- ✓ Injury, risk for (adverse reactions)
- ✓ Knowledge deficit (teaching)

Implementation

PO route

- Give in the presence of acid products only; do not use alkaline products or antacids within 2 hr of drug; may give coffee, tea, acidic fruit juices; give with food to decrease GI symptoms
- Give with hydrochloric acid if achlorhydria is present
- Store in tight container at room temp

Top route

- Use enough medication to cover fungally infected area and surrounding area; rub in; do not use occlusive dressing; do not get in eyes

Shampoo

• Hair should be wet; apply shampoo, lather, rub gently into scalp and hair for 1 min; rinse; reapply × 3 min; continue treatment 2 times/wk for 1 mo, no more than once q3 days

Patient/family education

• Advise patient that long-term therapy may be needed to clear infection (1 wk-6 mo depending on infection)
• Advise patient to avoid hazardous activities if dizziness occurs
• Instruct patient to take 2 hr before administration of other drugs that increase gastric pH (antacids, H_2-blockers, anticholinergics)
• Stress the importance of compliance with drug regimen
• Advise patient to notify prescriber of GI symptoms, signs of liver dysfunction (fatigue, nausea, anorexia, vomiting, dark urine, pale stools)
• Teach patient proper hygiene: hand washing, nail care, use of concomitant top agents if prescribed
• Caution patient to avoid alcohol, since nausea, vomiting, hypertension may occur
• Advise patient to use sunscreen or avoid direct sunlight to prevent photosensitivity
• Advise patient to notify prescriber of sore throat, fever, skin rash, which may indicate superinfection

Evaluation

Positive therapeutic outcome

• Decreased oral candidiasis, fever, malaise, rash
• Negative C&S for infectious organism
• Absence of dandruff, scaling

ketoprofen (℞)

(ke-to-proe'fen)

Ketoprofen, Orudis, Orudis-E ♣, Oruvail

Func. class.: NSAID; nonnarcotic analgesic

Chem. class.: Propionic acid derivative

Pregnancy category B

Action: Inhibits prostaglandin synthesis by decreasing enzyme needed for biosynthesis; analgesic, antiinflammatory

➔ **Therapeutic Outcome:** Decreased pain, inflammation

Uses: Mild to moderate pain, osteoarthritis, rheumatoid arthritis, dysmenorrhea

Dosage and routes

Antiinflammatory

Adult: PO 150-300 mg in divided doses tid-qid, not to exceed 300 mg/day

Analgesic

Adult: PO 25-50 mg q6-8h

Available forms: Caps 25, 50, 75 mg

Adverse effects

CNS: Dizziness, drowsiness, fatigue, tremors, confusion, insomnia, anxiety, depression
CV: Tachycardia, peripheral edema, palpitations, dysrhythmias, hypertension
EENT: Tinnitus, hearing loss, blurred vision
GI: Nausea, anorexia, vomiting, diarrhea, jaundice, ***cholestatic hepatitis,*** constipation, flatulence, cramps, dry mouth, peptic ulcer
GU: Nephrotoxicity: dysuria, hematuria, oliguria, azotemia
HEMA: Blood dyscrasias

K

INTEG: Purpura, rash, pruritus, sweating

Contraindications: Hypersensitivity, asthma, severe renal disease, severe hepatic disease, ulcer disease

Precautions: Pregnancy **B**, **P** lactation, children, bleeding disorders, GI disorders, cardiac disorders, hypersensitivity to other antiinflammatory agents, **G** elderly

Pharmacokinetics

Absorption	Well absorbed
Distribution	Not known
Metabolism	Liver
Excretion	Kidneys
Half-life	3-3½ hr

Pharmacodynamics

Onset	Unknown
Peak	2 hr
Duration	Unknown

Interactions

Individual drugs

Acetaminophen (long-term use): ↑ renal reactions
Alcohol: ↑ adverse reactions
Aspirin: ↓ effectiveness, ↑ adverse reactions
Coumadin: ↑ anticoagulant effects
Digoxin: ↑ toxicity, levels
Insulin: ↓ insulin effect
Lithium: ↑ toxicity
Methotrexate: ↑ toxicity
Phenytoin: ↑ toxicity
Probenecid: ↑ toxicity
Sulfonylurea: ↑ toxicity

Drug classifications

Anticoagulants: ↑ risk of bleeding
Antihypertensives: ↓ effect of antihypertensives
Antineoplastics: ↑ risk of hematologic toxicity
β-Blockers: ↑ antihypertension
Cephalosporins: ↑ risk of bleeding
Diuretics: ↓ effectiveness of diuretics
Glucocorticoids: ↑ adverse reactions
Hypoglycemics: ↓ hypoglycemic effect
NSAIDs: ↑ adverse reactions
Potassium supplements: ↑ adverse reactions
Radiation: ↑ risk of hematologic toxicity
Sulfonamides: ↑ toxicity

Lab test interferences

↑ Bleeding time, ↑ liver function studies, ↑ serum uric acid, ↑ amylase, ↑ CO_2, ↑ urinary protein
↓ Serum potassium, ↓ PBI, ↓ cholesterol
Interference: Urine catecholamines, pregnancy test, urine glucose tests (Clinistix, Tes-Tape)

NURSING CONSIDERATIONS

Assessment

- Monitor liver function, renal function, studies: AST (SGOT), ALT (SGPT), bilirubin, creatinine BUN, urine creatinine, CBC Hct, Hgb, pro-time if patient is on long-term therapy
- Check I&O ratio; decreasing output may indicate renal failure (long-term therapy)
- Assess hepatotoxicity: dark urine, clay-colored stools, yellowing of skin and sclera, itching, abdominal pain, fever, diarrhea if patient is on long-term therapy
- Assess for allergic reactions: rash, urticaria; if these occur, drug may have to be discontinued
- Assess for ototoxicity: tinnitus, ringing, roaring in ears;

audiometric testing needed before, after long-term therapy
• Assess for visual changes: blurring, halos; may indicate corneal, retinal damage
• Check edema in feet, ankles, legs
• Identify prior drug history; there are many drug interactions
• Monitor pain: location, duration, type, intensity, before dose and 1 hr after; ROM before dose and after

Nursing diagnoses

✓ Pain (uses)
✓ Mobility, impaired physical (uses)
✓ Injury, risk for (adverse reactions)
✓ Knowledge deficit (teaching)

Implementation

⊘ • Administer to patient whole; do not crush, break, or open cap
• Give with food or milk to decrease gastric symptoms; give 30 min ac or 2 hr pc; absorption may be slowed

Patient/family education

• Teach patient to report any symptoms of hepatotoxicity, renal toxicity, visual changes, ototoxicity, allergic reactions, bleeding (long-term therapy)
• Advise patient to take with 8 oz of water and sit upright for 30 min after dose to prevent ulceration
• Caution patient not to exceed recommended dosage; acute poisoning may result; to take as prescribed; do not double dose
• Advise patient to read label on other OTC drugs; many contain other antiinflammatories
• Inform patient that the therapeutic response takes 2 wk (arthritis)
• Teach patient to report tinnitus, confusion, diarrhea, sweating, hyperventilation, blurred vision, fever, joint aches
• Caution patient to avoid alcohol ingestion; GI bleeding may occur

Evaluation

Positive therapeutic outcome

• Decreased pain
• Decreased inflammation
• Increased mobility

ketorolac (℞)

(kee'toe role-ak)

Acular, Toradol

Func. class.: NSAID, nonnarcotic analgesic

Chem. class.: Pyrrolopyrrole

Pregnancy category C

Action: Inhibits prostaglandin synthesis by decreasing an enzyme needed for biosynthesis; analgesic, needed for biosynthesis; analgesic, antiinflammatory, antipyretic effects

➡ **Therapeutic Outcome:** Decreased pain, inflammation, ocular itching

Uses: Mild to moderate pain (short term); decreased ocular itching in seasonal allergic conjunctivitis

Dosage and routes

Adult (multiple dosing): **IV** bol/IM 30 mg q6h; max 120 mg/day, with transition of 20 mg PO (1st dose) then 10 mg q4-6h; ≥65 yr, renal impairment or weight <50 kg 15 mg q6hr, max 60 mg

Adult (single dose): **IV** bol/IM 30 mg **IV** or 60 mg IM, then 20 mg transition dose, not to exceed 40 mg/day; then 10 mg q4-6hr; ≥65 yr, renal impairment or weight <50 kg IM 30 mg **IV** 15 mg

Ophth

Adult: 1 gtt (0.25 mg) qid × 7 days

Available forms: Inj 15, 30 mg/ml (prefilled syringes); ophth 0.5% sol; tab 10 mg

Adverse effects

CV: Hypertension, flushing, syncope, pallor

CNS: Dizziness, drowsiness, tremors

EENT: Tinnitus, hearing loss, blurred vision

GI: Nausea, anorexia, vomiting, diarrhea, constipation, flatulence, cramps, dry mouth, peptic ulcer

GU: Nephrotoxicity: dysuria, hematuria, oliguria, azotemia

HEMA: Blood dyscrasias

INTEG: Purpura, rash, pruritus, sweating

Contraindications: Hypersensitivity, asthma, severe renal disease, severe hepatic disease, peptic ulcer disease

Precautions: Pregnancy **C,** P lactation, children, bleeding disorders, GI disorders, cardiac disorders, hypersensitivity to other antiinflammatory agents, G elderly

Pharmacokinetics

Absorption	Rapidly, completely absorbed
Distribution	Bound to plasma proteins (99%)
Metabolism	Liver (<50%)
Excretion	Kidney, metabolites (92%); breast milk (6%); feces
Half-life	6 hr; increased in renal disease

Pharmacodynamics

	IM	OPHTH/PO
Onset	Up to 10 min	Unknown
Peak	50 min	Unknown
Duration	4-6 hr	Unknown

Interactions

Individual drugs

Heparin: ↑ bleeding
Methotrexate: ↑ effects
Phenytoin: ↑ effects
Sulfinpyrazone: ↓ effects

Drug classifications

Anticoagulants: ↑ effects
NSAIDs: ↑ gastric ulcers
Salicylates: ↓ blood sugar levels
Sulfonamides: ↓ effects

Lab test interferences

↑ Coagulation studies, ↑ liver function studies, ↑ serum uric acid, ↑ amylase, ↑ CO_2, ↑ urinary protein
↓ Serum potassium, ↓ PBI, ↓ cholesterol

Interference: Urine catecholamines, pregnancy test, urine glucose tests (Clinistix, Tes-Tape)

NURSING CONSIDERATIONS

Assessment

- Monitor blood counts during therapy; watch for decreasing platelets; if low, therapy may need to be discontinued and restarted after hematologic recovery; assess for blood dyscrasia (thrombocytopenia):

bruising, fatigue, bleeding, poor healing
Assess patient's eyes: redness swelling, tearing, itching

Nursing diagnoses
- ✓ Pain (uses)
- ✓ Mobility, impaired physical (uses)
- ✓ Injury, risk for (adverse reactions)
- ✓ Knowledge deficit (teaching)

Implementation
PO route
- Administer to patient crushed or whole
- Give with food or milk to decrease gastric symptoms; give 30 min ac or 2 hr pc; absorption may be slowed

Y-site compatibility: Sufentanil

Syringe incompatibilities: Morphine, meperidine, promethazine, hydroxyzine

Patient/family education
- Teach patient that drug must be continued for prescribed time to be effective; to avoid aspirin, alcoholic beverages
- Caution patient to report bleeding, bruising, fatigue, malaise, since blood dyscrasias do occur
- Instruct patient to use caution when driving; drowsiness, dizziness may occur
- Teach patient to take with a full glass of water to enhance absorption; do not crush, break, or chew
- Caution patient that this drug may cause eye redness, burning if soft contact lenses are worn

Evaluation
Positive therapeutic outcome
- Decreased pain
- Decreased inflammatory response
- Increased mobility
- Decreased ocular itching

labetalol (℞)
(la-bet'a-lole)
Normodyne, Trandate
Func. class.: Antihypertensive
Chem. class.: α- and β-blocker
Pregnancy category C

Action: Competitively blocks stimulation of β-adrenergic receptor within vascular smooth muscle; produces chronotropic, inotropic activity (decreases rate of SA node discharge, increases recovery time), slows conduction of AV node, decreases heart rate, which decreases O_2 consumption in myocardium; also has α-andrenergic blocking activity

➔ **Therapeutic Outcome:** Decreased B/P

Uses: Mild to moderate hypertension; treatment of severe hypertension (**IV**)

Investigational uses: Angina pectoris (PO), hypotension during surgery (**IV**)

Dosage and routes
Hypertension
Adult: PO 100 mg bid; may be given with a diuretic; may increase to 200 mg bid after 2 days; may continue to increase q1-3 days; max 400 mg bid

Hypertensive crisis
Adult: **IV** inf 200 mg/160 ml D_5W, run at 2 ml/min; stop inf after desired response obtained; repeat q6-8h as needed; **IV** bol 20 mg over 2

L

min; may repeat 40-80 mg q10 min, not to exceed 300 mg

Available forms: Tabs 100, 200, 300 mg; inj 5 mg/ml in 20 ml ampules

Adverse effects
CNS: Dizziness, mental changes, drowsiness, fatigue, headache, catatonia, depression, anxiety, nightmares, paresthesias, lethargy
CV: Orthostatic hypotension, bradycardia, ***CHF,*** chest pain, ***ventricular dysrhythmias,*** AV block
EENT: Tinnitus, visual changes, sore throat, double vision, dry burning eyes
GI: Nausea, vomiting, diarrhea
GU: Impotence, dysuria, ejaculatory failure
HEMA: ***Agranulocytosis, thrombocytopenia, purpura*** (rare)
INTEG: Rash, alopecia, urticaria, pruritus, fever
RESP: ***Bronchospasm,*** dyspnea, wheezing

Contraindications: Hypersensitivity to β-blockers, cardiogenic shock, heart block (2nd or 3rd degree), sinus bradycardia, CHF, bronchial asthma

Precautions: Major surgery, pregnancy **C,** lactation, diabetes mellitus, renal disease, thyroid disease, COPD, well-compensated heart failure, CAD, nonallergic bronchospasm, elderly (G), hepatic disease

Pharmacokinetics

Absorption	Bioavailability 25% (PO); complete (IV)
Distribution	Crosses placenta, CNS
Metabolism	Liver, extensively
Excretion	Breast milk, kidneys, bile
Half-life	6-8 hr

Pharmacodynamics

	PO	IV
Onset	1-2 hr	5 min
Peak	2-4 hr	15 min
Duration	8-12 hr	2-4 hr

Interactions
Individual drugs
Alcohol: ↑ hypotension (large amounts)
Cimetidine: ↑ effect of labetolol
Epinephrine: α-Adrenergic stimulation
Glutethimide: ↓ effect of labetolol
Hydralazine: ↑ hypotension, bradycardia
Indomethacin: ↓ antihypertensive effect
Insulin: ↑ hypoglycemia
Methyldopa: ↑ hypotension, bradycardia
Prazosin: ↑ hypotension, bradycardia
Reserpine: ↑ hypotension, bradycardia
Thyroid: ↓ effect of labetolol
Verapamil: ↑ myocardial depression
Drug classifications
Antihypertensives: ↑ hypertension
β_2-Agonists: ↓ bronchodilatation
Cardiac glycosides: ↑ bradycardia
Nitrates: ↑ hypotension
Theophyllines: ↓ bronchodilatation
Lab test interferences
False ↑ Urinary catecholamines

NURSING CONSIDERATIONS
Assessment
- Monitor B/P at beginning of treatment, periodically thereafter; pulse q4h; note rate, rhythm, quality: apical/

radial pulse before administration; notify prescriber of any significant changes (pulse <50 bpm)
- Check for baselines in renal, liver function tests before therapy begins
- Assess for edema in feet, legs daily, monitor I&O, daily weight; check for jugular vein distention, rales bilaterally, dyspnea (CHF)
- Monitor skin turgor, dryness of mucous membranes for hydration status, especially G elderly

Nursing diagnoses

- ✓ Cardiac output, decreased (uses)
- ✓ Injury, potential for physical (side effects)
- ✓ Knowledge deficit (teaching)
- ✓ Noncompliance (teaching)

Implementation

PO route

- Given ac, hs, tab may be crushed or swallowed whole; give with food to prevent GI upset; reduce dosage in renal dysfunction
- Store protected from light, moisture; place in cool environment

IV **IV route**

- Give **IV** undiluted 20 mg/2 min; may increase q10 min 40-80 mg until desired effect
- Give **IV** cont inf by diluting in LR, D_5W, D_5 in 0.2%, 0.9%, 0.33% NaCl or Ringer's inj; inf is titrated to patient response; 200 mg of drug/160 ml sol (1 mg/ml); 300 mg of drug/240 ml sol (1 mg/ml); 200 mg of drug/250 ml sol (2 mg/3ml); use inf pump
- Keep patient recumbent for 3 hr after inf

Y-site incompatibilities: Cefoperazone, nafcillin

Y-site compatibilities: Amikacin, aminophylline, amiodarone, ampicillin, butorphanol, calcium gluconate, cefazolin, ceftazidime, ceftizoxime, chloramphenicol, cimetidine, clindamycin, dobutamine, dopamine, enalaprilat, erythromycin, esmolol, famotidine, fentanyl, gentamicin, heparin, lidocaine, magnesium sulfate, meperidine, metronidazole, midazolam, morphine, nitroglycerin, nitroprusside, oxacillin, penicillin G potassium, piperacillin, potassium chloride, ranitidine, tobramycin, vancomycin

Solution incompatibility: Sodium bicarbonate 5%

Solution compatibilities: D_5R, D_5LR, $D_{2½}$/0.45% NaCl, D_5/0.2% NaCl, D_5/0.33% NaCl, D_5/0.9% NaCl, D_5W, Ringer's, LR

Patient/family education

- Teach patient not to discontinue drug abruptly, or precipitate angina might occur; taper over 2 wk
- Teach patient not to use OTC products containing α-adrenergic stimulants (such as nasal decongestants, cold preparations); to avoid alcohol, smoking and to limit sodium intake as prescribed
- Teach patient how to take pulse and B/P at home; advise when to notify prescriber
- Instruct patient to comply with weight control, dietary adjustments, modified exercise program
- Advise patient to carry/wear Medic Alert ID to identify drug being taken, allergies; teach patient drug controls symptoms but does not cure
- Caution patient to avoid

L

hazardous activities if dizziness, drowsiness are present
- Teach patient to report symptoms of CHF: difficult breathing, especially on exertion or when lying down, night cough, swelling of extremities, bradycardia, dizziness, confusion, depression, fever
- Teach patient to take drug as prescribed, not to double or skip doses; take any missed doses as soon as remembered if at least 4 hr until next dose

Evaluation

Positive therapeutic outcome
- Decreased B/P in hypertension (after 1-2 wk)
- Absence of dysrhythmias

Treatment of overdose: Lavage, **IV** atropine for bradycardia, **IV** theophylline for bronchospasm, digitalis, O_2, diuretic for cardiac failure, hemodialysis, **IV** glucose for hyperglycemia, **IV** diazepam (or phenytoin) for seizures

lactulose (℞)

(lak'tyoo-lose)

Cephulac, Cholac, Chronulac, Constilac, Constulose, Duphalac Emulose, Enulose, Lactulax ♣

Func. class.: Laxative (hyperosmotic/ammonia detoxicant)

Chem. class.: Lactose synthetic derivative

Pregnancy category C

Action: Increases osmotic pressure; draws fluid into colon; prevents absorption of ammonia in colon; increases water in stool

➔ **Therapeutic Outcome:** Decreased constipation, decreased blood ammonia level

Uses: Chronic constipation, portal-systemic encephalopathy in patients with hepatic disease

Dosage and routes

Constipation

Adult: PO 15-60 ml qd

Encephalopathy

Adult: PO 20-30 g tid or qid until stools are soft; retention enema 30-45 ml in 100 ml of fluid

Available forms: Oral sol, rec sol 3.33 g/5 ml

Adverse effects

GI: Nausea, vomiting, anorexia, abdominal cramps, diarrhea, flatulence, *distention, belching*

Contraindications: Hypersensitivity, low-galactose diet

Precautions: Pregnancy **C,** lactation, diabetes mellitus, G elderly and debilitated patient

Pharmacokinetics	
Absorption	Poorly absorbed
Distribution	Not known
Metabolism	Colonic bacteria to acids
Excretion	Kidneys, unchanged
Half-life	Unknown

Pharmacodynamics
Unknown

Interactions

Individual drugs

Neomycin: ↓ effectiveness (portal-systemic encephalopathy)

Drug classifications

Laxatives: Do not use together (portal-systemic encephalopathy)

NURSING CONSIDERATIONS

Assessment

• Monitor glucose levels in diabetic (increases)
• Monitor blood, urine, electrolytes if used often by patient; may cause diarrhea, hypokalemia, hypernatremia; check I&O ratio to identify fluid loss
• Assess cramping, rec bleeding, nausea, vomiting; if these symptoms occur, drug should be discontinued; identify cause of constipation; identify whether fluids, bulk, or exercise is missing from lifestyle
• Monitor blood ammonia level (30-70 mg/100 ml); monitor for clearing of confusion, lethargy, restlessness, irritability (hepatic encephalopathy); may decrease ammonia level by 50%

Nursing diagnoses

✓ Constipation (uses)
✓ Diarrhea (adverse reactions)
✓ Knowledge deficit (teaching)
✓ Noncompliance (teaching)

Implementation

PO route

• Give with full glass fruit juice, water, milk to increase palatability of oral form; give increased fluids of 2 L/day; do not give with other laxatives; if diarrhea occurs, reduce dosage

Rec route

• Administer retention enema by diluting 300 ml lactulose/700 ml of water or 0.9% NaCl; administer by rec balloon catheter; retain for 30-60 min; repeat if evacuated too quickly

Patient/family education

• Discuss with the patient that adequate fluid consumption is necessary
• Teach patient that normal bowel movements do not always occur daily
• Teach patient not to use in presence of abdominal pain, nausea, vomiting; tell patient to notify prescriber if constipation unrelieved or if symptoms of electrolyte imbalance occur: muscle cramps, pain, weakness, dizziness, excessive thirst
• Teach patient not to use laxatives for long-term therapy; bowel tone will be lost
• Do not give at hs as a laxative; may interfere with sleep
• Notify prescriber if diarrhea occurs; may indicate overdosage

Evaluation

Positive therapeutic outcome

• Decreased constipation
• Decreased blood ammonia level
• Clearing of mental state

lamivudine (3TC) (℞)

(lam-i'vue-dine)

Epivir

Func. class.: Antiviral

Pregnancy category C

Action: Inhibits replication of HIV virus by incorporating into cellular DNA by viral reverse transcriptase, thereby terminating the cellular DNA chain

➔ **Therapeutic Outcome:** Improved symptoms of HIV infection

Uses: HIV infection in combination with zidovudine

Dosage and routes

Adult/adolescents (12-16 yr): PO 150 mg bid with

zidovudine; <50 kg: PO 2 mg/kg bid with zidovudine

P ***Child 3 mo-12 yr:*** PO 4 mg/kg bid; may give 150 mg bid with zidovudine

Renal function impairment: Dosage adjustment required

Available forms: Tabs 150 mg; oral sol 10 mg/ml

Adverse effects

CNS: Fever, headache, malaise, dizziness, insomnia, depression
EENT: Taste change, hearing loss, photophobia
GI: Nausea, vomiting, diarrhea, anorexia, cramps, dyspepsia
HEMA: **Neutropenia,** anemia, **thrombocytopenia**
INTEG: Rash
MS: Myalgia, arthralgia, pain
RESP: Cough

Contraindications: Hypersensitivity

Precautions: Granulocyte count <1000/mm^3 or Hgb <9.5 g/dl, pregnancy **C,** lactation, P children, severe renal disease, severe hepatic function, pancreatitis

Pharmacokinetics	
Absorption	Rapidly absorbed
Distribution	Extravascular space
Metabolism	Unknown
Excretion	Unchanged in urine
Half-life	Unknown

Pharmacodynamics

Unknown

Interactions

Individual drugs

Trimethoprim sulfamethoxazole: ↑ level of lamivudine
Zidovudine: ↑ level of zidovudine when given with lamivudine

NURSING CONSIDERATIONS

Assessment

- Monitor blood counts q2wk; watch for neutropenia, thrombocytopenia, Hgb; if low, therapy may have to be discontinued and restarted after hematologic recovery; blood transfusions may be required

Nursing diagnoses

- ✓ Infection, risk for (uses)
- ✓ Injury, risk for (adverse reactions)
- ✓ Knowledge deficit (teaching)

Implementation

- Administer PO bid
- Give with zidovudine only
- Store in cool environment; protect from light

Patient/family education

- Teach patient that GI complaints and insomnia resolve after 3-4 wk of treatment
- Tell patient that drug is not a cure for AIDS but will control symptoms
- Inform patient to notify prescriber of sore throat, swollen lymph nodes, malaise, fever; other infections may occur
- Teach patient that patient is still infective, may pass AIDS virus to others
- Encourage patient that follow-up visits must be continued since serious toxicity may occur; blood counts must be done q2wk
- Teach patient that drug must be taken tid, even if feeling better
- Tell patient that other drugs may be necessary to prevent other infections
- Teach patient that drug may cause fainting or dizziness

Evaluation

Positive therapeutic outcome

- Absence of infection, symptoms of HIV infection

lamotrigine (℞)

(lam-o-trye′geen)

Lamictal

Func. class.: Anticonvulsant

Chem. class.: Phenyltriazine

Pregnancy category C

Action: Unknown; may inhibit voltage-sensitive sodium channels

Therapeutic Outcome: Decrease in intensity and amount of seizures

Uses: Adjunct in the treatment of partial seizures

Investigational uses: Refractory bipolar disorder generalized tonic-clonic, absence, atypical absence and myoclonic seizures; children with Lennox-Gastaut syndrome

Dosage and routes

Without valproic acid

Adult: PO 50 mg/day for weeks 1 and 2, then increase to 100 mg divided bid for weeks 3 and 4; maintenance 300-500 mg/day

With valproic acid

Adult: PO 25 mg every other day, weeks 1 through 4, then 150 mg/day in divided doses

Available forms: Tabs 25, 100, 150, 200 mg

Adverse effects

CNS: Fever, insomnia, tremor, depression, anxiety, **dizziness,** ataxia, **headache**

EENT: Nystagmus, **diplopia, blurred vision**

GI: **Nausea, vomiting, anorexia,** abdominal pain

GU: **Dysmenorrhea**

INTEG: ***Rash (potentially life-threatening),*** alopecia, photosensitivity

RESP: **Rhinitis,** pharyngitis, cough

Contraindications: Hypersensitivity

Precautions: Pregnancy **C,** lactation, children <16 yr, renal, hepatic disease

Pharmacokinetics

Absorption	Well absorbed
Distribution	Unknown
Metabolism	Unknown
Excretion	Unknown
Half-life	Varies, depending on dose

Pharmacodynamics

Unknown

Interactions

Individual drugs

Carbenazine: ↑ metabolic clearance of lamotrigine

Phenobarbital: ↑ metabolic clearance of lamotrigine

Phenytoin: ↑ metabolic clearance of lamotrigine

Valproic acid: ↓ metabolic clearance of lamotrigine

NURSING CONSIDERATIONS

Assessment

- Assess for rash (Stevens-Johnson Syndrome or toxic epidermal necrolysis) in pediatric patients, drug should be discontinued at first sign of rash
- Assess for seizure activity: duration, type, intensity, halo before seizure
- Assess for hypersensitive reactions

Nursing diagnoses
✓ Injury, risk for (uses)
✓ Knowledge deficit (teaching)

Implementation
• May be given with food or fluids

Patient/family education
• Teach patient to take PO doses divided with or after meals to decrease adverse effects
• Caution patient not to discontinue drug abruptly; seizures may occur
• Caution patient to avoid hazardous activities until stabilized on drug
• Advise patient to notify prescriber of skin rash or increased seizure activity
• Instruct patient to report to prescriber if pregnant or if patient intends to become pregnant
• Teach patient to use sunscreen and protective clothing, photosensitivity occurs
• Advise patient to carry Medic Alert ID stating drug use

Evaluation
Positive therapeutic outcome
• Decrease in severity of seizures

lansoprazole (℞)
(lan-soe′prah-zole)
Prevacid
Func. class.: Antisecretory compound-proton pump inhibitor
Chem. class.: Benzimidazole
Pregnancy category B

Action: Suppresses gastric secretion by inhibiting hydrogen/potassium ATPase enzyme system in gastric parietal cell; characterized as gastric acid pump inhibitor since it blocks final step of acid production

➡ **Therapeutic Outcome:** Reduction in gastric pain, swelling, fullness

Uses: Gastroesophageal reflux disease (GERD), severe erosive esophagitis, poorly responsive systemic GERD, pathologic hypersecretory conditions (Zollinger-Ellison syndrome, systemic mastocytosis, multiple endocrine adenomas); possibly effective for treatment of duodenal ulcers, maintenance of healed duodenal ulcers

Dosage and routes
NG tube
Adult: Use intact granules mixed in 40 ml of apple juice injected through NG Tube, then flush with apple juice

Duodenal ulcer
Adult: PO 15 mg qd ac for 4 wk

Erosive esophagitis
Adult: PO 30 mg qd ac for up to 8 wk, may use another 8 wk course if needed

Pathological hypersecretory conditions
Adult: PO 60 mg qd, may give up to 90 mg bid

Available forms: Caps, delayed rel 15, 30 mg

Adverse effects
CNS: Headache, dizziness, confusion, agitation, amnesia, depression
GI: Diarrhea, abdominal pain, vomiting, nausea, constipation, flatulence, acid regurgitation, anorexia, irritable colon
RESP: Upper respiratory

infections, cough, epistaxis, asthma, bronchitis, dyspnea
INTEG: Rash, urticaria, pruritus, alopecia
META: Weight gain/loss, gout
EENT: Tinnitus, taste perversion, deafness, eye pain, otitis media
CV: Chest pain, angina, tachycardia, bradycardia, palpitations, ***CVA,*** hypertension/hypotension, ***MI,*** shock, vasodilation
GU: Hematuria, glycosuria, impotence, kidney calculus, breast enlargement
HEMA: ***Hemolysis,*** anemia

Contraindications: Hypersensitivity

Precautions: Pregnancy B, lactation, children

Pharmacokinetics	
Absorption	Rapid after granules leave stomach
Distribution	Protein binding 97%
Metabolism	Liver extensively
Excretion	Urine, feces; clearance decreased in elderly, renal, hepatic disease
Half-life	Plasma 1.5 hr

Pharmacodynamics

Unknown

Interactions
Individual drugs
Ampicillin: ↓ absorption of ampicillin
Digoxin: ↓ absorption of digoxin
Iron: ↓ absorption of iron
Ketoconazole: ↓ absorption of ketoconazole
Sucralfate: Delayed absorption of lansoprazole
Theophylline: ↓ clearance of theophylline

NURSING CONSIDERATIONS
Assessment
- Assess GI system; bowel sounds q8h, abdomen for pain, swelling, anorexia
- Monitor hepatic enzymes: AST (SGOT), ALT (SGPT), alk phosphatase during treatment

Nursing diagnoses
✓ Pain (uses)
✓ Knowledge deficit (teaching)

Implementation
- Administer before eating; swallow capsule whole
- Do not open, chew, crush

Patient/family education
- Instruct patient to report severe diarrhea; drug may have to be discontinued
- Inform diabetic patient that hypoglycemia may occur
- Encourage patient to avoid hazardous activities; dizziness may occur
- Tell patient to avoid alcohol, salicylates, ibuprofen; may cause GI irritation

Evaluation
Positive therapeutic outcome
- Absence of gastric pain, swelling, fullness

leucovorin (℞)
(loo-koe-vor'in)
Citrovorum Factor, 5-Formyl Tetrahydrofolate, Folinic Acid, leucovorin calcium, Wellcovorin
Func. class.: Vitamin/folic acid antagonist antidote
Chem. class.: Tetrahydrofolic acid derivative
Pregnancy category C

Action: Needed for normal growth patterns; prevents

toxicity during antineoplastic therapy by protecting normal cells

Therapeutic Outcome: Reversal of severe toxic effects of folic acid antagonists

Uses: Megaloblastic or macrocytic anemia caused by folic acid deficiency, overdose of folic acid antagonist, methotrexate toxicity, toxicity caused by pyrimethamine or trimethoprim, pneumocystosis, toxoplasmosis

Dosage and routes

Megaloblastic anemia caused by enzyme deficiency

P ***Adult and child:*** PO/IM/**IV** up to 1 mg/day

Megaloblastic anemia caused by deficiency of folate

P ***Adult and child:*** IM 1 mg or less qd until adequate response

Methotrexate toxicity

P ***Adult and child:*** PO/IM/**IV** given 6-36 hr after dose of methotrexate 10 mg/m², then 10 mg/m² q6h × 72 hr

Pyrimethamine toxicity

P ***Adult and child:*** PO/IM 5 mg qd

Trimethoprim toxicity

P ***Adult and child:*** PO/IM 400 µg qd

Available forms: Tabs 5, 10, 15, 25 mg; inj 3, 5 mg/ml; powder for inj 10 mg/ml

Adverse effects

INTEG: Rash, pruritus, erythema, thrombocytosis, urticaria

RESP: Wheezing

Contraindications: Hypersensitivity, anemias other than megaloblastic not associated with vitamin B_{12} deficiency

Precautions: Pregnancy **C**

Pharmacokinetics

Absorption	Rapidly absorbed (PO); completely absorbed (IV)
Distribution	Widely distributed
Metabolism	Liver
Excretion	Kidney
Half-life	3½ hr

Pharmacodynamics

	PO/IM/IV
Onset	Up to 5 min
Peak	Unknown
Duration	4-6 hr

Interactions

Individual drugs

Chloramphenicol: ↓ folate levels

Phenobarbital: ↑ metabolism of phenobarbital, ↓ effect

Drug classifications

Hydantoins: ↑ metabolism of hydantoins, ↓ effect

NURSING CONSIDERATIONS

Assessment

- Obtain CrCl before leucovorin rescue and qd to detect nephrotoxicity
- Monitor I&O; watch for nausea and vomiting; if vomiting occurs IM or **IV** route may be necessary
- Assess diet for inclusion of bran, yeast, dried beans, nuts, fruits, fresh vegetables, asparagus, which have high folic acid levels
- Assess drugs currently taken: alcohol, hydantoins, trimethoprim may cause increased folic acid use by body
- Assess for allergic reactions: rash, dyspnea, wheezing

Nursing diagnoses

✓ Injury, risk for (uses)

☑ Nutrition, altered: less than body requirements (uses)
☑ Knowledge deficit (teaching)

Implementation

PO route

• Use PO route only if patient is not vomiting

IM route

• Give within 1 hr of folic acid antagonist

• Give increased fluid intake if used to treat folic acid inhibitor overdose

• Provide protection from light and heat when storing ampules

IV route

• Reconstitute 50 mg/5 ml bacteriostatic water or sterile water for inj (10 mg/ml) or 100 mg/10 ml; use immediately if sterile water for inj is used to reconstitute

• Give by direct **IV** over 160 mg/min or less

• Give by intermittent inf after diluting in 100-500 ml of 0.9% NaCl, D_5W, $D_{10}W$, LR, Ringer's

Syringe/Y-site compatibilities: Bleomycin, cisplatin, cyclophosphamide, doxorubicin, fluorouracil, furosemide, heparin, methotrexate, metoclopramide, mitomycin, vinblastine, vincristine

Syringe/Y-site incompatibility: Droperidol

Additive compatibilities: Cisplatin, floxuridine

Y-*site compatibilities:* Amifostine, thiotepa

Patient/family education

• Advise patient to take drug exactly as prescribed; to notify prescriber of side effects immediately

• Advise patient to report signs of hyposensitivity reaction immediately

• Instruct patient about leucovorin rescue; have patient drink 3 L of fluid each day of rescue

• Advise patient with folic acid deficiency to eat folic acid–rich foods: bran, yeast, dried beans, nuts, fruits, fresh green leafy vegetables, asparagus

Evaluation

Positive therapeutic outcome

• Increased weight

• Improved orientation, well-being

• Absence of fatigue

leuprolide (℞)

(loo-proe'lide)

Leupron Depo Ped, Lupron Depot, Lupron, Lupron Depot-3 month,

Func. class.: Antineoplastic hormone

Chem. class.: Gonadotropin-releasing hormone

Pregnancy category (depot) X

Action: Causes initial increase in circulating levels of LH, FSH; continuous administration results in decreased LH, FSH; in men testosterone is reduced to castration levels; in premenopausal women estrogen is reduced to menopausal levels

Therapeutic Outcome: Prevention of rapidly growing malignant cells in prostate cancer, decreased pain in endometriosis, resolution of central precocious puberty (CPP)

L

Uses: Metastatic prostate cancer, management of endometriosis (depot), CPP

Dosage and routes

Prostate cancer

Adult: SC 1 mg/day; IM 7.5 mg/mo

Endometriosis

Adult: IM 7.5 mg once a month

Central precocious puberty

P ***Child:*** SC 50 μg/kg/day; increase as needed by 10 μg/kg/day

P ***Child:*** IM 0.3 mg/kg/mo; may increase by 3.75 mg/mo

Available forms: Inj (depot) 3.75 mg, 7.5 mg single-dose, multiple-dose vials (5 mg/ml); single-use kit 11.25 mg vial; pediatric depot 7.5, 11.25, 15 mg

Adverse effects

GU: Edema, hot flashes, impotence, decreased libido, amenorrhea, vaginal dryness, gynecomastia

Contraindications: Hypersensitivity to GnRH or analogs, thromboembolic disorders, pregnancy **X,** lactation, undiagnosed vaginal bleeding

Precautions: Edema, hepatic disease, CVA, MI, seizures, hypertension, diabetes mellitus

Pharmacokinetics	
Absorption	Rapidly absorbed (SC); slowly absorbed (IM depot)
Distribution	Unknown
Metabolism	Unknown
Excretion	Unknown
Half-life	3-4 hr

Pharmacodynamics

Unknown

Interactions

Individual drugs

Megestrol: ↑ antineoplastic action

Flutamide: ↑ antineoplastic action

NURSING CONSIDERATIONS

Assessment

- Assess for symptoms of endometriosis including lower abdominal pain if drug is given for the diagnosis of endometriosis
- If giving this drug for CPP, the diagnosis should have been confirmed by development of secondary sex characteristics in P child <9 yr; also included to confirm the diagnosis of CPP is estradiol/testosterone, GnRH test, tomography of head, adrenal steroid, chorionic gonadotropin, wrist x-ray, height, weight; patients diagnosed with CPP display the signs of testicular growth, facial, body hair (males), breast development, menses (females)
- Monitor liver function tests before, during therapy (bilirubin, AST [SGOT], ALT [SGPT], LDH) as needed or monthly
- Monitor pituitary gonadotropic and gonadal function during therapy and 4-8 wk after therapy is decreased; check LH, FSH, acid phosphate at beginning of treatment
- Monitor worsening of signs and symptoms (normal during beginning therapy): fatigue, increased pulse, pallor, lethargy, edema in feet, joints, stomach pain, shaking
- Monitor renal status: I&O ratio, check for bladder distention daily during beginning therapy (renal obstruction)

Nursing diagnoses
- ✓ Sexual dysfunction (adverse reactions)
- ✓ Injury, risk for (adverse reactions)
- ✓ Knowledge deficit (teaching)

Implementation
- Use syringe and drug packaged together; give deep in large muscle mass; rotate sites
- Use depot only IM; never give SC
- Reconstitute vial (single dose)/1 ml of diluent; shake (appearance should be white); withdraw and use immediately
- Unused vials may be stored at room temp

Patient/family education
- Advise patient to notify prescriber if menstruation continues; menstruation should stop; to use a nonhormonal method of contraception during therapy
- Instruct patient to report any complaints, side effects to nurse or prescriber; hot flashes are common
- Teach patient how to prepare, administer; to rotate sites for SC inj; to keep accurate records of dosing (prostate cancer)
- Instruct patient that tumor flare may occur: increase in size of tumor, increased bone pain; tell patient that bone pain disappears after 1 wk; may take analgesics for pain; premenopausal women must use mechanical birth control; ovulation may be induced

Evaluation
Positive therapeutic outcome
- Decreased size, spread of malignancy
- Decreased pain in endometriosis
- Decreased signs of CPP

levamisole (℞)
(lee-vam′i-sol)
Ergamisol
Func. class.: Antineoplastic, immunomodulator
Pregnancy category C

Action: May increase the action of macrophages, monocytes, and T cells, which restore immune function; complete action is unknown; cholinergic properties

➡ **Therapeutic Outcome:** Prevention of rapid growth of malignant cells when used with fluorouracil

Uses: Treatment of Dukes' stage C colon cancer when given with fluorouracil after surgical resection

Investigational uses: Malignant melanoma (advanced)

Dosage and routes
Adult: PO 50 mg q8h × 3 days; begin treatment at least 1 wk but no more than 4 wk after resection; give with fluorouracil 450 mg/m^2/day

Available forms: Tab 50 mg (base)

Adverse effects
CNS: Dizziness, headache, paresthesia, somnolence, depression, anxiety, *fatigue,* fever, mental changes, ataxia, insomnia
CV: Chest pain, edema
EENT: Blurred vision, conjunctivitis
GI: Nausea, vomiting, anorexia, diarrhea, stomatitis, constipation, flatulence, dyspepsia, abdominal pain
HEMA: Granulocytopenia, leukopenia, thrombocytopenia

INTEG: Rash, pruritus, *alopecia, dermatitis,* urticaria
META: Hyperbilirubinemia
MISC: Rigors, infection, altered sense of smell, arthralgia, myalgia

Contraindications: Hypersensitivity

Precautions: Pregnancy **C,** P lactation, children, blood dyscrasias

Pharmacokinetics

Absorption	Rapidly absorbed
Distribution	Unknown
Metabolism	Liver, extensively
Excretion	Unknown
Half-life	3-4 hr

Pharmacodynamics

Onset	Unknown
Peak	1½-2 hr
Duration	Unknown

Interactions

Individual drugs

Alcohol: ↑ disulfiram reaction
Phenytoin: ↑ plasma levels
Radiation: ↑ bone marrow depression

Drug classifications

Antineoplastics: ↑ bone marrow depression

NURSING CONSIDERATIONS

Assessment

- ! Monitor CBC, differential, platelet count weekly; withhold drug if WBC is <4000 or platelet count is <100,000; notify prescriber of results; drug should be discontinued and restarted after recovery
- Monitor renal function studies: BUN, serum uric acid, urine CrCl before, during therapy; I&O ratio; report fall in urine output of 30 ml/hr; check for decreased hyperuricemia
- Monitor for cold, fever, sore throat (may indicate beginning infection)
- Assess for bleeding: hematuria, guaiac, bruising or petechiae, mucosa or orifices q8h; no rec temp
- Identify inflammation of mucosa, breaks in skin; use viscous lidocaine (Xylocaine) for oral pain

Nursing diagnoses

- ✓ Injury, risk for (adverse reactions)
- ✓ Body image disturbance (adverse reactions)
- ✓ Infection, risk for (adverse reactions)
- ✓ Knowledge deficit (teaching)

Implementation

- Give 7-20 days after surgery; start fluorouracil with 2nd course of levamisole; begin no sooner than 21 days and no later than 35 days after surgery; if levamisole therapy begins 21-30 days after resection, fluorouracil should be given with 1st course; apply pressure to venipuncture sites for 10 min, especially if platelets are low

Patient/family education

- Advise patient to call prescriber if sore throat, swollen lymph nodes, malaise, fever occur, since other infections may develop
- Advise patient that contraceptive measures are recommended during therapy and 4 mo after; teratogenic effects are possible
- Caution patient to avoid ingestion of alcohol, since disulfiram reaction may occur with flushing, severe nausea, vomiting, pounding headache; death can result; advise patient that tyramine-containing foods and cold, hay fever, weight-

reducing products may cause hypertensive crisis
- Caution patient to avoid use of products containing aspirin or ibuprofen, razors, commercial mouthwash, since bleeding may occur; to report symptoms of bleeding (hematuria, tarry stools)
- Advise patient to report signs of anemia (fatigue, headache, irritability, faintness, shortness of breath) and CNS reactions including confusion, psychosis, nightmares, seizures, severe headaches
- Inform patient that hair may be lost during treatment; a wig or hair piece may make patient feel better; new hair may be different in color, texture
- Teach patient the reason for medication use and expected results

Evaluation

Positive therapeutic outcome
- Decreased spread of malignant cells when used with fluorouracil

levodopa (℞)

(lee'voe-doe-pa)

Dopar, Larodopa, L-Dopa

Func. class.: Antiparkinsonian agent

Chem. class.: Catecholamine, dopamine agonist

Pregnancy category C

Action: Decarboxylation to dopamine, which increases dopamine levels in brain

Therapeutic Outcome: Decreased symptoms of Parkinson's disease (involuntary movements)

Uses: Parkinsonism

Dosage and routes

Adult: PO 0.5-1 g qd divided bid-qid with meals; may increase by up to 0.75 g q3-7 days, not to exceed 8 g/day unless closely supervised

Available forms: Caps 100, 250, 500 mg; tabs 100, 250, 500 mg

Adverse effects

CNS: Involuntary choreiform movements, hand tremors, fatigue, headache, anxiety, twitching, numbness, weakness, confusion, agitation, insomnia, nightmares, psychosis, hallucinations, hypomania, severe depression, dizziness

CV: Orthostatic hypotension, tachycardia, hypertension, palpitations

EENT: Blurred vision, diplopia, dilated pupils

GI: Nausea, vomiting, anorexia, abdominal distress, dry mouth, flatulence, dysphagia, bitter taste, diarrhea, constipation

HEMA: Hemolytic anemia, leukopenia, agranulocytosis

INTEG: Rash, sweating, alopecia

MISC: Urinary retention, incontinence, weight change, dark urine

Contraindications: Hypersensitivity, narrow-angle glaucoma, undiagnosed skin lesions

Precautions: Renal disease, cardiac disease, hepatic disease, respiratory disease, MI with dysrhythmias, convulsions, peptic ulcer, pregnancy **C,** asthma, endocrine disease, affective disorders, psychosis, P lactation, children <12 yr peptic ulcer

Pharmacokinetics

Absorption	Well absorbed
Distribution	Widely distributed
Metabolism	Liver, GI tract, extensively
Excretion	Kidneys to metabolites; breast milk
Half-life	1 hr

Pharmacodynamics

Onset	10-15 min
Peak	1-3 hr
Duration	Up to 24 hr

Interactions

Individual drugs

Haloperidol: ↓ effects of levodopa
Methyldopa: ↑ CNS toxicity
Papaverine: ↓ effects of levodopa
Phenytoin: ↓ effects of levodopa
Pyridoxine: ↓ effects of levodopa
Reserpine: ↓ effects of levodopa
Selegiline: ↑ adverse reaction

Drug classifications

Anticholinergics: ↓ effects of levodopa
Antihypertensives: ↑ hypotension
Hydantoins: ↓ effects of levodopa
MAOIs: Hypertensive crisis

Food

↓ effects of levodopa from pyridoxine foods

Lab test interferences

False positive: Urine ketones, urine glucose, Coombs' test, urine, norepinephrine
False negative: Urine glucose (glucose oxidase)
False ↑ Uric acid, false ↑ urine protein
↓ VMA

NURSING CONSIDERATIONS

Assessment

- Monitor B/P, respiration during initial treatment; hypotension or hypertension should be reported
- Assess mental status: affect, mood, behavioral changes, depression; complete suicide assessment
- Monitor liver function enzymes: AST (SGOT), ALT (SGPT), alkaline phosphatase; also check LDH, bilirubin, CBC
- Assess for involuntary movements in parkinsonism: akinesia, tremors, staggering gait, muscle rigidity, drooling; these symptoms should improve with levodopa therapy
- ❗ Assess for levodopa toxicity: mental, personality changes, increased twitching, grimacing, tongue protrusion; these should be reported to prescriber

Nursing diagnoses

- ☑ Mobility, impaired (uses)
- ☑ Injury, risk for (uses)
- ☑ Knowledge deficit (teaching)
- ☑ Noncompliance (teaching)

Implementation

- Levodopa/carbidopa should not be started until this drug is withheld for 8 hr; toxicity may result if the two drugs are taken close together
- Give drug until NPO before surgery
- Adjust dosage to patient response
- Give with meals to decrease GI upset; limit protein taken with drug
- Give only after MAOIs have been discontinued for 2 wk

Patient/family education

- Advise patient that therapeu-

tic effects may take several wk to a few mo
- Caution patient to change positions slowly to prevent orthostatic hypotension
- Instruct patient to report side effects: twitching, eye spasms; indicate overdose
- Instruct patient to use drug exactly as prescribed; if drug is discontinued abruptly, parkinsonian crisis may occur
- Inform patient that urine, sweat may darken
- Advise patient to avoid vitamin B_6 preparations, vitamin-fortified foods containing B_6; these foods can reverse effects of levodopa; also OTC preparations should be avoided unless approved by prescriber

Evaluation

Positive therapeutic outcome
- Decreased akathisia, other involuntary movements
- Increased mood

levofloxacin (℞)
(lev-o-floks'a-sin)

Levaquin

Func. class.: Antiinfective
Chem. class.: Fluoroquinolone antibacterial

Pregnancy category C

Action: Interferes with conversion of intermediate DNA fragments into high-molecular-weight DNA in bacteria; DNA gyrase inhibitor

Therapeutic Outcome: Bacterial action against the following: *S. pneumoniae, H. influenzae, m. catarrhalis, S. aureus, H. parainfluenzae, K. pneumonia, M. pneumoniae*

Uses: Adult urinary tract infections (including complicated); lower respiratory, skin infection

Dosage and routes

Adult: **IV** inf 500 mg by slow inf over 1 hr q24hr × 7-14 days depending on infection

Available forms: Single-use vials (500 mg), 25 mg/ml 20 ml vials, premixed flexible container

Adverse effects:

CNS: Headache, dizziness, insomnia, anxiety
GI: Nausea, abdominal pain, constipation, ***pseudomembranous colitis***
GU: Vaginitis, crystalluria
INTEG: Rash, puruitus, urticaria, photosensitivity

Contraindications: Hypersensitivity to quinolones

Precautions: Pregnancy **C**, lactation, children, renal disease

Pharmacokinetics	
Absorption	Unknown
Distribution	Unknown
Metabolism	Liver
Excretion	Kidneys unchanged
Half-life	6-8 hr

Pharmacodynamics	
Onset	Immediate
Peak	Infusion's end

Interactions None significant

Lab test interferences

Interference: ↓ glucose, ↓ lymphocytes

NURSING CONSIDERATIONS
Assessment
- Assess patient for previous sensitivity reaction
- Assess patient for signs and symptoms of infection including characteristics of wounds, sputum, urine, stool, WBC >10,000, fever; obtain baseline

information before and during treatment
• Obtain C&S before beginning drug therapy to identify if correct treatment has been initiated
• Assess for allergic reactions: rash, urticaria, pruritus, chills, fever, joint pain; may occur a few days after therapy begins; epinephrine and resuscitation equipment should be available for anaphylactic reaction
• Identify urine output; if decreasing, notify prescriber (may indicate nephrotoxicity); also check for increased BUN, creatinine
• Monitor blood studies: AST (SGOT), ALT (SGPT), CBC, Hct, bilirubin, LDH, alkaline phosphatase, Coombs' test monthly if patient is on long-term therapy
• Monitor electrolytes: potassium, sodium, chloride monthly if patient is on long-term therapy
• Assess bowel pattern qd; if severe diarrhea occurs, drug should be discontinued
• Monitor for bleeding: ecchymosis, bleeding gums, hematuria, stool guaiac daily if on long-term therapy
• Assess for overgrowth of infection: perineal itching, fever, malaise, redness, pain, swelling, drainage, rash, diarrhea, change in cough, sputum

Nursing diagnoses

✓ Infection, risk for (uses)
✓ Diarrhea (side effects)
✓ Injury, risk for (side effects)
✓ Knowledge deficit (teaching)
✓ Noncompliance (teaching)

Implementation

• Check for irritation, extravasation, phlebitis daily

Patient/family education

• Teach patient to report sore throat, bruising, bleeding, joint pain; may indicate blood dyscrasias (rare)
• Advise patient to contact prescriber if vaginal itching, loose foul-smelling stools, furry tongue occur, may indicate superinfection; report itching, rash, pruritus, urticaria
• Instruct patient to take all medication prescribed for the length of time ordered; drug must be taken around the clock to maintain blood levels; do not give medication to others
• Advise patient to notify prescriber of diarrhea with blood or pus

Evaluation

Positive therapeutic outcome

• Absence of signs/symptoms of infection (W <10,000, temp WNL)
• Reported improvement in symptoms of infection

levorphanol (℞)

(lee-vor′ fan-ole)

Levo-Dromoran, Levorphan

Func. class.: Narcotic analgesic (opioid analgesic agonist)

Chem. class.: Opiate, synthetic morphine derivative

Pregnancy category B

Controlled substance schedule II

Action: Inhibits ascending pain pathways in limbic system, thalamus, midbrain, hypothalamus by binding to opiate receptor sites, altering pain perception and response

➡ **Therapeutic Outcome:** Relief of pain

Uses: Moderate to severe pain

Dosage and routes

Adult: PO/SC/**IV** 2-3 mg q4-5h prn

Available forms: Inj 2 mg/ml; tab 2 mg

Adverse effects

CNS: Drowsiness, dizziness, confusion, headache, sedation, euphoria

CV: Palpitations, bradycardia, change in B/P

EENT: Tinnitus, blurred vision, miosis, diplopia

GI: Nausea, vomiting, anorexia, constipation, cramps

GU: Urinary retention, dysuria

INTEG: *Rash*, urticaria, diaphoresis, pruritus

RESP: ***Respiratory depression***

Contraindications: Hypersensitivity, addiction (narcotic)

Precautions: Addictive personality, pregnancy **B**, lactation, increased intracranial pressure, MI (acute), severe heart disease, respiratory depression, hepatic disease, renal disease, P child <18 yr

Pharmacokinetics

Absorption	Well absorbed (SC, PO); completely absorbed (IV)
Distribution	Unknown
Metabolism	Liver, extensively
Excretion	Kidneys
Half-life	12-16 hr

Pharmacodynamics

	PO	SC	IV
Onset	½-1½ hr	Unknown	Unknown
Peak	½-1 hr	½-1 hr	20 min
Duration	6-8 hr	6-8 hr	6-8 hr

Interactions

Individual drugs

Alcohol: ↑ respiratory depression, hypotension, sedation

Nalbuphine: ↓ analgesia

Pentazocine: ↓ analgesia

Drug classifications

Antihistamines: ↑ respiratory depression, hypotension

Antidepressants: ↑ respiratory depression, hypotension

CNS depressants: ↑ respiratory depression, hypotension

MAOIs: ↑ respiratory depression

Sedative/hypnotics: ↑ respiratory depression, hypotension

Lab test interferences

↑ Amylase

NURSING CONSIDERATIONS

Assessment

- Monitor VS after parenteral route; note muscle rigidity, drug history, liver, kidney function tests, respiratory dysfunction: respiratory depression, character, rate, rhythm; notify prescriber if respirations are <10/min
- Monitor CNS changes: dizziness, drowsiness, hallucinations, euphoria, LOC, pupil reaction
- Monitor allergic reactions: rash, urticaria

Nursing diagnoses

- ✓ Pain (uses)
- ✓ Sensory-perceptual alteration: visual, auditory (adverse reactions)
- ✓ Breathing pattern, ineffective (adverse reactions)
- ✓ Injury, risk for (adverse reactions)
- ✓ Knowledge deficit (teaching)

Implementation

- Give with antiemetic if nausea, vomiting occur
- Administer when pain is

L

beginning to return, determine dosage interval by patient response; continuous dosing of medication is more effective given prn; explain analgesic effect

- Medication should be slowly withdrawn after long-term use to prevent withdrawal symptoms
- Store in light-resistant container at room temp

PO route

- May be given with food or milk to lessen GI upset

IV **IV route**

- Give **IV** directly; give through Y-tube or 3-way stopcock over 5 min; do not administer rapidly or circulatory collapse may occur
- Store in light-resistant area at room temp

Syringe compatibility: Glycopyrrolate

Additive incompatibilities: Aminophylline, ammonium chloride, amobarbital, chlorothiazide, heparin, methicillin, pentobarbital, phenobarbital, phenytoin, secobarbital, sodium bicarbonate, sodium iodine, thiopental

Patient/family education

- Caution patients to avoid CNS depressants: alcohol, sedative/hypnotics for at least 24 hr after taking this drug
- Discuss with patient that dizziness, drowsiness, confusion are common; to avoid getting up without assistance
- Discuss in detail all aspects of the drug and what to expect after anesthesia
- Advise patient to make position changes carefully to lessen orthostatic hypotension

Evaluation

Positive therapeutic outcome

- Decreased pain

Treatment of overdose: Narcan 0.2-0.8 **IV**, O_2, **IV** fluids, vasopressors

levothyroxine 🔑 (℞)

(lee-voe-thye-rox'een)

Eltroxin ♣, Levothroid, levothyroxine sodium, Levoxine, Synthroid, T_4

Func. class.: Thyroid hormone

Chem. class.: Levoisomer of thyroxine

Pregnancy category A

Action: Controls protein synthesis; increases metabolic rate, cardiac output, renal blood flow, O_2 consumption, body temp, blood volume, growth, development at cellular level

➔ **Therapeutic Outcome:** Correction of lack of thyroid hormone

Uses: Hypothyroidism, myxedema coma, thyroid hormone replacement, cretinism, thyrotoxicosis, congenital hypothyroidism

Dosage and routes

Severe hypothyroidism

Adult: PO 12.5-50 μg qd, increased by 0.05-0.1 mg q1-4 wk until desired response; maintenance dosage 75-125 μg qd, IM/**IV** 50-100 μg/day as a single dose

P ***Child >12 yr:*** PO 2-3 μg/kg/day given as a single dose AM

P ***Child 6-12 yr:*** PO 4-5 μg/kg/day given as a single dose AM

P ***Child 1-5 yr:*** PO 5-6 μg/kg/day given as a single dose AM

P ***Child 6-12 mo:*** PO 6-8 μg/kg/day give as a single dose AM

P ***Child to 6 mo:*** PO 8-10 μg/kg/day given as a single dose AM

Myxedema coma

Adult: **IV** 200-500 μg; may increase by 100-300 μg after 24 hr; place on oral medication as soon as possible; maintenance 50-100 μg/day

Available forms: Inj 50, 200, 500 μg/vial; tabs 0.025, 0.05, 0.075, 0.088, 0.1, 0.112, 0.125, 0.15, 0.175, 0.2, 0.3 mg

Adverse effects

CNS: Anxiety, insomnia, tremors, headache, ***thyroid storm***

CV: Tachycardia, palpitations, angina, dysrhythmias, hypertension, ***cardiac arrest***

GI: Nausea, diarrhea, increased or decreased appetite, cramps

MISC: Menstrual irregularities, weight loss, sweating, heat intolerance, fever

Contraindications: Adrenal insufficiency, MI, thyrotoxicosis

G **Precautions:** Elderly, angina pectoris, hypertension, ischemia, cardiac disease, pregnancy **A,** lactation

Pharmacokinetics

Absorption	Erratic (PO); complete (IV)
Distribution	Widely distributed
Metabolism	Liver; enterohepatic recirculation
Excretion	Feces via bile; breast milk (small amounts)
Half-life	6-7 days

Pharmacodynamics

	PO	IV
Onset	Unknown	6-8 hr
Peak	12-48 hr	12-48 hr
Duration	Unknown	Unknown

Interactions

Individual drugs

Cholestyramine: ↓ absorption of thyroid hormone

Colestipol: ↓ absorption of levothyroxine

Digitalis: ↓ effect of digitalis

Insulin: ↑ requirement for insulin

Phenytoin (IV): ↑ release of thyroid hormone

Drug classifications

Amphetamines: ↑ CNS, cardiac stimulation

β-Adrenergic blockers: ↓ effect of β-blockers

Decongestants: ↑ CNS, cardiac stimulation

Oral anticoagulants: ↑ requirements for anticoagulants

Vasopressors: ↑ CNS, cardiac stimulation

Lab test interferences

↑ CPK, ↑ LDH, ↑ AST (SGOT), ↑ PBI, ↑ blood glucose

↓ TSH, ↓ ^{131}I uptake test, ↓ uric acid, ↓ triglycerides

NURSING CONSIDERATIONS

Assessment

- Identify if the patient is taking anticoagulants, antidiabetic agents; document on chart
- Take B/P, pulse before each dose; monitor I&O ratio and weight every day in same clothing, using same scale, at same time of day
- Monitor height, weight, psychomotor development and growth rate if given to a child
- Monitor T_3, T_4, FTIs, which

L

are decreased; radioimmunoassay of TSH, which is increased; radio uptake, which is increased if patient is on too low a dosage of medication
• Monitor pro-time (may require decreased anticoagulant); check for bleeding, bruising
• Assess for increased nervousness, excitability, irritability, which may indicate too high a dosage of medication, usually after 1-3 wk of treatment
• Assess cardiac status: angina, palpitations, chest pain, change in VS; **G** the elderly patient may have undetected cardiac problems and baseline ECG should be completed before treatment

Nursing diagnoses

✓ Knowledge deficit (teaching)
✓ Noncompliance (teaching)

Implementation

PO route

• Give in AM if possible as a single dose to decrease sleeplessness; give at same time each day to maintain drug level
• Give crushed and mixed with water, non-soy formula, or **P** breast milk for infants/children
• Give only for hormone imbalances; not to be used for obesity, male infertility, menstrual conditions, lethargy; give lowest dosage that relieves symptoms; lower dosage for **G** the elderly and in cardiac diseases
• Store in tight, light-resistant container
• Remove medication 4 wk before RAIU test

IV **IV route**

• Give **IV** after diluting with provided diluent (0.9% NaCl), 0.5 mg/5 ml; shake well; give through Y-tube or 3-way stopcock; give 0.1 mg or less over 1 min; do not add to IV inf; 0.1 mg = 1 ml; discard any unused portion

Patient/family education

• Teach patient that drug is not a cure but controls symptoms and treatment is long term
• Instruct patient to report excitability, irritability, anxiety, sweating, heat intolerance, chest pain, palpitations, which indicate overdose
• Advise patient not to switch brands unless approved by prescriber; bioavailability may differ; do not take with food; absorption will be decreased
• Teach patient that drug may be discontinued after giving birth; thyroid panel will be evaluated after 1-2 mo
• Teach patient or parent that **P** hyperthyroid child will show almost immediate behavior/personality change; that hair loss will occur in child but is temporary
• Caution patient that drug is not to be taken to reduce weight
• Caution patient to avoid OTC preparations with iodine; read labels; other medications should not be used unless approved by prescriber
• Teach patient to avoid iodine-rich food: iodized salt, soybeans, tofu, turnips, some seafood, some bread

Evaluation

Positive therapeutic outcome

• Absence of depression
• Weight loss, increased diuresis, pulse, appetite
• Absence of constipation, peripheral edema, cold intolerance, pale, cool dry skin, brittle nails, alopecia, coarse hair, menorrhagia, night blindness,

paresthesias, syncope, stupor, coma, rosy cheeks
- Improved levels of T_3, T_4 by laboratory tests
- P Child: age-appropriate weight, height and psychomotor development

Treatment of overdose: Withhold dose for up to 1 wk: acute overdose: gastric lavage or induced emesis, activated charcoal; provide supportive treatment to control symptoms

lidocaine (℞)

(lye'doe-kane)

Anestacon, Baylocaine, L-Caine, Lidocaine HCl IV for Cardiac Arrhythmias, Lidopen Auto-Injector, Xylocaine HCl IM for Cardiac Arrhythmias, Xylocaine HCl IV for Cardiac Arrhythmias

Func. class.: Antidysrhythmic (Class IB); local anesthetic

Chem. class.: Aminoacyl amide

Pregnancy category B

Action: Increases electrical stimulation threshold of ventricle and His-Purkinje system, which stabilizes cardiac membrane and decreases automaticity; locally produces anesthesia by preventing initiation and conduction of nerve impulses

→ **Therapeutic Outcome:** Decreased ventricular dysrhythmia; produces anesthesia locally

Uses: Ventricular tachycardia, ventricular dysrhythmias during cardiac surgery, MI, digitalis toxicity, cardiac catheterization; anesthesia locally

Dosage and routes

Adult: **IV** bol 50-100 mg (1 mg/kg) over 2-3 min; repeat q3-5 min, not to exceed 300 mg in 1 hr; begin **IV** inf 20-50 µg/kg/min; IM 200-300 mg (4.3 mg/kg) in deltoid muscle, may repeat in 1-1½ hr if needed

G ***Elderly with CHF, reduced liver function:*** **IV** bol give ½ adult dose

P ***Child:*** **IV** bol 1 mg/kg, then **IV** inf 30 µg/kg/min

P ***Adult and child:*** Top apply as needed to affected areas

Available forms: **IV** inf 0.2% (2 mg/ml), 0.4% (4 mg/ml), 0.8% (8 mg/ml); **IV** admixture 4% (40 mg/ml), 10% (100 mg/ml), 20% (200 mg/ml); **IV** dir 1% (10 mg/ml), 2% (20 mg/ml), IM 300 mg/3 ml; ointment (top) 2.5, 5%; cream (top) 0.5%; spray 10%; jelly 2%; viscous sol 2%; local infiltrative inj 0.5, 1%

Adverse effects

CNS: Headache, dizziness, involuntary movement, confusion, tremor, *drowsiness,* euphoria, ***convulsions***

CV: Hypotension, bradycardia, ***heart block, cardiovascular collapse, arrest***

EENT: Tinnitus, blurred vision

GI: Nausea, vomiting, anorexia

INTEG: Rash, urticaria, edema, swelling, burning, stinging

MISC: Febrile response, phlebitis at inj site

Contraindications: Hypersensitivity to amides, severe heart

L

block, supraventricular dysrhythmias, Adams-Stokes syndrome, Wolff-Parkinson-White syndrome

Precautions: Pregnancy **B,** P lactation, children, renal disease, liver disease, CHF, respiratory depression, malignant hyperthermia

Pharmacokinetics

Absorption	Complete bioavailability (IV)
Distribution	Erythrocytes, cardiovascular endothelium
Metabolism	Liver
Excretion	Kidneys
Half-life	Biphasic 8 min, 1-2 hr

Pharmacodynamics

	IV	IM	TOP
Onset	2 min	5-15 min	Unknown
Peak	Unknown	½ hr	5 min
Duration	20 min	1½ hr	½-1 hr

Interactions

Individual drugs

Cimetidine: ↓ metabolism, ↑ toxicity
Procainamide: ↑ toxicity
Propranolol: ↑ toxicity
Phenytoin: ↑ toxicity
Quinidine: ↑ toxicity

Drug classifications

β-Blockers: ↑ toxicity

Lab test interferences

↑ Liver function tests

NURSING CONSIDERATIONS

Assessment

- Assess for oxygenation or perfusion deficit: decreased B/P, chest pain, dizziness, loss of consciousness
- Assess respiratory status: auscultate lung fields for bibasilar crackles in patients with advanced CHF
- Assess for urinary retention: check for pain, abdominal absorption, palpate bladder; check males with benign prostatic hypertrophy; anticholinergic reaction may cause retention
- Monitor I&O ratio, electrolytes (potassium, sodium, chloride); watch for decreasing urinary output, possible retention
- Monitor liver function studies: AST (SGOT), ALT (SGPT), bilirubin, alkaline phosphatase
- Monitor ECG continuously to determine drug effectiveness, measure PR, QRS, QT intervals, check for PVCs, other dysrhythmias; monitor B/P continuously for hypotension, hypertension; check for rebound hypertension after 1-2 hr, prolonged PR/QT intervals, QRS complex; if QT or QRS increases by 50% or more, withhold next dose, notify prescriber
- Monitor for CNS symptoms: confusion, numbness, depression, involuntary movements; if these occur, drug should be discontinued
- Monitor blood levels (therapeutic level 1.5-5 μg/ml), notify prescriber of abnormal results

Nursing diagnoses

- ✓ Cardiac output, decreased (uses)
- ✓ Impaired gas exchange (adverse reactions)
- ✓ Knowledge deficit (teaching)

Implementation

IM route

- Administer in deltoid, aspirate to prevent **IV** administration
- Check site daily for extravasation

IV **IV route**

- Give **IV** bolus undiluted (1%, 2% only); give 6 mg or less over 1 min; if using an **IV** line, use port near insertion site, flush with normal saline (50 ml)
- Store at room temp; sol should be clear
- Give by cont inf after adding 1 g/250-1000 ml D_5W; give 1-4 mg/min; use inf pump for P correct dosage; pediatric inf is 120 mg of lidocaine/100 ml of D_5W; 1-2.5 ml/kg/hr = 20-50 µg/kg/min; use only 1%, 2% sol

Solution compatibilities: D_5W, D_5/0.9% NaCl, D_5/0.45% NaCl, D_5/LR, LR, 0.9% NaCl, 0.45% NaCl

Syringe compatibilities: Glycopyrrolate, heparin, hydroxyzine, methicillin, metoclopramide, milrinone, moxalactam, nalbuphine

Syringe incompatibility: Cefazolin

Y-site compatibilities: Alteplase, amiodarone, amrinone, cefazolin, ciprofloxacin, diltiazem, dobutamine, enalaprilat, famotidine, haloperidol, heparin with hydrocortisone, labetalol, meperidine, morphine, nitroglycerin, nitroprusside, potassium chloride, streptokinase, vitamin B with C

Additive compatibilities: Alteplase, aminophylline, amiodarone, atracurium, bretylium, calcium chloride, calcium gluceptate, calcium gluconate, chloramphenicol, chlorothiazide, cimetidine, dexamethasone, digoxin, diphenhydramine, dobutamine, dopamine, ephedrine, erythromycin, floxacillin, flumazenil, furosemide, heparin, hydrocortisone, hydroxyzine, regular insulin, mephentermine, metaraminol, nitroglycerin, penicillin G potassium, pentobarbital, phenylephrine, potassium chloride, procainamide, prochlorperazine, promazine, ranitidine, sodium bicarbonate, verapamil, vitamin B with C

Additive incompatibilities: Methohexital, phenytoin; do not admix with blood transfusions

Infiltration

Physician may order lidocaine with epinephrine to minimize systemic absorption and prolong local anesthesia

Patient/family education

- Teach patient or family reason for use of medication and expected results
- Instruct patient in at-home use of Lidopen Auto-Injector; patient should call prescriber before use if heart attack is imminent

Evaluation

Positive therapeutic outcome

- Decreased B/P, dysrhythmias
- Decreased heart rate
- Normal sinus rhythm

Treatment of overdose: Oxygen, artificial ventilation, ECG, administer dopamine for circulatory depression, diazepam or thiopental for convulsions, decreased drug or discontinuation may be required

L

lindane (OTC)

(lin-dane)

Bio-Well, GBH ♣, G-Well, Kwell, Kwellada ♣, Kwildane, lindane, Scabene, Thionex

Func. class.: Scabicide/ pediculicide

Chem. class.: Chlorinated hydrocarbon (synthetic)

Pregnancy category B

Action: Stimulates nervous system of arthropods, resulting in seizures, death of organism

➔ **Therapeutic Outcome:** Resolution of infestation

Uses: Scabies, lice (head/ pubic/body), nits

Dosage and routes

Lice

P ***Adult and child:*** Cream/ lotion: wash area with soap and water 8-12 hr after application; may reapply in 1 wk if needed; shampoo using 30 ml: work into lather, rub for 5 min, rinse, dry with towel; use fine-toothed comb to remove nits

Scabies

P ***Adult and child:*** Top apply 1% cream/lotion to skin from neck to bottom of feet, toes; repeat in 1 wk if necessary

Available forms: Lotion, shampoo, cream (1%)

Adverse effects

CNS: Tremors, ***convulsions,*** stimulation, dizziness (chronic inhalation of vapors)

*CV: **Ventricular fibrillation*** (chronic inhalation of vapors)

GI: Nausea, vomiting, diarrhea, liver damage (inhalation of vapors)

*HEMA: **Aplastic anemia*** (chronic inhalation of vapors)

INTEG: Pruritus, rash, irritation, contact dermatitis

Contraindications: Hypersensitivity, P premature neonate, patients with known seizure disorders, inflammation of skin, abrasions, or breaks in skin

Precautions: Pregnancy **B,** P children <10 yr, infants, lactation; avoid contact with eyes

Pharmacokinetics	
Absorption	20%
Distribution	Fat
Metabolism	Liver
Excretion	Kidneys
Half-life	18 hr

Pharmacodynamics	
Onset	Rapid
Peak	Rapid
Duration	3 hr

Interactions

Oil-based hair dressing: ↑ absorption; wash, rinse, and dry hair before using lindane

NURSING CONSIDERATIONS

Assessment

- Assess head, hair for lice and nits before and after treatment; if scabies are present, check all skin surfaces
- Identify source of infection: school, family members, sexual contacts

Nursing diagnoses

✓ Skin integrity, impaired (uses)

✓ Knowledge deficit (teaching)

Implementation

- Apply to body areas, scalp only; do not apply to face, lips, mouth, eyes, any mucous membrane, anus, or meatus
- Give top corticosteroids as ordered to decrease contact

dermatitis; provide antihistamines
• Apply menthol or phenol lotions to control itching
• Give top antibiotics for infection
• Provide isolation until areas on skin, scalp have cleared and treatment is completed
• Remove nits by using a fine-toothed comb rinsed in vinegar after treatment; use gloves

Patient/family education
• Advise patient to wash all inhabitants' clothing, using insecticide; preventive treatment may be required of all persons living in same house, using lotion or shampoo to decrease spread of infection; use rubber gloves when applying drug
• Instruct patient that itching may continue for 4-6 wk; that drug must be reapplied if accidently washed off, or treatment will be ineffective
• Advise patient not to apply to face; if accidental contact with eyes occurs, flush with water
• Advise patient that sexual contacts should be treated simultaneously

Evaluation
Positive therapeutic outcome
• Decreased crusts, nits, brownish trails on skin, itching papules in skinfolds
• Decreased itching after several wk

Treatment of ingestion: Gastric lavage, saline laxatives, **IV** diazepam (Valium) for convulsions (if taken orally)

liothyronine (T_3) (℞)
(lye-oh-thye'roe-neen)
Cytomel, L-Triiodothyronine, liothyronine sodium, Triostat, T_3
Func. class.: Thyroid hormone
Chem. class.: Synthetic T_3
Pregnancy category A

Action: Controls protein synthesis; increases metabolic rates, cardiac output, renal blood flow, O_2 consumption, body temp, blood volume, growth, development at cellular level

➡ **Therapeutic Outcome:** Correction of lack of thyroid hormone

Uses: Hypothyroidism, myxedema coma, thyroid hormone replacement, nontoxic goiter, T_3 suppression test, congenital hypothyroidism

Dosage and routes
Adult: PO 25 μg qd, increased by 12.5-25 μg q1-2 wk until desired response, maintenance dosage 25-75 μg qd

Congenital hypothyroidism
P ***Child >3 yr:*** PO 50-100 μg qd
P ***Child <3 yr:*** PO 5 μg qd, increased by 5 μg q3-4 days titrated to response

Myxedema, severe hypothyroidism
Adult: PO 5 μg qd; may increase by 5-10 μg q1-2 wk; maintenance dosage 50-100 μg qd

Myxedema coma/precoma
Adult: **IV** 25-50 μg initially; 5
G μg in elderly; 10-20 μg in cardiac disease; give doses q4-12h

Nontoxic goiter
Adult: PO 5 μg qd, increased by 12.5-25 μg q1-2 wk; maintenance dosage 75 μg qd

Suppression test (T_3)
Adult: PO 75-100 μg qd × 1 wk; ^{131}I is given before and after 1st wk dose

Available forms: Tabs 5, 25, 50 μg; inj 10 μg/ml

Adverse effects
CNS: Insomnia, tremors, headache, ***thyroid storm***
CV: Tachycardia, palpitations, angina, dysrhythmias, hypertension, cardiac arrest
GI: Nausea, diarrhea, increased or decreased appetite, cramps
MISC: Menstrual irregularities, weight loss, sweating, heat intolerance, fever

Contraindications: Adrenal insufficiency, MI, thyrotoxicosis

G **Precautions:** Elderly, angina pectoris, hypertension, ischemia, cardiac disease, pregnancy **A,** lactation

Pharmacokinetics

Absorption	Well (PO); complete (IV)
Distribution	Widely distributed; does not cross placenta
Metabolism	Liver
Excretion	Feces via bile, breast milk
Half-life	6-7 days

Pharmacodynamics

	PO/IV
Onset	Unknown
Peak	12-24 hr
Duration	72 hr

Interactions
Individual drugs
Cholestyramine: ↓ absorption of thyroid hormone
Colestipol: ↓ absorption of thyroid hormone
Digitalis: ↓ effect of digitalis
Insulin: ↑ requirement for insulin
Phenytoin (IV): ↑ release of thyroid hormone
Drug classifications
Amphetamines: ↑ CNS, cardiac stimulation
β-Adrenergic blockers: ↓ effect of β-blockers
Decongestants: ↑ CNS, cardiac stimulation
Oral anticoagulants: ↑ requirements for anticoagulants
Vasopressors: ↑ CNS, cardiac stimulation
Lab test interferences
↑ CPK, ↑ LDH, ↑ AST (SGOT), ↑ PBI, ↑ blood glucose
↓ TSH, ↓ RAIU, ↓ uric acid, ↓ triglycerides

NURSING CONSIDERATIONS
Assessment
- Identify if the patient is taking anticoagulants, antidiabetic agents; document on patient record
- Take B/P, pulse before each dose; monitor I&O ratio and weight every day in same clothing, using same scale, at same time of day
- Monitor height, weight, psychomotor development, and growth rate if given to a P child
- Monitor T_3, T_4, FTIs, which are decreased; radioimmunoassay of TSH, which is increased; RAIU, which is increased if patient is on too low a dosage of medication
- Monitor pro-time; may require decreased anticoagulant; check for bleeding, bruising
- Assess for increased nervous-

ness, excitability, irritability, which may indicate too high a dosage, usually after 1-3 wk of treatment

- Assess cardiac status: angina, palpitations, chest pain, change in VS; elderly patients may have undetected cardiac problems, and baseline ECG should be completed before treatment

Nursing diagnoses

✓ Knowledge deficit (teaching)
✓ Noncompliance (teaching)

Implementation

PO route

- Give in AM if possible as a single dose to decrease sleeplessness; give at same time each day to maintain drug level
- Give only for hormone imbalances; not to be used for obesity, male infertility, menstrual conditions, lethargy; give lowest dosage that relieves symptoms; give lower dosage to the elderly and for cardiac diseases
- Store in air-tight, light-resistant container

IV route

- Administer **IV** for myxedema coma and precoma; do not give IM or SC; give q4-12h; use PO dose as soon as feasible

Patient/family education

- Teach patient that drug is not a cure but controls symptoms, and treatment is long term
- Instruct patient to report excitability, irritability, anxiety, sweating, heat intolerance, chest pain, palpitations, which indicate overdose
- Advise patient not to switch brands unless approved by prescriber; bioavailability may differ; do not take with food or absorption will be decreased
- Teach patient that drug may be discontinued after giving birth; thyroid panel will be evaluated after 1-2 mo
- Teach patient that hyperthyroid child will show almost immediate behavior/personality change; that hair loss will occur in child but is temporary
- Caution patient that drug is not to be taken to reduce weight
- Caution patient to avoid OTC preparations with iodine; read labels; other medications should not be used unless approved by prescriber
- Teach patient to avoid iodine-rich food: iodized salt, soybeans, tofu, turnips, some seafood, some bread

Evaluation

Positive therapeutic outcome

- Absence of depression
- Weight loss
- Increased diuresis, pulse, appetite
- Absence of constipation, peripheral edema, cold intolerance, pale, cool dry skin, brittle nails, alopecia, coarse hair, menorrhagia, night blindness, paresthesias, syncope, stupor, coma, rosy cheeks
- Improved levels of T_3, T_4 by laboratory tests
- Child: age-appropriate weight, height, and psychomotor development

Treatment of overdose:

Withhold dose for up to 1 wk; for acute overdose: gastric lavage or induce emesis, then activated charcoal; provide supportive treatment to control symptoms

L

liotrix (℞)

(lye'oh-trix)

Euthroid, T_3/T_4, Thyrolar

Func. class.: Thyroid hormone

Chem. class.: Levothyroxine/liothyronine (synthetic T_4, T_3)

Pregnancy category A

Action: Controls protein synthesis; increases metabolic rates, cardiac output, renal blood flow, O_2 consumption, body temp, blood volume, growth, development at cellular level

➔ **Therapeutic Outcome:** Correction of lack of thyroid hormone

Uses: Hypothyroidism, thyroid hormone replacement

Dosage and routes

P ***Adult and child:*** PO 15-30 mg qd, increased by 15-30 mg q1-2 wk until desired response; may increase by 15-30 mg q2 wk in child

G ***Geriatric:*** PO 15-30 mg; double dose q6-8 wk until desired response

Available forms: Euthroid ½, 1, 2, 3 gr; Thyrolar ¼, ½, 1, 2, 3, gr; ½ grain = 30 mg

Adverse effects

CNS: Insomnia, tremors, headache, thyroid storm

CV: Tachycardia, palpitations, angina, dysrhythmias, hypertension, cardiac arrest

GI: Nausea, diarrhea, increased or decreased appetite, cramps

MISC: Menstrual irregularities, weight loss, sweating, heat intolerance, fever

Contraindications: Adrenal insufficiency, MI, thyrotoxicosis

G **Precautions:** Elderly, angina pectoris, hypertension, ischemia, cardiac disease, pregnancy **A,** lactation

Pharmacokinetics

Absorption	50%-80% (T_4); 95% (T_3)
Distribution	Widely distributed; does not cross placenta
Metabolism	Liver, tissues
Excretion	Feces via bile; breast milk
Half-life	6-7 days (T_4); 2 days (T_3)

Pharmacodynamics

	PO (T_4)	PO (T_3)
Onset	Unknown	Unknown
Peak	Unknown	24-72 hr
Duration	Unknown	72 hr

Interactions

Individual drugs

Cholestyramine: ↓ absorption of thyroid hormone

Colestipol: ↓ absorption of liotrix

Digitalis: ↓ effect of digitalis

Insulin: ↑ requirement for insulin

Phenytoin (IV): ↑ release of thyroid hormone

Drug classifications

Amphetamines: ↑ CNS, cardiac stimulation

β-Adrenergic blockers: ↓ effect of β-blockers

Decongestants: ↑ CNS, cardiac stimulation

Oral anticoagulants: ↑ requirements for anticoagulants

Vasopressors: ↑ CNS, cardiac stimulation

Lab test interferences

↑ CPK, ↑ LDH, ↑ AST (SGOT), ↑ PBI, ↑ blood glucose

↓ TSH, ↓ RAIU, ↓ uric acid, ↓ triglycerides

NURSING CONSIDERATIONS

Assessment

- Identify if the patient is taking anticoagulants, antidiabetic agents; document on chart
- Take B/P, pulse before each dose; monitor I&O ratio and weight every day in same clothing, using same scale, at same time of day
- Monitor height, weight, psychomotor development, and growth rate if given to a child
- Monitor T_3, T_4, FTIs, which are decreased; radioimmunoassay of TSH, which is increased; RAIU, which is increased if patient is on too low a dosage of medication
- Monitor pro-time; may require decreased anticoagulant; check for bleeding, bruising
- Assess for increased nervousness, excitability, irritability, which may indicate too high a dosage of medication, usually after 1-3 wk of treatment
- Assess cardiac status: angina, palpitations, chest pain, change in VS; the elderly patient may have undetected cardiac problems, and baseline ECG should be completed before treatment

Nursing diagnoses

✓ Knowledge deficit (teaching)
✓ Noncompliance (teaching)

Implementation

- Give in AM if possible as a single dose to decrease sleeplessness; give at same time each day to maintain drug level
- Give only for hormone imbalances; not to be used for obesity, male infertility, menstrual conditions, lethargy; give lowest dosage that relieves symptoms; give lower dosage to the elderly and for cardiac diseases
- Store in airtight, light-resistant container
- Remove medication 4 wk before RAIU test

Patient/family education

- Teach patient that drug is not a cure but controls symptoms, and treatment is long term
- Instruct patient to report excitability, irritability, anxiety, sweating, heat intolerance, chest pain, palpitations, which indicate overdose
- Advise patient not to switch brands unless approved by prescriber; bioavailability may differ; do not take with food or absorption will be decreased
- Teach patient that drug may be discontinued after giving birth; thyroid panel will be evaluated after 1-2 mo
- Teach patient that hyperthyroid child will show almost immediate behavior/personality change; that hair loss will occur in child but is temporary
- Caution patient that drug is not to be taken to reduce weight
- Caution patient to avoid OTC preparations with iodine; read labels; other medications should not be used unless approved by prescriber
- Teach patient to avoid iodine-rich food: iodized salt, soybeans, tofu, turnips, some seafood, some bread

Evaluation

Positive therapeutic outcome

- Absence of depression
- Weight loss

• Increased diuresis, pulse, appetite
• Absence of constipation, peripheral edema, cold intolerance, pale, cool dry skin, brittle nails, alopecia, coarse hair, menorrhagia, night blindness, paresthesias, syncope, stupor, coma, rosy cheeks
• Improved levels of T_3, T_4 by laboratory tests
P • Child: age-appropriate weight, height, and psychomotor development

Treatment of overdose: Withhold dose for up to 1 wk; acute overdose: gastric lavage or induce emesis, then activated charcoal; provide supportive treatment to control symptoms

lisinopril (℞)

(lyse-in′oh-pril)

Prinivil, Zestril

Func. class.: Angiotensin converting enzyme (ACE) inhibitor

Chem. class.: Enalaprilat lysine analog

Pregnancy category C

Action: Selectively suppresses renin-angiotensin-aldosterone system; inhibits ACE; prevents conversion of angiotensin I to angiotensin II; results in dilatation of arterial, venous vessels

Therapeutic Outcome: Decreased B/P in hypertension, decreased preload, afterload in CHF

Uses: Mild to moderate hypertension, adjunctive therapy of CHF

Dosage and routes

Hypertension

Adult: PO 10-40 mg qd; may increase to 80 mg qd if required

CHF

Adult: PO 2.5-5 mg initially with diuretics/digitalis

Available forms: Tabs 5, 10, 20, 40 mg

Adverse effects

CNS: Vertigo, depression, stroke, insomnia, paresthesias, *headache,* fatigue, asthenia

EENT: Blurred vision, nasal congestion

GI: Nausea, vomiting, anorexia, constipation, flatulence, GI irritation

GU: ***Proteinuria, renal insufficiency,*** sexual dysfunction, impotence

INTEG: Rash, pruritus

RESP: Cough, dyspnea

Contraindications: Hypersensitivity

Precautions: Pregnancy **C,** lactation, renal disease, hyperkalemia

Pharmacokinetics	
Absorption	Variable
Distribution	Unknown
Metabolism	Not metabolized
Excretion	Kidneys, unchanged
Half-life	12 hr

Pharmacodynamics	
Onset	1 hr
Peak	6-8 hr
Duration	24 hr

Interactions

Individual drugs

Alcohol: ↑ hypotension (large amounts)

Allopurinol: ↑ hypersensitivity

Digoxin: ↑ serum levels

Hydralazine: ↑ toxicity

Indomethacin: ↓ antihypertensive effect
Lithium: ↑ levels of lithium
Prazosin: ↑ toxicity

Drug classifications

Adrenergic blockers: ↑ hypotension
Antacids: ↓ absorption
Antihypertensives: ↑ hypotension
Diuretics: ↑ hypotension
Diuretics, potassium-sparing: ↑ toxicity
Ganglionic blockers: ↑ hypotension
Potassium supplements: ↑ toxicity
Sympathomimetics: ↑ toxicity

Food

High-potassium diet (bananas, orange juice, avocados, broccoli, nuts, spinach) should be avoided; hyperuricemia may occur

Lab test interferences

False positive: Urine acetone

NURSING CONSIDERATIONS

Assessment

- Monitor B/P, check for orthostatic hypotension, syncope; if changes occur, dosage change may be required
- Monitor renal studies: protein, BUN, creatinine; watch for increased levels that may indicate nephrotic syndrome and renal failure; monitor renal symptoms: polyuria, oliguria, frequency, dysuria
- Establish baselines in renal, liver function tests before therapy begins
- Check potassium levels throughout treatment, although hyperkalemia rarely occurs
- Check for edema in feet, legs daily
- Assess for allergic reactions: rash, fever, pruritus, urticaria; drug should be discontinued if antihistamines fail to help

Nursing diagnoses

- ✓ Cardiac output, decreased (uses)
- ✓ Injury, risk for (side effects)
- ✓ Knowledge deficit (teaching)
- ✓ Noncompliance (teaching)

Implementation

- Store in tight container at 86° F (30° C) or less
- Severe hypotension may occur after 1st dose of this medication; it may be prevented by reducing or discontinuing diuretic therapy 3 days before beginning lisinopril therapy

Patient/family education

- Caution patient not to discontinue drug abruptly; advise patient to inform all health care providers about taking this drug
- Teach patient not to use OTC products (cough, cold, allergy) unless directed by prescriber; serious side effects can occur
- Teach patient the importance of complying with dosage schedule, even if feeling better; to continue with medical regimen to decrease B/P: exercise, cessation of smoking, decreasing stress, diet modifications
- Teach patient to notify prescriber of mouth sores, sore throat, fever, swelling of hands or feet, irregular heartbeat, chest pain, coughing, shortness of breath
- Caution patient to report excessive perspiration, dehydration, vomiting, diarrhea; may lead to fall in B/P
- Emphasize the need to rise slowly to sitting or standing position to minimize orthostatic hypotension; not to

exercise in hot weather or increased hypotension can occur

- Caution patient that drug may cause dizziness, fainting, light-headedness; may occur during 1st few days of therapy; to avoid activities that may be hazardous
- Teach patient how to take B/P, and normal readings for age group; advise patient to take B/P regularly

Evaluation

Positive therapeutic outcome

- Decreased B/P in hypertension
- Decreased CHF symptoms

Treatment of overdose: 0.9% NaCl **IV** inf, hemodialysis

lithium (℞)

(li'thee-um)

Carbolith ✦, Cibalith-S, Duralith, Eskalith, Eskalith CR, Lithane, lithium carbonate, Lithizine ✦, Lithonate, Lithotabs

Func. class.: Antimanic

Chem. class.: Alkali metal ion salt

Pregnancy category D

Action: May alter sodium, potassium ion transport across cell membrane in nerve, muscle cells; may balance biogenic amines of norepinephrine, serotonin in CNS areas involved in emotional responses

➔ **Therapeutic Outcome:** Stable mood

Uses: Manic-depressive illness (manic phase), prevention of bipolar manic-depressive psychosis

Dosage and routes

Adult: PO 300-600 mg tid; maintenance 300 mg tid or qid; slow rel tab 300 mg bid; dosage should be individualized to maintain blood levels at 0.5-1.5 mEq/L

P ***Child:*** PO 15-20 mg (0.4-0.5 mEq)/kg/day in 2-3 divided doses

Available forms: Caps 300, 600 mg; tab 300 mg; controlled rel tab 450 mg; syrup 300 mg/5 ml (8 mEq/5 ml); slow rel caps 150, 300 mg ✦

Adverse effects

CNS: Headache, drowsiness, dizziness, tremors, twitching, ataxia, ***seizure,*** slurred speech, restlessness, *confusion,* stupor, memory loss, clonic movements, *fatigue*

CV: Hypotension, ECG changes, dysrhythmias, ***circulatory collapse, edema***

EENT: Tinnitus, blurred vision, aphasia, dysarthria

ENDO: Hypothyroidism, goiter, hyperglycemia, hyperthyroidism

GI: Dry mouth, anorexia, nausea, vomiting, diarrhea, incontinence, abdominal pain, metallic taste

GU: ***Polyuria, glycosuria, proteinuria, albuminuria,*** urinary incontinence, polydipsia, edema, ***renal toxicity***

HEMA: ***Leukocytosis***

INTEG: Drying of hair, alopecia, rash, pruritus, hyperkeratosis, *acneiform rash, folliculitis*

MS: Muscle weakness, rigidity

SYST: Hyponatremia

Contraindications: Hepatic disease, renal disease, brain trauma, OBS, pregnancy **D,**

lactation, schizophrenia, severe cardiac disease, severe renal disease, severe dehydration

G **Precautions:** Elderly, thyroid disease, seizure disorders, diabetes mellitus, syst infection, urinary retention, P children <12 yr

Pharmacokinetics

Absorption	Completely absorbed
Distribution	Reabsorbed by renal tubules (80%); crosses blood-brain barrier; crosses placenta
Metabolism	Unknown
Excretion	Urine, unchanged
Half-life	18-36 hr depending on age

Pharmacodynamics

Onset	Rapid
Peak	½-4 hr
Duration	Unknown

Interactions
Individual drugs
Acetazolamide: ↑ renal clearance
Aminophylline: ↑ renal clearance
Calcium iodide: ↑ hypothyroid effect
Haloperidol: Brain damage
Iodinated glycerol: ↑ hypothyroid effect
Indomethacin: ↑ toxicity
Mannitol: ↑ renal clearance
Potassium: ↑ hypothyroid effect
Sodium bicarbonate: ↑ renal clearance
Thioridazine: Brain damage
Urea: ↑ toxicity
Drug classifications
Phenothiazines: ↑ effect of phenothiazines
Theophyllines: ↓ effect of lithium
Lab test interferences
↑ Potassium excretion, ↑ urine glucose, ↑ blood glucose, ↑ protein, ↑ BUN
↓ VMA, ↓ T_3, ↓ T_4, ↓ PBI, ↓ ^{131}I

NURSING CONSIDERATIONS
Assessment
- Assess for minor lithium toxicity: vomiting, diarrhea, poor coordination, fine motor tremors, weakness, lassitude; major toxicity: course tremors, severe thirst, tinnitus, dilute urine
- Assess weight daily; check for edema in legs, ankles, wrists; report if present; check skin turgor at least daily
- Monitor sodium intake; decreased sodium intake with decreased fluid intake may lead to lithium retention; increased sodium and fluids may decrease lithium retention
- Monitor urine for albuminuria, glycosuria, uric acid during beginning treatment, q2 mo thereafter
- Assess neuro status: LOC, gait, motor reflexes, hand tremors
- Monitor serum lithium levels weekly initially, then q2 mo (therapeutic level: 0.5-1.5 mEq/L); toxicity and therapeutic levels are very close; toxicity may occur rapidly; blood levels are drawn before the AM dose

Nursing diagnoses
✓ Ineffective individual coping (uses)
✓ Thought processes, altered (uses)
✓ Knowledge deficit (teaching)
✓ Noncompliance (teaching)

Implementation
- Administer reduced dosage G to elderly; give with meals to avoid GI upset

• Provide adequate fluids (2-3 L/day) to prevent dehydration during initial treatment, 1-2 L/day during maintenance

Patient/family education

• Provide patient with written information on symptoms of minor toxicity: vomiting, diarrhea, poor coordination, fine motor tremors, weakness, lassitude; major toxicity: coarse tremors, severe thirst, tinnitus, dilute urine

• Advise patient to monitor urine sp gr; emphasize need for follow-up care to determine lithium effects

• Advise patient that contraception is necessary, since lithium may harm fetus

• Caution patient not to operate machinery until lithium levels are stable and response determined; that beneficial effects may take 1-3 wk

• Provide to the patient a list of drugs that interact with lithium and discuss need for adequate salt and fluid intake

• Advise patient not to crush, chew caps

Evaluation

Positive therapeutic outcome

• Decrease in excitement, poor judgment, insomnia (manic phase)

• Decreased mood swings and lability

Treatment of overdose: Induce emesis or lavage, maintain airway, respiratory function; dialysis for severe intoxication

lomefloxacin (℞)

(lome-flocks'a-sin)

Maxaquin

Func. class.: Antiinfective

Chem. class.: Fluoroquinolone

Pregnancy category C

Action: Interferes with conversion of intermediate DNA fragments into high-molecular-weight DNA in bacteria; DNA gyrase inhibitor

Therapeutic Outcome: Bactericidal for gram-negative organisms *Aeromonas, Citrobacter, Enterobacter, Escherichia coli, Haemophilus influenzae, Klebsiella, Legionella, Moraxella catarrhalis, Morganella morganii, Proteus vulgaris, P. mirabilis, Providencia alcalifaciens, P. rettgeri, Pseudomonas aeruginosa, Serratia;* gram-positive organisms *Staphylococcus aureus, S. epidermidis, S. saprophyticus* (methicillin-resistant strains also)

Uses: Treatment of lower respiratory tract infections (pneumonia, bronchitis), genitourinary tract infections (prostatitis, UTIs), preoperatively to reduce urinary tract infections in transurethral surgical procedures

Dosage and routes

Adult: PO 400 mg/day × 7-14 days depending on type of infection

In renal impairment

Adult: PO 200 mg/day

Prophylaxis of UTI

Adult: PO 400 mg 2-6 hr before surgery

Available forms: Tab 400 mg

Adverse effects

CNS: Dizziness, headache, somnolence, depression, insomnia, nervousness, confusion, agitation
EENT: Visual disturbances
GI: Diarrhea, nausea, vomiting, anorexia, flatulence, heartburn, dry mouth, increased AST (SGOT), ALT (SGPT), constipation, abdominal pain, oral thrush, glossitis, stomatitis
INTEG: Rash, pruritus, urticaria, photosensitivity

Contraindications: Hypersensitivity to quinolones

P G **Precautions:** Pregnancy **C**, lactation, children, elderly, renal disease, seizure disorders, excessive exposure to sunlight

Pharmacokinetics	
Absorption	Well absorbed
Distribution	Widely distributed
Metabolism	Unknown
Excretion	Kidney, unchanged
Half-life	6-8 hr; increased in renal disease

Pharmacodynamics	
Onset	Unknown
Peak	1-2 hr

Interactions

Individual drugs

Cimetidine: ↑ lomefloxacin levels
Probenicid: ↑ lomefloxacin levels
Warfarin: ↑ levels of warfarin
Cyclosporine: ↑ levels of cyclosporine
Nitrofurantoin: ↓ lomefloxacin levels
Sucralfate: ↓ lomefloxacin levels

Drug classifications

Antacids: ↓ levels of lomefloxacin
Iron sulfate: ↓ levels of lomefloxacin
Zinc sulfate: ↓ levels of lomefloxacin

NURSING CONSIDERATIONS

Assessment

- Assess patient for previous sensitivity reaction
- Assess patient for signs and symptoms of infection: characteristics of wounds, sputum, urine, stool, WBC >10,000, fever; obtain baseline information before and during treatment
- Obtain C&S before beginning drug therapy to identify if correct treatment has been initiated
- Assess for allergic reactions: rash, urticaria, pruritus
- Monitor blood studies: AST (SGOT), ALT (SGPT), CBC, Hct, bilirubin, LDH, alkaline phosphatase, Coombs' test monthly if patient is on long-term therapy
- Assess bowel pattern qd; if severe diarrhea occurs, drug should be discontinued
- Assess for overgrowth of infection: perineal itching, fever, malaise, redness, pain, swelling, drainage, rash, diarrhea, change in cough, sputum
- Assess for CNS symptoms: insomnia, vertigo, headaches, agitation, confusion

Nursing diagnoses

- ✓ Infection, risk for (uses)
- ✓ Diarrhea (adverse reactions)
- ✓ Injury, risk for (adverse reactions)
- ✓ Knowledge deficit (teaching)
- ✓ Noncompliance (teaching)

Implementation

- Give with food for GI symptoms; give with 8 oz of water
- Do not give with iron, calcium, magnesium products or

L

antacids, which decrease absorption

Patient/family education

• Instruct patient to take all medication prescribed for the length of time ordered; drug must be taken around the clock to maintain blood levels; do not give medication to others

• Teach patient to use sunscreen when outdoors to decrease phototoxicity

• Advise patient to increase fluids to 2 L/day to prevent crystalluria

• Caution patient to avoid driving and other hazardous activities until response is known; dizziness, confusion, drowsiness may occur

Evaluation

Positive therapeutic outcome

• Absence of signs/symptoms of infection (WBC <10,000, temp WNL)

• Reported improvement in symptoms of infection

lomustine (℞)

(loe-mus'teen)

CCNU, CeeNU

Func. class.: Antineoplastic alkylating agent

Chem. class.: Nitrosourea

Pregnancy category D

Action: Changes essential cellular ions to covalent bonding with resultant alkylation; this interferes with normal biologic function of DNA; activity is not phase specific; action is due to myelosuppression

Therapeutic Outcome: Prevention of rapid growth of malignant cells in chronic myelocytic leukemia

Uses: Hodgkin's disease, lymphomas, multiple myeloma

Investigational uses: Brain, breast, renal, GI tract, bronchogenic carcinoma; melanomas

Dosage and routes

Adult: PO 100, 130 mg/m^2 as a single dose q6 wk; titrate dosage to WBC level; do not give repeat dose unless WBCs are >4000/mm^3, platelet count >100,000/mm^3

Available forms: Caps 10, 40, 100 mg

Adverse effects

*GI: Nausea, vomiting, anorexia, stomatitis, **hepatotoxicity***

GU: Azotemia, renal failure

HEMA: Thrombocytopenia, leukopenia, myelosuppression, anemia

INTEG: Burning at inj site

RESP: Fibrosis, pulmonary infiltrate

Contraindications: Radiation, chemotherapy, lactation, pregnancy (3rd trimester) **D,** "blastic" phase of chronic myelocytic leukemia, hypersensitivity

Precautions: Childbearing age men and women, leukopenia, thrombocytopenia, anemia, hepatotoxicity, renal toxicity

Pharmacokinetics

Absorption	Rapidly absorbed
Distribution	Widely
Metabolism	Liver
Excretion	Kidneys, breast milk
Half-life	16-48 hr

Pharmacodynamics

Unknown

Interactions

Individual drugs

Radiation: ↑ toxicity, bone marrow suppression

Drug classifications

Antineoplastics: ↑ toxicity, bone marrow suppression

Lab test interferences

False positive: Cytology tests for breast, bladder, cervix, lung

NURSING CONSIDERATIONS

Assessment

- ❗ Monitor CBC, differential, platelet count weekly; withhold drug if WBC is <4000 or platelet count is <75,000; notify prescriber of results if WBC <20,000 /mm^3, platelets <150,000/mm^3
- Monitor pulmonary function tests, chest x-ray films before, during therapy; chest film should be obtained q2 wk during treatment; assess for dyspnea, rales, unproductive cough, chest pain, tachypnea
- Monitor renal function studies: BUN, serum uric acid, urine CrCl before, during therapy; I&O ratio; report fall in urine output of 30 ml/hr; check for decreased hyperuricemia
- Monitor for cold, fever, sore throat (may indicate beginning infection); identify edema in feet, joint and stomach pain, shaking; prescriber should be notified
- Assess for bleeding: hematuria, guaiac, bruising or petechiae, mucosa or orifices q8h, no rec temp

Nursing diagnoses

✓ Injury, risk for (adverse reactions)
✓ Body image disturbance (adverse reactions)
✓ Infection, risk for (adverse reactions)
✓ Knowledge deficit (teaching)

Implementation

- Give drug after evening meal, before hs; administer antiemetic 30-60 min before giving drug to prevent vomiting
- Antibiotics for prophylaxis of infection may be prescribed since infection potential is high
- Store in tight container

Patient/family education

- Teach patient to avoid use of products containing aspirin or ibuprofen, razors, commercial mouthwash, since bleeding may occur; to report symptoms of bleeding (hematuria, tarry stools)
- Advise patient to report signs of anemia (fatigue, headache, irritability, faintness, shortness of breath)
- Caution patient to report any changes in breathing or coughing even several mo after treatment; to avoid crowds and persons with respiratory tract or other infections
- Caution patient not to have any vaccinations without the advice of prescriber; serious reactions can occur
- Tell patient contraception is needed during treatment and for several mo after the completion of therapy

Evaluation

Positive therapeutic outcome

- Decreased tumor sizes
- Decreased spread of malignancy

L

loperamide (OTC), (℞)

(loe-per'a-mide)

loperamide solution, Imodium, Imodium A-D, Imodium A-D Caplet, Loperamide, A-D Kaopectate II Caplets, Maalox Antidiarrheal Caplets, Pepto Diarrhea Control

Func. class.: Antidiarrheal

Chem. class.: Piperidine derivative

Pregnancy category B

Action: Direct action on intestinal muscles to decrease GI peristalsis; reduces volume, increases bulk; electrolytes are not lost

➔ **Therapeutic Outcome:** Absence of diarrhea

Uses: Diarrhea (cause undetermined), chronic diarrhea, ileostomy discharge

Dosage and routes

Adult: PO 4 mg, then 2 mg after each loose stool, not to exceed 16 mg/day

P ***Child 2-5 yr:*** PO 1 mg on day 1, then 0.1 mg/kg after each loose stool

P ***Child 5-8 yr:*** PO 2 mg bid on day 1, then 0.1 mg/kg after each loose stool

P ***Child 8-12 yr:*** PO 2 mg tid on day 1, then 0.1 mg/kg after each loose stool

Available forms: Cap 2 mg; liq 1 mg/5 ml; tab 2 mg

Adverse effects

CNS: Dizziness, drowsiness, fatigue, fever

GI: Nausea, dry mouth, vomiting, constipation, abdominal pain, anorexia, ***toxic megacolon***

INTEG: Rash

Contraindications: Hypersensitivity, severe ulcerative colitis, pseudomembranous colitis, acute diarrhea associated with *E. coli*

Precautions: Pregnancy **B,** P lactation, children <2 yr, liver disease, dehydration, bacterial disease

Pharmacokinetics	
Absorption	Poor
Distribution	Unknown
Metabolism	Liver
Excretion	Feces, unchanged; small amount in urine
Half-life	7-14 hr

Pharmacodynamics	
Onset	½-1 hr
Peak	Unknown
Duration	4-5 hr

Interaction

Solutions: Do not mix with other oral sol

NURSING CONSIDERATIONS

Assessment

- Monitor electrolytes (potassium, sodium, chloride) if patient is on long-term therapy; check fluid status, skin turgor
- Assess bowel pattern before, during treatment; check for rebound constipation after termination of medication; check bowel sounds
- Check response after 48 hr; if no response, drug should be discontinued and other treatment initiated
- Assess for abdominal distention, toxic megacolon, which may occur in ulcerative colitis

Nursing diagnoses

✓ Diarrhea (uses)

✓ Constipation (adverse reactions)

✓ Knowledge deficit (teaching)
✓ Noncompliance (teaching)

Implementation

- Do not chew, crush caps
- Store in airtight containers

Patient/family education

- Caution patient to avoid alcohol and OTC products unless directed by prescriber; may cause increased CNS depression
- Advise patient not to exceed recommended dosage; drug may be habit forming
- Advise patient that drug may cause drowsiness and to avoid hazardous activities until response to drug is determined
- Teach patient that dry mouth can be decreased by frequent sips of water, hard candy, sugarless gum

Evaluation

Positive therapeutic outcome

- Decreased diarrhea

loracarbef (℞)

(lor-a-kar′beff)

Lorabid

Func. class.: Antiinfective
Chem. class.: Cephalosporin (2nd generation)

Pregnancy category B

Action: Inhibits bacterial cell wall synthesis, which renders cell wall osmotically unstable, leading to cell death

➔ **Therapeutic Outcome:** Bactericidal for the following organisms: gram-negative *Haemophilus influenzae, Escherichia coli, Proteus mirabilis, Klebsiella;* gram-positive *Streptococcus pneumoniae, S. pyogenes, Staphylococcus aureus*

Uses: Upper and lower respiratory tract, urinary tract, skin infections; otitis media, pharyngitis, tonsillitis

Dosage and routes

P *Adult and child >13 yr:* PO 200-400 mg q12h

P *Child to 12 yr:* PO 15-30 mg/kg/day in 2 divided doses given q12h

Available forms: Cap 200 mg; oral susp 100, 200 mg/5 ml

Adverse effects

CNS: Dizziness, headache, fatigue, paresthesia, fever, chills, confusion
GI: Diarrhea, nausea, vomiting, anorexia, dysgeusia, glossitis, bleeding, increased AST (SGOT), ALT (SGPT), bilirubin, LDH, alkaline phosphatase, abdominal pain, loose stools, flatulence, heartburn, stomach cramps, colitis, jaundice
GU: Vaginitis, pruritus, candidiasis, increased BUN, ***nephrotoxicity, renal failure,*** pyuria, dysuria, reversible interstitial nephritis
HEMA: ***Leukopenia, thrombocytopenia, agranulocytosis,*** anemia, ***neutropenia, lymphocytosis, eosinophilia, pancytopenia, hemolytic anemia, leukocytosis, granulocytopenia***
INTEG: Rash, urticaria, dermatitis
MISC: ***Anaphylaxis***
RESP: Dyspnea

Contraindications: Hypersensitivity to cephalosporins or related antibiotics, seizures

Precautions: Pregnancy **B,** P lactation, children, renal disease

Pharmacokinetics

Absorption	Well absorbed
Distribution	Widely distributed; crosses placenta
Metabolism	Not metabolized
Excretion	Kidneys, unchanged; enters breast milk
Half-life	1 hr; increased in renal disease

Pharmacodynamics

Onset	Rapid
Peak	1 hr

Interactions: None

Lab test interferences

False ↑ Creatinine (serum urine), false ↑ urinary 17-KS

False positive: Urinary protein, direct Coombs' test, urine glucose testing (Clinitest)

Interference: Cross-matching

NURSING CONSIDERATIONS

Assessment

- Assess patient for previous sensitivity reaction
- Assess patient for signs and symptoms of infection: characteristics of wounds, sputum, urine, stool, WBC >10,000, earache, fever; obtain baseline information and during treatment
- Obtain C&S before beginning drug therapy to identify if correct treatment has been initiated
- Assess for allergic reactions: rash, urticaria, pruritus, chills, fever, joint pain; angioedema may occur a few days after therapy begins; epinephrine, resuscitation equipment should be available for anaphylactic reaction
- Identify urine output; if decreasing, notify prescriber (may indicate nephrotoxicity); also check for increased BUN, creatinine
- Monitor blood studies: AST (SGOT), ALT (SGPT), CBC, Hct, bilirubin, LDH, alkaline phosphatase, Coombs' test monthly if patient is on long-term therapy
- Assess bowel pattern qd; if severe diarrhea occurs, drug should be discontinued; may indicate pseudomembranous colitis
- Assess for overgrowth of infection: perineal itching, fever, malaise, redness, pain, swelling, drainage, rash, diarrhea, change in cough, sputum

Nursing diagnoses

- ✓ Infection, risk for (uses)
- ✓ Diarrhea (adverse reactions)
- ✓ Injury, risk for (adverse reactions)
- ✓ Knowledge deficit (teaching)
- ✓ Noncompliance (teaching)

Implementation

- Give on an empty stomach, 1 hr ac or 2 hr pc
- Do not crush, chew caps
- Oral susp should be shaken before administration; store for 2 wk at room temp, discard after 2 wk

Patient/family education

- Teach patient to report sore throat, bruising, bleeding, joint pain; may indicate blood dyscrasias (rare)
- Advise patient to contact prescriber if vaginal itching, loose, foul-smelling stools, furry tongue occur; may indicate superinfection
- Advise patient to notify prescriber of diarrhea with blood or pus, which may indicate pseudomembranous colitis

Evaluation

Positive therapeutic outcome

- Absence of signs/symptoms of infection (WBC <10,000,

temp WNL, absence of red, draining wounds, earache)
- Reported improvement in symptoms of infection
- Negative C&S

Treatment of anaphylaxis: Epinephrine, antihistamines, resuscitate if needed

loratadine (℞)
(lor-a'ti-deen)
Claritin
Func. class.: Antihistamine (2nd-generation)
Chem. class.: Selective histamine (H_1) receptor antagonist
Pregnancy category B

Action: Binds to peripheral histamine receptors, which provides antihistamine action without sedation

Therapeutic Outcome: Decreased nasal stuffiness, itching, swollen eyes

Uses: Seasonal rhinitis

Dosage and routes
Adult and child ≥12 yr: PO 10 mg qd; tabs rapid-disintegrating 10 mg; syrup 1 mg/ml

Child 6-12 yr: PO 10 mg (10ml) qd

Available forms: Tab 10 mg

Adverse effects
CNS: Sedation (more common with increased dosages)

Contraindications: Hypersensitivity, acute asthma attacks, lower respiratory tract disease

Precautions: Pregnancy **B,** increased intraocular pressure, bronchial asthma

Pharmacokinetics

Absorption	Well absorbed
Distribution	Unknown
Metabolism	Liver, extensively, to active metabolites
Excretion	Kidneys
Half-life	8½-28 hr

Pharmacodynamics

Onset	Unknown
Peak	1½ hr
Duration	Unknown

Interactions
Individual drugs
Alcohol: ↑ CNS depression
Cimetidine: ↑ loratadine levels
Drug classifications
Antibiotics, macrolide: ↑ CV effects
Antifungals, azole: ↑ CV effects
CNS depressants: ↑ CNS depression
MAOIs: ↑ anticholinelgic sedative effects
Narcotics: ↑ CNS depression
Sedative/hypnotics: ↑ CNS depression
Food
↑ absorption
Lab test interferences
False negative: Skin allergy tests (discontinue antihistamine 3 days before testing)

NURSING CONSIDERATIONS
Assessment
- Assess respiratory status: rate, rhythm, increase in bronchial secretions, wheezing, chest tightness; provide fluids to 2 L/day to decrease secretion thickness

Nursing diagnoses
✓ Airway clearance, ineffective (uses)
✓ Knowledge deficit (teaching)
✓ Noncompliance (teaching, overuse)

Implementation

- Give on an empty stomach, 1 hr ac or 2 hr pc to facilitate absorption
- Place rapidly disintegrating tabs on tongue, then swallow after disintegrated with or without water
- Store in tight, light-resistant container

Patient/family education

- Teach all aspects of drug uses; to notify prescriber if confusion, sedation, hypotension occur; to avoid driving and other hazardous activity if drowsiness occurs; to avoid alcohol and other CNS depressants that may potentiate effect
- Teach patient to take 1 hr ac or 2 hr pc to facilitate absorption
- Caution patient not to exceed recommended dosage; dysrhythmias may occur
- Teach patient hard candy, gum, frequent rinsing of mouth may be used for dryness

Evaluation

Positive therapeutic outcome

- Absence of running or congested nose

lorazepam (℞)

(lor-az'e-pam)

Alzapam, Apo-Lorazepam ✦, Ativan, Loraz, lorazepam, Novolorazem ✦

Func. class.: Sedative/hypnotic, antianxiety agent

Chem. class.: Benzodiazepine

Pregnancy category D

Controlled substance schedule IV

Action: Potentiates the actions of GABA, an inhibitory neurotransmitter, especially in the limbic system and reticular formation, which depresses the CNS

➔ **Therapeutic Outcome:** Decreased anxiety, relaxation

Uses: Anxiety, irritability in psychiatric or organic disorders, preoperatively, insomnia

Dosage and routes

Anxiety

Adult: PO 2-6 mg/day in divided doses, not to exceed 10 mg/day

G ***Elderly:*** PO 0.5-2 mg/day in divided doses

Insomnia

Adult: PO 2-4 mg hs; only minimally effective after 2 wk continuous therapy

G ***Elderly:*** PO 1-2 mg initially

Preoperatively

Adult: IM 50 μg/kg 2 hr before surgery; **IV** 44 μg/kg 15-20 min before surgery

Available forms: Tabs 0.5, 1, 2 mg; inj 2, 4 mg/ml; conc sol 0.2 mg/ml

Adverse effects

CNS: Dizziness, drowsiness, confusion, headache, anxiety, tremors, stimulation, fatigue, depression, insomnia, hallucinations, weakness, unsteadiness
CV: Orthostatic hypotension, ***ECG changes, tachycardia,*** hypotension
EENT: Blurred vision, tinnitus, mydriasis
GI: Constipation, dry mouth, nausea, vomiting, anorexia, diarrhea
INTEG: Rash, dermatitis, itching

Contraindications: Hypersensitivity to benzodiazepines, narrow-angle glaucoma, psychosis, pregnancy **D,** child <12 yr, history of drug abuse, COPD

Precautions: Elderly, debilitated patients, hepatic disease, renal disease

Pharmacokinetics

Absorption	Well absorbed (PO); completely absorbed (IM)
Distribution	Widely distributed; crosses placenta, blood-brain barrier
Metabolism	Liver, extensively
Excretion	Kidneys, breast milk
Half-life	14 hr

Pharmacodynamics

	PO	IM	IV
Onset	½ hr	15-30 min	5-15 min
Peak	1-3 hr	1-1½ hr	Unknown
Duration	3-6 hr	3-6 hr	3-6 hr

Interactions

Individual drugs

Alcohol: ↑ CNS depression
Cimetidine: ↑ action
Disulfiram: ↑ action
Fluoxetine: ↑ action
Levodopa: ↓ action of levodopa

Drug classifications

Analgesics, opioid: ↑ CNS depression
Antidepressants: ↑ CNS depression
Antihistamines: ↑ CNS depression

Smoking

↑ metabolism, ↓ effect

Lab test interferences

↑ AST (SGOT), ↑ ALT (SGPT), ↑ serum bilirubin
False ↑ 17-OHCS
↓ RAIU

NURSING CONSIDERATIONS

Assessment

- Assess degree of anxiety; what precipitates anxiety and whether drug controls symptoms; other signs of anxiety: dilated pupils, inability to sleep, restlessness, inability to focus
- Assess for alcohol withdrawal symptoms, including hallucinations (visual, auditory), delirium, irritability, agitation, fine to coarse tremors
- Monitor B/P (with patient lying/standing), pulse, check respiratory rate; if systolic B/P drops 20 mm Hg, hold drug, notify prescriber; respirations q5-15 min if given **IV**
- Monitor CBC during long-term therapy; blood dyscrasias have occurred (rarely)
- Monitor for seizure control; type, duration, and intensity of convulsions; what precipitates seizures
- Monitor hepatic studies: AST (SGOT), ALT (SGPT), bilirubin, creatinine, LDH, alkaline phosphatase
- Assess mental status: mood, sensorium, affect, sleeping pattern, drowsiness, dizziness,

suicidal tendencies, and ability of drug to control these symptoms; check for tolerance, withdrawal symptoms: headache, nausea, vomiting, muscle pain, weakness after long-term use

Nursing diagnoses

- ✓ Sleep pattern disturbance (uses)
- ✓ Coping, ineffective individual (uses)
- ✓ Knowledge deficit (teaching)
- ✓ Noncompliance (teaching)

Implementation

PO route

• Give with food or milk for GI symptoms; crush tab if patient is unable to swallow medication whole; provide sugarless gum, hard candy, frequent sips of water for dry mouth

• Use by SL route for rapid response (investigational use)

IM route

• Give deep in muscle mass; if using for preoperative sedation, give 2 hr or more before surgical procedure

IV **IV route**

• Dilute with sterile water for inj, 0.9% NaCl, or D_5W just before using; give by Y-site or 3-way stopcock at 2 mg/min

• Do not use sol that is discolored or contains a precipitate

Syringe compatibilities: Cimetidine, hydromorphone

Y-site incompatibilities: Idarubicin, ondansetron, sargramostim

Y-site compatibilities: Acyclovir, allopurinol, amifostine, amsacrine, atracurium, cefepime, cisplatin, cyclophosphamide, cytarabine, diltiazem, doxorubicin, etomidate, filgrastim, fludarabine, granisetron, melphalan, morphine, paclitaxel, pancuronium, tacrolimus, teniposide, vecuronium, vinorelbine, zidovudine

Patient/family education

• Advise patient that drug may be taken with food; that drug is not to be used for everyday stress or used longer than 4 mo unless directed by a prescriber; to take no more than prescribed amount; may be habit forming

• Caution patient to avoid OTC preparations unless approved by prescriber; to avoid alcohol, other psychotropic medications unless prescribed by physician; not to discontinue medication abruptly after long-term use

• Inform patient to avoid driving and activities that require alertness; drowsiness may occur; to rise slowly or fainting G may occur, especially in elderly

• Inform patient that drowsiness may worsen at beginning of treatment

Evaluation

Positive therapeutic outcome

• Decreased anxiety, restlessness, insomnia

Treatment of overdose: Lavage, VS, supportive care

losartan (℞)

(low-sar'tan)

Cozaar

Func. class.: Antihypertensive

Chem. class.: Angiotensin II receptor (Type AT_1)

Pregnancy category
C (1st trimester);
D (2nd/3rd trimester)

Action: Blocks the vasoconstrictor and aldosterone-secreting effects of angiotensin II; selectively blocks the binding of angiotensin II to the AT_1 receptor found in tissues

➔ **Therapeutic Outcome:** Decreased B/P

Uses: Hypertension, alone or in combination

Dosage and routes

Adult: PO mg qd alone or 25 mg qd when used in combination

Available forms: Tabs 25, 50 mg

Adverse effects

CNS: Dizziness, insomnia, anxiety, confusion, abnormal dreams, migraine, tremor, vertigo

CV: Angina pectoris, 2nd-degree AV block, ***cerebrovascular accident,*** hypotension, *myocardial infarction, dysrhythmias*

EENT: Blurred vision, burning eyes, conjunctivitis, task perversion

GI: Diarrhea, dyspepsia, anorexia, constipation, dry mouth, flatulence, gastritis, vomiting

GU: Impotence, nocturia, urinary frequency, urinary tract infection

HEMA: Anemia

INTEG: Alopecia, dermatitis, dry skin, flushing, photosensitivity, rash, pruritus, sweating

META: Gout

MS: Cramps, myalgia, pain, stiffness

RESP: Cough, upper respiratory infection, congestion, dyspnea, bronchitis

Contraindications: Hypersensitivity

Precautions: Hypersensitivity to ACE inhibitors; Pregnancy category **C** 1st trimester, **D** 2nd, 3rd trimester; lactation, children, elderly

Pharmacokinetics

Absorption	Well
Distribution	Bound to plasma proteins
Metabolism	Extensive
Excretion	Feces, urine
Half-life	Biphasic, 2 hr, 6-9 hr

Pharmacodynamics

Unknown

Interactions: None significant

NURSING CONSIDERATIONS

Assessment

- Assess B/P, pulse q4h; note rate, rhythm, quality
- Monitor electrolytes: potassium, sodium, chloride
- Obtain baselines in renal, liver function tests before therapy begins
- Monitor for edema in feet, legs daily
- Assess for skin turgor, dryness of mucous membranes for hydration status

Nursing diagnoses

- ✓ Fluid volume deficit (side effects)
- ✓ Noncompliance (teaching)
- ✓ Knowledge deficit (teaching)

Implementation

- Administer without regard to meals

Patient/family education

- Teach patient to avoid sunlight or wear sunscreen if in sunlight; photosensitivity may occur
- Advise patient to comply with dosage schedule, even if feeling better
- Teach patient to notify prescriber of mouth sores, fever, swelling of hands or feet, irregular heartbeat, chest pain

• Advise patient excessive perspiration, dehydration, vomiting, diarrhea may lead to fall in blood pressure—consult prescriber if these occur
• Inform patient that drug may cause dizziness, fainting; light-headedness may occur
• Caution patient to rise slowly to sitting or standing position to minimize orthostatic hypotension

Evaluation

Positive therapeutic outcome
• Decreased B/P

lovastatin ◆ (℞)

(loe'va-sta-tin)

Mevacor

Func. class.: Cholesterol-lowering agent

Chem. class.: Aspergillus terreus strain derivative

Pregnancy category X

Action: By inhibiting HMG-CoA reductase, inhibits biosynthesis of VLDL and LDL, which are responsible for cholesterol development

➔ **Therapeutic Outcome:** Decreased cholesterol levels and LDLs, increased HDLs

Uses: As an adjunct in primary hypercholesterolemia (types IIa, IIb), mixed hyperlipidemia, other osclerosis

Dosage and routes

(Patient should first be placed on a cholesterol-lowering diet)

Adult: PO 20 mg qd with evening meal; may increase to 20-80 mg/day in single or divided doses; not to exceed 80 mg/day; dosage adjustments should be made monthly; reduce dose in renal disease

Available forms: Tabs 10, 20, 40 mg

Adverse effects

CNS: Dizziness, headache, tremor

EENT: Blurred vision, dysgeusia, lens opacities

GI: Nausea, constipation, diarrhea, dyspepsia, flatus, abdominal pain, heartburn, ***liver dysfunction***

INTEG: Rash, pruritus, photosensitivity

MS: Muscle cramps, myalgia, ***myositis, rhabdomyolysis***

Contraindications: Hypersensitivity, pregnancy **X,** lactation, active liver disease

Precautions: Past liver disease, alcoholism, severe acute infections, trauma, hypotension, uncontrolled seizure disorders, severe metabolic disorders, electrolyte imbalances, visual condition, **P** children

Pharmacokinetics

Absorption	Poorly absorbed, erratic
Distribution	Crosses placenta, blood-brain barrier
Metabolism	Liver, extensively
Excretion	Feces, kidneys
Half-life	3-4 hr

Pharmacodynamics

Onset	Unknown
Peak	2-4 hr
Duration	Unknown

Interactions

Individual drugs

Cholestyramine: ↓ action of lovastatin

Cyclosporine: ↑ risk of myopathy

Erythromycin: ↑ risk of myopathy

Gemfibrozil: ↑ risk of myopathy
Niacin: ↑ risk of myopathy
Propranolol: ↓ antihyperlipidemic effect
Warfarin: ↑ bleeding

Food
↑ levels of lovastatin with food

Lab test interferences
↑ CPK, ↑ liver function tests

NURSING CONSIDERATIONS

Assessment

- Assess nutrition: fat, protein, carbohydrates; nutritional analysis should be completed by dietician before treatment
- Monitor bowel pattern daily; diarrhea may be a problem
- Monitor triglycerides, cholesterol at baseline and throughout treatment; LDL and VLDL should be watched closely; if increased, drug should be discontinued

Nursing diagnoses

✓ Diarrhea (adverse reactions)
✓ Knowledge deficit (teaching)
✓ Noncompliance (teaching)

Implementation

- Give with evening meal; if dosage is increased, take with breakfast and evening meal
- Store in cool environment in airtight, light-resistant container

Patient/family education

- Inform patient that compliance is needed for positive results to occur; not to double doses
- Teach patient that risk factors should be decreased: high-fat diet, smoking, alcohol consumption, absence of exercise
- Advise patient to notify prescriber if the GI symptoms of diarrhea, abdominal or epigastric pain, nausea, vomiting occur; or if chills, fever, sore throat occur

Evaluation

Positive therapeutic outcome

- Decreased cholesterol levels, serum triglyceride
- Improved ratio of HDLs

loxapine (℞)

(lox'a-peen)

Loxapac ✱, loxapine succinate, Loxitane IM, Loxitane, Loxitane-C

Func. class.: Antipsychotic/neuroleptic
Chem. class.: Dibenzoxazepine

Pregnancy category C

Action: Depresses cerebral cortex, hypothalamus, limbic system, which control activity and aggression; blocks neurotransmission produced by dopamine at synapse; exhibits strong α-adrenergic, anticholinergic blocking action; mechanism for antipsychotic effects is unclear

➔ **Therapeutic Outcome:** Decreased psychotic behavior

Uses: Psychotic disorders

Investigational uses: Depression, anxiety

Dosage and routes

Adult: PO 10 mg bid-qid initially; may be rapidly increased depending on severity of condition; maintenance 60-100 mg/day; IM 12.5-50 mg q4-6h or more until desired response, then start PO form

Available forms: Caps 5, 10,

25, 50 mg; conc 25 mg/ml; inj 50 mg/ml

Adverse effects

CNS: Extrapyramidal symptoms: pseudoparkinsonism, akathisia, dystonia, tardive dyskinesia, drowsiness, headache, ***seizures,*** confusion, neuroleptic malignant syndrome

CV: Orthostatic hypotension, ***cardiac arrest,*** ECG changes, tachycardia

EENT: Blurred vision, glaucoma

GI: Dry mouth, nausea, vomiting, anorexia, constipation, diarrhea, jaundice, weight gain

GU: Urinary retention, urinary frequency, enuresis, impotence, amenorrhea, gynecomastia

HEMA: Anemia, leukopenia, leukocytosis, agranulocytosis

INTEG: Rash, photosensitivity, dermatitis

RESP: Laryngospasm, dyspnea, ***respiratory depression***

Contraindications: Hypersensitivity, blood dyscrasias, coma, brain damage, bone marrow depression, alcohol and barbiturate withdrawal states

Precautions: Pregnancy **C,** lactation, seizure disorders, hepatic disease, cardiac disease, prostatic hypertrophy, cardiac conditions child <16 yr, glaucoma, GI obstruction

Pharmacokinetics

Absorption	Well absorbed (PO)
Distribution	Unknown
Metabolism	Liver, extensively
Excretion	Kidneys
Half-life	Biphasic 5 hr, 19 hr

Pharmacodynamics

	PO	IM
Onset	½ hr	15-30 min
Peak	2-4 hr	15-20 min
Duration	12 hr	12 hr

Interactions

Individual drugs

Alcohol: ↑ effects of both drugs, oversedation
Aluminum hydroxide: ↓ absorption
Epinephrine: ↑ toxicity
Guanethidine: ↓ antihypertensive response
Guanadrel: ↓ antihypertensive response
Magnesium hydroxide: ↓ absorption

Drug classifications

Analgesics, narcotic: ↑ CNS depression
Anticholinergics: ↑ anticholinergic effects
Antidepressants: ↑ CNS depression
Antihistamines: ↑ CNS depression
Barbiturate anesthetics: ↑ CNS depression
MAOIs: ↑ CNS depression
Sedatives/hypnotics: ↑ CNS depression

NURSING CONSIDERATIONS

Assessment

- Assess mental status: orientation, mood, behavior, presence and type of hallucinations before initial administration and monthly; this drug should significantly reduce psychotic behavior
- Check for swallowing of PO medication; check for hoarding or giving of medication to other patients
- Monitor I&O ratio; palpate bladder if low urinary output occurs, especially in elderly; urinalysis recommended before, during prolonged therapy
- Monitor bilirubin, CBC, liver function studies monthly
- Assess affect, orientation, LOC, reflexes, gait, coordination, sleep pattern disturbances

• Monitor B/P with patient sitting, standing, and lying; take pulse and respirations q4h during initial treatment; establish baseline before starting treatment; report drops of 30 mm Hg

• Check for dizziness, faintness, palpitations, tachycardia on rising; severe orthostatic hypotension is common

• Identify for neuroleptic malignant syndrome: hyperpyrexia, muscle rigidity, increased CPK, altered mental status; drug should be discontinued

• Assess for EPS including akathisia (inability to sit still, no pattern to movements), tardive dyskinesia (bizarre movements of the jaw, mouth, tongue, extremities), pseudoparkinsonism (ragged tremors, pill rolling, shuffling gate); an antiparkinsonian drug should be prescribed

• Assess for constipation, urinary retention daily; if these occur, increase bulk, water in diet

Nursing diagnoses

✓ Thought processes, altered (uses)
✓ Coping, ineffective individual (uses)
✓ Knowledge deficit (teaching)
✓ Noncompliance (teaching)

Implementation

PO route

• Administer drug in liq form mixed in glass of juice or cola if hoarding is suspected; do not mix in caffeine drinks, tannics, pectins

• Administer lowered dose in elderly, since metabolism is slowed

• Administer with full glass of water or milk; or give with food to decrease GI upset

• Store in airtight, light-resistant container, oral sol in amber bottle

IM route

• Inject deep in muscle mass; do not give SC; do not administer sol with a precipitate; amber-colored sol can be used

Patient/family education

• Teach patient to use good oral hygiene; suggest frequent rinsing of mouth, sugarless gum for dry mouth

• Caution patient to avoid hazardous activities until drug response is determined; dizziness, blurred vision may occur

• Inform patient that orthostatic hypotension occurs often and to rise from sitting or lying position gradually; to remain lying down after IM inj for at least 30 min; caution patient to avoid hot tubs, hot showers, tub baths, since hypotension may occur; tell patient that in hot weather heat stroke may occur; take extra precautions to stay cool

• Advise patient to avoid abrupt withdrawal of this drug, or EPS may result; drug should be withdrawn slowly

• Teach patient to avoid OTC preparations (cough, hay fever, cold) unless approved by prescriber, since serious drug interactions may occur; avoid use with alcohol, CNS depressants; increased drowsiness may occur

• Advise patient to use a sunscreen and sunglasses to prevent burns

• Teach patient about EPS and necessity of meticulous oral hygiene, since oral candidiasis may occur

• Suggest patient take antacids

2 hr before or after taking this drug

• Instruct patient to report sore throat, malaise, fever, bleeding, mouth sores; if these occur, CBC should be drawn and drug discontinued

Evaluation

Positive therapeutic outcome

• Decrease in emotional excitement, hallucinations, delusions, paranoia

• Reorganization of patterns of thought, speech

Treatment of overdose: Lavage if orally ingested; barbiturates; provide airway, **IV** fluids; do not use epinephrine, which may increase hypotension

magaldrate (OTC)

(mag'al-drate)

Antiflux ✦**, Lowsium, Riopan, Riopan Extra Strength**

Func. class.: Antacid

Chem. class.: Aluminum/magnesium hydroxide

Pregnancy category C

Action: Neutralizes gastric acidity; drug is dissolved in gastric contents; this drug is a combination of aluminum and magnesium

➔ **Therapeutic Outcome:** Decreased pain of ulcers

Uses: Antacid, peptic ulcer disease (adjunct), indigestion/heartburn, duodenal and gastric ulcers, reflex esophagitis, hyperacidity

Dosage and routes

Adult: PO 1-2 tab (480-1080 mg) between meals, hs, not to exceed 20 tab/day; 1-2 chew tab (480-960 mg) between meals, hs, not to exceed 20 tab/day; susp 5-10 ml (400-800 mg) with water between meals, hs, not to exceed 100 ml/day

Available forms: Tab 480 mg; chew tab 480 mg; susp 480 mg/5ml, 540 mg/5 ml, 1080 mg/5 ml

Adverse effects

GI: Constipation, diarrhea

META: Hypermagnesemia, hypophosphatemia

Contraindications: Hypersensitivity to this drug or aluminum products

G **Precautions:** Elderly, fluid restriction, decreased GI motility, GI obstruction, dehydration, renal disease, sodium-restricted diets, pregnancy **C**

Pharmacokinetics	
Absorption	Not absorbed
Distribution	Not distributed
Metabolism	Not metabolized
Excretion	Kidneys
Half-life	Unknown

Pharmacodynamics	
Onset	Unknown
Peak	½ hrs
Duration	1 hr

Interactions

Individual drugs

Chlordiazepoxide: ↓ absorption of chlordiazapoxide

Cimetidine: ↓ absorption of cimetidine

Ketoconazole: ↓ effect of ketoconazole

Phenytoin: ↓ absorption of phenytoin

Tetracycline: ↓ effect of tetracycline

Drug classifications
Anticholinergics: ↓ absorption of anticholinergics
Corticosteroids: ↓ absorption of corticosteroids
Iron salts: ↓ absorption of iron salts
Phenothiazines: ↓ absorption of phenothiazines
Salicylates: ↓ absorption of salicylates

NURSING CONSIDERATIONS
Assessment
- Assess GI status: location of pain, intensity, characteristics, what aggravates, ameliorates pain; heartburn/indigestion; hematemesis
- Monitor serum magnesium levels with impaired renal function
- Assess for constipation: increase bulk in diet if needed or obtain order for stool softener

Nursing diagnoses
✓ Pain (uses)
✓ Knowledge deficit (teaching)

Implementation
- Give laxatives or stool softeners if constipation occurs
- Give susp after shaking; give between meals and hs
- Give when stomach is empty pc and hs

Patient/family education
- Advise patient to separate ingestion of enteric-coated drugs and antacid by 1 hr
- Advise patient to use 2 wk or less; drug should not be used for long periods
- Teach patient to notify prescriber immediately if coffee-ground emesis, emesis with frank blood, or black tarry stools occur

Evaluation
Positive therapeutic outcome
- Absence of abdominal pain
- Decreased acidity

magnesium hydroxide (OTC)
Concentrated Phillip's Milk of Magnesia, Milk of Magnesia, Phillip's Milk of Magnesia
Func. class.: Laxative, saline; antacid
Pregnancy category B

Action: Increases osmotic pressure; draws fluid into the lumen of the colon; neutralizes hydrochloric acid

Therapeutic Outcome: Decreased constipation, decreased gastric acidity

Uses: Constipation, bowel preparation before surgery or examination; antacid

Dosage and routes
Laxative
Adult: PO 30-60 ml hs (milk of magnesia)
P ***Adult and child >6 yr:*** PO 15 g in 8 oz water; PO 10-20 ml (conc milk of magnesia)
Antacid
P ***Adult and child >12 yr:*** PO 5-15 ml (liq), 650-1300 mg (tab) qid
P ***Child 2-6 yr:*** PO 5-15 ml (milk of magnesia)

Available forms: Liq 395 mg/5 ml; chew tabs 300, 600 mg; conc liq 1.2 gm/5 ml

Adverse effects
CNS: Muscle weakness, flushing, sweating, confusion, seda-

tion, depressed reflexes, ***flaccid paralysis***, hypothermia
CV: Hypotension, heart block, ***circulatory collapse***
GI: Nausea, vomiting, anorexia, cramps
META: Electrolyte, fluid imbalances

Contraindications: Hypersensitivity, renal diseases, abdominal pain, nausea/vomiting, obstruction, acute surgical abdomen, rec bleeding

Precautions: Pregnancy **B**

Pharmacokinetics	
Absorption	Up to 30%
Distribution	Widely distributed, crosses placenta
Metabolism	Not metabolized
Excretion	Kidneys, breast milk
Half-life	Unknown

Pharmacodynamics	
Onset	Unknown
Peak	1-2 hr
Duration	Unknown

Interactions

Drug classifications

Neuromuscular blockers: ↑ action if absorbed systemically

Fluoroquinolones: ↓ absorption of fluoroquinolones

NURSING CONSIDERATIONS

Assessment

- Monitor blood, urine electrolytes if used often by patient; check I&O ratio to identify fluid loss
- Assess for cramping, rec bleeding, nausea, vomiting; if these symptoms occur, drug should be discontinued; identify cause of constipation; identify whether fluids, bulk, or exercise is missing from lifestyle
- Assess stool for color, consistency, amount, presence of flatulence
- Assess for magnesium toxicity: thirst, confusion, decrease in reflexes

Nursing diagnoses

- ✓ Constipation (uses)
- ✓ Diarrhea (adverse reaction)
- ✓ Knowledge deficit (teaching)
- ✓ Noncompliance (teaching)

Implementation

- Chew tab well before swallowing; follow with 4 oz of water to prevent undissolved tab entering small intestine
- Susp should be shaken before use

Patient/family education

- Discuss with the patient that adequate fluid consumption is necessary
- Teach patient that normal bowel movements do not always occur daily
- Caution patient not to use in presence of abdominal pain, nausea, vomiting; tell patient to notify prescriber if constipation is unrelieved or if symptoms of electrolyte imbalance occur (muscle cramps, pain, weakness, dizziness, excessive thirst)
- Teach patient not to use laxatives for long-term therapy; bowel tone will be lost and will decrease
- Instruct patient to shake susp well before use
- Teach patient not to take at hs as a laxative; may interfere with sleep
- Teach patient not to use with food or vitamin preparations; delays digestion and absorption of fat-soluble vitamins

Evaluation
Positive therapeutic outcome
- Decreased constipation in 4-6 hr
- Absence of GI symptoms

magnesium sulfate (℞)

Func. class.: Anticonvulsant
Chem. class.: Magnesium product
Pregnancy category C

Action: Decreases acetylcholine in motor nerve terminals, which is responsible for anticonvulsant properties; osmotically retains fluid, which increases amount of water in feces when used as laxative; reduces SA node impulse formation, prolongs conduction time in myocardium

➔ **Therapeutic Outcome:** Absence of seizures

Uses: Hypomagnesemic seizures, control of seizures in pregnancy-induced hypertension, seizures in acute nephritis

Dosage and routes
Hypomagnesemic seizures
Adult: **IV** 1-2 g over 15 min, then 1 g IM q4-6h, depending on response

Nephritis
P ***Child:*** IM 20-40 mg/kg in 20% sol; repeat as needed

Preeclampsia/eclampsia
Adult: **IV** 4 g/250 ml D_5W and 4 g IM, then 4 g (50% sol) IM q4h prn; or 4 g (10-20% sol) **IV** loading dose, then 1-4 g (5% sol) **IV** inf hourly, not to exceed 3 ml/min

Available forms: Inj 10%, 12.5%, 25%, 50%; granules

Adverse effects
CNS: Sweating, depressed deep tendon reflexes, flushing, drowsiness, flaccid paralysis, hypothermia, weakness, sedation
CV: Hypotension, ***circulatory collapse, heart block,*** decreased cardiac function
RESP: ***Paralysis***

Contraindications: Hypersensitivity, 2 hr preceding delivery in PIH

Precautions: Pregnancy **A**

Pharmacokinetics

Absorption	Well absorbed (IM); 15%-30% (PO)
Distribution	Widely distributed; crosses placenta
Metabolism	Unknown
Excretion	Kidneys, breast milk
Half-life	Unknown

Pharmacodynamics

	PO	IM	IV
Onset	3-6 hr	1 hr	1-5 min
Peak	Unknown	Unknown	Unknown
Duration	Unknown	3-4 hr	½ hr

M

Interactions
Drug classifications
Antipsychotics: ↑ CNS depression
Barbiturates: ↑ CNS depression
Fluoroquinolones: ↓ absorption of fluoroquinolones
Narcotics: ↑ CNS depression
Neuromuscular blockers: ↑ effect

NURSING CONSIDERATIONS
Assessment
- Monitor VS q15 min after **IV** dose; also check pulse, respirations

• Monitor cardiac function: magnesium levels; 2.5-7.5 mEq/L (therapeutic)
• Monitor timing of contractions; determine intensity; monitor fetal heart rate, reactivity; may decrease with this drug if using during labor
• Monitor I&O: should remain at 30 ml/hr or more; if less than this, notify prescriber; check urine output before each dose; output should be 100 ml/4 hr or more
• Assess mental status: mood, sensorium, affect, memory (long, short)
• Assess respiratory dysfunction: respiratory depression, character, rate, rhythm; hold drug if respirations are <16/min
• Assess for hypermagnesemia: depressed patellar reflex, flushing, polydipsia, confusion, weakness, flaccid paralysis, hypothermia, dyspnea begin to appear at blood levels of 4 mEq/L
• Assess respiratory rate, **P** rhythm of newborn if drug was given 24 hr before delivery or less; check reflexes of newborn whose mother received this drug before delivery
• Monitor reflexes: knee jerk, patellar; decreased signals in magnesium toxicity; mild depression will occur in therapeutic range

Nursing diagnoses

✓ Injury, risk for (uses)
✓ Knowledge deficit (teaching)

Implementation

IV route

• Give only when calcium gluconate available for magnesium toxicity
• Give **IV** undiluted 1.5 ml of 10% sol over 1 min; may dilute to 20% sol; inf over 3 hr; use inf pump to regulate rate accurately

Y-site compatibilities: Acyclovir, aldesleukin, amifostine, amikacin, ampicillin, aztreonam, cefamandole, cefazolin, cefoperazone, ceforanide, cefotaxime, cefoxitin, cephalothin, cephapirin, chloramphenicol, clindamycin, dobutamine, doxycycline, enalaprilat, erythromycin lactobionate, esmolol, famotidine, fludarabine, granisetron, gentamicin, heparin, hydrocortisone, hydromorphone, idarubicin, insulin, kanamycin, labetalol, meperidine, metronidazole, minocycline, morphine, nafcillin, ondansetron, oxacillin, paclitaxel, penicillin G potassium, piperacillin, potassium chloride, sargramostim, thiotepa, ticarcillin, tobramycin, trimethoprim/sulfamethoxazole, vancomycin, vitamin B complex with C

Additive compatibilities: Calcium gluconate, cephalothin, chloramphenicol, cisplatin, hydrocortisone, methyldopate, penicillin G potassium, potassium phosphate, verapamil

Additive incompatibilities: Calcium gluceptate, polymyxin, sodium bicarbonate, tobramycin

Patient/family education

• Teach patient symptoms of hypermagnesemia

Evaluation

Positive therapeutic outcome

• Absence of seizures

Treatment of overdose: Stop administration of drug; administer calcium gluconate, monitor reflexes, magnesium levels; ECG monitoring if calcium is administered

mannitol (℞)

(man′i-tole)

mannitol, Osmitrol, Resectisol

Func. class.: Osmotic diuretic

Chem. class.: Hexahydric alcohol

Pregnancy category C

Action: Increases osmolarity of glomerular filtrate, which raises osmotic pressure of fluid in renal tubules; there is a decrease in reabsorption of water, electrolytes; increases in urinary output, sodium, chloride, potassium, calcium, phosphorus, uric acid, urea, magnesium

Uses: Edema; promote systemic diuresis in cerebral edema, decrease intraocular pressure, improve renal function in acute renal failure, chemical poisoning

Dosage and routes

Oliguria, prevention

Adult: **IV** 50-100 g of a 5%-25% sol

Oliguria, treatment

Adult: **IV** 300-400 mg/kg of a 20%-25% sol up to 100 g of a 15%-20% sol over 30-60 min

P ***Child:*** **IV** 0.25-2 g/kg as a 15%-20% sol, run over 2-6 hr

Intraocular pressure/ intracranial pressure

Adult: **IV** 1.5-2 g/kg of a 15%-25% sol over 30-60 min

P ***Child:*** **IV** 1-2 g/kg (30-60 g/m^2) as a 15%-20% sol run over 30-60 min

Renal failure

Adult: **IV** 50-200 g/24 hr, adjusting to maintain output of 30-50 mg/hr

Diuresis in drug intoxication

P ***Adult and child >12 yr:*** 5%-10% sol continuously up to 200 g **IV**, while maintaining 100-500 ml urine output/hr

Available forms: Inj 5%, 10%, 15%, 20%, 25%

Adverse effects

CNS: Dizziness, headache, ***convulsions, rebound increased intracranial pressure,*** confusion

CV: Edema, hypotension, hypertension, tachycardia, *CHF,* thrombophlebitis

EENT: Loss of hearing, blurred vision, nasal congestion, decreased intraocular pressure

ELECT: Fluid, electrolyte imbalances, acidosis, electrolyte loss, dehydration

GI: Nausea, vomiting, dry mouth, diarrhea

GU: Marked diuresis, urinary retention, thirst

RESP: Pulmonary congestion

Contraindications: Active intracranial bleeding, hypersensitivity, anuria, severe pulmonary congestion, edema, severe dehydration, progressive heart, renal failure

Precautions: Dehydration, pregnancy **C,** severe renal disease, CHF, lactation

Pharmacokinetics	
Absorption	Complete
Distribution	Extracellular spaces
Metabolism	Minimal
Excretion	Renal
Half-life	100 min

M

Pharmacodynamics	
Onset	½-1 hr
Peak	1 hr
Duration	6-8 hr

Interactions
Individual drugs
EDTA: ↑ effects
Lithium: ↓ action, ↑ excretion
Food
Potassium foods: ↑ hyperkalemia
Lab test interferences
Interference: Inorganic phosphorus, ethylene glycol

NURSING CONSIDERATIONS
Assessment
• Assess neurologic status: LOC, intracranial pressure reading, pupil size and reaction when drug is given for increased intracranial pressure
• Assess for visual changes or eye discomfort or pain
• Assess patient for tinnitus, hearing loss, ear pain; periodic testing of hearing is needed when high doses of this drug are given by **IV** route
• Monitor manifestations of hypokalemia: acidic urine, reduced urine osmolality, nocturia, polyuria, polydipsia; hypotension, broad T wave, U wave, ectopy, tachycardia, weak pulse; muscle weakness, altered LOC, drowsiness, apathy, lethargy, confusion, depression; anorexia, nausea, cramps, constipation, distention, paralytic ileus; hypoventilation, respiratory muscle weakness
• Monitor for manifestations of hyponatremia: increased B/P, cold, clammy skin, hypovolemia or hypervolemia; anorexia, nausea, vomiting, diarrhea, abdominal cramps; lethargy, increased intracranial pressure, confusion, headache, seizures, coma, fatigue, tremors, hyperreflexia
• Assess fluid volume status: check I&O ratios and record hourly urine values, CVP, breath sounds, weight, distended red veins, crackles in lung, color, quality and sp gr of urine, skin turgor, adequacy of pulses, moist mucous membranes, bilateral lung sounds, peripheral pitting edema
• Assess for dehydration; symptoms of decreasing output, thirst, hypotension, dry mouth and mucous membranes should be reported
• Monitor electrolytes: potassium, sodium, calcium, magnesium; also include BUN, ABGs, CBC; regularly monitor serum and urine levels of sodium and potassium
• Assess B/P before and during therapy with patient lying, standing, and sitting as appropriate; orthostatic hypotension can occur rapidly
• Monitor for rebound intracranial pressure: headache, confusion

Nursing diagnoses
✓ Urinary elimination, altered (adverse reactions)
✓ Fluid volume deficit (adverse reactions)
✓ Fluid volume excess (uses)
✓ Knowledge deficit (teaching)

Implementation
• Administer potassium replacement if potassium level is whole, or use oral sol lightly; drug may be crushed if patient is unable to swallow
• Use an in-line filter for 15%, 20%, 25% give with inf pump; check **IV** patency at inf site before and during administration; do not use sol

that is yellow or has a precipitate or crystals; to redissolve, run bottle in hot water and shake vigorously; cool to body temp before giving
• Run at 30-50 ml/hr in oliguria
• Run over 30-60 min in increased intracranial pressure
• Run over 30 min for intraocular pressure; 60-90 min after surgery

Y-site incompatibilities: Allopurinol, amifostine, amsacrine, aztreonam, bleomycin sulfate, doxorubicin HCl, fluconazole, gentamicin sulfate, quinidine gluconate, vinblastine sulfate, vincristine sulfate

Y-site compatibilities: Ondansetron, fluorouracil, idarubicin, melphalan, paclitaxel, sargramostim, thiotepa, vinorelbine

Additive compatibilities: Amikacin, bretylium, cefamandole, cefoxitin, cimetidine, cisplatin, dopamine, gentamicin, metoclopramide, netilmicin, nizatidine, ofloxacin, ondansetron, tobramycin, verapamil

Additive incompatibilities: Blood, blood products, imipenem/cilastatin, potassium chloride, sodium chloride

Patient/family education
• Teach patient reason for and method of treatment

Evaluation

Positive therapeutic outcome
• Decreased intracranial pressure
• Decreased intraocular pressure
• Prevention of hypokalemia (diuretic use)
• Decreased edema
• Increased diuresis of >30 ml/hr
• Increased excretion of toxic substances

Treatment of overdose: Discontinue inf, correct fluid, electrolyte imbalances, hemodialysis, monitor hydration, CV, renal function

maprotiline (℞)

(ma-proe'ti-leen)

Ludiomil, maprotiline

Func. class.: Antidepressant

Chem. class.: Tetracyclic

Pregnancy category B

Action: Blocks reuptake of norepinephrine, serotonin into nerve endings, increasing action of norepinephrine, serotonin in nerve cells; has anticholinergic action

➔ **Therapeutic Outcome:** Decreased symptoms of depression after 2-3 wk

Uses: Depression, dysthymic disorder, bipolar disorder: depression, agitated depression

Dosage and routes

Adult: PO 75 mg/day in moderate depression; may increase to 150 mg/day; not to exceed 225 mg in hospitalized patients; severely depressed patients who are hospitalized may be given 300 mg/day

G ***Elderly:*** 50-75 mg/day

Available forms: Tabs 25, 50, 75 mg

Adverse effects

CNS: Dizziness, drowsiness, confusion, headache, anxiety,

M

tremors, stimulation, weakness, insomnia, nightmares, EPS (elderly), increased psychiatric symptoms, ***seizures***
CV: Orthostatic hypotension, ECG changes, tachycardia, ***hypertension,*** palpitations
EENT: Blurred vision, tinnitus, mydriasis
GI: Diarrhea, dry mouth, nausea, vomiting, ***paralytic ileus,*** increased appetite, cramps, epigastric distress, jaundice, ***hepatitis,*** stomatitis
GU: Retention, ***acute renal failure***
HEMA: ***Agranulocytosis, thrombocytopenia, eosinophilia, leukopenia***
INTEG: Rash, urticaria, sweating, pruritus, photosensitivity

Contraindications: Hypersensitivity to tricyclic antidepressants, recovery phase of MI, convulsive disorders, prostatic hypertrophy

Precautions: Suicidal patients, severe depression, increased intraocular pressure, narrow-angle glaucoma, urinary retention, cardiac disease, hepatic disease, hypothyroidism, hyperthyroidism, electroshock therapy, elective surgery, elderly, pregnancy **B**

Pharmacokinetics

Absorption	Slow, complete
Distribution	Widely distributed; crosses placenta
Metabolism	Liver, extensively
Excretion	Feces; breast milk
Half-life	21-25 hr

Pharmacodynamics

Onset	15-30 min
Peak	12 hr
Duration	3 wk

Interactions

Individual drugs

Alcohol: ↑ CNS depression
Cimetidine: ↑ levels, ↑ toxicity
Clonidine: Severe hypotension; avoid use
Disulfiram: Organic brain syndrome
Fluoxetine: ↑ levels, toxicity
Guanethidine: ↓ effects

Drug classifications

Analgesics: ↑ CNS depression
Anticholinergics: ↑ side effects
Antihistamines: ↑ CNS depression
Antihypertensives: May block antihypertensive effect
Barbiturates: ↑ effects
Benzodiazepines: ↑ effects
CNS depressants: ↑ effects
MAOIs: Hypertensive crisis, convulsions
Oral contraceptives: ↑ effects, toxicity
Phenothiazines: ↑ toxicity
Sedative/hypnotics: ↑ CNS depression
Sympathomimetics, indirect acting: ↓ effects

Smoking

↑ metabolism, ↓ effects

Lab test interferences

↑ Serum bilirubin, ↑ blood glucose, ↑ alkaline phosphatase
↓ VMA, ↓ 5-HIAA
False ↑ Urinary catecholamines

NURSING CONSIDERATIONS

Assessment

- Monitor B/P (with patient lying, standing), pulse q4h during beginning treatment; if systolic B/P drops 20 mm Hg, hold drug, notify prescriber; take VS q4h in patients with cardiovascular disease
- Monitor blood studies: CBC, leukocytes, differential,

cardiac enzymes if patient is receiving long-term therapy

- Monitor hepatic studies: AST (SGOT), ALT (SGPT), bilirubin
- Check weight weekly; drug may increase appetite
- Assess ECG for flattening of T wave, bundle branch block, AV block, dysrhythmias in cardiac patients
- Assess for EPS primarily in G elderly: rigidity, dystonia, akathisia
- Assess mental status: mood, sensorium, affect, suicidal tendencies; assess increase in psychiatric symptoms: depression, panic
- Monitor urinary retention, constipation; constipation is P more likely to occur in children G and elderly
- ◆! Assess for withdrawal symptoms: headache, nausea, vomiting, muscle pain, weakness; do not usually occur unless drug was discontinued abruptly
- Identify alcohol consumption; if alcohol is consumed, hold dose until AM

Nursing diagnoses

✓ Coping, ineffective individual (uses)
✓ Injury, risk for (side effects)
✓ Knowledge deficit (teaching)
✓ Noncompliance (teaching)

Implementation

- Give with food or milk for GI symptoms; crush if patient is unable to swallow medication whole
- Give dose hs if oversedation occurs during day; may take G entire dose hs; elderly may not tolerate once/day dosing
- Store at room temp; do not freeze

Patient/family education

- Inform patient that therapeutic effects may take 2-3 wk
- Advise patient to use caution in driving and other activities requiring alertness because of drowsiness, dizziness, blurred vision; to avoid rising quickly from sitting to standing, espe- G cially elderly
- Caution patient to avoid alcohol ingestion, other CNS depressants
- Caution patient not to discontinue medication quickly after long-term use: may cause nausea, headache, malaise
- Teach patient to wear sunscreen or large hat, since photosensitivity occurs
- Teach patient to increase fluids, bulk in diet if constipation, urinary retention occur, G especially elderly
- Teach patient to take gum, hard sugarless candy, or frequent sips of water for dry mouth

Evaluation

Positive therapeutic outcome

- Decrease in depression
- Absence of suicidal thoughts

Treatment of overdose: ECG monitoring, induce emesis, lavage, activated charcoal, administer anticonvulsant

mebendazole (℞)

(me-ben'da-zole)

Nemasole ✣, Vermox

Func. class.: Anthelmintic

Chem. class.: Carbamate

Pregnancy category C

Action: Inhibits glucose uptake, degeneration of cytoplasmic microtubules in the cell;

M

interferes with absorption, secretory function

➔ **Therapeutic Outcome:** Parasite, cyst, egg death

Uses: Infestation with pinworms, roundworms, hookworms, whipworms, threadworms, pork tapeworms, dwarf tapeworms, beef tapeworms; hydatid cyst

Dosage and routes

P ***Adult and child >2 yr:*** PO 100 mg as a single dose or bid × 3 days, depending on type of infestation; course may be repeated in 3 wk if needed

Available forms: Chew tab 100 mg

Adverse effects

CNS: Dizziness, fever

GI: Transient diarrhea, abdominal pain

Contraindication: Hypersensitivity

P **Precautions:** Child <2 yr, lactation, pregnancy (1st trimester) **C**

Pharmacokinetics	
Absorption	Minimal
Distribution	Highly bound to plasma proteins
Metabolism	Liver
Excretion	Feces in metabolites (>95%); urine, unchanged
Half-life	2½-9 hr; increased in hepatic disease

Pharmacodynamics	
Onset	Unknown
Peak	½-7 hr
Duration	Unknown

Interactions

Individual drugs

Carbamazepine: ↓ effect of mebendazole

Drug classifications

Hydantoins: ↓ effect of hydantoins

Food

High-fat foods: ↑ absorption

NURSING CONSIDERATIONS

Assessment

- Assess stools during entire treatment; specimens must be sent to lab while still warm, also 1-3 wk after treatment is completed; monitor for diarrhea during expulsion of worms; avoid self-contamination with patient's feces
- Assess for allergic reaction: rash (rare)
- Identify infestation in other family members, since transmission from person to person is common
- If pinworms are suspected, place a piece of cellophane tape over the anal area at night for 1 wk after treatment at night to identify ova; negative perianal swabs taken every AM for 3 days confirm that the patient is no longer infested
- Monitor blood studies: AST (SGOT), ALT (SGPT), alkaline phosphatase, BUN, CBC during treatment

Nursing diagnoses

✓ Infection, risk for (uses)
✓ Knowledge deficit (teaching)

Implementation

- Tabs may be chewed if patient is unable to swallow whole
- Give PO after meals to avoid GI symptoms, since absorption is not decreased by food
- Give second course after 3 wk if needed; usually recommended (pinworms)
- Store in airtight container

Patient/family education

- Teach patient proper hygiene after BM, including hand-washing technique; tell patient to avoid putting fingers in mouth; clean fingernails
- Advise patient that infested person should sleep alone; do not shake bed linen; wash bed linen daily in hot water; change and wash undergarments daily
- Advise patient to clean toilet daily with disinfectant (green soap sol)
- Inform patient that compliance is needed with dosage schedule, duration of treatment
- Tell patient to wear shoes, wash all fruits and vegetables well before eating, use commercial fruit and vegetable cleaner solution

Evaluation

Positive therapeutic outcome

- Expulsion of worms
- Three negative stool cultures after completion of treatment

mechlorethamine (℞)

(me-klor-eth'a-meen)

Mustargen, Nitrogen Mustard

Func. class.: Antineoplastic alkylating agent

Chem. class.: Nitrogen mustard

Pregnancy category D

Action: Alkylates DNA, RNA; inhibits enzymes that allow synthesis of amino acids in proteins; activity is not cell cycle phase specific; a vesicant

➔ **Therapeutic Outcome:** Prevention of rapidly growing malignant cells

Uses: Hodgkin's disease, lymphomas, leukemias, lymphosarcoma; ovarian, breast, lung carcinoma; neoplastic effusions

Dosage and routes

Adult: **IV** 0.4 mg/kg as 1 dose or 2-4 divided doses over 2-4 days; second course after 3 wk depending on blood cell count

Neoplastic effusions

Adult: Intracavity 10-20 mg (may be 200-400 μg/kg)

Available forms: Inj 10 mg/vial

Adverse effects

CNS: Headache, dizziness, drowsiness, paresthesia, peripheral neuropathy, ***coma***

EENT: Tinnitus, hearing loss

GI: Nausea, vomiting, diarrhea, stomatitis, weight loss, colitis, ***hepatotoxicity***

HEMA: ***Thrombocytopenia, leukopenia, agranulocytosis,*** anemia

INTEG: Alopecia, pruritus, herpes zoster, extravasation

Contraindications: Lactation, pregnancy (1st trimester) **D,** myelosuppression, acute herpes zoster

Precautions: Radiation therapy, chronic lymphocytic leukopenia

Pharmacokinetics	
Absorption	Complete (IV)
Distribution	Unknown
Metabolism	Tissues/fluids
Excretion	Kidneys
Half-life	Unknown

Pharmacodynamics	IV
Onset	1 day
Peak	1-2 wk
Duration	1-3 wk

M

Interactions

Individual drugs

Radiation: ↑ toxicity, bone marrow suppression

Drug classifications

Antineoplastics: ↑ toxicity, bone marrow suppression
Bone marrow–suppressing drugs: ↑ bone marrow suppression
Live vaccines: ↑ adverse reactions, ↓ antibody reaction

Lab test interferences

↑ Uric acid

NURSING CONSIDERATIONS

Assessment

- Monitor CBC, differential, platelet count weekly; withhold drug if WBC is <4000 or platelet count is <75,000; notify prescriber of results if WBC <20,000/mm^3, platelets <150,000/mm^3
- Monitor pulmonary function tests, chest x-ray films before, during therapy; chest film should be obtained q2 wk during treatment; assess for dyspnea, rales, unproductive cough, chest pain, tachypnea
- Assess for increased uric acid levels, swelling, joint pain primarily in extremities; patient should be well hydrated to prevent urate deposits
- Monitor renal function studies: BUN, serum uric acid, urine CrCl before, during therapy; I&O ratio; report fall in urine output of 30 ml/hr; for decreased hyperuricemia
- Monitor for cold, fever, sore throat (may indicate beginning infection); identify edema in feet, joint and stomach pain, shaking; prescriber should be notified
- Assess for bleeding: hematuria, guaiac, bruising or petechiae, mucosa or orifices q8h; no rec temp

Nursing diagnoses

- ✓ Injury, risk for (adverse reactions)
- ✓ Body image disturbance (adverse reactions)
- ✓ Infection, risk for (adverse reactions)
- ✓ Knowledge deficit (teaching)

Implementation

- Give fluids **IV** or PO before chemotherapy to hydrate patient
- Give antacid before oral agent; give drug after evening meal, before hs; administer antiemetic 30-60 min before giving drug and prn to prevent vomiting; give antibiotics for prophylaxis of infection
- Give top or syst analgesics for pain
- Give in AM so drug can be eliminated before hs
- Use a liq diet: carbonated beverages; gelatin may be added if patient is not nauseated or vomiting

IV IV route

- Give **IV** after diluting 10 mg/10 ml sterile water or 0.9% NaCl; leave needle in vial, shake, withdraw dose, give through Y-tube or 3-way stopcock or directly over 3-5 min into running **IV** of 0.9% NaCl

Y-site compatibilities: Amifostine, aztreonam, filgrastim, fludarabine, granisetron, melphalan, ondansetron, sargramostim, teniposide, vinorelbine

Additive incompatibility: Methohexital

Solution incompatibilities: D_5W, 0.9% NaCl (**IV** only)

Intracavity route
- Further dilute in 100 ml 0.9% NaCl; administration is completed by prescriber
- Watch for infiltration; if infiltration occurs, infiltrate area with isotonic sodium thiosulfate or 1% lidocaine; apply ice for 6-12 hr

Patient/family education
- Teach patient to avoid use of products containing aspirin or ibuprofen, razors, commercial mouthwash, since bleeding may occur; to report symptoms of bleeding (hematuria, tarry stools)
- Teach patient to report signs of anemia (fatigue, headache, irritability, faintness, shortness of breath)
- Advise patient to report any changes in breathing or coughing even several mo after treatment; to avoid crowds and persons with respiratory tract or other infections
- Tell patient hair loss is common; discuss the use of wigs or hair pieces
- Caution patient not to have any vaccinations without the advice of the presciber, serious reactions can occur
- Advise patient contraception is needed during treatment and for several mo after the completion of therapy
- Have patient rinse mouth tid-qid with water, club soda; brush teeth bid-qid with soft brush or cotton-tipped applicators for stomatitis; use unwaxed dental floss

Evaluation
Positive therapeutic outcome
- Decreased size of tumor
- Decreased spread of malignancy
- Improved blood values
- Absence of sweating at night
- Increased appetite, increased weight

meclofenamate (℞)
(me-kloe-fen-am'ate)
meclofenamate, Meclofen, Meclomen
Func. class.: Nonsteroidal antiinflammatory; analgesic (nonopioid)
Chem. class.: Anthranilic acid derivative
Pregnancy category B

Action: Inhibits prostaglandin synthesis by decreasing an enzyme needed for biosynthesis; analgesic, antiinflammatory

Therapeutic Outcome: Decreased pain, inflammation

Uses: Mild to moderate pain, osteoarthritis, rheumatoid arthritis, dysmenorrhea

Dosage and routes
Antiinflammatory
Adult: PO 200-400 mg/day in divided doses tid-qid

Analgesic
Adult: PO 50-100 mg q4-6h

Dysmenorrhea
Adult: PO 100 mg tid

Available forms: Caps 50, 100 mg

Adverse effects
CNS: Dizziness, drowsiness, fatigue, tremors, confusion, insomnia, anxiety, depression
CV: Tachycardia, hypertension, peripheral edema, palpitations, dysrhythmias
EENT: Tinnitus, hearing loss, blurred vision
GI: Nausea, anorexia, vomit-

M

ing, diarrhea, jaundice, ***cholestatic hepatitis,*** constipation, flatulence, cramps, dry mouth, peptic ulcer, ***ulceration, perforation***
GU: Nephrotoxicity: dysuria, hematuria, oliguria, azotemia
HEMA: Blood dyscrasias
INTEG: Purpura, rash, pruritus, sweating
SYST: Anaphylaxis, Stevens-Johnson syndrome

Contraindications: Hypersensitivity, asthma, severe renal disease, severe hepatic disease, ulcer disease

Precautions: Pregnancy **B,** lactation, children, bleeding disorders, GI disorders, cardiac disorders, hypersensitivity to other antiinflammatory agents

Pharmacokinetics	
Absorption	Well absorbed
Distribution	Unknown
Metabolism	Liver, extensively
Half-life	½-2 hr

Pharmacodynamics	
Onset	Unknown
Peak	2 hr
Duration	Unknown

Interactions
Individual drugs
Acetaminophen (long-term use): ↑ renal reactions
Alcohol: ↑ adverse reactions
Aspirin: ↓ effectiveness, ↑ adverse reactions
Coumadin: ↑ anticoagulant effects
Digoxin: ↑ toxicity, levels
Insulin: ↓ insulin effect
Lithium: ↑ toxicity
Methotrexate: ↑ toxicity
Phenytoin: ↑ toxicity
Probenecid: ↑ toxicity
Sulfonylurea: ↑ toxicity

Drug classifications
Anticoagulants: ↑ risk of bleeding
Antihypertensives: ↓ effect of antihypertensives
Antineoplastics: ↑ risk of hematologic toxicity
β-Blockers: ↑ antihypertension
Cephalosporins: ↑ risk of bleeding
Glucocorticoids: ↑ adverse reactions
Gold preparations: ↑ renal toxicity
Hypoglycemics: ↓ hypoglycemic effect
Diuretics: ↓ effectiveness of diuretics
NSAIDs: ↑ adverse reactions
Potassium supplements: ↑ adverse reactions
Radiation: ↑ risk of hematologic toxicity
Sulfonamides: ↑ toxicity

NURSING CONSIDERATIONS
Assessment
- Monitor blood counts during therapy; watch for decreasing platelets; if low, therapy may need to be discontinued, restarted after hematologic recovery; assess for blood dyscrasia (thrombocytopenia): bruising, fatigue, bleeding, poor healing
- Assess pain: intensity, area involved
- Assess joint pain, range of motion, inflammation before and during treatment in arthritis

Nursing diagnoses
✓ Pain (uses)
✓ Pain, chronic (uses)
✓ Mobility, impaired physical (uses)
✓ Injury, risk for (adverse reaction)
✓ Knowledge deficit (teaching)

Implementation

- Administer to patient whole
- Do not crush, chew caps
- Give with food or milk to decrease gastric symptoms; give 30 min ac or 2 hr pc; absorption may be slowed

Patient/family education

- Teach patient that drug must be continued for prescribed time to be effective; to avoid aspirin, alcoholic beverages, acetaminophen, ibuprofen
- Caution patient to report bleeding, bruising, fatigue, malaise, since blood dyscrasias do occur
- Instruct patient to use caution when driving; drowsiness, dizziness may occur
- Teach patient to take with a full glass of water to enhance absorption; do not crush, break or chew; patient should remain sitting up to prevent gastric irritation

Evaluation

Positive therapeutic outcome

- Decreased pain
- Decreased inflammation
- Increased mobility

medroxyprogesterone (Rx)

(me-drox-ee-proe-jess'te-rone)

Amen, Curretab, Cycrin, Depo-Provera, medroxyprogesterone acetate, Provera

Func. class.: Hormone—progestogen; contraceptive; antineoplastic

Chem. class.: Progesterone derivative

Pregnancy category X

Action: Inhibits secretion of pituitary gonadotropins, which prevents follicular maturation and ovulation; stimulates growth of mammary tissue; antineoplastic action against endometrial cancer

Therapeutic Outcome: Decreased abnormal uterine bleeding, absence of amenorrhea

Uses: Uterine bleeding (abnormal), secondary amenorrhea, endometrial cancer, renal cancer, contraceptive

Investigational uses: Pickwickian syndrome, sleep apnea

Dosage and routes

Secondary amenorrhea

Adult: PO 5-10 mg qd × 5-10 days

Endometrial/renal cancer

Adult: IM 400-1000 mg/wk

Uterine bleeding

Adult: PO 5-10 mg qd × 5-10 days starting on 16th day of menstrual cycle

Contraceptive

Adult: Inj q3 mo

M

Available forms: Tabs 2.5, 5, 10 mg; inj susp 100, 150, 400 mg/ml; contraceptive injectable

Adverse effects

CNS: Dizziness, headache, migraines, depression, fatigue
CV: Hypotension, thrombophlebitis, edema, ***thromboembolism, stroke, pulmonary embolism, myocardial infarction***
EENT: Diplopia
GI: Nausea, vomiting, anorexia, cramps, increased weight, ***cholestatic jaundice***
GU: Amenorrhea, cervical erosion, breakthrough bleeding, dysmenorrhea, vaginal candidiasis, breast changes, *gynecomastia, testicular atrophy, impotence,* endometriosis, ***spontaneous abortion***
INTEG: Rash, urticaria, acne, hirsutism, alopecia, oily skin, seborrhea, purpura, melasma, photosensitivity
META: Hyperglycemia

Contraindications: Breast cancer, hypersensitivity, thromboembolic disorders, reproductive cancer, genital bleeding (abnormal, undiagnosed), pregnancy **X**

Precautions: Lactation, hypertension, asthma, blood dyscrasias, gallbladder disease, CHF, diabetes mellitus, bone disease, depression, migraine headache, convulsive disorders, hepatic disease, renal disease, family history of cancer of breast or reproductive tract

Pharmacokinetics

Absorption	Unknown
Distribution	Unknown
Metabolism	Unknown
Excretion	Unknown
Half-life	Unknown

Pharmacodynamics

	PO	IM
Onset	Unknown	Unknown
Peak	Unknown	Unknown
Duration	2-4 hr	Unknown

Interactions

Individual drugs

Aminoglutethimide: ↓ contraceptive effect
Bromocriptine: ↓ effectiveness

Lab test interferences

↑ Alkaline phosphatase, ↑ pregnanediol, ↑ amino acids
↓ GTT, ↓ HDL

NURSING CONSIDERATIONS

Assessment

- Monitor B/P at beginning of treatment and periodically; check weight daily; notify prescriber of weekly weight gain >5 lb
- Monitor I&O ratio: be alert for decreasing urinary output, increasing edema, hypertension
- Assess liver function studies: ALT (SGPT), AST (SGOT), bilirubin, periodically during long-term therapy
- Assess for edema, hypertension, cardiac symptoms, jaundice
- Assess mental status: affect, mood, behavioral changes, depression

Nursing diagnoses

- ✓ Sexual dysfunction (uses)
- ✓ Tissue perfusion, altered (adverse reactions)
- ✓ Injury, risk for (adverse reactions)
- ✓ Knowledge deficit (teaching)

Implementation

PO route

- Give with food or milk to decrease GI symptoms; give in one dose in AM

IM route

- Store in dark area

- Give titrated dosage; use lowest effective dosage; give oil sol deep in large muscle mass (IM); rotate sites; use after warming to dissolve crystals

Patient/family education

- Advise patient to avoid sunlight or use sunscreen; photosensitivity and melasma (brown patches on the face) can occur
- Teach patient about cushingoid symptoms
- Teach patient to report breast lumps, vaginal bleeding, edema, jaundice, dark urine, clay-colored stools, dyspnea, headache, blurred vision, abdominal pain, numbness or stiffness in legs, chest pain; male to report impotence or gynecomastia
- Teach patient to report suspected pregnancy immediately

Evaluation

Positive therapeutic outcome

- Decreased abnormal uterine bleeding
- Absence of amenorrhea
- Prevented pregnancy
- Arrested spread of malignant cells

megestrol (℞)

(me-jess'trole)

Megace, megestrol acetate

Func. class.: Antineoplastic

Chem. class.: Hormone, progestin

Pregnancy category X

Action: Affects endometrium by antiluteinizing effect; this is thought to bring about cell death

Therapeutic Outcome: Prevention of rapidly growing malignant cells; weight gain, increased appetite in AIDS

Uses: Breast, endometrial, renal cell cancer; increase weight, decrease cachexia and anorexia associated with AIDS

Dosage and routes

Endometrial/ovarian carcinoma

Adult: PO 40-320 mg/day in divided doses

Breast carcinoma

Adult: PO 40 mg qid

Anorexia (AIDS)

Adult: PO 40 mg qid

Available forms: Tabs 20, 40 mg; oral susp 40 mg/ml

Adverse effects

CNS: Mood swings

CV: ***Thrombophlebitis***

GI: Nausea, vomiting, anorexia, diarrhea, abdominal cramps

GU: Gynecomastia, fluid retention, ***hypercalcemia***

INTEG: Alopecia, rash, pruritus, purpura, itching

Contraindications: Hypersensitivity, pregnancy **X**

Pharmacokinetics

Absorption	Well absorbed
Distribution	Unknown
Metabolism	Liver, completely
Excretion	Unknown
Half-life	1 hr

Pharmacodynamics

Onset	Several wk-mo
Peak	Unknown
Duration	1-3 days

Interactions: None

Lab test interferences

↑ Alkaline phosphatase, ↑ urinary pregnanediol, ↑ plasma amino acids

False positive: Urine glucose

M

↓ HDL, ↓ glucose tolerance test

NURSING CONSIDERATIONS

Assessment

- Monitor effects of alopecia on body image; discuss feelings about body changes
- In AIDS patients monitor calorie counts, weight, appetite
- Assess for thrombophlebitis: pain, redness, swelling in legs; notify prescriber if these occur

Nursing diagnoses

✓ Knowledge deficit (teaching)

Implementation

- Administer with meals for GI symptoms
- Oral susp is usually used for AIDS patients

Patient/family education

- Teach patient to report any complaints or side effects to prescriber
- Advise patient that contraceptive measures must be used during and several mo after treatment; drug is teratogenic
- Explore with patient the need for wig or hair piece for hair loss
- Caution patient to report vaginal bleeding to prescriber
- Review with patient the need to comply with dosage schedule, not to miss or double doses; missed doses may be taken up to 1 hr before next dose

Evaluation

Positive therapeutic outcome

- Decreased spread of malignant cells
- Weight gain, increased appetite in AIDS patients

melphalan (℞)

(mel′fa-lan)

Alkeran, Alkeran IV, L-Pam, L-Sarcolysin

Func. class.: Antineoplastic alkylating agent

Chem. class.: Nitrogen mustard

Pregnancy category D

Action: Alkylates DNA, RNA; inhibits enzymes that allow synthesis of amino acids in proteins; activity is not cell cycle phase specific

➔ **Therapeutic Outcome:** Prevention of rapidly growing malignant cells

Uses: Multiple myeloma, breast carcinoma, reticulum cell sarcoma, testicular seminoma, malignant melanoma, advanced ovarian cancer

Investigational uses: Breast, testicular, prostate carcinoma; osteogenic sarcoma, chronic myelogenous leukemia

Dosage and routes

Multiple myeloma

Adult: PO 6 mg qd × 2-3 wk; stop drug for 4 wk or until WBC level begins to rise; do not administer if WBC <3000/mm^3 or platelets <100,000/mm^3; may be given 0.15 mg/kg/day × 7 days; wait until platelets and WBCs rise, then 0.05 mg/kg/day

Ovarian carcinoma

Adult: **IV** inf 16 mg/m^2; reduce in renal insufficiency; give over 15 20 min; give at 2-wk intervals × 4 doses, then at 4-wk intervals

Available forms: Tabs 2 mg; inj 50 mg

Adverse effects

GI: Nausea, vomiting, stomatitis, diarrhea
GU: Amenorrhea, hyperuricemia, gonadal suppression
HEMA: Thrombocytopenia, neutropenia, leukopenia, anemia
INTEG: Rash, urticaria, alopecia, pruritus
RESP: Fibrosis, dysplasia
SYST: Anaphylaxis, allergic reaction

Contraindications: Lactation, pregnancy **D,** hypersensitivity to this drug or other nitrogen mustards

Precautions: Radiation therapy, bone marrow depression, infection, renal disease, P children

Pharmacokinetics	
Absorption	Variable; incompletely absorbed
Distribution	Rapidly distributed
Metabolism	Bloodstream
Excretion	Kidneys, unchanged (10%)
Half-life	1½ hr

Pharmacodynamics
Unknown

Interactions

Individual drugs

Radiation: ↑ toxicity, bone marrow suppression

Drug classifications

Antineoplastics: ↑ toxicity, bone marrow suppression
Bone marrow–suppressing drugs: ↑ bone marrow suppression
Live vaccines: ↑ adverse reactions, ↓ antibody reaction

Lab test interferences

Increase: Uric acid

NURSING CONSIDERATIONS

Assessment

- Monitor CBC, differential, platelet count weekly; withhold drug if WBC is <4000 or platelet count is <75,000; notify prescriber of results if WBC <20,000/mm^3, platelets <100,000/mm^3
- Monitor pulmonary function tests, chest x ray films before, during therapy; chest film should be obtained q2 wk during treatment; check for dyspnea, rales, unproductive cough, chest pain, tachypnea
- Assess for increased uric acid levels, swelling, joint pain primarily in extremities; patient should be well hydrated to prevent urate deposits
- Monitor renal function studies: BUN, serum uric acid, urine CrCl before, during therapy; check I&O ratio; report fall in urine output of 30 ml/hr; check for decreased hyperuricemia; monitor AST (SGOT), ALT (SGPT)
- Monitor for cold, fever, sore throat (may indicate beginning infection); identify edema in feet, joint and stomach pain, shaking; prescriber should be notified
- Assess for bleeding: hematuria, guaiac, bruising or petechiae, mucosa or orifices q8h; no rec temp

Nursing diagnoses

- ✓ Injury, risk for (adverse reactions)
- ✓ Body image disturbance (adverse reactions)
- ✓ Infection, risk for (adverse reactions)
- ✓ Knowledge deficit (teaching)

Implementation

- Give fluids **IV** or PO before

M

chemotherapy to hydrate patient
• Give antacid before oral agent; give drug after evening meal, before hs; provide antiemetic 30-60 min before giving drug and prn to prevent vomiting; give antibiotics for prophylaxis of infection
• Give top or syst analgesics for pain
• Give in AM so drug can be eliminated before hs
• Use a liq diet: carbonated beverages; gelatin may be added if patient is not nauseated or vomiting

PO route
• Give 1 hr ac or 2 hr pc to prevent nausea/vomiting

IV route
• Give as intermittent inf: reconstitute with provided diluent (10 ml) to 5 mg/ml; shake until clear; further dilute with 0.9% NaCl to <0.45 mg/ml; give over 15 min

Y-site compatibilities: Acyclovir, amikacin, aminophylline, ampicillin, aztreonam, bleomycin, calcium gluconate, carboplatin, carmustine, cimetidine, cisplatin, cyclophosphamide, cytarabine, doxycycline, droperidol, enalaprilat, etoposide, famotidine, floxuridine, furosemide, ganciclovir, gentamicin, heparin, hydrocortisone, idarubicin, ifosfamide, mannitol, meperidine, methotrexate, metronidazole, mitomycin, mitoxantrone, morphine, ondansetron, plicamycin, ranitidine, teniposide, thiotepa, vinblastine, vincristine, vinorelbine, zidovudine

Patient/family education
• Teach patient to avoid use of products containing aspirin or ibuprofen, razors, commercial mouthwash, since bleeding may occur; to report symptoms of bleeding (hematuria, tarry stools)
• Instruct patient to report signs of anemia (fatigue, headache, irritability, faintness, shortness of breath)
• Instruct patient to report any changes in breathing or coughing even several mo after treatment; to avoid crowds and persons with respiratory tract or other infections
• Tell patient hair loss is common; discuss the use of wigs or hair pieces
• Caution patient not to have any vaccinations without the advice of the prescriber, serious reactions can occur
• Advise patient that contraception is needed during treatment and for several mo after the completion of therapy
• Teach patient to rinse mouth tid-qid with water, club soda; brush teeth bid-qid with soft brush or cotton-tipped applicators for stomatitis; use unwaxed dental floss

Evaluation

Positive therapeutic outcome
• Decreased size of tumor
• Decreased spread of malignancy

menotropins (℞)
(men-oh-troe′pinz)
HMG, Pergonal
Func. class.: Gonadotropin
Chem. class.: Exogenous gonadotropin
Pregnancy category C

Action: In women, increases follicular growth, maturation;

in men, when given with HCG, stimulates spermatogenesis; contains FSH and LH

Therapeutic Outcome: Pregnancy, ovulation

Uses: Infertility, anovulation in women; stimulates spermatogenesis in men; usually used with HCG

Dosage and routes

Infertility

Adult (men): IM 1 ampule 3 times a wk with HCG 2000 U 2 times a wk × 4 mo

Anovulation

Adult (women): IM 75 IU of FSH, LH qd × 9-12 days, then 10,000 U HCG 1 day after these drugs, repeat × 2 menstrual cycles, then increase to 150 IU of FSH, LH qd × 9-12 days, then 10,000 U HCG 1 day after these drugs × 2 menstrual cycles

Available forms: Powder for inj 17 IU/ampule

Adverse effects

CNS: Fever

CV: ***Hypovolemia,*** thrombophlebitis, ***pulmonary embolism, thromboembolism***

GI: Nausea, vomiting, diarrhea, anorexia, abdominal distention/pain

GU: Ovarian enlargement, multiple births, ovarian hyperstimulation, sudden ovarian enlargement, ascites with or without pain, pleural effusion, gynecomastia in men

HEMA: Hemoperitoneum, arterial thromboembolism

Contraindications: Primary ovarian failure, abnormal bleeding, thyroid/adrenal dysfunction, organic intracranial lesion, ovarian cysts, primary testicular failure

Precautions: Pregnancy **C**

Pharmacokinetics	
Absorption	Well absorbed
Distribution	Unknown
Metabolism	Unknown
Excretion	Kidneys, unchanged (8%)
Half-life	70 hr (FSH); 4 hr (LH)

Pharmacodynamics
Unknown

Interactions: None

NURSING CONSIDERATIONS

Assessment

- Monitor weight qd; notify prescriber if weight gain increases rapidly
- Monitor estrogen excretion level; if >100 μg/24 hr, drug is withheld; hyperstimulation syndrome may occur
- Monitor I&O ratio; be alert for decreasing urinary output
- Assess for ovarian enlargement, abdominal distention/pain; report symptoms immediately

Nursing diagnoses

✓ Sexual dysfunction (uses)
✓ Knowledge deficit (teaching)

Implementation

- Give after reconstituting with 1-2 ml sterile saline inj; use immediately

Patient/family education

- Advise patient that multiple births are possible; if pregnancy occurs, it is usually 4-6 wk after start of treatment
- Instruct patient to keep daily appointment for 2 wk during treatment
- Tell patient that daily intercourse is necessary from day preceding administration of

M

gonadotropin until ovulation occurs

Evaluation

Positive therapeutic outcome

- Pregnancy

meperidine ⊶ (℞)

(me-per'i-deen)

Demerol, meperidine HCl, Pethandol, Pethidine

Func. class.: Narcotic analgesic

Chem. class.: Opiate, phenylpiperidine derivative

Pregnancy category B

Controlled substance schedule II

Action: Depresses pain impulse transmission at the spinal cord level by interacting with opioid receptors; produces CNS depression

➔ **Therapeutic Outcome:** Relief of pain

Uses: Moderate to severe pain, preoperatively, during labor

Dosage and routes

Pain

Adult: PO/SC/IM 50-150 mg q3-4h prn; dosage should be decreased if given **IV**

P ***Child:*** PO/SC/IM 1 mg/kg q4-6h prn, not to exceed 100 mg q4h

Preoperatively

Adult: IM/SC 50-100 mg q30-90 min before surgery; dosage should be reduced if given **IV**

P ***Child:*** IM/SC 1-2.2 mg/kg 30-90 min before surgery

Labor analgesia

Adult: SC/IM 50-100 mg given when contractions are regulary spaced, repeat q1-3h prn

Available forms: Inj 10, 50, 75, 100 mg/ml; tabs 50, 100 mg; syr 50 mg/5 ml

Adverse effects

CNS: Drowsiness, dizziness, confusion, headache, sedation, euphoria, **increased intracranial pressure**

CV: Palpitations, bradycardia, change in B/P, tachycardia (**IV**)

EENT: Tinnitus, blurred vision, miosis, diplopia, depressed corneal reflex

GI: Nausea, vomiting, anorexia, constipation, cramps

GU: Urinary retention, dysuria

INTEG: Rash, urticaria, bruising, flushing, diaphoresis, pruritus

RESP: **Respiratory depression**

Contraindications: Hypersensitivity, addiction (narcotic)

Precautions: Addictive personality, pregnancy **B,** lactation, increased intracranial pressure, MI (acute), severe heart disease, respiratory depression, hepatic disease, renal disease, P child <18 yr

Pharmacokinetics	
Absorption	Well absorbed (IM, SC); 50% (PO)
Distribution	Widely distributed; crosses placenta
Metabolism	Liver, extensively
Excretion	Kidneys; breast milk
Half-life	3-4 hr

Pharmacodynamics	PO	IM/SC	IV
Onset	15 min	10 min	Rapid
Peak	½-1 hr	½-1 hr	5-7 min
Duration	2-4 hr	2-4 hr	2-4 hr

Interactions

Individual drugs

Alcohol: ↑ respiratory depression, hypotension, sedation
Cimetidine: ↑ recovery
Erythromycin: ↑ recovery
Nalbuphine: ↓ analgesia
Pentazocine: ↓ analgesia

Drug classifications

Antihistamines: ↑ respiratory depression, hypotension
Barbiturates: ↑ respiratory depression
CNS depressants: ↑ respiratory depression, hypotension
MAOIs: Do not use for 2 wk before taking meperidine
Phenothiazines: ↑ respiratory depression, hypotension
Sedative/hypnotics: ↑ respiratory depression, hypotension

Lab test interferences

↑ Amylase

NURSING CONSIDERATIONS

Assessment

- Assess pain: location, duration, intensity before and 1 hr after administration
- Monitor VS after parenteral route; note muscle rigidity, drug history, liver, kidney function tests, respiratory dysfunction: respiratory depression, character, rate, rhythm; notify prescriber if respirations are <10/min
- Monitor CNS changes: dizziness, drowsiness, hallucinations, euphoria, LOC, pupil reaction; these are due to metabolite produced
- Monitor allergic reactions: rash, urticaria

Nursing diagnoses

- ✓ Pain (uses)
- ✓ Sensory perceptual alteration: visual, auditory (adverse reactions)
- ✓ Breathing pattern, ineffective (adverse reactions)
- ✓ Injury, risk for (adverse reactions)
- ✓ Knowledge deficit (teaching)

Implementation

- Give with antiemetic if nausea, vomiting occur
- Administer when pain is beginning to return; determine dosage interval by patient response; continuous dosing of medication is more effective given prn
- Medication should be slowly withdrawn after long-term use to prevent withdrawal symptoms
- Store in light-resistant container at room temp

PO route

- May be given with food or milk to lessen GI upset
- Syrup should be mixed with 4 oz of water

IM/SC route

- Do not give if cloudy or a precipitate has formed
- Patient should remain recumbent for 1 hr after administration

IV route

- Give by direct **IV** after diluting to 10 mg/ml with sterile water, 0.9% NaCl for inj; give slowly at 25 mg/1 min; rapid administration may cause respiratory depression, hypotension, circulatory collapse
- Give cont inf after diluting to 1 mg/ml with D_5W, $D_{10}W$, dextrose/saline combinations, dextrose/Ringer's, inj combinations, 0.45% NaCl, 0.9% NaCl, Ringer's, LR; give by inf

M

pump; titrate according to response

Syringe compatibilities: Atropine, benzquinamide, butorphanol, chlorpromazine, cimetidine, dimenhydrinate, diphenhydramine, droperidol, fentanyl, glycopyrrolate, hydroxyzine, metoclopramide, midazolam, pentazocine, perphenazine, prochlorperazine, promazine, promethazine, ranitidine, scopolamine

Syringe incompatibilities: Heparin, morphine, pentobarbital

Additive compatibilities: Dobutamine, ondansetron, scopolamine, triflupromazine

Y-site compatibilities: Amifostine, amikacin, ampicillin, bumetanide, cefamandole, cefazolin, cefotaxime, cefotetan, cefoxitin, ceftizoxime, ceftriaxone, cefuroxime, cephalothin, cephapirin, chloramphenicol, clindamycin, dexamethasone, diphenhydramine, dobutamine, dopamine, doxycycline, droperidol, erythromycin lactobionate, famotidine, filgrastim, fluconazole, fludarabine, gentamicin, heparin, hydrocortisone, regular insulin, kanamycin, labetalol, lidocaine, methyldopate, magnesium sulfate, melphalan, methylprednisolone, metoclopramide, metoprolol, metronidazole, ondansetron, oxacillin, oxytocin, paclitaxel, penicillin G potassium, piperacillin, potassium chloride, propranolol, ranitidine, sargramostim, teniposide, thiotepa, ticarcillin, ticarcillin/clavulanate, tobramycin, trimethoprim/sulfamethoxazole, vancomycin, verapamil, vinorelbine

Y-site incompatibilities: Cefoperazone, idarubicin, imipenem/cilastatin, mezlocillin, minocycline

Patient/family education

- Advise patients to avoid CNS depressants (alcohol, sedative/hypnotics) for at least 24 hr after taking this drug
- Discuss with patient that dizziness, drowsiness, and confusion are common; to avoid getting up without assistance
- Discuss in detail with the patient all aspects of the drug, including its purpose and what to expect
- Caution patient to make position changes carefully to lessen orthostatic hypotension

Evaluation

Positive therapeutic outcome

- Decreased pain

Treatment of overdose: Narcan 0.2-0.8 **IV**, O_2, **IV** fluids, vasopressors

meprobamate (℞)

(me-proe-ba'mate)

Apo-Meprobamate ✥, Equanil, Meditran ✥, meprobamate, Meprospan, Miltown, Miltown 600, Neuramate, Neo-Tran ✥, Novomepro ✥, Sedabamate, Trancot

Func. class.: Sedative/hypnotic; antianxiety

Chem. class.: Propanediol carbamate derivative

Pregnancy category D

Controlled substance schedule IV

Action: Produces widespread depression of the CNS

Therapeutic Outcome: Decreased anxiety, sedation

Uses: Anxiety, sedation

Dosage and routes

Adult: PO 1.2-1.6 g/day in 2-3 divided doses, not to exceed 2.4 g/day or 800-1600 mg/day in 2 divided doses (sus rel); max 2.4 g/day

P ***Child 6-12 yr:*** PO 100-200 mg bid-tid or 200 mg (sus rel) bid

Available forms: Tabs 200, 400, 600 mg; sus rel caps 200, 400 mg

Adverse effects

CNS: Dizziness, drowsiness, headache, ***convulsions,*** ataxia

CV: Hypotension, tachycardia, palpitations, ***hyperthermia***

EENT: Blurred vision, tinnitus, mydriasis, slurred speech

GI: Nausea, vomiting, anorexia, diarrhea, stomatitis

HEMA: Thrombocytopenia, leukopenia, eosinophilia

INTEG: Urticaria, pruritus, maculopapular rash

Contraindications: Hypersensitivity, renal failure, porphyria, pregnancy **D,** history of drug abuse or dependence

Precautions: Suicidal patients, severe depression, renal disease, hepatic disease, elderly G

Pharmacokinetics

Absorption	Well absorbed
Distribution	Widely distributed; crosses placenta
Metabolism	Liver
Excretion	Kidneys, feces, breast milk
Half-life	6-16 hr

Pharmacodynamics

	PO	PO–SUS REL
Onset	1 hr	Unknown
Peak	1-3 hr	Unknown
Duration	6-12 hr	Up to 12 hr

Interactions

Individual drugs

Alcohol: ↑ CNS depression

Fluoxetine: ↑ action

Propoxyphene: ↑ action

Drug classifications

Analgesics, opioid: ↑ CNS depression

Antidepressants: ↑ CNS depression

Antihistamines: ↑ CNS depression

Sedative/hypnotics: ↑ CNS depression

Lab test interferences

False ↑ 17-OHCS

False positive: Phentolamine test

NURSING CONSIDERATIONS

Assessment

- Assess patient's sleep pattern and note physical (sleep apnea, obstructed airway, pain/discomfort, urinary frequency) and psychologic (fear, anxiety) circumstances that interrupt sleep
- Assess patient's bedtime routine, presleep cues, props
- Assess potential for abuse; this drug may lend to physical and psychologic dependency; amount of drug should be limited
- Monitor blood studies: Hct, Hgb, RBCs, serum folate (if on long-term therapy), pro-time in patients receiving anticoagulants, since action of anticoagulant may be increased
- Monitor mental status: mood, sensorium, affect, memory (long, short)

M

- Monitor physical dependency: more frequent requests for medication, shakes, anxiety, pinpoint pupils
- Monitor respiratory dysfunction: respiratory depression, character, rate, rhythm; hold drug if respirations are <10/min or if pupils are dilated (rare)
- Assess for blood dyscrasias: fever, sore throat, bruising, rash, jaundice, epistaxis (rare)
- Assess previous history of substance abuse, cardiac disease, or gastritis

Nursing diagnoses

✓ Anxiety (uses)
✓ Knowledge deficit (teaching)
✓ Noncompliance (teaching)

Implementation

- Give with food to minimize GI symptoms
- Do not break, crush, or chew sus rel cap
- Store in tight container in cool environment

Patient/family education

- Advise patient to avoid driving and other activities requiring alertness; to avoid alcohol and CNS depressants; serious CNS depression may result, as well as tachycardia, flushing, headache, hypotension
- Caution patient not to discontinue medication quickly after long-term use; drug should be tapered over 1-2 wk; effects may take 2 nights for benefits to be noticed; withdrawal symptoms include tremors, anxiety, hallucinations, delirium
- Teach patient alternate measures to improve sleep (reading, exercise several hr before hs, warm bath, warm milk, TV, self-hypnosis, deep breathing)
- Instruct patient that hangover is common in elderly but less common than with barbiturates
- Teach patient symptoms of withdrawal: nausea, vomiting, anxiety, hallucinations, insomnia, tachycardia, fever, cramps, tremors, seizures
- Teach patient to watch for blood dyscrasias: fever, sore throat, bruising, rash, jaundice (rare)
- Teach patient to watch for allergic reaction (rash); discontinue drug if rash occurs

Evaluation

Positive therapeutic outcome

- Decreased anxiety, restlessness, insomnia

Treatment of overdose: Lavage, VS, supportive care

mercaptopurine (℞)

(mer-kap-toe-pyoor'een)

6-MP, Purinethol

Func. class.: Antineoplastic, antimetabolite

Chem. class.: Purine analog

Pregnancy category D

Action: Inhibits purine metabolism at multiple sites, which inhibits DNA and RNA synthesis S phase of cell cycle

Therapeutic Outcome: Prevention of rapidly growing malignant cells

Uses: Chronic myelocytic leukemia, acute lymphoblastic leukemia in children, acute myelogenous leukemia

Investigational Uses: Polycythemia vera, psoriatic arthritis, colitis, lymphoma

Dosage and routes

Adult: PO 2.5 mg/kg/day, not to exceed 5 mg/kg/day; maintenance 1.5-2.5 mg/kg/day

P ***Child:*** 75 mg/m^2/day (2.5 mg/kg/day)

Available forms: Tab 50 mg

Adverse effects

CNS: Fever, headache, weakness

GI: Nausea, vomiting, anorexia, diarrhea, stomatitis, ***hepatotoxicity*** (with high doses), jaundice, gastritis

GU: ***Renal failure,*** hyperuricemia, ***oliguria,*** crystalluria, ***hematuria***

HEMA: ***Thrombocytopenia, leukopenia, myelosuppression, anemia***

INTEG: Rash, dry skin, urticaria

Contraindications: Patients with prior drug resistance, leukopenia (<2500/mm^3), thrombocytopenia (<100,000/mm^3), anemia, pregnancy **D**

Precautions: Renal disease

Pharmacokinetics

Absorption	Variable
Distribution	Widely-body water
Metabolism	Liver-extensively
Excretion	Kidneys unchanged (small amounts)
Half-life	Unknown

Pharmacodynamics

Unknown

Interactions

Individual drugs

Allopurinol: ↑ toxicity
Cyclophosphamide: ↑ cardiotoxicity, CHF
Radiation: ↑ toxicity, bone marrow suppression
Warfarin: ↑ or ↓ effect of warfarin

Drug classifications

Antineoplastics: ↑ toxicity, bone marrow suppression
Hepatotoxic agents: ↑ hepatotoxicity
Live virus vaccines: ↓ antibodies
Nondepolarizing muscle relaxants: Reversal of neuromuscular blockade

NURSING CONSIDERATIONS

Assessment

- Assess buccal cavity q8h for dryness, sores or ulceration, white patches, oral pain, bleeding, dysphagia; obtain prescription for viscous lidocaine (Xylocaine)
- ! Assess symptoms indicating severe allergic reaction: rash, pruritus, urticaria, purpuric skin lesions, itching, flushing
- Monitor CBC, differential, platelet count weekly; withhold drug if WBC count is <4000/mm^3 or platelet count is <100,000/mm^3; notify prescriber of results if WBC <20,000/mm^3, platelets <150,000/mm^3
- Assess for increased uric acid levels, swelling, joint pain primarily in extremities; patient should be well hydrated to prevent urate deposits
- Monitor renal function studies: BUN, creatinine, serum uric acid, urine CrCl before and during therapy; check I&O ratio; report fall in urine output to <30 ml/hr
- Monitor temp q4h (may indicate beginning of infection)
- Monitor liver function tests before and during therapy (bilirubin, AST [SGOT], ALT [SGPT], LDH) as needed or

M

monthly; check for yellowing of skin or sclera, dark urine, clay-colored stools, itchy skin, abdominal pain, fever, diarrhea
- Assess for bleeding: hematuria, stool guaiac, bruising or petechiae, mucosa or orifices q8h; check for inflammation of mucosa, breaks in skin
- Identify inflammation of mucosa, breaks in skin

Nursing diagnoses

- ✓ Injury, risk for (adverse reactions)
- ✓ Body image disturbance (adverse reactions)
- ✓ Infection, risk for (adverse reactions)
- ✓ Knowledge deficit (teaching)

Implementation

- Give fluids **IV** or PO before chemotherapy to hydrate patient
- Give antiemetic 30-60 min before giving drug and prn to prevent vomiting; give antibiotics for prophylaxis of infection
- Give top or syst analgesics for pain
- Give in AM so drug can be eliminated before hs
- Provide liq diet: carbonated beverages; gelatin may be added if patient is not nauseated or vomiting
- Encourage patient to rinse mouth tid-qid with water, club soda; brush teeth bid-qid with soft brush or cotton-tipped applicators for stomatitis; use unwaxed dental floss
- Tab may be crushed and added to fluids or food to facilitate swallowing

Patient/family education

- Advise patient that contraceptive measures are recommended during therapy; serious teratogenic effects may occur
- Teach patient to avoid use of products containing aspirin or ibuprofen, razors, commercial mouthwash, since bleeding may occur; to report symptoms of bleeding (hematuria, tarry stools)
- Instruct patient to report signs of anemia (fatigue, headache, irritability, faintness, shortness of breath)
- Instruct patient to report any changes in breathing or coughing even several mo after treatment; to avoid crowds and persons with respiratory tract or other infections
- Caution patient not to have any vaccinations without the advice of the prescriber; serious reactions can occur

Evaluation

Positive therapeutic outcome

- Prevention of rapid division of malignant cells

meropenem (℞)

(mer-oh-pen′em)

Merrem **IV**

Func. class.: Antiinfective; miscellaneous carbapenem

Pregnancy category B

Action: Interferes with cell wall replication of susceptible organisms; osmotically unstable cell wall swells and bursts from osmotic pressure

⇒ Therapeutic Outcome: Bactericidal action against the following: *Streptococcus pneumoniae,* group A β-hemolytic streptococci, *viridans* group *streptococci,* enterococcus; gram-negative organisms:

Klebsiella, Proteus, Escherichia coli, Pseudomonas aeruginosa, B. fragilis, B.thetaiotamicron, P bacterial meningitis (>3 mo old)

Uses: Serious infections caused by gram-positive or gram-negative organisms (appendicitis, peritonitis)

Dosage and routes

Adult: **IV** 1 g q8h, given over 15-30 min or as an **IV** bolus 5-20 ml given over 3-5 min

P ***Child >3 mo:*** **IV** 20-40 mg/kg q8h, max 2 gm q8h

P ***Child >50 kg:*** **IV** 1 g q8h (intraabdominal infection) or 2 g q8h (meningitis) given over 15-30 min or as an **IV** bolus 5-20 ml over 3-5 min

Available forms: Inj 500 mg

Adverse effects

CNS: Fever, somnolence, *seizures,* dizziness, weakness

CV: Hypotension, palpitations

GI: Diarrhea, nausea, vomiting, *pseudomembranous colitis, hepatitis,* glossitis

HEMA: Eosinophilia, neutropenia, decreased Hgb, Hct

INTEG: Rash, urticaria, pruritus, pain at inj site, phlebitis, erythema at inj site

RESP: Chest discomfort, dyspnea, hyperventilation

SYST: Anaphylaxis

Contraindications: Hypersensitivity

Precautions: Pregnancy **B,** G lactation, elderly, renal disease

Pharmacokinetics

Absorption	Complete bioavailability
Distribution	Widely distributed
Metabolism	Liver
Excretion	Kidneys
Half-life	1 hr; increased in renal disease

Pharmacodynamics

Onset	Rapid
Peak	Dose dependent

Interactions

Individual drugs

Probenecid: ↓ renal excretion, ↑ blood level

Lab test interferences

False ↑ Creatinine (serum urine), false ↑ urinary 17-KS

False positive: Urinary protein, direct Coombs' test, urine glucose

Interference: Cross-matching

NURSING CONSIDERATIONS

Assessment

- Assess patient for previous sensitivity reaction to carbapenem antibiotics
- Assess patient for signs and symptoms of infection, including characteristics of wounds, sputum, urine, stool, WBC >10,000, fever; obtain baseline information before and during treatment
- Complete C&S tests before beginning drug therapy to identify if correct treatment has been initiated
- Assess for allergic reactions: rash, urticaria, pruritus, chills, fever, joint pain; angioedema may occur a few days after therapy begins; epinephrine, resuscitation equipment should be available for anaphylactic reaction
- Identify urine output; if decreasing, notify prescriber (may indicate nephrotoxicity); also check for increased BUN, creatinine
- Monitor blood studies: AST (SGOT), ALT (SGPT), CBC, Hct, bilirubin, LDH, alkaline phosphatase, Coombs' test

monthly if patient is on long-term therapy
- Monitor electrolytes: potassium, sodium, chloride monthly if patient is on long-term therapy
- Assess bowel pattern qd; if severe diarrhea occurs, drug should be discontinued; may indicate pseudomembranous colitis
- Monitor for bleeding: ecchymosis, bleeding gums, hematuria, stool guaiac daily if on long-term therapy
- Assess for overgrowth of infection: perineal itching, fever, malaise, redness, pain, swelling, drainage, rash, diarrhea, change in cough, sputum

Nursing diagnoses

- ✓ Infection, risk for (uses)
- ✓ Diarrhea (adverse reactions)
- ✓ Injury, risk for (adverse reactions)
- ✓ Knowledge deficit (teaching)
- ✓ Noncompliance (teaching)

Implementation

IV **IV route**

Patient/family education

- Teach patient to report sore throat, bruising, bleeding, joint pain; may indicate blood dyscrasias (rare)
- Advise patient to contact prescriber if vaginal itching, loose foul-smelling stools, furry tongue occur; may indicate superinfection
- Advise patient to notify prescriber of diarrhea with blood or pus, may indicate pseudomembranous colitis

Evaluation

Positive therapeutic outcome

- Absence of signs/symptoms of infection (WBC <10,000, temp WNL, absence of red draining wounds)
- Reported improvement in symptoms of infection

Treatment of anaphylaxis: Epinephrine, antihistamines, resuscitate if needed

mesalamine (℞)

(mez-al'a-meen)

Asacol, Pentusa, Rowasa, Salofulk ✤

Func class.: GI antiinflammatory

Chem class.: 5-Aminosalicylic acid

Pregnancy category B

Action: May diminish inflammation by blocking cyclooxygenase, inhibiting prostaglandin production in colon, local action only

➔ **Therapeutic Outcome:** Decreased cramping, pain in GI conditions

Uses: Mild to moderate active distal ulcerative colitis, proctosigmoiditis, proctitis

Dosage and routes

Adult: Rec 60 ml (4 g) hs, retained for 8 hr × 3-6 wk; PO 800 mg tid for 6 wk; supp 500 mg bid for 3-6 wk

Available forms: Rec susp 4 g/60 ml; supp 500 mg; delayed rel tab 400 mg

Adverse effects

CNS: Headache, fever, dizziness, insomnia, asthenia, weakness, fatigue

CV: Pericarditis, myocarditis

EENT: Sore throat, cough, pharyngitis, rhinitis

GI: Cramps, gas, nausea, diarrhea, rec pain, constipation

INTEG: Rash, itching, acne

SYST: Flu, malaise, back pain,

peripheral edema, leg and joint pain, arthralgia, dysmenorrhea

Contraindications: Hypersensitivity to this drug or salicylates

Precautions: Renal disease, pregnancy **B,** lactation, children, sulfite sensitivity

Pharmacokinetics

Absorption	20%-30% (PO), 10%-25% (rec)
Distribution	Unknown
Metabolism	Unknown
Excretion	Feces
Half-life	1 hr; metabolite 5-10 hr

Pharmacodynamics

Unknown

Interactions: None

NURSING CONSIDERATIONS

Assessment

• Assess for GI symptoms: cramping, gas, nausea, diarrhea, rec pain, abdominal pain; if severe, the drug should be discontinued

Nursing diagnoses

- Pain (uses)
- Diarrhea (uses)
- Knowledge deficit (teaching)

Implementation

PO route

• Do not crush, chew tabs
• May give orally

Rec route (susp)

• Give hs, retained until AM
• Store at room temp
• Usual course of therapy is 3-6 wk
• Give after shaking bottle well

Patient/family education

• Advise patient to notify prescriber if abdominal pain, cramping, diarrhea with blood, headache, fever, rash occur; drug should be discontinued
• Teach correct administration for PO, or enema

Evaluation

Positive therapeutic outcome

• Absence of pain, bleeding from GI tract

mesoridazine (℞)

(mez-oh-rid'a-zeen)

Serentil

Func. class.: Antipsychotic/neuroleptic

Chem. class.: Phenothiazine, piperidine

Pregnancy category C

Action: Depresses cerebral cortex, hypothalamus, limbic system, which control activity, aggression; blocks neurotransmission produced by dopamine at synapse; exhibits strong α-adrenergic, anticholinergic blocking action; mechanism for antipsychotic effects is unclear

Therapeutic Outcome: Decreased signs and symptoms of psychosis, reorganization of thought patterns

Uses: Psychotic disorders, schizophrenia, anxiety, alcoholism, behavioral problems in mental deficiency, chronic brain syndrome

Dosage and routes

Schizophrenia

Adult: PO 50 mg tid; optimum dosage 100-400 mg/day; IM 25 mg; may repeat in 30-60 min; dosage range 25-200 mg/day

Behavior problems

Adult: PO 25 mg tid; optimum dosage 75-300 mg/day

Alcoholism
Adult: PO 25 mg bid; optimum dosage 50-200 mg/day

Schizoaffective disorders
Adult: PO 10 mg tid; optimum dosage 30-150 mg/day

Available forms: Tabs 10, 25, 50, 100 mg; conc 25 mg/ml; inj 25 mg/ml

Adverse effects
CNS: Extrapyramidal symptoms: pseudoparkinsonism, akathisia, dystonia, tardive dyskinesia, drowsiness, headache, ***neuroleptic malignant syndrome***
CV: Orthostatic hypotension, hypertension, ***cardiac arrest,*** ECG changes, tachycardia
EENT: Blurred vision, glaucoma
GI: Dry mouth, nausea, vomiting, anorexia, constipation, diarrhea, jaundice, weight gain
GU: Urinary retention, urinary frequency, enuresis, impotence, amenorrhea, gynecomastia
HEMA: ***Anemia, leukopenia, leukocytosis, agranulocytosis***
INTEG: Rash, photosensitivity, dermatitis
RESP: ***Laryngospasm,*** dyspnea, ***respiratory depression***

Contraindications: Hypersensitivity, circulatory collapse, liver damage, cerebral arteriosclerosis, coronary disease, severe hypertension/hypotension, blood dyscrasias, coma, brain damage, bone marrow depression, narrow-angle glaucoma

Precautions: Pregnancy **C,** lactation, seizure disorders, hypertension, hepatic disease, cardiac disease, prostatic hypertrophy, intestinal obstruction, respiratory conditions

Pharmacokinetics	
Absorption	Well absorbed (PO, IM)
Distribution	Widely distributed; crosses placenta, blood-brain barrier
Metabolism	Liver, extensively
Excretion	Kidneys, breast milk
Half-life	Unknown

Pharmacodynamics	PO	IM
Onset	Erratic	15-30 min
Peak	2 hr	30 min
Duration	4-6 hr	6-8 hr

Interactions
Individual drugs
Alcohol: ↑ effects of both drugs, oversedation
Aluminum hydroxide: ↓ absorption
Bromocriptine: ↓ antiparkinsonian activity
Disopyramide: ↑ anticholinergic effects
Epinephrine: ↑ toxicity
Guanethidine: ↓ antihypertensive response
Levodopa: ↓ antiparkinsonian activity
Lithium: ↓ mesoridazine levels, ↑ extrapyramidal symptoms, masking of lithium toxicity
Magnesium hydroxide: ↓ absorption
Norepinephrine: ↓ vasoresponse, ↑ toxicity
Phenobarbital: ↓ effectiveness, ↑ metabolism
Drug classifications
Antacids: ↓ absorption
Anticholinergics: ↑ anticholinergic effects
Antidepressants: ↑ CNS depression
Antidiarrheals, adsorbent: ↓ absorption
Antihistamines: ↑ CNS depression

Antihypertensives: ↑ hypotension
Barbiturate anesthetics: ↑ CNS depression
β-Adrenergics: ↑ effects of both drugs
General anesthetics: ↑ CNS depression
MAOIs: ↑ CNS depression
Narcotics: ↑ CNS depression
Sedative/hypnotics: ↑ CNS depression

Lab test interferences
↑ Liver function tests, ↑ cardiac enzymes, ↑ cholesterol, ↑ blood glucose, ↑ prolactin, ↑ bilirubin, ↑ PBI, ↑ cholinesterase ^{131}I, ↑ alkaline phosphatase, ↑ leukocytes, ↑ granulocytes, ↑ platelets
↓ Hormones (blood and urine)
False positive: Pregnancy tests, PKU
False negative: Urinary steroids, 17-OHCS

NURSING CONSIDERATIONS

Assessment

- Assess mental status: orientation, mood, behavior, presence and type of hallucinations before initial administration and monthly; this drug should significantly reduce psychotic behavior
- Check for swallowing of PO medication; check for hoarding or giving of medication to other patients
- Monitor I&O ratio; palpate bladder if low urinary output occurs, especially in elderly; urinalysis recommended before, during prolonged therapy
- Monitor bilirubin, CBC, liver function studies monthly
- Assess affect, orientation, LOC, reflexes, gait, coordination, sleep pattern disturbances
- Monitor B/P with patient sitting, standing, and lying; take pulse and respirations q4h during initial treatment; establish baseline before starting treatment; report drops of 30 mm Hg; obtain baseline ECG, Q wave and T wave changes
- Check for dizziness, faintness, palpitations, tachycardia on rising; severe orthostatic hypotension is common
- Identify for neuroleptic malignant syndrome: hyperpyrexia, muscle rigidity, increased CPK, altered mental status; drug should be discontinued
- Assess for EPS including akathisia (inability to sit still, no pattern to movements), tardive dyskinesia (bizarre movements of the jaw, mouth, tongue, extremities), pseudoparkinsonism (ragged tremors, pill rolling, shuffling gate); an antiparkinsonism drug should be prescribed
- Assess for constipation, urinary retention daily; if these occur, increase bulk, water in diet

Nursing diagnoses

- ✓ Thought processes, altered (uses)
- ✓ Coping, ineffective individual (uses)
- ✓ Knowledge deficit (teaching)
- ✓ Noncompliance (teaching)

Implementation

PO route

- Administer drug in liq form mixed in glass of juice or cola if hoarding is suspected; do not mix in caffeine drinks or with tannics, pectins
- Administer decreased dosage in elderly, since metabolism is slowed
- Administer PO with full glass of water, milk; or give with food to decrease GI upset
- Store in airtight, light-

resistant container, oral sol in bottle

IM route

- Inject deeply in large muscle mass; do not give SC; do not administer sol with a precipitate

Patient/family education

- Teach patient to use good oral hygiene; frequent rinsing of mouth, sugarless gum for dry mouth
- Tell patient to avoid hazardous activities until drug response is determined; dizziness, blurred vision may occur
- Inform patient that orthostatic hypotension occurs often and to rise from sitting or lying position gradually; to remain lying down after IM inj for at least 30 min; tell patient to avoid hot tubs, hot showers, tub baths, since hypotension may occur; tell patient that in hot weather heat stroke may occur; take extra precautions to stay cool
- Caution patient to avoid abrupt withdrawal of this drug, or EPS may result; drug should be withdrawn slowly
- Teach patient to avoid OTC preparations (cough, hay fever, cold) unless approved by prescriber, since serious drug interactions may occur; avoid use with alcohol, CNS depressants; increased drowsiness may occur
- Caution patient to use a sunscreen and sunglasses in case of photosensitivity
- Teach patient about EPS and necessity of meticulous oral hygiene, since oral candidiasis may occur
- Advise patient to take antacids 2 hr before or after taking this drug
- Instruct patient to report sore throat, malaise, fever, bleeding, mouth sores; if these occur, CBC should be drawn and drug discontinued
- Teach patient that urine may turn pink or red

Evaluation

Positive therapeutic outcome

- Decrease in emotional excitement, hallucinations, delusions, paranoia
- Reorganization of patterns of thought, speech

Treatment of overdose: Lavage if orally ingested; provide airway; *do not induce vomiting or use epinephrine*

metaproterenol (℞)

(met-a-proe-ter′e-nole)

Alupent, Arm-A-Med metaproterenol sulfate, Metaprel

Func. class.: Selective β_2-agonist, bronchodilator

Pregnancy category C

Action: Relaxes bronchial smooth muscle by direct action on β_2-adrenergic receptors, with increased levels of cAMP and increased bronchodilatation, diuresis, and cardiac and CNS stimulation

Therapeutic Outcome: Bronchodilatation with ease of breathing

Uses: Bronchial asthma, bronchospasm

Dosage and routes

P ***Adult and child >12 yr:*** Inh 2-3 puffs; may repeat q3-4h, not to exceed 12 puffs/day

Asthma/bronchospasm

Adult: PO 20 mg q6-8h

P *Child >9 yr or >27 kg:* PO 20 mg q6-8h or 0.4-0.9 mg/kg tid

P *Child 6-9 yr or <27 kg:* PO 10 mg q6-8h or 0.4-0.9 mg/kg tid

Available forms: Tabs 10, 20 mg; aerosol 0.65 mg/dose; syr 10 mg/5 ml; sol nebulizer 0.4%, 0.6%, 5%

Adverse effects

CNS: Tremors, anxiety, insomnia, headache, dizziness, stimulation

CV: Palpitations, tachycardia, hypertension, dysrhythmias, ***cardiac arrest***

GI: Nausea, vomiting

Contraindications: Hypersensitivity to sympathomimetics, narrow-angle glaucoma

Precautions: Pregnancy **C**, cardiac disorders, hyperthyroidism, diabetes mellitus, prostatic hypertrophy

Pharmacokinetics

Absorption	Well absorbed (PO)
Distribution	Unknown
Metabolism	Liver, tissues
Excretion	Unknown
Half-life	2-4 hr

Pharmacodynamics

	PO	INH
Onset	15 min	5 min
Peak	1 hr	1 hr
Duration	4 hr	4 hr

Interactions

Drug classifications

β-Adrenergic blockers: Block therapeutic effect

Bronchodilators, aerosol: ↑ action of bronchodilator

MAOIs: ↑ chance of hypertensive crisis

Sympathomimetics: ↑ adrenergic side effects

NURSING CONSIDERATIONS

Assessment

- Monitor respiratory function: vital capacity, FEV, ABGs, lung sounds, heart rate, rhythm (baseline)
- Determine that patient has not received theophylline therapy before giving dose; identify client's ability to self-medicate
- Monitor for evidence of allergic reactions; paradoxic bronchospasm; withhold dose; notify prescriber

Nursing diagnoses

✓ Airway clearance, ineffective (uses)
✓ Impaired gas exchange (uses)
✓ Knowledge deficit (teaching)

Implementation

Aerosol route

- Give after shaking, exhale, place mouthpiece in mouth, inhale slowly, hold breath, remove, exhale slowly; allow at least 1 min between inh
- Store in light-resistant container, do not expose to temp over 86° F (30° C)

PO route

- Give PO with meals to decrease gastric irritation; syrup P to children (no alcohol, sugar)

Patient/family education

- Advise patient not to use OTC medications; extra stimulation may occur; to use this medication before other medications and allow at least 5 min between each to prevent overstimulation
- Teach patient use of inhaler; review package insert with patient; teach patient to avoid getting aerosol in eyes, since blurring may result; to wash inhaler in warm water qd and dry; to avoid smoking, smoke-filled rooms, persons with

M

respiratory tract infections
- Advise patient that paradoxic bronchospasm may occur and to stop drug immediately and notify prescriber; to limit caffeine products such as chocolate, coffee, tea, and colas
- Instruct patient on administration of dose; not to use more than prescribed; serious side effects may occur

Evaluation

Positive therapeutic outcome
- Absence of dyspnea, wheezing after 1 hr
- Improved airway exchange
- Improved ABGs

Treatment of overdose: Administer a β_1-adrenergic blocker

metformin (℞)
(met-for′min)
glucophage
Func. class.: Antidiabetic, oral
Chem. class.: Biguanide
Pregnancy category B

Action: Inhibits hepatic glucose production and increases sensitivity of peripheral tissue to insulin

Therapeutic Outcome Blood glucose in normal levels

Uses: Stable adult-onset diabetes mellitus (type II) NIDDM

Dosage and routes
Adult: PO 500 mg bid initially, then increase to desired response 1-3 g; dosage adjustment q2-3wk or 850 mg qd with morning meal with dosage increased every other week, max 2550 mg/day

Available forms: Tabs 500, 850 mg

Adverse effects:
CNS: Headache, weakness, dizziness, drowsiness, tinnitus, fatigue, vertigo, *agitation*
ENDO: Lactic acidosis
GI: Nausea, vomiting, diarrhea, heartburn, anorexia, metallic taste
HEMA: Thrombocytopenia
INTEG: Rash

Contraindications: Hypersensitivity, hepatic, renal disease, alcoholism, cardiopulmonary disease

Precautions: Pregnancy **B,** elderly, thyroid disease, previous hypersensitivity to phenformin or buformin

Pharmacokinetics	
Absorption	
Distribution	
Metabolism	
Excretion	Kidneys, unchanged (35-50%)
Half-life	1½-5,Terminal 9-17 hr

Pharmacodynamics	
Onset	
Peak	1-3 hr
Duration	

Interactions
Individual drugs
Acetazolamide: ↑ blood glucose levels
Cimetidine: ↑ hypoglycemia
Ethanol: ↑ risk of lactic acidosis
Drug classifications
Glucocorticoids: ↑ risk of lactic acidosis

NURSING CONSIDERATIONS
Assessment
- Assess for hypoglycemic reactions (sweating, weakness, dizziness, anxiety, tremors,

hunger), hyperglycemic reactions soon after meals

• Monitor CBC (baseline, q3mo) during treatment; check liver function tests periodically AST (SGOT), LDH, renal studies: BUN, creatinine during treatment

• Monitor for lactic acidosis

Nursing diagnoses

✓ Knowledge deficit (teaching)

Implementation

• Conversion from other oral hypoglycemic agents; change may be made without gradual dosage change; monitor serum or urine glucose and ketones tid during conversion

• Give twice a day with meals to decrease GI upset and provide best absorption

• Give tabs crushed and mixed with meal or fluids for patients with difficulty swallowing

• Store in tight container in cool environment

Patient/family education

• Teach patient to use capillary blood glucose test or Chemstrip tid

• Teach patient symptoms of hypo/hyperglycemia, what to do about each

• Advise patient that drug must be continued on daily basis; explain consequence of discontinuing drug abruptly

• Advise patient to take drug in morning to prevent hypoglycemic reactions at night

• Advise patient to avoid OTC medications unless approved by the prescriber

• Teach patient that diabetes is a lifelong illness; that this drug is not a cure; only controls symptoms

• Teach patient that all food included in diet plan must be eaten to prevent hypoglycemia

• Teach patient to carry Medic Alert ID and glucagon emergency kit for emergencies

Evaluation

• Therapeutic response: decrease in polyuria, polydipsia, polyphagia; clear sensorium; absence of dizziness; stable gait, blood glucose at normal level

Treatment of overdose: Glucose 25 g IV via dextrose 50% sol, 50 ml or 1 mg glucagon

methadone (℞)

(meth′a-done)

Dolophine HCl, methadone HCl, methadone HCl Diskets, methadone HCl Intensol, Methadose

Func. class.: Narcotic analgesic

Chem. class.: Opiate, synthetic diphenylheptane derivative

Pregnancy category B

Controlled substance schedule II

Action: Depresses pain impulse transmission at the spinal cord level by interacting with opioid receptors; produces CNS depression

➡ **Therapeutic Outcome:** Relief of pain; successful narcotic withdrawal

Uses: Severe pain, narcotic withdrawal

Dosage and routes

Pain

Adult: PO/SC/IM 2.5-10 mg q4-12h prn

M

Narcotic withdrawal
Adult: PO 15-40 mg/day individualized initially, then 20-120 mg/day titrated to patient response

Available forms: Inj 10 mg/ml; tabs 5, 10 mg; oral sol 5, 10 mg/5 ml; dispersible tab 40 mg; oral cap 10 mg/ml

Adverse effects
CNS: Drowsiness, dizziness, confusion, headache, sedation, euphoria
CV: Palpitations, bradycardia, change in B/P
EENT: Tinnitus, blurred vision, miosis, diplopia
GI: Nausea, vomiting, anorexia, constipation, cramps, biliary tract spasm
GU: Increased urinary output, dysuria, urinary retention
INTEG: Rash, urticaria, bruising, flushing, diaphoresis, pruritus
RESP: Respiratory depression

Contraindications: Hypersensitivity to this drug, or hypersensitivity to chlorobutanol (inj route), addiction (narcotic)

Precautions: Addictive personality, pregnancy **B,** lactation, increased intracranial pressure, MI (acute), severe heart disease, respiratory depression, hepatic disease, renal disease, P child <18 yr

Pharmacokinetics

Absorption	Well absorbed (PO, SC, IM)
Distribution	Widely distributed; crosses placenta
Metabolism	Liver, extensively
Excretion	Kidneys, breast milk
Half-life	15-30 hr

Pharmacodynamics

	PO	IM/SC
Onset	½-1hr	20 min
Peak	½-1 hr	½-1 hr
Duration	4-12 hr	4-6 hr

Interactions
Individual drugs
Alcohol: ↑ respiratory depression, hypotension, sedation
Cimetidine: ↑ recovery
Erythromycin: ↑ recovery
Nalbuphine: ↓ analgesia
Pentazocine: ↓ analgesia
Drug classifications
Antihistamines: ↑ respiratory depression, hypotension
CNS depressants: ↑ respiratory depression, hypotension
MAOIs: Do not use for 2 wk before taking methadone
Phenothiazines: ↑ respiratory depression, hypotension
Sedative/hypnotics: ↑ respiratory depression, hypotension
Lab test interferences
↑ Amylase, ↑ lipase

NURSING CONSIDERATIONS
Assessment
- Monitor VS after parenteral route; note muscle rigidity, drug history, liver, kidney function tests, respiratory dysfunction: respiratory depression, character, rate, rhythm; notify prescriber if respirations are <10/min
- Monitor CNS changes: dizziness, drowsiness, hallucinations, euphoria, LOC, pupil reaction
- Monitor allergic reactions: rash, urticaria

Nursing diagnoses
✓ Pain (uses)
✓ Sensory-perceptual alteration: visual, auditory (adverse reactions)

✓ Breathing pattern, ineffective (adverse reactions)
✓ Knowledge deficit (teaching)

Implementation

- Medication should be slowly withdrawn after long-term use to prevent withdrawal symptoms

PO route

- May be given with food or milk to lessen GI upset
- Store in light-resistant container at room temp

IM/SC route

- Do not give if cloudy or a precipitate has formed
- Give deeply in large muscle mass; rotate inj sites

Patient/family education

- Instruct patient to report any symptoms of CNS changes, allergic reactions; to avoid CNS depressants: alcohol, sedative/hypnotics for at least 24 hr after taking this drug
- Discuss with patient that dizziness, drowsiness, and confusion are common; to avoid getting up without assistance
- Discuss in detail with patient all aspects of the drug
- Caution patient to make position changes slowly to prevent orthostatic hypotension

Evaluation

Positive therapeutic outcome

- Decreased pain
- Successful narcotic withdrawal

Treatment of overdose: Naloxone (Narcan) 0.2-0.8 **IV**, O_2, **IV** fluids, vasopressors

methicillin (℞)

(meth-i-sill'in)
Staphcillin
Func. class.: Broad-spectrum antibiotic
Chem. class.: Penicillinase-resistant penicillin
Pregnancy category B

Action: Interferes with cell wall replication of susceptible organisms; osmotically unstable cell wall swells, bursts from osmotic pressure

➔ **Therapeutic Outcome:** Bactericidal for the following gram-positive cocci: *Staphylococcus aureus, Streptococcus pyogenes, S. viridans, S. faecalis, S. bovis, S. pneumoniae;* improvement of infections caused by penicillinase-producing *staphylococci*

Uses: Penicillinase-producing staphylococci, streptococci; infections of respiratory tract, skin, skin structures, urinary tract, bone, joint; sinusitis, endocarditis, septicemia, meningitis

Dosage and routes

Adult: IM/**IV** 4-12 g/day in divided doses q4-6h

P ***Child:*** IM/**IV** 50-300 mg/kg/day in divided doses q4-12h

Available forms: Powder for inj 1, 4, 6, 10 g; **IV** inf only 1 g

Adverse effects

CNS: Lethargy, hallucinations, anxiety, depression, twitching, ***coma, convulsions***

GI: Nausea, vomiting, diarrhea, increased AST (SGOT), ALT (SGPT), abdominal pain,

M

glossitis, colitis, interstitial nephritis
GU: Oliguria, ***proteinuria, hematuria, vaginitis, moniliasis, glomerulonephritis***
HEMA: Anemia, increased bleeding time, ***bone marrow depression, granulocytopenia***

Contraindications: Hypersensitivity to penicillins

Precautions: Pregnancy **B**, hypersensitivity to cephalosporins, P neonates

Pharmacokinetics

Absorption	Well absorbed
Distribution	Widely distributed; crosses placenta
Metabolism	Not metabolized
Excretion	Kidneys, unchanged; breast milk
Half-life	20-30 min; increased in renal disease

Pharmacodynamics

	IM	IV
Onset	Rapid	Rapid
Peak	½-1 hr	15 min
Duration	4 hr	4 hr

Interactions

Individual drugs

Probenecid: ↑ methicillin levels, ↓ renal excretion

Drug classifications

Erythromycins: ↓ antimicrobial effectiveness
Oral anticoagulants: ↑ anticoagulant effects
Oral contraceptives: ↓ contraceptive effectiveness
Tetracyclines: ↓ antimicrobial effectiveness

Lab test interferences

False positive: Urine glucose, urine protein

NURSING CONSIDERATIONS
Assessment

- Assess patient for previous sensitivity reaction to penicillins or other cephalosporins; cross-sensitivity between penicillins and cephalosporins is common
- Assess patient for signs and symptoms of infection including characteristics of wounds, sputum, urine, stool, WBC >10,000, fever; obtain baseline information and during treatment
- Obtain C&S before beginning drug therapy to identify if correct treatment has been initiated
- Assess for allergic reactions: rash, urticaria, pruritus, chills, fever, joint pain; angioedema may occur a few days after therapy begins; epinephrine, resuscitation equipment should be available for anaphylactic reaction
- Identify urine output; if decreasing, notify prescriber (may indicate nephrotoxicity); also check for increased BUN, creatinine
- Monitor blood studies: AST (SGOT), ALT (SGPT), CBC, Hct, bilirubin, LDH, alkaline phosphatase, Coombs' test monthly if patient is on long-term therapy
- Monitor electrolytes: potassium, sodium, chloride monthly if patient is on long-term therapy
- Assess bowel pattern qd; if severe diarrhea occurs, drug should be discontinued
- Monitor for bleeding: ecchymosis, bleeding gums, hematuria, stool guaiac daily if on long-term therapy
- Assess for overgrowth of infection: perineal itching, fever, malaise, redness, pain, swelling, drainage, rash, diarrhea, change in cough, sputum

Nursing diagnoses

- ✓ Infection, risk for (uses)
- ✓ Diarrhea (adverse reactions)
- ✓ Injury, risk for (adverse reactions)
- ✓ Knowledge deficit (teaching)
- ✓ Noncompliance (teaching)

Implementation

IM route

- Reconstitute 1 g/1.5 ml sterile water or 0.9% NaCl; 5 g/5.7 ml; 6 g/8.6 ml yielding conc of 500 mg/ml
- Give slowly in deep muscle mass; well tolerated by deep intragluteal inj; may be painful

IV route

- Reconstitute 1 g/1.5 ml sterile water or 0.9% NaCl; 5 g/5.7 ml; 6 g/8.6 ml yielding conc of 500 mg/ml
- Give by direct IV by further diluting in 20-25 ml of sterile water, 0.9% NaCl; give 10 ml/min
- Give by intermittent inf after diluting in D_5W, $D_{10}W$, 0.9% NaCl, D_5/0.9% NaCl, D_5/LR, LR, Ringer's, run over ½-8 hr; stable for 8 hr at room temp
- Do not admix with other drugs

Syringe incompatibilities: Heparin, kanamycin, oxytetracycline, tetracycline

Syringe compatibilities: Chloramphenicol, colistimethate, erythromycin, gentamicin, lidocaine, polymyxin B, procaine, streptomycin

Y-site compatibilities: Heparin, hydrocortisone, potassium chloride, verapamil, vitamin B with C

Additive incompatibilities: Amikacin, chlorpromazine, codeine, levorphanol, meperidine, metaraminol, methadone, methohexital, morphine, oxytetracycline, promethazine, tetracycline, vancomycin

Additive compatibilities: Aminophylline, ascorbic acid, calcium chloride, gluconate, cephalothin, chloramphenicol, colistimethate, corticotropin, dimenhydrinate, diphenhydramine, erythromycin, gentamicin, penicillin G potassium, polymyxin B, potassium chloride, prednisolone, procaine, vancomycin, verapamil

Patient/family education

- Teach patient to report sore throat, bruising, bleeding, joint pain; may indicate blood dyscrasias (rare)
- Advise patient to contact prescriber if vaginal itching, loose, foul-smelling stools, furry tongue occur; may indicate superinfection
- Advise patient to notify prescriber of diarrhea with blood or pus, which may indicate pseudomembranous colitis

Evaluation

Positive therapeutic outcome

- Absence of signs/symptoms of infection (WBC <10,000, temp WNL, absence of red, draining wounds)
- Reported improvement in symptoms of infection

Treatment of anaphylaxis:

Withdraw drug, maintain airway, administer epinephrine, aminophylline, O_2, **IV** corticosteroids

M

methimazole (℞)
(meth-im'a-zole)
Tapazole
Func. class.: Thyroid hormone antagonist (antithyroid)
Chem. class.: Thioamide
Pregnancy category D

Action: Inhibits synthesis of thyroid hormones by decreasing iodine use in the manufacture of thyroglobin and iodothyronine; does not affect already formed hormones

➔ Therapeutic Outcome: Decreased T_4 levels, hyperthyroid symptoms

Uses: Hyperthyroidism, preparation for thyroidectomy, thyrotoxic crisis, thyroid storm

Dosage and routes
Hyperthyroidism
Adult: PO 5-20 mg tid depending on severity of condition; continue until euthyroid; maintenance dosage 5-10 mg qd-tid; max dosage 150 mg qd

P ***Child:*** PO 0.4 mg/kg/day in divided doses q8h; continue until euthyroid; maintenance dosage 0.2 mg/kg/day in divided doses q8h

Preparation for thyroidectomy
P ***Adult and child:*** PO same as above; iodine may be added for 10 days before surgery

Thyrotoxic crisis
P ***Adult and child:*** PO same as hyperthyroidism with iodine and propranolol

Available forms: Tabs 5, 10 mg

Adverse effects
CNS: Drowsiness, headache, vertigo, fever, paresthesias, neuritis
ENDO: Enlarged thyroid
GI: Nausea, diarrhea, vomiting, ***jaundice, hepatitis,*** loss of taste
GU: Nephritis
HEMA: Agranulocytosis, leukopenia, thrombocytopenia, hypothrombinemia, lymphadenopathy, bleeding, vasculitis
INTEG: Rash, urticaria, pruritus, alopecia, hyperpigmentation, lupuslike syndrome
MS: Myalgia, arthralgia, nocturnal muscle cramps

Contraindications: Hypersensitivity, pregnancy (3rd trimester) **D,** lactation

Precautions: Infection, bone marrow depression, hepatic disease, pregnancy (1st, 2nd trimester), patient >40 yr

Pharmacokinetics	
Absorption	Rapidly absorbed
Distribution	Crosses placenta
Metabolism	Liver, extensively
Excretion	Kidneys, unchanged; breast milk
Half-life	1-2 hr

Pharmacodynamics	
Onset	½ hr
Peak	Unknown
Duration	2-4 hr

Interactions
Individual drugs
Lithium: ↑ antithyroid effect
Potassium iodide: ↑ antithyroid effect
Radiation: ↑ bone marrow depression
Drug classifications
Antineoplastics: ↑ bone marrow depression
Phenothiazines: ↑ granulocytosis

Lab test interferences

↑ Pro-time, ↑ AST (SGOT), ↑ ALT (SGPT), ↑ alkaline phosphatase

NURSING CONSIDERATIONS

Assessment

- Monitor pulse, B/P, temp; check I&O ratio; check for edema (puffy hands, feet, periorbits); indicates hypothyroidism
- Check weight qd; same clothing, scale, time of day
- Monitor T_3, T_4, which are increased; serum TSH, which is decreased; free thyroxine index, which is increased if dosage is too low; discontinue drug 3-4 wk before RAIU
- Monitor blood work: CBC for blood dyscrasias (leukopenia, thrombocytopenia, agranulocytosis); liver function tests
- ❗ Assess for overdose (peripheral edema, heat intolerance, diaphoresis, palpitations, dysrhythmias, severe tachycardia, increased temp, delirium, CNS irritability); drug should be discontinued
- Assess for hypersensitivity (rash, enlarged cervical lymph nodes); drug may have to be discontinued
- Assess for hypoprothrombinemia (bleeding, petechiae, ecchymosis)
- Monitor clinical response: after 3 wk should include increased weight, pulse, decreased T_4
- Assess for bone marrow depression: sore throat, fever, fatigue

Nursing diagnoses

✓ Knowledge deficit (teaching)
✓ Noncompliance (teaching)

Implementation

- Give with meals to decrease GI upset; give at same time each day to maintain drug level
- Give lowest dosage that relieves symptoms
- Store in light-resistant container
- Increase fluids to 3-4 L/day, unless contraindicated

Patient/family education

- Advise patient to abstain from breastfeeding after delivery; drug appears in breast milk
- Instruct patient to take pulse daily; to keep graph of weight, pulse, mood
- Advise patient to report redness, swelling, sore throat, mouth lesions, which indicate blood dyscrasias
- Caution patient to avoid OTC products that contain iodine; that seafood and other iodine-containing products may be restricted by prescriber
- Caution patient not to discontinue this medication abruptly; thyroid crisis may occur; stress patient compliance
- Advise patient that response may take several mo if thyroid is large
- Teach patient symptoms/signs of overdose: periorbital edema, cold intolerance, mental depression; notify prescriber at once
- Teach patient symptoms of inadequate dosage: tachycardia, diarrhea, fever, irritability; prescriber should be notified to adjust
- Teach patient to take medication exactly as prescribed, not to skip or double doses; missed doses should be taken

M

when remembered up to 1 hr before next dose
- Instruct patient to carry identification (Medic Alert) describing medication taken and condition being treated

Evaluation

Positive therapeutic outcome
- Decreased weight gain
- Decreased pulse
- Decreased T_4
- Decreased B/P

methocarbamol (℞)
(meth-oh-kar'ba-mole)
Delaxin, Marbaxin 750, methocarbamol, Robaxin, Robaxin-750, Robomol-500, Robomol-750, Tresortil ✦
Func. class.: Skeletal muscle relaxant, central acting
Chem. class.: Carbamate derivative
Pregnancy category C

Action: Depresses multisynaptic pathways in the spinal cord, causing skeletal muscle relaxation

➡ **Therapeutic Outcome:** Decreased pain, spasm

Uses: Adjunct for relief of spasm and pain in musculoskeletal conditions, tetanus management

Dosage and routes

Pain of muscle spasm
Adult: PO 1.5 g × 2-3 days, then 1 g qid; IM 500 mg in each gluteal region; may repeat q8h; **IV** bol 1-3 g/day at 3 ml/min; **IV** inf 1 g/250 ml D_5W or NS, not to exceed 3 g/day

Tetanus
Adult: **IV** inf 1-3 g/L of sol q6h; **IV** bol 1-2 g injected into running **IV**
P ***Child:*** **IV** 15 mg/kg q6h

Available forms: Tabs 500, 750 mg; inj 100 mg/ml

Adverse effects
CNS: Dizziness, weakness, drowsiness, headache, tremor, depression, insomnia, ***seizures***
CV: Postural hypotension, bradycardia
EENT: Diplopia, temporary loss of vision, blurred vision, nystagmus
GI: Nausea, vomiting, hiccups, anorexia, metallic taste
GU: Brown, black, green urine
HEMA: Hemolysis, increased hemoglobin (**IV** only)
INTEG: Rash, pruritus, fever, facial flushing, urticaria

Contraindications: Hypersensitivity, P child <12 yr, intermittent porphyria

Precautions: Renal disease, hepatic disease, addictive personalities, pregnancy **C,** myasthenia gravis, epilepsy

Pharmacokinetics

Absorption	Rapidly absorbed (PO)
Distribution	Widely distributed; crosses placenta
Metabolism	Liver, partially
Excretion	Kidney, unchanged
Half-life	1-2 hr

Pharmacodynamics

	PO	IM	IV
Onset	½ hr	Rapid	Rapid
Peak	1-2 hr	Unknown	Inf end
Duration	>8 hr	Unknown	Unknown

Interactions

Individual drugs
Alcohol: CNS depression

Drug classifications
Antidepressants, tricyclic: ↑ CNS depression
Barbiturates: ↑ CNS depression
Narcotics: ↑ CNS depression
Sedative/hypnotics: ↑ CNS depression
Lab test interferences
False ↑ VMA, false ↑ urinary 5 HIAA

NURSING CONSIDERATIONS

Assessment

- Assess for pain and spasm: location, duration, intensity, range of motion
- Monitor during and after inj: CNS effects, rash, conjunctivitis, and nasal congestion may occur
- Monitor ECG in epileptic patients; poor seizure control has occurred in patients taking this drug
- Assess allergic reactions: rash, fever, respiratory distress; check for severe weakness, numbness in extremities
- Assess for tolerance: increased need for medication, more frequent requests for medication, increased pain
- Assess for CNS depression: dizziness, drowsiness, psychiatric symptoms

Nursing diagnoses

✓ Physical mobility, impaired (uses)
✓ Injury, risk for (adverse reactions)
✓ Knowledge deficit (teaching)

Implementation

PO route

- Give with meals if GI symptoms occur
- Store in tight container at room temp

IV **IV route**

- Give **IV** undiluted over 1 min or more; give 300 mg or less/1 min or longer; may be diluted in 250 ml or less D_5 or isotonic NaCl sol
- Give by slow **IV** to prevent phlebitis; keep recumbent for 15 min to prevent orthostatic hypotension; check for extravasation

IM route

- Give deep in large muscle mass; rotate sites

Patient/family education

- Advise patient not to discontinue medication quickly; insomnia, nausea, headache, spasticity, tachycardia will occur; drug should be tapered off over 1-2 wk
- Inform patient that urine may turn green, black, or brown
- Caution patient not to take with alcohol, other CNS depressants; increased CNS depression can occur
- Advise patient to avoid altering activities while taking this drug
- Caution patient to avoid hazardous activities if drowsiness, dizziness occur; driving should be avoided until drug response is known
- Advise patient to avoid using OTC medications that are CNS depressants (cough preparations, antihistamines) unless directed by prescriber; CNS depression can occur

Evaluation

Positive therapeutic outcome

- Decreased pain, spasticity

Treatment of overdose:

Induce emesis in conscious patient; lavage, dialysis; have epinephrine, antihistamines, and corticosteroids available

M

methohexital (℞)

(meth-oh-hex′i-tal)

Brevital Sodium, Brietal Sodium ✱

Func. class.: General anesthetic

Chem. class.: Barbiturate

Pregnancy category C

Controlled substance schedule IV

Action: Acts in reticular activating system in the CNS to produce anesthesia; may be potentiated by GABA

➔ **Therapeutic Outcome:** Anesthesia

Uses: General anesthesia for electroshock therapy, reduction of fractures, adjunct with other anesthetics, balanced anesthesia

Dosage and routes

Induction

P ***Adult and child:*** **IV** 50-120 mg given 1 ml/5 sec

Maintenance

P ***Adult and child:*** **IV** 20-40 mg q4-7 min of a 0.1% sol

Available forms: Powder for inj 500 mg, 2.5, 5g; powder for inj 10mg/ml ✱

Adverse effects

CNS: Retrograde amnesia, prolonged somnolence, seizures

CV: Tachycardia, hypotension, ***myocardial depression, dysrhythmias***

EENT: Sneezing, coughing

GI: Nausea, vomiting, abdominal pain, hiccups

INTEG: Chills, ***shivering***, necrosis, pain at inj site

MS: Muscle irritability

RESP: Respiratory depression, bronchospasm, **dyspnea**

Contraindications: Hypersensitivity, status asthmaticus, hepatic/intermittent porphyrias

Precautions: Severe cardiovascular disease, renal disease, pregnancy **C**, hypotension, liver disease, myxedema, myasthenia gravis, asthma, increased intracranial pressure

Pharmacokinetics

Absorption	Well absorbed (IM); completely absorbed (IV)
Distribution	Fatty tissues
Metabolism	Liver, kidneys, brain
Excretion	Kidneys, breast milk
Half-life	4 hr; increased in elderly

Pharmacodynamics

	IM	IV
Onset	Unknown	30-40 sec
Peak	Unknown	Unknown
Duration	Unknown	6 min

Interactions

Individual drugs

Alcohol: ↑ action, CNS depression

Drug classifications

Analgesics, narcotics: ↑ action, CNS depression

Antihistamines: ↑ action, CNS depression

CNS depressants: ↑ action, CNS depression

NURSING CONSIDERATIONS

Assessment

- Monitor VS q10 min during **IV** administration, q30 min after IM dose
- Assess for hallucinations, delusions, separation from environment
- Assess for extrapyramidal reactions: dystonia, akathisia
- Check for increasing heart rate or decreasing B/P; notify prescriber at once

Nursing diagnoses
✓ Sensory-perceptual alterations (adverse reactions)
✓ Knowledge deficit (teaching)

Implementation
IV **IV route**
- Give by direct **IV** at 10 mg/5 sec or more
- Give by cont inf by reconstituting 2.5 g/15 ml or 5 g/30 ml sterile water, 0.9% NaCl, D_5W

Syringe incompatibility: Glycopyrrolate

Additive incompatibilities: Atropine, chlorpromazine, cimetidine, clindamycin, droperidol, fentanyl, hydralazine, kanamycin, lidocaine, mechlorethamine, metaraminol, methicillin, methyldopate, metocurine, oxytetracycline, pancuronium, penicillin G potassium, pentazocine, prochlorperazine, promazine, promethazine, propiomazine, scopolamine, succinylcholine, streptomycin, tetracycline, tubocurarine

Patient/family education
- Instruct patient to avoid CNS depressants for 24 hr after methohexital
- Teach patient reason for medication and expected results

Evaluation
Positive therapeutic outcome
- Maintenance of anesthesia

methotrexate (℞)
(meth-oh-trex'ate)
Amethopterin, Folex PFS, methotrexate, methotrexate LPF, Rheumatrex Dose Pack
Func. class.: Antineoplastic, antimetabolite
Chem. class.: Folic acid antagonist
Pregnancy category X

Action: Inhibits an enzyme that reduces folic acid, which is needed for nucleic acid synthesis in all cells; S phase of cell cycle specific; immunosuppressive

➔ **Therapeutic Outcome:** Prevention of rapidly growing malignant cells; immunosuppression

Uses: Acute lymphocytic leukemia, in combination for breast, lung, head, neck carcinoma, lymphosarcoma, gestational choriocarcinoma, hydatidiform mole, psoriasis, rheumatoid arthritis, mycosis fungoides

Dosage and routes
Leukemia
P ***Adult and child:*** PO 3.3 $mg/m^2/day$ given with prednisone IT 12 mg/m^2; maintenance 30 $mg/m^2/day$ 2 times a wk; **IV** 2.5 mg/kg q2 wk

Choriocarcinoma
P ***Adult and child:*** PO 15-30 mg/m^2 qd × 5 days, then off 1 wk; may repeat

Osteosarcoma
P ***Adult and child:*** **IV** 12 g/m^2 given over 4 hr, then leucovorin rescue is given

Mycosis fungoides
Adult: PO 2.5-10 mg/day

M

until cleared (may be many mo); IM 50 mg q wk or 25 mg 2 times a wk

Psoriasis

Adult: PO/IM/**IV** 10 mg q wk; may increase to 25 mg q wk

Available forms: Tab 2.5 mg; inj 25 mg/ml; powder for inj 20, 25, 50, 100, 250 mg/g; sodium inj 2.5, 25 mg/ml

Adverse effects

CNS: Dizziness, ***convulsions,*** headache, confusion, hemiparesis, malaise, fatigue, chills, fever

GI: Nausea, vomiting, anorexia, diarrhea, stomatitis, ***hepatotoxicity,*** cramps, ulcer, gastritis, ***GI hemorrhage,*** abdominal pain, hematemesis

GU: Urinary retention, ***renal failure,*** menstrual irregularities, defective spermatogenesis, ***hematuria, azotemia, uric acid nephropathy***

HEMA: ***Leukopenia, thrombocytopenia, myelosuppression, anemia***

INTEG: Rash, alopecia, dry skin, urticaria, photosensitivity, folliculitis, vasculitis, petechiae, ecchymosis, acne, alopecia

Contraindications: Hypersensitivity, leukopenia (<2500/mm^3), thrombocytopenia (<100,000/mm^3), anemia, psoriatic patients with severe renal/hepatic disease, pregnancy **X**

Precautions: Renal disease, lactation

Pharmacokinetics

Absorption	Well absorbed (GI)
Distribution	Widely distributed; crosses placenta
Metabolism	Not metabolized
Excretion	Kidneys, unchanged; breast milk (minimal)
Half-life	2-4 hr; increased in renal disease

Pharmacodynamics

	PO	IM/IV	IT
Onset	Unknown	Unknown	Unknown
Peak	1-4 hr	½-2 hr	Unknown
Duration	Unknown	Unknown	Unknown

Interactions

Individual drugs

Acyclovir: ↑ neurologic reactions (IT route)
Allopurinol: ↑ toxicity
Asparaginase: ↓ effects of methotrexate
Chloramphenicol: ↑ toxicity
Cyclophosphamide: ↑ cardiotoxicity, CHF
Phenylbutazone: ↑ toxicity,
Phenytoin: ↑ toxicity
Probenecid: ↑ toxicity
Radiation: ↑ toxicity, bone marrow suppression
Warfarin: ↑ or ↓ effect of warfarin

Drug classifications

Antineoplastics: ↑ toxicity, bone marrow suppression
Hepatotoxic agents: ↑ hepatotoxicity
Live virus vaccines: ↓ antibodies
Nephrotoxic drugs: ↑ toxicity
Nondepolarizing muscle relaxants: Reversal of neuromuscular blockade
NSAIDs: ↑ toxicity
Salicylates: ↑ toxicity
Sulfonylureas: ↑ toxicity
Tetracylines: ↑ toxicity

NURSING CONSIDERATIONS

Assessment

- Assess buccal cavity q8h for dryness, sores or ulceration, white patches, oral pain, bleeding, dysphagia; obtain prescription for viscous lidocaine (Xylocaine)
- Assess symptoms indicating severe allergic reaction: rash, pruritus, urticaria, purpuric skin lesions, itching, flushing
- Assess tachypnea, ECG changes, dyspnea, edema, fatigue; identify dyspnea, rales, unproductive cough, chest pain, tachypnea
- Monitor CBC, differential, platelet count weekly; withhold drug if WBC count is <4000/mm^3 or platelet count is <100,000/mm^3; notify prescriber of results if WBC <20,000/mm^3, platelets <150,000/mm^3
- Assess for increased uric acid levels, swelling, joint pain primarily in extremities; patient should be well hydrated to prevent urate deposits
- Monitor renal function studies: BUN, creatinine, serum uric acid, urine CrCl before and during therapy; check I&O ratio; report fall in urine output to <30 ml/hr
- Monitor temp q4h (may indicate beginning of infection)
- Monitor liver function tests before and during therapy (bilirubin, AST [SGOT], ALT [SGPT], LDH) as needed or monthly; check for yellowing of skin and sclera, dark urine, clay-colored stools, itchy skin, abdominal pain, fever, diarrhea (hepatotoxicity)
- Assess for bleeding: hematuria, stool guaiac, bruising or petechiae, mucosa or orifices q8h; check for inflammation of mucosa, breaks in skin
- Identify effects of alopecia on body image; discuss feelings about body changes
- Identify edema in feet, joint and stomach pain, shaking; prescriber should be notified
- Identify inflammation of mucosa, breaks in skin

Nursing diagnoses

- ✓ Injury, risk for (adverse reactions)
- ✓ Body image disturbance (adverse reactions)
- ✓ Infection, risk for (adverse reactions)
- ✓ Knowledge deficit (teaching)

Implementation

- Avoid contact with skin, since drug is very irritating, wash completely to remove
- ◆ Administer leucovorin calcium within 12 hr of giving this drug to prevent tissue damage; check agency policy
- Give fluids **IV** or PO before chemotherapy to hydrate patient
- Give antacid before oral agent; give drug after evening meal, before hs; give antiemetic 30-60 min before giving drug and prn to prevent vomiting; administer antibiotics for prophylaxis of infection
- Give in AM so drug can be eliminated before hs
- Provide liq diet: carbonated beverages; gelatin may be added if patient is not nauseated or vomiting
- Encourage patient to rinse mouth tid-qid with water, club soda; brush teeth bid-qid with soft brush or cotton-tipped applicators for stomatitis; use unwaxed dental floss

PO route
• Give 1 hr ac or 2 hr pc to prevent vomiting

IM route
• Give deeply in large muscle mass

IV **IV route**
• Give **IV** after diluting 5 mg/2 ml of sterile water for inj; give through Y-tube or 3-way stopcock at 10 mg or less/min
• Give **IV** inf after diluting in 0.9% NaCl, D_5W, D_5/0.9% NaCl and give as prescribed

Syringe incompatibilities:
Droperidol, ranitidine

Syringe compatibilities:
Bleomycin, cisplatin, cyclophosphamide, doxapram, doxorubicin, fluorouracil, furosemide, leucovorin, mitomycin, vinblastine, vincristine

Y-site incompatibilities:
Droperidol, idarubicin

Y-site compatibilities:
Allopurinol, amifostine, asparaginase, aztreonam, bleomycin, cisplatin, cyclophosphamide, doxorubicin, etoposide, famotidine, filgrastim, fludarabine, fluorouracil, furosemide, granisetron, heparin, leucovorin, metoclopramide, melphalan, mitomycin, ondansetron, paclitaxel, sargramostim, teniposide, thiotepa, vancomycin, vinblastine, vincristine, vinorelbine

Additive incompatibilities:
Bleomycin, prednisolone

Additive compatibilities:
Cephalothin, cyclophosphamide, cytarabine, fluorouracil, hydroxyzine, mercaptopurine, ondansetron, sodium bicarbonate, vincristine

Solution compatibilities:
Amino acids, 4.25%/D_{25}, D_5W, sodium bicarbonate 0.05 mol/L

Patient/family education
• Advise patient that contraceptive measures are recommended during therapy; drug is teratogenic; contraception should be used for 3 mo (male) and 4-6 wk (female)
• Teach patient to avoid use of products containing aspirin or ibuprofen, razors, commercial mouthwash, since bleeding may occur; to report symptoms of bleeding (hematuria, tarry stools)
• Caution patient to report signs of anemia (fatigue, headache, irritability, faintness, shortness of breath)
• Advise patient to report any changes in breathing or coughing even several mo after treatment; to avoid crowds and persons with respiratory tract or other infections
• Teach patient that hair may be lost during treatment; a wig or hair piece may make patient feel better; new hair may be different in color, texture
• Caution patient not to have any vaccinations without the advice of the prescriber; serious reactions can occur

Evaluation

Positive therapeutic outcome
• Prevention of rapid division of malignant cells

methotrimeprazine (℞)

(meth-oh-trye-mep′ra-zeen)

Levoprome, Nozinan ✦

Func. class.: Nonopioid analgesic

Chem. class.: Aliphatic (propylamine phenothiazine derivative)

Pregnancy category C

Action: Depresses cerebral cortex, hypothalamus, limbic system; blocks neurotransmission produced by dopamine at synapse; exhibits strong α-adrenergic, anticholinergic blocking action; antihistamine

Therapeutic Outcome: Decreased pain; analgesia

Uses: Sedation, analgesia, preoperative and postoperative analgesia, obstetric analgesia in nonambulatory patients

Dosage and routes

Analgesia/sedation

P ***Adult and child >12 yr:*** IM 10-20 mg q4-6h prn

G ***Elderly:*** IM 5-10 mg q4-6h

Preoperative medication

P ***Adult and child >12 yr:*** IM 2-20 mg 45 min to 3 hr before surgery

Postoperative medication

P ***Adult and child >12 yr:*** IM 2.5-7.5 mg q4-6h titrated to patient's needs

Obstetric analgesia

Adult: 15-20 mg; may be repeated

Available forms: Inj 20 mg/ml

Adverse effects

CNS: Weakness, dizziness, drowsiness, confusion, delirium, euphoria, headache, sedation, EPS

CV: Orthostatic hypotension, palpitations, tachycardia, bradycardia

EENT: Nasal congestion, blurred vision, slurred speech

GI: Nausea, vomiting, abdominal pain, dry mouth, jaundice (long-term use)

GU: ***Hematuria,*** dysuria, hesitancy, retention, uterine inertia (rare)

HEMA: Thrombocytopenia, agranulocytosis, leukopenia, neutropenia, hemolytic anemia (long-term use, high dosage)

INTEG: Pain, edema at inj site, fever, chills

Contraindications: Hypersensitivity to this drug, phenothiazines, bisulfite; seizures, severe hepatic disease, severe renal disease, severe cardiac disease, coma

G **Precautions:** Elderly, pregnancy **C**

Pharmacokinetics	
Absorption	Well absorbed
Distribution	CSF, placenta
Metabolism	Liver, extensively; to active metabolites
Excretion	Kidneys, unchanged (1%)
Half-life	15-30 hr

Pharmacodynamics	
Onset	20-30 min
Peak	1-2 hr
Duration	4 hr

Interactions

Individual drugs

Alcohol: ↑ sedation, hypotension

Atropine: ↑ anticholinergic effect

Disopyramide: ↑ anticholinergic effect

M

Epinephrine: ↓ vasopressor effect
Meprobamate: ↑ sedation
Reserpine: ↑ sedation
Scopolamine: ↑ anticholinergic effect

Drug classifications

Antidepressants: ↑ CNS depression, anticholinergic effect
Antihistamines: ↑ CNS depression, anticholinergic effect
Antihypertensives: ↑ hypotension
MAOIs: ↑ hypotension
Narcotic analgesics: ↑ CNS depression
Nitrates: ↑ hypotension
Phenothiazines: ↑ anticholinergic effect
Sedatives/hypnotics: ↑ CNS depression

NURSING CONSIDERATIONS

Assessment

- Assess pain: location, duration, intensity
- Monitor blood counts during therapy; watch for decreasing platelets; if low, therapy may need to be discontinued, restarted after hematologic recovery; check for blood dyscrasia (thrombocytopenia): bruising, fatigue, bleeding, poor healing
- Assess for effect on uterine contractions, fetal heart tones if drug is used for labor
- Assess patient for EPS (akathisia, dystonia), since drug is a phenothiazine derivative

Nursing diagnoses

✓ Pain (uses)
✓ Injury, risk for (adverse reactions)
✓ Knowledge deficit (teaching)

Implementation

- Give after removal of cigarettes to prevent fires
- Give lowest dosage, then gradually increase; lower dosages are required after general anesthesia
- Provide bed rest for several hours after inj if orthostatic hypotension occurs
- Provide safety measures: low side rails, night light, call bell within easy reach if drowsiness or dizziness occurs

IM route

- Give deeply in large muscle mass; rotate inj sites; do not give by **IV** or SC inj
- Do not allow to come in contact with skin, contact dermatitis may occur
- Store in darkness; product expires after 5 yr

Syringe compatibilities: Atropine, hydroxyzine, metoclopramide, scopolamine

Syringe incompatibility: Ranitidine

Patient/family education

- Teach patient that drug must be continued for prescribed time to be effective; to avoid aspirin, alcoholic beverages and other CNS depressants
- Caution patient to report bleeding, bruising, fatigue, malaise, since blood dyscrasias do occur
- Instruct patient to use caution when driving; drowsiness, dizziness may occur; to ask for assistance with ambulation for 6 hr after inj

Evaluation

Positive therapeutic outcome

- Decreased pain
- Increased sedation

Treatment of overdose: Monitor electrolytes, VS

methyldopa/ methyldopate (℞)

(meth-ill-doe′pa)

Aldomet, methyldopa/ methyldopate HCl

Func. class.: Antihypertensive

Chem. class.: Centrally acting α-adrenergic inhibitor

Pregnancy category C

Action: Stimulates central α_2-adrenergic receptors in the CNS, resulting in decreased sympathetic outflow from the brain with decreased peripheral resistance

Therapeutic Outcome: Decreased B/P in hypertension

Uses: Hypertension

Dosage and routes

Adult: PO 250-500 mg bid or tid, then adjusted q2 days prn, 0.5-2 g qd in 2-4 divided doses (maintenance), not to exceed 3 g/day; **IV** 250-500 mg in 100 ml D_5W q6h, run over 30-60 min, not to exceed 1 g q6h

P ***Child:*** PO 10 mg/kg/day in 2-4 divided doses, not to exceed 65 mg/kg or 3 g/day, whichever is less; **IV** 20-40 mg/kg/day in 4 divided doses, not to exceed 65 mg/kg or 3g, whichever is less

Available forms: Methyldopa tabs 125, 250, 500 mg; oral susp 50 mg/ml; methydopate inj 50 mg/ml (250 mg/5 ml)

Adverse effects

CNS: Drowsiness, weakness, dizziness, sedation, headache, depression, psychosis, paresthesias, parkinsonism, Bell's palsy, nightmares

CV: Bradycardia, myocarditis, orthostatic hypotension, angina, edema, weight gain, CHF

EENT: Nasal congestion, eczema

GI: Nausea, vomiting, diarrhea, constipation, hepatic dysfunction, sore or "black" tongue, pancreatitis

GU: Impotence, failure to ejaculate

HEMA: ***Leukopenia, thrombocytopenia, hemolytic anemia, granulocytopenia,*** positive Coombs' test

INTEG: Lupuslike syndrome, rash, toxic epidural necrolysis

ENDO: Breast enlargement, gynecomastia, lactation, amenorrhea

Contraindications: Active hepatic disease, hypersensitivity, blood dyscrasias

Precautions: Pregnancy **C,** liver disease, eclampsia, severe cardiac disease

M

Pharmacokinetics

Absorption	50% (PO)
Distribution	Crosses placenta, blood-brain barrier
Metabolism	Liver, moderately
Excretion	Kidneys, unchanged (partially)
Half-life	1½ hr

Pharmacodynamics

	PO	IV
Onset	Unknown	Unknown
Peak	2-4 hr	2 hr
Duration	12-24 hr	10-16 hr

Interactions

Individual drugs

Alcohol: ↑ hypotension

Antidepressants, tricyclic: ↓ effects of methyldopa

Barbiturates: ↓ effects of methyldopa

Haloperidol: ↑ psychosis

Levodopa: ↑ hypotension, toxicity
Lithium: ↑ lithium toxicity
Tolbutamide: ↑ hypoglycemia

Drug classifications

Amphetamines: ↓ antihypertensive effect
Antihypertensives: ↑ hypotension
Antidepressants, tricyclic: ↓ antihypertensive effect
β-blockers: ↑ B/P
NSAIDs: ↓ antihypertensive effect
Nitrates: ↑ hypotension
Phenothiazines: ↓ antihypertensive effect

Lab test interferences

Interference: Urinary uric acid, serum creatinine, AST
False ↑ Urinary Catecholamines

NURSING CONSIDERATIONS

Assessment

- Monitor blood studies: neutrophils, decreased platelets
- Monitor renal studies: protein, BUN, creatinine; watch for increased levels that may indicate nephrotic syndrome: polyuria, oliguria, frequency
- Obtain baselines in renal, liver function tests before therapy begins; check potassium levels, although hyperkalemia rarely occurs
- Monitor B/P, pulse if the drug is being used for hypertension; notify prescriber of changes
- Monitor edema in feet, legs daily; monitor I&O; check weight for decreasing output
- Assess for allergic reaction: rash, fever, pruritus, urticaria; drug should be discontinued if antihistamines fail to help

Nursing diagnoses

✓ Cardiac output, decreased (uses)
✓ Injury, risk for (side effects)
✓ Knowledge deficit (teaching)
✓ Noncompliance (teaching)

Implementation

PO route

- Give ac
- Shake susp before using
- Store in tight container at room temp

IV **IV route**

- Give by intermittent inf after diluting in 100 ml 0.9% NaCl, D_5W, D_5/0.9% NaCl, 5% sodium bicarbonate, Ringer's sol; administer over 30-60 min

Y-site compatibilities:
Esmolol, heparin, meperidine, morphine, theophylline

Additive incompatibilities:
Amphotericin B, barbiturates, methohexital, sulfonamides

Additive compatibilities:
Aminophylline, ascorbic acid, chloramphenicol, diphenhydramine, heparin, magnesium sulfate, multivitamins, netilmicin, potassium chloride, promazine, sodium bicarbonate, succinylcholine, verapamil, vitamin B with C

Solution compatibilities:
D_5W, D_5/0.9% NaCl, Ringer's, sodium bicarbonate 5%, 0.9% NaCl, amino acids 4.25%/D_{25}, $Dextran_6$/0.9% NaCl, Normosol R, Normosol M/D_5W

Patient/family education

- Instruct patient not to discontinue drug abruptly, or withdrawal symptoms may occur: anxiety, increased B/P, headache, insomnia, increased pulse, tremors, nausea, sweating
- Caution patient not to use OTC (cough, cold, or allergy) products unless directed by prescriber

• Teach patient to comply with dosage schedule even if feeling better; drug controls symptoms, does not cure
• Caution patient to change position slowly, to rise slowly to sitting or standing position to minimize orthostatic hypotension, especially elderly
• Teach patient about excessive perspiration, dehydration, vomiting, diarrhea, may lead to fall in B/P; consult prescriber if these occur
• Advise patient that drug may cause dizziness, fainting; lightheadedness may occur during 1st few days of therapy; that drug may cause dry mouth; use hard candy, saliva product, or frequent rinsing of mouth
• Caution patient that compliance is necessary; not to skip or stop drug unless directed by prescriber
• Teach patient that drug may cause skin rash
• Teach patient to avoid hazardous activities, since drug may cause drowsiness, dizziness
• Teach patient to take ac

Evaluation
Positive therapeutic outcome
• Decreased B/P

Treatment of overdose: Gastric evacuation, sympathomimetics, may be indicated if severe-hemodialysis

methylergonovine (℞)
(meth-ill-er-goe-noe'veen)
Methergine, Methylergobasine ✦, Methylergonovine
Func. class.: Oxytocic
Chem. class.: Ergot alkaloid
Pregnancy category C

Action: Stimulates uterine and vascular smooth muscle, causing contractions, decreased bleeding

Therapeutic Outcome: Absence of hemorrhage

Uses: Treatment of hemorrhage post partum or after abortion

Dosage and routes
Adult: IM 0.2 mg q2-5h, not to exceed 5 doses; **IV** 0.2 mg given over 1 min; PO 0.2 mg given over 1 min; PO 0.2-0.4 mg q6-12h × 2-7 days after initial IM or **IV** dose

Available forms: Inj 0.2 mg/ml; tab 0.2 mg

Adverse effects
CNS: Headache, dizziness
CV: Chest pain, palpitations, hypertension, *hypotension,* dysrhythmias
EENT: Tinnitus
GI: Nausea, vomiting
GU: Cramping
INTEG: Sweating, rash, allergic reactions
RESP: Dyspnea

Contraindications: Hypersensitivity to ergot preparations, indication of labor, before delivery of placenta, hypertension, pelvic inflammatory disease, respiratory disease, cardiac disease, peripheral vascular disease

Precautions: Pregnancy **C,** severe hepatic disease, severe renal disease, jaundice, diabetes mellitus, convulsive disorders

Pharmacokinetics

Absorption	Well absorbed (PO, IM)
Distribution	Unknown
Metabolism	Liver, possibly
Excretion	Unknown
Half-life	½-2 hr

Pharmacodynamics

	PO	IM	IV
Onset	5-15 min	5 min	Immediate
Peak	Unknown	Unknown	Unknown
Duration	3 hr	3 hr	Unknown

Interactions

Individual drugs

Cyclopropane anesthesia: ↑ hypotension

Drug classifications

Vasopressors: ↑ hypertension

Smoking

↑ vasoconstriction

NURSING CONSIDERATIONS

Assessment

- Monitor B/P, pulse; watch for change that may indicate hemorrhage; check respiratory rate, rhythm, depth; notify prescriber of abnormalities
- Assess fundal tone, nonphasic contractions; check for relaxation or severe cramping
- Assess for ergotism or overdose: nausea, vomiting, weakness, muscular pain, insensitivity to cold, paresthesia of extremities; drug should be decreased or inf discontinued
- Before administering ergonovine, check calcium levels; if hypocalcemia is present, correction should be made to increase effectiveness of this drug
- Monitor prolactin levels and for decreased breast milk production

Nursing diagnoses

- ✓ Tissue perfusion, decreased (uses)
- ✓ Injury, risk for (adverse reactions)
- ✓ Knowledge deficit (teaching)

Implementation

PO route

- PO is the preferred route

IM route

- Give deeply in large muscle mass

IV **IV route**

- Give by this route for severe, life-threatening hemorrhage
- Give directly undiluted or diluted with 5 ml 0.9% NaCl given through Y-site or 3-way stopcock; give 0.2 mg/min; use clear, colorless sol
- Store up to 2 mo if unused

Y-site compatibilities: Heparin, hydrocortisone sodium succinate, potassium chloride, vitamin B with C

Patient/family education

- Advise patient to stop smoking, since increased vasoconstriction will result
- Inform patient that abdominal cramps are a side effect of this medication
- Instruct patient to notify prescriber if chest pain, nausea, vomiting, headache, muscle pain, weakness or cold, numb extremities occur

Evaluation

Positive therapeutic outcome

- Prevention of hemorrhage

methylphenidate 🔑 (℞)

(meth-ill-fen′i-date)

Methidate, Ritalin, Ritalin SR

Func. class.: Cerebral stimulant

Chem. class.: Piperidine derivative

Pregnancy category C

Controlled substance schedule II

Action: Increases release of norepinephrine and dopamine in cerebral cortex to reticular activating system; exact action not known

Therapeutic Outcome: Increased alertness, decreased fatigue, ability to stay awake (narcolepsy), increased attention span, decreased hyperactivity (ADHD)

Uses: Attention deficit disorder with hyperactivity, narcolepsy

Investigational uses: Depression in the elderly, cancer, stroke

Dosage and routes

ADHD

Adult: PO 5-20 bid-tid

Child >6 yr: PO 5 mg before breakfast and lunch, increasing by 5-10 mg/wk, not to exceed 60 mg/day

Narcolepsy

Adult: PO 10 mg bid-tid, 30-45 min ac; may increase up to 40-60 mg/day

Available forms: Tabs 5, 10, 20 mg; sus rel tab 20 mg

Adverse effects

CNS: Hyperactivity, insomnia, restlessness, talkativeness, dizziness, headache, akathisia, dyskinesia, Gilles de la Tourette's syndrome

CV: Palpitations, tachycardia, B/P changes, angina, dysrhythmias, ***thrombocytopenic purpura***

ENDO: Growth retardation

GI: Nausea, anorexia, dry mouth, weight loss, abdominal pain

*GU: **Uremia***

HEMA: Leukopenia, anemia

*INTEG: **Exfoliative dermatitis**,* urticaria, rash, erythema multiforme

MISC: Fever, arthralgia, scalp hair loss

Contraindications: Hypersensitivity, anxiety, history of Gilles de la Tourette's syndrome; children <6 yr, glaucoma

Precautions: Hypertension, depression, pregnancy **C**, seizures, lactation, drug abuse

Pharmacokinetics

Absorption	Well absorbed (PO); delayed (sus rel)
Distribution	Widely distributed; crosses placenta
Metabolism	Liver
Excretion	Kidneys
Half-life	1-3 hr

Pharmacodynamics

	PO	PO–SUS REL
Onset	½-1 hr	2 hr
Peak	1-3 hr	4 hr
Duration	4-6 hr	6-8 hr

Interactions

Drug classifications

Anticonvulsants: ↑ effects

Antidepressants, tricyclics: ↑ effects

MAOIs: Hypertensive crisis

Oral anticoagulants: ↑ effects

Sympathomimetics: ↑ effects

Vasopressors: Hypertensive crisis

NURSING CONSIDERATIONS

Assessment

- Monitor VS, B/P, since this drug may reverse antihypertensives; check patients with cardiac disease more often for increased B/P
- Perform CBC, urinalysis; for diabetic patients monitor blood sugar, urine sugar; insulin changes may be required, since eating will decrease
- Monitor height and weight q3 mo since growth rate in P children may be decreased; appetite is suppressed, weight loss is common during the first few mo of treatment
- Monitor mental status: mood sensorium, affect, stimulation, insomnia; aggressiveness may occur; depression with crying spells may occur after drug has worn off
- Assess for tolerance; should not be used for extended time except in ADHD; dosage should be discontinued gradually to prevent withdrawal symptoms
- Assess for narcoleptic symptoms before medication and after; ability to stay awake should increase significantly
- P In children or adults with ADHD, monitor for improved organizational skills, attention span, attending to tasks, impulse control, socialization, and ability to get along better with others
- Assess for withdrawal symptoms: headache, nausea, vomiting, muscle pain, weakness; drug tolerance will develop after long-term use; dosage should not be increased if tolerance develops
- Assess appetite, sleep, speech patterns

Nursing diagnoses

- ✓ Thought processes, altered (uses, adverse reactions)
- ✓ Coping, ineffective individual (uses)
- ✓ Knowledge deficit (teaching)
- ✓ Family coping, impaired (uses)

Implementation

- Give at least 6 hr before hs to avoid sleeplessness; titrate to patient's response; lowest dosage should be used to control symptoms
- Do not chew, crush time-rel tabs
- Give gum, hard candy, frequent sips of water for dry mouth at beginning of treatment; these symptoms tend to lessen with time

Patient/family education

- Teach patient to decrease caffeine consumption (coffee, tea, cola, chocolate), which may increase irritability and stimulation; to avoid OTC preparations unless approved by prescriber; to avoid alcohol ingestion; these may cause serious drug interactions
- Advise patient to taper off drug over several wk, or depression, increased sleeping, lethargy may occur
- Caution patient to avoid hazardous activities until stabilized on medication
- Instruct patient not to double doses if medication is missed; prescriber may suggest drug holidays (ADHD) during the school year to assess progress and determine continued drug necessity
- Instruct patient/family to notify presciber if significant side effects occur: tremors, insomnia, palpitations,

restlessness; drug changes may be needed
• Inform patient that if dry mouth occurs to use frequent sips of water, sugarless gum, hard candy during beginning therapy; dry mouth lessens with continued treatment
• Encourage patient to get needed rest; patients will feel more tired at end of day; to take last dose at least 6 hr before hs to avoid insomnia

Evaluation

Positive therapeutic outcome
• Decreased activity in ADHD
• Improved attention span in ADHD
• Absence of sleeping during day in narcolepsy

Treatment of overdose: Administer fluids, hemodialysis, peritoneal dialysis, antihypertensives for increased B/P

methylprednisolone/ methylprednisolone acetate/ methylprednisolone sodium succinate (℞)

(meth-ill-pred-niss′oh-lone)

Medrol/Depo-Medrol, Duralone, Medralone, Rep-Pred/A-Methapred, Solu-Medrol

Func. class.: Corticosteroid

Chem. class.: Glucocorticoid, immediate acting

Pregnancy category C

Action: Decreases inflammation by suppression of migration of polymorphonuclear leukocytes, fibroblasts; reverses increased capillary permeability and lysosomal stabilization; antipruritic, antiinflammatory (top)

Therapeutic Outcome: Decreased inflammation

Uses: Severe inflammation, shock, adrenal insufficiency, collagen disorders, psoriasis, eczema, contact dermatitis, pruritus (top)

Dosage and routes

Adrenal insufficiency/ inflammation

Adult: PO 2-60 mg in 4 divided doses; IM 40-80 mg (acetate); IM/**IV** 10-250 mg (succinate); intraarticular 4-30 mg (acetate)

P ***Child:*** **IV** 117 μg-1.66 mg/kg in 3-4 divided doses (succinate)

Shock

Adult: **IV** 100-250 mg q2-6h (succinate)

Pruritus

P ***Adult and child:*** TOP apply to affected area qd-qid

Available forms: Tabs 2, 4, 6, 8, 16, 24, 32 mg; inj 20, 40, 80 mg/ml acetate; inj 40, 125, 500, 1000 mg/vial succinate; oint 0.25%, 1%

Adverse effects

CNS: Depression, flushing, sweating, headache, mood changes
CV: Hypertension, ***circulatory collapse, thrombophlebitis, embolism,*** tachycardia
EENT: Fungal infections, increased intraocular pressure, blurred vision
GI: Diarrhea, nausea, abdominal distention, GI hemorrhage, increased appetite, pancreatitis
HEMA: ***Thrombocytopenia***
INTEG: Burning, dryness, itching, irritation, acne, follicu-

M

litis, hypertrichosis, perioral dermatitis, hypopigmentation, atrophy, striae, miliaria, allergic contact dermatitis, secondary infection, poor wound healing, ecchymosis, petechiae
MS: Fractures, osteoporosis, weakness

Contraindications: Hypersensitivity to corticosteroids, fungal infections, psychosis, idiopathic thrombocytopenia, acute glomerulonephritis, amebiasis, nonasthmatic bronchial disease, **P** child <2 yr, AIDS, TB

Precautions: Pregnancy **C**, lactation, viral or bacterial infections, diabetes mellitus, glaucoma, osteoporosis

Pharmacokinetics

Absorption	Well absorbed (PO); systemic (top)
Distribution	Crosses placenta
Metabolism	Liver, extensively
Excretion	Kidney
Half-life	3-5 hr; adrenal suppression 3-4 days

Pharmacodynamics

	PO	IM	IV	TOP
Onset	Unknown	Unknown	Rapid	Min to hr
Peak	2 hr	4-8 days	Unknown	Hr to days
Duration	1½ days	1-4 wk	Unknown	Hr to days

Interactions

Individual drugs

Amphotericin B: ↑ hypokalemia
Insulin: ↑ need for insulin
Mezlocillin: ↑ hypokalemia
Phenytoin: ↓ action, ↑ metabolism
Rifampin: ↓ action, ↑ metabolism
Ticarcillin: ↑ hypokalemia

Drug classifications

Barbiturates: ↓ action, ↑ metabolism
Diuretics: ↑ hypokalemia
Hypoglycemic agents: ↑ need for hypoglycemic agents

Lab test interferences

↑ Cholesterol, ↑ sodium, ↑ blood glucose, ↑ uric acid, ↑ calcium, ↑ urine glucose
↓ Calcium, ↓ potassium, ↓ T_4, ↓ T_3, ↓ thyroid RAIU test, ↓ urine 17-OHCS, ↓ 17-KS, ↓ PBI
False negative: Skin allergy tests

NURSING CONSIDERATIONS

Assessment

- Monitor potassium, blood sugar, urine glucose while patient is on long-term therapy; hypokalemia and hyperglycemia
- Monitor weight daily; notify prescriber of weekly gain >5 lb
- Monitor B/P q4h, pulse; notify prescriber if chest pain occurs
- Monitor I&O ratio; be alert for decreasing urinary output and increasing edema
- Monitor plasma cortisol levels during long-term therapy (normal level 138-635 nmol/L when drawn at 8 AM)
- Monitor adrenal function periodically for HPA axis suppression
- Assess for infection: increased temp, WBC even after withdrawal of medication; drug masks infection symptoms
- Assess for potassium depletion: paresthesias, fatigue, nausea, vomiting, depression, polyuria, dysrhythmias, weakness
- Assess for edema, hypertension, cardiac symptoms
- Assess mental status: affect,

mood, behavioral changes, aggression
• Check temp; if fever develops, drug should be discontinued
• Assess for syst absorption: increased temp, inflammation, irritation (top)

Nursing diagnoses

✓ Infection, risk for (adverse reactions)
✓ Knowledge deficit (teaching)
✓ Noncompliance (teaching)

Implementation

IV **IV route**
• Give **IV**, use only sodium phosphate product; give >1 min; may be given by **IV** inf in compatible sol
• Give after shaking susp (parenteral)
• Give titrated dosage; use lowest effective dosage

Y-site compatibilities: Acyclovir, allopurinol, amifostine, amrinone, aztreonam, cefepime, cisplatin, cyclophosphamide, enalaprilat, famotidine, fludarabine, heparin, melphalan, meperidine, midazolam, morphine, tacrolimus, teniposide, theophylline, thiotepa, vitamin B with C

Y-site incompatibilities: Ondansetron, paclitaxel, sargramostim, vinorelbine

Syringe compatibility: Metoclopramide

Additive compatibilities: Aminophylline, chloramphenicol, cimetidine, clindamycin, dopamine, granisetron, heparin, ranitidine, theophylline

IM route
• Give IM inj deep in large muscle mass; rotate sites; avoid deltoid; use 21 G needle
• Give in one dose in AM to prevent adrenal suppression; avoid SC administration; may damage tissue

PO route
• Give with food or milk to decrease GI symptoms

Inh route
• Give inh with water to decrease possibility of fungal infections
• Give titrated dosage; use lowest effective dosage
• Clean aerosol top daily with warm water; dry thoroughly
• Store in cool environment; do not puncture or incinerate container

Top route
• Cleanse area before applying drug
• Apply only to affected areas; do not get in eyes
• Apply medication, then cover with occlusive dressing (only if prescribed); seal to normal skin; change q12h; syst absorption may occur
• Apply only to dermatoses; do not use on weeping, denuded, or infected area
• Apply treatment for a few days after area has cleared
• Store at room temp

Patient/family education

• Teach patient that ID as steroid user should be carried
• Advise patient to notify prescriber if therapeutic response decreases; dosage adjustment may be needed
• Caution patient not to discontinue abruptly; adrenal crisis can result
• Caution patient to avoid OTC products: salicylates, alcohol in cough products, cold preparations unless directed by prescriber
• Teach patient all aspects of drug usage including cushingoid symptoms

M

• Teach patient symptoms of adrenal insufficiency: nausea, anorexia, fatigue, dizziness, dyspnea, weakness, joint pain
• Inform patient that long-term therapy may be needed to clear infection (1-2 mo depending on type of infection)

Nasal route
• Advise patient to clear nasal passages if sneezing attack occurs; repeat dose
• Advise patient to continue using product even if mild nasal bleeding occurs; is usually transient
• Teach patient method of instillation after providing written instructions from manufacturer

Top route
• Advise patient to avoid sunlight on affected area; burns may occur

Evaluation
Positive therapeutic outcome
• Ease of respirations, decreased inflammation
• Absence of severe itching, patches on skin, flaking (top)

methysergide (℞)
(meth-i-ser′jide)
Sansert
Func. class.: Serotonin antagonist
Chem. class.: Ergot derivative
Pregnancy category C

Action: Competitively blocks serotonin hydroxytryptamine receptors in CNS and periphery; potent vasoconstrictor

Therapeutic Outcome: Absence of migraines and other vascular headaches

Uses: Prophylaxis for migraine and other vascular headaches

Dosage and routes
Adult: PO 2 mg bid with meals

Available forms: Tab 2 mg

Adverse effects
CNS: ***Tremors, anxiety,*** insomnia, headache, dizziness, euphoria, confusion, depersonalization, hallucinations, paresthesias, drowsiness
CV: ***Retroperitoneal fibrosis,*** valvular thickening, palpitations, tachycardia, postural hypertension, angina, thrombophlebitis, ECG changes, ***cardiac fibrosis***
GI: Nausea, vomiting, weight gain
HEMA: ***Blood dyscrasias***
INTEG: Flushing, rash, alopecia
MS: Arthralgia, myalgia

Contraindications: Hypersensitivity to ergot, tartrazine, peripheral vascular occlusion, CAD, hepatic disease, renal disease, peptic ulcer, hypertension, connective tissue disease, fibrotic pulmonary disease

Precautions: Pregnancy **C**, P lactation, children

Pharmacokinetics	
Absorption	Rapidly absorbed
Distribution	Widely distributed
Metabolism	Liver
Excretion	Kidneys, breast milk
Half-life	10 hr

Pharmacodynamics
Unknown

Interactions
Drug classifications
β-Blockers: ↑ vasoconstriction
Narcotic analgesics: ↓ effect of narcotics
Smoking
↑ vasoconstriction

NURSING CONSIDERATIONS
Assessment
- Monitor stress level, activity, reaction, coping mechanisms of patient
- Assess neurologic status: LOC, blurring vision, nausea, vomiting, tingling in extremities preceding headache
- Assess for ingestion of tyramine-containing foods (pickled products, beer, wine, aged cheese), food additives, preservatives, colorings, artificial sweeteners, chocolate, caffeine, which may precipitate these types of headaches

Nursing diagnoses
✓ Pain, chronic (uses)
✓ Injury, risk for (adverse reactions)
✓ Knowledge deficit (teaching)

Implementation
- Provide quiet, calm environment with decreased stimulation; no noise, bright lights, or excessive talking
- Give with or pc to avoid GI symptoms
- Store in dark area

Patient/family education
- Caution patient to avoid OTC medications and alcohol; serious drug interactions may occur
- Caution patient to maintain dosage at approved level; not to increase even if drug does not relieve headache
- Advise patient that an increase in headaches may occur when this drug is discontinued after long-term use
- Caution patient to keep drug out of the reach of children; death may occur
- Caution patient to use drug for less than 6 mo unless a 3-4 wk rest period has been taken

Evaluation
Positive therapeutic outcome
- Decrease in frequency, severity of headache

metoclopramide (℞)
(met-oh-kloe-pra′mide)
Clopra, Emex ✦, Maxeran ✦, Maxolon, metoclopramide HCl, Octamide PFS, Reclomide, Reglan
Func. class.: Cholinergic, antiemetic
Chem. class.: Central dopamine receptor antagonist
Pregnancy category B

Action: Enhances response to acetylcholine of tissue in upper GI tract, which causes contraction of gastric muscle, relaxes pyloric, duodenal segments, increases peristalsis without stimulating secretions

Therapeutic Outcome: Decreased symptoms of delayed gastric emptying, decreased nausea, vomiting

Uses: Prevention of nausea, vomiting induced by chemotherapy, radiation; delayed gastric emptying, gastroesophageal reflux

Dosage and routes
Nausea/vomiting
Adult: **IV** 2 mg/kg q2h × 5

doses 30 min before administration of chemotherapy

Delayed gastric emptying
Adult: PO 10 mg 30 min ac, hs × 2-8 wk

Gastroesophageal reflux
Adult: PO 10-15 mg qid 30 min ac

Available forms: Tabs 5, 10 mg; syr 5 mg/5 ml; inj 5 mg/ml

Adverse effects
CNS: Sedation, fatigue, restlessness, headache, sleeplessness, dystonia, dizziness, drowsiness
CV: Hypotension, supraventricular tachycardia
GI: Dry mouth, constipation, nausea, anorexia, vomiting
GU: Decreased libido, prolactin secretion, amenorrhea, galactorrhea
INTEG: Urticaria, rash

Contraindications: Hypersensitivity to this drug or procaine or procainamide, seizure disorder, pheochromocytoma, breast cancer (prolactin dependent), GI obstruction

Precautions: Pregnancy **B**, lactation, GI hemorrhage, CHF

Pharmacokinetics

Absorption	Well absorbed (PO)
Distribution	Widely distributed; crosses blood-brain barrier, placenta
Metabolism	Liver, minimally
Excretion	Kidneys, breast milk
Half-life	4 hr

Pharmacodynamics

	PO	IM	IV
Onset	½-1 hr	10-15 min	1-3 min
Peak	Unknown	Unknown	Unknown
Duration	1-2 hr	1-2 hr	1-2 hr

Interactions
Individual drugs
Alcohol: ↓ action of metoclopramide
Haloperidol: ↑ extrapyramidal reaction
Drug classifications
Anticholinergics: ↓ action of metoclopramide
Antidepressants: ↑ CNS depression
Antihistamines: ↑ CNS depression
CNS depressants: ↑ sedation
MAOIs: ↑ catecholamine levels
Opiates: ↑ sedation
Phenothiazines: ↑ extrapyramidal reaction
Sedative/hypnotics: ↑ CNS depression
Lab test interferences
↑ Prolactin, ↑ aldosterone, ↑ thyrotropin

NURSING CONSIDERATIONS
Assessment
- Assess GI complaints: nausea, vomiting, anorexia, constipation, abdominal distention before and after administration
- Assess for EPS and tardive dyskinesia: rigidity, grimacing, shuffling gait, tremors, rhythmic involuntary movements of tongue, mouth, jaw, feet, hands; these side effects should be reported to prescriber immediately; some effects may be irreversible
- Assess mental status: depression, anxiety, irritability during treatment

Nursing diagnoses
✓ Injury, risk for (adverse reactions)
✓ Knowledge deficit (teaching)

Implementation
IV route
- Give **IV** undiluted if dose is <10 mg; give over 2 min

• Dilute 10 mg or more in 50 ml or more D_5W, NaCl, Ringer's, LR and given over 15 min or more
• Discard open ampules

Syringe compatibilities: Aminophylline, ascorbic acid, atropine, benztropine, bleomycin, chlorpromazine, cisplatin, cyclophosphamide, cytarabine, dexamethasone, dimenhydrinate, diphenhydramine, doxorubicin, droperidol, fentanyl, fluorouracil, heparin, hydrocortisone, hydroxyzine, regular insulin, leucovorin, lidocaine, magnesium sulfate, meperidine, methylprednisolone, midazolam, mitomycin, morphine, pentazocine, perphenazine, prochlorperazine, promazine, promethazine, ranitidine, scopolamine, vinblastine, vincristine

Syringe incompatibilities: Ampicillin, calcium gluconate, cephalothin, chloramphenicol, furosemide, penicillin G potassium, sodium bicarbonate

Y-site incompatibility: Furosemide

Additive compatibilities: Clindamycin, multivitamins, potassium acetate/chloride/phosphate, verapamil

Additive incompatibilities: Cisplatin, erythromycin, tetracycline

Y-site compatibilities: Aldesleukin, amifostine, thiotepa

PO route
• Give 30-60 min ac for better absorption and at hs
• Use gum, hard candy, frequent rinsing of mouth for dryness of oral cavity

Patient/family education
• Instruct patient to avoid driving, other hazardous activities until stabilized on this medication
• Advise patient to avoid alcohol and other CNS depressants that enhance sedating properties of this drug
• Advise patient to notify prescriber if involuntary movements occur

Evaluation
Positive therapeutic outcome
• Absence of nausea, vomiting, anorexia, fullness

metocurine (℞)
(me-toe-cure'een)
Metubine
Func. class.: Neuromuscular blocker (nondepolarizing)
Chem. class.: Methyl analog of tubocurarine
Pregnancy category C

M

Action: Inhibits transmission of nerve impulses by binding with cholinergic receptor sites, antagonizing action of acetylcholine; no analgesic response

➔ **Therapeutic Outcome:** Paralysis of all skeletal muscles

Uses: Facilitation of endotracheal intubation, skeletal muscle relaxation during mechanical ventilation, surgery, or general anesthesia, reduction of fractures/dislocations

Dosage and routes
Surgery
***Adult:* IV** 2-4 mg if given cyclopropane as an anesthetic; 1.5-3 mg if given ether as an

anesthetic; 4-7 mg if given nitrous oxide

Electroconvulsive therapy adjunct
Adult: **IV** 2-3 mg

Available forms: Inj 2 mg/ml

Adverse effects
CV: Bradycardia, tachycardia, increased, decreased B/P
EENT: Increased secretions, salivation
INTEG: Rash, flushing, pruritus, urticaria
RESP: ***Prolonged apnea, bronchospasm, cyanosis, respiratory depression***

Contraindications: Hypersensitivity to iodides

Precautions: Pregnancy **C**, cardiac disease, hepatic disease, renal disease, lactation, P children <2 yr, electrolyte imbalances, dehydration, neuromuscular disease (myasthenia gravis), respiratory disease, when histamine release is a definite hazard (e.g., asthma)

Pharmacokinetics	
Absorption	Completely absorbed
Distribution	Widely distributed; crosses placenta
Metabolism	Plasma
Excretion	Kidneys, unchanged (50%)
Half-life	3½ hr

Pharmacodynamics	
Onset	2-2½ min
Peak	5 min
Duration	½-1½ hr

Interactions
Individual drugs
Clindamycin: ↑ paralysis length and intensity
Colistin: ↑ paralysis length and intensity
Lidocaine: ↑ paralysis length and intensity
Lithium: ↑ paralysis length and intensity
Magnesium sulfate: ↑ paralysis length and intensity
Polymyxin B: ↑ paralysis length and intensity
Procainamide: ↑ paralysis length and intensity
Quinidine: ↑ paralysis length and intensity
Succinylcholine: ↑ paralysis length and intensity
Drug classifications
Aminoglycosides: ↑ paralysis length and intensity
β-Blockers: ↑ paralysis length and intensity
Diuretics, potassium-losing: ↑ paralysis length and intensity
General anesthesia: ↑ paralysis length and intensity

NURSING CONSIDERATIONS
Assessment
- Monitor VS (B/P, pulse, respirations, airway) until fully recovered; rate, depth, pattern of respirations, strength of hand grip; patient should be intubated before use
- Monitor for electrolyte imbalances (potassium, magnesium) before drug is used; electrolyte imbalances may lead to increased action of this drug
- Monitor for recovery: decreased paralysis of face, diaphragm, leg, arm, rest of body; residual weakness and respiratory problems may occur during recovery period
- Assess for hypersensitive reactions: rash, fever, respiratory distress, pruritus; drug should be discontinued

Nursing diagnoses
✓ Breathing pattern, ineffective (uses)

☑ Communication, impaired verbal (adverse reactions)
☑ Fear (adverse reactions)
☑ Knowledge deficit (teaching)

Implementation

- Use peripheral nerve stimulator (anesthesiologist) to determine neuromuscular blockade; deep tendon reflexes should be monitored during extended periods
- Give direct **IV** undiluted over 1 min; may give doses of 0.5-1 mg titrated to patient response; should be administered only by qualified person, usually an anesthesiologist; do not administer IM
- Store in light-resistant container
- Give anticholinesterase to reverse neuromuscular blockade

Patient/family education

- Provide reassurance if communication is difficult during recovery from neuromuscular blockade
- Provide explanation to patients regarding all procedures or treatments; patient will remain conscious if anesthesia is not given also

Evaluation

Positive therapeutic outcome

- Paralysis of jaw, eyelid, head, neck, rest of body as evaluated by peripheral nerve stimulator

Treatment of overdose: Edrophonium or neostigmine, atropine, monitor VS; may require mechanical ventilation

metolazone (℞)

(me-tole'a-zone)

MyKrox, Zaroxolyn

Func. class.: Diuretic, antihypertensive

Chem. class.: Thiazide-like quinazoline derivative

Pregnancy category B

Action: Acts on the distal tubule and cortical thick ascending limb of the loop of Henle in the kidney, increasing excretion of sodium, water, chloride, magnesium, potassium, and bicarbonate

➔ **Therapeutic Outcome:** Decreased B/P, decreased edema in lung tissue and peripherally

Uses: Edema in CHF, nephrotic syndrome; may be used alone or as adjunct with antihypertensives for mild to moderate hypertension

Dosage and routes

Edema

Adult: PO 5-20 mg/day

Hypertension

Adult: PO 2.5-5 mg/day (Diulo, Zaroxolyn);
PO 0.5 mg (MyKrox) qd in AM: may increase to 1 mg

Available forms: MyKrox tab 0.5; Zaroxolyn 2.5, 5, 10 mg

Adverse effects

CNS: Drowsiness, paresthesia, anxiety, depression, headache, *dizziness, fatigue, weakness*
CV: Irregular pulse, orthostatic hypotension, palpitations, volume depletion, chest pain
EENT: Blurred vision
ELECT: Hypokalemia, hypercalcemia, hyponatremia, hypochloremia, hypomagnesemia, hypophosphatemia

M

GI: Nausea, vomiting, anorexia, constipation, diarrhea, cramps, pancreatitis, GI irritation, ***hepatitis***
GU: Frequency, polyuria, ***uremia,*** glucosuria
HEMA: ***Aplastic anemia, hemolytic anemia, leukopenia, agranulocytosis, neutropenia***
INTEG: Rash, urticaria, purpura, photosensitivity, fever
META: Hyperglycemia, hypomagnesemia, increased creatinine, BUN

Contraindications: Hypersensitivity to thiazides or sulfonamides, anuria, renal decompensation

Precautions: Hypokalemia, renal disease, hepatic disease, gout, COPD, lupus erythematosus, diabetes mellitus, elderly, pregnancy **B,** lactation

Pharmacokinetics	
Absorption	GI tract (10%-20%)
Distribution	Crosses placenta
Metabolism	Urine, unchanged
Excretion	Breast milk
Half-life	8 hr (extended); 14 hr (prompt)

Pharmacodynamics	
Onset	1 hr
Peak	2 hr
Duration	12-24 hr

Interactions
Individual drugs
Cholestyramine: ↓ absorption of metolazone
Colestipol: ↓ absorption of metolazone
Diazoxide: ↓ hyperglycemia, hyperuricemia, hypotension
Digitalis: ↑ toxicity
Indomethacin: ↓ hypotensive response
Lithium: ↑ toxicity
Mezlocillin: ↑ hypokalemia
Piperacillin: ↑ hypokalemia
Ticarcillin: ↑ hypokalemia
Drug classifications
Antidiabetics: ↓ effect of antidiabetic agent
Antihypertensives: ↑ antihypertensive effect
Cardiac glycosides: ↑ hypokalemia
Glucocorticoids: ↑ hypokalemia
Sulfonylureas: ↓ effect of sulfonylurea
Nondepolarizing skeletal muscle relaxants: ↑ toxicity
Food
↑ absorption
Lab test interferences
Interference: Urine steroid tests
↑ BSP retention, ↑ calcium, ↑ amylase, ↑ parathyroid test
↓ PBI, ↓ PSP

NURSING CONSIDERATIONS
Assessment
- Monitor glucose in urine if patient is diabetic
- Check for rashes, temp elevation qd
- Monitor patients that receive cardiac glycosides for increased hypokalemia
- Monitor manifestations of hypokalemia; acidic urine, reduced urine, osmolality, nocturia; hypotension, broad T wave, U wave, ectopy, tachycardia, weak pulse; muscle weakness, altered LOC, drowsiness, apathy, lethargy, confusion, depression; anorexia, nausea, cramps, constipation, distention, paralytic ileus; hypoventilation, respiratory muscle weakness
- Monitor for manifestations of hypomagnesemia: agitation, muscle twitching, paresthesias, hyperactive reflexes, positive Babinski reflex, dysphagia, nystagmus seizures, tetany;

nausea, vomiting, diarrhea, anorexia, abdominal distention; ectopy, tachycardia, broad, flat, or inverted T waves, depressed ST segment, prolonged QT, decreased cardiac output, hypotension

- Monitor for manifestations of hyponatremia; increased B/P, cold, clammy skin, hypovolemia or hypervolemia; anorexia, nausea, vomiting, diarrhea, abdominal cramps; lethargy, increased ICP, confusion, headache, seizures, coma, fatigue, tremors, hyperreflexia
- Monitor for manifestations of hyperchloremia: weakness, lethargy, coma, deep rapid breathing
- Assess and record fluid volume status: I&O ratios; monitor weight, distended red veins, crackles in lung, color, quality and sp gr of urine, skin turgor, adequacy of pulses, moist mucous membranes, bilateral lung sounds, peripheral pitting edema; dehydration symptoms of decreasing output, thirst, hypotension, dry mouth and mucous membranes should be reported
- Monitor electrolytes: potassium, sodium, calcium, magnesium; also include BUN, blood pH, ABGs, uric acid, CBC, blood sugar
- Assess B/P before and during therapy with patient lying, standing, and sitting as appropriate; orthostatic hypotension can occur rapidly

Nursing diagnoses

✓ Altered urinary elimination (adverse reactions)
✓ Fluid volume deficit (adverse reactions)
✓ Fluid volume excess (uses)
✓ Knowledge deficit (teaching)

Implementation

- Give in AM to avoid interference with sleep
- Provide potassium replacement if potassium level is 3.0; drug may be crushed if patient is unable to swallow
- Give with food; if nausea occurs, absorption may be increased; extended release products are Diulo, Zaroxolyn; prompt action product is MyKrox; the two formulations are not equivalent

Patient/family education

- Teach patient to take the medication early in the day to prevent nocturia
- Instruct patient to take with food or milk if GI symptoms of nausea and anorexia occur
- Teach patient to maintain a weekly record of weight and notify prescriber of weight loss >5 lb
- Caution patient that this drug causes a loss of potassium, so food rich in potassium should be added to the diet; refer to a dietician for assistance in planning
- Caution the patient not to exercise in hot weather or stand for prolonged periods, since orthostatic hypotension will be enhanced
- Teach patient not to use alcohol or any OTC medications without prescriber's approval; serious drug reactions may occur
- Emphasize the need to contact prescriber immediately if muscle cramps, weakness, nausea, dizziness or numbness occurs
- Teach patient to take own B/P and pulse and record

- Advise patient to use sunscreen to prevent burns
- Caution the patient that orthostatic hypotension may occur and to rise slowly from sitting or reclining positions, lie down if dizziness occurs
- Teach patient to continue taking medication even if feeling better; this drug controls symptoms but does not cure the condition
- Advise patient with hypertension to continue other medical treatment (exercise, weight loss, relaxation techniques, cessation of smoking)

Evaluation

Positive therapeutic outcome

- Decreased edema
- Decreased B/P

Treatment of overdose: Lavage if taken orally, monitor electrolytes; administer dextrose in saline; monitor hydration, CV, renal status

metoprolol (℞)

(met-oh-proe'lole)

Apo-Metoprolol ✤, Betaloc ✤, Betaloc Durules ✤, Lopressor, Lopressor SR ✤, Novometoprol ✤, Toprol XL

Func. class.: Antihypertensive, antianginal

Chem. class.: β_1-Blocker

Pregnancy category C

Action: Competitively blocks stimulation of β_1-adrenergic receptor within vascular smooth muscle; produces chronotropic, inotropic activity (decreases rate of SA node discharge, increases recovery time), slows conduction of AV node, decreases heart rate, which decreases O_2 consumption in myocardium; also decreases renin-aldosterone-angiotensin system at high doses

Therapeutic Outcome: Decreased B/P, heart rate, AV conduction

Uses: Mild to moderate hypertension, acute MI to reduce cardiovascular mortality, angina pectoris

Investigational uses: Dysrhythmias, hypertrophic cardiomyopathy, mitral valve prolapse, pheochromocytoma, tremors, prevention of vascular headaches, aggression

Dosage and routes

Hypertension

Adult: PO 50 mg bid, or 100 mg qd; may give 200-450 mg in divided doses; ext rel tabs give qd

MI

Adult: Early treatment, **IV** bol 5 mg q2 min × 3 doses, then 50 mg PO 15 min after last dose and q6h × 48 hr; late treatment, PO maintenance 100 mg bid for 3 mo

Available forms: Tabs 50, 100 mg; inj 1 mg/ml; ext rel tabs 50, 100, 200 mg

Adverse effects

CNS: Insomnia, dizziness, mental changes, hallucinations, ***depression,*** anxiety, headaches, nightmares, confusion, fatigue

CV: Hypotension, *bradycardia, CHF: Palpitations,* dysrhythmias, ***cardiac arrest, AV block***

EENT: Sore throat, dry burning eyes

GI: Nausea, vomiting, colitis, cramps, *diarrhea,* constipation, flatulence, dry mouth, *hiccups*

GU: Impotence
HEMA: Agranulocytosis, *eosinophilia,* ***thrombocytopenic purpura***
INTEG: Rash, purpura, alopecia, dry skin, urticaria, pruritus
RESP: Bronchospasm, *dyspnea, wheezing*

Contraindications: Hypersensitivity to β-blockers, cardiogenic shock, heart block (2nd-3rd-degree), sinus bradycardia, CHF, bronchial asthma

Precautions: Major surgery, pregnancy C, lactation, diabetes mellitus, renal disease, thyroid disease, COPD, heart failure, CAD, nonallergic bronchospasm, hepatic disease

Pharmacokinetics

Absorption	Well absorbed (PO); completely absorbed (IV)
Distribution	Crosses blood-brain barrier, placenta
Metabolism	Liver, extensively
Excretion	Kidneys, breast milk
Half-life	3-4 hr

Pharmacodynamics

	PO	IV
Onset	15 min	Immediate
Peak	2-4 hr	20 min
Duration	6-19 hr	5-8 hr

Interactions

Individual drugs

Alcohol: ↑ hypotension (large amounts)
Epinephrine: α-Adrenergic stimulation
Hydralazine: ↑ hypotension, bradycardia
Indomethacin: ↓ antihypertensive effect
Insulin: ↑ hypoglycemia
Methyldopa: ↑ hypotension, bradycardia
Prazosin: ↑ hypotension, bradycardia
Reserpine: ↑ hypotension, bradycardia
Thyroid: ↓ effectiveness
Verapamil: ↑ myocardial depression

Drug classifications

Amphetamines: ↑ hypertension, bradycardia
Antihypertensive: ↑ hypotension
β_2-Agonists: ↓ bronchodilatation
Cardiac glycosides: ↑ bradycardia
Nitrates: ↑ hypotension
Sulfonylureas: ↓ hypoglycemic effect
Theophyllines: ↓ bronchodilatation

Lab test interferences

False ↑ Urinary catecholamines

NURSING CONSIDERATIONS

Assessment

- Monitor B/P during beginning treatment, periodically thereafter; pulse q4h; note rate, rhythm, quality; check apical/radial pulse before administration; notify prescriber of any significant changes (pulse <50 bpm)
- Check for baselines in renal, liver function tests before therapy begins and periodically thereafter
- Assess for edema in feet, legs daily; monitor I&O, daily weight; check for jugular vein distention, rales bilaterally, dyspnea (CHF)
- Monitor skin turgor, dryness of mucous membranes for hydration status, especially G elderly

Nursing diagnoses

- ✓ Cardiac output, decreased (uses)
- ✓ Injury, risk for (adverse reactions)

M

☑ Knowledge deficit (teaching)
☑ Noncompliance (teaching)

Implementation

PO route

- Given ac, hs; tab may be crushed or swallowed whole; give with food to prevent GI upset; reduced dosage in renal dysfunction
- Do not crush or chew ext rel tab
- Store protected from light, moisture; place in cool environment

IV route

- Give by direct **IV** 5 mg/2 min or more; keep patient recumbent for 3 hr

Y-site compatibilities: Alteplase, meperidine, morhpine

Patient/family education

- Teach patient not to discontinue drug abruptly; taper over 2 wk; may cause precipitate angina if stopped abruptly
- Teach patient not to use OTC products containing α-adrenergic stimulants (such as nasal decongestants, cold preparations); to avoid alcohol, smoking and to limit sodium intake as prescribed
- Teach patient how to take pulse and B/P at home; advise when to notify prescriber
- Instruct patient to comply with weight control, dietary adjustments, modified exercise program
- Tell patient to carry/wear Medic Alert ID to identify drug being taken, allergies; tell patient drug controls symptoms but does not cure
- Caution patient to avoid hazardous activities if dizziness, drowsiness is present, to avoid driving until drug response is known
- Teach patient to report symptoms of CHF; difficult breathing, especially on exertion or when lying down, night cough, swelling of extremities or bradycardia, dizziness, confusion, depression, fever
- Teach patient to take drug as prescribed, not to double doses or skip doses; take any missed doses as soon as remembered if at least 4 hr until next dose

Evaluation

Positive therapeutic outcome

- Decreased B/P in hypertension (after 1-2 wk)
- Absence of dysrhythmias

Treatment of overdose: Lavage, **IV** atropine for bradycardia, **IV** theophylline for bronchospasm, digitalis, O_2, diuretic for cardiac failure, hemodialysis, **IV** glucose for hyperglycemia, **IV** diazepam (or phenytoin) for seizures

metronidazole (℞)

(me-troe-ni'da-zole)

Apo-Metronidazole ♣, Flagyl, Flagyl IV, Flagyl IV RTU, Metro IV, Metronidazole, Metronidazole Redi-Infusion, Metryl, Neo-Metric ♣, Novonidazole ♣, PMS-Metronidazole ♣, Protostat, Satric, Trikacide ♣

Func. class.: Trichomonacide, amebicide, antiinfective

Chem. class.: Nitroimidazole derivative

Pregnancy category B

Action: Direct-acting amebicide/trichomonacide;

binds, degrades DNA in organism

Therapeutic Outcome: Trichomonacidal, amebicidal, bactericidal for the following susceptible organisms: *Bacteroides, Clostridium, Trichomonas vaginalis, Giardia lamblia, Entamoeba histolytica*

Uses: Intestinal amebiasis, amebic abscess, trichomoniasis, refractory trichomoniasis, bacterial anaerobic infections, giardiasis; septicemia, endocarditis, bone, joint, and lower respiratory tract infections

Dosage and routes

Trichomoniasis

Adult: PO 250 mg tid × 7 days or 2 g in single dose; do not repeat treatment for 4-6 wk

P ***Child:*** PO 15 mg/kg/day in divided doses × 7-10 days

Refractory trichomoniasis

Adult: PO 250 mg bid × 10 days

Amebic abscess

Adult: PO 500-750 mg tid × 5-10 days

P ***Child:*** PO 35-50 mg/kg/day in 3 divided doses × 10 days

Intestinal amebiasis

Adult: PO 750 mg tid × 5-10 days

P ***Child:*** PO 35-50 mg/kg/day in 3 divided doses × 10 days; then oral iodoquinol

Anaerobic bacterial infections

Adult: **IV** inf 15 mg/kg/over 1 hr, then 7.5 mg/kg **IV** or PO q6h, not to exceed 4 g/day; first maintenance dose should be administered 6 hr following loading dose

Giardiasis

Adult: PO 250 mg tid × 5 days

P ***Child:*** PO 5 mg/kg tid × 5 days

Available forms: Tabs 250, 500 mg; film-coated tabs 250, 1500 mg; inj 5 mg/vial; HCl inj 500 mg

Adverse effects

CNS: Headache, dizziness, confusion, irritability, restlessness, ataxia, depression, fatigue, drowsiness, insomnia, paresthesia, peripheral neuropathy, ***convulsions,*** incoordination, depression

CV: Flat T waves

EENT: Blurred vision, sore throat, retinal edema, dry mouth, metallic taste, furry tongue, glossitis, stomatitis

GI: Nausea, vomiting, diarrhea, epigastric distress, *anorexia,* constipation, *abdominal cramps,* metallic taste, ***pseudomembranous colitis***

GU: Darkened urine, vaginal dryness, polyuria, ***albuminuria,*** dysuria, cystitis, decreased libido, ***nephrotoxicity,*** incontinence, dyspareunia

HEMA: ***Leukopenia, bone marrow depression, aplasia***

INTEG: Rash, pruritus, urticaria, flushing

SYST: Superinfection

Contraindications: Hypersensitivity to this drug, renal disease, hepatic disease, contracted visual or color fields, blood dyscrasias, pregnancy (1st trimester), lactation, CNS disorders

Precautions: Candidal infections, pregnancy (2nd, 3rd trimesters) **B**

M

Pharmacokinetics

Absorption	80% (PO)
Distribution	Widely distributed, crosses placenta
Metabolism	Liver
Excretion	Urine, unchanged; feces
Half-life	6-11 hr

Pharmacodynamics

	PO	IV
Onset	Rapid	Immediate
Peak	1-2 hr	Infusion's end

Interactions
Individual drugs
Alcohol: ↑ disulfiram-like reaction
Azathioprine: ↑ leukopenia
Cimetidine: ↓ action of metronidazole
Phenobarbital: ↓ effect of metronidazole
Disulfiram: ↑ risk of psychosis
Fluorouracil: ↑ leukopenia
Drug classifications
Anticoagulants, oral: ↑ risk of bleeding
Lab test interferences
↓ AST (SGOT), ↓ ALT (SGPT)

NURSING CONSIDERATIONS
Assessment
• Assess patient for signs and symptoms of infection including characteristics of wounds, WBC >10,000, vaginal secretions, fever; obtain baseline information and during treatment
• Obtain C&S before beginning drug therapy to identify if correct treatment has been initiated
• Assess for allergic reactions: rash, urticaria, pruritus
• Identify urine output; if decreasing, notify prescriber (may indicate nephrotoxicity); also check for increased BUN, creatinine
• Assess bowel pattern qd; if severe diarrhea occurs, drug should be discontinued
• Assess for overgrowth of infection: perineal itching, fever, malaise, redness, pain, swelling, drainage, rash, diarrhea, change in cough, sputum

Nursing diagnoses
✓ Infection, risk for (uses)
✓ Diarrhea (adverse reactions)
✓ Injury, risk for (adverse reactions)
✓ Knowledge deficit (teaching)
✓ Noncompliance (teaching)

Implementation
IV IV route
• Give intermittent **IV** prediluted; for Flagyl **IV** dilute with 4.4 ml sterile water or 0.9% NaCl; must be diluted further with 8 mg/ml or more 0.9% NaCl, D_5W, or LR; must neutralize with 5 mEq $NaHCO_3$/500 mg; CO_2 gas will be generated and may require venting; run over 1 hr; primary **IV** must be discontinued; may be given as cont inf; do not use aluminum products; **IV** may require venting

Additive compatibilities:
Cefazolin, cefotaxime, cefotiam, ceftazidime, cefuroxime, chloramphenicol, ciprofloxacin, clindamycin, floxacillin, fluconazole, gentamicin, heparin, moxalactam, multivitamins, netilmicin, penicillin G potassium, tobramycin

Y-site compatibilities:
Acyclovir, allopurinol, amifostine, amiodarone, cefepime, cyclophosphamide, diltiazem, enalaprilat, esmolol, fluconazole, foscarnet, heparin, hydromorphone, labetalol, lorazepam, magnesium sul-

fate, melphalan, meperidine, midazolam, morphine, perphenazine, sargramostim, tacrolimus, teniposide, theophylline, thiotepa, vinorelbine

Top route

• A thin coating should be applied to affected area after cleaning with soap and water and patting dry

PO route

• Give with or pc to avoid GI symptoms, metallic taste; crush tab if needed

• Store in light-resistant container; do not refrigerate

Patient/family education

• Teach patient to report sore throat, bruising, bleeding, joint pain; may indicate blood dyscrasias (rare)

• Advise patient to contact prescriber if vaginal itching, loose, foul-smelling stools, furry tongue occur; may indicate superinfection

• Teach trichomoniasis patient that both partners need to be treated; condoms should be used during intercourse to prevent reinfection

• Advise patient of disulfiram-like reaction to alcohol ingestion; alcohol should not be used when taking this anti-infective

• Inform patient drug has a metallic taste and urine may turn dark

• Advise patient to contact prescriber if pregnancy is suspected

Evaluation

Positive therapeutic outcome

• Decreased symptoms of infection

mexiletine (℞)

(mex-il′e-teen)

Mexitil

Func. class.: Antidysrhythmic (Class IB)

Chem. class.: Lidocaine analog

Pregnancy category C

Action: Increases electrical stimulation threshold of ventricle and His-Purkinje system, which stabilizes cardiac membrane and decreases automaticity

➔ **Therapeutic Outcome:** Decreased ventricular dysrhythmia

Uses: Ventricular tachycardia, ventricular dysrhythmias during cardiac surgery, MI

Dosage and routes

Adult: PO 400 mg (loading dose), then 200 mg q8h, then 200-400 mg q8h

Available forms: Caps 150, 200, 250 mg

Adverse effects

CNS: Headache, dizziness, confusion, ***convulsions,*** tremors, psychosis, nervousness, paresthesias, weakness, fatigue, coordination difficulties, change in sleep habits

CV: Hypotension, bradycardia, angina, PVCs, ***heart block, cardiovascular collapse, arrest,*** sinus node slowing, ***left ventricular failure,*** syncope, ***cardiogenic shock***

EENT: Blurred vision, hearing loss, tinnitus

GI: Nausea, vomiting, anorexia, diarrhea, abdominal pain, ***hepatitis,*** dry mouth, peptic ulcer, altered taste, GI bleeding

M

GU: Urinary hesitancy, decreased libido
HEMA: ***Thrombocytopenia, leukopenia, agranulocytosis, hypoplastic anemia,*** SLE syndrome
INTEG: Rash, alopecia, dry skin
MISC: Edema, arthralgia, fever
RESP: Dyspnea, ***fibrosis, embolism,*** pneumonia

Contraindications: Hypersensitivity to amides, cardiogenic shock, blood dyscrasias, severe heart block

Precautions: Pregnancy **C**, lactation, children, renal disease, liver disease, CHF, respiratory depression, myasthenia gravis

Pharmacokinetics	
Absorption	Well absorbed
Distribution	Body tissues
Metabolism	Liver, extensively
Excretion	Kidneys, unchanged (10%)
Half-life	12 hr

Pharmacodynamics	
Onset	½-2 hr
Peak	2-3 hr
Duration	8-12 hr

Interactions

Individual drugs

Cimetidine: ↑ toxicity
Digoxin: ↑ blood levels, toxicity
Disopyramide: ↑ levels, toxicity
Flecainide: ↑ levels, toxicity
Lidocaine: Bradycardia, cardiac arrest
Metoclopramide: ↑ effects of mexiletine
Phenobarbital: ↓ effectiveness
Phenytoin: ↑ effectiveness
Procainamide: ↑ levels, toxicity
Quinidine: ↑ levels, toxicity
Rifampin: ↓ effectiveness
Warfarin: ↑ level, bleeding

Drug classifications

Antacids: ↓ absorption
Analgesics, opioid: ↓ absorption

Smoking

↓ effectiveness

Lab test interferences

↑ CPK

NURSING CONSIDERATIONS

Assessment

- Assess for oxygenation or perfusion deficit: decreased B/P, chest pain, dizziness, loss of consciousness
- Assess respiratory status: auscultate lung fields for bibasilar crackles in patients with advanced CHF
- Assess for urinary retention: check for pain, abdominal absorption, palpate bladder; check males with benign prostatic hypertrophy; anticholinergic reaction may cause retention
- Monitor I&O ratio; electrolytes potassium, sodium, chloride; watch for decreasing urinary output, possible retention
- Monitor liver function studies: AST (SGOT), ALT (SGPT), bilirubin, alkaline phosphatase
- Monitor ECG periodically to determine drug effectiveness; measure PR, QRS, QT intervals; check for PVCs, other dysrhythmias; assess B/P for hypotension, hypertension, for rebound hypertension after 1-2 hr; for prolonged PR/QT intervals, QRS complex, if QT or QRS increase by 50% or more, withhold next dose, notify prescriber
- Monitor for dehydration and hypovolemia
- Monitor blood levels (thera-

peutic level 0.5-2 μg/ml), notify prescriber of abnormal results

- Assess pulmonary toxicity: dyspnea, fatigue, cough, fever, chest pain; drug should be discontinued
- Assess cardiac rate, respiration: rate, rhythm, character, chest pain, ventricular tachycardia, supraventricular tachycardia, fibrillation

Nursing diagnoses

✓ Cardiac output, decreased (uses)
✓ Impaired gas exchange (adverse reactions)
✓ Knowledge deficit (teaching)

Implementation

- Give with meals for GI upset

Patient/family education

- Teach patient to report side effects immediately to prescriber; to take exactly as prescribed; if dose is missed, take when remembered if within 3-4 hr of next dose; do not double doses
- Caution patient to avoid temp extremes; impairment of heat-regulating mechanism can occur
- Encourage patient to complete follow-up appointment with health care provider, including pulmonary function studies, chest x-ray
- Instruct patient that dry mouth may be relieved by frequent sips of water, hard candy, sugarless gum
- Caution patient to make position changes from lying to standing slowly to prevent orthostatic hypotension

Evaluation

Positive therapeutic outcome

- Decreased B/P, dysrhythmias
- Decreased heart rate
- Normal sinus rhythm

Treatment of overdose: O_2, artificial ventilation, ECG, administer dopamine for circulatory depression, administer diazepam or thiopental for convulsions, isoproterenol

mezlocillin (℞)

(mez-loe-sill'in)

Mezlin

Func. class.: Broad-spectrum antiinfective

Chem. class.: Extended-spectrum penicillin

Pregnancy category B

Action: Interferes with cell wall replication of susceptible organisms; osmotically unstable cell wall swells, bursts from osmotic pressure

Uses: Infection due to penicillinase-producing staphylococci, streptococci; respiratory tract, skin, skin structure, urinary tract, bone, joint infections; sinusitis, endocarditis, septicemia, meningitis; may be combined with an aminoglycoside for *Pseudomonas* infection

➔ **Therapeutic Outcome:** Bactericidal effects on the following: gram-positive cocci *Staphylococcus aureus, Streptococcus viridans, S. faecalis, S. pneumoniae,* gram-negative coccus *Neisseria gonorrhoeae,* gram-positive bacilli *Clostridium perfringens, C. tetani,* gram-negative bacilli *Bacteroides, Escherichia coli, Haemophilus influenzae, Klebsiella, Proteus mirabilis, Pepto-*

M

coccus, Peptostreptococcus, Morganella morganii, Enterobacter, Serratia, Pseudomonas, Proteus vulgaris, P. rettgeri, Shigella, Citrobacter, Veillonella

Dosage and routes

Adult: IM/**IV** 200-300 mg/kg/day in divided doses q4-6h; may give up to 24 g/day for severe infections

P ***Child:*** IM/**IV** 50 mg/kg q4-6h

P ***Infants >8 days:*** >2000 g, 75 mg/kg q6h; <2000 g, 75 mg/kg q8h

P ***Infants <8 days:*** 75 mg/kg q12h

Available forms: Powder for inj 1, 2, 3, 4 g; **IV** inf 2, 3, 4 g

Adverse effects

CNS: Lethargy, hallucinations, anxiety, depression, twitching, ***coma, convulsions***

GI: Nausea, vomiting, diarrhea, increased AST (SGOT), ALT (SGPT), abdominal pain, glossitis, colitis, abnormal taste

GU: Oliguria, proteinuria, hematuria vaginitis, moniliasis, ***glomerulonephritis,*** increased BUN, creatinine

HEMA: Anemia, increased bleeding time, ***bone marrow depression, granulocytopenia***

META: Hyperkalemia, hypokalemia, alkalosis, hypernatremia

Contraindications: Hypersensitivity to penicillins

Precautions: Pregnancy **B,** hypersensitivity to cephalosporins, P neonates

Pharmacokinetics

Absorption	Well absorbed
Distribution	Widely distributed; crosses placenta
Metabolism	Liver, small amounts
Excretion	Kidneys, unchanged (40%-70%); breast milk, bile (15%-30%)
Half-life	50-55 min; increased in renal disease

Pharmacodynamics

	IM	IV
Onset	Rapid	Rapid
Peak	5 min	Inf end

Interactions

Individual drugs

Aspirin: ↑ mezlocillin levels, ↓ renal excretion

Cholestyramine: ↓ effectiveness of mezlocillin

Chloramphenicol: ↑ half-life of chloramphenicol, ↓ effectiveness of mezlocillin

Colestipol: ↓ effectiveness of mezlocillin

Lithium: ↓ excretion, ↑ toxicity

Probenecid: ↑ mezlocillin levels, ↓ renal excretion

Drug classifications

Diuretics: ↑ hypokalemia

Erythromycins: ↓ antimicrobial effectiveness

Oral anticoagulants: ↑ anticoagulant effects

Oral contraceptives: ↓ contraceptive effectiveness

Tetracyclines: ↓ antimicrobial effectiveness

Food

Food, carbonated drinks, citrus fruit juices: ↓ absorption

Lab test interferences

False positive: Urine glucose, urine protein

NURSING CONSIDERATIONS

Assessment

- Assess patient for previous

sensitivity reaction to penicillins or other cephalosporins; cross-sensitivity between penicillins and cephalosporins is common

- Assess patient for signs and symptoms of infection including characteristics of wounds, sputum, urine, stool, WBC >10,000, fever; obtain baseline information and during treatment
- Obtain C&S before beginning drug therapy to identify if correct treatment has been initiated
- Assess for allergic reactions: rash, urticaria, pruritus, chills, fever, joint pain; angioedema may occur a few days after therapy begins; epinephrine, resuscitation equipment should be available for anaphylactic reaction
- Identify urine output; if decreasing, notify prescriber (may indicate nephrotoxicity); also check for increase BUN, creatinine
- Monitor blood studies: AST (SGOT), ALT (SGPT), CBC, Hct, bilirubin, LDH, alkaline phosphatase, Coombs' test monthly if patient is on long-term therapy
- Monitor electrolytes: potassium, sodium, chloride monthly if patient is on long-term therapy
- Assess bowel pattern qd; if severe diarrhea occurs, drug should be discontinued; may indicate pseudomembranous colitis
- Monitor for bleeding: ecchymosis, bleeding gums, hematuria, stool guaiac daily if on long-term therapy
- Assess for overgrowth of infection: perineal itching, fever, malaise, redness, pain, swelling, drainage, rash, diarrhea, change in cough, sputum

Nursing diagnoses

- ✓ Infection, risk for (uses)
- ✓ Diarrhea (adverse reactions)
- ✓ Injury, risk for (adverse reactions)
- ✓ Knowledge deficit (teaching)
- ✓ Noncompliance (teaching)

Implementation

IV route

- Dilute 1g or less/10 ml of sterile water, for inj; D_5, 0.9% NaCl, for inj; shake, dilute further with D_5W or 0.45 NaCl, give over 3-5 min

Syringe compatibility:
Heparin

Y-site compatibilities:
Amifostine, aztreonam, cyclophosphamide, famotidine, fludarabine, granisetron, hydromorphone, morphine, perphenazine, sargramostim, tacrolimus, teniposide, thiotepa

Patient/family education

- Teach patient to report sore throat, bruising, bleeding, joint pain; may indicate blood dyscrasias (rare)
- Advise patient to contact prescriber if vaginal itching, loose, foul-smelling stools, furry tongue occur; may indicate superinfection
- Advise patient to notify prescriber of diarrhea with blood or pus, which may indicate pseudomembranous colitis

Evaluation

Positive therapeutic outcome

- Absence of signs/symptoms of infection (WBC <10,000, temp WNL, absence of red, draining wounds)
- Reported improvement in symptoms of infection

M

Treatment of anaphylaxis: Withdraw drug, maintain airway, administer epinephrine, aminophylline, O_2, **IV** corticosteroids

miconazole 🔑 (OTC)

(mi-kon'a-zole)

Monistat, Monistat IV; topical: Micatin, Micatin Liquid, miconazole Nitrate, Monistat-Derm, Monistat 3, Monistat 7, Monistat Dual-Pak

Func. class.: Antifungal
Chem. class.: Imidazole

Pregnancy category B

Action: Alters cell membranes, inhibits fungal enzymes, inhibits sterols so intracellular contents are lost, prevents biosynthesis of phospholipids/triglycerides

Therapeutic Outcome: Fungistatic/fungicidal against: *Aspergillus, Coccidioides, Cryptococcus, Candida, Dermatophytes, Histoplasma*

Uses: Coccidioidomycosis, candidiasis, cryptococcosis, paracoccidioidomycosis, chronic mucocutaneous candidiasis, fungal meningitis; **IV** used for severe infections only; (top) tinea pedis, tinea cruris, tinea corporis, tinea versicolor, vaginal or vulva candidal infections

Dosage and routes

Adult: **IV** inf 200-3600 mg/day; may be divided in 3 inf at 200-1200 mg/inf; may have to repeat course; IT 20 mg given simultaneously with **IV** for fungal meningitis q3-7 days

P ***Child:*** **IV** 20-40 mg/kg/day, not to exceed 15 mg/kg/day

P ***Adult and child:*** Top apply to affected area bid × 2-4 wk

Adult: Intravag give 1 applicator or suppository × 7 days hs

Available forms: Inj 10 mg/ml; aerosol 2%; cream 2%; lotion 2%; powder 2%; spray 2%; vag cream 2%; vag supp 100, 200 mg

Adverse effects

CNS: Drowsiness, headache, lethargy
CV: Tachycardia, dysrhythmias (rapid **IV**)
GI: Nausea, vomiting, anorexia, diarrhea, cramps
GU: Vulvovaginal burning, itching, hyponatremia, pelvic cramps (topical forms)
HEMA: Decreased Hct, thrombocytopenia, hyperlipidemia
INTEG: Pruritus, rash, fever, flushing, hives
SYST: Anaphylaxis

Contraindications: Hypersensitivity

Precautions: Renal disease, hepatic disease, pregnancy **B**

Pharmacokinetics

Absorption	Poorly absorbed (PO)
Distribution	Widely distributed (IV); bound to serum proteins (90%)
Metabolism	Liver, extensively
Excretion	Unknown
Half-life	Triphasic: 0.4, 2.1, 24 hr

Pharmacodynamics

	IV	TOP	VAG
Onset	Rapid	Unknown	Unknown
Peak	Infusion's end	Unknown	Unknown

Interactions
Individual drugs
Amphotericin B: ↓ effect of miconazole
Coumadin: ↑ anticoagulant effect
Isoniazid: ↓ effect of miconazole
Rifampin: ↓ effect of miconazole
Lab test interferences
False positive: Urine glucose, urine protein

NURSING CONSIDERATIONS
Assessment
- Assess for signs and symptoms of infection: drainage, sore throat, urinary pain, hematuria, fever
- Obtain cultures for C&S before beginning treatment; therapy may be started after culture is taken; monitor signs of infection before and throughout treatment
- Monitor bowel pattern before and during treatment; diarrhea may occur
- Monitor cardiac system: B/P, pulse; watch for increasing pulse, cardiac dysrhythmias; drug should be discontinued
- Monitor blood studies: WBC, RBC, Hgb, Hct, bleeding time; patients taking anticoagulants may need a decreased dosage; monitor liver and renal studies periodically for patients on long-term therapy
- Monitor I&O ratio; watch for decreasing urinary output, change in sp gr; discontinue drug to prevent renal damage; patients with renal disease may require lowered dose
- Monitor **IV** for thrombophlebitis; site should be changed q48-72h
- Monitor for allergies before initiation of treatment and reaction to each medication; highlight allergies on chart; check for allergic reaction: burning, stinging, swelling, redness (top); observe for skin eruptions after administration of drug to 1 wk after discontinuing drug

Nursing diagnoses
- ✓ Skin integrity, impaired (uses)
- ✓ Infection, risk (uses)
- ✓ Injury, risk for (adverse reactions)
- ✓ Knowledge deficit (teaching)

Implementation
- Have adrenalin, suction, tracheostomy set, endotracheal intubation equipment available

IV route
- Give 200 mg initially to prevent severe hypersensitive reaction
- Give by intermittent **IV** after diluting in 200 ml or more, D_5W or 0.9% NaCl; give over 30-60 min
- Store at room temp; reconstituted sol is stable for 24 hr refrigerated

Y-site incompatibility:
Fludarabine

Y-site compatibilities:
Allopurinol, filgrastim, foscarnet, melphalan, ondansetron, sargramostim, teniposide, thiotepa, vinorelbine

Top route
- Apply after cleansing area with soap and water before each application; use enough medication to cover lesions completely; dry well
- Store at room temp in dry place

Vag route
- Administer 1 applicatorful

every night high into the vagina
• Store at room temp in dry place

Patient/family education
• Inform patient that culture may be taken after completed course of medication
• Advise patient to notify nurse of diarrhea, symptoms of candidal vaginitis

Top route
• Teach patient to use medical asepsis (hand washing) before, after each application; to apply with glove to prevent further infection; to avoid contact with eyes; not to use occlusive dressings
• Caution patient to avoid use of OTC creams, ointments, lotions unless directed by prescriber
• Instruct patient to notify prescriber if no improvement in condition in 4 wk or if symptoms return in 2 mo; pregnancy or a serious medical condition may be the cause
• Teach patient to use for full prescribed treatment time, or reinfection may occur

Vag route
• Instruct patient in asepsis (hand washing) before, after each application
• Teach patient to apply with applicator only; to avoid use of any other vag product unless directed by prescriber; sanitary napkin may prevent soiling of undergarments; to abstain from sexual intercourse until treatment is completed; reinfection and irritation may occur
• Instruct patient to notify prescriber if symptoms persist

Evaluation

Positive therapeutic outcome
• Decreasing oral candidiasis, fever, malaise, rash
• Negative C&S for infectious organism
• Decrease in size, number of lesions
• Decrease in itching or white discharge (vaginal)

Treatment of overdose: Withdraw drug; maintain airway; administer epinephrine, aminophylline, O_2, **IV** corticosteroids for anaphylaxis

midazolam (℞)
(mid′ay-zoe-lam)
Versed
Func. class.: Sedative/hypnotic
Chem. class.: Benzodiazepine, short-acting
Pregnancy category D
Controlled substance schedule IV

Action: Depresses subcortical levels in CNS; may act on limbic system, reticular formation; may potentiate GABA by binding to specific benzodiazepine receptors

➡ **Therapeutic Outcome:** Sedation for anesthesia induction and procedures

Uses: Preoperative sedation, general anesthesia induction, sedation for diagnostic endoscopic procedures, intubation

Investigational uses: Epileptic seizures, refractory status epilepticus

Dosage and routes

Preoperative sedation

Adult: IM 0.07-0.08 mg/kg

30-60 min before general anesthesia

Child: IM 0.1-0.15 mg/kg, may give up to 0.5 mg/kg if needed

Induction of general anesthesia
Adult and child 12-16 yr: Unpremedicated patients, **IV** 0.3-0.35 mg/kg over 30 sec, wait 2 min, follow with 25% of initial dose if needed; premedicated patients, 0.15-0.35 mg/kg over 20-30 sec, allow 2 min for effect

Child 6-12 yr: **IV** 0.025-0.05 mg/kg, total dose up to 0.4 mg/kg if needed

Child 6 mo-5 yr: **IV** 0.05-0.1 mg/kg, total dose up to 0.6 mg/kg may be needed

Child <6 mo: Titrate with small increments

Available forms: Inj 1, 5 mg/ml

Adverse effects
CNS: Retrograde amnesia, euphoria, confusion, headache, anxiety, insomnia, slurred speech, paresthesia, tremors, weakness, chills
CV: Hypotension, PVCs, tachycardia, bigeminy, nodal rhythm
EENT: Blurred vision, nystagmus, diplopia, blocked ears, loss of balance
GI: Nausea, vomiting, increased salivation, hiccups
INTEG: Urticaria, pain, swelling at inj site, rash, pruritus
RESP: Coughing, ***apnea, bronchospasm, laryngospasm,*** dyspnea

Contraindications: Pregnancy **D,** hypersensitivity to benzodiazepines, shock, coma, alcohol intoxication, acute narrow-angle glaucoma

Precautions: COPD, CHF, chronic renal failure, chills, G debilitated, elderly, children, P lactation

Pharmacokinetics

Absorption	Well absorbed
Distribution	Crosses placenta, blood-brain barrier
Metabolism	Liver
Excretion	Kidneys, breast milk
Half-life	1-12 hr

Pharmacodynamics

	IM	IV
Onset	15 min	3-5 min
Peak	½-1 hr	Unknown
Duration	2-6 hr	2-6 hr

Interactions
Individual drugs
Alcohol: ↑ CNS depression
Cimetidine: ↑ levels of midazolam
Fluvoxamine: ↑ respiratory depression
Indinavir: ↑ respiratory depression
Propofol: ↑ effect of propofol
Ritonavir: ↑ respiratory depression
Valproic acid: ↓ metabolism of midazolam
Verapamil: ↑ respiratory depression
Drug classifications
Analgesics, opioid: ↑ CNS depression
Antifungals, azole: ↑ levels of midalozam
Antihistamines: ↑ CNS depression
Antihypertensives: ↑ hypotension
Nitrates: ↑ hypotension
Oral contraceptives: half-life of midazolam
Rifamycins: ↑ clearance and ↓ half-life of midazolam

M

Sedative/hypnotics: ↑ CNS depression
Theophyllines: ↓ effect of midazolam

NURSING CONSIDERATIONS

Assessment

- Monitor B/P, pulse, respiration during **IV**; O_2 and emergency equipment should be nearby
- Monitor inj site for redness, pain, swelling
- Assess degree of amnesia in G elderly; may be increased
- Assess anterograde amnesia
- Assess vital signs for recovery period in obese patient, since half-life may be extended

Nursing diagnoses

✓ Knowledge deficit (teaching)

Implementation

IV **IV route**

- Give **IV** undiluted or after diluting with D_5W or 0.9% NaCl to a conc of 0.25 mg/ml; give over 2 min (conscious sedation) or over 30 sec (anesthesia induction)
- Ensure immediate availability of resuscitation equipment, O_2 to support airway; do not give by rapid bol

Syringe compatibilities: Atracurium, atropine, benzquinamide, buprenorphine, butorphanol, chlorpromazine, cimetadine, diphenhydramine, droperidol, fentanyl, glycopyrrolate, hydromorphine, hydroxyzine, meperidine, metoclopramide, morphine, nalbuphine, promazine, promethazine, scopolamine, thiethylperazine, trimethobenzamide

Syringe incompatibilities: Dimenhydrinate, pentobarbital, perphenazine, prochlorperazine, ranitidine

Y-site compatibilities: Amiodarone, atracurium, famotidine, fentanyl, fluconazole, morphine, pancuronium, vecuronium

Y-site incompatibility: Foscarnet

IM route

- Give IM deep in large muscle mass
- Store at room temp

Patient/family education

- Instruct patient to avoid hazardous activities until drowsiness, weakness subside
- Inform patient that amnesia occurs; events may not be remembered
- Caution patient to avoid CNS depressants including alcohol for 24 hr after taking this drug

Evaluation

Positive therapeutic outcome

- Induction of sedation, amnesia

Treatment of overdose: O_2, vasopressors, physostigmine, resuscitation; flumazenil will reverse effects

midodrine (℞)

(mye'doh-dreen)
ProAmatine
Func. class.: Prodrug
Pregnancy category C

Action: Activates α-adrenergic receptors of arteriolar venous vasculature

⇒ **Therapeutic Outcome:** Decreased feeling of faintness upon rising, absence of significant change in B/P

Uses: Orthostatic hypotension

Dosage and routes
Adult: PO 10 mg

Available forms: Tabs 2.5, 5 mg

Adverse effects
CNS: Drowsiness, restlessness, headache, paresthesia, pain, chills
EENT: Dry mouth, blurred vision
GI: Nausea, anorexia
INTEG: Pruritus, piloerection, rash

Contraindications: Hypersensitivity, severe organic heart disease, acute renal disease, urinary retention, pheochromocytoma, thyrotoxicosis, persistent/excessive supine hypertension

P **Precautions:** Children, urinary retention, lactation, prostatic hypertrophy, pregnancy **C**

Pharmacokinetics	
Absorption	Unknown
Distribution	Unknown
Metabolism	Unknown
Excretion	Unknown
Half-life	3-4 hr

Pharmacodynamics	
Onset	Unknown
Peak	1-2 hr
Duration	Unknown

Interactions
Drug classifications
α-Agonists: ↑ pressor effects
β-Blockers: ↑ bradycardia
Psychopharmacologics: ↑ bradycardia
Cardiac glycosides: ↑bradycardia
Steroids: ↑ intraocular pressure

NURSING CONSIDERATIONS
Assessment
- Monitor VS, B/P
- Observe for drowsiness, dizziness, LOC

Implementation
- Tablets may be swallowed whole, chewed, or allowed to dissolve

Nursing diagnoses
✓ Knowledge deficit (teaching)

Patient/family education
- Advise to avoid hazardous activities; activities requiring alertness; dizziness may occur; instruct patient to request assistance with ambulation
- Advise to avoid alcohol, other depressants

Evaluation
Positive therapeutic outcome
- Decreased orthostatic hypotension

miglitol (℞)
(mig′le-tol)
Glyset
Func. class.: Oral hypoglycemic
Chem. class.: α-glucosidase inhibitor
Pregnancy cateogry B

Action: Delays the digestion of ingested carbohydrates, results in a smaller rise in blood glucose after meals; does not increase insulin production

➔ **Therapeutic Outcome:** Decreased blood glucose levels in diabetes mellitus

Uses: Stable adult-onset diabetes mellitus (type II) NIDDM

Dosage and routes
Initial dose
Adult: PO 25 mg tid with first bite of meal
Maintenance dose
Adult: PO may be increased to

50 mg tid; may increase to 100 mg tid if needed only in patients >60 kg; dosage adjustment at 4-8 wk intervals

Available forms: Tabs 25, 50, 100 mg

Adverse effects

*GI: Abdominal pain, diarrhea, flatulence, **hepatotoxicity***
HEMA: Low iron
INTEG: Rash

Contraindications: Hypersensitivity, diabetic ketoacidosis, cirrhosis, inflammatory bowel disease, colonic ulceration, partial intestinal obstruction, chronic intestinal disease

P **Precautions:** Pregnancy **B,** renal disease, lactation, children, hepatic disease

Pharmacokinetics

Absorption	Unknown
Distribution	Unknown
Metabolism	Not metabolized
Excretion	Kidneys, unchanged drug
Half-life	2 hr

Pharmacodynamics

Unknown

Interactions

Individual drugs

Digoxin: ↓ levels of digoxin
Insulin: ↑ hypoglycemia
Propranolol: ↓ levels of propranolol
Ranitidine: ↓ levels of ranitidine

Drug classifications

Adsorbents, intestinal: ↓ miglitol levels; do not use together
Enzymes, digestive: ↓ miglitol levels; do not use together
Sulfonylureas: ↑ hypoglycemia

NURSING CONSIDERATIONS

Assessment

• Assess for hypoglycemia, hyperglycemia; even though this drug does not cause hypoglycemia, if on a sulfonylurea or insulin, hypoglycemia may be additive
• Monitor blood glucose levels, glycosylated hemoglobin, LFTs

Nursing diagnoses

✓ Nutrition altered, more than body requirements (uses)
✓ Nutrition altered, less than body requirements (adverse reactions)
✓ Knowledge deficit (teaching)
✓ Noncompliance (teaching)

Implementation

• Give tid with first bite of each meal
• Provide storage in tight container in cool environment

Patient/family education

• Teach patient the symptoms of hypoglycemia, hyperglycemia and what to do about each
• Instruct that medication must be taken as prescribed; explain consequences of discontinuing the medication abruptly
• Tell patient to avoid OTC medications unless approved by prescriber
• Teach patient that diabetes is a life-long illness; drug will not cure condition
• Instruct patient to carry/wear Medic Alert ID as diabetic
• Teach patient that diet and exercise regimen must be followed

Evaluation

Positive therapeutic outcome

• Decreased signs, symptoms of diabetes mellitus (polyuria, polydipsia, polyphagia, clear sensorium, absence of dizziness, stable gait)

milrinone (℞)

(mill-re'none)

Primacor

Func. class.: Inotropic/vasodilator agent with phosphodiesterase activity

Chem. class.: Bipyridine derivative

Pregnancy category C

Action: Positive inotropic agent with vasodilator properties; reduces preload and afterload by direct relaxation of vascular smooth muscle; increases myocardial contractility

➔ **Therapeutic Outcome:** Increased inotropic effect resulting in increased cardiac output

Uses: Short-term management of CHF that has not responded to other medication; can be used with digitalis products

Dosage and routes

***Adult:* IV** bol 50 μg/kg given over 10 min; start inf of 0.375-0.75 μg/kg/min; reduce dosage in renal impairment

Available forms: Inj 1 mg/ml

Adverse effects

CV: Dysrhythmias, hypotension, chest pain

GI: Nausea, vomiting, anorexia, abdominal pain, ***hepatotoxicity,*** jaundice

HEMA: Thrombocytopenia

MISC: Headache, hypokalemia, tremor

Contraindications: Hypersensitivity to this drug, severe aortic disease, severe pulmonic valvular disease, acute MI

Precautions: Lactation, pregnancy **C,** children, renal disease, hepatic disease, atrial flutter/fibrillation, elderly

Pharmacokinetics

Absorption	Completely absorbed
Distribution	Unknown
Metabolism	Liver (50%)
Excretion	Kidney, unchanged and metabolites (60%-90%)
Half-life	3½-6 hr; increased in CHF

Pharmacodynamics

Onset	2-5 min
Peak	10 min
Duration	Variable

Interactions: None

NURSING CONSIDERATIONS

Assessment

- Monitor manifestations of hypokalemia: acidic urine, reduced urine, osmolality, nocturia; hypotension, broad T wave, U wave, ectopy, tachycardia, weak pulse; muscle weakness, altered LOC, drowsiness, apathy, lethargy, confusion, depression; anorexia, nausea, cramps, constipation, distention, paralytic ileus; hypoventilation, respiratory muscle weakness
- Assess fluid volume status: complete I&O ratio and record; note weight, distended red veins, crackles in lung, color, quality and sp gr of urine, skin turgor, adequacy of pulses, moist mucous membranes, bilateral lung sounds, peripheral pitting edema; dehydration symptoms of decreasing output, thirst, hypotension, dry mouth and mucous membranes should be reported
- Monitor electrolytes: potassium, sodium, calcium, magnesium; also include BUN, blood pH, ABGs

• Monitor B/P and pulse, PCWP, CVP, index, often during inf; if B/P drops 30 mm Hg, stop inf and call prescriber
• Monitor ALT (SGPT), AST (SGOT), bilirubin daily; if these are elevated, hepatoxicity is suspected
• Monitor platelets; if <150,000/mm^3, drug is usually discontinued and another drug started
• Assess for extravasation: change site q48h

Nursing diagnoses

✓ Cardiac output, decreased (uses)
✓ Fluid volume excess (uses)
✓ Knowledge deficit (teaching)

Implementation

• Do not mix directly with glucose sol; chemical reaction occurs over 24 hr; precipitate forms if milrinone and furosemide come in contact
• Administer by direct **IV** into inf through Y-connector or directly into tubing; may give undiluted over 2-3 min
• Give by cont inf diluted with normal saline to conc of 1-3 mg/ml, run at prescribed rate; give by inf pump for doses other than bol
• Administer potassium supplements if ordered for potassium levels <3.0

Additive compatibility: Quinidine

Syringe compatibilities: Atropine, calcium chloride, digoxin, epinephrine, lidocaine, morphine, propranolol

Y-site compatibilities: Digoxin, propranolol, quinidine

Patient/family education

• Teach patient reason for medication and expected results
• Instruct patient to make position changes slowly; orthostatic hypotension may occur
• Teach patient signs and symptoms of hypersensitivity reactions and hypokalemia

Evaluation

Positive therapeutic outcome

• Increased cardiac output
• Decreased PCWP, adequate CVP
• Decreased dyspnea, fatigue, edema, ECG

Treatment of overdose: Discontinue drug, support circulation

minocycline (℞)

(min-oh-sye'kleen)
Minocin, Minocin IV
Func. class.: Antiinfective
Chem. class.: Tetracycline
Pregnancy category D

Action: Inhibits protein synthesis and phosphorylation in microorganisms by binding to 30S ribosomal subunits and reversibly binding to 50S ribosomal subunits; bacteriostatic

➔ **Therapeutic Outcome:** Bactericidal action against susceptible organisms, including *Neisseria meningitidis, N. gonorrhoeae, Treponema pallidum, Chlamydia trachomatis, Ureaplasma urealyticum, Mycoplasma pneumoniae, Nocardia, Rickettsia*

Uses: Syphilis, chlamydial infection, gonorrhea, lymphogranuloma venereum, rickettsial infections, inflammatory acne, meningitis carriers

Dosage and routes

Adult: PO/**IV** 200 mg, then 100 mg q12h or 50 mg q6h, not to exceed 400 mg/24h **IV**

P ***Child >8 yr:*** PO/**IV** 4 mg/kg then 4 mg/kg/day PO in divided doses q12h

Gonorrhea

Adult: PO 200 mg, then 100 mg q12h × 4 days

Chlamydia trachomatis infection

Adult: PO 100 mg bid × 7 days

Syphilis

Adult: PO 200 mg, then 100 mg q12h × 10-15 days

Available forms: Tabs 50, 100 mg; caps 50, 100 mg; oral susp 50 mg/5 ml; powder for inj 100 mg/vial

Adverse effects

CNS: Dizziness, fever, lightheadedness, vertigo

CV: Pericarditis

EENT: Dysphagia, glossitis, decreased calcification, permanent discoloration of deciduous teeth, oral candidiasis

GI: Nausea, abdominal pain, *vomiting, diarrhea,* anorexia, enterocolitis, ***hepatotoxicity,*** flatulence, abdominal cramps, epigastric burning, stomatitis

GU: Increased BUN, polyuria, polydipsia, ***renal failure, nephrotoxicity***

HEMA: ***Eosinophilia, neutropenia, thrombocytopenia, hemolytic anemia***

INTEG: Rash, urticaria, photosensitivity, increased pigmentation, ***exfoliative dermatitis,*** pruritus, angioedema, blue-gray color of skin and mucous membranes

Contraindications: Hypersensitivity to tetracyclines,
P children <8 yr, pregnancy **D**

Precautions: Hepatic disease, lactation

Pharmacokinetics

Absorption	Well absorbed (PO)
Distribution	Widely distributed (55%-88% protein bound); some distribution in CSF, crosses placenta
Metabolism	Liver, some
Excretion	Kidneys, unchanged (20%), bile, feces
Half-life	11-17 hr

Pharmacodynamics

	PO	IV
Onset	Rapid	Rapid
Peak	2-3 hr	Infusion's end

Interactions

Individual drugs

Calcium: Forms chelates, ↓ absorption

Carbamazepine: ↑ effect of carbamazepine

Iron: Forms chelates, ↓ absorption

Magnesium: Forms chelates, ↓ absorption

Drug classifications

Antidiarrheals, adsorbent: ↓ absorption

Anticoagulants, oral: ↑ effect of anticoagulants

Contraceptives, oral: ↓ effect of oral contraception

Lab test interferences

False negative: Urine glucose with Clinistix, Tes-Tape

NURSING CONSIDERATIONS

Assessment

- Assess patient for previous sensitivity reaction
- Assess patient for signs and symptoms of infection including characteristics of wounds, sputum, urine, stool, WBC >10,000, fever; obtain baseline

information, before and during treatment

- Obtain C&S before beginning drug therapy to identify if correct treatment has been initiated
- Assess for allergic reactions: rash, urticaria, pruritus
- Monitor blood studies: AST (SGOT), ALT (SGPT), CBC, Hct, bilirubin, alkaline phosphatase, amylase monthly if patient is on long-term therapy
- Assess bowel pattern qd; if severe diarrhea occurs, drug should be discontinued
- Monitor for bleeding: ecchymosis, bleeding gums, hematuria, stool guaiac daily if on long-term therapy; blood dyscrasias may occur
- Assess for overgrowth of infection: perineal itching, fever, malaise, redness, pain, swelling, drainage, rash, diarrhea, change in cough, sputum; black, furry tongue

Nursing diagnoses

- ✓ Infection, risk for (uses)
- ✓ Diarrhea (adverse reactions)
- ✓ Knowledge deficit (teaching)
- ✓ Noncompliance (teaching)

Implementation

PO route

- Give around the clock to maintain proper blood levels; give with food to increase absorption of drug; do not give within 3 hr of other agents; drug interactions may occur
- Give with 8 oz of water 1 hr before hs to prevent ulceration
- Shake liquid preparation well before giving; use calibrated device for proper dosing
- Do not give with iron, calcium, magnesium products or antacids, which decrease absorption and form insoluble chelate

IV IV route

- Check for irritation, extravasation, phlebitis daily; change site q72hr
- For intermittent inf, dilute each 100 mg/10 ml 0.9% NaCl, sterile water for inj; further dilute in 500-1000 ml 0.9% NaCl, D_5W, Ringer's, LR, D_5/LR; give over 6 hr

Y-site incompatibilities: Aztreonam, filgrastim, hydromorphone, meperidine, morphine, teniposide

Y-site compatibilities: Cyclophosphamide, fludarabine, heparin, hydrocortisone, magnesium sulfate, melphalan, perphenazine, potassium chloride, sargramostim, sodium succinate, vinorelbine, vitamin B with C

Patient/family education

- Teach patient to use sunscreen when outdoors to decrease photosensitivity reaction
- Teach patient to report sore throat, bruising, bleeding, joint pain; may indicate blood dyscrasias (rare)
- Advise patient to contact prescriber if vaginal itching, loose, foul-smelling stools, furry tongue occur; may indicate superinfection; report itching, rash, pruritus, urticaria
- Instruct patient to take all medication prescribed for the length of time ordered; drug must be taken around the clock to maintain blood levels; do not give medication to others; take with a full glass of water; may take with food or milk
- Advise patient to use a form of contraception other than hormonal

Evaluation

Positive therapeutic outcome

- Absence of signs/symptoms of infection (WBC <10,000, temp WNL, absence of red, draining wounds)
- Reported improvement in symptoms of infection

minoxidil (℞)

(mi-nox'i-dill)

Loniten, Minodyl, minoxidil, Rogaine

Func. class.: Antihypertensive, hair growth stimulant

Chem. class.: Vasodilator, peripheral

Pregnancy category C

Action: Directly relaxes arteriolar smooth muscle, causing vasodilatation; increased cutaneous blood flow; stimulation of hair follicles

➔ **Therapeutic Outcome:** Decreased B/P in hypertension; hair growth

Uses: Severe hypertension unresponsive to other therapy (use with diuretic); topically to treat alopecia

Dosage and routes

Adult: PO 5 mg/day not to exceed 100 mg daily; usual range 10-40 mg/day in single doses

P ***Child <12 yr:*** Initial, 0.2 mg/kg/day; effective range, 0.25-1 mg/kg/day; max, 50 mg/day

Alopecia

Adult: Apply top, rub into scalp daily

Available forms: Tabs 2.5, 10 mg; top 20 mg/ml

Adverse effects

CNS: Drowsiness, dizziness, sedation, headache, depression, fatigue

CV: Severe rebound hypertension, tachycardia, angina, increased T wave, ***CHF, pulmonary edema, pericardial effusion,*** edema, sodium retention, water retention

GI: Nausea, vomiting

GU: Gynecomastia, breast tenderness

HEMA: Hct, Hgb, erythrocyte count may decrease initially

INTEG: Pruritus, ***Stevens-Johnson syndrome,*** rash, hirsutism

Contraindications: Acute MI, dissecting aortic aneurysm, hypersensitivity, pheochromocytoma

Precautions: Pregnancy **C,** P lactation, children, renal disease, CAD, CHF

Pharmacokinetics

Absorption	Well absorbed (PO); minimally absorbed (top)
Distribution	Widely distributed
Metabolism	Liver
Excretion	Kidneys, breast milk
Half-life	4.2 hr

Pharmacodynamics

	PO	TOP
Onset	½ hr	4 mo
Peak	2-3 hr	Unknown
Duration	75 hr	4 mo

Interactions

Individual drugs

Alcohol: ↑ hypotension

Drug classifications

Antihypertensives: ↑ hypotension

Glucocorticoids (top route): ↑ absorption

Nitrates: ↑ nitrates

M

NSAIDs: ↓ antihypertensive effect
Retinoids (top route): ↑ absorption

NURSING CONSIDERATIONS

Assessment

- Monitor B/P, pulse, jugular venous distention periodically throughout treatment
- Monitor electrolytes, blood studies: potassium, sodium, chloride, carbon dioxide, CBC, serum glucose
- Monitor weight daily, I&O; assess edema in feet, legs daily; check skin turgor, dryness of mucous membranes for hydration status
- Assess for rales, dyspnea, orthopnea, peripheral edema, fatigue, weight gain, jugular vein distention (CHF)
- Assess for signs of hyperglycemia: acetone breath, increased urinary output, severe thirst, lethargy, dizziness

Nursing diagnoses

✓ Cardiac output, decreased (adverse reactions)
✓ Injury, risk for (side effects)
✓ Knowledge deficit (teaching)

Implementation

PO route

- Give with meals to decrease GI symptoms
- Give with β-blockers and/or diuretic for hypertension
- Store protected from light and heat

Top route

- Administer 1 ml dose no matter how much balding has occurred; increasing dose does not speed hair growth
- Treatment must continue long term or new hair will be lost again

Patient/family education

Top route

- Teach patient that new hair will be soft and hardly visible
- Caution patient not to use on other parts of the body; drug is to be used on the scalp only
- Instruct patient that hair should be clean before applying medication; do not get on clothing
- Caution patient not to get medication near mucous membranes (mouth, nose, eyes) and to contact prescriber if burning, stinging or rash occurs

Evaluation

Positive therapeutic outcome

- Decreased B/P in hypertension
- Hair growth (top)

mirtazapine (℞)

(mer-ta'za-peen)
Remeron
Func. class.: Antidepressant
Chem. class.: Tetracyclic
Pregnancy category B

Action: Blocks reuptake of norepinephrine, serotonin into nerve endings, increasing action of norepinephrine, serotonin in nerve cells; has anticholinergic action

➔ **Therapeutic Outcome:** Decreased symptoms of depression after 2-3 wk

Uses: Depression, dysthymic disorder, bipolar disorder: depression, agitated depression

Dosage and routes
Adult: PO 15 mg/day at hs, maintenance to continue for 6 mo

Available forms: Tabs 15, 30 mg

Adverse effects

CNS: Dizziness, drowsiness, confusion, headache, anxiety, tremors, stimulation, weakness, insomnia, nightmares, EPS G (elderly), increased psychiatric symptoms, *seizures*

CV: Orthostatic hypotension, ECG changes, tachycardia, hypertension, palpitations

EENT: Blurred vision, tinnitus, mydriasis

GI: Diarrhea, dry mouth, nausea, vomiting, ***paralytic ileus,*** increased appetite; cramps, epigastric distress, jaundice, *hepatitis,* stomatitis

GU: Retention, acute renal failure

HEMA: Agranulocytosis, thrombocytopenia, eosinophilia, leukopenia

INTEG: Rash, urticaria, sweating, pruritus, photosensitivity

Contraindications: Hypersensitivity to tricyclic antidepressants, recovery phase of MI, convulsive disorders, prostatic hypertrophy

Precautions: Suicidal patients, severe depression, increased intraocular pressure, narrow-angle glaucoma, urinary retention, cardiac disease, hepatic disease, hypothyroidism, hyperthyroidism, electroshock therapy, elective surgery, G elderly, pregnancy **B**

Pharmacokinetics

Absorption	Slow, complete
Distribution	Widely distributed; crosses placenta
Metabolism	Liver, extensively
Excretion	Feces; breast milk
Half-life	20-40 hr

Pharmacodynamics

Onset	Unknown
Peak	12 hr
Duration	Unknown

Interactions

Individual drugs

Alcohol: ↑ CNS depression
Cimetidine: ↑ levels, ↑ toxicity
Clonidine: Severe hypotension; avoid use
Disulfiram: Organic brain syndrome
Fluoxetine: ↑ levels, toxicity
Guanethidine: ↓ effects

Drug classifications

Analgesics: ↑ CNS depression
Anticholinergics: ↑ side effects
Antihistamines: ↑ CNS depression
Antihypertensives: May block antihypertensive effect
Barbiturates: ↑ effects
CNS depressants: ↑ effects
MAOIs: Hypertensive crisis, convulsions
Oral contraceptives: ↑ effects, toxicity
Phenothiazines: ↑ toxicity
Sedative/hypnotics: ↑ CNS depression
Sympathomimetics, indirect acting: ↓ effects

Smoking

↑ metabolism, ↓ effects

Lab test interferences

↑ Serum bilirubin, ↑ blood gluclose, ↑ alkaline phosphatase
↓ VMA, ↓ 5-HIAA
False ↑ Urinary catecholamines

NURSING CONSIDERATIONS

Assessment

• Monitor B/P (with patient lying, standing), pulse q4h during beginning treatment; if systolic B/P drops 20 mm Hg,

M

hold drug, notify prescriber; take VS q4h in patients with cardiovascular disease
• Monitor blood studies: CBC, leukocytes, differential, cardiac enzymes if patient is receiving long-term therapy
• Monitor hepatic studies: AST (SGOT), ALT (SGPT), bilirubin
• Check weight weekly, drug may increase appetite
• Assess ECG for flattening of T wave, bundle branch block, AV block, dysrhythmias in cardiac patients
• Assess for EPS primarily in G elderly: rigidity, dystonia, akathisia
• Assess mental status: mood, sensorium, affect, suicidal tendencies; assess increase in psychiatric symptoms: depression, panic
• Monitor urinary retention, constipation, constipation is P more likely to occur in children G and elderly
• Assess for withdrawal symptoms: headache, nausea, vomiting, muscle pain, weakness; do not usually occur unless drug was discontinued abruptly
• Identify alcohol consumption; if alcohol is consumed, hold dose until AM

Nursing diagnoses

✓ Coping, ineffective individual (uses)
✓ Injury, risk for (side effects)
✓ Knowledge deficit (teaching)
✓ Noncompliance (teaching)

Implementation

• Give with food or milk for GI symptoms; crush if patient is unable to swallow medication whole
• Give dose hs if oversedation occurs during day; may take G entire dose hs; elderly may not tolerate once/day dosing
• Store at room temp; do not freeze

Patient/family education

• Inform patient that therapeutic effects may take 2-3 wk
• Advise patient to use caution in driving and other activities requiring alertness because of drowsiness, dizziness, blurred vision; to avoid rising quickly from sitting to standing, espe- G cially elderly
• Caution patient to avoid alcohol ingestion, other CNS depressants
• Caution patient not to discontinue medication quickly after long-term use: may cause nausea, headache, malaise
• Teach patient to wear sunscreen or large hat, since photosensitivity occurs
• Teach patient to increase fluids, bulk in diet if constipation, urinary retention occur, G especially elderly
• Teach patient to take gum, hard sugarless candy, or frequent sips of water for dry mouth

Evaluation

Positive therapeutic outcome
• Decrease in depression
• Absence of suicidal thoughts

Treatment of overdose:

ECG monitoring, induce emesis, lavage, activated charcoal, administer anticonvulsant

misoprostol (℞)

(mye-soe-prost'ole)

Cytotec

Func. class.: Gastric mucosa protectant; antiulcer

Chem. class.: Prostaglandin E_1 analog

Pregnancy category X

Action: Inhibits gastric acid secretion; may protect gastric mucosa; can increase bicarbonate, mucus production

➔ **Therapeutic Outcome:** Prevention of gastric ulcers

Uses: Prevention of NSAID-induced gastric ulcers

Dosage and routes

Adult: PO 200 μg qid with food for duration of NSAID therapy; if 200 μg is not tolerated, 100 μg may be given

Available forms: Tabs 100, 200 μg

Adverse effects

GI: Diarrhea, nausea, vomiting, flatulence, constipation, dyspepsia, abdominal pain

GU: Spotting, cramps, hypermenorrhea, menstrual disorders

Contraindications: Hypersensitivity, pregnancy **X**

P G **Precautions:** Lactation, children, elderly, renal disease

Pharmacokinetics

Absorption	Well absorbed
Distribution	Unknown
Metabolism	Liver
Excretion	Kidneys
Half-life	½-1 hr

Pharmacodynamics

Onset	½ hr
Peak	Unknown
Duration	3 hr

Interactions

Drug classifications

Antacids, magnesium: ↑ diarrhea

NURSING CONSIDERATIONS

Assessment

- Assess patient for GI symptoms: hematemesis, occult or frank blood in stools, also severe abdominal pain, cramping, severe diarrhea
- Obtain a negative pregnancy test in women of childbearing age before starting medication; miscarriages are common

Nursing diagnoses

✓ Pain (uses)

✓ Knowledge deficit (teaching)

Implementation

- Give with meals for prolonged drug effect; avoid use of magnesium antacids

Patient/family education

- Advise patient to avoid black pepper, caffeine, alcohol, harsh spices, extremes in temp of food, which may aggravate condition
- Caution patient to avoid OTC preparations: aspirin, cough, cold preparations; condition may worsen
- Teach patient that drug must be continued for prescribed time to be effective and taken exactly as prescribed; doses are not to be doubled
- Instruct patient to report to prescriber diarrhea, black tarry stools, abdominal pain, cramping, menstrual disorders
- Caution patient to prevent pregnancy while taking this drug; spontaneous abortion may occur

Evaluation

Positive therapeutic outcome

- Prevention of ulcers

mitomycin (℞)

(mye-toe-mye'sin)

Mutamycin

Func. class.: Antineoplastic, antibiotic

Pregnancy category D

Action: Inhibits DNA synthesis, primarily; derived from *Streptomyces caespitosus;* appears to cause cross-linking of DNA, a vesicant

Therapeutic Outcome: Prevention of rapidly growing malignant cells

Uses: Pancreas, stomach, head and neck, breast cancer

Investigational uses: Palliative treatment of head, neck, colon, breast, biliary, cervical, lung malignancies

Dosage and routes

Adult: **IV** 20 mg/m^2/day × 5 days, stop drug for 2 days, then repeat cycle; or 10-20 mg/m^2 as a single dose; repeat cycle in 6-8 wk; stop drug if platelets are <75,000/mm^3 or WBC is <3000/mm^3

Available forms: Inj 5, 20, 40 mg/vial

Adverse effects

CNS: Fever, headache, confusion, drowsiness, syncope, fatigue

EENT: Blurred vision, drowsiness, syncope

GI: Nausea, vomiting, anorexia, stomatitis, ***hepatotoxicity,*** diarrhea

GU: Urinary retention, ***renal failure,*** edema

HEMA: ***Thrombocytopenia, leukopenia, anemia***

INTEG: Rash, alopecia, ***extravasation***

RESP: ***Fibrosis, pulmonary infiltrate,*** dyspnea

Contraindications: Hypersensitivity, pregnancy (1st trimester) **D,** as a single agent, thrombocytopenia, coagulation disorders

Precautions: Renal disease, bone marrow depression

Pharmacokinetics

Absorption	Complete bioavailability
Distribution	Widely distributed; concentrates in tumor
Metabolism	Liver, extensively
Excretion	Kidneys, unchanged
Half-life	1 hr

Pharmacodynamics

Unknown

Interactions

Individual drugs

Radiation: ↑ toxicity, bone marrow suppression

Drug classifications

Antineoplastics: ↑ toxicity, bone marrow suppression

NURSING CONSIDERATIONS

Assessment

- Assess buccal cavity q8h for dryness, sores or ulceration, white patches, oral pain, bleeding, dysphagia; obtain prescription for viscous lidocaine (Xylocaine)
- Assess symptoms indicating severe allergic reaction: rash, pruritus, urticaria, purpuric skin lesions, itching, flushing
- Monitor CBC, differential, platelet count weekly; withhold drug if WBC count is <4000/mm^3 or platelet count is <100,000/mm^3, notify prescriber of results if WBC <20,000/mm^3, platelets <150,000/mm^3

• Monitor renal function studies: BUN, creatinine, serum uric acid, urine CrCl before and during therapy; check I&O ratio; report fall in urine output to <30 ml/hr
• Monitor temp q4h (may indicate beginning of infection)
• Monitor liver function tests before and during therapy (bilirubin, AST [SGOT], ALT [SGPT], LDH) as needed or monthly; check for yellowing of skin and sclera, dark urine, clay-colored stools, itchy skin, abdominal pain, fever, diarrhea
• Assess for bleeding: hematuria, stool guaiac, bruising or petechiae, mucosa or orifices q8h, inflammation of mucosa, breaks in skin
• Identify effects of alopecia on body image; discuss feelings about body changes
• Identify edema in feet, joint pain, stomach pain, shaking; check for inflammation of mucosa, breaks in skin

Nursing diagnoses

✓ Injury, risk for (adverse reactions)
✓ Body image disturbance (adverse reactions)
✓ Infection, risk for (adverse reactions)
✓ Knowledge deficit (teaching)

Implementation

• Avoid contact with skin, since medication is very irritating; wash completely to remove
• Give fluids **IV** or PO before chemotherapy to hydrate patient
• Provide antacid before oral agent; give drug after evening meal, before hs; administer antiemetic 30-60 min before giving drug and prn to prevent vomiting; use antibiotics for prophylaxis of infection
• Give top or syst analgesics for pain
• Give in AM so drug can be eliminated before hs
• Provide a liq diet: carbonated beverages; gelatin may be added if patient is not nauseated or vomiting
• Encourage patient to rinse mouth tid-qid with water, club soda, brush teeth bid-qid with soft brush or cotton-tipped applicators for stomatitis, use unwaxed dental floss
• Drug should be prepared by experienced personnel using proper precautions in a biologic cabinet using gown, gloves, mask
• Give by direct **IV** after diluting 5 mg/10 sterile water for inj; shake, allow to stand, give through Y-tube or 3 way stopcock; give over 5-10 min through running D_5W, 0.9% NaCl **IV**
• Apply ice compress for extravasation

Syringe compatibilities: Bleomycin, cisplatin, cyclophosphamide, doxorubicin, droperidol, fluorouracil, furosemide, heparin, leucovorin, methotrexate, metoclopramide, vinblastine, vincristine

Y-site compatibilities: Allopurinol, bleomycin, cisplatin, cyclophosphamide, doxorubicin, droperidol, fluorouracil, furosemide, heparin, leucovorin, melphalan, methotrexate, metoclopramide, ondansetron, teniposide, vinblastine, vincristine

Y-site incompatibilities: Sargramostim, vinorelbine

M

Additive incompatibility:
Bleomycin

Solution compatibilities:
LR, 0.3% NaCl, 0.5% NaCl

Patient/family education

- Teach patient to avoid use of products containing aspirin or ibuprofen, razors, commercial mouthwash, since bleeding may occur; to report symptoms of bleeding (hematuria, tarry stools)
- Caution patient to report signs of anemia (fatigue, headache, irritability, faintness, shortness of breath)
- Advise patient to report any changes in breathing or coughing even several mo after treatment; to avoid crowds and persons with respiratory tract or other infections
- Inform patient that hair may be lost during treatment; a wig or hair piece may make patient feel better; new hair may be different in color, texture
- Advise patient not to have any vaccinations without the advice of the prescriber, serious reactions can occur
- Teach patient that contraception is needed during treatment and for several mo after completion of therapy

Evaluation

Positive therapeutic outcome

- Prevention of rapid division of malignant cells

mitotane (℞)

(mye'toe-tane)

Lysodren, p'-DDD

Func. class.: Antineoplastic

Chem. class.: Hormone, adrenal cytotoxic agent

Pregnancy category C

Action: Cytotoxic and suppressive activity without cellular destruction in the adrenal cortex; related to DDT

➔ **Therapeutic Outcome:** Prevention of rapid growth of malignant cells

Uses: Adrenocortical carcinoma

Investigational uses: Pituitary disorders with cushingoid symptoms

Dosage and routes

Adult: PO 9-10 g/day in divided doses tid or qid; may have to decrease dosage if severe reactions occur

Available forms: Tab 500 mg

Adverse effects

CNS: Lightheadedness, flushing, sedation, vertigo
CV: Hypertension, orthostatic hypotension
EENT: Lethargy, blurring, retinopathy
GI: Nausea, vomiting, anorexia, diarrhea
GU: ***Proteinuria, hematuria***
INTEG: Rash
RESP: ***Fibrosis, pulmonary infiltrate***

Contraindications: Hypersensitivity

Precautions: Lactation, hepatic disease, pregnancy **C**

Pharmacokinetics

Absorption	40%
Distribution	Widely distributed
Metabolism	Liver, extensively
Excretion	Kidneys (10%), bile (15%)
Half-life	18 days-6 mo

Pharmacodynamics

Unknown

Interactions

Individual drugs

Alcohol: ↑ CNS depression
Phenytoin: ↓ effectiveness of phenytoin
Spironolactone: Blocked response in Cushing's disease
Warfarin: ↓ effectiveness of warfarin

Drug classifications

Antidepressants: ↑ CNS depression
Antihistamines: ↑ CNS depression
CNS depressants: ↑ CNS depression
Opioid analgesics: ↑ CNS depression
Sedative/hypnotics: ↑ CNS depression

Lab test interferences

↓ PBI, ↓ urinary 17-OHCS, ↓ uric acid

NURSING CONSIDERATIONS

Assessment

- Assess for adrenal insufficiency: fatigue, orthostatic hypotension, weight loss, weakness, nausea, vomiting, diarrhea
- Monitor renal function studies: BUN, serum uric acid, urine CrCl electrolytes before, during therapy; determine I&O ratio, urinary 17-OHCS, 8-hr plasma cortisol, before, during treatment
- Assess for dyspnea, chest pain, tachypnea, fatigue, increased pulse, pallor, lethargy, muscular weakness, fatigue, oliguria, hypoglycemia
- Assess for frequency of stools, and characteristics of stool: cramping, acidosis, signs of dehydration (rapid respirations, poor skin turgor, decreased urine output, dry skin, restlessness, weakness)
- Assess for symptoms indicating severe allergic reactions: rash, pruritus, itching, flushing
- Assess for signs of infection: increased temp, cough, fatigue, malaise

Nursing diagnoses

- ✓ Injury, risk for (adverse reactions)
- ✓ Body image disturbance (adverse reactions)
- ✓ Infection, risk for (adverse reactions)
- ✓ Knowledge deficit (teaching)

Implementation

- Give 1 hr ac or 2 hr pc to lessen nausea and vomiting or give antacid before oral agent; give drug after evening meal, before hs; administer anti emetic 30-60 min before giving drug to prevent vomiting
- Store in tight container

Patient/family education

- Instruct patient to report any complaints, side effects to the prescriber
- Instruct patient to report any changes in breathing, coughing, signs of wheezing
- Caution patient to avoid driving and other activities requiring alertness until response to drug is known
- Advise patient that a mechanical barrier method of contraception is needed to prevent pregnancy; drug is teratogenic
- Advise patient to use a

M

Medic Alert bracelet or other form of identification to identify treatment and drug used
- Advise patient that if lethargy, somnolence, dizziness, tremors, or weakness occur the prescriber should be contacted
- Caution patient not to use alcohol or OTC drugs unless approved by prescriber; serious adverse reactions may result

Evaluation

Positive therapeutic outcome
- Prevention of rapid division of malignant cells

mitoxantrone (℞)

(mye-toe-zan′trone)

Novantrone

Func. class.: Antineoplastic-antibiotic

Chem. class.: Synthetic anthraquinone

Pregnancy category D

Action: DNA reactive agent; cytocidal effect on both proliferating and nonproliferating cells, suggesting lack of cell cycle phase specificity; a vesicant

Therapeutic Outcome: Prevention of rapidly growing malignant cells

Uses: Acute nonlymphocytic leukemia (adult), relapsed leukemia, breast cancer

Investigational uses: Breast and liver malignancies, non-Hodgkin's lymphoma

Dosage and routes

Induction

Adult: **IV** inf 12 mg/m^2/day on days 1-3, and 100 mg/m^2 cytosine arabinoside × 7 days as a cont 24-hr inf; if complete remission occurs, 2nd inductor may be used

Consolidation

Adult: **IV** inf 12 mg/m^2/day × 2 days, given with cytosine arabinoside 100 mg/m^2/day × 5 days as cont inf usually 6 wk after induction

Available forms: Inj 2 mg/ml

Adverse effects

CNS: Headache, seizures
CV: ***CHF, cardiomyopathy, dysrhythmias,*** ECG changes
EENT: Conjunctivitis, blue-green sclera
GI: Nausea, vomiting, diarrhea, anorexia, mucositis, ***hepatoxicity***
HEMA: ***Thrombocytopenia, leukopenia, myelosuppression, anemia***
INTEG: Rash, necrosis at inj site, alopecia, dermatitis, thrombophlebitis at inj site
MISC: Fever, hypersensitivity, hyperuricemia
RESP: Cough, dyspnea

Contraindications: Hypersensitivity

Precautions: Myelosuppression, lactation, cardiac disease, P children, pregnancy **D,** renal, hepatic disease, gout

Pharmacokinetics

Absorption	Completely absorbed
Distribution	Widely distributed
Metabolism	Liver
Excretion	Bile; kidneys, unchanged (<10%)
Half-life	24-72 hr

Pharmacodynamics

Unknown

Interactions

Individual drugs

Radiation: ↑ toxicity, bone marrow suppression

Drug classifications
Antineoplastics: ↑ toxicity, bone marrow suppression
Live virus vaccines: ↑ adverse reactions

NURSING CONSIDERATIONS

Assessment

- Monitor ECG; watch for ST-T wave changes, low QRS and T, possible dysrhythmias (sinus tachycardia, heart block, PVCs)
- Assess buccal cavity q8h for dryness, sores or ulceration, white patches, oral pain, bleeding, dysphagia; obtain prescription for viscous lidocaine (Xylocaine)
- Assess symptoms indicating severe allergic reaction: rash, pruritus, urticaria, purpuric skin lesions, itching, flushing
- Assess tachypnea, ECG changes, dyspnea, edema, fatigue
- Monitor CBC, differential, platelet count weekly; withhold drug if WBC count is <4000/mm^3 or platelet count is <100,000/mm^3, notify prescriber of results if WBC <20,000/mm^3, platelets <150,000/mm^3
- Assess for increased uric acid levels, swelling, joint pain primarily in extremities; patient should be well hydrated to prevent urate deposits
- Monitor renal function studies: BUN, creatinine, urine CrCl before and during therapy; determine I&O ratio
- Monitor temp q4h (may indicate beginning of infection)
- Monitor liver function tests before and during therapy (bilirubin, AST [SGOT], ALT [SGPT], LDH) as needed or monthly; check for yellowing of skin and sclera, dark urine, clay-colored stools, itchy skin, abdominal pain, fever, diarrhea
- Assess for bleeding: hematuria, stool guaiac, bruising or petechiae, mucosa or orifices q8h; check for inflammation of mucosa, breaks in skin
- Identify effects of alopecia on body image; discuss feelings about body changes

Nursing diagnoses

- ✓ Injury, risk for (adverse reactions)
- ✓ Body image disturbance (adverse reactions)
- ✓ Infection, risk for (adverse reactions)
- ✓ Knowledge deficit (teaching)

Implementation

- Avoid contact with skin, since medication is very irritating; wash completely to remove
- Give fluids **IV** or PO before chemotherapy to hydrate patient
- Give antacid before oral agent; give drug after evening meal, before hs; provide antiemetic 30-60 min before giving drug and prn to prevent vomiting; administer antibiotics for prophylaxis of infection
- Give top or syst analgesics for pain
- Liq diet: carbonated beverages; gelatin may be added if patient is not nauseated or vomiting
- Encourage patient to rinse mouth tid-qid with water, club soda, brush teeth bid-qid with soft brush or cotton-tipped applicators for stomatitis, use unwaxed dental floss
- Sol should be prepared by qualified personnel only under controlled conditions in a

M

biologic cabinet using mask, gloves, gown
• Use Luer-Lok tubing to prevent leakage; do not let sol come in contact with skin; if contact occurs wash well with soap and water
• Give by direct **IV** after diluting with 50 ml or more normal saline or D_5W; give over 3-5 min, running **IV** of D_5W or 0.9% NaCl
• Intermittent inf may be diluted further in D_5W, 0.9% NaCl and run over 15-30 min; check for extravasation

Y-site compatibilities: Allopurinol, amifostine, filgrastim, fludarabine, melphalan, ondansetron, sargramostim, teniposide, thiotepa, vinorelbine

Y-site incompatibility: Paclitaxel

Additive incompatibility: Heparin

Additive compatibilities: Cyclophosphamide, cytarabine, fluorouracil, potassium chloride

Solution compatibilities: D_5/0.9 NaCl, D_5W, 0.9% NaCl

Patient/family education
• Teach patient to avoid use of products containing aspirin or ibuprofen, razors, commercial mouthwash, since bleeding may occur; to report symptoms of bleeding (hematuria, tarry stools)
• Caution patient to report signs of anemia (fatigue, headache, irritability, faintness, shortness of breath)
• Inform patient that hair may be lost during treatment; a wig or hair piece may make patient feel better; new hair may be different in color, texture
• Caution patient not to have any vaccinations without the advice of the prescriber; serious reactions can occur
• Advise patient that contraception is needed during treatment and for several mo after completion of therapy

Evaluation
Positive therapeutic outcome
• Prevention of rapid division of malignant cells

mivacurium (℞)
(mi-va-kure'ee-um)
Mivacron
Func. class.: Nondepolarizing neuromuscular blocker
Pregnancy category C

Action: Inhibits transmission of nerve impulses by binding with cholinergic receptor sites, antagonizing action of acetylcholine; no analgesic response

Therapeutic Outcome: Paralysis of all skeletal muscles

Uses: Facilitation of endotracheal intubation; skeletal muscle relaxation during mechanical ventilation, surgery, or general anesthesia; reduction of fractures/dislocations

Dosage and routes
Adult: **IV** 0.15 mg/kg; maintenance q15 min
P ***Child 2-12:*** **IV** 0.2 mg/kg for a 10-min block

Available forms: 5, 10 ml single-use vial (2 mg/ml); premixed inf in D_5W 50 ml flex container

Adverse effects

CV: Decreased B/P, bradycardia, tachycardia
EENT: Diplopia
INTEG: Rash, urticaria
MS: Weakness, prolonged skeletal muscle relaxation, ***paralysis***
RESP: ***Prolonged apnea, bronchospasm, wheezing, respiratory depression***

Contraindications: Hypersensitivity

Precautions: Pregnancy **C**, renal or hepatic disease, lactation, children <3 mo, fluid and electrolyte imbalances, neuromuscular disease, respiratory disease, obesity, elderly

P G

Pharmacokinetics

Absorption	Completely absorbed
Distribution	Extracellular spaces; crosses placenta
Metabolism	Plasma
Excretion	Kidneys
Half-life	2 hr

Pharmacodynamics

Onset	2-2½ min
Peak	2-3 min
Duration	20-30 min

Interactions

Individual drugs

Clindamycin: ↑ paralysis length and intensity
Colistin: ↑ paralysis length and intensity
Lidocaine: ↑ paralysis length and intensity
Lithium: ↑ paralysis length and intensity
Magnesium: ↑ paralysis length and intensity
Polymyxin B: ↑ paralysis length and intensity
Procainamide: ↑ paralysis length and intensity
Quinidine: ↑ paralysis length and intensity
Succinylcholine: ↑ paralysis length and intensity

Drug classifications

Aminoglycosides: ↑ paralysis length and intensity
β-Blockers: ↑ paralysis length and intensity
Diuretics, potassium-losing: ↑ paralysis length and intensity
General anesthesia: ↑ paralysis length and intensity

NURSING CONSIDERATIONS

Assessment

- Monitor VS (B/P, pulse, respirations, airway) until fully recovered; rate, depth, pattern of respirations, strength of hand grip; patient should be intubated before use
- Monitor for electrolyte imbalances (potassium, magnesium) before drug is used; electrolyte imbalances may lead to increased action of this drug
- Monitor for recovery: decreased paralysis of face, diaphragm, leg, arm, rest of body; residual weakness and respiratory problems may occur during recovery period
- Assess for hypersensitive reactions: rash, fever, respiratory distress, pruritus; drug should be discontinued

Nursing diagnoses

- ✓ Breathing pattern, ineffective (uses)
- ✓ Communication, impaired verbal (adverse reactions)
- ✓ Fear (adverse reactions)
- ✓ Knowledge deficit (teaching)

Implementation

- Use peripheral nerve stimulator (anesthesiologist) to determine neuromuscular blockade; deep tendon reflexes should be monitored during extended periods

M

• Give direct **IV** undiluted over 5-15 min
• Give cont **IV** diluted to 0.5 mg ml in D_5W, 0.9% NaCl, D_5/0.9% NaCl, LR, D_5/LR and give as an inf at prescribed rate (only by qualified person, usually an anesthesiologist); do not administer IM
• Store in light-resistant container
• Give anticholinesterase to reverse neuromuscular blockade

Y-site compatibilities: Alfentanil, droperidol, etomidate, fentanyl, midazolam, sufentanil, thiopental

Y-site incompatibility: Barbiturates

Patient/family education
• Provide reassurance if communication is difficult during recovery from neuromuscular blockade
• Provide explanation to patients regarding all procedures or treatments; patient will remain conscious if anesthesia is not given also

Evaluation

Positive therapeutic outcome
• Paralysis of jaw, eyelid, head, neck, rest of body as evaluated by peripheral nerve stimulator

Treatment of overdose: Edrophonium or neostigmine, atropine; monitor VS; may require mechanical ventilation

moexipril (℞)

(moe-ex'i-pril)

Univasc

Func. class.: Antihypertensive

Chem. class.: Angiotensin-converting enzyme inhibitor

Pregnancy category C

Action: Selectively suppresses renin-angiotensin-aldosterone system; inhibits ACE; prevents conversion of angiotensin I to angiotensin II; results in dilation of arterial, venous vessels

Therapeutic Outcome: Decreased B/P in hypertension

Uses: Hypertension, alone or in combination with thiazide diuretics

Dosage and routes

Initial treatment

Adult: PO 7.5 mg 1 hr ac, may be increased or divided depending on B/P response

Maintenance

Adult: PO 7.5-30 mg qd in 1-2 divided doses 1 hr ac

Available forms: Tabs 7.5, 15 mg

Adverse effects

CNS: Fever, chills
CV: Hypotension, postural hypotension
GI: Loss of taste
GU: Impotence, dysuria, nocturia, proteinura, nephrotic syndrome, acute reversible renal failure, polyuria, oliguria, frequency
HEMA: **Neutropenia**
INTEG: Rash
META: Hypokalemia

RESP: **Bronchospasm,** dyspnea, cough
SYST: **Angioedema**

Contraindications: Hypersensitivity, children, lactation, heart block, bilateral renal stenosis, K-sparing diuretics

P

Precautions: Dialysis patients, hypovolemia, leukemia, scleroderma, lupus erythematosus, blood dyscrasias, CHF, diabetes mellitus, renal disease, thyroid disease, COPD, asthma, pregnancy **C**

Pharmacokinetics

Absorption	Unknown
Distribution	Unknown
Metabolism	Liver to metabolites
Excretion	Via kidneys, crosses placenta; excreted in breast milk
Half-life	Unknown

Pharmacodynamics

Unknown

Interactions

Drug classification

Adrenergic blockers: ↑ hypotension
Antihypertensives: ↑ hypotension
Diuretics: ↑ hypotension
Diuretics, potassium-sparing: Do not use together
Ganglionic blockers: ↑ hypotension
Potassium supplements: Do not use together
Sympathomimetics: Do not use together

Lab test interferences

False positive: Urine acetone

NURSING CONSIDERATIONS

Assessment

- Monitor blood studies: neutrophils, decreased platelets
- Monitor B/P
- Monitor renal studies: protein, BUN, creatinine; watch for increased levels that may indicate nephrotic syndrome
- Monitor baselines in renal, liver function tests before therapy begins
- Monitor K levels, although hyperkalemia rarely occurs
- Assess edema in feet, legs daily
- Assess allergic reaction: rash, fever, pruritus, urticaria; drug should be discontinued if antihistamines fail to help
- Assess for symptoms of CHF: edema, dyspnea, wet rales, B/P
- Monitor for renal symptoms: polyuria, oliguria, frequency

Implementation

- Give PO 1 hr ac
- Store in tight container at 86° F or less

Nursing diagnoses

✓ Knowledge deficit (teaching)

M

Patient/family education

- Teach patient to take 1 hr ac
- Instruct patient not to discontinue drug abruptly
- Tell patient not to use OTC (cough, cold, allergy) products unless directed by prescriber
- Teach patient to comply with dosage schedule, even if feeling better
- Encourage patient to rise slowly to sitting or standing position to minimize orthostatic hypotension
- Teach patient to notify prescriber of mouth sores, sore throat, fever, swelling of hands or feet, irregular heartbeat, chest pain, signs of angioedema
- Tell patient that excessive perspiration, dehydration, vomiting, diarrhea may lead to fall in B/P; consult prescriber if this occurs

- Teach patient that dizziness, fainting, lightheadedness may occur during first few days of therapy
- Tell patient that skin rash or impaired perspiration may occur
- Teach patient how to take B/P

Evaluation

Positive therapeutic outcome

- Decreased B/P in hypertension

Treatment of overdose: 0.9% NaCl **IV** inf, hemodialy sis

moricizine (℞)

(more-i'siz-een)

Ethmozine

Func. class.: Antidysrhythmic, group I

Chem. class.: Phenothiazine

Pregnancy category B

Action: Decreased rate of rise of action potential, prolonging refractory period and shortening the action potential duration; depression of inward influx if sodium mediates the effects; may slow atrial and AV nodal conduction

Therapeutic Outcome: Resolution of life-threatening dysrhythmias

Uses: Life-threatening dysrhythmias

Dosage and routes

Adult: PO 10-15 mg/kg/day in 2-3 divided doses or 600-900 mg/day given in 2-3 divided doses

Available forms: Film-coated tabs 200, 250, 300 mg

Adverse effects

CNS: ***Dizziness, headache, fatigue, perioral numbness, euphoria,*** nervousness, sleep disorders, depression, tinnitus, fatigue

CV: Palpitations, chest pain, CHF, hypertension, syncope, ***dysrythmias,*** bradycardia, ***MI,*** thrombophlebitis

GI: Nausea, abdominal pain, vomiting, diarrhea

GU: Sexual dysfunction, difficult urination, dysuria, incontinence

MISC: Sweating, musculoskeletal pain

RESP: Dyspnea, hyperventilation, ***apnea,*** asthma, pharyngitis, cough

Contraindications: 2nd- to 3rd-degree AV block, right bundle branch block, cardiogenic shock, hypersensitivity

Precautions: CHF, hypokalemia, hyperkalemia, sick sinus syndrome, pregnancy **B,** lactation, [P] children, impaired hepatic and renal function, cardiac dysfunction

Pharmacokinetics

Absorption	Well absorbed
Distribution	Plasma protein binding (95%)
Metabolism	Liver, extensively
Excretion	Kidneys, breast milk
Half-life	1½-3½ hr

Pharmacodynamics

Onset	Unknown
Peak	½-2 hr
Duration	8-12 hr

Interactions

Individual drugs

Cimetidine: ↑ effect of moricizine

Theophylline: ↓ effect of theophylline

NURSING CONSIDERATIONS
Assessment
- Monitor ECG at baseline and periodically to determine drug effectiveness; measure PR, QRS, QT intervals, check for PVCs, other dysrhythmias; check B/P for hypotension, hypertension and for rebound hypertension after 1-2 hr; check for dehydration or hypovolemia
- Monitor I&O ratio and electrolytes: potassium, sodium, chloride; check weight daily and for signs of CHF or pulmonary toxicity: dyspnea, fatigue, cough, fever, chest pain; drug should be discontinued
- Monitor liver function studies: AST (SGOT), ALT (SGPT), bilirubin, alkaline phosphatase
- Monitor cardiac rate; monitor respiration rate, rhythm, character, and chest pain; watch for ventricular tachycardia, supraventricular tachycardia, or fibrillation

Nursing diagnoses
- ✓ Cardiac output, decreased (uses)
- ✓ Impaired gas exchange (adverse reactions)
- ✓ Knowledge deficit (teaching)

Implementation
- Give with meals for GI upset; may be given in 2 divided doses if adverse reactions are minimal
- Make dosage adjustment q 3 days or more

Patient/family education
- Instruct patient to report side effects immediately to prescriber
- Instruct patient to complete follow-up appointment with health care provider including pulmonary function studies, chest x-ray, ophth and otoscopic examinations
- Advise patient to carry identification (Medic Alert) indicating condition and treatment
- Caution patient to avoid driving and other hazardous activities until drug response is determined
- Instruct patient to take medication as prescribed, not to double doses; missed doses may be taken up to 6 hr after previous dose

Treatment of overdose: O_2, artificial ventilation, ECG, administer dopamine for circulatory depression, administer diazepam or thiopental for convulsions, isoproterenol

morphine (℞)
(mor'feen)
Astramorph PF, Duramorph, Epimorph ✤, Infumorph 200, Infumorph 500, Morphine H.P. ✤, morphine sulfate, Morphitec ✤, M.O.S. ✤, M.O.S.-S.R. ✤, MS Contin, MSIR, MSIR, OMS Concentrate, Oramorph SR, RMS, Roxanol, Roxanol 100, Roxanol Rescudose, Roxanol SR

Func. class.: Opioid analgesic

Pregnancy category B

Controlled substance schedule II

Action: Depresses pain impulse transmission at the spinal cord level by interacting with opioid receptors, produces CNS depression

Pharmacodynamics

	PO	PO–EXT REL	IM	SC	REC	IV	IT
Onset	Variable	Unknown	10-30 min	20 min	Unknown	Rapid	Rapid
Peak	1 hr	Unknown	½-1 hr	1-1½ hr	½-1 hr	20 min	Unknown
Duration	4-5 hr	8-12 hr	3-7 hr	4-5 hr	4-5 hr	4-5 hr	Ext

➔ **Therapeutic Outcome:** Decreased pain

Uses: Severe pain; often given after or during an MI

Dosage and routes

Adult: SC/IM 4-15 mg q4h prn; PO 10-30 mg q4h prn; ext rel q8-12h; rec 10-20 mg q4h prn; **IV** 4-10 mg diluted in 4-5 ml water for inj, over 5 min; epidural 2-10 mg/day

P ***Child:*** SC 0.1-0.2 mg/kg, not to exceed 15 mg; IM/**IV** 50-100 μg/kg, max 10 mg/dose initially

Available forms: Inj 2, 4, 5, 8, 10, 15 mg/ml; sol tabs 10, 15, 30 mg; oral sol 10, 20 mg/5 ml, 20 mg/10 ml, 20 mg/ml; oral tabs 15, 30 mg; rec supp 5, 10, 20 mg; ext rel tab 30 mg; caps 15, 30 mg

Adverse effects

CNS: Drowsiness, dizziness, *confusion,* headache, *sedation,* euphoria, hallucinations, dysphoria
CV: Palpitations, bradycardia, *hypotension*
EENT: Tinnitus, blurred vision, miosis, diplopia
GI: Nausea, vomiting, anorexia, *constipation,* cramps, biliary tract pressure
GU: Urinary retention

Pharmacokinetics

Absorption	Variably absorbed (PO); well absorbed (IM, SC, rec); completely absorbed (IV)
Distribution	Widely distributed; crosses placenta
Metabolism	Liver, extensively
Excretion	Kidneys
Half-life	1½-2 hr

INTEG: Rash, urticaria, bruising, flushing, diaphoresis, pruritus
RESP: Respiratory depression

Contraindications: Hypersensitivity, addiction (narcotic), hemorrhage, bronchial asthma, increased intracranial pressure

Precautions: Addictive personality, pregnancy **B,** lactation, acute MI, severe heart G disease, elderly, respiratory depression, hepatic disease, P renal disease, child <18 yr

Interactions

Individual drugs

Alcohol: ↑ respiratory depression, hypotension, sedation
Nalbuphine: ↓ analgesia
Pentazocine: ↓ analgesia

Drug classifications

Antihistamines: ↑ respiratory depression, hypotension
CNS depressants: ↑ respiratory depression, hypotension
MAOIs: Reduce dosage; unpredictable reaction may occur

Sedative/hypnotics: ↑ respiratory depression, hypotension

Lab test interferences

↑ Amylase

NURSING CONSIDERATIONS

Assessment

- Assess pain: location, type, character, intensity; give dose before pain becomes extreme
- Monitor I&O ratio; check for decreasing output; may indicate urinary retention; check for constipation; increase fluids, bulk in diet if needed or stool softeners may be prescribed
- Monitor CNS changes: dizziness, drowsiness, hallucinations, euphoria, LOC, pupil reactions
- Monitor allergic reactions: rash, urticaria
- Assess respiratory dysfunction: depression, character, rate, rhythm; notify prescriber if respirations are <10/min

Nursing diagnoses

- ✓ Pain (uses)
- ✓ Sensory-perceptual alteration: visual, auditory (adverse reactions)
- ✓ Breathing pattern, ineffective (adverse reactions)
- ✓ Knowledge deficit (teaching)

Implementation

- Give with antiemetic if nausea, vomiting occur
- Administer when pain is beginning to return; determine dosage interval by patient response; continuous dosing of medication is more effective than giving prn
- Withdraw medication slowly after long-term use to prevent withdrawal symptoms
- Store in light-resistant container at room temp

PO route

- May be given with food or milk to lessen GI upset; may be crushed and mixed with food or fluids; ext rel tabs should be swallowed whole

IM/SC route

- Do not give if cloudy or a precipitate has formed

IV IV route

- Give direct **IV** by diluting with ≥5 ml of sterile water or 0.9% NaCl for inj; give 2.5-15 mg/4-5 min; rapid administration may lead to increased respiratory depression, death
- Give cont inf by adding to D_5W, $D_{10}W$, 0.9% NaCl, 0.45% NaCl, Ringer's, LR, any dextrose/saline sol, or any dextrose/Ringer's, 0.1-1 mg/ml
- Give by inf pump to deliver correct dosage; titrate to provide adequate pain relief without serious sedation, respiratory depression, hypotension
- May be given by patient-controlled analgesia (PCA) pump in terminal illnesses; patient is able to control amount of morphine

Syringe compatibilities: Atropine, benzquinamide, butorphanol, chlorpromazine, cimetidine, dimenhydrinate, diphenhydramine, droperidol, fentanyl, glycopyrrolate, hydroxyzine, metoclopramide, midazolam, perphenazine, promazine, ranitidine, scopolamine

Syringe incompatibilities: Meperidine, thiopental

Y-site compatibilities: Allopurinol, amikacin, aminophylline, ampicillin, ampicillin/sulbactam, atracurium, calcium

M

chloride, cefamandole, cefazolin, cefoperazone, ceforanide, cefotaxime, cefotetan, cefoxitin, ceftizoxime, cefuroxime, cephalothin, cephapirin, chloramphenicol, cisplatin, clindamycin, doxycycline, enalaprilat, erythromycin, esmolol, famotidine, foscarnet, gentamicin, heparin, hydrocortisone, IL-2, insulin, kanamycin, labetalol, magnesium sulfate, melphalan, metronidazole, mezlocillin, moxalactam, nafcillin, ondansetron, oxacillin, oxytocin, paclitaxel, pancuronium, penicillin G potassium, piperacillin, potassium chloride, ranitidine, sodium bicarbonate, ticarcillin, ticarcillin/clavulanate, tobramycin, trimethoprim-sulfamethoxazole, vancomycin, vecuronium, vinorelbine, vitamin B with C, zidovudine

Y-site incompatibilities: Furosemide, minocycline, tetracycline

Additive compatibilities: Alteplase, amifostine, amiodarone, dobutamine, granisetron, insulin (reg), lorazepam, midazolam, nitroprusside, succinylcholine, thiotepa, verapamil

Additive incompatibility: Aminophylline

Patient/family education

- Advise patient to report any symptoms of CNS changes, allergic reactions
- Caution patients to avoid CNS depressants (alcohol, sedative/hypnotics) for at least 24 hr after taking this drug
- Discuss with patient that dizziness, drowsiness, and confusion are common; to avoid getting up without assistance
- Discuss in detail all aspects of the drug and expected response

Evaluation

Positive therapeutic outcome

- Decreased pain

Treatment of overdose: Naloxone (Narcan) 0.2-0.8 **IV**, O_2, **IV** fluids, vasopressors

multivitamins

(PO, OTC; IV, ℞)

Adavite, Dayalets, LKV Drops, Multi-75, Multi-Day, One-A-Day, Optilets, Poly-Vi-Sol, Quintabs, Rulets, Sesame Street Vitamins, Tab-A-Vite, Therabid, Theragran, Unicaps, Vita-Bob, Vita-Kid, many other brands; Berocca Parenteral, M.V.C. 9+3, M.V.I. Pediatric

Func. class.: Vitamins, multiple

Pregnancy category A

Action: Needed for adequate metabolism

➡ **Therapeutic Outcome:** Prevention and treatment of vitamin deficiencies

Uses: Prevention and treatment of vitamin deficiencies

Dosage and routes

P ***Adult and child:*** PO depends on brand

Available forms: Many forms available

Adverse effects

Rare at recommended dosage

Precautions: Pregnancy **A**

Pharmacokinetics

Absorption	Well absorbed (PO)
Distribution	Widely distributed; crosses placenta
Metabolism	Widely metabolized
Excretion	Kidney, unchanged (water soluble)
Half-life	Unknown

Pharmacodynamics

Unknown

Interactions
Individual drugs
Levodopa: ↓ effect of levodopa (large amounts of B_6)

NURSING CONSIDERATIONS
Assessment
- Assess patient for vitamin deficiency; usually more than one vitamin is deficient

Nursing diagnoses
✓ Nutrition, less than body requirements (uses)
✓ Knowledge deficit (teaching)

Implementation
PO route
- Liq multivitamins can be diluted or dropped into patients' mouth using dropper provided with some brands
- Chew tab should be chewed and not swallowed whole

IV **IV route**
- Give by cont inf only after diluting 5-10 ml (multivitamins)/500-1000 ml of D_5W, $D_{10}W$, $D_{20}W$, LR, D_5/LR, D_5/0.9% NaCl, 0.9% NaCl, 3% NaCl
- Do not use sol with crystals, precipitate or color other than bright yellow

Y-site compatibilities:
Acyclovir, ampicillin, cefazolin, cephalothin, cephapirin, erythromycin, fludarabine, gentamicin, tacrolimus, tetracycline

Additive compatibilities:
Cefoxitin, isoproterenol, methyldopate, metoclopramide, metronidazole, netilmicin, norepinephrine, sodium bicarbonate, verapamil

Additive incompatibilities:
Penicillin G, erythromycin, tetracycline, kanamycin, streptomycin, doxycycline, lincomycin should not be admixed

Patient/family education
- Advise patient that adequate nutrition must be maintained to prevent further deficiencies; to comply with treatment regimen
- Advise patient to avoid treating flavored multivitamins as P candy; child may overdose
- Caution patient to store P vitamins out of children's reach

Evaluation
Positive therapeutic outcome
- Check each individual vitamin for guidelines
- Absence of vitamin deficiencies

M

muromonab-CD3 (℞)
(mur-oe-mone'ab)
Orthoclone OKT3
Func. class.: Immunosuppressive
Chem. class.: Murine monoclonal antibody
Pregnancy category C

Action: Reverses graft rejection by blocking T cell function

➔ **Therapeutic Outcome:** Prevention of graft rejection

Uses: Acute allograft rejection

in renal, cardiac/hepatic transplant patients

Dosage and routes

Adult: **IV** bol 5 mg/day × 10-14 days; usually methylprednisolone sodium succinate, 1 mg/kg **IV**, is given before muromonab-CD3, 100 mg **IV** hydrocortisone sodium succinate is given 30 min after muromonab-CD3

P ***Child:*** **IV** 100 µg/kg/day × 10-14 day

Cardiac/hepatic allograft rejection, steroid resistant

Adult: **IV** bol 5 mg/day × 10-14 days; begin when it is known that rejection has not been reversed by steroids

Available forms: Inj 5 mg/5 ml

Adverse effects

CNS: Pyrexia, chills, tremors
CV: Chest pain
GI: Vomiting, nausea, diarrhea
MISC: Infection
RESP: Dyspnea, wheezing, pulmonary edema

Contraindications: Hypersensitivity to murine origin, fluid overload

Precautions: Pregnancy **C,**
P child <2 yr, fever

Pharmacokinetics	
Absorption	Completely absorbed
Distribution	Unknown
Metabolism	Unknown
Excretion	Unknown
Half-life	Unknown

Pharmacodynamics
Unknown

Interactions

Individual drugs

Allopurinol: ↑ toxicity
Cyclosporine: ↑ myelosuppression

Drug classifications

Antineoplastics: ↑ myelosuppression

NURSING CONSIDERATIONS

Assessment

- ❗ Assess for cytosine release syndrome (CRS): nausea, vomiting, chills, fever, joint pain, weakness, dizziness, diarrhea, tremors, abdominal pain; occurs 30-60 min after first dose; methylprednisolone sodium succinate may be prescribed to lessen this reaction
- Assess for hypersensitivity reaction: dyspnea, bronchospasm, urticaria, tachycardia, hypotension, angioedema; discontinue drug; all emergency equipment must be nearby
- Assess for headache, photophobia, fever, rigidity; indicate aseptic meningitis has developed
- Assess for sore throat, fever, chills, rash, dysuria which may indicate infection; therapy may be discontinued
- Assess for fluid overload: edema, pulmonary edema, increasing weight
- Monitor blood studies: CBC with differential, platelets, BUN, creatinine, alkaline phosphatase, bilirubin during treatment monthly
- Monitor AST (SGOT), ALT (SGPT), BUN, creatinine, alkaline phosphatase, bilirubin
- Obtain human-mouse antibody; if titer is over 1:1000, this drug should not be used
- Monitor T cell with CD_3 antigen qd; report should be CD_3 positive and T cells <25/mm^3

Nursing diagnoses

- ✓ Infection, risk for (uses)
- ✓ Knowledge deficit (teaching)

Implementation

• Give by direct **IV** undiluted; withdraw with a 0.2-0.22 low–protein binding µm filter; discard and use new needle for administration; give over 1 min
• Give for several days before transplant surgery

Patient/family education

• Instruct patient to report fever, chills, sore throat, fatigue, since serious infections may occur
• Advise patient to use contraceptive measures during treatment for 12 wk after ending therapy; drug is mutagenic
• Advise patient to avoid crowds and persons with known infections to reduce risk of infection

Evaluation

Positive therapeutic outcome
• Absence of graft rejection

mycophenolate mofetil (℞)

(mie-koe-feen'oh-late moe-feh-til)

CellCept

Func. class.: Immunosuppressive

Pregnancy category C

Action: Inhibits inflammatory responses that are mediated by the immune system; prolongs survival of allogenic transplants

➔ **Therapeutic Outcome:** Absence of graft rejection

Uses: Organ transplants to prevent rejection

Dosage and routes

Adult: PO; give initial dose 72 hr prior to transplantation; 1 gm bid given to renal transplant patients in combination with corticosteroids and cyclosporine

Available forms: Cap 250 mg; tab 500 mg

Adverse effects

CNS: Tremor, dizziness, insomnia, headache, fever
GI: Nausea, vomiting, stomatitis
GU: UTI, hematuria, ***renal tubular necrosis***
HEMA: ***Leukopenia, thrombocytopenia, anemia, pancytopenia***
INTEG: Rash
META: Peripheral edema, hypercholesteremia, hypophosphatemia, edema, hyperkalemia, hypokalemia, hyperglycemia
MS: Arthralgia, muscle wasting
RESP: Dyspnea, respiratory infection, increased cough, pharyngitis, bronchitis, pneumonia

Contraindications: Hypersensitivity to this drug or mycophenolic acid

Precautions: Lymphomas, malignancies, neutropenia, renal disease, pregnancy **C**, lactation

Pharmacokinetics	
Absorption	Rapidly and completely absorbed
Distribution	Unknown
Metabolism	To active metabolite (MPA)
Excretion	Urine, feces
Half-life	Unknown

Pharmacodynamics

Unknown

M

Interactions

Individual drugs

Acyclovir: ↑ concentration of both drugs
Cholestyramine: ↓ levels of mycophenolate
Ganciclovir: ↑ concentration of both drugs
Phenytoin: ↑ binding of phenytoin
Probenecid: ↑ levels of mycophenolate
Theophylline: ↓ binding of theophylline

Drug classifications

Antacids: ↓ levels of mycophenolate
Salicylates: ↑ levels of mycophenolate

NURSING CONSIDERATIONS

Assessment

- Monitor blood studies: CBC during treatment monthly
- Monitor liver function studies: alk phosphatase, AST (SGOT), ALT (SGPT), bilirubin

Nursing diagnoses

✓ Infection, risk for (uses)
✓ Knowledge deficit (teaching)

Implementation

- Give 72 hrs prior to transplantation; may be given in combination with corticosteroids and cyclosporine
- Give alone for better absorption
- ⊘ Do not crush, chew caps

Patient/family education

- Teach patient to report fever, rash, severe diarrhea, chills, sore throat, fatigue, since serious infections may occur
- Instruct patient to avoid crowds to reduce risk of infection

Evaluation

Positive therapeutic outcome

- Absence of graft rejection

nabumetone (℞)

(na-byoo′me-tone)
Relafen
Func. class.: Nonsteroidal antiinflammatory
Chem. class.: Acetic acid derivative

Pregnancy category C

Action: Inhibits prostaglandin synthesis by decreasing an enzyme needed for biosynthesis; analgesic, antiinflammatory

➔ **Therapeutic Outcome:** Decreased pain, swelling of joints

Uses: Osteoarthritis, rheumatoid arthritis, acute or chronic treatment

Dosage and routes

Adult: PO 1 g as a single dose; may increase to 1.5-2 g/day if needed; may give qd or bid (as a divided dose)

Available forms: Tabs 500, 750 mg

Adverse effects

CNS: Dizziness, headache, drowsiness, fatigue, tremors, confusion, insomnia, anxiety, depression, nervousness
CV: Tachycardia, peripheral edema, palpitations, dysrhythmias, CHF
EENT: Tinnitus, hearing loss, blurred vision
GI: Nausea, anorexia, vomiting, diarrhea, jaundice, cholestatic hepatitis, constipation, flatulence, cramps, dry mouth, peptic ulcer, gastritis, ***ulceration, perforation***
GU: ***Nephrotoxicity, dysuria, hematuria, oliguria, azotemia,*** cystitis
HEMA: ***Blood dyscrasias***
INTEG: Purpura, rash, pruri-

tus, sweating, photosensitivity
RESP: Dyspnea, pharyngitis, ***bronchospasm***

Contraindications: Hypersensitivity to this drug or aspirin, iodides, NSAIDs, asthma, severe renal disease

Precautions: Pregnancy **C** 1st and 2nd trimester, lactation, P children, bleeding disorders, GI disorders, cardiac disorders, renal disorders hepatic dysfunction, G elderly

Pharmacokinetics

Absorption	Well absorbed
Distribution	Unknown
Metabolism	Liver, extensively, to inactive metabolite
Excretion	Unknown
Half-life	22-30 hr

Pharmacodynamics

Onset	Unknown
Peak	2½-4 hr
Duration	Unknown

Interactions

Individual drugs

Acetaminophen (long-term use): ↑ renal reactions
Alcohol: ↑ adverse reactions
Aspirin: ↓ effectiveness, ↑ adverse reactions
Cefamandole: ↑ bleeding
Cefoperazone: ↑ bleeding
Cefotetan: ↑ bleeding
Coumadin: ↑ anticoagulant effects
Digoxin: ↑ toxicity, levels
Insulin: ↓ insulin effect
Lithium: ↑ toxicity
Methotrexate: ↑ toxicity
Phenytoin: ↑ toxicity
Probenecid: ↑ toxicity
Sulfonylurea: ↑ toxicity
Valproic acid: ↑ bleeding

Drug classifications

Anticoagulants: ↑ risk of bleeding
Antihypertensives: ↓ effect of antihypertensives
Antineoplastics: ↑ risk of hematologic toxicity
Cephalosporins: ↑ risk of bleeding
Diuretics: ↓ effectiveness of diuretics
Glucocorticoids: ↑ adverse reactions
Hypoglycemics, oral: ↓ hypoglycemic effect
NSAIDs: ↑ adverse reactions
Potassium supplements: ↑ adverse reactions
Radiation: ↑ risk of hematologic toxicity
Sulfonamides: ↑ toxicity

NURSING CONSIDERATIONS

Assessment

- Assess for pain: location, duration, intensity; and for inflammation of joints, ROM
- Monitor blood counts during therapy; watch for decreasing platelets; if low, therapy may need to be discontinued, restarted after hematologic recovery; check for blood dyscrasias (thrombocytopenia): brusing, fatigue, bleeding, poor healing; monitor liver function tests: AST (SGOT), ALT (SGPT), alkaline phosphatase

Nursing diagnoses

- ✓ Pain (uses)
- ✓ Mobility, impaired (uses)
- ✓ Injury, risk for (adverse reactions)
- ✓ Knowledge deficit (teaching)

Implementation

- Administer tab to patient crushed or whole
- Give with food or milk to decrease gastric symptoms

Patient/family education

- Tell patient that drug must be continued for prescribed

N

time to be effective; to avoid aspirin, alcoholic beverages, ibuprofen, and OTC medications unless approved by prescriber

- Caution patient to report bleeding, bruising, fatigue, malaise, since blood dyscrasias do occur
- Instruct patient to use caution when driving; drowsiness, dizziness may occur
- Advise patient to use sunscreen, hat, and other protective clothing to prevent burning

Evaluation

Positive therapeutic outcome

- Decreased pain
- Decreased inflammation
- Increased mobility

nadolol (℞)

(nay-doe'lole)

Corgard

Func. class.: Antihypertensive, antianginal

Chem. class.: β-Adrenergic receptor blocker

Pregnancy category C

Action: Competitively blocks stimulation of β-adrenergic receptor within vascular smooth muscle; produces chronotropic, inotropic activity (decreases rate of SA node discharge, increases recovery time), slows conduction of AV node, decreases heart rate, which decreases O_2 consumption in myocardium; also decreases renin-aldosterone-angiotensin system at high doses, inhibits β_2-receptors in bronchial system

Therapeutic Outcome: Decreased B/P, heart rate

Uses: Chronic stable angina pectoris, mild to moderate hypertension

Investigational uses: Tachydysrhythmias, aggression, anxiety, tremors, esophageal varices (rebleeding only), prophylaxis of migraine headaches

Dosage and routes

Adult: PO 40 mg qd; increase by 40-80 mg q3-7 days; maintenance 40-240 mg/day for angina, 40-320 mg/day for hypertension

Available forms: Tabs 20, 40, 80, 120, 160 mg

Adverse effects

CNS: Depression, hallucinations, dizziness, fatigue, lethargy, paresthesia, headache

*CV: **Bradycardia, hypotension, CHF,*** palpitations, AV block, chest pain, peripheral ischemia, flushing, edema, vasodilatation, conduction disturbances

EENT: Sore throat

GI: Nausea, vomiting, diarrhea, colitis, constipation, cramps, dry mouth, flatulence, hepatomegaly, pancreatitis, taste distortion

*HEMA: **Agranulocytosis, thrombocytopenia***

INTEG: Rash, pruritus, fever

RESP: Dyspnea, respiratory dysfunction, ***bronchospasm,*** cough, wheezing, nasal stuffiness, pharyngitis, ***laryngospasm***

Contraindications: Hypersensitivity to this drug, cardiac failure, cardiogenic shock, 2nd- or 3rd-degree heart block, bronchospastic disease, sinus bradycardia, CHF, COPD

Precautions: Diabetes mellitus, pregnancy **C,** renal disease, lactation, hyperthyroidism, peripheral vascular disease, myasthenia gravis

Pharmacokinetics

Absorption	Variably absorbed
Distribution	Crosses placenta; minimal concentration in CNS
Excretion	Kidneys, unchanged
Half-life	10-24 hr; increased in renal disease

Pharmacodynamics

Onset	Variable
Peak	3-4 hr
Duration	17-24 hr

Interactions

Individual drugs

Alcohol: ↑ hypotension (large amounts)
Epinephrine: α-Adrenergic stimulation
Hydralazine: ↑ hypotension, bradycardia
Indomethacin: ↓ antihypertensive effect
Insulin: ↑ hypoglycemia
Methyldopa: ↑ hypotension, bradycardia
Prazosin: ↑ hypotension, bradycardia
Reserpine: ↑ hypotension, bradycardia
Thyroid: ↓ effect of nadolol
Verapamil: ↑ myocardial depression

Drug classifications

Amphetamines: ↑ hypotension, bradycardia
Antihypertensives: ↑ hypertension
β_2-Agonists: ↓ bronchodilatation
Cardiac glycosides: ↑ bradycardia
MAOIs: ↑ bradycardia
Nitrates: ↑ hypotension
NSAIDs: ↓ effect
Theophyllines: ↓ bronchodilatation

Lab test interferences

False ↑ Urinary catecholamines

NURSING CONSIDERATIONS

Assessment

- Monitor B/P at beginning of treatment, periodically thereafter; note rate, rhythm, quality of apical/radial pulse before administration; notify prescriber of any significant changes (pulse <55 bpm)
- Check for baselines in renal, liver function tests before therapy begins
- Assess for edema in feet, legs daily; monitor I&O, daily weight; check for jugular vein distention and rales bilaterally, dyspnea (CHF)
- Monitor skin turgor, dryness of mucous membranes for hydration status, especially G elderly

Nursing diagnoses

✓ Cardiac output, decreased (uses)
✓ Injury, potential for (adverse reactions)
✓ Knowledge deficit (teaching)
✓ Noncompliance (teaching)

Implementation

- Given ac, hs, tab may be crushed or swallowed whole; give with food to prevent GI upset; give reduced dosage in renal dysfunction
- Store protected from light, moisture; placed in cool environment

Patient/family education

- Teach patient not to discontinue drug abruptly; taper over 2 wk; may cause precipitate angina if stopped abruptly
- Teach patient not to use OTC products containing

α-adrenergic stimulants (such as nasal decongestants, cold preparations); to avoid alcohol, smoking and to limit sodium intake as prescribed

- Teach patient how to take pulse and B/P at home; advise when to notify prescriber
- Instruct patient to comply with weight control, dietary adjustments, modified exercise program
- Advise patient to carry/wear Medic Alert ID to identify drug being taken, allergies; teach patient drug controls symptoms but does not cure condition
- Caution patient to avoid hazardous activities if dizziness, drowsiness present
- Teach patient to report symptoms of CHF: difficult breathing, especially on exertion or when lying down, night cough, swelling of extremities or bradycardia, dizziness, confusion, depression, fever
- Teach patient to take drug as prescribed, not to double doses, skip doses; take any missed doses as soon as remembered if at least 4 hr until next dose

Evaluation

Positive therapeutic outcome

- Decreased B/P in hypertension

nafcillin (℞)

(naf-sill'in)

Nafcil, nafcillin sodium, Nallpen, Unipen

Func. class.: Broad-spectrum antiinfective

Chem. class.: Penicillinase-resistant penicillin

Pregnancy category B

Action: Interferes with cell wall replication of susceptible organisms; osmotically unstable cell wall swells, bursts from osmotic pressure

Therapeutic Outcome: Bactericidal effects for gram-positive cocci *Staphylococcus aureus, Streptococcus viridans, S. pneumoniae* and infections caused by penicillinase-producing *Staphylococcus*

Uses: Infections caused by penicillinase-producing staphylococci, streptococci; respiratory tract, skin, skin structure, urinary tract, bone, joint infections, sinusitis, endocarditis, septicemia, meningitis

Dosage and routes

Adult: IM/**IV** 2-6 g/day in divided doses q4-6h; PO 2-6 g/day in divided doses q4-6h

P ***Child:*** IM 25 mg/kg q12h; PO 25-50 mg/kg/day in divided doses q6h

P ***Neonates:*** IM 10 mg/kg bid

Available forms: Cap 250 mg; tab 500 mg; powder for oral susp 250 mg/5 ml; powder for inj 500 mg, 1, 2, 10 g; **IV** 1, 1.5, 2, 4 g

Adverse effects

CNS: Lethargy, hallucinations, anxiety, depression, muscle twitching, ***coma, convulsions***

GI: Nausea, vomiting, diarrhea, increased AST (SGOT), ALT (SGPT), abdominal pain, glossitis, ***pseudomembranous colitis***
GU: Oliguria, ***proteinuria, hematuria, vaginitis, moniliasis, glomerulonephritis,*** interstitial nephritis
HEMA: Anemia, increased bleeding time, ***bone marrow depression, granulocytopenia***

Contraindications: Hypersensitivity to penicillins

Precautions: Pregnancy **B**, hypersensitivity to cephalosporins, P neonates

Pharmacokinetics

Absorption	Well absorbed (IM); erratic (PO)
Distribution	Widely distributed; crosses placenta
Metabolism	Not metabolized
Excretion	Kidneys, unchanged; breast milk
Half-life	1 hr; increased in renal disease

Pharmacodynamics

	PO	IM	IV
Onset	½ hr	½ hr	Immediate
Peak	1-2 hr	1-2 hr	Inf end

Interactions
Individual drugs
Aspirin: ↑ nafcillin levels, ↓ renal excretion
Probenecid: ↑ nafcillin levels, ↓ renal excretion
Drug classifications
Oral anticoagulants: ↑ anticoagulant effects
Oral contraceptives: ↓ contraceptive effectiveness
Food
Food, carbonated drinks, citrus fruit juices: ↓ absorption
Lab test interferences
False positive: Urine glucose, urine protein

NURSING CONSIDERATIONS
Assessment
- Assess patient for previous sensitivity reaction to penicillins or other cephalosporins; cross-sensitivity between penicillins and cephalosporins is common
- Assess patient for signs and symptoms of infection including characteristics of wounds, sputum, urine, stool, WBC >10,000, earache, fever; obtain baseline information and during treatment
- Obtain C&S before beginning drug therapy to identify if correct treatment has been initiated
- Assess for allergic reactions: rash, urticaria, pruritus, chills, fever, joint pain; angioedema may occur a few days after therapy begins; epinephrine, resuscitation equipment should be available for anaphylactic reaction
- Identify urine output; if decreasing, notify prescriber (may indicate nephrotoxicity); also check for increased BUN, creatinine
- Monitor blood studies: AST (SGOT), ALT (SGPT), CBC, Hct, bilirubin, LDH, alkaline phosphatase, Coombs' test monthly if patient is on long-term therapy
- Monitor electrolytes: potassium, sodium, chloride monthly if patient is on long-term therapy
- Assess bowel pattern qd; if severe diarrhea occurs, drug should be discontinued; may indicate pseudomembranous colitis
- Monitor for bleeding: ecchymosis, bleeding gums, hematuria, stool guaiac daily if on long-term therapy

N

• Assess for overgrowth of infection: perineal itching, fever, malaise, redness, pain, swelling, drainage, rash, diarrhea, change in cough, sputum

Nursing diagnoses

✓ Infection, risk for (uses)
✓ Diarrhea (adverse reactions)
✓ Injury, risk for (adverse reactions)
✓ Knowledge deficit (teaching)
✓ Noncompliance (teaching)

Implementation

PO route

• Give in even doses around the clock; if GI upset occurs, give with food; drug must be given for 10-14 days to ensure organism death and prevent superinfection; store in tight container.
• Do not crush, chew caps
• Shake susp; store in refrigerator for 2 wk, 1 wk at room temp

IM route

• Reconstitute 500 mg/1.7-1.8 ml; 1 g/3.4 ml; 2 g/6.6-6.8 ml with sterile water or bacteriostatic water for a conc of 250 mg/ml; store unused portion in refrigerator for up to 7 days
• Give deep in large muscle mass

IV route

• Reconstitute 500 mg/1.7 ml; 1 g/3.4 ml; 2 g/6.6-6.8 ml with sterile water or bacteriostatic water for a conc of 250 mg/ml; store unused portion in refrigerator for up to 7 days
• Give by direct **IV** by diluting reconstituted sol with 15-30 ml of sterile water or 0.9% NaCl; give over 5-10 min
• Give by intermittent inf by diluting to a conc of 2-40 mg/ml with 0.9% NaCl, D_5W, $D_{10}W$, D_5/0.9% NaCl, D_5/LR, LR, Ringer's; store in refrigerator for up to 96 hr or 24 hr room temp; run over 30-60 min

Syringe compatibilities: Cimetidine, heparin

Y-site incompatibilities: Droperidol, fentanyl/droperidol, labetalol, nalbuphine, pentazocine, regular insulin, verapamil

Y-site compatibilities: Acyclovir, atropine, cyclophosphamide, diazepam, enalaprilat, esmolol, famotidine, fentanyl, fluconazole, foscarnet, hydromorphone, magnesium sulfate, morphine, perphenazine, zidovudine

Additive incompatibilities: Ascorbic acid, aztreonam, bleomycin, cytarabine, gentamicin, hydrocortisone sodium succinate, methylprednisolone sodium succinate, promazine

Additive compatibilities: Chloramphenicol, chlorothiazide, dexamethasone, diphenhydramine, ephedrine, heparin, hydroxyzine, potassium chloride, prochlorperazine, sodium bicarbonate, sodium lactate

Patient/family education

• Teach patient to report sore throat, bruising, bleeding, joint pain; may indicate blood dyscrasias (rare)
• Advise patient to contact prescriber if vaginal itching, loose, foul-smelling stools, furry tongue occur; may indicate superinfection
• Instruct patient to take all medication prescribed for the length of time ordered
• Advise patient to notify prescriber of diarrhea with

blood or pus, which may indicate pseudomembranous colitis

Evaluation

Positive therapeutic outcome

- Absence of signs/symptoms of infection (WBC <10,000, temp WNL, absence of red, draining wounds, earache)
- Reported improvement in symptoms of infection

Treatment of anaphylaxis: Withdraw drug, maintain airway, administer epinephrine, aminophylline, O_2, **IV** corticosteroids

nalbuphine (℞)

(nal'byoo-feen)

Nubain, nalbuphine HCl

Func. class.: Opioid analgesic

Chem. class.: Synthetic opioid agonist/antagonist

Pregnancy category C

Action: Inhibits ascending pain pathways in limbic system, thalamus, midbrain, hypothalamus by binding to opiate receptor sites, thus altering pain perception and response

➔ **Therapeutic Outcome:** Relief of pain

Uses: Moderate to severe pain, labor analgesia, balanced anesthesia (adjunct)

Dosage and routes

Analgesic

Adult: SC/IM/**IV** 10-20 mg q3-6h prn, not to exceed 160 mg/day

Balanced anesthesia supplement

Adult: **IV** 0.3-3 mg/kg given over 10-15 min; may give 0.25-0.5 mg/kg as needed (maintenance)

Available forms: Inj 10, 20 mg/ml

Adverse effects

CNS: Drowsiness, dizziness, confusion, headache, sedation, euphoria, dysphoria (high doses), hallucinations, dreaming, tolerance, physical and psychologic dependency

CV: Palpitations, bradycardia, change in B/P, orthostatic hypotension

EENT: Tinnitus, blurred vision, miosis (high doses), diplopia

GI: Nausea, vomiting, anorexia, constipation, cramps

GU: Increased urinary output, dysuria, urinary retention, urgency

INTEG: Rash, urticaria, bruising, flushing, *diaphoresis,* pruritus

RESP: Respiratory depression

Contraindications: Hypersensitivity, addiction (narcotic)

Precautions: Addictive personality, pregnancy **C,** lactation, increased intracranial pressure, MI (acute), severe heart disease, respiratory depression, hepatic disease, renal disease

Pharmacokinetics	
Absorption	Well absorbed (SC, IM); completely absorbed (IV)
Distribution	Crosses placenta
Metabolism	Liver, extensively
Excretion	Feces, kidneys, unchanged (small amounts); breast milk
Half-life	5 hr

Pharmacodynamics

	IM	SC	IV
Onset	Up to 15 min	Up to 15 min	Rapid
Peak	1 hr	Unknown	½ hr
Duration	3-6 hr	3-6 hr	3-6 hr

Interactions

Individual drugs

Alcohol: ↑ respiratory depression, hypotension, sedation

Drug classifications

Antihistamines: ↑ respiratory depression, hypotension
CNS depressants: ↑ respiratory depression, hypotension
MAOIs: Use cautiously, results are unpredictable
Phenothiazines: ↑ respiratory depression, hypotension
Opioid agonists: ↑ opioid withdrawals (dependency)
Sedative/hypnotics: ↑ respiratory depression, hypotension

Lab test interferences

↑ Amylase, ↑ lipase

NURSING CONSIDERATIONS

Assessment

- Assess pain characteristics (location, intensity, type) before medication administration and following treatment
- Monitor VS after parenteral route; note muscle rigidity, drug history, liver, kidney function tests; respiratory dysfunction: respiratory depression, character, rate, rhythm; notify prescriber if respirations are <10/min
- Monitor CNS changes: dizziness, drowsiness, hallucinations, euphoria, LOC, pupil reaction
- Monitor allergic reactions: rash, urticaria

Nursing diagnoses

- ✓ Pain (uses)
- ✓ Sensory-perceptual alteration: visual, auditory (adverse reactions)
- ✓ Breathing pattern, ineffective (adverse reactions)
- ✓ Knowledge deficit (teaching)

Implementation

- Give by inj (IM, **IV**), only with resuscitative equipment available; give slowly to prevent rigidity
- Store in light-resistant area at room temp

IM route

- Give deeply in large muscle mass; rotate inj sites

IV **IV route**

- Give direct **IV** undiluted 10 mg or less over 3-5 min or more

Syringe incompatibilities: Diazepam, pentobarbital

Syringe compatibilities: Atropine, cimetidine, droperidol, hydroxyzine, lidocaine, midazolam, prochlorperazine, promethazine, ranitidine, scopolamine, trimethobenzamide

Y-site incompatibilities: Nafcillin, sargramostim

Y-site compatibilities: Amifostine, aztreonam, filgrastim, fludarabine, melphalan, paclitaxel, teniposide, thiotepa, vinorelbine

Patient/family education

- Instruct patient to report any symptoms of CNS changes, allergic reactions
- Caution patients to avoid CNS depressants: alcohol, sedative/hypnotics for at least 24 hr after taking this drug
- Discuss with patient that dizziness, drowsiness, confusion are common; to avoid getting up without assistance
- Discuss in detail all aspects of

the drug: reason for taking drug and expected results
• Instruct patient to change position slowly to prevent orthostatic hypotension
• Teach patient to turn, cough, deep breathe after surgery to prevent atelectasis

Evaluation

Positive therapeutic outcome
• Relief of pain

Treatment of overdose: Naloxone (Narcan) 0.2-0.8 **IV**, O_2, **IV** fluids, vasopressors

nalmefene (℞)

(nahl'meh-feen)

Revex

Func. class.: Opioid antagonist

Chem. class.: Analog of naltrexone

Pregnancy category B

Action: Competes with opioids at opioid receptor sites; prevents or reverses the effects of opioids

Therapeutic Outcome: Absence of opioid overdose

Uses: Reversal of opioid effects, management of known or suspected opioid overdose

Dosage and routes

Opioid overdose

Adult: (Green label) Titrate to reverse effects of opioids 0.5 mg/70 kg, may give 1 mg/70 kg at 2-5 min intervals; since this drug is longer-acting use incremental dosing to avoid over-reversal

Postoperative opioid depression

Adult: (Blue label) 0.25 mcg/kg, then 0.25 mcg/kg at 2-5 min intervals

Available forms: Inj 1 mg/ml

Adverse effects

CNS: Drowsiness, nervousness, dizziness, headache, chills, fever

CV: Tachycardia, hypertension, hypotension, vasodilation, bradycardia

GI: Nausea, vomiting, diarrhea

Contraindications: Hypersensitivity

Precautions: Pregnancy **B**, P children, opioid dependency, lactation, respiratory depression, renal, hepatic disease, G elderly

Pharmacokinetics

Absorption	Complete
Distribution	Rapidly distributed
Metabolism	Liver
Excretion	Via kidneys
Half-life	Terminal biphasic 40 min, 10-15 hr

Pharmacodynamics

Unknown

Interactions

Individual drugs

Flumazenil: ↑ seizures

NURSING CONSIDERATIONS

Assessment

• Assess for opioid withdrawal; cramping hypertension, anxiety, vomiting
• Monitor VS q3-5 min
• Monitor ABGs, including PaO_2, $PaCO_2$
• Assess cardiac status: tachycardia, hypertension; monitor ECG
• Assess for respiratory dysfunction: respiratory depression, character, rate, rhythm; if respirations are <10 min, administer this drug;

N

probably due to opioid overdose; monitor LOC

Implementation

- Give only with resuscitative equipment, O_2 nearby
- Store at room temp

Nursing diagnoses

✓ Injury, potential (side effects)

Evaluation

Positive therapeutic outcome

- Reversal of respiratory depression; LOC-alert

naloxone (℞)

(nal-oks'one)

naloxone HCl, Narcan

Func. class.: Opioid antagonist

Chem. class.: Thebaine derivative

Pregnancy category B

Action: Competes with narcotics at narcotic receptor sites

➡ **Therapeutic Outcome:** Absence of opioid overdose

Uses: Respiratory depression induced by narcotics, pentazocine, propoxyphene; refractory circulatory shock

Dosage and routes

Opioid-induced respiratory depression, CNS depression

Adult: **IV**/SC/IM 0.4-2 mg; repeat q2-3 min if needed

Postoperative respiratory depression

Adult: **IV** 0.1-0.2 mg q2-3 min prn

P ***Child:*** **IV**/IM/SC 0.01 mg/kg q2-3 min prn

Asphyxia neonatorum

P ***Neonates:*** **IV** 0.01 mg/kg given into umbilical vein after delivery; may repeat in q2-3 min × 3 doses

Available forms: Inj 0.4, 1 mg/ml; P neonatal inj 0.02 mg/ml

Adverse effects

CNS: Drowsiness, nervousness

CV: Ventricular tachycardia, fibrillation, increased systolic B/P (high doses)

GI: Nausea, vomiting

RESP: Hyperpnea

Contraindications: Hypersensitivity, respiratory depression

Precautions: Pregnancy **B,** P children, cardiovascular disease, opioid dependency, lactation

Pharmacokinetics

Absorption	Well absorbed (SC, IM); completely absorbed (IV)
Distribution	Rapidly distributed; crosses placenta
Metabolism	Liver
Excretion	Kidneys
P **Half-life**	1 hr; up to 3 hr (neonates)

Pharmacodynamics

	IV	IM/SC
Onset	1 min	2-5 min
Peak	Unknown	Unknown
Duration	45 min	45-60 min

Interactions

Drug classifications

Analgesics, opioids: ↑ withdrawal in those addicted to opioids

Lab test interferences

Interference: Urine VMA, 5-HIAA, urine glucose

NURSING CONSIDERATIONS

Assessment

- Assess for opioid withdrawal: cramping, hypertension, anxiety, vomiting in drug-dependent individuals

• Monitor VS q3-5 min; ABGs including Po_2, Pco_2
• Assess cardiac status: tachycardia, hypertension; monitor ECG
• Assess for respiratory dysfunction: respiratory depression, character, rate, rhythm; if respirations are <10/min, administer naloxone; probably due to opioid overdose; monitor LOC

Nursing diagnoses

✓ Breathing pattern, ineffective (uses)
✓ Coping, ineffective individual (uses)
✓ Pain (adverse reactions)
✓ Knowledge deficit (teaching)

Implementation

IV **IV route**

• Give by direct **IV** undiluted; give 0.4 mg or less over 15 sec or titrate inf to response
• Give cont **IV** further diluted with 0.9% NaCl and D_5 and give as an inf
• Give only with resuscitative equipment, O_2 nearby
• Use only sol prepared within 24 hr
• Store at room temp in darkness

Patient/family education

• Explain reason for and expected results of medication when patient alert

Evaluation

Positive therapeutic outcome

• Reversal of respiratory depression
• LOC: alert

naproxen (℞)

(na-prox'en)

Apo-Naproxen ✤, Naxen, Novonaprox ✤, Naprosyn, naproxen sodium, Anaprox, Anaprox DS, Apo-Napro-Na ✤, Novonaprox Sodium ✤, Synflex ✤

Func. class.: Nonsteroidal antiinflammatory, nonopioid analgesic

Chem. class.: Propionic acid derivative

Pregnancy category B

Action: Inhibits prostaglandin synthesis by decreasing enzyme needed for biosynthesis; analgesic, antiinflammatory

➔ **Therapeutic Outcome:** Decreased pain, inflammation

Uses: Mild to moderate pain, osteoarthritis, rheumatoid arthritis, gouty arthritis, juvenile arthritis, primary dysmenorrhea

Dosage and routes

Adult: PO 250-500 mg bid, not to exceed 1 g/day (base); 525 mg, then 275 mg q6-8h prn, not to exceed 1475 mg (sodium)

P ***Child:*** PO 10 mg/kg in 2 divided doses

Available forms: Naproxen, tabs 250, 375, 500 mg; oral susp 125 mg/5 ml; naproxen sodium, tabs 275, 550 mg

Adverse effects

CNS: Dizziness, drowsiness, fatigue, tremors, confusion, insomnia, anxiety, depression
CV: Tachycardia, peripheral edema, palpitations, dysrhythmias

N

EENT: Tinnitus, hearing loss, blurred vision
GI: Nausea, anorexia, vomiting, diarrhea, jaundice, ***cholestatic hepatitis,*** constipation, flatulence, cramps, dry mouth, peptic ulcer, ***GI ulceration, bleeding, perforation***
GU: ***Nephrotoxicity: dysuria, hematuria, oliguria, azotemia***
HEMA: ***Blood dyscrasias***
INTEG: Purpura, rash, pruritus, sweating

Contraindications: Hypersensitivity, asthma, severe renal disease, severe hepatic disease, ulcer disease

Precautions: Pregnancy **B**, **P** lactation, children <2 yr, bleeding disorders, GI disorders, cardiac disorders, hypersensitivity to other antiinflammatory agents, **G** elderly

Pharmacokinetics	
Absorption	Completely absorbed
Distribution	Crosses placenta, 99% protein binding
Metabolism	Liver, extensively
Excretion	Breast milk
Half-life	10-20 hr

Pharmacodynamics	
Onset	1 hr
Peak	2-4 hr
Duration	<7 hr

Interactions
Individual drugs
Acetaminophen (long-term use): ↑ renal reactions
Alcohol: ↑ adverse reactions
Aspirin: ↓ effectiveness, ↑ adverse reactions
Cefamandole: ↑ bleeding
Cefoperazone: ↑ bleeding
Cefotetan: ↑ bleeding
Coumadin: ↑ anticoagulant effects
Digoxin: ↑ toxicity, levels
Insulin: ↓ insulin effect
Lithium: ↑ toxicity
Methotrexate: ↑ toxicity
Phenytoin: ↑ toxicity
Probenecid: ↑ toxicity
Sulfonylurea: ↑ toxicity
Valproic acid: ↑ bleeding
Drug classifications
Anticoagulants: ↑ risk of bleeding
Antihypertensives: ↓ effect of antihypertensives
Antineoplastics: ↑ risk of hematologic toxicity
β-Blockers: ↑ antihypertension
Cephalosporins: ↑ risk of bleeding
Diuretics: ↓ effectiveness of diuretics
Glucocorticoids: ↑ adverse reactions
Hypoglycemics, oral: ↓ hypoglycemic effect
NSAIDs: ↑ adverse reactions
Potassium supplements: ↑ adverse reactions
Radiation: ↑ risk of hematologic toxicity
Sulfonamides: ↑ toxicity
Lab test interferences
↑ BUN, ↑ alkaline phosphatase
False ↑ 5-HIAA, false ↑ 17KS

NURSING CONSIDERATIONS
Assessment

- Monitor liver function, renal function, other blood studies: AST (SGOT), ALT (SGPT), bilirubin, creatinine BUN, CBC, Hct, Hgb, pro-time if patient is on long-term therapy
- Check I&O ratio; decreasing output may indicate renal failure (long-term therapy)
- Assess hepatotoxicity: dark urine, clay-colored stools, yellowing of the skin and sclera, itching, abdominal pain, fever, diarrhea if patient is on long-term therapy

• Assess for allergic reactions: rash, urticaria; if these occur, drug may have to be discontinued
• Assess for ototoxicity: tinnitus, ringing, roaring in ears; audiometric testing needed before, after long-term therapy
• Assess for visual changes: blurring, halos; may indicate corneal, retinal damage
• Check for edema in feet, ankles, legs
• Identify prior drug history; there are many drug interactions
• Monitor pain: location, duration, type, intensity before dose and 1 hour after; assess ROM before dose and after

Nursing diagnoses
✓ Pain (uses)
✓ Mobility, impaired (uses)
✓ Injury, risk for (adverse reactions)
✓ Knowledge deficit (teaching)

Implementation
• Administer to patient crushed or whole
• Give with food or milk to decrease gastric symptoms; give ½ hr ac or 2 hr pc for better absorption

Patient/family education
• Teach patient to report any symptoms of hepatotoxicity, renal toxicity, visual changes, ototoxicity, allergic reactions, bleeding (long-term therapy)
• Advise patient to take with 8 oz of water and sit upright for 30 min after dose to prevent ulceration
• Caution patient not to exceed recommended dosage; acute poisoning may result; to take as prescribed, do not double dose
• Teach patient to read label on other OTC drugs; many contain other antiinflammatories; caution patient to avoid alcohol ingestion; GI bleeding may occur
• Inform patient that the therapeutic response takes 2 wk (arthritis)
• Teach patient to report tinnitus, confusion, diarrhea, sweating, hyperventilation, blurred vision, fever, joint aches

Evaluation
Positive therapeutic outcome
• Decreased pain
• Decreased inflammation
• Increased mobility

nedocromil (℞)
(ned-o-kroe'mil)
Tilade
Func. class.: Antiasthmatic
Chem. class.: Mast cell stabilizer
Pregnancy category B

N

Action: Stabilizes the membrane of the sensitized mast cell, preventing release of chemical mediators after an antigen-IgE interaction

➔ **Therapeutic Outcome:** Reduced symptoms of asthma

Uses: Allergic rhinitis, severe perennial bronchial asthma, exercise-induced bronchospasm (prevention), prevention of acute bronchospasm induced by environmental pollutants, mastocytosis

Dosage and routes
Bronchospasm
P ***Adult and child >12 yr:*** 2 inh 2-4 times a day at regular intervals to provide 14 g/day

Bronchial asthma
P ***Adult and child >12 yr:*** Same as above

Available forms: 1.75 mg nedocromil per activation in 16.2-g canisters providing at least 112 metered inh

Adverse effects
CNS: Headache, dizziness, neuritis, dysphonia
EENT: Throat irritation, cough, nasal congestion, burning eyes, rhinitis
GI: Nausea, vomiting, anorexia, dry mouth, bitter taste

Contraindications: Hypersensitivity to this drug or lactose, status asthmaticus

Precautions: Pregnancy **B**, P lactation, children

Pharmacokinetics	
Absorption	Poorly, 3%
Distribution	Unknown
Metabolism	Not usually metabolized
Excretion	Small amounts in bile, urine unchanged
Half-life	80 min

Pharmacodynamics	
Onset	Unknown
Peak	15 min
Duration	4-6 hr

Interactions: None

NURSING CONSIDERATIONS
Assessment
- Monitor eosinophil count during treatment
- Assess respiratory status: respiratory rate, rhythm, characteristics, cough, wheezing, dyspnea

Nursing diagnoses
✓ Airway clearance, ineffective (uses)
✓ Knowledge deficit (teaching)

Implementation
- Give by inh only
- Encourage patient to gargle, sip water to decrease irritation in throat

Patient/family education
- Instruct patient to clear mucus before using
- Teach patient proper inh technique: exhale; using inhaler, inhale deeply with head tipped back to open airway; remove, hold breath, exhale; repeat until all of drug is inhaled
- Inform patient that therapeutic effect may take up to 4 wk
- Teach patient that drug is preventive only, not restorative

Evaluation
Positive therapeutic outcome
- Decrease in asthmatic symptoms

nefazodone (℞)
(nef-az′oe-done)
Serzone
Func. class.: Second-generation antidepressant
Chem. class.: Phenylpiperazine
Pregnancy category C

Action: Selectively inhibits serotonin uptake by brain, potentiates behavioral changes, occupies central HT_2 receptors

➔ **Therapeutic Outcome:** Decreased symptoms of depression after 2-3 wk

Uses: Major depression

Dosage and routes
Adult: PO 200 mg/day (100 mg bid); dosage may be in-

creased to 300 mg/day (150 bid); max 600 mg/day

G *Elderly:* PO 100 mg/day (50 mg bid)

Available forms: Tabs 100, 150, 200, 250 mg

Adverse effects

CNS: Dizziness, headache, insomnia

CV: **Postural hypotension**

GI: **Nausea, constipation, dry mouth**

EENT: **Blurred vision**

GU: **Urinary frequency,** retention, UTI

RESP: Pharyngitis, cough

Contraindications: Hypersensitivity to this drug or phenylpiperazines

Precautions: Pregnancy C, P lactation, children, elderly, G cardiovascular disease, seizure disorder

Pharmacokinetics	
Absorption	Well absorbed
Distribution	Widely distributed; crosses placenta
Metabolism	Liver, extensively, to metabolites
Excretion	Kidneys, breast milk
Half-life	2-4 hr

Pharmacodynamics	
Onset	Unknown
Peak	1-3 hr
Duration	Unknown

Interactions

Individual drugs

Alcohol: ↑ CNS depression

Drug classifications

Antihistamines, nonsedating: Fatal reaction

Benzodiazepines: ↑ plasma concentrations

Barbiturates: ↑ effects

CNS depressants: ↑ effects

Smoking

↑ metabolism, ↓ effects

NURSING CONSIDERATIONS

Assessment

- Monitor B/P (with patient lying, standing), pulse q4h; if systolic B/P drops 20 mm Hg hold drug, notify prescriber; take vital signs q4h in patients with cardiovascular disease
- Monitor blood studies: CBC, leukocytes, differential, cardiac enzymes if patient is receiving long-term therapy
- Monitor hepatic studies: AST (SGOT), ALT (SGPT), bilirubin
- Assess mental status: mood, sensorium, affect, suicidal tendencies; increase in psychiatric symptoms: depression, panic
- Monitor urinary retention, constipation; constipation is more likely to occur in the G elderly
- ! Assess for withdrawal symptoms: headache, nausea, vomiting, muscle pain, weakness; do not usually occur unless drug was discontinued abruptly
- Identify alcohol consumption; if alcohol is consumed, hold dose until AM

Nursing diagnoses

✓ Coping, ineffective individual (uses)

✓ Knowledge deficit (teaching)

✓ Noncompliance (teaching)

Implementation

- Give with food or milk for GI symptoms
- Give crushed if patient is unable to swallow medication whole
- Store at room temp; do not freeze

Patient/family education

- Teach patient that therapeutic effects may take 3-4 wk
- Teach patient to use caution

N

in driving and other activities requiring alertness because of drowsiness, dizziness; to avoid rising quickly from sitting to G standing, especially elderly

- Teach patient to avoid alcohol ingestion, other CNS depressants
- Teach patient not to discontinue medication quickly after long-term use; may cause nausea, headache, malaise
- Teach patient to increase bulk in diet if constipation G occurs, especially elderly
- Teach patient to take gum, hard sugarless candy, or frequent sips of water for dry mouth

Evaluation

Positive therapeutic outcome

- Decrease in depression
- Absence of suicidal thoughts

Treatment of overdose: ECG monitoring, induce emesis, lavage, activated charcoal, administer anticonvulsant

neomycin (℞)

(nee-oh-mye'sin)

Mycifradin Sulfate, Myciguent

Func. class.: Antiinfective

Chem. class.: Aminoglycoside

Pregnancy category C

Action: Interferes with protein synthesis in bacterial cell by binding to 30S ribosomal subunit causing inaccurate peptide sequence to form in protein chain, resulting in bacterial death

➔ **Therapeutic Outcome:** Bactericidal effects for *Pseudomonas aeruginosa, Escherichia coli, Enterobacter,* enteropathogenic *E. coli, Klebsiella pneumoniae, Proteus vulgaris*

Uses: Severe systemic infections of CNS, respiratory tract, GI tract, urinary tract, eye, bone, skin, soft tissues, also used for hepatic coma, preoperatively to sterilize bowel, infectious diarrhea; minor skin infections (top)

Dosage and routes

Severe systemic infections

Adult: IM 15 mg/kg/day in 4 divided doses; not to exceed 1 g/day

Hepatic coma

Adult: PO 4-12 g/day in divided doses times 5-6 days

P ***Child:*** PO 50-100 mg/kg/day in divided doses

Preoperative bowel sterilization

Adult: PO on 3rd day of a 3-day regimen; give 1 g early PM; repeat in 1 hr; repeat at hs (given with erythromycin); give saline cathartic before giving this drug

Skin infection

P ***Adult and child:*** Top 0.5% cream or ointment qd-tid

Available forms: Tab 500 mg; top 500 mg; oral sol 125 ml/5 ml; inj 500 mg

Adverse effects

CNS: Confusion, depression, numbness, tremors, ***convulsions,*** muscle twitching, ***neurotoxicity,*** dizziness, vertigo

CV: Hypotension, hypertension, palpitations

EENT: ***Ototoxicity,*** deafness, visual disturbances, tinnitus

GI: Nausea, vomiting, anorexia, increased ALT (SGPT), AST (SGOT), bilirubin, hepa-

tomegaly, ***hepatic necrosis,*** splenomegaly
GU: ***Oliguria, hematuria, renal damage, azotemia, renal failure, nephrotoxicity***
HEMA: ***Agranulocytosis, thrombocytopenia,*** leukopenia, eosinophilia, anemia
INTEG: Rash, burning, urticaria, photosensitivity, dermatitis, alopecia

Contraindications: Bowel obstruction (oral use), severe renal disease, hypersensitivity, P infants, children

Precautions: Mild renal disease, pregnancy **C**, hearing deficits, lactation, myasthenia gravis, Parkinson's disease

Pharmacokinetics

Absorption	Well absorbed (IM); minimally absorbed (top)
Distribution	Unknown
Metabolism	Liver, minimal
Excretion	Feces, unchanged
Half-life	2-3 hr

Pharmacodynamics

	IM
Onset	Rapid
Peak	1-2 hr
Duration	6-8 hr

Interactions

Individual drugs

Amphotericin B: ↑ ototoxicity, neurotoxicity, nephrotoxicity
Cisplatin: ↑ ototoxicity, neurotoxicity, nephrotoxicity
Ethacrynic acid: ↑ ototoxicity, neurotoxicity, nephrotoxicity
Furosemide: ↑ ototoxicity, neurotoxicity, nephrotoxicity
Mannitol: ↑ ototoxicity, neurotoxicity, nephrotoxicity
Methoxyflurane: ↑ ototoxicity, neurotoxicity, nephrotoxicity
Polymyxin: ↑ ototoxicity, neurotoxicity, nephrotoxicity
Succinylcholine: ↑ neuromuscular blockade, respiratory depression
Vancomycin: ↑ ototoxicity, neurotoxicity, nephrotoxicity

Drug classifications

Aminoglycosides: ↑ otoxicity, neurotoxicity, nephrotoxicity
Anesthetics, inhalation: ↑ neuromuscular blockade, respiratory depression
Nondepolarizing neuromuscular blockers: ↑ neuromuscular blockade, respiratory depression

NURSING CONSIDERATIONS

Assessment

- Assess patient for previous sensitivity reaction
- Assess patient for signs and symptoms of infection: characteristics of skin; obtain baseline information and during treatment
- Obtain C&S before beginning drug therapy to identify if correct treatment has been initiated
- Assess for allergic reactions: rash, urticaria, pruritus, chills, fever, joint pain

Nursing diagnoses

✓ Infection, risk for (uses)
✓ Knowledge deficit (teaching)
✓ Noncompliance (teaching)

Implementation

PO route

- Give as a preoperative medication before bowel surgery

Patient/family education

- Instruct patient to take all medication prescribed for the length of time ordered
- Advise patient to report headache, dizziness, symptoms of overgrowth of infection and

N

loss of hearing, ringing or roaring in ears

Evaluation

Positive therapeutic outcome

- Reported improvement in symptoms of infection (top)

Treatment of overdose: Withdraw drug; hemodialysis; monitor serum levels of drug

neostigmine (℞)

(nee-oh-stig'meen)

neostigmine methylsulfate, Prostigmin

Func. class.: Cholinergic stimulant; anticholinesterase

Chem. class.: Quaternary compound

Pregnancy category C

Action: Inhibits destruction of acetylcholine, which increases concentration at sites where acetylcholine is released; this facilitates transmission of impulses across the myoneural junction

Therapeutic Outcome: Increased strength in myasthenia gravis, reversal of nondepolarizing muscular blockers

Uses: Myasthenia gravis, nondepolarizing neuromuscular blocker, antagonist, bladder distention, postoperative ileus

Dosage and routes

Myasthenia gravis

Adult: PO 15-375 mg/day; IM/**IV** 0.5-2 mg q1-3h

P ***Child:*** PO 2 mg/kg/day q3-4h

Nondepolarizing neuromuscular blocker antagonist

Adult: **IV** 0.5-2 mg slowly; may repeat if needed (give 0.6-1.2 mg atropine before this drug)

Abdominal distention/ postoperative ileus

Adult: IM/SC 0.25-1 mg (1:4000) q4-6h depending on condition x 2-3 days

Available forms: Tab 15 mg; inj 1:400, 1:1000, 1:2000, 1:4000

Adverse effects

CNS: Dizziness, headache, sweating, weakness, ***convulsions,*** incoordination, ***paralysis,*** drowsiness, LOC

CV: Tachycardia, dysrhythmias, bradycardia, hypotension, AV block, ECG changes, ***cardiac arrest,*** syncope

EENT: Miosis, blurred vision, lacrimation, visual changes

GI: Nausea, diarrhea, vomiting, cramps, increased peristalsis, salivary and gastric secretions

GU: Frequency, incontinence, urgency

INTEG: Rash, urticaria, flushing

RESP: ***Respiratory depression, bronchospasm, constriction, laryngospasm, respiratory arrest,*** dyspnea

Contraindications: Obstruction of intestine, renal system, pregnancy **C**, bromide sensitivity, peritonitis

Precautions: Bradycardia, hypotension, seizure disorders, bronchial asthma, coronary occlusion, hyperthyroidism, dysrhythmias, peptic ulcer, megacolon, poor GI motility, P lactation, children

Pharmacokinetics

Absorption	Poorly absorbed (PO), completely absorbed (IV)
Distribution	Unknown
Metabolism	Liver
Excretion	Kidneys
Half-life	40-90 min

Pharmacodynamics

	PO	IM	IV
Onset	45-75 min	10-30 min	4-8 min
Peak	Unknown	30 min	30 min
Duration	2½-4 hr	2½-4 hr	2-4 hr

Interactions

Individual drugs

Atropine: ↓ action of atropine
Mecamylamine: ↓ action of neostigmine
Polymyxin: ↓ action of neostigmine
Procainamide: ↓ action of neostigmine
Quinidine: ↓ action of neostigmine

Drug classifications

Antidepressants: ↑ antagonism
Antihistamines: ↑ antagonism
Cholinesterase inhibitors: ↑ toxicity
Phenothiazines: ↑ antagonism
Muscle relaxants, depolarizing: ↑ action of muscle relaxants

NURSING CONSIDERATIONS

Assessment

- Monitor VS, respiration during rest
- Monitor for bradycardia, hypotension, bronchospasm, headache, dizziness, convulsions, respiratory depression; drug should be discontinued if toxicity occurs

Nursing diagnoses

✓ Breathing pattern, ineffective (uses)
✓ Knowledge deficit (teaching)

Implementation

PO route

- Give only after all other cholinergics have been discontinued
- Increased dosage may be needed if tolerance develops
- Give larger doses after exercise or fatigue
- Administer on empty stomach for better absorption
- Store at room temp

IV route

- Give direct **IV** undiluted, through Y-tube or 3-way stopcock; give 0.5 mg or less over 1 min
- Give only with atropine sulfate available for cholinergic crisis

Syringe compatibilities: Glycopyrrolate, heparin, pentobarbital, thiopental

Y-site compatibilities: Heparin, hydrocortisone sodium succinate, potassium chloride

Additive compatibility: Netilmicin

Patient/family education

- Teach patient to wear Medic Alert ID specifying myasthenia gravis, drugs taken, prescriber's phone number

Evaluation

Positive therapeutic outcome

- Increased muscle strength, hand grasp
- Improved gait
- Absence of labored breathing (if severe)

Treatment of overdose:

Respiratory support, **IV** atropine 1-4 mg

N

netilmicin (℞)

(ne-til-mye′sin)

Netromycin

Func. class.: Antibiotic

Chem. class.: Aminoglycoside

Pregnancy category D

Action: Interferes with protein synthesis in bacterial cell by binding to 30S ribosomal subunit, causing inaccurate peptide sequence to form in protein chain, resulting in bacterial death

→ **Therapeutic Outcome:** Bactericidal effects for the organisms *Pseudomonas aeruginosa, Escherichia coli, Enterobacter, Citrobacter, Staphylococcus, Klebsiella pneumoniae, Proteus mirabilis, Serratia, Shigella, Salmonella, Acinetobacter, Neisseria*

Uses: Severe systemic infections of CNS, respiratory tract, GI tract, urinary tract, bone, skin, soft tissues

Dosage and routes

Normal renal function

P ***Adult and child >12 yr:*** IM/**IV** 3-6.5 mg/kg/day; may give q8-12h for severe infections

P ***Child and infant 6 wk-12 yr:*** IM/**IV** 5.5-8 mg/kg/day in divided doses q8-12h

P ***Neonate <6 wk:*** IM/**IV** 4-6.5 mg/kg/day in divided doses q12h

Available forms: Inj 100 mg/ml

Adverse effects

CNS: Confusion, depression, numbness, tremors, ***convulsions,*** muscle twitching, ***neurotoxicity,*** dizziness, vertigo

CV: Hypotension, hypertension, palpitations

EENT: ***Ototoxicity,*** deafness, visual disturbances, tinnitus

GI: Nausea, vomiting, anorexia, increased ALT (SGPT), AST (SGOT), bilirubin, hepatomegaly, ***hepatic necrosis,*** splenomegaly

GU: ***Oliguria, hematuria, renal damage, azotemia, renal failure, nephrotoxicity***

HEMA: ***Agranulocytosis, thrombocytopenia, leukopenia, eosinophilia, anemia***

INTEG: Rash, burning, urticaria, dermatitis

Contraindications: Severe renal disease, hypersensitivity, pregnancy **D**

Precautions: Neonates, mild P renal disease, children <12 yr, lactation, myasthenia gravis, hearing deficit, Parkinson's disease, severe burns, cystic fibrosis

Pharmacokinetics

Absorption	Well absorbed (IM)
Distribution	Widely distributed in extracellular fluids, poor in CSF; crosses placenta
Metabolism	Liver, minimal
Excretion	Kidneys, unchanged (90%); breast milk
Half-life	2-3 hr; increased in renal disease

Pharmacodynamics

	IM	IV
Onset	Rapid	Immediate
Peak	1-2 hr	1-2 hr

Interactions

Individual drugs

Amphotericin B: ↑ ototoxicity, neurotoxicity, nephrotoxicity

Cisplatin: ↑ ototoxicity, neurotoxicity, nephrotoxicity

Ethacrynic acid: ↑ ototoxicity, neurotoxicity, nephrotoxicity
Furosemide: ↑ ototoxicity, neurotoxicity, nephrotoxicity
Mannitol: ↑ ototoxicity, neurotoxicity, nephrotoxicity
Methoxyflurane: ↑ ototoxicity, neurotoxicity, nephrotoxicity
Polymyxin: ↑ ototoxicity, neurotoxicity, nephrotoxicity
Succinylcholine: ↑ neuromuscular blockade, respiratory depression
Vancomycin: ↑ ototoxicity, neurotoxicity, nephrotoxicity

Drug classifications

Anesthetics: ↑ neuromuscular blockade, respiratory depression
Aminoglycosides: ↑ otoxicity, neurotoxicity, nephrotoxicity
Nondepolarizing neuromuscular blockers: ↑ neuromuscular blockade, respiratory depression

NURSING CONSIDERATIONS

Assessment

- Assess patient for previous sensitivity reaction
- Assess patient for signs and symptoms of infection including characteristics of wounds, sputum, urine, stool, WBC >10,000, fever; obtain baseline information and during treatment
- Obtain C&S before beginning drug therapy to identify if correct treatment has been initiated
- Assess for allergic reactions: rash, urticaria, pruritus, chills, fever, joint pain
- Identify urine output; if decreasing, notify prescriber (may indicate nephrotoxicity); also check for increased BUN, creatinine, urine CrCl <80 ml/min
- Monitor blood studies: AST (SGOT), ALT (SGPT), CBC, Hct, bilirubin, LDH, alkaline phosphatase, Coombs' test monthly if patient is on long-term therapy
- Monitor electrolytes: potassium, sodium, chloride, magnesium monthly if patient is on long-term therapy
- Assess for overgrowth of infection: perineal itching, fever, malaise, redness, pain, swelling, drainage, rash, diarrhea, change in cough, sputum
- Obtain weight before treatment; calculation of dosage is usually based on ideal body weight, but may be calculated on actual body weight
- Monitor I&O ratio; perform urinalysis daily for proteinuria, cells, casts; report sudden change in urine output
- Monitor VS during inf; watch for hypotension, change in pulse
- Assess **IV** site for thrombophlebitis including pain, redness, swelling q30 min; change site if needed; apply warm compresses to discontinued site
- Obtain serum peak, drawn at 30-60 min after **IV** inf or 60 min after IM inj; trough level drawn just before next dose; blood level should be 2-4 times bacteriostatic level
- Monitor urine pH if drug is used for UTI; urine should be kept alkaline
- Monitor for dehydration: high sp gr, decrease in skin turgor, dry mucous membranes, dark urine
- Assess for vestibular dysfunction: nausea, vomiting, dizziness, headache; drug should be discontinued if severe; monitor deafness by

N

audiometric testing, ringing, roaring in ears, vertigo; assess hearing before, during, after treatment

Nursing diagnoses

- ✓ Infection, risk for (uses)
- ✓ Knowledge deficit (teaching)
- ✓ Noncompliance (teaching)
- ✓ Sensory-perceptual alteration: auditory (uses)

Implementation

IM route

• Give deeply in large muscle mass

IV **IV route**

• Dilute intermittent inf dose in 50-200 ml D_5W, $D_{10}W$, D_5/LR, D_5/0.9% NaCl, LR, 0.9% NaCl, 3% NaCl, 5% NaCl, or Ringer's; give over ½-2 hr

• Separate aminoglycosides and penicillins by ≥1 hr

• Diluted sol is stable for 72 hr at room temp

Additive compatibilities: Aminocaproic acid, atropine, cefuroxime, chlorpromazine, clindamycin, dexamethasone, diazepam, diphenhydramine, hydrocortisone, iron dextran, isoproterenol, methyldopate, metronidazole, multivitamins, potassium chloride, vitamin B complex

Y-site incompatibilities: Furosemide, heparin

Y-site compatibilities: Amifostine, aminophylline, aztreonam, calcium gluconate, filgrastim, fludarabine, melphalan, sargramostim, teniposide, thiotepa, vinorelbine

Patient/family education

• Teach patient to report sore throat, bruising, bleeding, joint pain; may indicate blood dyscrasias (rare); ringing, roaring in the ears or a feeling of dullness in the head

• Advise patient to contact prescriber if vaginal itching, loose, foul-smelling stools, furry tongue occur; may indicate superinfection

Evaluation

Positive therapeutic outcome

• Absence of signs/symptoms of infection (WBC <10,000, temp WNL, absence of red, draining wounds)

• Reported improvement in symptoms of infection

Treatment of overdose: Withdraw drug; hemodialysis; exchange transfusion in the P newborn; monitor serum levels of drug; may give ticarcillin or carbenicillin

nevirapine (℞)

(ne-veer'a-peen)

Viramune

Func. class.: Non-nucleoside reverse transcriptase inhibitor (NNRII)

Pregnancy category C

Action: Binds directly to reverse transcriptase and blocks RNA, DNA causing a disruption of the enzyme's site

➔ **Therapeutic Outcome:** Improvement off HIV-1 infection

Uses: HIV-1 in combination with nucleoside analogs in those experiencing deterioration

Dosage and routes

Adult: PO 200 mg qd × 2 wk, then 200 mg bid in combination with nucleoside analogs

Available forms: Tabs 200 mg

Adverse effects

CNS: Paresthesia, headache, fever, peripheral neuropathy
GI: Diarrhea, abdominal pain, nausea, stomatitis, hepatitis
INTEG: Rash
MS: Pain, myalgia

Contraindications: Hypersensitivity

Precautions: Liver disease, P pregnancy **C,** lactation, children, renal disease

Pharmacokinetics

Absorption	Rapid
Distribution	60% bound to plasma proteins
Metabolism	Liver
Excretion	Unknown
Half-life	Unknown

Pharmacodynamics

Unknown

Interactions

Drug classifications

Oral contraceptives: ↓ action
Protease inhibitors: ↓ action
Rifamycins: ↓ nevirapine levels

NURSING CONSIDERATIONS

Assessment

- Assess signs of infection, anemia
- Assess liver studies: ALT, AST; renal studies
- Assess C&S before drug therapy; drug may be taken as soon as culture is taken; repeat C&S after treatment; determine the presence of other sexually transmitted disease
- Assess bowel pattern before, during treatment; if severe abdominal pain with bleeding occurs, drug should be discontinued; monitor hydration
- Assess skin eruptions; rash, urticaria, itching
- Assess allergies before treatment, reaction to each medication; place allergies on chart

Nursing diagnoses

✓ Infection, risk for (uses)
✓ Diarrhea (side effects)
✓ Knowledge deficit (teaching)

Patient/family education

- Advise patient to take as prescribed; if dose is missed, take as soon as remembered up to 1 hr before next dose; do not double dose
- Advise patient that drug must be taken in equal intervals around the clock to maintain blood levels for duration of therapy

niacin (vitamin B_3/ nicotinic acid)/ niacinamide (PO, OTC; IV/IM/SC, ℞)

(nye'a-sin) (nye-a-sin'a-mide)

Nia-Bid, Niac, Niacels, Niacin TD, SpaN Niacin, Niacin TR, Niacor, Niaspan, Nico-400, Nicobid, Nicolar, Nicotinex, nicotinic acid, Novaniacin ✤, Slo-Niacin, Tri-B_3 ✤, Vitamin B_3, Nicothamide

Func. class.: Vitamin B_3
Chem. class.: Water-soluble vitamin, lipid-lowering drug

Pregnancy category C

Action: Needed for conversion of fats, protein, carbohydrates by oxidation-reduction; acts directly on vascular smooth muscle, causing vasodilatation; high dosages decrease serum lipids

Therapeutic Outcome: Decreasing cholesterol and low-density lipoprotein levels, vitamin B_3 supplementation

Uses: Pellagra, hyperlipidemias, peripheral vascular disease

Dosage and routes

Niacin deficiency

Adult: PO up to 500 mg/day in divided doses; IM/SC 5-100 mg 5 or more times a day; **IV** 25-100 mg bid or tid

P ***Child:*** PO up to 300 mg/day in divided doses

Adjunct in hyperlipidemia

Adult: PO 500 mg qd in 3 divided doses pc; may be increased to 2 g/day

Pellagra

Adult: PO 300-500 mg, qd in divided doses

P ***Child:*** PO 100-300 mg qd in divided doses

Peripheral vascular disease

Adult: PO 250-800 mg qd in divided doses

Available forms: Nicotinic acid, tabs 20, 25, 50, 100, 500 mg; time rel caps 125, 250, 300, 400, 500 mg; time rel tabs 150, 375 mg; elix 50 mg/5 ml; inj 100 mg/ml; nicotinamide, tabs 50, 100, 500 mg; time rel tab 1000 mg

Adverse effects

CNS: Paresthesias, headache, dizziness, anxiety
CV: Postural hypotension, vasovagal attacks, dysrhythmias, vasodilatation
EENT: Blurred vision, ptosis
GI: Nausea, vomiting, anorexia, flatulence, xerostomia, ***jaundice***, diarrhea, peptic ulcer
GU: Hyperuricemia, ***glycosuria, hypoalbuminemia***
INTEG: Flushing, dry skin, rash, pruritus
RESP: Wheezing

Contraindications: Hypersensitivity, peptic ulcer, hepatic disease, lactation, hemorrhage, severe hypotension

Precautions: Glaucoma, cardiovascular disease, CAD, diabetes mellitus, gout, schizophrenia, pregnancy **C**

Pharmacokinetics

Absorption	Well absorbed (PO)
Distribution	Widely distributed
Metabolism	Converted to niacinamide
Excretion	Urine, unchanged (30%); breast milk
Half-life	45 min

Pharmacodynamics

	PO	IV
Onset	Unknown	Unknown
Peak	30-70 min	Unknown
Duration	Unknown	Unknown

Interactions

Individual drugs

Guanadrel: ↑ hypotension
Guanethidine: ↑ hypotension
Lovastatin: ↑ myopathy
Probenecid: ↑ uricosuric effects
Sulfinpyrazone: ↑ uricosuric effects

Lab test interferences

↑ Bilirubin, ↑ alkaline phosphatase, ↑ liver enzymes, ↑ LDH, ↑ uric acid
↓ Cholesterol
False ↑ Urinary catecholamines
False positive: Urine glucose

NURSING CONSIDERATIONS

Assessment

- Assess for niacin deficiency (pellagra): nausea, vomiting, stomatitis, confusion, hallucinations before and throughout treatment

• Assess nutrition: fat, protein, carbohydrates, nutritional analysis should be completed by dietician
• Monitor liver function studies: AST (SGOT), ALT (SGPT), bilirubin, alkaline phosphatase; blood glucose before and during treatment; liver dysfunction: clay-colored stools, itching, dark urine, jaundice
• Monitor niacin levels during administration of this drug
• Monitor cardiac status: rate, rhythm, quality; postural hypotension, dysrhythmias
• Monitor nutritional status: liver, yeast, legumes, organ meat, lean poultry; high-level niacin products should be included in the diet
• Assess for CNS symptoms: headache, paresthesias, blurred vision

Nursing diagnoses
✓ Nutrition, less than body requirements (uses)
✓ Knowledge deficit (teaching)
✓ Noncompliance (teaching)

Implementation
PO route
• Give with meals or milk for GI symptoms
⊘ • Do not crush, break, or chew time rel products

IV route
• Give by direct **IV** after diluting to 2 mg/ml at a rate of ≤2 mg/min
• Give by inf by adding 500 ml of 0.9% NaCl at a rate of ≤2 mg/min

Additive incompatibilities: Acids (strong), alkalis, erythromycin, kanamycin, streptomycin

Additive compatibility: TPN sol

Patient/family education
• Advise patient that flushing and increase in feelings of warmth will occur several hr after taking drug (PO); time rel product minimizes flushing
• Instruct patient to remain recumbent if postural hypotension occurs; to rise slowly from sitting or recumbent
• Caution patient to abstain from alcohol if drug is prescribed for hyperlipidemia
• Caution patient to avoid sunlight if skin lesions are present

Evaluation
Positive therapeutic outcome
• Decreased lipid levels
• Warm extremities
• Absence of numbness in extremities

nicardipine (℞)
(nye-card′i-peen)
Cardene, Cardene SR
Func. class.: Calcium channel blocker
Chem. class.: Dihydropyridine
Pregnancy category C

Action: Inhibits calcium ion influx across cell membrane during cardiac depolarization, produces relaxation of coronary vascular smooth muscle and peripheral vascular smooth muscle, dilates coronary arteries, increases myocardial oxygen delivery in patients with vasospastic angina

Therapeutic Outcome: Decreased angina pectoris, decreased B/P in hypertension

Uses: Chronic stable angina pectoris, hypertension

Dosage and routes

Adult: PO 20 mg tid initially; may increase after 3 days (range 20-40 mg tid) or 30 mg bid sus rel, may increase to 60 mg bid

Available forms: Caps 20, 30 mg; sus rel caps 30, 45, 60 mg

Adverse effects

CNS: Headache, fatigue, drowsiness, dizziness, anxiety, depression, weakness, insomnia, confusion, paresthesia, somnolence

CV: Dysrhythmia, edema, CHF, bradycardia, hypotension, palpitations, ***MI, pulmonary edema***

GI: Nausea, vomiting, diarrhea, gastric upset, constipation, ***hepatitis,*** abdominal cramps

GU: Nocturia, polyuria, ***acute renal failure***

INTEG: Rash, pruritus, urticaria, photosensitivity, hair loss

MISC: Blurred vision, flushing, nasal congestion, sweating, shortness of breath, gynecomastia, hyperglycemia, sexual difficulties

Contraindications: Sick sinus syndrome, 2nd- or 3rd-degree heart block, hypotension less than 90 mm Hg systolic, hypersensitivity

Precautions: CHF, hypotension, hepatic injury, pregnancy [P] **C,** lactation, children, renal [G] disease, elderly

Pharmacokinetics

Absorption	Well absorbed (PO); bioavailability poor
Distribution	Unknown
Metabolism	Liver, extensively
Excretion	Kidneys, minimal
Half-life	2-5 hr

Pharmacodynamics

	PO	PO–SUS REL
Onset	½ hr	Unknown
Peak	1-2 hr	2-6 hr
Duration	8 hr	10-12 hr

Interactions

Individual drugs

Alcohol: ↑ hypotension

Digoxin: ↑ digoxin levels, bradycardia, CHF

Phenobarbital: ↓ effectiveness

Phenytoin: ↓ effectiveness

Propranolol: ↑ toxicity

Drug classifications

Antihypertensives: ↑ hypotension

β-Adrenergic blockers: ↑ bradycardia, CHF

Nitrates: ↑ nitrates

NURSING CONSIDERATIONS

Assessment

- Assess fluid volume status (I&O ratio) and record weight, color, quality and sp gr of urine, skin turgor, adequacy of pulses, moist mucous membranes, bilateral lung sounds, peripheral pitting edema; dehydration symptoms of decreasing output, thirst, hypotension, dry mouth, and mucous membranes should be reported
- Monitor B/P and pulse

Nursing diagnoses

✓ Cardiac output, decreased (uses)

✓ Knowledge deficit (teaching)

Implementation

- Give ac, hs on an empty stomach 1 hr ac or 2 or more hr pc
- Store in tight container at room temp

Patient/family education

- Advise patient to avoid hazardous activities until stabilized

on drug and dizziness is no longer a problem
- Instruct patient to limit caffeine consumption; to avoid alcohol and OTC drugs unless directed by a prescriber
- Instruct patient to comply in all areas of medical regimen: diet, exercise, stress reduction, drug therapy; to notify prescriber of irregular heart beat, shortness of breath, swelling of feet and hands, pronounced dizziness, constipation, nausea, hypotension
- Teach patient to use medication as directed even if feeling better; may be taken with other cardiovascular drugs (nitrates, β-blockers)
- Teach patient to take medication exactly as prescribed
- Advise patient to contact prescriber if anginal attacks continue or become worse

Evaluation

Positive therapeutic outcome
- Decreased angina attacks
- Decreased B/P

Treatment of overdose: Defibrillation, atropine for AV block, vasopressor for hypotension

nicotine polacrilex gum (℞), OTC

(nik'o-teen)

Nicorette, Nicorette DS

Func. class.: Smoking deterrent

Chem. class.: Ganglionic cholinergic agonist

Pregnancy category X

Action: Agonist at nicotinic receptors in the peripheral and central nervous systems; acts at sympathetic ganglia, on chemoreceptors of the aorta and carotid bodies; also affects adrenalin-releasing catecholamines

Therapeutic Outcome: Decreased withdrawal effects when smoking cessation is attempted

Uses: Deter cigarette smoking

Dosage and routes

Adult: Gum 1 piece chewed × 30 min as needed to abstain from smoking; not to exceed 30/day

Available forms: Gum 2 mg/piece of gum

Adverse effects

CNS: Dizziness, vertigo, insomnia, headache, confusion, convulsions, depression, euphoria, numbness, tinnitus

CV: Dysrhythmias, tachycardia, palpitations, edema, flushing, hypertension

EENT: Jaw ache, irritation in buccal cavity

GI: Nausea, vomiting, anorexia, indigestion, diarrhea, abdominal pain, constipation, eructation

RESP: Breathing difficulty, cough, hoarseness, sneezing, wheezing

Contraindications: Hypersensitivity, immediate post-MI recovery period, severe angina pectoris, pregnancy **X**

Precautions: Vasospastic disease, dysrhythmias, diabetes mellitus, hyperthyroidism, pheochromocytoma, coronary disease, esophagitis, peptic ulcer, lactation, hepatic/renal disease

N

Pharmacokinetics

Absorption	Slowly absorbed, buccal cavity
Distribution	Unknown
Metabolism	Liver; some by lungs, kidneys
Excretion	Kidneys, unchanged (20%); breast milk
Half-life	1-2 hr

Pharmacodynamics

Onset	Rapid
Peak	½ hr
Duration	Unknown

Interactions

Individual drugs

Acetaminophen: ↑ effects of acetaminophen
Caffeine: ↑ effects of caffeine
Furosemide: ↑ effects of furosemide
Imipramine: ↑ effects of imipramine
Oxazepam: ↑ effects of oxazepam
Pentazocine: ↑ effects of pentazocine
Propranolol: ↑ effects of propranolol

NURSING CONSIDERATIONS

Assessment

- Assess for adverse reaction to gum: irritation of buccal cavity, dislike of taste, jaw ache
- Assess for withdrawal symptoms: headache, fatigue, drowsiness, restlessness, irritability, severe cravings for nicotine products before, during, and after treatment
- Obtain a nicotine assessment: brand of cigarettes, chewing tobacco, cigars, number of each used per day; what increases need or activities performed when each is used
- Gum should not be used if temporomandibular condition exists
- Assess for nicotine toxicity: GI symptoms (nausea, vomiting, diarrhea), cardiopulmonary symptoms (decreased B/P, dyspnea, change in pulse), weakness, abdominal cramping, headache, blurred vision, tinnitus; drug should be discontinued

Nursing diagnoses

- ✓ Coping, ineffective individual (uses)
- ✓ Knowledge deficit (teaching)
- ✓ Noncompliance (teaching)

Implementation

- Give only prescribed amount, or toxicity may occur
- Protect gum from light and heat

Patient/family education

- Instruct patient to chew gum slowly for 30 min to promote buccal absorption of the drug; do not chew over 45 min
- Advise patient to begin drug withdrawal after 3 mo use; do not exceed 6 mo
- Teach patient all aspects of drug; give package insert to patient and explain; caution patient not to exceed prescribed dose
- Inform patient that gum will not stick to dentures, dental appliances
- Caution patient that gum is as toxic as cigarettes; it is to be used only to deter smoking
- Caution patient not to use during pregnancy; birth defects may occur

Evaluation

Positive therapeutic outcome

- Decrease in urge to smoke
- Decreased need for gum after 3-6 mo

nicotine transdermal system (℞), OTC

Habitrol, Nicoderm, Nicotrol, Prostep

Func. class.: Smoking deterrent

Chem. class.: Ganglionic cholinergic agonist

Pregnancy category D

Action: Binds to acetylcholine receptors at autonomic ganglia in the adrenal medulla, at neuromuscular junctions, and in the brain

➔ **Therapeutic Outcome:** Decreased withdrawal efforts when smoking cessation is attempted

Uses: Deter cigarette smoking

Dosage and routes

Nicotrol

Adult: Transdermal 15 mg/day × 12 wk; 10 mg/day × 2 wk; 5 mg/day × 2 wk

Prostep

Adult: Transdermal 22 mg/day × 4-8 wk; 11 mg/day × 2-4 wk

Nicoderm/Habitrol

Adult: Transdermal 21 mg/day × 6 wk; 14 mg/day × 14 days; 7 mg/day × 14 days

Available forms: Transdermal patch delivering 7, 14, 21 mg; 15 mg, 10 mg, 5 mg, 22 mg, 11 mg/day patches depending on product

Adverse effects

CNS: Abnormal dreams, *insomnia*, nervousness, *headache*, dizziness, paresthesia, poor concentration, weakness

EENT: Dry mouth, abnormal taste

GI: Diarrhea, dyspepsia, constipation, nausea, abdominal pain, vomiting, dry mouth, abnormal taste

INTEG: Erythema, pruritus, burning at application site, hypersensitivity, sweating, rash

MISC: Chest pain, dysmenorrhea

MS: Arthralgia, myalgia, back pain

RESP: Cough, sinusitis

Contraindications: Hypersensitivity, children, pregnancy **D**, nonsmokers, during immediate post-MI period, life-threatening dysrhythmias, severe or worsening angina pectoris

Precautions: Skin disease, angina pectoris, MI, renal or hepatic insufficiency, peptic ulcer, accelerated hypertension, serious cardiac dysrhythmias, hyperthyroidism, pheochromocytoma, insulin-dependent diabetes, elderly

Pharmacokinetics

Absorption	Slowly absorbed
Distribution	Unknown
Metabolism	Liver
Excretion	Kidneys, unchanged (20%)
Half-life	1-2 hr

Pharmacodynamics

Onset	Rapid
Peak	½ hr
Duration	Unknown

Interactions

Individual drugs

Acetaminophen: ↑ effects of acetaminophen

Caffeine: ↑ effects of caffeine

Furosemide: ↑ effects of furosemide

Imipramine: ↑ effects of imipramine

Oxazepam: ↑ effects of oxazepam

Pentazocine: ↑ effects of pentazocine
Propranolol: ↑ effects of propranolol

NURSING CONSIDERATIONS

Assessment

- Monitor for adverse reaction: irritation of buccal cavity, dislike of taste, jaw ache
- Assess for withdrawal symptoms: headache, fatigue, drowsiness, restlessness, irritability, severe cravings for nicotine products before, during, and after treatment
- Obtain a nicotine assessment: brand of cigarettes, chewing tobacco, cigars, number of each used per day; what increases need or activities performed when each is used
- Assess for nicotine toxicity: GI symptoms (nausea, vomiting, diarrhea), cardiopulmonary symptoms (decreased B/P, dyspnea, change in pulse), weakness, abdominal cramping, headache, blurred vision, tinnitus; drug should be discontinued

Nursing diagnoses

- ✓ Coping, ineffective individual (uses)
- ✓ Knowledge deficit (teaching)
- ✓ Noncompliance (teaching)

Implementation

- Protect from heat
- Some patches are worn during the waking hr only (Nicotrol); other patches are worn 24 hr

Patient/family education

- Teach patient all aspects of drug; give package insert to patient and explain
- Caution patient that patch is as toxic as cigarettes; it is to be used only to deter smoking
- Caution patient not to use during pregnancy; birth defects may occur
- Caution patient to keep used and unused system out of reach of children and pets
- Instruct patient to apply once a day to a nonhairy, clean, dry area of skin on upper body or upper outer arm; some products are used during waking hr, some 24 hr/day; to rotate sites to prevent skin irritation
- Instruct patient to stop smoking immediately when beginning treatment with patch
- Teach patient to apply promptly after removing from protective pouch; system may lose strength

Evaluation

Positive therapeutic outcome

- Decrease in urge to smoke
- Decreased need for gum, patch

nifedipine (℞)

(nye-fed'i-peen)

Adalat, Adalat CC, Adalat P.A. ✤, Apo-Nifed ✤, Novo-Nifedin ✤, NuNifed ✤, nifedipine, Procardia, Procardia XL

Func. class.: Calcium channel blocker, antihypertensive

Chem. class.: Dihydropyridine

Pregnancy category C

Action: Inhibits calcium ion influx across cell membrane during cardiac depolarization, produces relaxation of coronary vascular smooth muscle and peripheral vascular smooth muscle, dilates coronary vascular arteries, increases myocardial oxygen delivery in patients with vasospastic angina

➔ **Therapeutic Outcome:** Decreased angina pectoris, decreased B/P in hypertension

Uses: Chronic stable angina pectoris, vasospastic angina, hypertension (sus rel only)

Investigational uses: Hypertension (acute), migraines, CHF, Raynaud's disease

Dosage and routes

Adult: PO immediate release, 10 mg tid; increase in 10-mg increments q4-6h, not to exceed 180 mg/24 hr or single dose of 30 mg

Adult: PO sus rel, 30-60 mg/day; may increase q7-14 days; doses >120 mg not recommended

Available forms: Caps 5 ✦, 10, 20 mg; sus rel tabs 30, 60, 90 mg

Adverse effects

CNS: *Headache,* fatigue, drowsiness, *dizziness,* anxiety, depression, weakness, insomnia, *lightheadedness,* paresthesia, tinnitus, blurred vision, nervousness
CV: Dysrhythmias, edema, ***CHF,*** hypotension, palpitations, ***MI, pulmonary edema,*** tachycardia
GI: *Nausea,* vomiting, diarrhea, gastric upset, constipation, increased liver function studies, dry mouth
GU: Nocturia, polyuria
INTEG: Rash, pruritus, *flushing,* photosensitivity, hair loss
MISC: Sexual difficulties, cough, fever, chills

Contraindications: Hypersensitivity

Precautions: CHF, hypotension, sick sinus syndrome, 2nd- or 3rd-degree heart block, hypotension less than 90 mm Hg systolic, hepatic injury, pregnancy **C,** lactation, P children, renal disease

Pharmacokinetics

Absorption	Well absorbed (PO)
Distribution	Unknown
Metabolism	Liver, extensively
Excretion	Unknown
Half-life	2-5 hr

Pharmacodynamics

	PO	PO–SUS REL
Onset	½ hr	Unknown
Peak	Unknown	Unknown
Duration	6-8 hr	24 hr

Interactions

Individual drugs
Alcohol: ↑ hypotension
Digoxin: ↑ digoxin levels, bradycardia, CHF
Propranolol: ↑ toxicity
Drug classifications
Antihypertensives: ↑ hypotension
β-Adrenergic blockers: ↑ bradycardia, CHF
Nitrates: ↑ nitrates

NURSING CONSIDERATIONS
Assessment

- Assess fluid volume status (I&O ratio) and record weight, distended red veins, crackles in lung, color, quality and sp gr of urine, skin turgor, adequacy of pulses, moist mucous membranes, bilateral lung sounds, peripheral pitting edema; dehydration symptoms of decreasing output, thirst, hypotension, dry mouth, and mucous membranes should be reported

N

• Monitor ALT (SGPT), AST (SGOT), bilirubin daily; if these are elevated, hepatotoxicity is suspected
• Monitor cardiac status: B/P, pulse, respirations, ECG

Nursing diagnoses
- ✓ Cardiac output, decreased (uses)
- ✓ Pain (uses)
- ✓ Knowledge deficit (teaching)

Implementation
PO route
• Give ac, at hs, or with meals for GI symptoms
• Store in tight container at room temp
Sublingual route
• Using a sterile needle puncture the cap and squeeze medication in buccal area (not an FDA-approved use)

Patient/family education
• Advise patient to avoid hazardous activities until stabilized on drug and dizziness is no longer a problem
• Instruct patient to limit caffeine consumption; to avoid alcohol and OTC drugs unless directed by prescriber
• Instruct patient to comply in all areas of medical regimen: diet, exercise, stress reduction, drug therapy; to notify prescriber of irregular heart beat, shortness of breath, swelling of feet and hands, pronounced dizziness, constipation, nausea, hypotension
• Teach patient to use as directed even if feeling better; may be taken with other cardiovascular drugs (nitrates, β-blockers)

Evaluation
Positive therapeutic outcome
• Decreased angina attacks
• Decreased B/P

Treatment of overdose: Defibrillation, atropine for AV block, vasopressor for hypotension

nilutamide (℞)
(nil-u'ta-mide)
Nilandron, Anandron ♣
Func. class.: Antineoplastic, hormone
Chem. class.: Antiandrogen
Pregnancy category C

Action: Interferes with testosterone uptake in the nucleus or testosterone activity in target tissues; arrests tumor growth in androgen-sensitive tissue, i.e., prostate gland, prostatic carcinoma is androgen-sensitive, so tumor growth is arrested

➡ **Therapeutic Outcome:** Decreased tumor size

Uses: Metastatic prostatic carcinoma, stage D2 in combination with surgical castration

Dosage and routes
Adult: PO 300 mg qd × 30 days, then 150 mg qd

Available forms: Tabs 50, 100 mg ♣

Adverse effects
CNS: Hot flashes, drowsiness, insomnia, dizziness, hyperthesia, depression
EENT: Delay in adaptation to dark
GU: Decreased libido, impotence, testicular atrophy, UTI, hematuria, nocturia, gynecomastia
GI: Diarrhea, nausea, vomiting, increased liver function studies, constipation, dyspepsia
HEMA: Anemia

INTEG: Rash, sweating, alopecia, dry skin
RESP: Dyspnea, URI, pneumonia, ***interstitial pneumonitis***
MISC: Edema

Contraindications: Hypersensitivity, severe hepatic impairment, severe respiratory disease

Precautions: Pregnancy **C**

Pharmacokinetics

Absorption	Rapidly, completely
Distribution	Unknown
Metabolism	Unknown
Excretion	Urine, feces
Half-life	Unknown

Pharmacodynamics

Unknown

Interactions

Individual drugs

Phenytoin: ↑ toxicity
Theophylline: ↑ toxicity
Vitamin K: ↑ toxicity

NURSING CONSIDERATIONS

Assessment

- Monitor liver function studies: AST (SGOT), ALT (SGPT), alk phosphatase, which may be elevated
- Monitor for CNS symptoms: drowsiness, insomnia, dizziness
- Monitor chest x-rays, routinely; dyspnea, cough, which may indicate interstitial pneumonitis, discontinue treatment if this condition is suspected

Nursing diagnoses

✓ Infection, risk of (side effects)
✓ Knowledge deficit (teaching)

Patient/family education

- Advise to report side effects: decreased libido, impotence, breast enlargement, hot flashes, diarrhea, dyspnea, cough
- Advise to wear tinted lens to alleviate delay in adapting to the dark

Evaluation

Positive therapeutic outcome

- Decrease in prostatic tumor size, decrease in spread of cancer

Treatment of overdose: Induce vomiting, provide supportive care

nimodipine (℞)

(ni-moe′dip-een)

Nimotop

Func. class.: Calcium channel blocker

Chem. class.: Dihydropyridine

Pregnancy category C

Action: Inhibits calcium ion influx across cell membrane during cardiac depolarization, produces relaxation of coronary vascular smooth muscle and peripheral vascular smooth muscle, dilates coronary vascular arteries, increases myocardial oxygen delivery in patients with vasospastic angina

➔ **Therapeutic Outcome:** Prevention of vascular spasm (subarachnoid hemorrhage)

Uses: Prevention of cerebral vascular spasm in subarachnoid hemorrhage

Dosage and routes

Adult: PO 20 mg tid initially; may increase after 3 days (range 20-40 mg tid)

Available forms: Caps 20, 30 mg; sus rel caps 30, 45, 60 mg

Adverse effects

CNS: Headache, fatigue, drowsiness, dizziness, anxiety,

N

depression, weakness, insomnia, confusion, paresthesia, somnolence
CV: Dysrhythmia, edema, CHF, bradycardia, hypotension, palpitations, ***MI, pulmonary edema***
GI: Nausea, vomiting, diarrhea, gastric upset, constipation, ***hepatitis,*** abdominal cramps
GU: Nocturia, polyuria, ***acute renal failure***
INTEG: Rash, pruritus, urticaria, photosensitivity, hair loss
MISC: Blurred vision, flushing, nasal congestion, sweating, shortness of breath, gynecomastia, hyperglycemia, sexual difficulties

Contraindications: Sick sinus syndrome, 2nd- or 3rd-degree heart block, hypotension less than 90 mm Hg systolic, hypersensitivity

Precautions: CHF, hypotension, hepatic injury, pregnancy P **C,** lactation, children, renal G disease, elderly

Pharmacokinetics

Absorption	Well absorbed, bioavailability poor
Distribution	Crosses blood-brain barrier
Metabolism	Liver, extensively
Excretion	Kidneys
Half-life	1-2 hr

Pharmacodynamics

Onset	Unknown
Peak	1 hr
Duration	Unknown

Interactions
Individual drugs
Alcohol: ↑ hypotension
Digoxin: ↑ digoxin levels, bradycardia
Phenobarbital: ↓ effectiveness
Phenytoin: ↓ effectiveness
Propranolol: ↑ toxicity
Drug classifications
Antihypertensives: ↑ hypotension
β-Adrenergic blockers: ↑ bradycardia
Nitrates: ↑ nitrates

NURSING CONSIDERATIONS
Assessment
- Assess fluid volume status (I&O ratio) and record weight, distended red veins, crackles in lung, color, quality and sp gr of urine, skin turgor, adequacy of pulses, moist mucous membranes, bilateral lung sounds, peripheral pitting edema; dehydration symptoms of decreasing output, thirst, hypotension, dry mouth and mucous membranes should be reported
- Monitor B/P and pulse; if B/P drops 30 mm Hg, call prescriber
- Monitor ALT (SGPT), AST (SGOT), bilirubin daily; if these are elevated, hepatotoxicity is suspected

Nursing diagnoses
✓ Injury, risk for (uses)
✓ Knowledge deficit (teaching)

Implementation
- May puncture cap and dilute in water and give through nasogastric tube; flush tube with 0.90% NaCl
- Store in airtight container at room temp

Patient/family education
- Teach patient to comply in all areas of medical regimen: diet, exercise, stress reduction, drug therapy; to notify prescriber of irregular heart beat, shortness of breath, swelling of feet and hands, pronounced dizziness, constipation, nausea, hypotension

Evaluation

Positive therapeutic outcome
- Decreased angina
- Decreased B/P

Treatment of overdose: Defibrillation, atropine for AV block, vasopressor for hypotension

nisoldipine (℞)

(nye'sol-dye-peen)

Sular

Func. class.: Calcium channel blocker

Chem. class.: Dihydropyridine

Pregnancy category C

Action: Inhibits calcium ion influx across cell membrane, resulting in dilation of peripheral arteries

Therapeutic Outcome: Decreased B/P in hypertension

Uses: Essential hypertension, alone or with other antihypertensives

Dosage and routes

Adult: PO 20 mg qd initially, may increase by 10 mg/wk, usual dose 20-40 mg qd

Available forms: Tabs, ext rels 10, 20, 30, 40 mg

Adverse effects

CNS: Headache, fatigue, drowsiness, dizziness, anxiety, depression, nervousness, insomnia, light-headedness, paresthesia, tinnitus, psychosis, somnolence

CV: Dysrhythmias, edema, CHF, hypotension, palpitations, ***MI, pulmonary edema,*** tachycardia, syncope, AV block, angina

GI: Nausea, vomiting, diarrhea, gastric upset, constipation, increased liver function studies, dry mouth

HEMA: Anemia

INTEG: Rash, pruritus

MISC: Flushing, sexual difficulties, cough, nasal congestion, shortness of breath, wheezing, epistaxis, respiratory infection, chest pain

Contraindications: Hypersensitivity, sick sinus syndrome, 2nd- or 3rd-degree heart block

Precautions: CHF, hypotension <90 mm Hg systolic, hepatic injury, pregnancy **C**, P lactation, children, renal disease, G elderly

Pharmacokinetics

Absorption	Well absorbed
Distribution	Unknown
Metabolism	Liver
Excretion	Kidneys
Half-life	Unknown

Pharmacodynamics

Unknown

Interactions

Individual drugs

Alcohol: ↑ hypotension
Carbamazepine: ↑ toxicity
Digoxin: ↑ digoxin levels, ↑ bradycardia, CHF
Phenobarbital: ↓ effectiveness
Phenytoin: ↓ effectiveness
Propranolol: ↑ toxicity

Drug classifications

Antihypertensives: ↑ hypotension
β-Adrenergic blockers: ↑ bradycardia, CHF
Nitrates: ↑ nitrates

NURSING CONSIDERATIONS

Assessment
- Assess fluid volume status: I&O ratio and record; weight; skin turgor; adequacy of pulses;

moist mucous membranes; bilateral lung sounds; peripheral pitting edema—dehydration symptoms of decreasing output, thirst, hypotension, dry mouth, and mucous membranes should be reported

- Monitor ALT (SGPT), AST (SGOT), bilirubin daily; if these are elevated
- Monitor cardiac status: B/P, pulse, respiration, ECG

Nursing diagnoses

✓ Cardiac output, decreased (uses)

✓ Knowledge deficit (teaching)

Implementation

- Give once a day, with food for GI symptoms, avoid high-fat foods, grapefruit

Patient/family education

- Caution patient to avoid hazardous activities until stabilized on drug, and dizziness is no longer a problem
- Instruct patient to limit caffeine consumption; to avoid alcohol and OTC drugs unless directed by prescriber
- Urge patient to comply in all areas of medical regimen: diet, exercise, stress reduction, drug therapy; to notify prescriber of irregular heart beat, shortness of breath, swelling of feet and hands, pronounced dizziness, constipation, nausea, hypotension
- Teach patient to use as directed even if feeling better; may be taken with other cardiovascular drugs (nitrates, beta blockers)

Evaluation

Positive therapeutic outcome

- Decreased B/P

nitroglycerin 🔑 (℞)
(nye-troe-gli'ser-in)
Nitro-Bid IV, nitroglycerin, Tridil, Nitrostat, Nitro-Bid Plateau Caps, Nitrocine Timecaps, Nitroglyn, Nitrong, Nitro-Bid, Nitrol, Deponit, Minitran, Nitrek, Nitrodisc, Nitro-Dur, nitroglycerin transdermal, Nitrocine, Transderm-Nitro, Nitrolingual, Nitrogard

Func. class.: Coronary vasodilator, antianginal

Chem. class.: Nitrate

Pregnancy category C

Action: Decreases preload and afterload, which thus decreases left ventricular end-diastolic pressure and systemic vascular resistance; dilates coronary arteries and improves blood flow

➔ **Therapeutic Outcome:** Prevention of anginal attack

Uses: Chronic stable angina pectoris, prophylaxis of angina pain, CHF associated with acute MI, controlled hypotension in surgical procedures

Dosage and routes

Adult: SL dissolve tab under tongue when pain begins; may repeat q5 min until relief occurs; take no more than 3 tab/15 min; use 1 tab prophylactically 5-10 min before activities; sus rel cap q6-12h on empty stomach; top 1-2 in q8h; increase to 4 in q4h as needed; **IV** 5 μg/min, then increase by 5 μg/min q3-5 min; if no response after 20 μg/min, increase by 10-20 μg/min until desired response; trans apply a pad qd to a site free from hair

Available forms: Buccal tab 1, 2, 3 mg; aero 0.4 mg/meter spray; sus rel caps 2.5, 6.5, 9, 13 mg; sus rel tabs 2.6, 6.5, 9 mg; inj 0.5, 5 mg/ml; SL tabs 0.15, 0.3, 0.4, 0.6 mg; trans oint 2%; trans syst 0.1, 0.2, 0.3, 0.4, 0.6 mg/24 hr; inj 25 mg/250 ml, 50 mg/250 ml, 50 mg/500 ml, 100 mg/250 ml, 200 mg/500 ml; patches 22.4, 44.8, 67.2 mg

Adverse effects

CNS: Headache, flushing, dizziness

CV: Postural hypotension, tachycardia, ***collapse,*** syncope

GI: Nausea, vomiting

INTEG: Pallor, sweating, rash

Contraindications: Hypersensitivity to this drug or nitrites, severe anemia, increased intracranial pressure, cerebral hemorrhage

Precautions: Postural hypotension, pregnancy **C,** lactation

Interactions

Individual drugs

Alcohol: ↑ hypotension

Haloperidol: ↑ hypotension

Drug classifications

Antidepressants, tricyclic: ↓ absorption of SL, transmucosal

Antihistamines: ↓ absorption of SL, transmucosal

Antihypertensives: ↑ hypotension

β-Blockers: ↑ hypotension

Calcium channel blockers: ↑ hypotension

Phenothiazines: ↓ absorption of SL, transmucosal

Pharmacokinetics	
Absorption	Well absorbed (PO, buccal, SL)
Distribution	Unknown
Metabolism	Liver, extensively
Excretion	Kidney
Half-life	1-4 min

NURSING CONSIDERATIONS

Assessment

- Monitor orthostatic B/P, pulse
- Assess pain: duration, time started, activity being performed, character; check for tolerance if taken over long period
- Monitor for headache, lightheadedness, decreased B/P; may indicate a need for decreased dosage

Nursing diagnoses

- ✓ Cardiac output, decreased (uses)
- ✓ Poisoning (uses)
- ✓ Tissue perfusion, decreased (uses)
- ✓ Knowledge deficit (teaching)
- ✓ Noncompliance (teaching)

Implementation

IV IV route

- Give **IV** diluted in amount specified D_5 or NS for inf; use glass inf bottles, non–polyvinyl chloride inf tubing, titrate to

N

Pharmacodynamics

	SUS REL	SL	TRANS	IV	TRANSMUCOSAL	AEROSOL	TOP OINT
Onset	20-45 min	1-3 min	½-1 hr	1-2 min	3 min	2 min	½-1 hr
Peak	Unknown	Unknown	Unknown	Unknown	Unknown	Unknown	Unknown
Duration	3-8 hr	½ hr	12-24 hr	3-5 min	3-5 hr	½-1 hr	2-12 hr

patient response; do not use filters

Syringe compatibility:
Heparin

Y-site compatibilities:
Amiodarone, amrinone, atracurium, diltiazem, dobutamine, dopamine, esmolol, famotidine, fluconazole, haloperidol, heparin, regular insulin, labetalol, lidocaine, nitroprusside, pancuronium, ranitidine, streptokinase, tacrolimus, theophylline, vecuronium

Y-site incompatibility:
Alteplase

Additive incompatibilities:
Manufacturer recommends that nitroglycerin not be admixed with other medications

Additive compatibility:
Alteplase

SL route

- Keep tab in original container
- If 3 SL tab in 15 min do not relieve pain, consider diagnosis of MI
- SL tab should be held under tongue until dissolved (a few min); do not take anything by mouth when SL tab is in place

PO route

- Give 1 hr ac or 2 hr pc with 8 oz of water
- Sus rel tab should not be chewed or crushed

Transmucosal route

- Tab should be placed between cheek and gum line
- Do not take anything by PO when tab is in place

Top route

- Apply ointment using dose-measuring papers supplied; apply to an area without hair; ointment should cover 2-3 in area; may apply an occlusive dressing as directed
- Apply trans patches to area without hair; press hard to adhere; if patch becomes dislodged, apply a new one

Patient/family education

- Teach patient to place buccal tab between lip and gum above incisors or between cheek and gum; sus rel tab must be swallowed whole, do not chew; SL should be dissolved under tongue, do not swallow; aerosol should be sprayed under tongue, do not inhale; use inhaler only when lying down; do not inhale spray
- Instruct patient to avoid alcohol
- Advise patient that drug may cause headache; tolerance usually develops; use nonnarcotic analgesic
- Teach patient that drug may be taken before stressful activity, exercise, sexual activity
- Inform patient that SL may sting when drug comes in contact with mucous membranes
- Caution patient to avoid hazardous activities if dizziness occurs
- Instruct patient to comply with complete medical regimen
- Advise patient to make position changes slowly to prevent fainting

Evaluation

Positive therapeutic outcome

- Decreased, prevention of anginal pain

nitroprusside (℞)

(nye-troe-pruss'ide)

Nitropress, Sodium nitroprusside

Func. class.: Antihypertensive

Chem. class.: Peripheral vasodilator

Pregnancy category C

Action: Directly relaxes arteriolar, venous smooth muscle, resulting in reduction in cardiac preload, afterload

Therapeutic Outcome: Decreased B/P in hypertensive crisis, decreased preload, afterload

Uses: Hypertensive crisis, to decrease bleeding by creating hypotension during surgery, acute CHF

Dosage and routes

Adult: **IV** inf dissolve 50 mg in 2-3 ml of D_5W, then dilute in 250-1000 ml of D_5W; run at 0.5 8 μg/kg/min

Available forms: Inj 50 mg

Adverse effects

CNS: Dizziness, headache, agitation, twitching, decreased reflexes, ***LOC,*** restlessness

CV: Palpitations, severe hypotension, dyspnea

EENT: Tinnitus, blurred vision

GI: Nausea, vomiting, abdominal pain

GU: Impotence

INTEG: Pain, irritation at inj site, sweating

MISC: Cyanide, thiocyanate toxicity

Contraindications: Hypersensitivity, hypertension (compensatory)

Precautions: Pregnancy **C,** P lactation, children, fluid, electrolyte imbalances, hepatic disease, renal disease, hypothy- G roidism, elderly

Pharmacokinetics

Absorption	Complete bioavailability
Distribution	Not known
Metabolism	RBCs, tissues
Excretion	Kidneys
Half-life	Unknown

Pharmacodynamics

Onset	1-2 min
Peak	Rapid
Duration	1-10 min

Interactions

Drug classifications

Antihypertensives: ↑ hypotension

Ganglionic blockers: ↑ hypotension

NURSING CONSIDERATIONS

Assessment

- Monitor B/P q5 min × 2 hr, then q1h × 2 hr; monitor pulse q4h; monitor jugular venous distention q4h; ECG should be monitored continuously; monitor PCWP
- Monitor electrolytes, blood studies: potassium, sodium, chloride, CO_2, CBC, serum glucose, serum methemoglobin if pulmonary oxygen levels are decreased
- Check weight, I&O, edema in feet and legs daily; assess skin turgor, dryness of mucous membranes for hydration status
- Assess for signs of CHF: dyspnea, edema, wet rales
- Monitor for increased lactate, cyanide, thiocyanate levels
- Monitor for decrease in bicarbonate, Pco_2 and blood

N

pH; acidosis may occur with this drug

Nursing diagnoses

- ✓ Tissue perfusion, altered (uses)
- ✓ Injury, risk for (adverse reactions)
- ✓ Knowledge deficit (teaching)

Implementation

• Give by cont inf after diluting 50 mg/2-3 ml of D_5W; further dilute in 250 ml of D_5W; use an inf pump only; wrap bottle with aluminum foil to protect from light; observe for color change in the inf; discard if highly discolored (blue, green, red); titrate to patient response; avoid extravasation

Additive incompatibilities: Do not give with any other drugs

Syringe compatibility: Heparin

Y-site compatibilities: Amrinone, atracurium, diltiazem, dobutamine, dopamine, enalaprilat, famotidine, lidocaine, nitroglycerin, pancuronium, tacrolimus, theophylline, vecuronium

Patient/family education

• Teach patient to report headache, dizziness, loss of hearing, blurred vision, dyspnea, faintness; may indicate adverse reactions

Evaluation

Positive therapeutic outcome

• Decreased B/P in hypertension

• Absence of bleeding in surgery

Treatment of overdose: Administer amyl nitrite inh until 3% sodium nitrate sol can be prepared for **IV** administration, then inject sodium thiosulfate **IV**; correct drop in B/P with vasopressor

nizatidine (℞)

(ni-za'ti-deen)

Axid

Func. class.: H_2-Receptor antagonist

Chem. class.: Substituted thiazole

Pregnancy category C

Action: Blocks H_2 receptors thereby reducing gastric acid output

➔ **Therapeutic Outcome:** Healing of duodenal ulcers or gastric ulcers; prevention of duodenal ulcers; decreases symptoms of GERD

Uses: Benign gastric and duodenal ulceration, prevention of duodenal ulcer recurrence, symptomatic relief of gastroesophageal reflux

Dosage and routes

Gastric and duodenal ulcer disease

Adult: PO 300 mg at night or 150 mg bid for 4-8 weeks; maintenance 150 mg at night for up to 1 yr

Gastroesophageal reflux

Adult: PO 150-300 mg bid for up to 12 weeks

Available forms: Caps 150, 300 mg

Adverse effects

CNS: Headache, somnolence, confusion, abnormal dreams

ENDO: Gynecomastia

GI: Elevated liver enzymes, hepatitis, jaundice, nausea

HEMA: ***Thrombocytopenia***

INTEG: Pruritus, sweating, urticaria, exfoliative dermatitis
METAB: Hyperuricemia
MS: Myalgia
RESP: ***Bronchospasm, laryngeal edema***

Contraindications: Hypersensitivity

Precautions: Renal or hepatic impairment (reduce dose in renal impairment), pregnancy **C**, lactation

Pharmacokinetics

Absorption	PO 70%
Distribution	Breast milk, crosses placenta
Metabolism	Liver, partially
Excretion	Kidney
Half-life	1½ hr

Pharmacodynamics

Onset	Variable
Peak	½-3 hr
Duration	Unknown

NURSING CONSIDERATIONS

Assessment

- Assess patient with ulcers or suspected ulcers: epigastric or abdominal pain, hematemesis, occult blood in stools, blood or gastric aspirate prior to and throughout treatment, monitor gastric pH (5 should be maintained)
- Monitor I&O ratio, BUN, creatinine, CBC with differential monthly

Nursing diagnoses

- ✓ Pain (uses)
- ✓ Knowledge deficit (teaching)

Implementation

- May be given with or without meals
- Give antacids 1 hr before or 1 hr after this drug

Patient/family education

- Caution patient that gynecomastia, impotence may occur and are reversible after treatment is discontinued
- Advise patient to avoid driving, other hazardous activities until stabilized on this medication; drowsiness or dizziness may occur
- Caution patient to avoid black pepper, caffeine, alcohol, harsh spices, extremes in temp of food; tell patient to avoid OTC preparations: aspirin, cough, cold preparations because condition may worsen
- Inform patient that smoking decreases the effectiveness of the drug; that smoking cessation should be considered
- Instruct patient that drug must be continued for prescribed time to be effective and taken exactly as prescribed; doses should not be doubled; a missed dose should be taken as soon as remembered up to 1 hr before next dose
- Advise patient to report bruising, fatigue, malaise; blood dyscrasias may occur
- Advise patient to report diarrhea, black tarry stools, sore throat, rash, dizziness, confusion, or delirium to prescriber immediately

Evaluation

Positive therapeutic outcome

- Decreased pain in abdomen
- Healing of ulcers
- Absence of gastroesophageal reflux

N

norfloxacin (℞)

(nor-flox'a-sin)

Chibroxin, Noroxin

Func. class.: Urinary anti-infective

Chem. class.: Fluoroquinolone antibacterial

Pregnancy category C

Action: Interferes with conversion of intermediate DNA fragments into high-molecular-weight DNA in bacteria

Therapeutic Outcome: Bactericidal action against the gram-positive *Staphylococcus epidermidis,* methicillin-resistant strains of *Staphylococcus aureus,* group D streptococci; gram-negative *Escherichia coli, Klebsiella pneumoniae, Enterobacter cloacae, Proteus mirabilis, P. vulgaris, Providencia rettgeri, Morganella morganii, Pseudomonas aeruginosa, Citrobacter freundii*

Uses: Adult UTIs (including complicated), uncomplicated gonorrhea, ocular infections

Dosage and routes

Uncomplicated infections

Adult: PO 400 mg bid × 7-10 days 1 hr ac or 2 hr pc

Complicated infections

Adult: PO 400 mg bid × 10-21 days; 400 mg qd × 7-10 days in impaired renal function

Uncomplicated gonorrhea

Adult: PO 800 mg as a single dose

Occular infection

P ***Adult and child:*** Ophth i gtt qid; may increase to i gtt q2h for severe infections

Available forms: Tabs 400 mg; ophth sol 3 mg/ml

Adverse effects

CNS: Headache, dizziness, fatigue, somnolence, depression, insomnia

EENT: Visual disturbances

GI: Nausea, constipation, increased ALT (SGPT), AST (SGOT), flatulence, heartburn, vomiting, diarrhea, dry mouth

INTEG: Rash

Contraindications: Hypersensitivity to quinolones

Precautions: Pregnancy **C,** P lactation, children, renal disease, seizure disorders

Pharmacokinetics

Absorption	30% (PO)
Distribution	Concentration in urinary system
Metabolism	Liver (minimal)
Excretion	Kidneys, unchanged (30%)
Half-life	3-4 hr; increased in renal disease

Pharmacodynamics

	PO
Onset	Unknown
Peak	1 hr

Interactions

Individual drugs

Nitrofurantoin: ↓ effectiveness

Probenecid: ↑ blood levels

Sucralfate: ↓ absorption of norfloxacin

Theophylline: ↑ toxicity

Zinc sulfate: ↓ absorption of norfloxacin

Drug classifications

Antacids: ↓ absorption of norfloxacin

Anticoagulants, oral: ↑ effect of anticoagulants

Antineoplastics: ↓ norfloxacin levels

Iron salts: ↓ absorption of norfloxacin

Lab test interferences

↑ AST (SGOT), ↑ ALT (SGPT), ↑ BUN, ↑ creatinine, ↑ alkaline phosphatase

NURSING CONSIDERATIONS

Assessment

- Assess patient for previous sensitivity reaction
- Assess patient for signs and symptoms of infection including characteristics of urine, WBC >10,000, temp; obtain baseline information before and during treatment
- Obtain C & S before beginning drug therapy to identify if correct treatment has been initiated
- Assess for allergic reactions: rash, urticaria, pruritus
- Monitor blood studies: AST (SGOT), ALT (SGPT), BUN, creatinine, alkaline phosphatase monthly if patient is on long-term therapy
- Assess bowel pattern qd; if severe diarrhea occurs, drug should be discontinued
- Assess for overgrowth of infection: perineal itching, fever, malaise, redness, pain, swelling, drainage, rash, diarrhea, change in cough, sputum

Nursing diagnoses

✓ Infection, risk for (uses)
✓ Diarrhea (adverse reactions)
✓ Injury, risk for (adverse reactions)
✓ Knowledge deficit (teaching)
✓ Noncompliance (teaching)

Implementation

PO route

- Give in equal intervals q12h around the clock to maintain proper blood levels; give with food to increase absorption of drug; do not give within 3 hr of other agents; drug interactions may occur; give with 8 oz of water
- Do not give with iron, zinc products, or antacids, which decrease absorption

Patient/family education

- Instruct patient to take all medication prescribed for the length of time ordered; drug must be taken around the clock to maintain blood levels; do not give medication to others; do not double doses; take any missed dose when remembered
- Advise patient to increase fluids to 2 L/day to prevent crystalluria
- Caution patient to avoid driving and other hazardous activities until response is known; dizziness may occur
- Instruct patient to use sunglasses to prevent photophobia
- Have patient use hard candy, frequent sips of water for dry mouth
- Teach patient correct instillation procedure (ophth)

Evaluation

Positive therapeutic outcome

- Reported improvement in symptoms of infection
- Absence of red or itching eyes (ophth)

N

nortriptyline (℞)

(nor-trip′ti-leen)

Aventyl, Pamelor

Func. class.: Antidepressant, tricyclic

Chem. class.: Dibenzocycloheptene, secondary amine

Pregnancy category C

Action: Blocks reuptake of norepinephrine, serotonin into nerve endings, increasing action of norepinephrine, serotonin in nerve cells; has anticholinergic effects

➔ **Therapeutic Outcome:** Decreased symptoms of depression after 2-3 wk

Uses: Major depression

Investigational uses: Chronic pain management

Dosage and routes

Adult: PO 25 mg tid or qid; may increase to 150 mg/day; may give daily dose hs

Available forms: Caps 10, 25, 50, 75 mg; sol 10 mg/5 ml

Adverse effects

CNS: Dizziness, drowsiness, confusion, headache, anxiety, tremors, stimulation, weakness, insomnia, nightmares, EPS G (elderly), increased psychiatric symptoms

CV: Orthostatic hypotension, ECG changes, tachycardia, ***hypertension,*** palpitations

EENT: Blurred vision, tinnitus, mydriasis

GI: Constipation, dry mouth, nausea, vomiting, ***paralytic ileus,*** increased appetite, cramps, epigastric distress, jaundice, ***hepatitis,*** stomatitis

GU: Retention, ***acute renal failure***

HEMA: ***Agranulocytosis, thrombocytopenia, eosinophilia, leukopenia***

INTEG: Rash, urticaria, sweating, pruritus, photosensitivity

Contraindications: Hypersensitivity to tricyclic antidepressants, recovery phase of MI, convulsive disorders, prostatic hypertrophy

Precautions: Suicidal patients, severe depression, increased intraocular pressure, narrow-angle glaucoma, urinary retention, cardiac disease, hepatic disease, hyperthyroidism, electroshock therapy, elective surgery, pregnancy **C**

Pharmacokinetics

Absorption	Well absorbed
Distribution	Widely distributed; crosses placenta
Metabolism	Liver, extensively
Excretion	Kidneys, breast milk
Half-life	18-28 hr; steady state 4-19 days

Pharmacodynamics

Unknown

Interactions

Individual drugs

Alcohol: ↑ CNS depression

Cimetidine: ↑ levels, toxicity

Clonidine: Severe hypotension; avoid use

Disulfiram: Organic brain syndrome

Fluoxetine: ↑ levels, toxicity

Guanethidine: ↓ effects

Drug classifications

Analgesics: ↑ CNS depression

Anticholinergics: ↑ side effects

Antihistamines: ↑ CNS depression

Antihypertensives: May block antihypertensive effect

Barbiturates: ↑ effects
Benzodiazepines: ↑ effects
CNS depressants: ↑ effects
MAOIs: Hypertensive crisis, convulsions
Oral contraceptives: ↑ effects, toxicity
Phenothiazines: ↑ toxicity
Sedative/hypnotics: ↑ CNS depression
Sympathomimetics, indirect-acting: ↓ effects

Smoking
↑ metabolism, ↓ effects

Lab test interferences
↑ Serum bilirubin, ↑ blood glucose, ↑ alkaline phosphatase
↓ VMA, ↓ 5-HIAA, ↓ blood glucose
False ↑ Urinary catecholamines

NURSING CONSIDERATIONS

Assessment

- Monitor B/P (with patient lying, standing), pulse q4h; if systolic B/P drops 20 mm Hg, hold drug, notify prescriber; take VS q4h of patients with cardiovascular disease
- Monitor blood studies: CBC, leukocytes, differential, cardiac enzymes if patient is receiving long-term therapy
- Monitor hepatic studies: AST (SGOT), ALT (SGPT), bilirubin
- Check weight weekly; appetite may increase with drug
- Assess ECG for flattening of T wave, bundle branch block, AV block, dysrhythmias in cardiac patients
- Assess for EPS primarily in [G] elderly: rigidity, dystonia, akathisia
- Assess mental status: mood, sensorium, affect, suicidal tendencies; increase in psychiatric symptoms: depression, panic
- Monitor urinary retention, constipation; constipation is [P] more likely to occur in children [G] or elderly
- [!] Assess for withdrawal symptoms: headache, nausea, vomiting, muscle pain, weakness; do not usually occur unless drug was discontinued abruptly
- Identify alcohol consumption; if alcohol is consumed, hold dose until AM

Nursing diagnoses

- ✓ Coping, ineffective individual (uses)
- ✓ Injury, risk for (adverse reactions)
- ✓ Knowledge deficit (teaching)
- ✓ Noncompliance (teaching)

Implementation

- Give with food or milk for GI symptoms; mix conc with water, milk, fruit juice to disguise taste
- Give dose hs if oversedation occurs during day; may take [G] entire dose hs; elderly may not tolerate once/day dosing
- Store at room temp; do not freeze

Patient/family education

- Teach patient that therapeutic effects may take 2-3 wk
- Teach patient to use caution in driving and other activities requiring alertness because of drowsiness, dizziness, blurred vision; to avoid rising quickly from sitting to standing, espe- [G] cially elderly
- Teach patient to avoid alcohol ingestion, other CNS depressants; teach patient not to discontinue medication quickly after long-term use; may cause nausea, headache, malaise
- Teach patient to wear sun-

N

screen or large hat, since photosensitivity occurs

- Teach patient to increase fluids, bulk in diet if constipation, urinary retention occur, **G** especially elderly
- Teach patient to take gum, hard sugarless candy, or frequent sips of water for dry mouth

Evaluation

Positive therapeutic outcome

- Decrease in depression
- Absence of suicidal thoughts

Treatment of overdose: ECG monitoring, induce emesis, lavage, activated charcoal, administer anticonvulsant

nystatin (℞, OTC)

(nis′ta-tin)

Mycostatin, Mycostatin Pastilles, Nadostine ✤, Nyaderm ✤, nystatin, Nystex; topical: Mycostatin, Nilstat, Nodostine ✤, Nyoderm ✤, Nystatin, Nystex; vaginal: Mycostatin, Nilstat, Nadostine ✤, Nyoderm ✤, O-V Statin

Func. class.: Antiinfective

Chem. class.: Antifungal

Pregnancy category B; A vaginal

Action: Interferes with fungal DNA replication; binds sterols in fungal cell membrane, which increases permeability, resulting in leaking of cell nutrients

➔ Therapeutic Outcome: Fungistatic/fungicidal against *Candida* organisms

Uses: *Candida* species causing oral, vaginal, intestinal infections; vag: cutaneous vulvovaginal candidiasis, top: mucocutaneous fungal infec- **P** tions, infant eczema, pruritus ani and vulvae

Dosage and routes

Oral infection

Adult: Susp 400,000-600,000 U qid

P ***Child and infants >3 mo:*** Susp 250,000-500,000 U qid

P ***Newborn and premature infants:*** Susp 100,000 U qid

GI infection

Adult: PO 500,000-1,000,000 U tid

Top

P ***Adult and child:*** Top apply to affected area bid-tid × 14 days

Vag: 1-2 tabs (100,000 U each) inserted into vagina

Available forms: Tab 500,000 U; powder 50 mill, 150 mill, 500 mill, 1 bill, 2 bill, 5 bill U; susp 100,000 U; cream, oint, powder, spray, vag tab 100,000 U; vag cream, lotion 2%

Adverse effects

GI: Nausea, vomiting, anorexia, diarrhea, cramps

INTEG: Rash, urticaria, stinging, burning

Contraindication: Hypersensitivity

Precautions: Pregnancy **B,** lactation

Pharmacokinetics	
Absorption	Poorly absorbed
Distribution	Unknown
Metabolism	Not metabolized
Excretion	Feces, unchanged
Half-life	Unknown

Pharmacodynamics	
Onset	Rapid
Peak	Unknown
Duration	6-12 hr

Interactions: None

NURSING CONSIDERATIONS

Assessment

- Assess for allergic reaction: rash, urticaria; drug may have to be discontinued
- Assess for predisposing factors for candidal infection: antibiotic therapy, pregnancy, diabetes mellitus, sexual partner infection (vag infections), AIDS

Nursing diagnoses

✓ Skin integrity, impaired (uses)
✓ Infection, risk for (uses)
✓ Knowledge deficit (teaching)

Implementation

PO route

- Give oral susp dose by placing ½ in each cheek, swish for several min, then swallow; shake susp before use
- Store oral susp in refrigerator, tab in tight, light-resistant containers at room temp

Top route

- Administer by moistening lesions with a swab coated with cream or ointment; use enough medication to cover lesions completely; give after cleansing with soap, water before each application; dry well

Vag route

- Insert vag tab high into vagina with applicator provided; administer in gravid client 3-6 wk before term to decrease candidiasis in the P newborn
- Store at room temp in dry place; protect from light, air, heat

Patient/family education

- Instruct patient that long-term therapy may be needed to clear infection; to complete entire course of medication
- Teach patient proper hygiene: use no commercial mouthwashes for mouth infection
- Advise patient to avoid getting preparation on hands
- Instruct patient to wear light-day pad for vag preparations to avoid soiling clothing; to avoid sexual contact during treatment to minimize reinfection
- Instruct patient to notify prescriber if irritation occurs; drug may have to be discontinued
- Inform patient that relief from itching may occur after 24-72 hr

Top

- Advise patient to discontinue use and notify prescriber if irritation occurs
- Teach patient to apply with glove to prevent further infection; drug may stain
- Caution patient not to use occlusive dressings; to avoid use of OTC creams, ointments, lotions unless directed by prescriber

N

Evaluation

Positive therapeutic outcome

- Culture negative for *Candida*
- Decrease in size, number of lesions
- Decreased itching, white patches on vulva (vag)

ofloxacin (℞)

(o-flox'a-sin)

Floxin, Floxin IV, Ocuflox

Func. class.: Antiinfective

Chem. class.: Fluoroquinolone

Pregnancy category C

Action: Interferes with conversion of intermediate DNA fragments into high-molecular-weight DNA in bacteria

Therapeutic Outcome: Bactericidal action against the following gram-positive pathogens: *Staphylococcus epidermidis,* methicillin-resistant strains of *S. aureus, Streptococcus pyogenes, S. pneumoniae;* gram-negative pathogens *Escherichia coli, Klebsiella* species, *Enterobacter, Salmonella, Shigella, Proteus vulgaris, Providencia stuartii, P. rettgeri, Morganella morganii, Pseudomonas aeruginosa, Serratia, Haemophilus* species, *Acinetobacter, Neisseria gonorrhoeae, N. meningitidis, Yersinia, Vibrio, Brucella, Campylobacter,* and *Aeromonas* species; anaerobic pathogens: *Bacteroides fragilis intermedius, Clostridium perfrigens, Gardnerella vaginalis, Peptococcus niger, Peptostreptococcus* species; *Chlamydia pneumoniae, C. trachomatis, Legionella pneumoniae, Mycobacterium tuberculosis, Mycoplasma pneumoniae*

Uses: Treatment of lower respiratory tract infections (pneumonia, bronchitis), genitourinary infections (prostatitis, UTIs), skin and skin structure infections, conjunctivitis (ophth)

Dosage and routes

Lower respiratory tract infection/skin and skin structure infections

Adult: PO/**IV** 200-400 mg q12h × 10 days

Cervicitis, urethritis

Adult: PO/**IV** 300 mg q12h × 7 days

Prostatitis

Adult: PO 300 mg q12h × 6 wk

Acute, uncomplicated gonorrhea

Adult: PO/**IV** 400 mg as a single dose

Conjunctivitis

P ***Adult and child:*** Ophth 1-2 gtt q2-4h × 2 days, then qid × 5 days

Available forms: Tabs 200, 300, 400 mg; inj 200, 400 mg; ophth sol 0.3%

Adverse effects

CNS: Dizziness, headache, fatigue, somnolence, depression, insomnia, lethargy, malaise

EENT: Visual disturbances

GI: Diarrhea, nausea, vomiting, anorexia, flatulence, heartburn, dry mouth, increased AST (SGOT), ALT (SGPT), abdominal pain, constipation

INTEG: Rash, pruritus

Contraindication: Hypersensitivity to quinolones

Precautions: Pregnancy **C,** P lactation, children, elderly, G renal disease, seizure disorders, excessive sunlight

Pharmacokinetics	
Absorption	Well absorbed (PO)
Distribution	Widely distributed
Excretion	Kidneys, unchanged; breast milk
Half-life	5-9 hr; increased in renal disease

Pharmacodynamics

	PO	IV	OPHTH
Onset	Rapid	Rapid	Unknown
Peak	1-2 hr	Inf end	Unknown

Interactions

Individual drugs

Nitrofurantoin: ↓ effectiveness
Probenecid: ↑ blood levels
Sucralfate: ↓ absorption of ofloxacin
Theophylline: ↑ toxicity
Zinc sulfate: ↓ absorption of ofloxacin

Drug classifications

Antacids: ↓ absorption of ofloxacin
Anticoagulants, oral: ↑ effect of anticoagulants
Antineoplastics: ↓ ofloxacin levels
Iron salts: ↓ absorption of ofloxacin

Lab test interferences

Increase: AST (SGOT), ALT (SGPT), BUN, creatinine, alkaline phosphatase

NURSING CONSIDERATIONS

Assessment

- Assess patient for previous sensitivity reaction
- Assess patient for signs and symptoms of infection including characteristics of wounds, sputum, urine, stool, WBC >10,000, fever; obtain baseline information before and during treatment
- Obtain C&S before beginning drug therapy to identify if correct treatment has been initiated
- Assess for allergic reactions: rash, urticaria, pruritus
- Monitor blood studies: AST (SGOT), ALT (SGPT), CBC, serum glucose monthly if patient is on long-term therapy
- Assess bowel pattern qd; if severe diarrhea occurs, drug should be discontinued
- Assess for overgrowth of infection: perineal itching, fever, malaise, redness, pain, swelling, drainage, rash, diarrhea, change in cough, sputum
- Assess for CNS symptoms: seizures, vertigo, drowsiness, agitation, confusion, tremors

Nursing diagnoses

- ✓ Infection, risk for (uses)
- ✓ Diarrhea (adverse reactions)
- ✓ Injury, risk for (adverse reactions)
- ✓ Knowledge deficit (teaching)
- ✓ Noncompliance (teaching)

Implementation

PO route

- Give in equal intervals q12h around the clock to maintain proper blood levels; do not give within 3 hr of other agents, since drug interactions are possible: give with 8 oz of water
- Do not give with iron, aluminum, zinc products or antacids, which decrease absorption and form insoluble chelate

O

IV IV route

- For intermittent inf, dilute to 4 mg/ml with D_5W, D_5/0.9% NaCl, 0.9% NaCl, D_5/LR, sodium bicarbonate, sodium lactate, D_5/Plasmalyte 56; give over 1 hr or more

Additive compatibilities: Amoxicillin, ceftazidime, clindamycin, gentamicin, piperacillin, tobramycin, vancomycin

Syringe compatibility: cefotaxime

Y-site compatibilities: Ampicillin, thiotepa

Patient/family education

- Store for 2 wk refrigerated or

6 mo frozen, after reconstitution

• Instruct patient to take all medication prescribed for the length of time ordered; drug must be taken around the clock to maintain blood levels; do not give medication to others

• Teach patient to use sunscreen when outdoors to decrease phototoxicity

• Advise patient to increase fluids to 2 L/day to prevent crystalluria

• Caution patient to avoid driving and other hazardous activities until response is known; dizziness, confusion, drowsiness may occur

Evaluation

Positive therapeutic outcome

• Absence of signs/symptoms of infection (WBC <10,000, temp WNL)

• Reported improvement in symptoms of infection

• Absence of red or itching eyes (ophth)

olanzapine (℞)

(oh-lanz'a-peen)

Zyprexa

Func. class.: Antipsychotic/neuroleptic

Chem. class.: Thienbenzodiazepine

Pregnancy category C

Action: Unknown; may mediate antipsychotic activity by both dopamine and serotonin type 2 (5HT2) antagonism; also, may antagonize muscarinic receptors, histaminic (H_1)- and α-adrenergic receptors

Therapeutic Outcome: Decreased psychotic symptoms

Uses: Psychotic disorders

Dosage and routes

Adult: PO 5-10 mg initially qd, may increase dosage by 5 mg at 1 wk or more intervals

G ***Elderly:*** PO 5 mg, may increase cautiously at 1 wk intervals

Available forms: Tabs 5, 7.5, 10 mg

Adverse effects

CNS: EPS: pseudoparkinsonism, akathisia, dystonia, tardive dyskinesia, seizures, headache, ***neuroleptic malignant syndrome (rare),*** fever, insomnia, somnolence, agitation, nervousness, hostility, dizziness, hypertonia, tremor, euphoria

CV: Orthostatic hypotension, tachycardia, chest pain

EENT: Blurred vision

GI: Dry mouth, nausea, vomiting, anorexia, constipation, abdominal pain, weight gain

GU: Urinary retention, urinary frequency, enuresis, impotence, amenorrhea, gynecomastia, breast engorgement, premenstrual syndrome

INTEG: Rash

MS: Joint pain, twitching

RESP: Dyspnea, rhinitis, cough, pharyngitis

Contraindications: Hypersensitivity

Precautions: Pregnancy **C,** lactation, hypertension, hepatic disease, cardiac disease, elderly G

Pharmacokinetics

Absorption	Well
Distribution	93% plasma protein binding
Metabolism	Liver
Excretion	Kidneys
Half-life	Unknown

Pharmacodynamics

Onset	Unknown
Peak	6 hr
Duration	Unknown

Interactions

Individual drugs

Alcohol: ↑ sedation
Bromocriptine: ↓ antiparkinson activity
Carbamazepine: ↓ levels of olanzapine
Levodopa: ↓ antiparkinson activity

Drug classifications

Anesthetics, barbiturates: ↑ sedation
Antihistamines: ↑ sedation
Antidepressants: ↑ sedation
Antihypertensives: ↑ hypotension
Anticholinergics: ↑ anticholinergic effects

Lab test interferences

↑ Liver function test, ↑ prolactin, ↑ CPK

NURSING CONSIDERATIONS

Assessment

- Assess mental status, orientation, mood, behavior, presence of hallucinations and type before initial administration and monthly
- Monitor swallowing of PO medication: check for hoarding or giving of medication to other patients
- Monitor I&O ratio; palpate bladder if low urinary output occurs, especially in elderly [G]
- Monitor bilirubin, CBC, liver function studies monthly
- Monitor urinalysis; recommended before, during prolonged therapy
- Assess affect, orientation, LOC, reflexes, gait, coordination, sleep pattern disturbances
- Monitor B/P sitting, standing, lying; take pulse and respirations q4h during initial treatment; establish baseline before starting treatment; report drops of 30 mm Hg; obtain baseline ECG
- Assess dizziness, faintness, palpitations, tachycardia on rising
- Assess for neuroleptic malignant syndrome: hyperpyrexia, muscle rigidity, increased CPK, altered mental status, for acute dystonia (check chewing, swallowing, eyes, pin rolling)
- EPS, including akathisia (inability to sit still, no pattern to movements), tardive dyskinesia (bizarre movements of the jaw, mouth, tongue, extremities), pseudoparkinsonism (rigidity, tremors, pill rolling, shuffling gait)
- Monitor skin turgor daily
- Monitor constipation, urinary retention daily; increase bulk, H_2O in diet

Nursing diagnoses

- ✓ Thought processes, altered (uses)
- ✓ Knowledge deficit (teaching)
- ✓ Noncompliance (teaching)

Implementation

- Give antiparkinsonian agent for EPS
- [G] Give decreased dose in elderly
- Give PO with full glass of water, milk; or with food to decrease GI upset
- Provide decreased stimuli by dimming light, avoiding loud noises
- Provide supervised ambula-

O

tion until stabilized on medication; do not involve in strenuous exercise program because fainting is possible; patients should not stand still for long periods
• Give increased fluids to prevent constipation
• Give sips of water, candy, gum for dry mouth
• Store in tight, light-resistant container

Patient/family education
• Teach patient to use good oral hygiene; frequent rinsing of mouth, sugarless gum for dry mouth
• Advise patient to avoid hazardous activities until drug response is determined
• Advise patient that orthostatic hypotension occurs often and to rise from sitting or lying position gradually
• Advise patient to avoid hot tubs, hot showers, tub baths, since hypotension may occur
• Advise patient to avoid abrupt withdrawal of this drug, or EPS may result; drug should be withdrawn slowly
• Advise patient to avoid OTC preparations (cough, hay fever, cold) unless approved by prescriber, since serious drug interactions may occur; avoid use with alcohol, CNS depressants, increased drowsiness may occur
• Advise patient that in hot weather, heat stroke may occur; take extra precautions to stay cool

Evaluation
Positive therapeutic outcome
• Decrease in emotional excitement, hallucinations, delusion, paranoia, reorganization of patterns of thought, speech

Treatment of overdose: Lavage if orally ingested; provide airway; do not induce vomiting or use epinephrine

omeprazole (℞)
(oh-mep′ra-zole)
Losec ✱, Prilosec
Func. class.: Antisecretory compound
Chem. class.: Benzimidazole
Pregnancy category C

Action: Suppresses gastric secretion by inhibiting hydrogen/potassium ATPase enzyme system in the gastric parietal cell; characterized as a gastric acid pump inhibitor, since it blocks the final step of acid production

➔ **Therapeutic Outcome:** Absence of duodenal ulcers; decreased gastroesophageal reflux

Uses: Gastroesophageal reflux disease (GERD), severe erosive esophagitis, poorly responsive systemic GERD, pathologic hypersecretory conditions (Zollinger-Ellison syndrome, systemic mastocytosis, multiple endocrine adenomas); possibly effective for treatment of duodenal ulcers

Dosage and routes
Severe erosive esophagitis/poorly responsive gastroesophageal reflux disease
Adult: PO 20 mg qd × 4-8 wk
Pathologic hypersecretory conditions
Adult: PO 60 mg/day; may increase to 120 mg tid; daily doses >80 mg should be divided

Available forms: Sus rel cap 20 mg

Adverse effects

CNS: Headache, dizziness, asthenia

CV: Chest pain, angina, tachycardia, bradycardia, palpitations, peripheral edema

EENT: Tinnitus, taste perversion

GI: Diarrhea, abdominal pain, vomiting, nausea, constipation, flatulence, acid regurgitation, abdominal swelling, anorexia, irritable colon, esophageal candidiasis, dry mouth

GU: UTI, frequency, increased creatinine, ***proteinuria, hematuria,*** testicular pain, glycosuria

HEMA: Pancytopenia, thrombocytopenia, neutropenia, leukocytosis, anemia

INTEG: Rash, dry skin, urticaria, pruritus, alopecia

META: Hypoglycemia, increased hepatic enzymes, weight gain

MISC: Back pain, fever, fatigue, malaise

RESP: Upper respiratory tract infections, cough, epistaxis

Contraindications: Hypersensitivity

Precautions: Pregnancy **C,**
P lactation, children

Pharmacokinetics

Absorption	Rapidly absorbed
Distribution	Protein binding (95%); gastric parietal cells
Metabolism	Liver, extensively
Excretion	Kidneys, feces
Half-life	½-1 hr; increased in the G elderly, hepatic disease

Pharmacodynamics

Onset	1 hr
Peak	½-3½ hr
Duration	3-4 days

Interactions

Individual drugs

Ampicillin: ↓ absorption of omeprazole

Diazepam: ↑ serum levels of diazepam

Ketoconazole: ↓ absorption of ketoconazole

Phenytoin: ↑ serum levels of phenytoin

Warfarin: ↑ bleeding tendencies

Drug classification

Iron products: ↓ absorption of iron

NURSING CONSIDERATIONS

Assessment

- Assess GI system: bowel sounds q8h, abdomen for pain and swelling, anorexia
- Monitor hepatic enzymes: AST (SGOT), ALT (SGPT), increased alkaline phosphatase during treatment

Nursing diagnoses

✓ Pain (uses)
✓ Knowledge deficit (teaching)

Implementation

- Give before patient eats; patient should swallow cap whole
- ⊘ Do not open, chew, or crush; may give with antacids

Patient/family education

- Advise patient to report severe diarrhea; drug may have to be discontinued
- Caution patient to avoid driving and other hazardous activities until response to drug is known
- Caution patient to avoid alcohol, salicylates, ibuprofen; may cause GI irritation

Evaluation

Positive therapeutic outcome

- Absence of epigastric pain, swelling, fullness

O

ondansetron (℞)

(on-dan'sa-tron)

Zofran

Func. class.: Antiemetic

Chem. class.: 5-HT receptor antagonist

Pregnancy category B

Action: Prevents nausea, vomiting by blocking serotonin peripherally, centrally, and in the small intestine

Therapeutic Outcome: Control of nausea, vomiting

Uses: Prevention of nausea, vomiting associated with cancer chemotherapy and prevention of postopertive nausea, vomiting

Dosage and routes

Prevention of nausea/vomiting associated with cancer chemotherapy

Adult/child 4-18 yr: **IV** 0.15 mg/kg infused over 15 min, 30 min before start of cancer chemotherapy; 0.15 mg/kg is given 4 hr and 8 hr after first dose or 32 mg as a single dose; dilute in 50 ml of D_5W or 0.9% NaCl before giving

Prevention of nausea/vomiting of radiotherapy

Adult: PO 8 mg tid

Prevention of postoperative nausea/vomiting

Adult: **IV** 4 mg undiluted over >30 sec

Available forms: Inj 2 mg/ml, 32 mg/50 ml (premixed); tabs 4, 8 mg

Adverse effects

CNS: Headache, dizziness, drowsiness, fatigue, extrapyramidal syndrome

GI: Diarrhea, constipation, abdominal pain

MISC: Rash, ***bronchospasm*** (rare), *MS pain, wound problems, shivering, fever, hypoxia, urinary retention*

Contraindications: Hypersensitivity

Precautions: Pregnancy **B,** lactation, children, elderly

Pharmacokinetics	
Absorption	Completely absorbed (IV)
Distribution	Unknown
Metabolism	Liver, extensively
Excretion	Kidneys
Half-life	3.5-4.7 hr

Pharmacodynamics

Unknown

Interactions: Unknown

NURSING CONSIDERATIONS

Assessment

- Assess for absence of nausea, vomiting during chemotherapy
- Assess for hypersensitivity reaction: rash, bronchospasm

Nursing diagnoses

- Knowledge deficit (teaching)
- Noncompliance (teaching)

Implementation

IV route

- Give **IV** after diluting a single dose in 50 ml 0.9% NaCl or D_5W, 0.45%; give over 15 min
- Store at room temp for 48-hr dilution

Y-site compatibilities: Aldesleukin, amifostine, amikacin, aztreonam, bleomycin, carboplatin, carmustine, cefazolin, ceforanide, cefotazime, cefoxitin, ceftazidime, ceftizoxime, cefuroxime, chlorpromazine, cimetidine, cisplatin, clindamycin, cyclophosphamide, cytarabine, dacarbazine, dactinomycin, daunorubicin, dexamethasone, diphenhydramine, doxorubicin, doxycycline, droperidol, etoposide, famotidine, filgrastim, floxuridine, fluconazole, fludarabine, gentamicin, haloperidol, heparin, hydrocortisone, hydromorphone, hydroxyzine, ifosfamide, imipenem/cilastatin, magnesium sulfate, mannitol, mechlorethamine, melphalan, meperidine, mesna, methotrexate, metoclopramide, miconazole, mitomycin, mitoxantrone, morphine, paclitaxel, pentostatin, potassium chloride, prochlorperazine, ranitidine, streptozocin, teniposide, thiotepa, ticarcillin, ticarcillin/clavulanate, vancomycin, vinblastine, vincristine, vinorelbine, zidovudine

Y-site incompatibilities:
Acyclovir, aminophylline, amphotericin B, ampicillin, ampicillin/sulbactam, cefoperazone, furosemide, ganciclovir, lorazepam, methylprednisolone, mezlocillin, piperacillin, sargramostim, sodium bicarbonate

Additive compatibilities:
Cisplatin, cyclophosphamide, cytarabine, dacarbazine, dexamethasone, doxorubicin, etoposide, meperidine, methotrexate

Solution compatibilities:
May also be diluted with D_5W, Lactated Ringers, $D_5/0.9\%$ NaCl, $D_5/0.45\%$ NaCl

Patient/family education
- Instruct patient to report diarrhea, constipation, rash, or changes in respirations
- Teach patient reason for medication and expected results

Evaluation
Positive therapeutic outcome
- Absence of nausea, vomiting during cancer chemotherapy

oral contraceptives
(℞)
Func. class.: Hormone
Chem. class.: Estrogen/progestin combinations
Pregnancy category X

Action: Prevents ovulation by suppressing FSH, LH; **monophasic:** estrogen/progestin (fixed dose) used during a 21-day cycle; ovulation is inhibited by suppression of FSH and LH; thickness of cervical mucus and endometrial lining prevents pregnancy; **biphasic:** ovulation is inhibited by suppression of FSH and LH; alteration of cervical mucus, endometrial lining prevents pregnancy; **triphasic:** ovulation is inhibited by suppression of FSH and LH; change of cervical mucus, endometrial lining prevents pregnancy; variable doses of estrogen/progestin combinations may be similar to natural hormonal fluctuations; **progestin-only pill and implant:** change of cervical mucus and endometrial lining prevents pregnancy; ovulation may be suppressed

Therapeutic Outcome: Prevention of pregnancy, decreased severity of endometriosis, hypermenorrhea

Uses: To prevent pregnancy,

endometriosis, hypermenorrhea

Dosage and routes

Adult: PO 1 qd starting on day 5 of menstrual cycle; day 1 is 1st day of period

20/21-tab packs

Adult: PO 1 qd starting on day 7 of menstrual cycle; day 1 is 1st day of period; then on 20 or 21 days, off 7 days

28-tab packs

Adult: PO 1 qd continuously

Biphasic

Adult: 1 qd × 10 days, then next color 1 qd × 11 days

Triphasic

Adult: 1 qd; check package insert for each brand

Implant

Adult: Subdermal 6 cap implanted during the first wk of menses

Endometriosis

Adult: PO 1 qd × 20 days from day 5 to day 24 of cycle

Adult: PO 1 qd; check package insert for specific instructions

Available forms: Check specific brand

Adverse effects

CNS: Depression, fatigue, dizziness, nervousness, anxiety, headache

CV: Increased B/P, thromboembolic conditions, fluid retention, edema

EENT: Optic neuritis, retinal thrombosis, cataracts

ENDO: Decreased glucose tolerance, increased TBG, PBI, T_4, T_3

GI: Nausea, vomiting, cramps, diarrhea, bloating, constipation, change in appetite, ***cholestatic jaundice***

GU: Breakthrough bleeding, amenorrhea, spotting, dysmenorrhea, galactorrhea, endocervical hyperplasia, vaginitis, cystitis-like syndrome, breast change

HEMA: Increased fibrinogen, clotting factor

INTEG: Chloasma, melasma, acne, rash, urticaria, erythema, pruritus, hirsutism, alopecia, photosensitivity

Contraindications: Pregnancy **X,** lactation, reproductive cancer, thrombophlebitis, MI, hepatic tumors, hepatic disease, CAD, women 40 yr and over, CVA

Precautions: Depression, hypertension, renal disease, seizure disorders, lupus erythematosus, rheumatic disease, migraine headache, amenorrhea, irregular menses, breast cancer (fibrocystic), gallbladder disease, diabetes mellitus, heavy smoking, acute mononucleosis, sickle cell disease

Pharmacokinetics

Absorption	Well absorbed
Distribution	Unknown
Metabolism	Liver, extensively
Excretion	Kidneys
Half-life	Unknown

Pharmacodynamics

	PO	IM	IMPLANT
Onset	1 mo	1 mo	1 mo
Peak	1 mo	1 mo	1 mo
Duration	1 mo	3 mo	5 yr

Interactions

Individual drugs

Aminocaproic acid: ↑ clotting

Bromocriptine: ↓ effectiveness of bromocriptine

Carbamazepine: ↓ effectiveness of oral contraceptive

Chenodiol: ↓ effectiveness of oral contraceptive

Chloramphenicol: ↓ effectiveness of oral contraceptive
Dantrolene: ↑ hepatic toxicity (estrogen only)
Dihydroergotamine: ↓ effectiveness of oral contraceptive
Griseofulvin: ↓ effectiveness of oral contraceptive
Mineral oil: ↓ effectiveness of oral contraceptive
Phenylbutazone: ↓ effectiveness of oral contraceptive
Phenytoin: ↓ effectiveness of oral contraceptive
Primidone: ↓ effectiveness of oral contraceptive
Rifampin: ↓ effectiveness of oral contraceptive
Warfarin: ↑ or ↓ effect of warfarin

Drug classifications

Analgesics: ↓ action of oral contraceptives
Antibiotics: ↓ action of oral contraceptives
Anticonvulsants: ↓ action of oral contraceptives
Antihistamines: ↓ action of oral contraceptives
Glucocorticoids: ↓ action of oral contraceptives
Oral anticoagulants: ↓ action of oral anticoagulants
Tricyclic antidepressants: ↑ toxicity

Lab test interferences

↑ Pro-time; ↑ clotting factors VII, VIII, IX, X; ↑ TBG, ↑ PBI, ↑ T_4, ↑ platelet aggregation, ↑ BSP, ↑ triglycerides, ↑ bilirubin, ↑ AST (SGOT), ↑ ALT (SGPT)
↓ T_3, ↓ antithrombin III, ↓ folate, ↓ metyrapone test, ↓ GTT, ↓ 17-OHCS

NURSING CONSIDERATIONS

Assessment

- Assess for reproductive changes: change in breasts, tumors, positive Pap smear; drug should be discontinued if changes occur
- Monitor glucose, thyroid function, liver function tests, B/P

Nursing diagnoses

- ✓ Injury, risk for (adverse reactions)
- ✓ Body image disturbance (adverse reactions)
- ✓ Knowledge deficit (teaching)
- ✓ Noncompliance (teaching)

Implementation

PO route

- If GI symptoms occur, medication may be taken with food; take at same time each day

Implant route

- Inject 6 cap subdermally
- Implant is effective for 5 yr, should be removed after that

IM route

- Administer deep in large muscle mass after shaking susp well; ensure pregnancy has not occurred if inj are 2 wk or more apart

Patient/family education

- Teach patient about detection of clots using Homans' sign; teach monitoring technique for heat, redness, pain, swelling
- Teach patient to use sunscreen or to avoid sunlight; photosensitivity can occur
- Teach patient to take at same time each day to ensure equal drug level; to take another tab as soon as possible if one is missed; teach patient that after drug is discontinued, pregnancy may not occur for several mo
- Instruct patient to report GI symptoms that occur after 4 mo
- Advise patient to use another birth control method during

first 3 wk of oral contraceptive use

• Teach patient to report abdominal pain, change in vision, shortness of breath, change in menstrual flow, spotting, breakthrough bleeding, breast lumps, swelling, headache, severe leg pain, mental changes; that continuing medical care is needed: PAP smear and gynecologic examinations q6 mo

• Teach patient to notify physicians and dentist of oral contraceptive use

Evaluation

Positive therapeutic outcome

• Absence of pregnancy

• Decreased severity of endometriosis

• Decreased severity of hypermenorrhea

oxacillin (℞)

(ox-a-sill'in)

Bactocill, oxacillin sodium, Prostaphilin

Func. class.: Broad-spectrum antiinfective

Chem. class.: Penicillinase-resistant penicillin

Pregnancy category B

Action: Interferes with cell wall replication of susceptible organisms; osmotically unstable cell wall swells, bursts from osmotic pressure

Therapeutic Outcome: Bactericidal effects for gram-positive cocci *Staphylococcus aureus, Streptococcus pneumoniae,* infections caused by penicillinase-producing *staphylococci*

Uses: Infections caused by penicillinase-producing staphylococci, streptococci; respiratory tract, skin, skin structure, urinary tract, bone, joint infections, sinusitis, endocarditis, septicemia, meningitis

Dosage and routes

Adult: PO 2-6 g/day in divided doses q4-6h; IM/**IV** 2-12 g/day in divided doses q4-6h

P ***Child:*** PO 50-100 mg/kg/day in divided doses q6h; IM/**IV** 50-100 mg/kg/day in divided doses q4-6h

Available forms: Caps 250, 500 mg; powder for oral susp 250 mg/5 ml; powder for inj 250, 500 mg, 1, 2, 4, 10 g; inf 1, 2 g

Adverse effects

CNS: Lethargy, hallucinations, anxiety, depression, twitching, ***coma, convulsions***

GI: Nausea, vomiting, diarrhea, increased AST (SGOT), ALT (SGPT), abdominal pain, glossitis, colitis

GU: Oliguria, proteinuria, hematuria, vaginitis, moniliasis, glomerulonephritis

HEMA: Anemia, increased bleeding time, ***bone marrow depression, granulocytopenia***

Contraindications: Hypersensitivity to penicillins

Precautions: Pregnancy **B,** hypersensitivity to cephalosporins, P neonates

Pharmacokinetics

Absorption	Rapid, incomplete (PO); well absorbed (IM); completely (IV)
Distribution	Widely distributed; crosses placenta
Metabolism	Liver
Excretion	Kidneys, unchanged (51%); breast milk
Half-life	20-50 min; increased in severe hepatic disease

Pharmacodynamics

	PO	IM	IV
Onset	Rapid	Rapid	Rapid
Peak	½-1 hr	½ hr	Inf end

Interactions

Individual drugs

Aspirin: ↑ oxacillin levels, ↓ renal excretion
Chloramphenicol: ↑ half-life of chloramphenicol, ↓ effectiveness of oxacillin
Cholestyramine: ↓ effectiveness of oxacillin
Colestipol: ↓ effectiveness of oxacillin
Probenecid: ↑ oxacillin levels, ↓ renal excretion

Drug classifications

Erythromycins: ↓ antimicrobial effectiveness
Oral anticoagulants: ↑ anticoagulant effects
Oral contraceptives: ↓ contraceptive effectiveness
Tetracyclines: ↓ antimicrobial effectiveness

Food

Food, carbonated drinks, citrus fruit juices: ↓ absorption

Lab test interferences

False positive: Urine glucose, urine protein

NURSING CONSIDERATIONS

Assessment

• Assess patient for previous sensitivity reaction to penicillins or other cephalosporins; cross-sensitivity between penicillins and cephalosporins is common
• Assess patient for signs and symptoms of infection including characteristics of wounds, sputum, urine, stool, WBC >10,000, fever; obtain baseline information and during treatment
• Obtain C&S before beginning drug therapy to identify if correct treatment has been initiated
• Assess for allergic reactions: rash, urticaria, pruritus, chills, fever, joint pain; angioedema may occur a few days after therapy begins; epinephrine, resuscitation equipment should be available for anaphylactic reaction
• Assess urine output; if decreasing, notify prescriber (may indicate nephrotoxicity); also check for increased BUN, creatinine
• Monitor blood studies: AST (SGOT), ALT (SGPT), CBC, Hct, bilirubin, LDH, alkaline phosphatase, Coombs' test monthly if patient is on long-term therapy
• Monitor electrolytes: potassium, sodium, chloride monthly if patient is on long-term therapy
• Assess bowel pattern qd; if severe diarrhea occurs, drug should be discontinued; may indicate pseudomembranous colitis
• Monitor for bleeding: ecchymosis, bleeding gums, hematuria, stool guaiac daily if on long-term therapy
• Assess for overgrowth of infection: perineal itching, fever, malaise, redness, pain, swelling, drainage, rash, diarrhea, change in cough, sputum

O

Nursing diagnoses

- ✓ Infection, risk for (uses)
- ✓ Diarrhea (adverse reactions)
- ✓ Injury, risk for (adverse reactions)
- ✓ Knowledge deficit (teaching)
- ✓ Noncompliance (teaching)

Implementation

PO route

- Give in even doses around the clock; if GI upset occurs, give with food; drug must be given for 10-14 days to ensure organism death and prevent superinfection; store in tight container
- Shake susp; store in refrigerator for 2 wk, 1 wk at room temp

IM route

- Reconstitute 250 mg/1.4 ml, 500 mg/2.7-2.8 ml, 1 g/5.7 ml, 2 g/11.4-11.5 ml, 4 g/21.8-23 ml of sterile water for a conc of 250 mg/1.5 ml; store unused portion in refrigerator for 1 wk or 3 days at room temp
- Inject deeply in large muscle mass

IV IV route

- Reconstitute 250 mg/1.4 ml, 500 mg/2.7-2.8 ml, 1 g/5.7 ml, 2 g/11.4-11.5 ml, 4 g/21.8-23 ml of sterile water for a conc of 250 mg/1.5 ml; store unused portion in refrigerator for 1 week or 3 days at room temp
- Give direct **IV** by diluting reconstituted sol with 250-500 mg/5 ml, 1 g/10 ml, 2 g/20 ml, 4 g/40 ml of sterile water or 0.9% NaCl, give over 10 min
- Give by intermittent inf by diluting to a conc of 0.5-40 mg/ml with D_5W, 0.9% NaCl, D_5/0.9% NaCl, LR; give over 6 hr or less

Y-site incompatibility:
Verapamil

Y-site compatibilities:
Acyclovir, cyclophosphamide, diltiazem, famotidine, fluconazole, foscarnet, heparin, hydrocortisone, hydromorphone, labetalol, magnesium sulfate, meperidine, morphine, perphenazine, potassium chloride, tacrolimus, vitamin B with C, zidovudine

Additive incompatibilities:
Cytarabine, tetracycline

Additive compatibilities:
Cephapirin, chloramphenicol, dopamine, potassium chloride, sodium bicarbonate

Patient/family education

- Teach patient to report sore throat, bruising, bleeding, joint pain; may indicate blood dyscrasias (rare)
- Advise patient to contact prescriber if vaginal itching, loose, foul-smelling stools, furry tongue occur; may indicate superinfection
- Instruct patient to take all medication prescribed for the length of time ordered
- Advise patient to notify prescriber of diarrhea with blood or pus, which may indicate pseudomembranous colitis

Evaluation

Positive therapeutic outcome

- Absence of signs/symptoms of infection (WBC <10,000, temp WNL, absence of red, draining wounds)
- Reported improvement in symptoms of infection

Treatment of anaphylaxis: Withdraw drug, maintain airway, administer epinephrine, aminophylline, O_2, **IV** corticosteroids

oxaprozin (℞)
(ox-a-proe'zin)
Daypro
Func. class.: Nonsteroidal antiinflammatory
Chem. class.: Propionic acid derivative
Pregnancy category C

Action: Inhibits prostaglandin synthesis by decreasing an enzyme needed for biosynthesis; analgesic, antiinflammatory

➔ **Therapeutic Outcome:** Decreased pain, inflammation

Uses: Acute and long-term management of osteoarthritis, rheumatoid arthritis

Dosage and routes
Adult: PO 600-1200 mg qd; maximum dose 1800 mg/day or 26 mg/kg, whichever is lower in divided doses

Available forms: Tab 600 mg

Adverse effects
CNS: Dizziness, headache, drowsiness, fatigue, tremors, confusion, insomnia, anxiety, malaise, depression
CV: Tachycardia, peripheral edema, palpitations, dysrhythmias
EENT: Tinnitus, hearing loss, blurred vision
GI: Nausea, *anorexia,* vomiting, *diarrhea,* jaundice, ***cholestatic hepatitis,*** constipation, flatulence, *cramps,* dry mouth, peptic ulcer, ***bleeding,*** melena, gastroenteritis
GU: Nephrotoxicity: dysuria, hematuria, oliguria, azotemia
HEMA: Increased bleeding time
INTEG: Purpura, rash, pruritus, sweating, photosensitivity
SYST: Anaphylaxis, angioneurotic edema

Contraindications: Hypersensitivity, asthma, patients in whom aspirin and iodides have induced symptoms of allergic reactions or asthma

Precautions: Pregnancy **C** 1st and 2nd trimester, lactation, P children, bleeding disorders, GI disorders, cardiac disorders, hypersensitivity to other antiinflammatory agents, severe renal G and hepatic disease, elderly

Pharmacokinetics

Absorption	Well absorbed
Distribution	Unknown
Metabolism	Liver, extensively
Excretion	Breast milk
Half life	40-50 hr

Pharmacodynamics

Onset	Unknown
Peak	2 hr
Duration	Unknown

Interactions
Individual drugs
Acetaminophen (long-term use): ↑ renal reactions
Alcohol: ↑ adverse reactions
Aspirin: ↓ effectiveness, ↑ adverse reactions
Coumadin: ↑ anticoagulant effects
Digoxin: ↑ toxicity, levels
Insulin: ↑ insulin effect
Lithium: ↑ toxicity
Methotrexate: ↑ toxicity
Sulfonylurea: ↑ toxicity
Drug classifications
Anticoagulants: ↑ risk of bleeding
Antihypertensives: ↓ effect of antihypertensives
Antineoplastics: ↑ risk of hematologic toxicity
β-Blockers: ↑ antihypertension

Cephalosporins: ↑ risk of bleeding
Glucocorticoids: ↑ adverse reactions
Hypoglycemics: ↓ hypoglycemic effect
Diuretics: ↓ effectiveness of diuretics
NSAIDs: ↑ adverse reactions
Potassium supplements: ↑ adverse reactions
Radiation: ↑ risk of hematologic toxicity
Sulfonamides: ↑ toxicity

Lab test interferences
↑ BUN, ↑ alkaline phosphatase
False ↑ 5-HIAA, false ↑ 17KS

NURSING CONSIDERATIONS

Assessment

- Assess for pain and ROM: intensity, location, duration
- Monitor blood studies: alkaline phosphatase, LDH, AST (SGOT), ALT (SGPT), and bleeding time (may be increased)

Nursing diagnoses

- ✓ Pain (uses)
- ✓ Mobility, impaired (uses)
- ✓ Injury, risk for (adverse reactions)
- ✓ Knowledge deficit (teaching)

Implementation

- Give with food or milk to decrease gastric symptoms

Patient/family education

- Teach patient that drug must be continued for prescribed time to be effective; to avoid aspirin, alcoholic beverages
- Instruct patient to use caution when driving; drowsiness, dizziness may occur
- Teach patient to take with a full glass of water to enhance absorption; patient should sit upright for 30 min to prevent stomach irritation and ulceration
- ⊘ Do not crush, break, or chew
- Instruct patient to use sunscreen and protective clothing to prevent burns
- Advise patient to report to prescriber severe abdominal pain, rash, itching, yellowing of skin or eyes, depression

Evaluation

Positive therapeutic outcome

- Decreased pain
- Decreased inflammation
- Increased mobility

---

oxazepam (℞)

(ox-az′e-pam)

Apo-Oxazepam ✦, Novoxapam ✦, oxazepam, Ox-Pam ✦, Serax, Zapex ✦

Func. class.: Sedative/hypnotic; antianxiety

Chem. class.: Benzodiazepine

Pregnancy category D

Controlled substance schedule IV

Action: Depresses subcortical levels of CNS, including limbic system, reticular formation; potentiates GABA

➔ **Therapeutic Outcome:** Decreased anxiety, successful alcohol withdrawal, relaxation

Uses: Anxiety, alcohol withdrawal

Dosage and routes

Anxiety
Adult: PO 10-30 mg tid-qid

Alcohol withdrawal
Adult: PO 15-30 mg tid-qid

Available forms: Caps 10, 15, 30 mg; tab 15 mg

Adverse effects

CNS: Dizziness, drowsiness, confusion, headache, anxiety, tremors, fatigue, depression, insomnia, hallucinations, paradoxic excitement, transient amnesia

CV: Orthostatic hypotension, ECG changes, tachycardia, hypotension

EENT: Blurred vision, tinnitus, mydriasis

GI: Nausea, vomiting, anorexia

INTEG: Rash, dermatitis, itching

Contraindications: Hypersensitivity to benzodiazepines, narrow-angle glaucoma, psychosis, pregnancy **D,** child <12 yr

Precautions: Elderly, debilitated, hepatic disease, renal disease

Pharmacokinetics

Absorption	Well absorbed
Distribution	Widely distributed; crosses placenta, blood-brain barrier
Metabolism	Liver
Excretion	Kidneys, breast milk
Half-life	5-15 hr

Pharmacodynamics

Onset	½-1½ hr
Peak	Unknown
Duration	6-12 hr

Interactions

Individual drugs

Alcohol: ↑ CNS depression
Cimetidine: ↑ action
Fluoxetine: ↑ action
Levodopa: ↓ action of levodopa
Metoprolol: ↑ action
Phenytoin: ↓ effect
Propoxyphene: ↑ action
Theophylline: ↓ sedative effects

Drug classifications

Analgesics, opioid: ↑ CNS depression
Antidepressants: ↑ CNS depression
Antihistamines: ↑ CNS depression
Oral contraceptives: ↑ effect

Lab test interferences

↑ AST (SGOT), ↑ ALT (SGPT), ↑ serum bilirubin
False ↑ 17-OHCS
↓ RAIU

NURSING CONSIDERATIONS

Assessment

- Assess mental status: mood, sensorium, anxiety, affect, sleeping pattern, drowsiness, dizziness, especially elderly; physical dependency, withdrawal symptoms: anxiety, panic attacks, agitation, convulsions, headache, nausea, vomiting, muscle pain, weakness; suicidal tendencies; indications of increasing tolerance and abuse
- Monitor B/P with patient lying, standing, pulse; if systolic B/P drops 20 mm Hg, hold drug, notify prescriber
- Monitor blood studies: CBC during long-term therapy; blood dyscrasias have occurred rarely; decreased hematocrit, neutropenia may occur
- Monitor hepatic studies: AST (SGOT), ALT (SGPT), bilirubin, creatinine LDH, alkaline phosphatase
- Monitor I&O; indicate renal dysfunction

Nursing diagnoses

✓ Anxiety (uses)
✓ Depression (uses)
✓ Injury, risk for (adverse reactions)
✓ Knowledge deficit (teaching)

Implementation

• Give with food or milk for GI symptoms; tab may be crushed if patient is unable to swallow medication whole; give sugarless gum, hard candy, frequent sips of water for dry mouth

Patient/family education

• Teach patient that drug may be taken with food or fluids; tab may be crushed or swallowed whole
• Caution patient not to use for everyday stress or longer than 3 mo unless directed by prescriber; not to take more than prescribed amount; may be habit forming; not to double doses or skip doses
• Advise patient to avoid OTC preparations unless approved by prescriber; alcohol and CNS depressants will increase CNS depression
• Caution patient to avoid driving and activities that require alertness, since drowsiness may occur; to avoid alcohol and other psychotropic medications; to rise slowly or fainting may occur, especially G elderly; that drowsiness may worsen at beginning of treatment
• Caution patient not to discontinue medication abruptly after long-term use; withdrawal symptoms include vomiting, cramping, tremors, seizures

Evaluation

Positive therapeutic outcome
• Decreased anxiety, restlessness, sleeplessness (short-term treatment only)

Treatment of overdose: Lavage, VS, supportive care

oxtriphylline (℞)

(ox-trye′fi-lin)
Apo-Oxtriphylline ✦, Choledyl, Choledyl SA, Novotriphyl ✦, oxtriphylline
Func. class.: Bronchodilator, spasmolytic
Chem. class.: Choline salt of theophylline
Pregnancy category C

Action: Relaxes smooth muscle of respiratory system by blocking phosphodiesterase, which increases cAMP; 64% theophylline

➔ **Therapeutic Outcome:** Bronchodilatation with ease of breathing

Uses: Acute bronchial asthma, reversible bronchospasm in chronic bronchitis and COPD

Dosage and routes

P ***Adult and child >12 yr:*** PO 200 mg qid or sus action q12h
P ***Child 2-12 yr:*** PO 4 mg/kg q6h; may be increased to desired response, therapeutic level

Available forms: Elix 100 mg/5 ml; syr 50 mg/5 ml; tabs 100, 200, 400, 600 mg; sus action tabs 400, 600 mg

Adverse effects

CNS: Anxiety, restlessness, insomnia, dizziness, ***convulsions,*** headache, lightheadedness
CV: Palpitations, sinus tachycardia, hypotension
GI: Nausea, vomiting, anorexia, diarrhea, bitter taste, dyspepsia
INTEG: Flushing, urticaria, alopecia
RESP: Increased rate

Contraindications: Hypersensitivity to xanthines, tachydysrhythmias

G **Precautions:** Elderly, CHF, cor pulmonale, hepatic disease, active peptic ulcer disease, diabetes mellitus, hyperthyroidism, hypertension, children, pregnancy **C**, glaucoma, prostatic hypertrophy P

Pharmacokinetics

Absorption	Well absorbed (PO); slow (PO-SA)
Distribution	Widely distributed; crosses placenta
Metabolism	Liver to caffeine
Excretion	Kidneys, breast milk
Half-life	3-13 hr; increased in renal disease, CHF

Pharmacodynamics

	PO	PO-SA
Onset	15-60 min	Unknown
Peak	1-5 hr	4-8 hr
Duration	6-8 hr	8-12 hr

Interactions

Individual drugs

Allopurinol: ↓ metabolism, ↑ toxicity
Carbamazepine: ↑ or ↓ oxtriphylline levels
Cimetidine: ↓ metabolism, ↑ toxicity
Disulfiram: ↓ metabolism, ↑ toxicity
Erythromycin: ↓ metabolism, ↑ toxicity
Halothane: ↑ risk of dysrhythmias
Interferon: ↓ metabolism, ↑ toxicity
Isoniazid: ↑ or ↓ oxtriphylline level
Ketoconazole: ↑ metabolism, ↓ effect
Lithium: ↓ effect of lithium
Mexiletine: ↓ metabolism, ↑ toxicity
Phenytoin: ↑ metabolism, ↓ effect
Rifampin: ↑ metabolism, ↓ effect
Thiabendazole: ↓ metabolism, ↑ toxicity

Drug classifications

Barbiturates: ↓ effect of oxtriphylline
β-Adrenergic blockers: ↓ metabolism, ↑ toxicity
Diuretics, loop: ↑ or ↓ oxtriphylline levels
Fluoroquinolones: ↓ metabolism, ↑ toxicity
Glucocorticoids: ↓ metabolism, ↑ toxicity
Sympathomimetics: ↑ CNS, CV adverse reactions

Food

Caffeinated foods (cola, coffee, tea, chocolate): ↑ CNS, CV adverse reactions

Smoking

↑ metabolism, ↓ effect

Lab test interferences

↑ Plasma free fatty acids

NURSING CONSIDERATIONS

Assessment

- Monitor blood levels (therapeutic level is 10-20 μg/ml); toxicity may occur with small increase above 20 μg/ml, G especially elderly; check whether theophylline was given recently (24 hr)
- Monitor I&O; diuresis can G occur; dehydration may result P in elderly or children
- Monitor respiratory rate, rhythm, depth; auscultate lung fields bilaterally; notify prescriber of abnormalities
- Monitor allergic reactions: rash, urticaria; if these occur, drug should be discontinued

Nursing diagnoses

✓ Airway clearance, ineffective (uses)
✓ Activity intolerance (uses)

O

- ✓ Injury, risk for (uses, adverse reactions)
- ✓ Knowledge deficit (teaching)

Implementation

- Give PO pc to decrease GI symptoms; absorption may be affected with a full glass of water; do not crush or chew enteric coated or SA tab

Patient/family education

- Teach patient to take doses as prescribed, not to skip dose; to check OTC medications, current prescription medications for ephedrine, which will increase CNS stimulation; not to drink alcohol or caffeine products (tea, coffee, chocolate, colas)
- Caution patient to avoid hazardous activities; dizziness may occur
- Instruct patient if GI upset occurs, to take drug with 8 oz water or food
- Teach patient to notify prescriber of change in smoking habit; a change in dosage may be required
- Teach patient to increase fluids to 2L/day to decrease viscosity of secretions

Evaluation

Positive therapeutic outcome

- Decreased dyspnea
- Clear lung fields bilaterally

oxybutynin (℞)

(ox-i-byoo'ti-nin)

Ditropan, oxybutynin chloride

Func. class.: Spasmolytic, urinary

Chem. class.: Synthetic tertiary amine

Pregnancy category B

Action: Relaxes smooth muscles in urinary tract by inhibiting acetylcholine at postganglionic sites

➔ **Therapeutic Outcome:** Decreased symptoms of urgency, nocturia, incontinence

Uses: Antispasmodic for neurogenic bladder

Dosage and routes

Adult: PO 5 mg bid-tid, not to exceed 5 mg qid

P ***Child >5 yr:*** PO 5 mg bid, not to exceed 5 mg tid

Available forms: Syrup 5 mg/5 ml; tab 5 mg

Adverse effects

CNS: Anxiety, restlessness, dizziness, ***convulsions,*** headache, drowsiness, confusion

CV: Palpitations, sinus tachycardia, hypotension

EENT: Blurred vision, increased intraocular tension, dry mouth, throat

GI: Nausea, vomiting, anorexia, abdominal pain, constipation

GU: Dysuria, retention, hesitancy

Contraindications: Hypersensitivity, GI obstruction, GI hemorrhage, GU obstruction, glaucoma, severe colitis, myasthenia gravis, unstable CV status in acute hemorrhage

Precautions: Pregnancy **B**, P lactation, suspected glaucoma, G children <12 yr, elderly

Pharmacokinetics

Absorption	Rapidly absorbed
Distribution	Unknown
Metabolism	Liver
Excretion	Unknown
Half-life	Unknown

Pharmacodynamics

Onset	½-1 hr
Peak	3-4 hr
Duration	6-10 hr

Interactions

Individual drugs

Acetaminophen: ↓ levels of acetaminophen
Alcohol: ↑ CNS depression
Atenolol: ↑ levels of atenolol
Digoxin: ↑ levels of digoxin
Disopyramide: ↑ anticholinergic effects
Haloperidol: ↑ anticholinergic effects
Levodopa: ↓ levels of levodopa
Nitrofurantoin: ↑ levels of nitrofurantoin
Oxybutynin: ↑ levels of oxybutynin

Drug classifications

Analgesics, narcotic: ↑ CNS depressants
Antidepressants: ↑ anticholinergic effects
Antihistamines: ↑ CNS depression
Phenothiazines: ↑ anticholinergic effects
Sedative/hypnotics: ↑ CNS depressants

NURSING CONSIDERATIONS

Assessment

- Assess for allergic reactions: rash, urticaria; if these occur, drug should be discontinued
- Assess urinary patterns: distention, nocturia, frequency, urgency, incontinence; catheterization may be required to remove residual urine

Nursing diagnoses

✓ Urinary elimination, altered patterns (uses)
✓ Pain (uses)
✓ Knowledge deficit (teaching)

Implementation

- May be given with meals or fluids or given on an empty stomach

Patient/family education

- Advise patient to avoid hazardous activities until response to drug is known; dizziness may occur
- Caution patient to avoid OTC medication with alcohol or other CNS depressants
- Advise patient to prevent photophobia by wearing sunglasses
- Caution patient to stay cool, since overheating may occur
- Teach patient to use frequent rinsing of mouth, sips of water

Evaluation

Positive therapeutic outcome

- Absence of dysuria, frequency, nocturia, incontinence

O

oxycodone (℞)

(ox-i-koe'done)

Roxicodone Supeudol ✱; ***oxycodone/aspirin:*** Endodan ✱, Oxycodan ✱, Percodan, Percodan-Demi, Roxiprin; ***oxycodone/acetaminophen:*** Endocet ✱, Oxycocet ✱, OxylR, Percocet, Roxicet, Roxilox, Tylox

Func. class.: Narcotic analgesic

Chem. class.: Opiate, semisynthetic derivative

Pregnancy category B

Controlled substance schedule II

Action: Inhibits ascending pain pathways in CNS, increases pain threshold, alters pain perception

➔ **Therapeutic Outcome:** Decreased pain

Uses: Moderate to severe pain

Dosage and routes

Adult: PO 5 mg q4-6h or 10 mg tid or qid prn

Available forms: *Oxycodone:* supp 10, 20 mg; tabs 5 mg; caps, immediate rel 5 mg; oral sol conc 20 mg/ml; *oxycodone with acetaminophen:* tab 5 mg/325 mg; cap 5 mg/500 mg; oral sol 5 mg/325 mg/5 ml; *oxycodone with aspirin:* 2.44 mg/325 mg, 4.88/325 mg

Adverse effects

CNS: Drowsiness, dizziness, confusion, headache, sedation, euphoria

CV: Palpitations, bradycardia, change in B/P

EENT: Tinnitus, blurred vision, miosis, diplopia

GI: Nausea, vomiting, anorexia, constipation, cramps

GU: Increased urinary output, dysuria, urinary retention

INTEG: Rash, urticaria, bruising, flushing, diaphoresis, pruritus

RESP: Respiratory depression

Contraindications: Hypersensitivity, addiction (narcotic)

Precautions: Addictive personality, pregnancy **B,** lactation, increased intracranial pressure, MI (acute), severe heart disease, respiratory depression, hepatic disease, renal disease, **P** child <18 yr

Pharmacokinetics

Absorption	Well absorbed
Distribution	Widely distributed; crosses placenta
Metabolism	Liver, extensively
Excretion	Kidneys, breast milk
Half-life	2-3 hr

Pharmacodynamics

	PO	REC
Onset	15-30 min	Unknown
Peak	½-1 hr	Unknown
Duration	4-6 hr	4-6 hr

Interactions

Individual drugs

Alcohol: ↑ respiratory depression, hypotension, sedation

Nalbuphine: ↓ analgesia

Pentazocine: ↓ analgesia

Drug classifications

Antihistamines: ↑ respiratory depression, hypotension

CNS depressants: ↑ respiratory depression, hypotension

MAOIs: Do not use 2 wk before oxycodone

Phenothiazines: ↑ respiratory depression, hypotension

Sedative/hypnotics: ↑ respiratory depression, hypotension

Lab test interferences

↑ Amylase

NURSING CONSIDERATIONS

Assessment

- Monitor VS after parenteral route; note muscle rigidity, drug history, liver, kidney function tests, respiratory dysfunction: respiratory depression, character, rate, rhythm; notify prescriber if respirations are <10/min
- Monitor CNS changes: dizziness, drowsiness, hallucinations, euphoria, LOC, pupil reaction
- Monitor allergic reactions: rash, urticaria

Nursing diagnoses

- ✓ Pain (uses)
- ✓ Sensory-perceptual alteration: visual, auditory (adverse reactions)
- ✓ Breathing pattern, ineffective (adverse reactions)
- ✓ Injury, risk for (adverse reactions)
- ✓ Knowledge deficit (teaching)

Implementation

- Give with antiemetic if nausea, vomiting occur
- Give when pain is beginning to return; determine dosage interval by patient response; continuous dosing of medication is more effective than when given prn
- Medication should be slowly withdrawn after long-term use to prevent withdrawal symptoms
- Store in light-resistant container at room temp

PO route

- May be given with food or milk to lessen GI upset

Rec route

- Store supp in the refrigerator; run under warm water before insertion

Patient/family education

- Advise patients to avoid CNS depressants: alcohol, sedative/hypnotics
- Discuss with patient that dizziness, drowsiness, and confusion are common; to avoid getting up without assistance
- Discuss in detail all aspects of the drug, including purpose and what to expect
- Advise patient to make position changes slowly to lessen orthostatic hypotension

Evaluation

Positive therapeutic outcome

- Decreased pain

Treatment of overdose:

Narcan 0.2-0.8 **IV**, O_2, **IV** fluids, vasopressors

oxymorphone (℞)

(ox-i-mor′fone)

Numorphan

Func. class.: Narcotic analgesic

Chem. class.: Opiate, semisynthetic phenanthrene derivative

Pregnancy category B

Controlled substance schedule II

Action: Depresses pain impulse transmission at the spinal cord level by interacting with opioid receptors

➔ **Therapeutic Outcome:** Decreased pain

Uses: Moderate to severe pain

Dosage and routes

Adult: IM/SC 1-1.5 mg q4-6h prn; **IV** 0.5 mg q4-6h prn; rec 2.5-5 mg q4-6h prn

Labor analgesia

Adult: IM 0.5-1 mg

Available forms: Inj 1, 1.5 mg/ml; supp 5 mg

Adverse effects

CNS: ***Drowsiness, dizziness, confusion, headache, sedation, euphoria***

CV: Palpitations, bradycardia, change in B/P

EENT: Tinnitus, blurred vision, miosis, diplopia

GI: ***Nausea, vomiting, anorexia, constipation, cramps***

GU: Increased urinary output, dysuria, urinary retention

INTEG: ***Rash,*** urticaria, bruising, flushing, diaphoresis, pruritus

RESP: ***Respiratory depression***

Contraindications: Hypersensitivity, addiction (narcotic)

Precautions: Addictive personality, pregnancy **B,** lactation, increased intracranial pressure, MI (acute), severe heart disease, respiratory depression, hepatic disease, renal disease, P child <18 yr

Pharmacokinetics

Absorption	Well absorbed (rec, IM, SC); completely absorbed (IV)
Distribution	Widely distributed; crosses placenta
Metabolism	Liver, extensively
Excretion	Kidneys
Half-life	2½-4 hr

Pharmacodynamics

	IM/SC	IV	REC
Onset	15 min	10 min	30 min
Peak	1-1½ hr	15-30 min	Unknown
Duration	3-6 hr	3-4 hr	3-6 hr

Interactions

Individual drugs

Alcohol: ↑ respiratory depression, hypotension, sedation
Nalbuphine: ↓ analgesia
Pentazocine: ↓ analgesia

Drug classifications

Antihistamines: ↑ respiratory depression, hypotension
CNS depressants: ↑ respiratory depression, hypotension
MAOIs: Do not use 2 wk before oxymorphone
Sedative/hypnotics: ↑ respiratory depression, hypotension

Lab test interferences

↑ Amylase, ↑ lipase

NURSING CONSIDERATIONS

Assessment

- Monitor VS after parenteral route; note muscle rigidity, drug history, liver, kidney function tests, respiratory dysfunction: respiratory depression, character, rate, rhythm; notify prescriber if respirations are <10/min
- Monitor CNS changes: dizziness, drowsiness, hallucinations, euphoria, LOC, pupil reaction
- Monitor allergic reactions: rash, urticaria

Nursing diagnoses

- ✓ Pain (uses)
- ✓ Sensory-perceptual alteration: visual, auditory (adverse reactions)
- ✓ Breathing pattern, ineffective (adverse reactions)
- ✓ Injury, risk for (adverse reactions)
- ✓ Knowledge deficit (teaching)

Implementation

- Give with antiemetic if nausea, vomiting occur
- Give when pain is beginning to return; determine dosage interval by patient response; continuous dosing of medication is more effective than when given prn
- Medication should be slowly withdrawn after long-term use

to prevent withdrawal symptoms
• Store in light-resistant container at room temp

Rec route
• Store in refrigerator

IV route
• Give by direct **IV** undiluted over 2-3 min

Y-site compatibilities: Glycopyrrolate, hydroxyzine, ranitidine

Patient/family education
• Advise patients to avoid CNS depressants: alcohol, sedative/hypnotics
• Discuss with patient that dizziness, drowsiness, and confusion are common; to avoid getting up without assistance
• Discuss in detail all aspects of the drug, including purpose and what to expect
• Advise patient to make position changes slowly to lessen orthostatic hypotension

Evaluation

Positive therapeutic outcome
• Decreased pain

Treatment of overdose: Naloxone (Narcan) 0.2-0.8 **IV**, O_2, **IV** fluids, vasopressors

oxytocin (℞)

(ox-i-toe'sin)

Pitocin, Syntocinon

Func. class.: Oxytocic hormone

Pregnancy category N/A

Action: Acts directly on myofibrils, producing uterine contraction; stimulates breast milk letdown

Therapeutic Outcome: Stimulation of labor, control of bleeding; stimulation of milk letdown

Uses: Stimulation, induction of labor; missed or incomplete abortion, postpartum bleeding, postpartum breast engorgement, initial milk letdown

Dosage and routes

Labor induction

Adult: **IV** 0.5-2 μU/min, increase by 1-2 μU q15-60 min until regular contractions occur, then decrease dosage

Postpartum hemorrhage

Adult: **IV** 10 U infused at 20-40 μU/min

Adult: IM 10 U after placenta delivery

Incomplete abortion

Adult: **IV** 10 U at a rate of 20-40 μU/min

Fetal stress test

Adult: **IV** 0.5 μU/min; increase q20 min until 3 contractions occur at 10 min; not to exceed 20 μU only with fetal monitoring

Milk letdown

Adult: Instill 1 spray into one or both nostrils q2-3 min before breastfeeding; instill 3 gtt into one or both nostrils q2-3 min before breastfeeding

Available forms: Nasal spray 40 U/ml; inj 10 U/ml

Adverse effects

CNS: Hypertension, ***convulsions, tetanic contractions***

CV: Hypotension, dysrhythmias, increased pulse, bradycardia, tachycardia, PVC

FETUS: Dysrhythmias, jaundice, hypoxia, ***intracranial hemorrhage***

GI: Anorexia, nausea, vomiting, constipation

O

GU: Abruptio placentae, decreased uterine blood flow
HEMA: Increased hyperbilirubinemia
INTEG: Rash
RESP: Asphyxia

Contraindications: Hypersensitivity, PIH, cephalopelvic disproportion, fetal distress, hypertonic uterus

Precautions: Cervical/uterine surgery, uterine sepsis, primipara >35 yr, 1st, 2nd stage of labor

Pharmacokinetics

Absorption	Well absorbed (nasal); completely absorbed (IV)
Distribution	Widely distributed (extracellular fluid)
Metabolism	Liver, rapidly
Excretion	Kidneys
Half-life	3-12 min

Pharmacodynamics

	NASAL	IV	IM
Onset	5 min	Rapid	3-7 min
Peak	Unknown	Unknown	Unknown
Duration	20 min	1 hr	1 hr

Interactions

Individual drugs

Cyclopropane anesthesia: ↑ hypotension

Drug classifications

Vasopressors: ↑ hypertension

NURSING CONSIDERATIONS

Assessment

- Assess labor contractions: fetal heart tones, frequency, duration, intensity of contractions; if fetal heart tones increase or decrease significantly or if contractions are longer than 1 min, notify prescriber; turn patient on left side to increase oxygen to fetus
- Assess for water intoxication: confusion, anuria, drowsiness, headache; notify prescriber
- Watch for fetal distress, acceleration, deceleration, fetal presentation, pelvic dimensions
- Monitor B/P, pulse, respiratory rate, rhythm, depth
- Monitor I&O ratio
- Provide an environment conducive to letdown reflex

Nursing diagnoses

- ✓ Breastfeeding (uses)
- ✓ Injury, risk for (uses)
- ✓ Knowledge deficit (teaching)

Implementation

IV route

- Use an inf pump; rotate sol for mixing; have magnesium sulfate available
- For labor induction administer after diluting 10 U/1 L of D_5W, 0.9% NaCl, 0.45% NaCl, LR, Ringer's for a conc of 10 μU/ml; start at 1-2 μU/min (0.1-0.2 ml); may increase by 1-2 μU/min q15-30 min until labor begins
- For threatened abortion administer after diluting 10 U/500 ml of D_5W, $D_{10}W$, 0.9% NaCl, 0.45% NaCl, LR, Ringer's for a conc of 20 μU/ml; give at 10-40 μU/m
- For postpartum bleeding administer after diluting 10-40 U/L of D_5W, $D_{10}W$, 0.9% NaCl, 0.45% NaCl, LR, Ringer's for a conc of 10-40 μU/ml; may titrate to response

Additive incompatibilities: Fibrinolysin, warfarin

Additive compatibilities: Chloramphenicol, metaraminol, netilmicin, sodium bicarbonate, thiopental, verapamil

Y-site compatibilities: Heparin, regular insulin, hydrocortisone, meperidine, morphine, potassium chloride, vitamin B with C

Nasal route

• Have patient clear nasal passages before use; use product while holding upright

Patient/family education

Nasal route

• Advise patient to blow nose before administering; not to overuse

• Teach patient to report increased blood loss, abdominal cramps, increased temp or foul-smelling lochia

• Advise patient that contractions will be similar to menstrual cramps, gradually increasing in intensity

Evaluation

Positive therapeutic outcome

• Stimulation of milk letdown (nasal)

• Induction of labor

• Decreased postpartum bleeding

paclitaxel (℞)

(pa-kli-tax'el)

Taxol

Func. class.: Miscellaneous antineoplastic

Chem. class.: Natural diterpene, antimicrotubule

Pregnancy category D

Action: Inhibits the reorganization of the microtubule network needed for interphase and mitotic cellular functions; also causes abnormal bundles of microtubules during cell cycle and multiple esters of microtubules during mitosis

➔ **Therapeutic Outcome:** Prevention of rapidly growing malignant cells

Uses: Metastatic carcinoma of the ovary unresponsive to other treatment, breast; AIDS-related Kaposi's sarcoma (2nd-line)

Investigational uses: Advanced head, neck, small-cell lung cancer; non-Hodgkin's lymphoma, adenocarcinoma of the upper GI tract, hormone-refractory prostate cancer

Dosage and routes

Ovarian carcinoma

Adults: **IV** inf 135 mg/m^2 given over 24 hr q 3 wk or 175 mg/m^2 over 3 hr q3wk

Breast carcinoma

Adult: **IV** inf 175 mg/m^2 over 3 hr q3wk

AIDS-related Kaposi's sarcoma

Adult: **IV** inf 135 mg/m^2 over 3 hr q3wk or 100 mg/m^2 over 3 hr q2wk

Available forms: Inj 30 mg/5 ml vial

Adverse effects

CV: Bradycardia, hypotension, abnormal ECG

GI: Nausea, vomiting, diarrhea, mucositis; increased bilirubin, alkaline phosphatase, AST (SGOT)

HEMA: ***Neutropenia, leukopenia, thrombocytopenia, anemia,*** bleeding, infections

INTEG: Alopecia

MS: ***Arthralgia, myalgia***

NEURO: Peripheral neuropathy

SYST: Hypersensitivity reactions, ***anaphylaxis***

Contraindications: Hypersensitivity to paclitaxel or other drugs with polyoxyethylated castor oil, neutropenia of <1500/mm^3, pregnancy **D**

P **Precautions:** Children, lac-

P

tation, hepatic disease, cardiovascular disease, CNS disorder

Pharmacokinetics

Absorption	Completely absorbed
Distribution	89%-98% protein binding
Metabolism	Liver, extensively
Excretion	Unknown
Half-life	5-17 hr

Pharmacodynamics

Onset	Unknown
Peak	1-2 wk
Duration	3 wk

Interactions

Individual drugs

Cisplatin: ↑ myelosuppression
Cyclosporine: ↓ metabolism of paclitaxel
Dexamethasone: ↓ metabolism of paclitaxel
Diazepam: ↓ metabolism of paclitaxel
Doxorubicin: ↑ levels of doxorubicin
Etoposide: ↓ metabolism of paclitaxel
Ketoconazole: ↑ toxicity
Quinidine: ↓ metabolism of paclitaxel
Teniposide:↓ metabolism of paclitaxel
Testosterone: ↓ metabolism of paclitaxel

NURSING CONSIDERATIONS

Assessment

- Assess CNS changes: confusion, paresthesias, psychosis, tremors, seizures, neuropathies; drug should be discontinued
- Check buccal cavity q8h for dryness, sores or ulceration, white patches, oral pain, bleed ing, dysphagia; obtain prescription for viscous lidocaine (Xylocaine) to use in mouth
- Assess symptoms indicating severe allergic reaction: rash, pruritus, urticaria, purpuric skin lesions, itching, flushing
- Monitor CBC, differential, platelet count weekly; withhold drug if WBC count is <4000/mm^3 or platelet count is <100,000/mm^3, notify prescriber of results
- Monitor renal function studies: BUN, creatinine, serum uric acid, urine CrCl before and during therapy; check I&O ratio; report fall in urine output to <30 ml/hr
- Monitor temp q4h (may indicate beginning of infection)
- Monitor liver function tests before and during therapy (bilirubin, AST [SGOT], ALT [SGPT], LDH) as needed or monthly; check for yellowing of skin and sclera, dark urine, clay-colored stools, itchy skin, abdominal pain, fever, diarrhea
- Assess for bleeding: hematuria, stool guaiac, bruising or petechiae, mucosa or orifices q8h; check for inflammation of mucosa, breaks in skin
- Assess effects of alopecia on body image; discuss feelings about body changes

Nursing diagnoses

✓ Injury, risk for (adverse reactions)
✓ Body image disturbance (adverse reactions)
✓ Infection, risk for (adverse reactions)
✓ Knowledge deficit (teaching)

Implementation

Y-site compatiblilities:
Acyclovir, amikacin, aminophylline, bleomycin, butorphanol, calcium chloride, carboplatin, cefepime, cefotetan, ceftazidime, ceftriaxone, cimetidine, cisplatin, cyclophosphamide, cytarabine, dacarbazine,

dexamethasone, etoposide, famotidine, floxuridine, fluconazole, heparin, mannitol, meperidine, mesna, metoclopramide, morphine, ondansetron, pentostatin, potassium chloride, ranitidine, sodium bicarbonate, vancomycin, vinblastine, vincristine, zidovudine
• Give fluids PO before chemotherapy to hydrate patient
• Give antacid before oral agent; give drug after evening meal, before hs; provide antiemetic 30-60 min before giving drug and prn to prevent vomiting; administer antibiotics for prophylaxis of infection
• Give top or syst analgesics for pain to lessen effects of stomatitis
• Give liq diet: carbonated beverages; gelatin may be added if patient is not nauseated or vomiting
• Encourage patient to rinse mouth tid-qid with water, club soda; brush teeth bid-qid with soft brush or cotton-tipped applicators for stomatitis; use unwaxed dental floss

Patient/family education
• Inform patient that contraceptive measures are recommended during therapy and >4 mo after; teratogenic effects are possible
• Teach patient to avoid use of products containing aspirin or ibuprofen, razors, commercial mouthwash, since bleeding may occur; to report symptoms of bleeding (hematuria, tarry stools)
• Instruct patient to report signs of anemia (fatigue, headache, irritability, faintness, shortness of breath) and CNS reactions (confusion, psychosis, nightmares, seizures, severe headaches)
• Inform patient that hair may be lost during treatment; a wig or hair piece may make patient feel better; new hair may be different in color, texture
• Inform patient that receiving vaccinations during therapy may cause serious reactions

Evaluation
Positive therapeutic outcome
• Prevention of rapid division of malignant cells

pamidronate (℞)
(pam-i-drone'ate)
Aredia
Func. class.: Bone resorption inhibitor
Chem. class.: Bisphosphonate
Pregnancy category C

Action: Absorbs calcium phosphate crystals in bone and may directly block dissolution of hydroxyapatite crystals of bone; inhibits bone resorption, apparently without inhibiting bone formation and mineralization

➔ **Therapeutic Outcome:** Serum calcium at normal level

Uses: Moderate to severe hypercalcemia associated with malignancy with or without bone metastases; osteolytic lesions in breast cancer patients

Dosage and routes
IV *Adult:* **IV** inf 60-90 mg in moderate hypercalcemia, 90 mg in severe hypercalcemia given over 24 hr

Available forms: Inj 30 mg

pamidronate disodium and 470 mg of mannitol

Adverse effects

CNS: Fatigue

CV: Hypertension, fluid overload, dysrhythmias, tachycardia

GI: Abdominal pain, anorexia, constipation, nausea, vomiting

GU: UTI, fluid overload

INTEG: Redness, swelling, induration, pain on palpation at site of catheter insertion

META: Anemia, hypokalemia, hypomagnesemia, hypophosphatemia

MS: Bone pain

Contraindications: Hypersensitivity to bisphosphonates

P **Precautions:** Children, nursing mothers, pregnancy **C**, renal dysfunction

Pharmacokinetics

Absorption	Rapidly cleared from circulation
Distribution	Mainly to bones
Metabolism	Unknown
Excretion	Kidneys, unchanged (50%)
Half-life	Biphasic 1½ hr; 27 hr; from bone to 300 days

Pharmacodynamics

Onset	1 day
Peak	1 wk
Duration	Unknown

Interactions: None

NURSING CONSIDERATIONS

Assessment

- Assess for hypocalcemia: Chvostek's, Trousseau's sign, paresthesia, twitching, laryngospasm
- Monitor manifestations of hypocalcemia: personality changes, anxiety, disturbances, depression, psychosis; nausea, vomiting, constipation, abdominal pain from muscle spasm; decreased contractility, decreased cardiac output, hypotension, lengthened ST segment, prolonged QT interval; scaling eczema, alopecia, hyperpigmentation; tetany, muscle twitching, cramping, grimacing, seizure, altered deep tendon reflexes, spasm
- Monitor manifestations of hypomagnesemia: agitation; muscle twitching, paresthesia, hyperactive reflexes, positive Babinski reflex, dysphagia, nystagmus, seizures, tetany; nausea, vomiting, diarrhea, anorexia, abdominal distention; ectopy, tachycardia, broad, flat or inverted T waves, depressed ST segment, prolonged QT, decreased cardiac output, hypotension
- Monitor manifestations of hypokalemia: acidic urine, reduced urine osmolality, nocturia, polyuria, polydipsia; hypotension, broad T wave, U wave, ectopy, tachycardia, weak pulse; muscle weakness, altered LOC, drowsiness, apathy, lethargy, confusion, depression; anorexia, nausea, cramps, constipation, distention, paralytic ileus; hypoventilation, respiratory muscle weakness
- Assess fluid volume status: check I&O ratio and record, assess for distended red veins, crackles in lung, color, quality and sp gr of urine, skin turgor, adequacy of pulses, moist mucous membranes, bilateral lung sounds, peripheral pitting edema
- Monitor electrolytes: phosphorus, potassium, sodium, calcium, magnesium; also include BUN, creatinine, CBC, platelets, hemoglobin
- Assess B/P before and during therapy

• Assess for pain: in joints or on exertion, duration and characteristics; analgesics may be ordered
• Assess for phlebitis at **IV** site: swelling, redness, pain, warmth

Nursing diagnoses

✓ Injury, risk for (uses, adverse reactions)
✓ Fluid excess (side effects)
✓ Knowledge deficit (teaching)

Implementation

• Give by **IV** inf after reconstituting by adding 10 ml of sterile water for inj to each vial, then adding to 1000 ml of sterile 0.45%, 0.9% NaCl, D_5W, run over 24 hr
• Store inf sol for up to 24 hr at room temp
• Reconstituted sol with sterile water may be stored under refrigeration for up to 24 hr

Additive incompatibilities: Calcium products, sol

Evaluation

Positive therapeutic outcome
• Decreased calcium levels to normal

pancrelipase (℞)

(pan-kre-li'pase)
Cotazym, Cotazym Capsules, Cotazym-S Capsules, Creon Capsules, Ilozyme, Ku-Zyme HP Capsules, Pancrease Capsules, Pancrease MT 4, Pancrease MT 10, Pancrease MT 16, Ultrase MT 12, Ultrase MT 20, Ultrase MT 24, Viokase Powder, Viokase Tablets, Zymase
Func. class.: Digestant
Chem. class.: Pancreatic enzyme (bovine/porcine)
Pregnancy category C

Action: Pancreatic enzyme needed for breakdown of substances released from the pancreas

Therapeutic Outcome: Increases protein, fat, carbohydrate digestion

Uses: Exocrine pancreatic secretion insufficiency, cystic fibrosis (digestive aid), steatorrhea, pancreatic enzyme deficiency

Dosage and routes

P ***Adult and child:*** PO 1-3 cap/tab ac or with meals, or 1 cap/tab with snack or 1-2 powder packets ac

Available forms: Tabs 8000, 11,000, 30,000 U; caps 8000, 30,000 U; enteric coated caps 4000, 5000, 20,000, 25,000 U; powder 16,800 U

Adverse effects

GI: Anorexia, nausea, vomiting, diarrhea
GU: Hyperuricuria, hyperuricemia

Contraindications: Allergy to pork, chronic pancreatic disease

P

Precautions: Pregnancy **C**

Pharmacokinetics	
Absorption	Unknown
Distribution	Unknown
Metabolism	Unknown
Excretion	Unknown
Half-life	Unknown

Pharmacodynamics

Unknown

Interactions
Individual drugs

Cimetidine: ↓ absorption of pancrelipase

Oral iron: ↓ absorption of pancrelipase

Drug classifications

Antacids: ↓ absorption of pancrelipase

Food
Alkaline foods: ↓ enteric coating

Lab test interferences
↑ Uric acid (serum, urine)

NURSING CONSIDERATIONS
Assessment
- Monitor I&O ratio; watch for increasing urinary output
- Monitor fecal fat, nitrogen, pro-time, during treatment
- Monitor for polyuria, polydipsia, polyphagia (may indicate diabetes mellitus)
- Assess for allergy to pork; patient may also be sensitive to this drug
- Assess for appropriate weight, height, development; there may be a developmental lag
- Check stools for steatorrhea, which signifies undigested fat content

Nursing diagnoses
✓ Nutrition, altered: less than body requirements (uses)
✓ Knowledge deficit (teaching)

Implementation
- Give after antacid or cimetidine; decreased pH inactivates drug
- P Give powder mixed in prepared fruit for infants, children
- ⊘ Give enteric coated caps whole; do not crush or chew
- Administer low-fat diet to decrease GI symptoms
- Store in tight container at room temp

Patient/family education
- Teach patient to take tab with 8 oz or more water, not to let tab sit in mouth; have patient take tab sitting up only
- Advise patient to notify prescriber of allergic reactions, abdominal pain, cramping, or hematuria

Evaluation
Positive therapeutic outcome
- Absence of steatorrhea
- Improved digestion of carbohydrates, proteins, fat

pancuronium (℞)
(pan-cure-oh'nee-yum)

pancuronium bromide, Pavulon

Func. class.: Neuromuscular blocker (nondepolarizing)

Chem. class.: Synthetic curariform

Pregnancy category C

Action: Inhibits transmission of nerve impulses by binding with cholinergic receptor sites, antagonizing action of acetylcholine; no analgesic response

➔ **Therapeutic Outcome:** Paralysis of all skeletal muscles

Uses: Facilitation of endotracheal intubation, skeletal muscle relaxation during mechanical ventilation, surgery, or general anesthesia

Dosage and routes

Adult: **IV** 0.04-0.1 mg/kg, then 0.01 mg/kg q30-60 min

P ***Child >10 yr:*** **IV** 0.04-0.1 mg/kg, then 1/5 initial dose q30-60 min

Available forms: Inj 1, 2 mg/ml

Adverse effects

CV: Bradycardia, tachycardia, increased, decreased B/P, ventricular extrasystoles

EENT: Increased secretions

INTEG: Rash, flushing, pruritus, urticaria, sweating, salivation

MS: Weakness to prolonged skeletal muscle relaxation

RESP: Prolonged apnea, bronchospasm, cyanosis, respiratory depression

Contraindications: Hypersensitivity to bromide ion

Precautions: Pregnancy **C**, renal disease, cardiac disease, P lactation, children <2 yr, electrolyte imbalances, dehydration, neuromuscular disease, respiratory disease

Pharmacokinetics	
Absorption	Complete bioavailability
Distribution	Extracellular space; crosses placenta
Metabolism	Plasma
Excretion	Kidneys, unchanged
Half-life	2 hr

Pharmacodynamics	
Onset	30-45 sec
Peak	3-5 min
Duration	35-40 min

Interactions

Individual drugs

Clindamycin: ↑ paralysis length and intensity
Colistin: ↑ paralysis length and intensity
Lidocaine: ↑ paralysis length and intensity
Lithium: ↑ paralysis length and intensity
Magnesium: ↑ paralysis length and intensity
Polymyxin B: ↑ paralysis length and intensity
Procainamide: ↑ paralysis length and intensity
Quinidine: ↑ paralysis length and intensity
Succinylcholine: ↑ paralysis length and intensity

Drug classifications

Aminoglycosides: ↑ paralysis length and intensity
β-Blockers: ↑ paralysis length and intensity
Diuretics, potassium-losing: ↑ paralysis length and intensity
General anesthesia: ↑ paralysis length and intensity

NURSING CONSIDERATIONS

Assessment

- Monitor vital signs (B/P, pulse, respirations, airway) until fully recovered; note rate, depth, pattern of respirations, strength of hand grip; patient should be intubated before use
- Monitor for electrolyte imbalances (potassium, magnesium) before drug is used; electrolyte imbalances may lead to increased action of this drug
- Monitor for recovery: decreased paralysis of face, diaphragm, leg, arm, rest of body; residual weakness and respiratory problems may occur during recovery period
- Assess for hypersensitive reactions: rash, fever, respira-

P

tory distress, pruritus; drug should be discontinued

Nursing diagnoses

- ✓ Breathing pattern, ineffective (uses)
- ✓ Communication, impaired verbal (adverse reactions)
- ✓ Fear (adverse reactions)
- ✓ Knowledge deficit (teaching)

Implementation

• Use peripheral nerve stimulator (anesthesiologist) to determine neuromuscular blockade; deep tendon reflexes should be monitored during extended periods

• Give direct **IV** undiluted over 1-2 min, or diluted in D_5W or 0.9% NaCl and give as an inf at prescribed rate; titrate to patient response; should be administered only by qualified person, usually an anesthesiologist; do not administer IM

• Store in light-resistant area

• Give anticholinesterase to reverse neuromuscular blockade

Syringe compatibility: Heparin

Y-site compatibilities: Aminophylline, cefazolin, cefuroxime, cimetidine, dobutamine, dopamine, epinephrine, esmolol, fentanyl, fluconazole, gentamicin, heparin, hydrocortisone, isoproterenol, lorazepam, midazolam, morphine, nitroglycerin, nitroprusside, ranitidine, sulfamethoxazole/trimethoprim, vancomycin

Y-site incompatibility: Diazepam

Additive compatibility: Verapamil

Additive incompatibility: Barbiturates

Patient/family education

• Provide reassurance if communication is difficult during recovery from neuromuscular blockade

• Provide explanation to patients regarding all procedures or treatments; patient will remain conscious if anesthesia is not given also

Evaluation

Positive therapeutic outcome

• Paralysis of jaw, eyelid, head, neck, rest of body as evaluated by peripheral nerve stimulator

Treatment of overdose: Edrophonium or neostigmine, atropine; monitor VS; may require mechanical ventilation

paroxetine (℞)

(par-ox'e-teen)

Paxil

Func. class.: Antidepressant, serotonin reuptake inhibitor

Chem. class.: Phenylpiperidine derivative

Pregnancy category B

Action: Inhibits CNS neuron reuptake of serotonin but not of norepinephrine or dopamine

➔ **Therapeutic Outcome:** Relief of depression

Uses: Major depressive disorder, obsessive-compulsive disorder, panic disorder

Investigational uses: Diabetic neuropathy, headache, premature ejaculation

Dosage and routes

Adult: PO 20 mg qd in AM;

after 4 wk if no clinical improvement is noted, dosage may be increased by 10 mg/day weekly to desired response; not to exceed 50 mg/day; G decrease dosage for elderly, max 40 mg/day

Obsessive-compulsive disorder
Adults: PO 40 mg/day in AM; start with 20 mg/day, increase 10 mg/day increments, max 60 mg/day

Panic disorder
Adults: PO 40 mg/day; start with 10 mg/day and increase in 10 mg/day increments, max 60 mg/day

Available forms: Tabs 10, 20, 30, 40 mg

Adverse effects
CNS: Headache, nervousness, insomnia, drowsiness, anxiety, tremor, dizziness, fatigue, sedation, abnormal dreams, agitation, apathy, euphoria, hallucinations, delusions, psychosis
CV: Vasodilatation, postural hypotension, palpitations
EENT: Visual changes, rhinitis, oropharyngeal disorder
GI: Nausea, diarrhea, constipation, dry mouth, anorexia, dyspepsia, vomiting, taste changes, flatulence, decreased appetite
GU: Dysmenorrhea, decreased libido, urinary frequency, UTI, amenorrhea, cystitis, impotence, *abnormal ejaculation, male genital disorders*
INTEG: Sweating, rash
MS: Pain, arthritis, myalgia, myopathy, myasthenia gravis
RESP: Infection, pharyngitis, nasal congestion, sinus headache, sinusitis, cough, dyspnea
SYST: Asthenia, fever, chills

Contraindications: Hypersensitivity, patients taking MAOIs

Precautions: Pregnancy **B**, P lactation, children, elderly, G seizure history, patients with history of mania, renal and hepatic disease

Pharmacokinetics

Absorption	Well absorbed
Distribution	Widely distributed; crosses blood-brain barrier, protein-binding 95%
Metabolism	Liver, mostly
Excretion	Kidneys, unchanged (2%); breast milk
Half-life	21 hrs

Pharmacodynamics

Onset	Unknown
Peak	5.2 hr
Duration	Unknown

Interactions
Individual drugs
Alcohol: ↑ CNS depression
Digoxin: ↓ effect of digoxin
Phenytoin: ↓ effect of paroxetine
Procycline: ↓ metabolism
Quinidine: ↓ metabolism
Theophylline: ↑ theophylline levels
Warfarin: ↑ warfarin levels
Drug classifications
Antidepressants: ↓ metabolism
Antidysrhythmics, IC: ↓ metabolism
Barbiturates: ↑ effects
Benzodiazepines: ↑ effects
CNS depressants: ↑ effects
MAOIs: Hypertensive crisis, convulsions; do not use together
Phenothiazines: ↓ metabolism
Lab test interferences
↑ Serum bilirubin, ↑ blood glucose, ↑ alkaline phosphatase
↓ VMA, ↓ 5-HIAA, ↓ blood glucose

P

False ↑ Urinary catecholamines

NURSING CONSIDERATIONS

Assessment

- Assess mental status: mood, sensorium, affect, suicidal tendencies; increase in psychiatric symptoms: depression, panic
- Assess for withdrawal symptoms: headache, nausea, vomiting, muscle pain, weakness; do not usually occur unless drug was discontinued abruptly
- Monitor B/P (with patient lying, standing), pulse q4h; if systolic B/P drops 20 mm Hg, hold drug, notify prescriber; take VS q4h in patients with cardiovascular disease
- Monitor blood studies: CBC, leukocytes, differential, cardiac enzymes if patient is receiving long-term therapy
- Monitor hepatic studies: AST (SGOT), ALT (SGPT), bilirubin
- Check weight weekly; appetite may increase with drug
- Assess ECG for flattening of T wave, bundle branch block, AV block, dysrhythmias in cardiac patients
- Assess for EPS primarily in **G** elderly: rigidity, dystonia, akathisia
- Monitor urinary retention, constipation; constipation is **P** more likely to occur in children **G** or elderly
- Identify alcohol consumption; if alcohol is consumed, hold dose until AM

Nursing diagnoses

✓ Coping, ineffective individual (uses)
✓ Injury, risk for (adverse reactions)
✓ Knowledge deficit (teaching)
✓ Noncompliance (teaching)

Implementation

- Give with food or milk for GI symptoms; store at room temp; do not freeze
- Give crushed if patient is unable to swallow whole

Patient/family education

- Advise patient that therapeutic effects may take 1-4 wk
- Teach patient to use caution in driving and other activities requiring alertness because of drowsiness, dizziness, blurred vision; to avoid rising quickly from sitting to standing, espe- **G** cially elderly
- Caution patient to avoid alcohol ingestion, other CNS depressants, and OTC medication unless prescribed
- Caution patient not to discontinue medication quickly after long-term use; may cause nausea, anxiety, headache, malaise; do not double doses if one is missed
- Advise patient to use gum, hard sugarless candy, or frequent sips of water for dry mouth; if dry mouth continues an artificial saliva may be used

Evaluation

Positive therapeutic outcome

- Decrease in depression
- Absence of suicidal thoughts

Treatment of overdose:

Maintain airway, for seizures give diazepam, symptomatic treatment

pegaspargase (℞)

(peg-as′per-gase)

Colaspase, Elspar, Kidrolase ♣

Func. class.: Antineoplastic

Chem. class.: Escherichia coli enzyme

Pregnancy category D

Action: Indirectly inhibits protein synthesis in tumor cells; without amino acid, DNA, RNA synthesis is halted; asparagine, protein synthesis is halted; G_1 phase of cell cycle specific; a nonvesicant

➔ **Therapeutic Outcome:** Prevention of rapidly growing malignant cells

Uses: Acute lymphocytic leukemia in combination with other antineoplastics unresponsive to other agents

Dosage and routes

In combination

Adult: **IV** 1000 IU/kg/day × 10 days given over 30 min; IM 6000 IU/m²/day

Sole induction

Adult: **IV** 200 IU/kg/day × 28 days

Available forms: Inj 10,000 IU

Adverse effects

CNS: Neuritis, dizziness, headache, ***coma,*** depression, fatigue, confusion, hallucinations

CV: Chest pain

ENDO: Hyperglycemia

GI: Nausea, vomiting, anorexia, cramps, stomatitis, ***hepatotoxicity, pancreatitis***

GU: Urinary retention, ***renal failure,*** glycosuria, polyuria, azotemia, uric acid neuropathy

HEMA: Thrombocytopenia, leukopenia, myelosuppression, anemia, decreased clotting factors

INTEG: Rash, urticaria, chills, fever

RESP: Fibrosis, pulmonary infiltrate

SYST: Anaphylaxis, hypersensitivity

Contraindications: Hypersensitivity, infants, pregnancy **D,** lactation, pancreatitis

Precautions: Renal disease, hepatic disease

Pharmacokinetics

Absorption	Complete bioavailability
Distribution	Intravascular spaces
Metabolism	Unknown
Excretion	Reticuloendothelial system
Half-life	Unknown

Pharmacodynamics

Unknown

Interactions

Individual drugs

Methotrexate: Blocking action of methotrexate

Vincristine: ↑ neurotoxicity

Drug classifications

Hepatotoxic agents: ↑ hepatotoxic agents

Glucocorticosteroids: ↑ hyperglycemia

Lab test interferences

↓ Thyroid function tests

↑ BUN

NURSING CONSIDERATIONS

Assessment

- Assess for signs and symptoms of pancreatitis (nausea, vomiting, severe abdominal pain), anaphylaxis (bronchospasm, dyspnea), cyanosis; monitor amylase, glucose
- Assess symptoms indicating severe allergic reaction: rash, pruritus, urticaria, purpuric

skin lesions, itching, flushing; monitor for joint pain, bronchospasm, hypotension; epinephrine and crash carts should be nearby

- Monitor for frequency of stools, characteristics: cramping, acidosis; signs of dehydration: rapid respirations, poor skin turgor, decreased urine output, dry skin, restlessness, weakness
- Monitor CBC, differential, platelet count weekly; withhold drug if WBC count is <4000/mm^3 or platelet count is <100,000/mm^3; notify physician of results; also assess PT, PTT and thrombin time, which may be increased
- Monitor renal function studies: BUN, creatinine, serum uric acid, urine CrCl before and during therapy; check I&O ratio; report fall in urine output to <30 ml/hr; patient should be well hydrated with 2-3 L/day to prevent urate deposits
- Monitor temp q4h (may indicate beginning of infection)
- Monitor liver function tests before and during therapy (bilirubin, AST [SGOT], ALT [SGPT], LDH) as needed or monthly; check for yellowing of skin and sclera, dark urine, clay-colored stools, itchy skin, abdominal pain, fever, diarrhea; also monitor cholesterol, alkaline phosphatase
- Assess for bleeding: hematuria, stool guaiac, bruising or petechiae, mucosa or orifices q8h; check for inflammation of mucosa, breaks in skin
- Identify edema in feet, joint pain, stomach pain, shaking

Nursing diagnoses

- ✓ Injury, risk for (adverse reactions)
- ✓ Infection, risk for (adverse reactions)
- ✓ Knowledge deficit (teaching)

Implementation

- Preparation by trained personnel is required in controlled environment
- Give fluids **IV** or PO before chemotherapy to hydrate patient
- Provide antiemetic 30-60 min before giving drug and PRN to prevent vomiting; administer antibiotics for prophylaxis of infection
- Provide a liq diet: carbonated beverages; gelatin may be added if patient is not nauseated or vomiting

Intradermal route

- After intradermal skin testing and desensitization, give 0.1 ml (2 IU) intradermally after reconstituting with 5 ml sterile water or 0.9% NaCl for inj; then add 0.1 ml of reconstituted drug to 9.9 ml diluent (20 IU/ml); observe for 1 hr, check for wheal; desensitization may be required
- For direct **IV** dilute 10,000 IU/5 ml sterile water for inj or 0.9% NaCl without preservatives; give through 5-μm filter if fibers are present; do not use if cloudy or discolored, give over 30 min through Y-site of full-flowing **IV** of 0.9% NaCl or D_5W; run **IV** sol for at least 2 hr after direct administration
- Give **IV** inf using 21G, 23G, 25G needle; administer by slow **IV** inf via Y-tube or 3-way stopcock of flowing D_5W or NS inf over 30 min after diluting 10,000 IU/5 ml of sterile

water or 0.9% NaCl (no preservatives) to 2000 IU/ml; filter may be necessary if fibers are present

- Provide allopurinol or sodium bicarbonate to reduce uric acid levels, alkalinization of urine

IM route

- Dilute 10,000 IU/2 ml 0.9% NaCl with preservatives; give 2 ml or less per site

Patient/family education

- Advise patient that contraceptive measures are recommended during therapy; drug is teratogenic
- Teach patient to avoid use of products containing aspirin or ibuprofen, razors, commercial mouthwash, since bleeding may occur; to report symptoms of bleeding (hematuria, tarry stools)
- Teach patient to report signs of anemia (fatigue, headache, irritability, faintness, shortness of breath)
- Tell patient to avoid crowds and persons with respiratory tract infections to prevent patient infection
- Advise patient to avoid vaccinations, since serious reactions can occur

Evaluation

Positive therapeutic outcome

- Prevention of rapid division of malignant cells

pemoline (℞)

(pem′oh-leen)

Cylert, Cylert Chewable

Func. class.: Cerebral stimulant

Chem. class.: Oxazolidinone derivative

Pregnancy category B

Controlled substance schedule IV

Action: Exact mechanism unknown; may act through dopaminergic mechanisms; produces CNS stimulation and a paradoxic effect in ADHD

➔ Therapeutic Outcome: Increased alertness, increased attention span, decreased hyperactivity (ADHD)

Uses: Attention deficit hyperactivity disorder for children >6 yr [P]

Investigational uses: Schizophrenia, fatigue, depression

Dosage and routes

[P] ***Child >6 yr:*** PO 37.5 mg in AM, increasing by 18.75 mg/wk, not to exceed 112.5 mg/day

Available forms: Tabs 18.75, 37.5, 75 mg; chewable tab 37.5 mg

Adverse effects

CNS: Hyperactivity, insomnia, restlessness, dizziness, depression, headache, stimulation, irritability, aggressiveness, hallucinations, ***seizures, Gilles de la Tourette's syndrome,*** drowsiness, dyskinetic movements

CV: Tachycardia

GI: Nausea, *anorexia,* diarrhea, abdominal pain, increased liver enzymes, hepatitis, jaundice, weight loss

MISC: Rashes, growth suppression in children

Contraindications: Hypersensitivity, hepatic insufficiency

Precautions: Renal disease, pregnancy **B,** lactation, drug abuse, child <6 yr, psychosis, tics, seizure disorders

Pharmacokinetics	
Absorption	Well absorbed
Distribution	Widely distributed; crosses placenta
Metabolism	Liver
Excretion	Kidneys, pH dependent; increased pH, increased reabsorption
Half-life	12 hr; increased when urine is alkaline

Pharmacodynamics	
Onset	Unknown
Peak	2-4 hr
Duration	8 hr

Interactions

Drug classifications

Adrenergics: ↑ stimulation

Decongestants: ↑ stimulation

Stimulants, CNS: ↑ stimulation

Food

Caffeine (coffee, teas, chocolate): ↑ stimulation

NURSING CONSIDERATIONS

Assessment

- Monitor VS, B/P, since this drug may reverse antihypertensives; check patients with cardiac disease more often for increased B/P
- Monitor height and weight q3 mo, since growth rate in children may be decreased; appetite is suppressed; weight loss is common during the first few mo of treatment
- Monitor mental status: mood, sensorium, affect, stimulation, insomnia; aggressiveness may occur; depression with crying spells may occur after drug has worn off
- Assess for tolerance; should not be used for extended time except in ADHD; dosage should be diminished gradually to prevent withdrawal symptoms
- In children or adults with ADHD, monitor for improved organizational skills, attention span, attending to tasks, impulse control, socialization, and ability to get along better with others
- Assess for withdrawal symptoms: headache, nausea, vomiting, muscle pain, weakness; drug tolerance will develop after long-term use; dosage should not be increased if tolerance develops

Nursing diagnoses

- ✓ Thought processes, altered (uses, adverse reactions)
- ✓ Coping, impaired individual (uses)
- ✓ Knowledge deficit (teaching)
- ✓ Family coping, impaired individual (uses)

Implementation

- Give at least 6 hr before hs to avoid sleeplessness; titrate to patient's response; lowest dosage should be used to control symptoms
- Provide gum, hard candy, frequent sips of water for dry mouth at beginning of treatment; these symptoms tend to lessen with time

Patient/family education

- Teach patient to decrease caffeine consumption (coffee, tea, cola, chocolate), which may increase irritability and stimulation; to avoid OTC preparations unless approved by prescriber; to avoid alcohol

ingestion; these may cause serious drug interactions
• Instruct patient to taper off drug over several wk, or depression, increased sleeping, lethargy may occur
• Caution patient to avoid hazardous activities until stabilized on medication
• Instruct patient not to double doses if medication is missed; prescriber may suggest drug holidays (ADHD) during the school year to assess progress and determine continued drug necessity
• Teach patient/family to notify prescriber if significant side effects occur: tremors, insomnia, palpitations, restlessness; drug changes may be needed
• Inform patient that if dry mouth occurs to use frequent sips of water, sugarless gum, hard candy during beginning therapy; dry mouth lessens with continued treatment
• Advise patient to get needed rest; patients will feel more tired at end of day; to take last dose at least 6 hr before hs to avoid insomnia

Evaluation

Positive therapeutic outcome
• Decreased activity in ADHD

Treatment of overdose: Administer fluids, hemodialysis, peritoneal dialysis, antihypertensives for increased B/P; ammonium chloride for increased excretion

penicillin G benzathine (℞)

(pen-i-sill'in)

Bicillin L-A, Megacillin ♣, Permapen, Bicillin C-R, Bicillin C-R 900/300

Func. class.: Broad-spectrum antiinfective

Chem. class.: Natural penicillin

Pregnancy category B

Action: Interferes with cell wall replication of susceptible organisms; osmotically unstable cell wall swells and bursts from osmotic pressure, resulting in cell death

Therapeutic Outcome: Bactericidal effects on the gram-positive cocci *Staphylococcus, Streptococcus pyogenes, S. viridans, S. faecalis, S. bovis, S. pneumoniae;* gram-negative cocci *Neisseria gonorrhoeae;* gram-positive bacilli *Bacillus anthracis, Clostridium perfringens, C. tetani, Corynebacterium diphtheriae, Listeria monocytogenes;* gram-negative bacilli *Escherichia coli, Proteus mirabilis, Salmonella, Shigella, Enterobacter, Streptobacillus moniliformis,* spirochete *Treponema pallidum; Actinomyces*

Uses: Respiratory tract infections, scarlet fever, erysipelas, otitis media, pneumonia, skin and soft tissue infections, gonorrhea; prevention of rheumatic fever, glomerulonephritis

Dosage and routes

Early syphilis

Adult: IM 2.4 million U in single dose

P

Congenital syphilis

P ***Child <2 yr:*** IM 50,000 U/kg in single dose

Prophylaxis of rheumatic fever, glomerulonephritis

P ***Adult and child >60 lb:*** IM 1.2 million U in single dose q mo or 600,000 U q2 wk

P ***Child <60 lb:*** IM 600,000 U in single dose

Upper respiratory tract infections (group A streptococcal)

Adult: IM 1.2 million U in single dose; PO 400,000-600,000 U q4-6h

P ***Child >27 kg:*** IM 900,000 U in single dose

P ***Child <27 kg:*** IM 300,000-600,000 U in single dose

Available forms: Inj 300,000, 600,000 U/ml; tab 200,000 U

Adverse effects

CNS: Lethargy, hallucinations, anxiety, depression, twitching, ***coma, convulsions***

GI: Nausea, vomiting, diarrhea, increased AST (SGOT), ALT (SGPT), abdominal pain, glossitis, colitis

GU: ***Oliguria, proteinuria, hematuria, vaginitis, moniliasis, glomerulonephritis***

HEMA: Anemia, increased bleeding time, ***bone marrow depression, granulocytopenia***

META: Hyperkalemia, hypokalemia, alkalosis, hypernatremia

MISC: Local pain, tenderness and fever with IM inj

Contraindications: Hypersensitivity to penicillins; P neonates

Precautions: Hypersensitivity to cephalosporins, pregnancy **B**, severe renal disease

Pharmacokinetics	
Absorption	Delayed; prolonged drug levels
Distribution	Widely distributed; crosses placenta
Metabolism	Liver, minimally
Excretion	Kidneys, unchanged; breast milk
Half-life	½-1 hr

Pharmacodynamics	
Onset	Slow
Peak	12-24 hr
Duration	1-4 wk

Interactions

Individual drugs

Aspirin: ↑ penicillin levels, ↓ renal excretion

Chloramphenicol: ↑ half-life of chloramphenicol, ↓ effectiveness of penicillin

Probenecid: ↑ penicillin levels, ↓ renal excretion

Drug classifications

Erythromycins: ↓ antimicrobial effectiveness

Oral anticoagulants: ↑ anticoagulant effects

Oral contraceptives: ↓ contraceptive effectiveness

Tetracyclines: ↓ antimicrobial effectiveness

Lab test interferences

False positive: Urine glucose, urine protein

NURSING CONSIDERATIONS

Assessment

- Assess patient for previous sensitivity reaction to penicillins or cephalosporins; cross-sensitivity between penicillins and cephalosporins is common
- Assess patient for signs and symptoms of infection including characteristics of wounds, sputum, urine, stool, WBC >10,000, earache, fever; obtain baseline information and during treatment
- Obtain C&S before begin-

ning drug therapy to identify if correct treatment has been initiated

- Assess for allergic reactions: rash, urticaria, pruritus, chills, fever, joint pain; angioedema may occur a few days after therapy begins; epinephrine, resuscitation equipment should be available for anaphylactic reaction
- Identify urine output; if decreasing, notify prescriber (may indicate nephrotoxicity); also check for increased BUN, creatinine
- Monitor blood studies: AST (SGOT), ALT (SGPT), CBC, Hct, bilirubin, LDH, alkaline phosphatase, Coombs' test monthly if patient is on long-term therapy
- Monitor electrolytes: potassium, sodium, chloride monthly if patient is on long-term therapy
- Assess bowel pattern daily; if severe diarrhea occurs, drug should be discontinued; may indicate pseudomembranous colitis
- Monitor for bleeding: ecchymosis, bleeding gums, hematuria, stool guaiac daily if on long-term therapy
- Assess for overgrowth of infection: perineal itching, fever, malaise, redness, pain, swelling, drainage, rash, diarrhea, change in cough, sputum

Nursing diagnoses

- ✓ Infection, risk for (uses)
- ✓ Diarrhea (adverse reactions)
- ✓ Injury, risk for (adverse reactions)
- ✓ Knowledge deficit (teaching)
- ✓ Noncompliance (teaching)

Implementation

PO route

- Give in even doses around the clock; if GI upset occurs, give with food, avoid acidic juices; carbonated beverages may decrease PO absorption; drug must be given for 10-14 days to ensure organism death and prevent superinfection
- Shake susp

IM route

- Do not give **IV**
- Give deep in large muscle mass
- Reconstitute with 0.9% NaCl, sterile water for inj, D_5W; refrigerate unused portion

Patient/family education

- Teach patient to report sore throat, bruising, bleeding, joint pain; may indicate blood dyscrasias (rare)
- Advise patient to contact prescriber if vaginal itching, loose, foul-smelling stools, furry tongue occur; may indicate superinfection
- Instruct patient to take all medication prescribed for the length of time ordered
- Advise patient to notify prescriber of diarrhea with blood or pus, which may indicate pseudomembranous colitis

Evaluation

Positive therapeutic outcome

- Absence of signs/symptoms of infection (WBC <10,000, temp WNL, absence of red, draining wounds, earache)
- Reported improvement in symptoms of infection

Treatment of anaphylaxis:

Withdraw drug, maintain airway, administer epinephrine, aminophylline, O_2, **IV** corticosteroids

penicillin G potassium (℞)

Acrocillin, Burcillin-G, Deltapen, Megacillin ✱, Novopen G ✱, Pentids, Pfizerpen

Func. class.: Broad-spectrum antiinfective
Chem. class.: Natural penicillin

Pregnancy category B

Action: Interferes with cell wall replication of susceptible organisms; osmotically unstable cell wall swells and bursts from osmotic pressure, resulting in cell death

➔ **Therapeutic Outcome:** Bactericidal effects for the non–penicillinase-producing gram-positive cocci *Staphylococcus aureus, Streptococcus pyogenes, S. viridans, S. faecalis, S. bovis, S. pneumoniae;* gram-negative cocci *Neisseria gonorrhoeae, N. meningitidis;* gram-positive bacilli *Bacillus anthracis, Clostridium perfringens, C. tetani, Corynebacterium diphtheriae, Listeria monocytogenes;* gram-negative bacilli *Bacteroides, Fusobacterium nucleatum, Pasteurella multocida, Streptobacillus moniliformis;* spirochetes *Treponema pallidum, T. pertenue, Borrelia recurrentis, Leptospira icterohaemorrhagiae; Actinomyces*

Uses: Emphysema, gangrene, anthrax, gonorrhea, mastoiditis, meningitis, osteomyelitis, pneumonia, tetanus, UTIs, prophylactically in rheumatic fever

Dosage and routes

Pneumococcal/streptococcal infections (mild to moderate)

Adult: PO 400,000-500,000 U q6-8h × 10 days (streptococcal infections) or afebrile × 2 days (pneumococcal infections); IM/**IV** 1.2-24 million U in divided doses q4h

P ***Child <12 yr:*** PO 25,000-90,000 U/kg/day in 3-6 divided doses; IM/**IV** 25,000-300,000 μ/kg/day in individual doses q4h

Prevention of recurrence of rheumatic fever

Adult: PO 200,000-250,000 U bid continuously

P ***Child <12 yr:*** PO 25,000-90,000 U/kg/day in 3-6 divided doses

Vincent's gingivitis/pharyngitis

Adult: PO 400,000-500,000 U q6-8h

Available forms: Tabs 200,000, 250,000, 400,000, 500,000, 800,000 U; powder for oral sol 200,000, 400,000 U/5 ml; inj

Adverse effects

CNS: Lethargy, hallucinations, anxiety, depression, twitching, ***coma, convulsions***

GI: Nausea, vomiting, diarrhea, increased AST (SGOT) and ALT (SGPT), abdominal pain, glossitis, colitis

HEMA: Anemia, ***increased bleeding time, bone marrow depression, granulocytopenia***

META: Hyperkalemia, hypokalemia, alkalosis, hypernatremia

Contraindications: Hypersensitivity to penicillins; P neonates

Precautions: Hypersensitivity to cephalosporins, pregnancy **B**

Pharmacokinetics

Absorption	Variably absorbed (PO); well absorbed (IM)
Distribution	Widely distributed; crosses placenta
Metabolism	Liver, minimally
Excretion	Kidneys unchanged; breast milk
Half-life	½-1 hr

Pharmacodynamics

	PO	IM	IV
Onset	Rapid	Rapid	Rapid
Peak	1 hr	¼-½ hr	Immediate

Interactions

Individual drugs

Aspirin: ↑ penicillin levels, ↓ renal excretion

Cholestyramine: ↓ effectiveness of penicillin

Chloramphenicol: ↑ half-life of chloramphenicol, ↓ effectiveness of penicillin

Colestipol: ↓ effectiveness of penicillin

Probenecid: ↑ penicillin levels, ↓ renal excretion

Drug classifications

Erythromycins: ↓ antimicrobial effectiveness

Oral anticoagulants: ↑ anticoagulant effects

Oral contraceptives: ↓ contraceptive effectiveness

Tetracyclines: ↓ antimicrobial effectiveness

Food

Food, carbonated drinks, citrus fruit juices: ↓ absorption

Lab test interferences

False positive: Urine glucose, urine protein

NURSING CONSIDERATIONS

Assessment

- Assess patient for previous sensitivity reaction to penicillins or cephalosporins; cross-sensitivity between penicillins and cephalosporins is common
- Assess patient for signs and symptoms of infection including characteristics of wounds, sputum, urine, stool, WBC >10,000, earache, fever; obtain baseline information and during treatment
- Obtain C&S before beginning drug therapy to identify if correct treatment has been initiated
- Assess for allergic reactions: rash, urticaria, pruritus, chills, fever, joint pain; angioedema may occur a few days after therapy begins; epinephrine, resuscitation equipment should be available for anaphylactic reaction
- Identify urine output; if decreasing, notify prescriber (may indicate nephrotoxicity); also check for increased BUN, creatinine
- Monitor blood studies: AST (SGOT), ALT (SGPT), CBC, Hct, bilirubin, LDH, alkaline phosphatase, Coombs' test monthly if patient is on long-term therapy
- Monitor electrolytes: potassium, sodium, chloride monthly if patient is on long-term therapy
- Assess bowel pattern daily; if severe diarrhea occurs, drug should be discontinued; may indicate pseudomembranous colitis
- Monitor for bleeding: ecchymosis, bleeding gums, hematuria, stool guaiac daily if on long-term therapy
- Assess for overgrowth of infection: perineal itching, fever, malaise, redness, pain, swelling, drainage, rash, diarrhea, change in cough, sputum

P

Nursing diagnoses

- ✓ Infection, risk for (uses)
- ✓ Diarrhea (adverse reactions)
- ✓ Injury, risk for (adverse reactions)
- ✓ Knowledge deficit (teaching)
- ✓ Noncompliance (teaching)

Implementation

PO route

• Give in even doses around the clock; if GI upset occurs, give with food; drug must be given for 10-14 days to ensure organism death and prevent superinfection

• Shake susp

IM route

• Reconstitute with D_5W, 0.9% NaCl, sterile water for inj; shake well

• Give deep in large muscle mass; massage

• Do not give SC; may cause severe pain

• If injected near a nerve, loss of function and severe pain may occur

IV **IV route**

• Change **IV** sites q48h to prevent pain and phlebitis

• Give by intermittent inf by diluting 3 million U or less/50 ml or more; dilute 3 million U or more/100 ml D_5W, $D_{10}W$, 0.45% NaCl, 0.9% NaCl, LR, Ringer's or any combination run over 1-2 hr (adult), 15-30 P min (child)

• Give by cont inf by diluting and infusing over 24 hr

Syringe incompatibility: Metoclopramide

Syringe compatibility: Heparin

Additive incompatibilities: Aminoglycosides, aminophylline, amphotericin B, chlorpromazine, dopamine, floxacillin, hydroxyzine, metaraminol, oxytetracycline, pentobarbital, prochlorperazine mesylate, promazine, tetracycline, thiopental

Additive compatibilities: Ascorbic acid, calcium chloride, calcium gluconate, cephapirin, chloramphenicol, cimetidine, clindamycin, colistimethate, corticotropin, dimenhydrinate, diphenhydramine, ephedrine, erythromycin, furosemide, hydrocortisone, kanamycin, lidocaine, magnesium sulfate, methicillin, methylprednisolone, metronidazole, polymyxin B, prednisolone, potassium chloride, procaine, prochlorperazine, verapamil

Y-site compatibilities: Acyclovir, amiodarone, cyclophosphamide, diltiazem, enalaprilat, esmolol, fluconazole, foscarnet, heparin, hydromorphone, labetalol, magnesium sulfate, meperidine, morphine, perphenazine, potassium chloride, tacrolimus, theophylline, verapamil, vitamin B with C

Patient/family education

• Teach patient to report sore throat, bruising, bleeding, joint pain; may indicate blood dyscrasias (rare)

• Advise patient to contact prescriber if vaginal itching, loose, foul-smelling stools, furry tongue occur; may indicate superinfection

• Instruct patient to take all medication prescribed for the length of time ordered

• Advise patient to notify prescriber of diarrhea with blood or pus, which may indicate pseudomembranous colitis

Evaluation

Positive therapeutic outcome

• Absence of signs/symptoms

of infection (WBC <10,000, temp WNL, absence of red, draining wounds, earache)
- Reported improvement in symptoms of infection

Treatment of anaphylaxis: Withdraw drug, maintain airway, administer epinephrine, aminophylline, O_2, **IV** corticosteroids

penicillin G procaine (℞)

Ayercillin ✱, Crysticillin A.S., Duracillin A.S., Wycillin, Pfizerpen-AS

Func. class.: Broad-spectrum long-acting antiinfective

Chem. class.: Natural penicillin

Pregnancy category B

Action: Interferes with cell wall replication of susceptible organisms; osmotically unstable cell wall swells and bursts from osmotic pressure, resulting in cell death

➔ **Therapeutic Outcome:** Bactericidal effects for the gram-positive cocci *Staphylococcus aureus, Streptococcus pyogenes, S. viridans, S. faecalis, S. bovis, S. pneumoniae;* gram-negative cocci *Neisseria gonorrhoeae, N. meningitidis;* gram-positive bacilli *Bacillus anthracis, Clostridium perfringens, C. tetani, Corynebacterium diphtheriae, Listeria monocytogenes;* gram-negative bacilli *Bacteroides, Fusobacterium nucleatum, Pasteurella multocida, Streptobacillus moniliformis;* spirochetes *Treponema pallidum, T. pertenue, Borrelia recurrentis, Leptospira icterohaemorrhagiae; Actinomyces*

Uses: Empyema, gangrene, anthrax, gonorrhea, mastoiditis, meningitis, osteomyelitis, pneumonia, tetanus, UTIs, prophylactically in rheumatic fever

Dosage and routes

Moderate to severe infections

P ***Adult and child:*** IM 600,000-1.2 million U in one or two doses/day × 10 days to 2 wk

P ***Newborn:*** IM 50,000 U/kg single dose

Gonorrhea

P ***Adult and child >12 yr:*** IM 4.8 million units in two inj given 30 min after probenecid 1 g

Pneumonia (pneumococcal)

P ***Adult and child >12 yr:*** IM 300,000-600,000 U q6-12h

Available forms: Inj 300,000, 500,000, 600,000 U/ml, 600,000 U/1.2 ml, 1.2 million U/dose, 2.4 million U/dose

Adverse effects

CNS: Lethargy, hallucinations, anxiety, depression, twitching, ***coma, convulsions***

GI: Nausea, vomiting, diarrhea, increased AST (SGOT), ALT (SGPT), abdominal pain, glossitis, colitis

GU: ***Oliguria, proteinuria, hematuria, vaginitis, moniliasis, glomerulonephritis***

HEMA: Anemia, increased bleeding time, ***bone marrow depression, granulocytopenia***

META: Hyperkalemia, hypokalemia, alkalosis, hypernatremia

Contraindications: Hypersen-

P

sitivity to penicillins, procaine, **P** neonates

Precautions: Hypersensitivity to cephalosporins, pregnancy **B,** lactation, severe renal disease

Pharmacokinetics	
Absorption	Delayed; prolonged drug levels
Distribution	Widely distributed; crosses placenta
Metabolism	Liver, minimally
Excretion	Kidneys, unchanged; breast milk
Half-life	½-1 hr

Pharmacodynamics	
Onset	Slow
Peak	1-4 hr
Duration	15 hr

Interactions

Individual drugs

Aspirin: ↑ penicillin levels, ↓ renal excretion
Chloramphenicol: ↑ half-life of chloramphenicol, ↓ effectiveness of penicillin
Probenecid: ↑ penicillin levels, ↓ renal excretion

Drug classifications

Erythromycins: ↓ antimicrobial effectiveness
Oral anticoagulants: ↑ anticoagulant effects
Oral contraceptives: ↓ contraceptive effectiveness
Tetracyclines: ↓ antimicrobial effectiveness

Lab test interferences

False positive: Urine glucose, urine protein

NURSING CONSIDERATIONS

Assessment

- Assess patient for previous sensitivity reaction to penicillins or cephalosporins; cross-sensitivity between penicillins and cephalosporins is common
- Assess patient for signs and symptoms of infection including characteristics of wounds, sputum, urine, stool, WBC >10,000, earache, fever; obtain baseline information and during treatment
- Obtain C&S before beginning drug therapy to identify if correct treatment has been initiated
- Assess for allergic reactions: rash, urticaria, pruritus, chills, fever, joint pain; angioedema may occur a few days after therapy begins; epinephrine, resuscitation equipment should be available for anaphylactic reaction
- ❗ Identify urine output; if decreasing, notify prescriber (may indicate nephrotoxicity); also check for increased BUN, creatinine
- Monitor blood studies: AST (SGOT), ALT (SGPT), CBC, Hct, bilirubin, LDH, alkaline phosphatase, Coombs' test monthly if patient is on long-term therapy
- Monitor electrolytes: potassium, sodium, chloride monthly if patient is on long-term therapy
- Assess bowel pattern daily; if severe diarrhea occurs, drug should be discontinued; may indicate pseudomembranous colitis
- Monitor for bleeding: ecchymosis, bleeding gums, hematuria, stool guaiac daily if on long-term therapy
- Assess for overgrowth of infection: perineal itching, fever, malaise, redness, pain, swelling, drainage, rash, diarrhea, change in cough, sputum

Nursing diagnoses

- ✓ Infection, risk for (uses)
- ✓ Diarrhea (adverse reactions)
- ✓ Injury, risk for (adverse reactions)
- ✓ Knowledge deficit (teaching)
- ✓ Noncompliance (teaching)

Implementation

- Do not give **IV**
- Give deeply in large muscle mass
- Reconstitute with 0.9% NaCl, sterile water for inj, D_5W; refrigerate unused portion
- Shake medication before administering
- IM route may include procaine reactions: fear of death, depression, convulsions, anxiety, confusion, hallucinations

Patient/family education

- Teach patient to report sore throat, bruising, bleeding, joint pain; may indicate blood dyscrasias (rare)
- Advise patient to contact prescriber if vaginal itching, loose, foul-smelling stools, furry tongue occur; may indicate superinfection
- Advise patient to notify prescriber of diarrhea with blood or pus, which may indicate pseudomembranous colitis

Evaluation

Positive therapeutic outcome

- Absence of signs/symptoms of infection (WBC <10,000, temp WNL, absence of red, draining wounds, earache)
- Reported improvement in symptoms of infection

Treatment of anaphylaxis: Withdraw drug, maintain airway, administer epinephrine, aminophylline, O_2, **IV** corticosteroids

penicillin G sodium 🗝 (℞)

Crystapen 🍁, Pfizerpen

Func. class.: Broad-spectrum antiinfective

Chem. class.: Natural penicillin

Pregnancy category B

Action: Interferes with cell wall replication of susceptible organisms; osmotically unstable cell wall swells and bursts from osmotic pressure, resulting in cell death

➔ **Therapeutic Outcome:** Bactericidal effects for the non–penicillinase-producing gram positive cocci *Staphylococcus aureus, Streptococcus pyogenes, S. viridans, S. faecalis, S. bovis, S. pneumoniae;* gram-negative cocci *Neisseria gonorrhoeae, N. meningitidis;* gram-positive bacilli *Bacillus anthracis, Clostridium perfringens, C. tetani, Corynebacterium diphtheriae, Listeria monocytogenes;* gram-negative bacilli *Bacteroides, Fusobacterium nucleatum, Pasteurella multocida, Streptobacillus moniliformis;* spirochetes *Treponema pallidum, T. pertenue, Borrelia recurrentis, Leptospira icterohaemorrhagiae; Actinomyces*

Uses: Empyema, gangrene, anthrax, gonorrhea, mastoiditis, meningitis, osteomyelitis, pneumonia, tetanus, UTIs, prophylactically in rheumatic fever

Dosage and routes

Moderate to severe infections

Adult: IM/**IV** 12 million-

P

30 million U/day in divided doses q4h

P *Child:* IM/**IV** 25,000-300,000 U/day in divided doses q4-12h

Dental surgery prophylaxis for endocarditis

Adult: IM/**IV** 2 million U 30-60 min before procedure, then 1 million U 6 hr after procedure

Available forms: Inj 1 million, 5 million, 20 million U

Adverse effects

CNS: Lethargy, hallucinations, anxiety, depression, twitching, ***convulsions***

GI: Nausea, vomiting, diarrhea, increased AST (SGOT), ALT (SGPT), abdominal pain, glossitis, colitis

GU: ***Oliguria, proteinuria, hematuria,*** vaginitis, moniliasis, ***glomerulonephritis***

HEMA: Anemia, increased bleeding time, ***bone marrow depression, granulocytopenia***

META: Hyperkalemia, hypokalemia, alkalosis, hypernatremia

Contraindications: Hypersen-
P sitivity to penicillins, neonates

Precautions: CHF caused by sodium retention, pregnancy **B**

Pharmacokinetics	
Absorption	Well absorbed
Distribution	Widely distributed; crosses placenta
Metabolism	Liver, minimally
Excretion	Kidneys, unchanged; breast milk
Half-life	½-1 hr

Pharmacodynamics	IM	IV
Onset	Rapid	Rapid
Peak	1-3 hr	Rapid

Interactions

Individual drugs

Aspirin: ↑ penicillin levels, ↓ renal excretion

Cholestyramine: ↓ effectiveness of penicillin

Chloramphenicol: ↑ half-life of chloramphenicol, ↓ effectiveness of penicillin

Colestipol: ↓ effectiveness of penicillin

Probenecid: ↑ penicillin levels, ↓ renal excretion

Drug classifications

Erythromycins: ↓ antimicrobial effectiveness

Oral anticoagulants: ↑ anticoagulant effects

Oral contraceptives: ↓ contraceptive effectiveness

Tetracyclines: ↓ antimicrobial effectiveness

Food

Food, carbonated drinks, citrus fruit juices: ↓ absorption

Lab test interferences

False positive: Urine glucose, urine protein

NURSING CONSIDERATIONS
Assessment

- Assess patient for previous sensitivity reaction to penicillins or cephalosporins; cross-sensitivity between penicillins and cephalosporins is common
- Assess patient for signs and symptoms of infection including characteristics of wounds, sputum, urine, stool, WBC >10,000, earache, fever; obtain baseline information and during treatment
- Obtain C&S before beginning drug therapy to identify if correct treatment has been initiated
- Assess for allergic reactions: rash, urticaria, pruritus, chills,

fever, joint pain; angioedema may occur a few days after therapy begins; epinephrine, resuscitation equipment should be available for anaphylactic reaction

- Identify urine output; if decreasing, notify prescriber (may indicate nephrotoxicity); also check for increased BUN, creatinine
- Monitor blood studies: AST (SGOT), ALT (SGPT), CBC, Hct, bilirubin, LDH, alkaline phosphatase, Coombs' test monthly if patient is on long-term therapy
- Monitor electrolytes: potassium, sodium, chloride monthly if patient is on long-term therapy
- Assess bowel pattern daily; if severe diarrhea occurs, drug should be discontinued; may indicate pseudomembranous colitis
- Monitor for bleeding: ecchymosis, bleeding gums, hematuria, stool guaiac daily if on long-term therapy
- Assess for overgrowth of infection: perineal itching, fever, malaise, redness, pain, swelling, drainage, rash, diarrhea, change in cough, sputum

Nursing diagnoses

- ✓ Infection, risk for (uses)
- ✓ Diarrhea (adverse reactions)
- ✓ Injury, risk for (adverse reactions)
- ✓ Knowledge deficit (teaching)
- ✓ Noncompliance (teaching)

Implementation

IM route

- Reconstitute with 0.9% NaCl, D_5W, sterile water
- May be diluted with lidocaine (1%, 2%) to prevent pain from inj (IM only); use lidocaine without epinephrine only
- Shake after reconstitution; give deep in large muscle mass; massage
- Do not give SC; severe pain may occur
- Inj near nerves can result in severe pain and loss of function of nerve that was injected

IV route

- Change **IV** sites q48h to prevent phlebitis and pain at site
- Give by intermittent inf by diluting 3 million U or less/50 ml or more; or doses of 73 million U/100 ml D_5W, 0.9% NaCl; give over 1-2 hr (adult) or 30 min (child)
- Give by cont inf by diluting in compatible sol and run over 24 hr

Syringe incompatibilities: Oxytetracycline, tetracycline

Syringe compatibilities: Aminoglycosides, chloramphenicol, cimetidine, colistimethate, gentamicin, heparin, kanamycin, lincomycin, polymyxin B, streptomycin

Additive incompatibilities: Amphotericin B, bleomycin, cephalothin, chlorpromazine, cytarabine, floxacillin, hydroxyzine, methylprednisolone, oxytetracycline, prochlorperazine, promethazine

Additive compatibilities: Calcium chloride, calcium gluconate, chloramphenicol, clindamycin, colistimethate, diphenhydramine, erythromycin, furosemide, gentamicin, hydrocortisone, kanamycin, methicillin, polymyxin B, prednisolone, procaine, ranitidine, verapamil, vitamin B with C

Patient/family education
- Teach patient to report sore throat, bruising, bleeding, joint pain; may indicate blood dyscrasias (rare)
- Advise patient to contact prescriber if vaginal itching, loose, foul-smelling stools, furry tongue occur; may indicate superinfection
- Advise patient to notify prescriber of diarrhea with blood or pus, which may indicate pseudomembranous colitis

Evaluation
Positive therapeutic outcome
- Absence of signs/symptoms of infection (WBC <10,000, temp WNL, absence of red, draining wounds, earache)
- Reported improvement in symptoms of infection

Treatment of anaphylaxis: Withdraw drug, maintain airway, administer epinephrine, aminophylline, O_2, **IV** corticosteroids

penicillin V potassium (℞)

Pen-Vee K ✤, Deltapen-VK, V-Cillin K, Veetids, PVFK ✤, Apo-Pen-VK ✤, Novopen-VK ✤, Ledercillin-VK, Uticillin-VK, Betapen-VK, Penapar-VK, Robicillin-VK

Func. class.: Broad-spectrum antiinfective
Chem. class.: Natural penicillin

Pregnancy category B

Action: Interferes with cell wall replication of susceptible organisms; osmotically unstable cell wall swells and bursts from osmotic pressure, resulting in cell death

Therapeutic Outcome: Bactericidal effects for gram-positive cocci *Staphylococcus aureus, Streptococcus pyogenes, S. viridans, S. faecalis, S. bovis, S. pneumoniae;* gram-negative cocci *Neisseria gonorrhoeae, N. meningitidis;* gram-positive bacilli *Bacillus anthracis, Clostridium perfringens, C. tetani, Corynebacterium diphtheriae, Listeria monocytogenes;* gram-negative bacillus *Streptobacillus moniliformis;* spirochete *Treponema pallidum; Actinomyces*

Uses: Emphysema, gangrene, anthrax, gonorrhea, mastoiditis, meningitis, osteomyelitis, pneumonia, tetanus, UTIs, prophylactically in rheumatic fever

Dosage and routes
Pneumococcal/ staphylococcal infections
Adult: PO 250-500 mg q6h
P ***Child <12 yr:*** PO 15-50 mg/kg/day in divided doses q6-8h

Streptococcal infections
Adult: PO 125-250 mg q6-8h × 10 days

Prevention of recurrence of rheumatic fever/chorea
Adult: PO 125-250 mg bid continuously

Vincent's infection of oropharynx
Adult: PO 500 mg q6h

Available forms: Tabs 125, 250, 500 mg; film-coated tabs 250, 500 mg; powder for oral susp 125, 250 mg/5 ml

Adverse effects
CNS: Lethargy, hallucinations, anxiety, ***depression***, twitching, ***coma, convulsions***

GI: Nausea, vomiting, diarrhea, increased AST (SGOT), ALT (SGPT), abdominal pain, glossitis, colitis
GU: ***Oliguria, proteinuria, hematuria, vaginitis, moniliasis, glomerulonephritis***
HEMA: Anemia, increased bleeding time, ***bone marrow depression, granulocytopenia***
META: Hyperkalemia, hypokalemia, alkalosis

Contraindications: Hypersensitivity to penicillins, neonates

Precautions: Hypersensitivity to cephalosporins, pregnancy **B**

Pharmacokinetics

Absorption	Widely absorbed
Distribution	Widely distributed; crosses placenta
Metabolism	Liver, minimally
Excretion	Kidneys, unchanged; breast milk
Half-life	½-1 hr

Pharmacodynamics

Onset	Rapid
Peak	½-1 hr

Interactions

Individual drugs

Aspirin: ↑ penicillin levels, ↓ renal excretion
Cholestyramine: ↓ effectiveness of penicillin
Chloramphenicol: ↑ half-life of chloramphenicol, ↓ effectiveness of penicillin
Colestipol: ↓ effectiveness of penicillin
Probenecid: ↑ penicillin levels, ↓ renal excretion

Drug classifications

Erythromycins: ↓ antimicrobial effectiveness
Oral anticoagulants: ↑ anticoagulant effects
Oral contraceptives: ↓ contraceptive effectiveness
Tetracyclines: ↓ antimicrobial effectiveness

Food

Food, carbonated drinks, citrus fruit juices: ↓ absorption

Lab test interferences

False positive: Urine glucose, urine protein

NURSING CONSIDERATIONS

Assessment

- Assess patient for previous sensitivity reaction to penicillins or cephalosporins; cross-sensitivity between penicillins and cephalosporins is common
- Assess patient for signs and symptoms of infection including characteristics of wounds, sputum, urine, stool, WBC >10,000, earache, fever; obtain baseline information and during treatment
- Obtain C&S before beginning drug therapy to identify if correct treatment has been initiated
- Assess for allergic reactions: rash, urticaria, pruritus, chills, fever, joint pain; angioedema may occur a few days after therapy begins; epinephrine, resuscitation equipment should be available for anaphylactic reaction
- Identify urine output; if decreasing, notify prescriber (may indicate nephrotoxicity); also check for increased BUN, creatinine
- Monitor blood studies: AST (SGOT), ALT (SGPT), CBC, Hct, bilirubin, LDH, alkaline phosphatase, Coombs' test monthly if patient is on long-term therapy
- Monitor electrolytes: potassium, sodium, chloride monthly if patient is on long-term therapy

• Assess bowel pattern daily; if severe diarrhea occurs, drug should be discontinued; may indicate pseudomembranous colitis
• Monitor for bleeding: ecchymosis, bleeding gums, hematuria, stool guaiac daily if on long-term therapy
• Assess for overgrowth of infection: perineal itching, fever, malaise, redness, pain, swelling, drainage, rash, diarrhea, change in cough, sputum

Nursing diagnoses

✓ Infection, risk for (uses)
✓ Diarrhea (adverse reactions)
✓ Injury, risk for (adverse reactions)
✓ Knowledge deficit (teaching)
✓ Noncompliance (teaching)

Implementation

• Give in even doses around the clock; if GI upset occurs, give with food; drug must be given for 10-14 days to ensure organism death and prevent superinfection; store in tight container
• Shake susp; store in refrigerator for 2 wk or for 1 wk at room temp

Patient/family education

• Teach patient to report sore throat, bruising, bleeding, joint pain; may indicate blood dyscrasias (rare)
• Advise patient to contact prescriber if vaginal itching, loose, foul-smelling stools, furry tongue occur; may indicate superinfection
• Instruct patient to take all medication prescribed for the length of time ordered
• Advise patient to notify prescriber of diarrhea with blood or pus, which may indicate pseudomembranous colitis

Evaluation

Positive therapeutic outcome

• Absence of signs/symptoms of infection (WBC <10,000, temp WNL, absence of red, draining wounds, earache)
• Reported improvement in symptoms of infection

Treatment of anaphylaxis: Withdraw drug, maintain airway, administer epinephrine, aminophylline, O_2, **IV** corticosteroids

pentamidine (℞)

(pen-tam'i-deen)

Nebupent, Pentam 300, Pentacarinat ✤, Pneumopent ✤

Func. class.: Antiprotozoal

Chem. class.: Aromatic diamide derivative

Pregnancy category C

Action: Interferes with DNA/RNA synthesis in protozoa; has direct effect on islet cells in the pancreas

➡ **Therapeutic Outcome:** Protozoa death

Uses: *Pneumocystis carinii* infections

Investigational uses: Babesiosis, leishmaniasis, African trypanosomiasis

Dosage and routes

P ***Adult and child:*** **IV**/IM 4 mg/kg/day × 2 wk; neb 600 mg/6 ml NS via specific nebulizer given q4wk for prevention

Available forms: Inj; aerosol 300 mg/vial

Adverse effects

CNS: Disorientation, hallucinations, dizziness, confusion

CV: Hypotension, ventricular tachycardia, ECG abnormalities
GI: Nausea, vomiting, anorexia, increased AST (SGOT), ALT (SGPT), ***acute pancreatitis,*** metallic taste
GU: Acute renal failure, increased serum creatinine, renal toxicity
HEMA: Anemia, ***leukopenia, thrombocytopenia***
INTEG: Sterile abscess, pain at inj site, pruritus, urticaria, rash
META: Hyperkalemia, hypocalcemia, *hypoglycemia, hyperglycemia*
MISC: Fatigue, chills, night sweats
RESP: Cough, shortness of breath, ***bronchospasm*** (with aerosol)

Precautions: Blood dyscrasias, hepatic disease, renal disease, diabetes mellitus, cardiac disease, hypocalcemia, pregnancy **C,** hypertension, hypotension, P lactation, children

Pharmacokinetics

Absorption	Well absorbed (IM); minimally absorbed (inh); completely absorbed (IV)
Distribution	Widely distributed; does not appear in CSF
Metabolism	Not known
Excretion	Kidneys, unchanged (up to 30%)
Half-life	6½-9½ hr; increased in renal disease

Pharmacodynamics

	IM	IV	INH
Onset	Unknown	Unknown	Unknown
Peak	½-1 hr	Inf end	Unknown

Interactions
Individual drugs
Amphotericin B: ↑ nephrotoxicity
Cisplatin: ↑ bone marrow depression
Colistin: ↑ nephrotoxicity
Methoxyflurane: ↑ bone marrow depression
Polymyxin B: ↑ bone marrow depression
Vancomycin: ↑ bone marrow depression
Drug classifications
Aminoglycosides: ↑ nephrotoxicity
Antineoplastics: ↑ nephrotoxicity, bone marrow depression
Radiation: ↑ nephrotoxicity, bone marrow depression

NURSING CONSIDERATIONS
Assessment
- ❗ Assess any patient with compromised renal system: drug is excreted slowly in poor renal system function; toxicity may occur rapidly
- Assess patient for infection including increased temp, thick sputum, WBC >10,000; monitor these signs of infection throughout treatment; obtain C&S before beginning therapy; treatment may begin after culture is obtained
- Assess respiratory system including rate, rhythm, bilateral lung sounds, shortness of breath, wheezing, dyspnea
- Monitor ECG for cardiac dysrhythmias; ECG and pulse should be checked frequently during treatment, since cardiotoxicity can occur
- Assess for hypoglycemia including nausea, tremors, anxiety, chills, diaphoresis, headache, hunger, cold, pale skin; this side effect can last for several mo after treatment is completed
- Monitor for hyperglycemia including flushed, dry skin, acetone breath, thirst, an-

P

orexia, drowsiness, polyuria; this side effect can last for several mo after treatment is completed

- Monitor renal studies including BUN, urinalysis, creatinine; obtain at baseline and frequently during treatment; nephrotoxicity may occur; check I&O, report hematuria, oliguria
- Monitor blood studies including blood glucose, CBC, platelets; blood glucose fluctuations are common; anemia, leukopenia, thrombocytopenia can occur
- Monitor liver studies including AST (SGOT), ALT (SGPT), alkaline phosphatase, bilirubin before beginning treatment and every 3 days during therapy
- Monitor calcium before beginning treatment and every 3 days during therapy; hypocalcemia may occur

Nursing diagnoses

- ✓ Infection, risk for (uses)
- ✓ Knowledge deficit (teaching)

Implementation

IM route

- Reconstitute 300 mg/3 ml sterile water for inj; give deep in large muscle mass; IM is a painful route

IV **IV route**

- For intermittent inf reconstitute 300 mg/3-5 ml sterile water for inj, D_5W; withdraw dose and further dilute in 50-250 ml D_5W; diluted sol is stable for 48 hr; discard unused sol; give over 1 hr or more

Y-site incompatibilities: Foscarnet, fluconazole

Y-site compatibility: Zidovudine

Inh route

- Dilute 300 mg/600 ml sterile water for inj; put reconstituted sol into nebulizer; do not use with other drugs or sol precipitate may occur; stable for 48 hr at room temp; protect from light; administer over 30-45 min

Patient/family education

- Teach patient to report sore throat, fever, fatigue; could indicate superinfection
- Advise patient not to drink alcohol or take aspirin, since gastric bleeding may occur
- Teach patient to make position changes slowly to prevent orthostatic hypotension

Evaluation

Positive therapeutic outcome

- Decreased signs and symptoms of protozoan infections
- Decreased signs and symptoms of *Pneumocystis carinii* pneumonia in HIV infections

pentazocine (℞)

(pen-taz'oh-seen)

Talwin, Talwin NX

Func. class.: Narcotic analgesic

Chem. class.: Synthetic benzomorphan (agonist/antagonist)

Pregnancy category C

Controlled substance schedule IV

Action: Inhibits ascending pain pathways in limbic system, thalamus, midbrain, hypothalamus by binding to opiate receptor sites, altering pain perception and response

Therapeutic Outcome: Relief of pain

Uses: Moderate to severe pain

Dosage and routes

Adult: PO 50-100 mg q3-4h prn, not to exceed 600 mg/day; **IV**/IM/SC 30 mg q34h prn, not to exceed 360 mg/day

Available forms: SC, IM, IV 30 mg/ml; tab 50 mg

Adverse effects

CNS: Drowsiness, dizziness, confusion, headache, sedation, euphoria, hallucinations, dreaming

CV: Palpitations, bradycardia, change in B/P, tachycardia, increased B/P (high doses)

EENT: Tinnitus, blurred vision, miosis (high doses), diplopia

GI: Nausea, vomiting, anorexia, constipation, cramps

GU: Urinary retention

INTEG: Rash, urticaria, bruising, flushing, diaphoresis, pruritus, severe irritation at inj sites

RESP: Respiratory depression

Contraindications: Hypersensitivity, addiction (narcotic)

Precautions: Addictive personality, pregnancy **C,** lactation, increased intracranial pressure, MI (acute), severe heart disease, respiratory depression, hepatic disease, renal disease, seizure disorder, child <18 yr

Pharmacokinetics

Absorption	Well absorbed (PO, SC, IM); completely absorbed (IV)
Distribution	Widely distributed; crosses placenta
Metabolism	Liver, extensively
Excretion	Kidneys, small amounts (unchanged)
Half-life	2-3 hr

Pharmacodynamics

	PO	SC/IM	IV
Onset	15-30 min	15-30 min	Rapid
Peak	1-3 hr	1-2 hr	15 min
Duration	3 hr	2-4 hr	1 hr

Interactions

Individual drugs

Alcohol: ↑ respiratory depression, hypotension, sedation

Drug classifications

Antihistamines: ↑ respiratory depression, hypotension

CNS depressants: ↑ respiratory depression, hypotension

MAOIs: Use cautiously; results are unpredictable

Phenothiazines: ↑ respiratory depression, hypotension

Opioid agonists: ↑ opioid withdrawals (dependency)

Sedative/hypnotics: ↑ respiratory depression, hypotension

Lab test interferences

↑ Amylase, ↑ lipase

NURSING CONSIDERATIONS

Assessment

- Assess pain characteristics: location, intensity, type of pain before medication administration and following treatment
- Monitor VS after parenteral route; note muscle rigidity, drug history, liver, kidney function tests, respiratory dysfunction: respiratory depression, character, rate, rhythm; notify prescriber if respirations are <10/min

- Monitor CNS changes: dizziness, drowsiness, hallucinations, euphoria, LOC, pupil reaction
- Monitor allergic reactions: rash, urticaria

Nursing diagnoses

☑ Pain (uses)
☑ Sensory-perceptual alteration: visual, auditory (adverse reactions)
☑ Breathing pattern, ineffective (adverse reactions)
☑ Knowledge deficit (teaching)

Implementation

- Give by inj (IM, **IV**), only when resuscitative equipment available; give slowly to prevent rigidity
- Store in light-resistant area at room temp

PO route

- Tab made in the United States contain naloxone 0.5 mg to prevent abuse if the PO preparation is used **IV**

IM route

- Give deeply in large muscle mass; rotate inj sites

IV **IV route**

- Give by direct **IV** after diluting 5 mg/ml of sterile water for inj; give 5 mg or less over 1 min

Syringe incompatibilities: Glycopyrrolate, heparin, pentobarbital, other barbiturates

Syringe compatibilities: Atropine, benzquinamide, butorphanol, chlorpromazine, cimetidine, dimenhydrinate, diphenhydramine, droperidol, fentanyl, hydromorphone, hydroxyzine, meperidine, metoclopramide, morphine, perphenazine, prochlorperazine, promazine, promethazine, propiomazine, ranitidine, scopolamine

Y-site incompatibility: Nafcillin

Y-site compatibilities: Heparin, hydrocortisone, potassium chloride, vitamin B with C

Additive incompatibilities: Aminophylline, amobarbital, pentobarbital, phenobarbital, secobarbital, sodium bicarbonate

Patient/family education

- Teach patient to report any symptoms of CNS changes, allergic reactions
- Advise patients to avoid CNS depressants: alcohol, sedative/hypnotics for at least 24 hr after taking this drug
- Discuss with patient that dizziness, drowsiness, and confusion are common; to avoid getting up without assistance
- Discuss in detail all aspects of the drug
- Instruct patient to change position slowly to prevent orthostatic hypotension
- Teach patient to turn, cough, deep breathe after surgery to prevent atelectasis

Evaluation

Positive therapeutic outcome

- Relief of pain

Treatment of overdose: Naloxone (Narcan) 0.2-0.8 **IV**, O_2, **IV** fluids, vasopressors

pentobarbital (℞)
(pen-toe-bar'bi-tal)
Nembutal, Nembutal Sodium, Nembutal Sodium Solution, Nova-Rectal ✤, pentobarbital sodium, Pentogen ✤
Func. class.: Sedative/hypnotic barbiturate
Chem. class.: Barbitone, short acting

Pregnancy category D
Controlled substance schedule II (USA), schedule G (Canada)

Action: Depresses activity in brain cells, primarily in reticular activating system in brainstem; also selectively depresses neurons in posterior hypothalamus, limbic structures; may decrease cerebral blood flow, intracranial pressure (**IV**) and cerebral edema; may potentiate GABA, an inhibitory neurotransmitter

→ **Therapeutic Outcome:** Sedation, sleep

Uses: Insomnia, sedation, preoperative medication, increased intracranial pressure, dental anesthetic

Dosage and routes
Adult: PO 100-200 mg hs; IM 150-200 mg hs; **IV** 100 mg initially, then up to 500 mg; rec 120-200 mg hs
P ***Child:*** IM 3-5 mg, not to exceed 100 mg
P ***Child 2 mo-1 yr:*** Rec 30 mg
P ***Child 1-4 yr:*** Rec 30-60 mg
P ***Child 5-12 yr:*** Rec 60 mg
P ***Child 12-14 yr:*** Rec 60120 mg

Available forms: Caps 50, 100 mg; elix 18.2 mg/5 ml; powder, rec supp 30, 60, 120, 200 mg; inj 50 mg/ml

Adverse effects
CNS: Lethargy, drowsiness, hangover, dizziness, paradoxic G stimulation in elderly and P children, lightheadedness, dependence, ***CNS depression,*** mental depression, slurred speech
CV: Hypotension, bradycardia
GI: Nausea, vomiting, diarrhea, constipation
HEMA: Agranulocytosis, thrombocytopenia, megaloblastic anemia (long-term treatment)
INTEG: Rash, urticaria, pain, abscesses at inj site, angioedema, thrombophlebitis, ***Stevens-Johnson syndrome***
RESP: Depression, apnea, laryngospasm, bronchospasm

Contraindications: Hypersensitivity to barbiturates, respiratory depression, addiction to barbiturates, severe liver, renal impairment, porphyria, uncontrolled pain

Precautions: Anemia, pregnancy **D,** lactation, hepatic disease, renal disease, hyper- G tension, elderly, acute/chronic pain

Pharmacokinetics	
Absorption	Well absorbed
Distribution	Widely distributed; crosses placenta, enters breast milk
Metabolism	Liver
Excretion	Kidneys, unchanged (minimally)
Half-life	15-48 hr

P

Pharmacodynamics

	PO	IM	IV	REC
Onset	15-30 min	10-25 min	Immediate	Slow
Peak	3-4 hr	Unknown	1 min	Unknown
Duration	4-6 hr	1-4 hr	15 min	4-6 hr

Interactions:

Individual drugs

Alcohol: ↑ CNS depression
Chloramphenicol: ↓ effectiveness
Cyclosporine: ↓ effectiveness
Dacarbazine: ↓ effectiveness
Cyclophosphamide: ↑ hematologic toxicity
Quinidine: ↓ effectiveness
Valproic acid: ↑ sedation

Drug classifications

Anticoagulants: ↓ effectiveness
Antidepressants: ↑ CNS depression
Antihistamines: ↑ CNS depression
Glucocorticoids: ↓ effectiveness
MAOIs: ↑ CNS depression
Narcotics: ↑ CNS depression
Oral contraceptives: ↓ effectiveness
Sedative/hypnotics: ↑ CNS depression
Tricyclic antidepressants: ↓ effectiveness

NURSING CONSIDERATIONS

Assessment

- Assess mental status: mood, sensorium, affect, memory (long, short), especially elderly [G]; if using as a hypnotic, assess sleep patterns during therapy; drug suppresses REM sleep with dreaming; withdrawal insomnia may occur after short-term use; do not start using drug again; insomnia will improve in 1-3 nights; may experience increased dreaming
- Monitor for respiratory dysfunction: respiratory depression, character, rate, rhythm (when using **IV**); hold drug if respirations are <10/min or if pupils are dilated; also check VS q30 min after parenteral route for 2 hr
- Assess for blood dyscrasias: fever, sore throat, bruising, rash, jaundice, epistaxis (long-term treatment only)
- Assess seizure activity including type, location, duration, and character; provide seizure precaution
- Assess for pain in postoperative patients; pain threshold is lowered when patients are taking this medication

Nursing diagnoses

✓ Injury, risk for (side effects)
✓ Knowledge deficit (teaching)

Implementation

- Administer only after removal of cigarettes, to prevent fires
- Reserve use until after trying conservative measures for insomnia

PO route

- Give 30 min before hs for expected sleeplessness
- May dilute elixir in juice, milk, or water if needed
- Give on empty stomach for best absorption

IM route

- Give deeply in muscle mass (gluteal) to minimize irritation to tissues; split inj of >5 ml into two since irritation to tissues may occur; do not administer SC

[IV] **IV route**

- Use large vein to prevent extravasation; if extravasation occurs, use moist heat to the area and 5% procaine sol injected into area; give at 50 mg/1 min or more

- Give **IV** only with resuscitative equipment available (and only by qualified personnel)

Syringe compatibilities: Aminophylline, ephedrine, hydromorphone, neostigmine, scopolamine, sodium bicarbonate, thiopental

Syringe incompatibilities: Benzquinamide, butorphanol, chlorpromazine, cimetidine, dimenhydrinate, diphenhydramine, droperidol, fentanyl, glycopyrrolate, hydroxyzine, meperidine, midazolam, nalbuphine, pentazocine, perphenazine, prochlorperazine, promazine, promethazine, ranitidine

Y-site compatibilities: Acyclovir, regular insulin

Additive compatibilities: Amikacin, aminophylline, calcium chloride, cephapirin, chloramphenicol, dimenhydrinate, erythromycin, lidocaine, thiopental, verapamil

Additive incompatibilities: Chlorpheniramine, codeine, ephedrine, erythromycin gluceptate, regular insulin, levorphanol, hydrocortisone, sodium succinate, hydroxyzine, methadone, norepinephrine, pentazocine, penicillin G potassium, phenytoin, promazine, promethazine, streptomycin, triflupromazine, vancomycin

Patient/family education

- Teach patient to carry ID card or Medic Alert bracelet stating name, drugs taken, condition, prescriber's name, phone number
- Caution patient to avoid driving and other activities that require alertness
- Caution patient to avoid alcohol ingestion and CNS depressants; increased sedation may occur
- Teach patient not to discontinue medication quickly after long-term use; taper off over several wk

Evaluation

Positive therapeutic outcome

- Improved sleeping patterns
- Decreased seizure activity
- Improved energy

Treatment of overdose: Lavage, activated charcoal, warming blanket, vital signs, hemodialysis

pentosan polysulfate sodium (℞)

(pen-toe-san' pol-ee-sul'fate)

Elmiron

Func. class.: Urinary analgesic

Pregnancy category B

P

Action: Low-molecular-weight heparin-like compound; mechanism of action for interstitial cystitis is unknown; may act as a buffer on bladder wall mucosal membrane

➔ **Therapeutic Outcome:** Decreased pain in cystitis

Uses: UTI used with a urinary antiinfective

Dosage and routes

Adult: PO 100 mg tid

Available forms: Cap 100 mg

Adverse effects

CNS: Headache, insomnia

GI: Nausea, vomiting, diarrhea, anorexia, ***hepatic toxicity***
HEMA: Thrombocytopenia, leukopenia, increased PT, PTT
INTEG: Rash, urticaria, alopecia, photosensitivity

Contraindications: Hypersensitivity

Precautions: Pregnancy **B**, renal disease

Pharmacokinetics

Absorption	Unknown
Distribution	Unknown
Metabolism	Liver
Excretion	Kidneys
Half-life	Unknown

Pharmacodynamics

Unknown

Interactions Unknown

NURSING CONSIDERATIONS

Assessment

- Assess urinary status: burning, pain, itching, urgency, frequency, hematuria; before and after completion of treatment
- Assess hepatotoxicity: dark urine, clay-colored stools, yellow skin and sclera, itching, abdominal pain, fever, diarrhea if patient is on long-term therapy
- Assess allergic reactions; rash, urticaria; drug may have to be discontinued

Nursing diagnoses

✓ Pain (uses)
✓ Knowledge deficit (teaching)

Implementation

- Give to patient whole, do not crush or chew capsule
- Give with food or milk to decrease gastric symptoms

Patient/family education

- Teach patient not to exceed recommended dosage and to take with meals
- Teach patient to discontinue after pain is relieved but continue to take concurrent prescribed antibiotic until finished

Evaluation

Positive therapeutic outcome

- Decreased pain of cystitis

pentostatin (℞)

(pen′toe-sta-tin)

Nipent

Func. class.: Antineoplastic, enzyme inhibitor
Chem. class.: Streptomyces antibioticus derivative

Pregnancy category C

Action: Inhibits the enzyme adenosine deaminase (ADA), which is able to block DNA synthesis and some RNA synthesis

Therapeutic Outcome: Prevention of rapidly growing malignant cells

Uses: α-Interferon–refractory hairy cell leukemia, chronic lymphocytic leukemia

Dosage and routes

Adult: **IV** 4 mg/m^2 every other wk; may be given **IV** bol or diluted in a larger volume and given over 20-30 min

Available forms: Inj 10 mg/vial

Adverse effects

CNS: Headache, anxiety, confusion, depression, dizziness, insomnia, nervousness, paresthesia
GI: Nausea, vomiting, anorexia, diarrhea, constipation,

flatulence, stomatitis, elevated liver function tests
GU: ***Hematuria,*** dysuria, increased BUN/creatinine
HEMA: ***Leukopenia, anemia, thrombocytopenia, ecchymosis, lymphadenopathy,*** petechiae
INTEG: Rash, eczema, dry skin, pruritus, sweating, herpes simplex/zoster
RESP: Cough, upper respiratory tract infection, bronchitis, dyspnea, epistaxis, pneumonia, pharyngitis, rhinitis, sinusitis
SYST: Fever, infection, fatigue, pain, allergic reaction, chills, ***death, sepsis,*** chest pain, flu syndrome

Contraindications: Hypersensitivity to this drug or mannitol

Precautions: Renal disease, pregnancy C, lactation, children, bone marrow depression

Pharmacokinetics

Absorption	Completely absorbed
Distribution	Unknown; low protein binding
Metabolism	Unknown
Excretion	Kidneys
Half-life	5-7 hr; increased in renal disease

Pharmacodynamics

Onset	4-5 mo
Peak	Unknown
Duration	1½-34 mo

Interactions
Individual drugs
Fludarabine: Fatal pulmonary reaction
Vidarabine: ↑ adverse reactions

NURSING CONSIDERATIONS
Assessment
- Assess CNS changes: confusion, paresthesias, psychosis, tremors, seizures, neuropathies; drug should be discontinued
- Assess for toxicity: facial flushing, epistaxis, increased pro-time, thrombocytopenia; drug should be discontinued
- Assess acidosis, signs of dehydration: rapid respirations, poor skin turgor, decreased urine output, dry skin, restlessness, weakness
- Check buccal cavity q8h for dryness, sores or ulceration, white patches, oral pain, bleeding, dysphagia; obtain prescription for viscous lidocaine (Xylocaine) to use in mouth
- Assess symptoms indicating severe allergic reaction: rash, pruritus, urticaria, purpuric skin lesions, itching, flushing
- Assess tachypnea, ECG changes, dyspnea, edema, fatigue; respiratory and cardiovascular reaction can be severe
- Monitor CBC, differential, platelet count weekly; withhold drug if WBC count is <4000/mm^3 or platelet count is <100,000/mm^3, notify prescriber of results
- Monitor renal function studies: BUN, creatinine, serum uric acid, urine CrCl before and during therapy; I&O ratio; report fall in urine output to <30 ml/hr
- Monitor temp q4h (may indicate beginning of infection)
- Monitor liver function tests before and during therapy (bilirubin, AST [SGOT], ALT [SGPT], LDH) as needed or monthly; check for yellowing of skin and sclera, dark urine, clay-colored stools, itchy skin, abdominal pain, fever, diarrhea
- Assess for bleeding: hematuria, stool guaiac, bruising or petechiae, mucosa or orifices

q8h; check for inflammation of mucosa, breaks in skin
- Assess effects of alopecia on body image; discuss feelings about body changes

Nursing diagnoses

- ✓ Injury, risk for (adverse reactions)
- ✓ Body image disturbance (adverse reactions)
- ✓ Infection, risk for (adverse reactions)
- ✓ Knowledge deficit (teaching)

Implementation

- Give fluids **IV** or PO before chemotherapy to hydrate patient
- Give antacid before oral agent, antiemetic 30-60 min before giving drug and prn to prevent vomiting; administer antibiotics for prophylaxis of infection
- Give top or syst analgesics for pain to lessen effects from stomatitis
- Give liq diet: carbonated beverages; gelatin may be added if patient is not nauseated or vomiting
- Encourage patient to rinse mouth tid-qid with water, club soda; brush teeth bid-qid with soft brush or cotton-tipped applicators for stomatitis; use unwaxed dental floss
- Preparation should be done by personnel knowledgeable in preparing antineoplastics wearing gloves, gown, mask in biologic cabinet
- Give by direct **IV** by reconstituting 10 mg/5 ml of sterile water for inj (2 mg/ml); shake well
- Give over 5 min
- Give by intermittent inf after diluting 10 mg/25-50 ml of 0.9% NaCl, D_5W; give over 30 min
- Diluted sol should be used within 8 hr at room temp

Y-site compatibilities: Fludarabine, melphalan, ondansetron, paclitaxel, sargramostim

Solution compatibilities: D_5W, 0.9% NaCl, LR

Patient/family education

- Teach patient to avoid use of products containing aspirin or ibuprofen, razors, commercial mouthwash, since bleeding may occur; to report symptoms of bleeding (hematuria, tarry stools)
- Advise patient to report signs of anemia (fatigue, headache, irritability, faintness, shortness of breath); CNS reactions including confusion, psychosis, nightmares, seizures, severe headaches
- Inform patient that hair may be lost during treatment; a wig or hair piece may make patient feel better; new hair may be different in color, texture
- Advise patient to use sunscreen and protective clothing to prevent photosensitive reactions

Evaluation

Positive therapeutic outcome

- Prevention of rapid division of malignant cells
- Decreased bone marrow hairy cells

pentoxifylline (℞)
(pen-tox-if'i-lin)
Trental
Func. class.: Hemorheologic agent
Chem. class.: Dimethylxanthine derivative
Pregnancy category C

Action: Decreases blood viscosity, stimulates prostacyclin formation, increases blood flow by increasing flexibility of RBCs; decreases RBC hyperaggregation; reduces platelet aggregation, decreases fibrinogen concentration

➡ **Therapeutic Outcome:** Decreased claudication and improved blood flow

Uses: Intermittent claudication related to chronic occlusive vascular disease

Investigational uses: Cerebrovascular insufficiency, diabetic neuropathies, TIAs, leg ulcers, strokes

Dosage and routes
Adult: PO 400 mg tid with meals

Available forms: Cont rel tab 400 mg

Adverse effects
CNS: Headache, anxiety, *tremors,* confusion, *dizziness*
CV: Angina, dysrhythmias, palpitations, hypotension, chest pain, dyspnea, edema
EENT: Blurred vision, earache, increased salivation, sore throat, conjunctivitis
GI: Dyspepsia, nausea, vomiting, anorexia, bloating, belching, constipation, cholecystitis, dry mouth, thirst, bad taste
INTEG: Rash, pruritus, urticaria, brittle fingernails
MISC: Epistaxis, flulike symptoms, laryngitis, nasal congestion, ***leukopenia,*** malaise, weight changes

Contraindications: Hypersensitivity to this drug or xanthines, retinal/cerebral hemorrhage

Precautions: Pregnancy C, angina pectoris, cardiac disease, P lactation, children, impaired renal function, recent surgery, peptic ulcer

Pharmacokinetics

Absorption	Well absorbed
Distribution	Unknown
Metabolism	Liver, degradation
Excretion	Kidneys
Half-life	½-1 hr

Pharmacodynamics

Onset	Unknown
Peak	1 hr
Duration	Unknown

Interactions
Individual drugs
Theophylline: ↑ theophylline level

NURSING CONSIDERATIONS
Assessment
- Monitor B/P, respirations in patient taking antihypertensives
- Assess for intermittent claudication during treatment

Nursing diagnoses
☑ Pain (uses)
☑ Activity intolerance (uses)
☑ Knowledge deficit (teaching)
☑ Noncompliance (teaching)

Implementation
- Give with meals to prevent GI upset
- ⊘ Tab should not be crushed or chewed

P

Patient/family education
- Teach patient that therapeutic response may take 2-4 wk
- Advise patient that decreased fats, cholesterol, increased exercise, decreased smoking are necessary to correct condition
- Instruct patient to observe feet for arterial insufficiency
- Instruct patient to use cotton socks, well-fitted shoes; not to go barefoot
- Advise patient to watch for bleeding, bruises, petechiae, epistaxis

Evaluation
Positive therapeutic outcome
- Decreased pain, cramping
- Increased ambulation

perphenazine (℞)
(per-fen'a-zeen)
Apo-Perphenazine ✤, Trilafon, perphenazine, Phenazine ✤, PMS Perphenazine ✤
Func. class.: Antipsychotic/neuroleptic
Chem. class.: Phenothiazine piperidine

Pregnancy category C

Action: Depresses cerebral cortex, hypothalamus, limbic system, which control activity, aggression; blocks neurotransmission produced by dopamine at synapse; exhibits strong α-adrenergic, anticholinergic blocking action; as antiemetic inhibits medullary chemoreceptor trigger zone; mechanism for antipsychotic effects is unclear

➡ **Therapeutic Outcome:** Decreased signs and symptoms of psychosis; decreased nausea and vomiting

Uses: Psychotic disorders, schizophrenia, nausea, vomiting

Dosage and routes
Nausea/vomiting/alcoholism
P ***Adult and child >12 yr:*** IM 5-10 mg prn, max 15 mg in ambulatory patients, 30 mg in hospitalized patients; PO 8-16 mg/day in divided doses, up to 24 mg; **IV** not to exceed 5 mg; give diluted or slow **IV** drip

Psychiatric use in hospitalized patients
Adults: PO 8-16 mg bid-qid, gradually increased to desired dose, not to exceed 64 mg/day; IM 5 mg q6h, not to exceed 30 mg/day

P ***Child >12 yr:*** PO 6-12 mg in divided doses

Nonhospitalized patients
Adult: PO 4-8 mg tid; IM 5 mg q6h

Available forms: Tabs 2, 4, 8, 16 mg; oral sol 16 mg/5ml; inj 5 mg/ml

Adverse effects
CNS: EPS: pseudoparkinsonism, akathisia, dystonia, tardive dyskinesia, ***seizures, headache***
CV: Orthostatic hypotension, ***cardiac arrest,*** ECG changes, ***tachycardia***
EENT: Blurred vision, glaucoma
GI: Dry mouth, nausea, vomiting, anorexia, constipation, diarrhea, jaundice, weight gain
GU: Urinary retention, urinary frequency, enuresis, impotence, amenorrhea, gynecomastia
HEMA: Anemia, ***leukopenia, leukocytosis, agranulocytosis***
INTEG: Rash, photosensitivity, dermatitis

*RESP: **Laryngospasm**,* dyspnea, ***respiratory depression***

Contraindications: Hypersensitivity, blood dyscrasias, coma, P child <12 yr, brain damage, bone marrow depression

Precautions: Pregnancy **C**, lactation, seizure disorders, hypertension, hepatic disease, cardiac disease

Pharmacokinetics

Absorption	Variably absorbed (PO); well absorbed (IM)
Distribution	Widely distributed; high concentrations in CNS; crosses placenta
Metabolism	Liver, extensively; GI mucosa
Excretion	Kidneys

Pharmacodynamics

	PO	IM	IV
Onset	Erratic	10 min	Rapid
Peak	2-4 hr	1-2 hr	Unknown
Duration	6-12 hr	6-12 hr	Unknown

Interactions

Individual drugs

Alcohol: ↑ effects of both drugs, oversedation
Aluminum hydroxide: ↓ absorption
Bromocriptine: ↓ antiparkinson activity
Disopyramide: ↑ anticholinergic effects
Epinephrine: ↑ toxicity
Guanethidine: ↓ antihypertensive response
Levodopa: ↓ antiparkinson activity
Lithium: ↓ perphenazine levels, ↑ EPS, masking of lithium toxicity
Magnesium hydroxide: ↓ absorption
Norepinephrine: ↓ vasoresponse, ↑ toxicity
Phenobarbital: ↓ effectiveness, ↑ metabolism

Drug classifications

Antacids: ↓ absorption
Anticholinergics: ↑ anticholinergic effects
Antidepressants: ↑ CNS depression
Antidiarrheals, adsorbent: ↓ absorption
Antihistamines: ↑ CNS depression
Antihypertensives: ↑ hypotension
Antithyroid agents: ↑ agranulocytosis
Barbiturate anesthetics: ↑ CNS depression
β-Adrenergics: ↑ effects of both drugs
General anesthetics: ↑ CNS depression
MAOIs: ↑ CNS depression
Narcotics: ↑ CNS depression
Sedative/hypnotics: ↑ CNS depression

Lab test interferences

↑ Liver function tests, ↑ cardiac enzymes, ↑ cholesterol, ↑ blood glucose, ↑ prolactin, ↑ bilirubin, ↑ PBI, ↑ cholinesterase, ↑ iodine, ↑ alkaline phosphatase, ↑ leukocytes, ↑ granulocytes, ↑ platelets
↓ Hormones (blood and urine)
False positive: Pregnancy tests, PKU
False negative: Urinary steroids, 17-OHCS

NURSING CONSIDERATIONS

Assessment

- Assess mental status: orientation, mood, behavior, presence and type of hallucinations before initial administration and monthly; this drug should significantly reduce psychotic behavior
- Check for swallowing of PO medication; check for hoarding

P

or giving medication to other patients
- Monitor I&O ratio; palpate bladder if low urinary output occurs, especially in elderly; urinalysis recommended before, during prolonged therapy
- Monitor bilirubin, CBC, liver function studies monthly
- Assess affect, orientation, LOC, reflexes, gait, coordination, sleep pattern disturbances
- Monitor B/P with patient sitting, standing, and lying; take pulse and respirations q4h during initial treatment; establish baseline before starting treatment; report drops of 30 mm Hg; obtain baseline ECG, Q wave and T wave changes
- Check for dizziness, faintness, palpitations, tachycardia on rising; severe orthostatic hypotension is common
- Identify for neuroleptic malignant syndrome: hyperpyrexia, muscle rigidity, increased CPK, altered mental status; drug should be discontinued
- Assess for EPS including akathisia (inability to sit still, no pattern to movements), tardive dyskinesia (bizarre movements of the jaw, mouth, tongue, extremities), pseudoparkinsonism (ragged tremors, pill rolling, shuffling gate); an antiparkinsonian drug should be prescribed
- Assess for constipation, urinary retention daily; if these occur, increase bulk, water in diet

Nursing diagnoses
- ✓ Thought processes, altered (uses)
- ✓ Coping, ineffective individual (uses)
- ✓ Knowledge deficit (teaching)
- ✓ Noncompliance (teaching)

Implementation

PO route
- Administer drug in liq form mixed in glass of juice or cola if hoarding is suspected; do not mix in caffeine drinks, tannics, pectins
- Repeat-action tab should be taken whole
- Administer decreased dose in elderly, in whom metabolism is slowed
- Administer PO with full glass of water, milk; or give with food to decrease GI upset
- Store in airtight, light-resistant container; oral sol in amber bottle

IM route
- Inject in deep muscle mass; do not give SC; do not administer sol with a precipitate

IV route
- Give by direct **IV** after diluting with 0.9% NaCl to a conc of 0.5 mg/1 ml; administer at 1 mg/min; may be further diluted and given as an inf

Syringe incompatibilities: Midazolam, opium alkaloids, pentobarbital, thiethylperazine

Syringe compatibilities: Atropine, benztropine, butorphanol, chlorpromazine, cimetidine, dimenhydrinate, diphenhydramine, droperidol, fentanyl, meperidine, metoclopramide, morphine, pentazocine, prochlorperazine, promethazine, scopolamine

Y-site compatibilities: Acyclovir, amikacin, ampicillin, azlocillin, cefamandole, cefazolin, ceforanide, cefotaxime, cefoxitin, cefuroxime, cephalothin, cephapirin, chloramphenicol, clindamycin, co-trimoxazole, doxycycline, erythromycin, famotidine, gentamicin, kanamycin, metronidazole, mezlocillin, minocycline, moxalactam, nafcillin, oxacillin, penicillin G potassium, piperacillin, sulfamethoxazole, tacrolimus, tetracycline, ticarcillin, ticarcillin/clavulanate, tobramycin, trimethoprim, vancomycin

Additive incompatibility: Cefoperazone

Additive compatibilities: Ascorbic acid, ethacrynate, netilmicin

Patient/family education

- Teach patient to use good oral hygiene; frequent rinsing of mouth, sugarless gum for dry mouth
- Advise patient to avoid hazardous activities until drug response is determined, dizziness, blurred vision may occur
- Inform patient that orthostatic hypotension occurs often and to rise from sitting or lying position gradually; to remain lying down after IM inj for at least 30 min; tell patient to avoid hot tubs, hot showers, tub baths, since hypotension may occur; teach patient that in hot weather heat stroke may occur; take extra precautions to stay cool
- Teach patient to avoid abrupt withdrawal of this drug, or EPS may result; drug should be withdrawn slowly
- Teach patient to avoid OTC preparations (cough, hay fever, cold) unless approved by prescriber, since serious drug interactions may occur; avoid use with alcohol, CNS depressants; increased drowsiness may result
- Caution patient to use a sunscreen and sunglasses to prevent burns
- Teach patient about EPS and necessity of meticulous oral hygiene, since oral candidiasis may occur
- Instruct patient to take antacids 2 hr before or after taking this drug
- Teach patient to report sore throat, malaise, fever, bleeding, mouth sores; if these occur, CBC should be drawn and drug discontinued
- Teach patient that urine may turn pink or red

Evaluation

Positive therapeutic outcome

- Decrease in emotional excitement, hallucinations, delusions, paranoia
- Reorganization of patterns of thought, speech

Treatment of overdose: Lavage if orally ingested; provide airway; *do not induce vomiting or use epinephrine*

phenazopyridine (℞)

(fen-az-o-peer′i-deen)

Azo-Standard, Baridium, Phenazo ✤, Phenazodine, phenazopyridine HCl, Prodium, Pyridiate, Pyridate No. 2, Pyridium, Urogesic

Func. class.: Nonnarcotic analgesic

Chem. class.: Azodye

Pregnancy category B

Action: Exerts analgesic, anesthetic action on the urinary tract mucosa

Uses: Urinary tract irritation, infection (for symptoms only of pain, burning, itching) used with urinary antiinfectives

Dosage and routes

Adult: PO 200 mg tid x 2 days

P

or less when used with antibacterial for UTI

P ***Child 6-12 yr:*** PO 12 mg/kg/24 hr in divided doses × 2 days

Available forms: Tabs 95, 100, 200 mg

Adverse effects

CNS: Headache

GI: ***Nausea, vomiting, diarrhea, heartburn,*** anorexia, ***hepatic toxicity***

GU: Renal toxicity, orange-red urine

HEMA: Thrombocytopenia, agranulocytosis, leukopenia, neutropenia, hemolytic anemia, methemoglobinemia

INTEG: Rash, pruritus, skin pigmentation

Contraindications: Hypersensitivity, renal insufficiency

Precautions: Pregnancy **B,** P renal disease, lactation, children <12 yr

Pharmacokinetics	
Absorption	Well absorbed
Distribution	Unknown; crosses placenta
Metabolism	Unknown
Excretion	Kidneys, unchanged
Half-life	Unknown

Pharmacodynamics	
Onset	Unknown
Peak	5-6 hr
Duration	8 hr

Interactions: None

Lab test interferences

Interference: Urinalysis

NURSING CONSIDERATIONS

Assessment

- Assess urinary status: burning, pain, itching, urgency, frequency, hematuria before, during and after completion of drug therapy
- Monitor liver function studies: AST (SGOT), ALT (SGPT), bilirubin if patient is on long-term therapy
- Assess for hepatotoxicity: dark urine, clay-colored stools, yellowing of skin and sclera, itching, abdominal pain, fever, diarrhea if patient is on long-term therapy
- Assess for allergic reactions: rash, urticaria; if these occur, drug may have to be discontinued

Nursing diagnoses

- ✓ Pain (uses)
- ✓ Urinary elimination, altered patterns (uses)
- ✓ Knowledge deficit (teaching)

Implementation

- Give to patient crushed or whole; chew tab may be chewed
- Give with food or milk to decrease gastric symptoms

Patient/family education

- Advise patient to report any symptoms of hepatotoxicity
- Caution patient not to exceed recommended dosage and to take with meals; to read label on other OTC drugs
- Teach patient not to discontinue after pain is relieved but continue to take concurrent prescribed antibiotic until finished
- Inform patient urine may turn red-orange, may stain clothing or contact lens

Evaluation

Positive therapeutic outcome

- Decrease in pain, burning, itching when urinating

Treatment of overdose: Methylene blue 1-2 mg/kg **IV** or 100-200 mg vitamin C PO

phenelzine (℞)

(fen′el-zeen)

Nardil

Func. class.: Antidepressant, MAOI

Chem. class.: Hydrazine

Pregnancy category C

Action: Increases concentrations of endogenous epinephrine, norepinephrine, serotonin, dopamine in storage sites in CNS by inhibition of MAO; increased concentration reduces depression

➔ **Therapeutic Outcome:** Decreased symptoms of depression after 2-3 wk

Uses: Depression, when uncontrolled by other means

Investigational uses: Bulimia, cocaine addiction, migraines, seasonal affective disorder, panic disorder

Dosage and routes

Adult: PO 45 mg/day in divided doses; may increase to 60 mg/day

Available forms: Tab 15 mg

Adverse effects

CNS: Dizziness, drowsiness, confusion, headache, anxiety, tremors, stimulation, weakness, hyperreflexia, mania, insomnia, fatigue, weight gain

CV: Orthostatic hypotension, hypertension, dysrhythmias, hypertensive crisis

EENT: Blurred vision

ENDO: SIADH-like syndrome

GI: Constipation, dry mouth, nausea, vomiting, *anorexia,* diarrhea, weight gain

GU: Change in libido, frequency of urination

HEMA: Anemia

INTEG: Rash, flushing, increased perspiration

Contraindications: Hypersensitivity to MAOIs, G elderly, hypertension, CHF, severe hepatic disease, pheochromocytoma, severe renal disease, severe cardiac disease

Precautions: Suicidal patients, convulsive disorders, severe depression, schizophrenia, hyperactivity, diabetes mellitus, pregnancy **C**

Pharmacokinetics

Absorption	Well absorbed
Distribution	Crosses placenta
Metabolism	Liver, extensively
Excretion	Kidneys, breast milk
Half-life	Unknown

Pharmacodynamics

Unknown

Interactions

Individual drugs

Alcohol: ↑ CNS depression

Clonidine: Severe hypotension; avoid use

Guanethidine: ↓ effects

L-**tryptophan:** ↑ confusion, shivering, hyperreflexia

Sulfonamide: ↑ toxicity

Sumatriptan: ↑ toxicity

Drug classifications

Analgesics: ↑ CNS depression

Anticholinergics: ↑ side effects

Antidiabetics: ↑ hypoglycemia

Antihistamines: ↑ CNS depression

Antihypertensives: May block antihypertensive effect

Barbiturates: ↑ effects of barbiturates

Benzodiazepines: ↑ effects of benzodiazepines

CNS depressants: ↑ effects of CNS depressants

P

Diuretics, thiazide: ↑ hypotension
Oral contraceptives: ↑ effects, toxicity
Phenothiazines: ↑ toxicity
Rauwolfias: ↓ seratonin, norepinephrine
Sedative/hypnotics: ↑ CNS depression
SSRIs: ↑ Hyperpyrectic crisis, convulsions, hypertensive
Sympathomimetics, indirect-acting or mixed: ↑ pressor effect

Food

Tyramine-containing foods: Hypertensive crisis

NURSING CONSIDERATIONS

Assessment

- Monitor B/P (with patient lying, standing), pulse q4h; if systolic B/P drops 20 mm Hg, hold drug, notify prescriber; take VS q4h in patients with cardiovascular disease
- Monitor hepatic studies: AST (SGOT), ALT (SGPT), bilirubin if patient is on long-term therapy
- Check weight weekly; appetite may increase with drug
- Assess ECG for flattening of T wave, bundle branch block, AV block, dysrhythmias in cardiac patients
- Assess mental status: mood, sensorium, affect, suicidal tendencies; increase in psychiatric symptoms: depression, panic
- Monitor urinary retention, constipation; constipation is G more likely to occur in elderly
- Assess for withdrawal symptoms: headache, nausea, vomiting, muscle pain, weakness; do not usually occur unless drug was discontinued abruptly
- Identify alcohol consumption; if alcohol is consumed, hold dose until AM

Nursing diagnoses

✓ Coping, ineffective individual (uses)
✓ Injury, risk for (adverse reactions)
✓ Knowledge deficit (teaching)
✓ Noncompliance (teaching)

Implementation

- Give with food or milk for GI symptoms; crush if patient is unable to swallow medication whole and mix with food or fluids
- Store at room temp; do not freeze

Patient/family education

- Teach patient that therapeutic effects may take 2-3 wk
- Advise patient to use caution in driving and other activities requiring alertness because of drowsiness, dizziness, blurred vision; to avoid rising quickly from sitting to standing, espe- G cially elderly
- Caution patient to avoid alcohol ingestion, other CNS depressants; serious reaction can occur
- Advise patient not to discontinue medication quickly after long-term use: may cause nausea, headache, malaise, sweating, hallucinations
- Instruct patient to increase fluids, bulk in diet if constipation, urinary retention occur, G especially elderly; a stool softener may be ordered
- Teach patient to take gum, hard sugarless candy, or frequent sips of water for dry mouth
- Teach patient that therapeutic effects may take 1-4 wk
- Teach patient to avoid alcohol ingestion, CNS depres-

sants, OTC medications: cold, weight loss, hay fever, cough syrup
• Teach patient not to discontinue medication quickly after long-term use
• Teach patient to avoid high-tyramine foods: cheese (aged), sour cream, beer, wine, pickled products, liver, raisins, bananas, figs, avocados, meat tenderizers, chocolate, yogurt; increased caffeine
• Teach patient to report headache, palpitations, neck stiffness, dizziness, constriction in chest, throat

Evaluation
Positive therapeutic outcome
• Decrease in depression
• Absence of suicidal thoughts

Treatment of overdose: Lavage, activated charcoal, monitor electrolytes, VS, diazepam **IV**, sodium bicarbonate

phenobarbital ⚷ (℞)
(fee-noe-bar′bit-tal)
Barbita, Luminal, Phenobarbital, phenobarbital sodium, Solfoton
Func. class.: Anticonvulsant, sedative/hypnotic
Chem. class.: Barbiturate
Pregnancy category D
Controlled substance schedule IV

Action: Depresses activity in brain cells primarily in reticular activating system in brainstem; also selectively depresses neurons in posterior hypothalamus, limbic structures; able to decrease seizure activity by inhibition of impulses in CNS; decreases motor activity

Therapeutic Outcome: Sedation, anticonvulsant, improved energy

Uses: All forms of epilepsy, status epilepticus, febrile seizures in children, sedation, insomnia

Investigational uses: Hyperbilirubinemia, chronic cholestasis

Dosage and routes
Seizures
Adult: PO 100-200 mg/day in divided doses tid or total dose hs
Child: PO 4-6 mg/kg/day in divided doses q12h; may be given as single dose

Status epilepticus
Adult: **IV** inf 10 mg/kg; run no faster than 50/mg/min; may give up to 20 mg/kg
Child: **IV** inf 5-10 mg/kg; may repeat q10-15 min up to 20 mg/kg; run no faster than 50 mg/min

Insomnia
Adult: PO/IM 100-320 mg
Child: PO/IM 3-6 mg/kg

Sedation
Adult: PO 30-120 mg/day in 2-3 divided doses
Child: PO 6 mg/kg/day in 3 divided doses

Preoperative sedation
Adult: IM 100-200 mg 1-1½ hr before surgery
Child: PO 6 mg/kg/day in 3 divided doses

Hyperbilirubinemia
Neonate: PO 7 mg/kg/day on days 1-5 after birth; IM 5 mg/kg/day on day 1, then PO on days 2-7 after birth

P

Chronic cholestasis
Adult: PO 90-180 mg/day in 2-3 divided doses

P ***Child <12 yr:*** PO 3-12 mg/kg/day in 2-3 divided doses

Available forms: Cap 16 mg; elix 15, 20 mg/5 ml; tabs 8, 15, 16, 30, 32, 60, 65, 100 mg; inj 30, 60, 130 mg/ml

Adverse effects
CNS: Paradoxic excitement G (elderly), drowsiness, lethargy, *hangover headache*, flushing, hallucinations, coma
GI: Nausea, vomiting, diarrhea, constipation
INTEG: Rash, urticaria, Stevens-Johnson syndrome, angioedema, local pain, swelling, necrosis, thrombophlebitis

Contraindications: Hypersensitivity to barbiturates, porphyria, hepatic disease, respiratory disease, nephritis, hyperthyroidism, diabetes mellitus, G elderly, lactation, pregnancy **D**

Precautions: Anemia

Pharmacokinetics

Absorption	Slow (70%-90%) (PO/IM/IV)
Distribution	Not known; crosses placenta
Metabolism	Liver (75%)
Excretion	Kidneys (25% unchanged)
Half-life	2-6 days

Pharmacodynamics

	PO	IM	IV
Onset	30-60 min	10-30 min	5 min
Peak	Unknown	Unknown	30 min
Duration	6-8 hr	4-6 hr	4-6 hr

Interactions
Individual drugs
Alcohol: ↑ CNS depression
Chloramphenicol: ↓ effectiveness
Cyclosporine: ↓ effectiveness
Cyclophosphamide: ↑ hematologic toxicity
Dacarbazine: ↓ effectiveness
Quinidine: ↓ effectiveness
Valproic acid: ↑ sedation
Drug classifications
Anticoagulants: ↓ effectiveness
Antidepressants: ↑ CNS depression
Antihistamines: ↑ CNS depression
Glucocorticoids: ↓ effectiveness
MAOIs: ↑ CNS depression
Narcotics ↑ CNS depression
Oral contraceptives: ↓ effectiveness
Sedative/hypnotics: ↑ CNS depression
Tricyclic antidepressants: ↓ effectiveness

NURSING CONSIDERATIONS
Assessment

- Assess mental status: mood, sensorium, affect, memory G (long, short), especially elderly; if using as a hypnotic, assess sleep patterns during therapy; drug suppresses REM sleep with dreaming
- Withdrawal insomnia may occur after short-term use; do not start using drug again; insomnia improves in 1-3 nights; may experience increased dreaming
- Assess respiratory dysfunction: respiratory depression, character, rate, rhythm when using **IV**; hold drug if respirations are <10/min or if pupils are dilated; also check VS q30 min after parenteral route for 2 hr
- Assess for barbiturate toxicity: hypotension, pulmo-

nary constriction, cold, clammy skin, cyanosis of lips, CNS depression, nausea, vomiting, hallucinations, delirium, weakness, coma, pupillary constriction; mild symptoms occur in 8-12 hr without drug

- Assess for pain in postoperative patients; pain threshold is lowered when patients are taking this medication
- Assess for blood dyscrasias: fever, sore throat, bruising, rash, jaundice, epistaxis (long-term treatment only)
- Assess seizure activity including type, location, duration, and character; provide seizure precaution

Nursing diagnoses

- ✓ Sleep pattern disturbance (uses)
- ✓ Injury, risk for (adverse reactions)
- ✓ Knowledge deficit (teaching)

Implementation

- Give medication after removal of cigarettes to prevent fires
- Give medication after trying conservative measures for insomnia

PO route

- Tab may be crushed and mixed with food if swallowing is difficult; also may be mixed with other fluids 30-60 min before hs for expected sleeplessness; on empty stomach for best absorption

IM route

- Give in deep muscle mass (gluteal) to minimize irritation to tissues
- Split inj of >5 ml into two, since irritation to tissues may occur

IV Direct IV route

- Use large vein to prevent extravasation; if extravasation occurs, use moist heat to the area and 5% procaine sol injected into area; give at 65 mg or less/min; titrate to patient response

Syringe compatibility: Heparin

Syringe incompatibilities: Benzquinamide, ranitidine

Y-site compatibilities: Enalaprilat, sufentanil

Y-site incompatibility: Hydromorphone

Solution compatibilities: D_5W, $D_{10}W$, 0.45% NaCl, 0.9% NaCl, Ringer's, dextrose/saline combinations, dextrose/Ringer's, dextrose/LR combinations, sodium lactate

Additive compatibilities: Amikacin, aminophylline, calcium chloride, calcium gluceptate, cephapirin, colistimethate, dimenhydrinate, polymyxin B, sodium bicarbonate, thiopental, verapamil

Additive incompatibilities: Cephalothin, chlorpromazine, codeine, ephedrine, hydralazine, hydrocortisone sodium succinate, hydroxyzine, insulin, levorphanol, meperidine, methadone, morphine, norepinephrine, pentazocine, procaine, prochlorazine mesylate, promazine, promethazine, streptomycin, vancomycin

Patient/family education

- Teach patient that hangover is common
- Instruct patient that drug is indicated only for short-term treatment of insomnia and is probably ineffective after 2 wk
- Inform patient that physical dependency may result when

P

used for extended time (45-90 days depending on dosage)

- Teach patient to avoid driving and other activities requiring alertness
- Caution patient to avoid alcohol ingestion and CNS depressants; serious CNS depression may result
- Instruct patient not to discontinue medication quickly after long-term use; may cause seizures; drug should be tapered over 1 wk; take exactly as prescribed
- Emphasize the need to tell all prescribers that a barbiturate is being taken
- Teach the patient to make position changes slowly; orthostatic hypotension may occur
- Teach patient that response may take from 4 days to 2 wk of therapy
- Instruct patient to notify prescriber immediately if bruising, bleeding occur, which may indicate blood dyscrasias

Evaluation

Positive therapeutic outcome

- Improved sleeping patterns
- Decreased seizure activity
- Sedative preoperatively

Treatment of overdose: Lavage, activated charcoal, warming blanket, VS, hemodialysis, alkalinize urine, give **IV** volume expanders, **IV** fluids

phenolphthalein (OTC)

(fee-nol-thay'leen)

Alophen, Correctol, Espotabs, Evac-U-Gen, Evac-U-Lax, Ex-Lax, Feen-A-Mint, Lax-Pills, Modane, Medilax, Phenolax, Prulet

Func. class.: Laxative, stimulant/irritant

Chem. class.: Diphenylmethane

Pregnancy category C

Action: Directly acts on intestinal smooth muscle by increasing motor activity; thought to irritate colonic intramural plexus; increases fluid in small intestine; alters fluid and electrolytes; action requires presence of bile

→ **Therapeutic Outcome:** Decreased constipation

Uses: Constipation, preparation for bowel surgery or examination

Dosage and routes

Adult: PO 30-270 mg hs

P ***Child >6 yr:*** 30-60 mg/day

P ***Child 2-5 yr:*** 15-20 mg/day

Available forms: Tabs 60, 90, 97.2, 130 mg; chew tabs 65, 90, 97.2 mg; chew gum 97.2 mg; wafers 64.8 mg; chew wafers 80 mg

Adverse effects

*GI: **Nausea, vomiting, anorexia, diarrhea**,* abdominal cramps, rectal burning

INTEG: Rash, urticaria, ***Stevens-Johnson syndrome***

META: Hypokalemia, electrolyte and fluid imbalances

Contraindications: Hypersensitivity, GI obstructions, abdominal pain, nausea/

vomiting, fecal impaction, rectal fissures, hemorrhoids (ulcerated)

Precautions: Pregnancy **C**, lactation

Pharmacokinetics	
Absorption	Minimally absorbed (15%)
Distribution	Unknown
Metabolism	Not metabolized
Excretion	Kidneys, feces
Half-life	Unknown

Pharmacodynamics	
Onset	6-8 hr
Peak	Unknown
Duration	3-4 days

Interactions

Drug classifications

Oral drugs (any): ↓ absorption

Lab test interferences

Interference: BSP test

NURSING CONSIDERATIONS

Assessment

- Monitor blood, urine electrolytes if used often by patient; check I&O ratio to identify fluid loss
- Assess for cramping, rec bleeding, nausea, vomiting; if these symptoms occur, drug should be discontinued; identify cause of constipation; identify whether fluids, bulk, or exercise is missing from lifestyle
- Assess stool for color, consistency, amount, presence of flatulence

Nursing diagnoses

✓ Constipation (uses)
✓ Diarrhea (adverse reaction)
✓ Knowledge deficit (teaching)
✓ Noncompliance (teaching)

Implementation

- Chew well before swallowing; follow with 4 oz of water to prevent undissolved tab entering small intestine
- Give with 8 oz water (tab); administer on empty stomach for more rapid results; do not give at hs

Patient/family education

- Discuss with the patient that adequate fluid consumption is necessary
- Teach patient that normal bowel movements do not always occur daily
- Caution patient not to use in presence of abdominal pain, nausea, vomiting; tell patient to notify prescriber if constipation is unrelieved or if symptoms of electrolyte imbalance occur (muscle cramps, pain, weakness, dizziness, excessive thirst)
- Teach patient not to use laxatives for long-term therapy; bowel tone will be lost and will decrease
- Shake susp well as needed
- Teach patient not to take at hs as a laxative; may interfere with sleep; also can cause problems with lipid pneumonia
- Teach patient not to use with food or vitamin preparations; delays digestion and absorption of fat-soluble vitamins

Evaluation

Positive therapeutic outcome

- Decreased constipation in 8-10 hr

P

phentolamine (℞)
(fen-tole'a-meen)
Regitine, Rogitine ✦
Func. class.: Antihypertensive
Chem. class.: α-Adrenergic blocker
Pregnancy category C

Action: α-Adrenergic blocker, binds to α-adrenergic receptors, dilating peripheral blood vessels, lowering peripheral resistances, lowering blood pressure

Therapeutic Outcome: Decreased B/P, reversal of vasoconstriction (dermal necrosis)

Uses: Hypertension, pheochromocytoma, prevention, treatment of dermal necrosis following extravasation of norepinephrine or dopamine, impotence

Dosage and routes
Treatment of hypertensive episodes in pheochromocytoma
Adult: **IV**/IM 5 mg; repeat if necessary
P ***Child:*** **IV**/IM 1 mg; repeat if necessary

Diagnosis of pheochromocytoma
Adult: **IV** 2.5 mg; if negative, repeat with 5 mg **IV**
P ***Child:*** **IV** 0.5 mg; if negative, repeat with 1 mg **IV**

Prevention of dermal necrosis
Adult: **IV** 10 mg/100 ml of **IV** fluids with norepinephrine

Impotence (adjunct)
Adult: Intracavernosal 0.5-1 mg with 30 mg papaverine given 1, 2, or 3 treatments/wk

Available forms: Inj 5 mg/ml; tabs 25, 50 mg (only injectable form available in US)

Adverse effects
CNS: Dizziness, flushing, weakness
CV: Hypotension, tachycardia, ***angina, dysrhythmias, MI***
EENT: Nasal congestion
GI: Dry mouth, nausea, vomiting, diarrhea, abdominal pain

Contraindications: Hypersensitivity, MI, coronary insufficiency, angina

Precautions: Pregnancy **C,** lactation

Pharmacokinetics

Absorption	Well absorbed (IM); completely absorbed (**IV**)
Distribution	Unknown
Metabolism	Unknown
Excretion	Kidneys, unchanged (10%)
Half-life	Unknown

Pharmacodynamics

	IM	IV	INTRACAVERNOSAL
Onset	Unknown	Rapid	Unknown
Peak	20 min	2 min	5-10 min
Duration	½-1 hr	½ hr	4 hr

Interactions
Individual drugs
Epinephrine: ↑ effects of epinephrine, hypotension
Guanethidine: ↑ hypotension, bradycardia
Guanadrel: ↑ hypotension, bradycardia
Dopamine: ↓ peripheral vasoconstriction
Ephedrine: ↓ pressor effect
Phenylephrine: ↓ pressor effect
Metaraminol: ↓ pressor effect

Methoxamine: ↑ effects of methoxamine, hypotension

Drug classifications

α-Adrenergics: Antagonistic effect

Antihypertensives: ↑ effects of antihypertensives

NURSING CONSIDERATIONS

Assessment

- Monitor B/P, orthostatic hypotension, syncope, pulse and ECG until stable

Nursing diagnoses

✓ Cardiac output, decreased (uses)

✓ Injury, potential for (adverse reactions)

✓ Knowledge deficit (teaching)

✓ Noncompliance (teaching)

Implementation

- Give with vasopressor nearby

IV IV route

- Give by direct **IV** after diluting 5 mg/1 ml sterile water for inj or 0.9% NaCl; give 5 mg or less/min
- Give by cont inf by further diluting 5-10 mg/500 ml D_5W

Y-site compatibility: Amiodarone

Syringe compatibility: Papaverine

Additive compatibilities: Dobutamine, verapamil

Prevention of dermal necrosis

- Add 10 mg/L to norepinephrine in **IV** sol

Patient/family education

- Caution patient not to discontinue drug abruptly
- Teach patient not to use OTC products (cough, cold, allergy) unless directed by prescriber
- Teach patient the importance of complying with dosage schedule, even if feeling better
- Emphasize the need to rise slowly to sitting or standing position to minimize orthostatic hypotension
- Teach patient to notify prescriber of mouth sores, sore throat, fever, swelling of hands or feet, irregular heartbeat, chest pain
- Caution patient to report excessive perspiration, dehydration, vomiting, diarrhea; may lead to fall in B/P
- Caution patient that drug may cause dizziness, fainting, lightheadedness; may occur during 1st few days of therapy
- Teach patient how to take B/P, and normal readings for age group

Evaluation

Positive therapeutic outcome

- Decreased B/P in hypertension
- Resolution of impotence
- Prevention of dermal necrosis

Treatment of overdose: Administer norepinephrine; discontinue drug

P

phenylbutyrate (℞)

(fen-ill-byoo′te-rate)

Buphenyl

Func. class.: Nitrogen excretion product

Pregnancy category C

Action: Provides an alternate method for waste nitrogen excretion; similar to urea

➔ Therapeutic Outcome: Decreased nitrogen levels

Uses: Cycle disorders; urea

cycle disorders with CPS, OTC, AAS

Dosage and routes

P ***Adult and child:*** PO 450-600 mg/kg/day <20 kg or 9.9-13 g/m^2/day in larger persons; may use powder via mouth, NG tube, gastrostomy tube, mixed with solid or liquid food

Available forms: Tabs 500 mg; powder 3.2 g (3 g phenylbutyrate) per tsp, 9.1 g (8.6 g phenylbutyrate) per tsp

Adverse effects

CNS: Depression, ***neutotoxicity,*** headache
CV: Dysrhythmias
GI: Decreased appetite; taste aversion, abdominal pain, nausea, vomiting, constipation, rectal bleeding, peptic ulcer
GU: Amenorrhea, menstrual changes
HEMA: Aplastic anemia
OTHER: Body odor

Contraindications: Hypersensitivity, acute hyperammonemia

Precautions: CHF, severe renal insufficiency, hepatic P disease, pregnancy **C,** lactation, children, preexisting neurologic impairment

Pharmacokinetics

Absorption	1 hr
Distribution	Unknown
Metabolism	Unknown
Excretion	Kidneys (24 hr)
Half-life	Unknown

Pharmacodynamics

Unknown

Interactions

Individual drugs

Haloperidol: ↑ plasma ammonia levels
Probenecid: Renal excretion may be affected
Valproate: ↑ plasma ammonia levels

Drug classifications

Corticosteroids: ↑ plasma ammonia levels

NURSING CONSIDERATIONS

Assessment

- Maintain levels of ammonia, arginine, branched-chain amino acids, and serum proteins: glutamine levels should be <1000 amol/L; monitor drug levels of: phenylbutyrate, phenylacetate, phenylactyl-glutamine
- Assess for neurotoxicity and aplastic anemia; drug should be discontinued

Nursing diagnoses

✓ Knowledge deficit (teaching)

Evaluation

Positive therapeutic outcome

- Decreased ammonia levels

phenylephrine

(℞; nasal, OTC)
(fen-ill-ef'rin)
AK-Dilate Ophthalmic, AK-Nefrin Ophthalmic, Alconefrin, Alconefrin-25, Alconefrin-50, Duration, Isopto Frin, Neo-Synephrine, Neo-Synephrine 2.5%, Neo-Synephrine 10% Plain, Neo-Synephrine Viscous, Nostril, Phenylephrine HCl, 2.5% Mydfrin Ophthalmic, Phenoptic, Relief, Rhinall-10 Prefrin, Sinex, St Joseph Measured Dose

Func. class.: Adrenergic, direct acting; ophthalmic vasoconstrictor
Chem. class.: Direct sympathomimetic amine (α-agonist)

Pregnancy category C

Action: Powerful and selective receptor agonist causing contraction of blood vessels, vasoconstriction of eye arterioles; decreases eye engorgement by stimulation of α-adrenergic receptors

➔ **Therapeutic Outcome:** Increased B/P, decreased nasal-congestion, decreased eye irritation

Uses: Hypotension, paroxysmal supraventricular tachycardia, shock, B/P maintenance during spinal anesthesia, top ocular vasoconstrictor in uveitis, open-angle glaucoma, preoperatively, diagnostic procedures, refraction without cycloplegia, nasal congestion

Dosage and routes

Eye irritation
Adult: Instill 2 gtt of a 0.12% sol; may repeat q3-4h

Refraction/ophthalmoscopic exam
Adult: Sol 1 gtt of 2.5%

Uveitis/glaucoma/surgery
P ***Adult and child:*** Instill 1 gtt of a 2.5% or 10% sol in upper surface of cornea

Nasal congestion
Adult: Instill 2-3 gtt or sprays to nasal mucosa bid (0.25%-1%); top apply to nasal mucosa q3-4h prn
P ***Child 6-12 yrs:*** Instill 1-2 gtt or sprays (0.25%) q3-4h prn
P ***Child <6 yrs:*** Instill 2-3 gtt or sprays (0.125%) q3-4h prn

Hypotension
Adult: SC/IM 2-5 mg; may repeat q10-15 min if needed; **IV** 0.1-0.5 mg; may repeat q10-15 min if needed

PVCs
Adult: **IV** bol 0.5 mg given rapidly, not to exceed prior dose by >0.1 mg; total dose >1 mg

Shock
Adult: **IV** inf 10 mg/500 ml D_5W given 100-180 gtt/min, then 40-60 gtt/min titrated to B/P

Available forms: Sol 10%, 2.5%, 1%, 0.12%, 0.125%, 0.16%, 0.2%, 0.25%, 0.5%, jelly 0.5%; inj **IV**, SC, IM, 1% (10 mg/ml)

Adverse effects
CNS: Headache, dizziness, weakness, anxiety, tremor, insomnia
CV: Reflex bradycardia, *hypertension, dysrhythmias,* ***tachycar-***

P

dia, CV collapse, palpitations, ectopic beats, angina
EENT: Stinging, lacrimation, blurred vision, conjunctival allergy
GI: Nausea, vomiting
INTEG: Necrosis, tissue sloughing with extravasation, ***gangrene***

Contraindications: Hypersensitivity, narrow-angle glaucoma, ventricular fibrillation, tachydysrhythmias, pheochromocytoma

Precautions: Severe hypertension, diabetes, hyperthyroidism, G elderly, severe arteriosclerosis, cardiac disease, P infants, pregnancy **C,** lactation, arterial embolism, peripheral vascular disease, bradycardia, myocardial disease

Pharmacokinetics

Absorption	Well absorbed (IM); completely absorbed (IV); minimally absorbed (nasal, ophth)
Distribution	Unknown
Metabolism	Liver
Excretion	Unknown
Half-life	Unknown

Pharmacodynamics

	IV	SC/IM	NASAL	OPHTH
Onset	Rapid	15 min	Unknown	Min
Peak	Unknown	Unknown	Unknown	1 hr
Duration	20-30 min	45-60 min	½-4 hr	½-7 hr

Interactions

Individual drugs

Bretylium: ↑ dysrhythmias
Guanethidine: ↑ pressor effect
Mecamylamine: ↑ hypotension
Methyldopa: ↑ hypotension
Reserpine: ↑ hypotension

Drug classifications

Antidepressants, tricyclic: ↑ pressor effect
β-Blockers: ↑ pressor effect
General anesthetics: ↑ dysrhythmias
H_1 antihistamines: ↑ pressor effect
MAOIs: ↑ pressor effect
Oxytocics: ↑ B/P

NURSING CONSIDERATIONS

Assessment

Syst route

- Monitor I&O ratio, notify prescriber if output <30 ml/hr
- Monitor ECG during administration continuously; if B/P increases, drug is decreased
- Monitor B/P and pulse q5 min after parenteral route; CVP or PWP during inf if possible
- Assess for paresthesias and coldness of extremities; peripheral blood flow may decrease

Nasal route

- Assess for redness, swelling, pain in nasal passages

Nursing diagnoses

✓ Tissue perfusion, altered (uses)
✓ Cardiac output, decreased (uses)
✓ Knowledge deficit (teaching)

Implementation

IV route

- Give plasma expanders for hypovolemia
- Give **IV** after diluting 1 mg/9 ml sterile water for inj; give dose over 30-60 sec; may be diluted 10 mg/500 ml of D_5W or NS; titrate to patient response; low normal B/P; check for extravasation; check site for infiltration; use inf pump
- Store reconstituted sol in refrigerator for no longer than 24 hr
- Do not use discolored sol

Y-site compatibilities: Amrinone, famotidine, haloperidol, zidovudine

Additive compatibilities: Chloramphenicol, dobutamine, lidocaine, potassium chloride, sodium bicarbonate

Nasal route

- Use no more than q4h for <4 consecutive days
- Use environmental humidification to decrease nasal congestion, dryness
- Store in light-resistant container; do not expose to high temp

Ophth route

- Store in tight, light-resistant container; do not use discolored sol

Patient/family education

- Inform patient of reason for drug administration and expected result
- Advise patient to report pain at inf site immediately
- Instruct patient to report change in vision, blurring, loss of sight; breathing trouble, sweating, flushing

Ophth route

- Teach patient method of instill: tilt head backward, hold dropper over eye, drop medication inside lower lid; using pressure on inside corner of eye hold 1 min; do not touch dropper to eye
- Teach patient that blurred vision will decrease with repeated use of drug
- Advise patient to notify prescriber of headache, spots, redness, pain; discontinue use
- Advise patient to use sunglasses if photophobia occurs
- Instruct patient to use exactly as prescribed

Nasal route

- Inform patient that stinging may occur for a few applications; drying of mucosa may be decreased by environmental humidification
- Teach patient to notify prescriber if irregular pulse, insomnia, dizziness, or tremors occur
- Teach patient proper administration to avoid syst absorption

Evaluation

Positive therapeutic outcome

- Increased B/P with stabilization
- Decreased nasal congestion
- Decreased eye irritation

phenytoin (℞)

(fen′i-toyn)

Diphenylhydantoin, Dilantin, Dilantin Capsules, Diphenylan, Phenytoin Oral Suspension

Func. class.: Anticonvulsant/antidysrhythmic (IB)

Chem. class.: Hydantoin

Pregnancy category D

Action: Inhibits spread of seizure activity in motor cortex by altering ion transport; increases AV conduction to decrease dysrhythmias

Therapeutic Outcome: Decreased seizures, absence of dysrhythmias

Uses: Generalized tonic-clonic seizures, status epilepticus, non-epileptic seizures associated with Reye's syndrome or after head trauma, migraines, trigeminal neuralgia, Bell's palsy, ventricular dysrhythmias uncontrolled by antidysrhythmics

Dosage and routes

Seizures

Adult: **IV** loading dose 900 mg-1.5 g run at 50 mg/min; if patient has received phenytoin, 100-300 mg run at 50 mg/min; PO loading dose 900 mg-1.5 g divided tid, then 300 mg/day (extended) or divided tid (extended/prompt)

P ***Child:*** **IV** loading dose 15 mg/kg run at 50 mg/min; if patient has received phenytoin, 5-7 mg/kg run at 50 mg/min; may repeat in 30 min; PO loading dose of 15 mg/kg divided q8-12h, then 5-7 mg/kg in divided doses q12h

Status epilepticus

Adult: **IV** 15-20 mg/kg, max 25-50 mg/min; may give 100 mg q6-8h thereafter

P ***Child:*** **IV** 15-20 mg/kg given 1-3 mg/kg/min

Neuritic pain

Adult: PO 200-400 mg/day in divided doses

Ventricular dysrhythmias

Adult: PO loading dose 1 g divided over 24 hr, then 500 mg/day × 2 days; **IV** 250 mg given over 5 min until dysrhythmias subside or 1 g is given, or 100 mg q15 min until dysrhythmias subside or 1 g is given

P ***Child:*** PO 3-8 mg/kg or 250 mg/m²/day as single dose or divided in 2 doses; **IV** 3-8 mg/kg given over several min, or 250 mg/m²/day as single dose or divided in 2 doses

Available forms: Susp 30, 125 mg/5 ml; chew tab 50 mg; inj 50 mg/ml; ext rel cap 100 mg; prompt caps 30 ✤, 100 mg

Adverse effects

CNS: Drowsiness, dizziness, insomnia, paresthesias, depression, suicidal tendencies, aggression, headache, confusion, slurred speech

CV: Hypotension, ***ventricular fibrillation***

EENT: Nystagmus, diplopia, blurred vision

GI: Nausea, vomiting, constipation, anorexia, weight loss, ***hepatitis,*** jaundice, gingival hyperplasia

GU: ***Nephritis,*** urine discoloration

HEMA: ***Agranulocytosis, leukopenia, aplastic anemia, thrombocytopenia, megaloblastic anemia***

INTEG: Rash, ***lupus erythematosus, Stevens-Johnson syndrome,*** hirsutism

SYST: Hypocalcemia

Contraindications: Hypersensitivity, psychiatric condition, pregnancy **D,** bradycardia, SA and AV block, Stokes-Adams syndrome

Precautions: Allergies, hepatic disease, renal disease

Pharmacokinetics

Absorption	Slowly absorbed from GI tract; erratic (IM)
Distribution	Crosses placenta
Metabolism	Liver, extensively
Excretion	Kidneys, minimally; enters breast milk
Half-life	22 hr

Pharmacodynamics

	PO	PO–EXT REL	IM	IV
Onset	2-24 hr	2-24 hr	Erratic	1-2 hr
Peak	1.5-3 hr	4-12 hr	Erratic	Unknown
Duration	6-12 hr	12-36 hr	12-24 hr	12-24 hr

Interactions

Individual drugs

Alcohol: ↑ CNS depression
Carbamazepine: ↓ effectiveness
Chloramphenicol: ↑ blood level
Cimetidine: ↓ metabolism, ↑ action, blood level
Disulfiram: ↓ metabolism, ↑ action
Felbamate: ↑ blood level
Fluconazole: ↑ blood level
Isoniazid: ↓ metabolism, ↑ action
Ketoconazole: ↓ metabolism, ↑ action
Metronidazole: ↑ blood level
Miconazole: ↑ blood level
Omeprazole: ↑ blood level
Phenylbutazone: ↑ blood level
Valproic acid: ↑ seizures
Warfarin: ↓ blood level of phenytoin

Drug classifications

Anticonvulsants: ↑ CNS depression
Antidepressants: ↑ CNS depression
Antihistamines: ↑ CNS depression
Barbiturates: ↑ CNS depression, ↓ effect of phenytoin
Benzodiazepines: ↑ blood levels
General anesthetics: ↑ CNS depression
Hypnotics: ↑ CNS depression
Narcotics: ↑ CNS depression
Oral contraceptives: ↓ metabolism, ↑ action
Sedatives: ↑ CNS depression
Sulfonamides: ↑ blood levels

Lab test interferences

↓ Dexamethasone, ↓ metyrapone test serum, ↓ PBI, ↓ urinary steroids
↑ Glucose, ↑ alkaline phosphatase, ↑ BSP

NURSING CONSIDERATIONS

Assessment

- Assess drug level: toxic level 30-50 μg/ml
- Assess mental status: mood, sensorium, affect, memory (long, short), especially elderly [G]
- Assess for blood dyscrasias: fever, sore throat, bruising, rash, jaundice, epistaxis (long-term treatment only)
- Assess seizure activity including type, location, duration, and character; provide seizure precaution
- Assess renal studies: urinalysis, BUN, urine creatinine
- Monitor blood studies: RBC, Hct, Hgb, reticulocyte counts weekly for 4 wk then monthly; also check thyroid function tests, serum calcium
- Monitor hepatic studies: ALT (SGPT), AST (SGOT), bilirubin, creatinine
- Assess for signs of physical withdrawal if medication suddenly discontinued
- Assess eye problems: need for ophth examinations before, during, after treatment (slit lamp, fundoscopy, tonometry)
- Assess allergic reaction: red raised rash; if this occurs, drug should be discontinued
- Monitor for toxicity: bone marrow depression, nausea, vomiting, ataxia, diplopia, cardiovascular collapse, slurred speech, confusion

Nursing diagnoses

- ✓ Injury, risk for (uses, adverse reactions)
- ✓ Knowledge deficit (teaching)
- ✓ Noncompliance (teaching)

Implementation

PO route

- Give with meals to decrease GI upset
- Chew tab can be crushed or

P

chewed; cap can be opened and mixed with foods or fluids; cap and tab are not interchangeable
- Shake oral susp well; use measuring device for correct dose

IV IV route
- Administer by direct **IV** after diluting with special diluent provided (1 ml/50 mg, 2.2 ml/100 mg, 5.2 ml/250 mg); shake; place vial in warm water to dissolve powder; give through Y-tube or 3-way stopcock; inject slowly <50 mg/min
- Give intermittent **IV** after diluting to a conc of 1-10 mg/ml
- Clear **IV** tubing first with 0.9% NaCl sol; use in-line filter; discard 4 hr after preparation; inject into large veins to prevent purple glove syndrome

Additive compatibilities: Bleomycin, verapamil

Y-site incompatibilities: Enalaprilat, potassium chloride, vitamin B with C

Y-site compatibilities: Esmolol, famotidine, fluconazole, foscarnet, tacrolimus

Patient/family education
- Teach patient to carry ID card or Medic Alert bracelet stating name, drugs taken, condition, prescriber's name and phone number
- Advise patient to avoid driving and other activities that require alertness until drug response is known; dizziness, drowsiness can occur
- Advise patient to avoid alcohol ingestion and CNS depressants unless approved by prescriber; increased sedation may occur
- Teach patient not to discontinue medication quickly after long-term use; taper off over several wk
- Advise patient that urine may turn pink, red, or brown, which is normal
- Caution patient to avoid antacids within 2-3 hr of taking phenytoin
- To prevent gingival hyperplasia, instruct patient in proper oral hygiene; a dentist should be seen routinely

Evaluation

Positive therapeutic outcome
- Decreased seizure activity
- Decreased dysrhythmias
- Relief of pain

physostigmine (℞)
(fi-zoe-stig'meen)

Antilerium, Isopto Eserine Solution, Eserine Sulfate Ointment, Fisostin

Func. class.: Antidote, reversible anticholinesterine, miotic

Chem. class.: Tertiary amine; cholinesterase inhibitor

Pregnancy category C

Action: Increases concentration of acetylcholine at cholinergic transmission sites, causing prolonged, exaggerated action; produces constriction of ciliary muscles, iris sphincter, causing iris to be pulled away from anterior chamber angle, aiding in aqueous humor drainage

➔ Therapeutic Outcome: Treatment of anticholinergic overdose, Alzheimer's disease, glaucoma

Uses: To reverse CNS effects of diazepam; anticholinergic, tricyclic antidepressant; Alzheimer's disease, hereditary ataxia, wide-angle glaucoma

Dosage and routes

Overdose of anticholinergics

Adult: IM/**IV** 2 mg; give no more than 1 mg/min; may repeat

P ***Child:*** IM/**IV** inj 0.02 mg/kg, not more than 0.5 mg/min; may repeat at 5-10 min intervals until max dose of 2 mg

Postanesthesia

Adult: IM/**IV** 0.5-1 mg; give no more than 1 mg/min (**IV**); can repeat at 10-30 min intervals

P ***Adult and child:*** Instill ¼-inch strip of 0.25% oint in conjunctival sac; instill 1-2 gtt of a 0.25%-0.5% sol in conjunctival sac qd-qid

Available forms: Inj IM, **IV** 1 mg/ml; oint 0.25% (sulfate); sol 0.25% (salicylate)

Adverse effects

CNS: ***Convulsions,*** headache, dizziness, sweating, weakness, incoordination, ***paralysis,*** hallucinations, delirium, drowsiness

CV: Hypertension, hypotension, bradycardia, irregular pulse, syncope

EENT: Blurred vision, conjunctivitis, allergic reactions, rhinorrhea, salivation, eye and brow pain, lacrimation, twitching of eyelids

GI: Nausea, vomiting, abdominal cramps, diarrhea, increased salivary and gastric secretions

GU: Frequency, incontinence, urgency

INTEG: Rash, urticaria

RESP: ***Bronchospasm,*** dyspnea, ***pulmonary edema, respiratory depression, constriction***

Contraindications: Hypotension, obstruction of intestine or renal system, asthma, gangrene, CV disease, choline esters, depolarizing neuromuscular blocking agents, diabetes, hypersensitivity, inflammatory disease of iris or ciliary body

Precautions: Epilepsy, parkinsonism, bradycardia, pregnancy **C**, asthma, bronchitis, diabetes mellitus, CV disease, seizure disorders, bronchial asthma, coronary occlusion, hyperthyroidism, dysrhythmias, peptic ulcer, megacolon, poor GI motility, Parkinson's disease, bradycardia, lactation

Pharmacokinetics

Absorption	Well absorbed
Distribution	Widely distributed; crosses blood-brain barrier
Metabolism	By cholinesterase
Excretion	Kidneys, unknown
Half-life	Unknown

Pharmacodynamics

	MIOSIS	INTRAOCULAR PRES	IV/IM
Onset	20-30 min	Unknown	Unknown
Peak	Unknown	2-6 hr	5 min
Duration	12-36 hr	12-36 hr	45-60 min

Interactions

Individual drugs

Decamethonium: ↑ action
Succinylcholine: ↑ action
Procainamide: ↓ action
Quinidine: ↓ action

Drug classifications

Aminoglycosides: ↓ action

P

Anesthetics: ↓ action
Neuromuscular blockers: ↓ action

NURSING CONSIDERATIONS
Assessment
- Monitor VS, respiration q8h
- Monitor I&O ratio; check for urinary retention or incontinence
- Discontinue drug if toxicity occurs

Nursing diagnoses
- ✓ Mobility, impaired physical (uses)
- ✓ Breathing pattern, ineffective (uses)
- ✓ Knowledge deficit (teaching)

Implementation
IV IV route
- Give **IV** undiluted through Y-tube or 3-way stopcock; give 1 mg or less/1-3 min or 0.5 mg or less over 1 min or more **P** (child)
- Give only with atropine sulfate available for cholinergic crisis
- Give only after all other cholinergics have been discontinued
- Give increased doses if tolerance occurs
- Store at room temp

Ophth route
- Give topically to conjunctival sac
- Give immediately after reconstituting; discard unused portion
- Give only clear sol, never pink or brown

Patient/family education
Ophth route
- Advise patient to report change in vision, blurring, or loss of sight, trouble breathing, sweating, flushing
- Teach patient method of instillation, including pressure on lacrimal sac for 1 min, not to touch dropper to eye
- Advise patient that long-term therapy may be required
- Advise patient that blurred vision will decrease with repeated use of drug
- Advise patient that drug is often irritating to eye, rarely tolerated for prolonged periods
- Advise patient that drug may be prescribed for bedtime use to prevent nocturnal rise in ocular tension
- Inform patient that maximal effect of top application is reached in 30 min, may last 12-36 hr
- Inform patient to observe eyes for irritation, development of cataracts

Evaluation
Positive therapeutic outcome
- Decreased intraocular pressure
- Alert

Treatment of overdose: Can cause cholinergic crisis; atropine is an antagonist

phytonadione (℞)
(fye-toe-na-dye'one)
AquaMEPHYTON, Konakion, Mephyton, vitamin K_1
Func. class.: Vitamin K_1, fat-soluble vitamin
Pregnancy category C

Action: Needed for adequate blood clotting (factors II, VII, IX, X)

➔ **Therapeutic Outcome:** Prevention of bleeding

Uses: Vitamin K malabsorption, hypoprothrombinemia,

prevention of hypoprothrombinemia caused by oral anticoagulants, prevention of hemorrhagic disease of the newborn

Dosage and routes

Hypoprothrombinemia caused by vitamin K malabsorption

Adult: PO/IM 2-25 mg; may repeat or increase to 50 mg

Child: PO/IM 5-10 mg

Infants: PO/IM 2 mg

Prevention of hemorrhagic disease of the newborn

Neonate: SC/IM 0.5-1 mg after birth; repeat in 6-8 hr if required

Hypoprothrombinemia caused by oral anticoagulants

Adult: PO/SC/IM 2.5-10 mg, may repeat 12-48 hr after PO dose or 6-8 hr after SC/IM dose, based on PT

Available forms: Tab 5 mg; inj 2 mg, 10 mg/ml; aqueous colloidal (IM, **IV**); inj aqueous dispersion 2, 10 mg/ml (IM)

Adverse effects

CNS: Headache, ***brain damage*** (large doses)

GI: Nausea, decreased liver function tests

HEMA: Hemolytic anemia, hemoglobinuria, hyperbilirubinemia

INTEG: Rash, urticaria

Contraindications: Hypersensitivity, severe hepatic disease, last few wk of pregnancy

Precautions: Pregnancy **C**, neonates

Pharmacokinetics

Absorption	Well absorbed (PO, IM, SC)
Distribution	Crosses placenta
Metabolism	Liver, rapidly
Excretion	Breast milk
Half-life	Unknown

Pharmacodynamics

	PO	SC/IM
Onset	6-12 hr	1-2 hr
Peak	Unknown	6 hr
Duration	Unknown	14 hr

Interactions

Individual drugs

Cholestyramine: ↓ action of phytonadione

Mineral oil: ↓ action of phytonadione

Sucralfate: ↓ phytonadione absorption

Drug classifications

Antiinfectives: ↑ phytonadione need

Oral anticoagulants: ↓ action of phytonadione

Salicylates: ↑ phytonadione need

NURSING CONSIDERATIONS

Assessment

- Monitor pro-time during treatment (2-sec deviation from control time, bleeding time, and clotting time); monitor for bleeding, pulse, and BP
- Assess nutritional status: liver (beef), spinach, tomatoes, coffee, asparagus, broccoli, cabbage, lettuce, greens
- Assess for bleeding or bruising: hematuria, black tarry stools, hematemesis

Nursing diagnoses

- ✓ Nutrition, altered: less than body requirements (uses)
- ✓ Tissue perfusion, altered (uses)
- ✓ Knowledge deficit (teaching)

P

Implementation

IV **IV route**

- Give **IV** after diluting with D_5 NS 10 ml or more; give 1 mg/min or more
- Give **IV** only when other routes not possible (deaths have occurred)
- Store in tight, light-resistant container

Additive compatibilities: Amikacin, calcium gluceptate, cephapirin, chloramphenicol, cimetidine, netilmicin, sodium bicarbonate

Syringe compatibility: Doxapram

Y-site compatibilities: Ampicillin, epinephrine, famotidine, heparin, hydrocortisone, potassium chloride, tolazoline, vit B/C

Patient/family education

- Teach patient not to take other supplements, unless directed by prescriber; to take this medication as directed
- Teach patient necessary foods to be included in diet high in vitamin K
- Advise patient to avoid IM inj, hard toothbrush, flossing; use electric razor until treatment is terminated
- Instruct patient to report symptoms of bleeding, bruising, nosebleeds, blood in urine, heavy menstruation, black tarry stools
- Caution patient not to use OTC medications unless approved by prescriber
- Stress the need for periodic lab tests to monitor coagulation levels
- Stress the need for patient to wear identification with condition, treatment, and medication taken

Evaluation

Positive therapeutic outcome

- Decreased bleeding tendencies
- Decreased pro-time
- Decreased clotting time

pindolol (℞)

(pin'doe-lole)

Visken

Func. class.: Antihypertensive

Chem. class.: Nonselective β-blocker

Pregnancy category B

Action: Competitively blocks stimulation of β-adrenergic receptor within vascular smooth muscle; produces chronotropic, inotropic activity (decreases rate of SA node discharge, increases recovery time), slows conduction of AV node, decreases heart rate, which decreases O_2 consumption in myocardium; also decreases renin-aldosterone-angiotensin system and at high doses inhibits β_2 receptors in bronchial system

Therapeutic Outcome: Increased B/P in hypertension, heart rate

Uses: Mild to moderate hypertension

Investigational uses: Mitral valve prolapse, hypertrophic cardiomyopathy, angina pectoris, ventricular dysrhythmias, anxiety

Dosage and routes

Adult: PO 5 mg bid; usual dose 15 mg/day (5 mg tid); may increase by 10 mg/day q3-4 wk to a max of 60 mg/day

Available forms: Tabs 5, 10 mg

Adverse effects

CNS: Insomnia, dizziness, hallucinations, anxiety, fatigue
CV: Hypotension, bradycardia, *CHF,* edema, chest pain, palpitations, claudication, tachycardia, ***AV block***
EENT: Visual changes, sore throat, *double vision,* dry burning eyes
GI: Nausea, vomiting, ***ischemic colitis,*** diarrhea, *abdominal pain,* ***mesenteric arterial thrombosis***
GU: Impotence, frequency
HEMA: Agranulocytosis, thrombocytopenia, purpura
INTEG: Rash, alopecia, pruritus, fever
MISC: Joint pain, muscle pain
RESP: Bronchospasm, *dyspnea,* cough, rales

Contraindications: Hypersensitivity to β-blockers, cardiogenic shock, 2nd-, 3rd-degree heart block, sinus bradycardia, CHF, cardiac failure, bronchial asthma

Precautions: Major surgery, pregnancy **B,** lactation, diabetes mellitus, renal disease, thyroid disease, COPD, well-compensated heart failure, CAD, nonallergic bronchospasm

Pharmacokinetics

Absorption	Well absorbed
Distribution	Crosses placenta; some penetration in CNS
Metabolism	Liver, moderately (60%-65%)
Excretion	Kidneys, unchanged (30%-45%)
Half-life	3-4 hr

Pharmacodynamics

Onset	Unknown
Peak	2-4 hr
Duration	8-24 hr

Interactions

Individual drugs

Alcohol: ↑ hypotension (large amounts)
Epinephrine: α-Adrenergic stimulation
Hydralazine: ↑ hypotension, bradycardia
Indomethacin: ↓ antihypertensive effect
Insulin: ↑ hypoglycemia
Methyldopa: ↑ hypotension, bradycardia
Prazosin: ↑ hypotension, bradycardia
Reserpine: ↑ hypotension, bradycardia
Thyroid: ↓ effect of β-blockers
Verapamil: ↑ cardiac depression

Drug classifications

Antihypertensives: ↑ hypertension
β_2-Agonist: ↓ bronchodilatation
Cardiac glycosides: ↑ bradycardia
Nitrates: ↑ hypotension
Sulfonylureas: ↓ hypoglycemic effect
Theophyllines: ↓ bronchodilatation

Lab test interferences

False ↑ Urinary catecholamines

NURSING CONSIDERATIONS

Assessment

- Monitor B/P during beginning treatment, periodically thereafter; pulse q4h; note rate, rhythm, quality: apical/radial pulse before administration; notify pre-

P

scriber of any significant changes (pulse <50 bpm)
• Check for baselines in renal, liver function tests before therapy begins
• Assess for edema in feet, legs daily; monitor I&O, daily weight; check for jugular vein distention, rales bilaterally, dyspnea (CHF)
• Monitor skin turgor, dryness of mucous membranes for hydration status, especially G elderly

Nursing diagnoses

✓ Cardiac output, decreased (uses)
✓ Injury, potential for (adverse reactions)
✓ Knowledge deficit (teaching)
✓ Noncompliance (teaching)

Implementation

• Given ac, hs, tab may be crushed or swallowed whole; give with food to prevent GI upset; reduced dosage in renal
• Store protected from light, moisture; place in cool environment

Patient/family education

• Teach patient not to discontinue drug abruptly; taper over 2 wk; may cause precipitate angina if stopped abruptly
• Teach patient not to use OTC products containing α-adrenergic stimulants (such as nasal decongestants, cold preparations); to avoid alcohol, smoking, and to limit sodium intake as prescribed
• Teach patient how to take pulse and B/P at home; advise when to notify prescriber
• Instruct patient to comply with weight control, dietary adjustments, modified exercise program
• Tell patient to carry/wear Medic Alert ID to identify drug being taken, allergies; tell patient drug controls symptoms but does not cure
• Caution patient to avoid hazardous activities if dizziness, drowsiness present
• Teach patient to report symptoms of CHF: difficult breathing, especially on exertion or when lying down, night cough, swelling of extremities or bradycardia, dizziness, confusion, depression, fever
• Teach patient to take drug as prescribed, not to double doses, skip doses; take any missed doses as soon as remembered if at least 4 hr until next dose

Evaluation

Positive therapeutic outcome
• Decreased B/P in hypertension (after 1-2 wk)

Treatment of overdose: Lavage, **IV** atropine for bradycardia, **IV** theophylline for bronchospasm, digitalis, O_2, diuretic for cardiac failure, hemodialysis, **IV** glucose for hyperglycemia, **IV** diazepam (or phenytoin) for seizures

pipecuronium (℞)

(pip-e-kyoor'oh'nee-um)
Arduran
Func. class.: Neuromuscular blocker (nondepolarizing)
Chem. class.: Synthetic curariform
Pregnancy category C

Action: Inhibits transmission of nerve impulses by binding with cholinergic receptor sites, antagonizing action of acetylcholine; no analgesic response

➔ **Therapeutic Outcome:** Paralysis of all skeletal muscles

Uses: Facilitation of endotracheal intubation, skeletal muscle relaxation during mechanical ventilation, surgery, or general anesthesia

Dosage and routes

Adult: **IV** dosage is individualized; in patients with normal renal function who are not obese, initial dose is 70-85 μg/kg; maintenance dose ranges from 10-15 μg/kg

P ***Child 1-14 yr:*** **IV** 57 μg/kg

P ***Child 3 mo-1 yr:*** **IV** 40 μg/kg

Available forms: Inj 10-mg vials

Adverse effects

CNS: Hypesthesia, CNS depression

CV: Bradycardia, tachycardia, increased or decreased B/P, ventricular extrasystole, ***myocardial ischemia, cardiovascular accident, thrombosis, atrial fibrillation***

EENT: Increased secretions

GU: Anuria

INTEG: Rash, urticaria

META: Hypoglycemia, hyperkalemia, increased creatinine

MS: Weakness to prolonged skeletal muscle relaxation

RESP: Prolonged apnea, bronchospasm, cyanosis, respiratory depression

Contraindications: Hypersensitivity to bromide ion

Precautions: Pregnancy **C**, renal disease, cardiac disease, P lactation, children <3 mo, fluid and electrolyte imbalances, neuromuscular diseases, respiratory disease, obesity

Pharmacokinetics	
Absorption	Complete bioavailability
Distribution	Unknown
Metabolism	Unknown
Excretion	Kidneys, unchanged (>75%)
Half-life	1½ hr; increased in renal disease

Pharmacodynamics	
Onset	30-45 sec
Peak	3-5 min
Duration	1-2 hr

Interactions

Individual drugs

Clindamycin: ↑ paralysis length and intensity

Colistin: ↑ paralysis length and intensity

Lidocaine: ↑ paralysis length and intensity

Lithium: ↑ paralysis length and intensity

Magnesium: ↑ paralysis length and intensity

Polymyxin B: ↑ paralysis length and intensity

Procainamide: ↑ paralysis length and intensity

Quinidine: ↑ paralysis length and intensity

Succinylcholine: ↑ paralysis length and intensity

Drug classifications

Aminoglycosides: ↑ paralysis length and intensity

β-Blockers: ↑ paralysis length and intensity

Diuretics, potassium-losing: ↑ paralysis length and intensity

General anesthesia: ↑ paralysis length and intensity

NURSING CONSIDERATIONS

Assessment

• Monitor vital signs (B/P, pulse, respirations, airway) until fully recovered; rate, depth, pattern of respirations,

P

strength of hand grip; patient should be intubated before use

- Monitor for electrolyte imbalances (potassium, magnesium) before drug is used; electrolyte imbalances may lead to increased action of this drug
- Monitor for recovery: decreased paralysis of face, diaphragm, leg, arm, rest of body; residual weakness and respiratory problems may occur during recovery period
- Assess for hypersensitive reactions: rash, fever, respiratory distress, pruritus; drug should be discontinued

Nursing diagnoses

- ✓ Breathing pattern, ineffective (uses)
- ✓ Communication, impaired verbal (adverse reactions)
- ✓ Fear (adverse reactions)
- ✓ Knowledge deficit (teaching)

Implementation

- Use peripheral nerve stimulator (anesthesiologist) to determine neuromuscular blockade; deep tendon reflexes should be monitored during extended periods
- Give **IV** after reconstituting with 0.9% NaCl, D_5W, D_5/0.9% NaCl, LR, sterile water for inj; sol with benzyl alcohol should not be used for newborns; should be administered only by qualified person, usually an anesthesiologist; do not administer IM
- Store in light-resistant area (powder); refrigerate unused portions (sterile water); use within 24 hr

Patient/family education

- Provide reassurance if communication is difficult during recovery from neuromuscular blockade
- Provide explanation to patients regarding all procedures or treatments; patient will remain conscious if anesthesia is not given also

Evaluation

Positive therapeutic outcome

- Paralysis of jaw, eyelid, head, neck, rest of body as evaluated by peripheral nerve stimulator

Treatment of overdose: Edrophonium or neostigmine, atropine, monitor VS; may require mechanical ventilation

piperacillin (℞)

(pi-per'a-sill-in)

Pipracil

Func. class.: Broad-spectrum antiinfective

Chem. class.: Extended-spectrum penicillin

Pregnancy category B

Action: Interferes with cell wall replication of susceptible organisms; osmotically unstable cell wall swells and bursts from osmotic pressure

Therapeutic Outcome: Bactericidal effects for gram-positive cocci *Staphylococcus aureus, Streptococcus pyogenes, S. viridans, S. faecalis, S. bovis, S. pneumoniae;* gram-negative cocci *Neisseria gonorrhoeae, N. meningitidis;* gram-positive bacilli *Clostridium perfringens, C. tetani;* gram-negative bacilli *Bacteroides, Fusobacterium nucleatum, Escherichia coli, Klebsiella, Proteus mirabilis, Morganella morganii, P. vulgaris, P. rettgeri, Enterobacter, Citrobacter, Pseudomonas aeruginosa, Serratia, Acineto-*

bacter, Peptococcus, Peptostreptococcus, Eubacterium

Uses: Respiratory tract, skin, skin structure, urinary tract, bone, and joint infections; gonorrhea, pneumonia, endocarditis, septicemia, meningitis, sinusitis; infections caused by penicillinase-producing staphylococci, streptococci; may be combined with an aminoglycoside for *Pseudomonas* infection

Dosage and routes

Systemic infections

P ***Adult and child >12 yr:*** IM/**IV** 100-300 mg/kg/day in divided doses q4-6h

Prophylaxis of surgical infections

Adult: **IV** 2 g 30-60 min before procedure; may be repeated during or after surgery

Available forms: Inj 2, 3, 4, 40 g; inf 2, 3, 4 g

Adverse effects

CNS: Lethargy, hallucinations, anxiety, depression, twitching, ***coma, convulsions***

GI: Nausea, vomiting, diarrhea, increased AST (SGOT), ALT (SGPT), abdominal pain, glossitis, colitis

GU: ***Oliguria, proteinuria, hematuria, vaginitis, moniliasis, glomerulonephritis***

HEMA: Anemia, increased bleeding time, ***bone marrow depression***

META: Hypokalemia, hypernatremia

P **Contraindications:** Hypersensitivity to penicillins; neonates

Precautions: Pregnancy **B**, hypersensitivity to cephalosporins, CHF

Pharmacokinetics

Absorption	Well absorbed (80%)
Distribution	Widely distributed; crosses placenta
Metabolism	Not metabolized
Excretion	Kidneys, unchanged (90%); bile (10%); breast milk
Half-life	0.7-1.3 hr

Pharmacodynamics

	IM	IV
Onset	Rapid	Rapid
Peak	30-50 min	Inf end

Interactions

Individual drugs

Aminoglycosides: ↓ half-life in renal disease
Amphotericin B: ↑ hypokalemia
Aspirin: ↑ piperacillin levels, ↓ renal excretion
Cholestyramine: ↓ effectiveness of piperacillin
Chloramphenicol: ↑ half-life of chloramphenicol, ↓ effectiveness of piperacillin
Colestipol: ↓ effectiveness of piperacillin
Diuretics: ↑ hypokalemia
Glucocorticoids: ↑ hypokalemia
Hepatotoxic agents: ↑ hepatotoxicity
Probenecid: ↑ piperacillin levels, ↓ renal excretion

Drug classifications

Erythromycins: ↓ antimicrobial effectiveness
Lithium: ↓ excretion, ↑ toxicity
Oral anticoagulants: ↑ anticoagulant effects
Oral contraceptives: ↓ contraceptive effectiveness
Tetracyclines: ↓ antimicrobial effectiveness

Food

Food, carbonated drinks, citrus fruit juices: ↓ absorption

P

Lab test interferences
False positive: Urine glucose, urine protein

NURSING CONSIDERATIONS
Assessment

- Assess patient for previous sensitivity reaction to penicillins or other cephalosporins; cross-sensitivity between penicillins and cephalosporins is common
- Assess patient for signs and symptoms of infection including characteristics of wounds, sputum, urine, stool, WBC >10,000, fever; obtain baseline information and during treatment
- Obtain C&S before beginning drug therapy to identify if correct treatment has been initiated
- Assess for allergic reactions: rash, urticaria, pruritus, chills, fever, joint pain; angioedema may occur a few days after therapy begins; epinephrine, resuscitation equipment should be available for anaphylactic reaction
- Identify urine output; if decreasing, notify prescriber (may indicate nephrotoxicity); also check for increased BUN, creatinine
- Monitor blood studies: AST (SGOT), ALT (SGPT), CBC, Hct, bilirubin, LDH, alkaline phosphatase, Coombs' test monthly if patient is on long-term therapy
- Monitor electrolytes: potassium, sodium, chloride monthly if patient is on long-term therapy
- Assess bowel pattern daily; if severe diarrhea occurs, drug should be discontinued; may indicate pseudomembranous colitis
- Monitor for bleeding: ecchymosis, bleeding gums, hematuria, stool guaiac daily if on long-term therapy
- Assess for overgrowth of infection: perineal itching, fever, malaise, redness, pain, swelling, drainage, rash, diarrhea, change in cough, sputum

Nursing diagnoses

- ✓ Infection, risk for (uses)
- ✓ Diarrhea (adverse reactions)
- ✓ Injury, risk for (adverse reactions)
- ✓ Knowledge deficit (teaching)
- ✓ Noncompliance (teaching)

Implementation

IM route

- Reconstitute 2 g/4 ml, 3 g/6 ml, 4 g/7.8 gm with sterile water, 0.9% NaCl, bacteriostatic water, 0.5% or 1% lidocaine without epinephrine
- Inject deep in large muscle mass, massage; split inj over 2 g into 2 inj

IV route

- Reconstitute with 5 ml or more 0.9% NaCl, bacteriostatic water; shake sol to dissolve
- Change **IV** sites q48h to prevent phlebitis and pain
- Give direct **IV** over 3-5 min
- Give by intermittent inf by diluting in 50 ml or more D_5W, 0.9% NaCl, D_5/0.9% NaCl, LR give over 20-30 min by Y-site; discontinue primary inf during intermittent inf

Syringe compatibility:
Heparin

Y-site incompatibilities:
Ondansetron, fluconazole, sargramostim, vinorelbine

Y-site compatibilities:
Acyclovir, aldesleukin, allopurinol, amifostine, aztreonam, ciprofloxacin, cyclophosphamide, diltiazem, enalaprilat,

esmolol, famotidine, fludarabine, foscarnet, heparin, hydromorphone, IL-2, labetalol, lorazepam, magnesium sulfate, melphalan, meperidine, midazolam, morphine, perphenazine, thiotepa, verapamil, zidovudine

Additive incompatibility: Aminoglycosides

Additive compatibilities: Ciprofloxacin, clindamycin, flucoxacillin, fluconazole, hydrocortisone sodium succinate, ofloxacin, potassium chloride, verapamil

Patient/family education

- Teach patient to report sore throat, bruising, bleeding, joint pain; may indicate blood dyscrasias (rare)
- Advise patient to contact prescriber if vaginal itching, loose, foul-smelling stools, furry tongue occur; may indicate superinfection
- Advise patient to notify prescriber of diarrhea with blood or pus, which may indicate pseudomembranous colitis

Evaluation

Positive therapeutic outcome

- Absence of signs/symptoms of infection (WBC <10,000, temp WNL, absence of red, draining wounds)
- Reported improvement in symptoms of infection

Treatment of anaphylaxis: Withdraw drug, maintain airway, administer epinephrine, aminophylline, O_2, **IV** corticosteroids

piperacillin/tazobactam (℞)

Pipracil

Func. class.: Broad-spectrum antiinfective

Chem. class.: Extended-spectrum penicillin

Pregnancy category B

Action: Interferes with cell wall replication of susceptible organisms; osmotically unstable cell wall swells and bursts from osmotic pressure

➔ **Therapeutic Outcome:** Bactericidal effects for piperacillin-resistant β-lactamase, *Escherichia coli, Staphylococcus aureus, Bacteroides fragilis, Haemophilus influenzae*

Uses: Respiratory tract, skin, skin structure, urinary tract, bone, and joint infections; gonorrhea, pneumonia, infections from penicillinase-producing staphylococci, streptococci

Dosage and routes

Adult: **IV** 3 g piperacillin with 0.375 g tazaobactam q6h before procedure; may be repeated during or after surgery

Nosocomial pneumonia

Adult: **IV** 3.375 g q4h with an aminoglycoside; continue aminoglycoside only if *P. aeruginosa* is isolated

Available forms: 2 g/0.25 g; 3 g/0.375 g; 4 g/0.5 g

Adverse effects

CNS: Headache, insomnia, agitation, dizziness

CV: Chest pain, edema, hypertension

EENT: Rhinitis

P

INTEG: Rash
MISC: Fever, superinfection
RESP: Dyspnea

Contraindications: Hypersensitivity to penicillins, cephalosporins, tazobactam; neonates P

Precautions: Pregnancy **B,** CHF, renal disease, lactation, sodium restriction

Pharmacokinetics

Absorption	Well absorbed (80%)
Distribution	Widely distributed; crosses placenta
Metabolism	Not metabolized
Excretion	Kidneys, unchanged (90%); bile (10%); breast milk
Half-life	0.7-1.3 hr

Pharmacodynamics

Onset	Rapid
Peak	Inf end

Interactions

Individual drugs

Aminoglycosides: ↓ half-life in renal disease
Amphotericin B: ↑ hypokalemia
Aspirin: ↑ piperacillin levels, ↑ renal excretion
Cholestyramine: ↓ effectiveness of piperacillin
Chloramphenicol: ↑ half-life of chloramphenicol, ↓ effectiveness of piperacillin
Colestipol: ↓ effectiveness of piperacillin
Diuretics: ↑ hypokalemia
Glucocorticoids: ↑ hypokalemia
Hepatotoxic agents: ↑ hepatotoxicity
Probenecid: ↑ piperacillin levels, ↓ renal excretion

Drug classifications

Erythromycins: ↓ antimicrobial effectiveness
Lithium: ↓ excretion, ↑ toxicity
Oral anticoagulants: ↑ anticoagulant effects
Oral contraceptives: ↓ contraceptive effectiveness
Tetracyclines: ↓ antimicrobial effectiveness

Food

Food, carbonated drinks, citrus fruit juices: ↓ absorption

Lab test interferences

False positive: Urine glucose, urine protein

NURSING CONSIDERATIONS

Assessment

- Assess patient for previous sensitivity reaction to penicillins or other cephalosporins, cross-sensitivity between penicillins and cephalosporins is common
- Assess patient for signs and symptoms of infection including characteristics of wounds, sptum, urine, stool, WBC >10,000, fever; obtain baseline information and during treatment
- Obtain C&S before beginning drug therapy to identify if correct treatment has been initiated
- Assess for allergic reactions: rash, urticaria, pruritus, chills, fever, joint pain; angioedema may occur a few days after therapy begins; epinephrine, resuscitation equipment should be available for anaphylactic reaction
- Identify urine output; if decreasing, notify prescriber (may indicate nephrotoxicity); also check for increased BUN, creatinine
- Monitor blood studies: AST (SGOT), ALT (SGPT), CBC, Hct, bilirubin, LDH, alkaline phosphatase, Coombs' test

monthly if patient is on long-term therapy

- Monitor electrolytes: potassium, sodium, chloride monthly if patient is on long-term therapy
- Assess bowel pattern daily; if severe diarrhea occurs, drug should be discontinued; may indicate pseudomembranous colitis
- Monitor for bleeding: ecchymosis, bleeding gums, hematuria, stool guaiac daily if on long-term therapy
- Assess for overgrowth of infection: perineal itching, fever, malaise, redness, pain, swelling, drainage, rash, diarrhea, change in cough, sputum

Nursing diagnoses

- ✓ Infection, risk for (uses)
- ✓ Diarrhea (adverse reactions)
- ✓ Injury, risk for (adverse reactions)
- ✓ Knowledge deficit (teaching)
- ✓ Noncompliance (teaching)

Implementation

- Reconstitute with 5 ml or more 0.9% NaCl, bacteriostatic water; shake sol to dissolve
- Give by intermittent inf by diluting in 50 ml or more D_5W, 0.9% NaCl, D_5/0.9% NaCl, LR; give over 20-30 min by Y-site; discontinue primary inf during intermittent inf
- Change **IV** sites q48h to prevent phlebitis and pain
- Give direct **IV** over 3-5 min

Y-site incompatibilities: Ondansetron, fluconazole, sargramostim, vinorelbine

Y-site compatibilities: Cyclophosphamide, enalaprilat, fludarabine, hydromorphone, magnesium sulfate, meperidine, morphine, zidovudine

Patient/family education

- Teach patient to report sore throat, bruising, bleeding, joint pain; may indicate blood dyscrasias (rare)
- Advise patient to contact prescriber if vaginal itching, loose, foul-smelling stools, furry tongue occur; may indicate superinfection
- Advise patient to notify prescriber of diarrhea with blood or pus, which may indicate pseudomembranous colitis

Evaluation

Positive therapeutic outcome

- Absence of signs/symptoms of infection (WBC <10,000, temp WNL, absence of red, draining wounds)
- Reported improvement in symptoms of infection

Treatment of anaphylaxis: Withdraw drug, maintain airway, administer epinephrine, aminophylline, O_2, **IV** corticosteroids

pirbuterol (℞)

(peer-byoo'ter-ole)

Maxair

Func. class.: Bronchodilator

Chem. class.: β-Adrenergic agonist

Pregnancy category C

Action: Relaxes bronchial smooth muscle by direct action on β_2-adrenergic receptors, with increased levels of cAMP and increased bronchodilatation, diuresis, and cardiac and CNS stimulation

➲ **Therapeutic Outcome:** Bron-

P

chodilatation with ease of breathing

Uses: Reversible bronchospasm (prevention, treatment), including asthma, may be given with theophylline or steroids

Dosage and routes

P ***Adult and child >12 yr:*** Aerosol 1-2 inh (0.4 mg) q4-6h; do not exceed 12 inh/day

Available forms: Aerosol delivers 0.2 mg pirbuterol/actuation

Adverse effects

CNS: Tremors, anxiety, insomnia, headache, dizziness, stimulation, restlessness, hallucinations, drowsiness, irritability
CV: Palpitations, tachycardia, hypertension, angina, hypotension, dysrhythmias
EENT: Dry nose and mouth, irritation of nose, throat
GI: Gastritis, nausea, vomiting, anorexia
MS: Muscle cramps
RESP: Bronchospasm, dyspnea, coughing

Contraindications: Hypersensitivity to sympathomimetics, tachycardia

Precautions: Lactation, pregnancy **C,** cardiac disorders, hyperthyroidism, diabetes mellitus, prostatic hypertrophy

Pharmacokinetics	
Absorption	Minimally absorbed
Distribution	Unknown
Metabolism	Liver
Excretion	Unknown
Half-life	2 hr

Pharmacodynamics	
Onset	5-15 min
Peak	1-1½ hr
Duration	5 hr

Interactions

Drug classifications

β-Adrenergic blockers: Block therapeutic effect
Bronchodilators, aerosol: ↑ action of bronchodilator
MAOIs: ↑ chance of hypertensive crisis
Sympathomimetics: ↑ adrenergic side effects

NURSING CONSIDERATIONS

Assessment

- Monitor respiratory function: vital capacity, FEV, ABGs, lung sounds, heart rate, rhythm (baseline)
- Monitor for evidence of allergic reactions; paradoxic bronchospasm; withhold dose; notify prescriber

Nursing diagnoses

✓ Airway clearance, ineffective (uses)
✓ Gas exchange, impaired (uses)
✓ Knowledge deficit (teaching)

Implementation

- Give after shaking; have patient exhale, place mouthpiece in mouth, inhale slowly, hold breath, remove, exhale slowly; allow at least 1 min between inh
- Store in light-resistant container; do not expose to temp over 86° F (30° C)

Patient/family education

- Advise patient not to use OTC medications; extra stimulation may occur; to use this medication before other medications and allow at least 1 min between each to prevent overstimulation
- Teach patient use of inhaler; review package insert with patient; to avoid getting aerosol in eyes; blurring may result; to wash inhaler in warm water and dry daily; to avoid smok-

ing, smoke-filled rooms, persons with respiratory tract infections

- Teach patient that paradoxic bronchospasm may occur and to stop drug immediately and notify prescriber; to limit caffeine products such as chocolate, coffee, tea, and colas
- Instruct patient on administration of dose; not to use more than prescribed; serious side effects may occur

Evaluation

Positive therapeutic outcome

- Absence of dyspnea, wheezing after 1 hr
- Improved airway exchange
- Improved ABGs

Treatment of overdose: Administer a β_2-adrenergic blocker

piroxicam (℞)

(peer-ox'i-kam)

Apo-Piroxicam ✦, Feldene, Novopirocam ✦

Func. class.: Nonsteroidal antiinflammatory

Chem. class.: Oxicam derivative

Pregnancy category C

Action: Inhibits prostaglandin synthesis by decreasing an enzyme needed for biosynthesis; analgesic, antiinflammatory

Therapeutic Outcome: Decreased pain, inflammation

Uses: Mild to moderate pain, osteoarthritis, rheumatoid arthritis

Dosage and routes

Adult: PO 20 qd or 10 mg bid

Available forms: Caps 10, 20 mg

Adverse effects

GI: Nausea, anorexia, vomiting, diarrhea, jaundice, ***cholestatic hepatitis,*** constipation, flatulence, cramps, dry mouth, peptic ulcer, ***bleeding, ulceration, perforation***

CNS: Dizziness, *drowsiness,* fatigue, tremors, confusion, insomnia, anxiety, depression, *headache*

CV: Tachycardia, peripheral edema, palpitations, dysrhythmias

EENT: Tinnitus, hearing loss, blurred vision

GU: Nephrotoxicity: dysuria, hematuria, oliguria, azotemia

HEMA: Blood dyscrasias

INTEG: Purpura, rash, pruritus, sweating, photosensitivity

Contraindications: Hypersensitivity, asthma, severe renal disease, severe hepatic disease, ulcer disease, cardiac disease

Precautions: Pregnancy **C**, lactation, children, bleeding disorders, GI disorders, cardiac disorders, hypersensitivity to other antiinflammatory agents

Pharmacokinetics	
Absorption	Well absorbed
Distribution	Unknown
Metabolism	Liver, extensively
Excretion	Kidneys, minimal; breast milk
Half-life	50 hr

Pharmacodynamics	
Onset	1 hr
Peak	Unknown
Duration	Unknown

Interactions

Individual drugs

Acetaminophen (long-term use): ↑ renal reactions

Alcohol: ↑ adverse reactions

Aspirin: ↓ effectiveness, ↑ adverse reactions
Coumadin: ↑ anticoagulant effects
Digoxin: ↑ toxicity, levels
Insulin: ↓ insulin effect
Lithium: ↑ toxicity
Methotrexate: ↑ toxicity
Phenytoin: ↑ toxicity
Probenecid: ↑ toxicity
Sulfonylurea: ↑ toxicity

Drug classifications
Anticoagulants: ↑ risk of bleeding
Antihypertensives: ↓ effect of antihypertensives
Antineoplastics: ↑ risk of hematologic toxicity
β-Blockers: ↑ antihypertension
Cephalosporins: ↑ risk of bleeding
Glucocorticoids: ↑ adverse reactions
Hypoglycemics: ↓ hypoglycemic effect
Diuretics: ↓ effectiveness of diuretics
NSAIDs: ↑ adverse reactions
Potassium supplements: ↑ adverse reactions
Radiation: ↑ risk of hematologic toxicity
Sulfonamides: ↑ toxicity

Lab test interferences
↑ Serum potassium, ↑ liver function studies
↓ Hct, ↓ Hgb, ↓ blood glucose

NURSING CONSIDERATIONS

Assessment

- Monitor blood counts during therapy; watch for decreasing platelets; if low, therapy may need to be discontinued, restarted after hematologic recovery; check for blood dyscrasia (thrombocytopenia): bruising, fatigue, bleeding, poor healing

Nursing diagnoses

- ✓ Pain (uses)
- ✓ Mobility, impaired (uses)
- ✓ Knowledge deficit (teaching)
- ✓ Injury, risk for (adverse reactions)

Implementation

- Administer to patient whole; give with food or milk to decrease gastric symptoms
- ⊘ Do not crush, chew caps

Patient/family education

- Teach patient that drug must be continued for prescribed time to be effective; to avoid aspirin, alcoholic beverages and other OTC medications unless approved by prescriber
- Caution patient to report bleeding, bruising, fatigue, malaise, since blood dyscrasias do occur
- Instruct patient to use caution when driving; drowsiness, dizziness may occur
- Teach patient to take with a full glass of water to enhance absorption; do not crush, break, or chew

Evaluation

Positive therapeutic outcome

- Decreased pain
- Decreased inflammation
- Increased mobility

plasma protein fraction (℞)

Plasmanate, Plasma Plex, Plasmatein, PPF Protenate
Func. class.: Blood derivative
Chem. class.: Human plasma in sodium chloride
Pregnancy category C

Action: Exerts similar oncotic pressure as human plasma, expands blood volume, shifts water from extravascular space to intravascular space

➔ **Therapeutic Outcome:** Shift of fluid from extravascular into intravascular space

Uses: Hypovolemic shock, hypoproteinemia, ARDS, preoperative cardiopulmonary bypass, acute liver failure, nephrotic syndrome

Dosage and routes

Hypovolemia

Adult: **IV** inf 250-500 ml (12.5-25 g protein), not to exceed 10 ml/min

P ***Child:*** **IV** inf 22-33 ml/kg at 5-10 ml/min

Hypoproteinemia

Adult: **IV** inf 1000-1500 ml qd, not to exceed 8 ml/min

Available forms: Inj 50 mg/ml

Adverse effects

CNS: Fever, chills, headache, paresthesias, flushing
CV: Fluid overload, hypotension, erratic pulse
GI: Nausea, vomiting, increased salivation
INTEG: Rash, urticaria, cyanosis
RESP: Altered respirations, dyspnea, pulmonary edema

Contraindications: Hypersensitivity, CHF, severe anemia, renal insufficiency

Precautions: Decreased salt intake, decreased cardiac reserve, lack of albumin deficiency, hepatic disease, renal disease, pregnancy **C**

Pharmacokinetics	
Absorption	Completely absorbed
Distribution	Intravascular space
Metabolism	Unknown
Excretion	Unknown
Half-life	Unknown

Pharmacodynamics	
Onset	15-30 min
Peak	Unknown
Duration	Unknown

Interactions: None

Lab test interferences

False ↑ Alkaline phosphatase

NURSING CONSIDERATIONS

Assessment

- Monitor blood studies: Hct, Hgb; electrolytes, serum protein, if serum protein declines, dyspnea, hypoxemia can result
- Monitor B/P (decreased), pulse (erratic), respiration during inf; CVP, pulmonary wedge pressure (increases if overload occurs)
- Monitor I&O ratio; urinary output may decrease
- Assess for allergy: fever, rash, itching, chills, flushing, urticaria, nausea, vomiting, or hypotension requires discontinuation of inf; use new lot if therapy reinstituted
- Monitor for increased CVP reading: distended neck veins indicate circulatory overload; SOB, anxiety, insomnia, expiratory rales, frothy blood-tinged cough, cyanosis indicate pulmonary overload

Nursing diagnoses

✓ Fluid volume deficit (uses)
✓ Cardiac output, decreased (uses)
✓ Fluid volume excess (adverse reactions)

Implementation

- Give by **IV**; no dilution required; use inf pump, large-

P

gauge needle (≥20 G); discard unused portion; infuse slowly within 4 hr of opening

- Provide adequate hydration before administration
- When storing, check type of albumin, date; may have to refrigerate

Additive compatibilities: Carbohydrate and electrolyte sol, whole blood, packed red blood cells, chloramphenicol, tetracycline

Additive incompatibilities: Protein hydrolysate sol, amino acids solution, alcohol, norepinephrine

Patient/family education

- Explain reason for and expected result of medication

Evaluation

Positive therapeutic outcome

- Increased B/P
- Decreased edema
- Increased serum albumin

plicamycin (℞)

(plik-a-mi′cin)

Mithramycin, Mithracin

Func. class.: Antineoplastic, antibiotic; hypocalcemic

Chem. class.: Crystalline aglycone

Pregnancy category X

Action: Inhibits DNA, RNA, protein synthesis; derived from *Streptomyces plicatus;* replication is decreased by binding to DNA; demonstrates calcium-lowering effect not related to its tumoricidal activity; also acts on osteoclasts and blocks action of parathyroid hormone; a vesicant

➔ Therapeutic Outcome: Prevention of rapidly growing malignant cells, decreased calcium levels

Uses: Testicular cancer, hypercalcemia, hypercalciuria, symptomatic treatment of advanced neoplasms

Dosage and routes

Testicular tumors

Adult: **IV** 25-30 μg/kg/day × 8-10 days, not to exceed 30 μg/kg/day

Hypercalcemia/hypercalciuria

Adult: **IV** 25 μg/kg/day × 3-4 days; repeat at intervals of 1 wk

Available forms: Inj 2.5 mg/vial powder

Adverse effects

CNS: Drowsiness, weakness, lethargy, headache, flushing, fever, depression

GI: Nausea, vomiting, anorexia, diarrhea, stomatitis, increased liver enzymes

GU: Increased BUN, creatinine, ***proteinuria***

HEMA: Hemorrhage, thrombocytopenia, decreased protime, WBC count

INTEG: Rash, cellulitis, ***extravasation,*** facial flushing

META: Decreased serum calcium, potassium, phosphorus

Contraindications: Hypersensitivity, thrombocytopenia, bone marrow depression, bleeding disorders, pregnancy **X**

Precautions: Renal disease, hepatic disease, electrolyte imbalances

Pharmacokinetics

Absorption	Completely absorbed
Distribution	Crosses blood-brain barrier; concentration in bone, liver, renal system
Metabolism	Unknown
Excretion	Kidneys
Half-life	Unknown

Pharmacodynamics

Unknown

Interactions

Individual drugs

Aspirin: ↑ risk of bleeding
Dextran: ↑ risk of bleeding
Heparin: ↑ risk of bleeding
Radiation: ↑ toxicity, bone marrow suppression
Sulfinpyrazone: ↑ risk of bleeding
Valproic acid: ↑ risk of bleeding

Drug classifications

Anticoagulants, oral: ↑ risk of bleeding
Antineoplastics: ↑ toxicity, bone marrow suppression
Cephalosporins: ↑ risk of bleeding
Hepatotoxic agents: ↑ hepatotoxicity
Neurotoxic agents: ↑ neurotoxicity
NSAIDs: ↑ risk of bleeding
Thrombolytics: ↑ risk of bleeding

NURSING CONSIDERATIONS

Assessment

- Assess buccal cavity q8h for dryness, sores or ulceration, white patches, oral pain, bleeding, dysphagia; obtain prescription for viscous lidocaine (Xylocaine)
- Assess symptoms indicating severe allergic reaction: rash, pruritus, urticaria, purpuric skin lesions, itching, flushing
- Monitor CBC, differential, platelet count weekly; withhold drug if WBC count is <4000/mm^3 or platelet count is <100,000/mm^3; notify prescriber of results if WBC <20,000/mm^3, platelets <150,000/mm^3
- Monitor renal function studies: BUN, creatinine, serum uric acid, urine CrCl before and during therapy; I&O ratio; report fall in urine output to <30 ml/hr
- Monitor temp q4h (may indicate beginning of infection)
- Monitor liver function tests before and during therapy (bilirubin, AST [SGOT], ALT [SGPT], LDH) as needed or monthly; check for yellowing of skin and sclera, dark urine, clay-colored stools, itchy skin, abdominal pain, fever, diarrhea
- Assess for bleeding: hematuria, stool guaiac, bruising or petechiae, mucosa or orifices q8h; check for inflammation of mucosa, breaks in skin

Nursing diagnoses

- ✓ Injury, risk for (adverse reactions)
- ✓ Body image disturbance (adverse reactions)
- ✓ Infection, risk for (adverse reactions)
- ✓ Knowledge deficit (teaching)

Implementation

- Avoid contact with skin; very irritating; wash completely to remove
- Give fluids **IV** or PO before chemotherapy to hydrate patient
- Give antacid before oral agent; give drug after evening meal, before hs; provide antiemetic 30-60 min before giving drug and prn to prevent

P

vomiting; administer antibiotics for prophylaxis of infection
• Give top or syst analgesics for pain
• Give in AM so drug can be eliminated before hs
• Provide liq diet: carbonated beverages; gelatin may be added if patient is not nauseated or vomiting
• Encourage patient to rinse mouth tid-qid with water, club soda; brush teeth bid-qid with soft brush or cotton-tipped applicators for stomatitis; use unwaxed dental floss
• Make sure drug is prepared by experienced personnel using proper precautions
• Give **IV** direct by **IV** push over 20-30 min
• Give **IV** intermittent inf by diluting 2.5 mg/4.9 ml of sterile water; (1 ml = 500 μg); dilute single dose in 1000 ml of D_5W run over 4-6 hr; give slow **IV** inf using 20 G, 21 G needle
• Administer EDTA for extravasation; apply ice compress

Y-site compatibilities: Allopurinol, amifostine, aztreonam, filgrastim, melphalan, piperacillin/tazobactam, teniposide, thiotepa, vinorelbine

Patient/family education
• Teach patient to avoid use of products containing aspirin or ibuprofen, razors, commercial mouthwash, since bleeding may occur; to report symptoms of bleeding (hematuria, tarry stools)
• Caution patient to report signs of anemia (fatigue, headache, irritability, faintness, shortness of breath)
• Advise patient to report any changes in breathing or coughing even several mo after treatment; to avoid crowds or persons with respiratory tract and other infections
• Advise patient that hair may be lost during treatment; a wig or hair piece may make patient feel better; new hair may be different in color, texture
• Caution patient not to have any vaccinations without the advice of the prescriber; serious reactions can occur
• Advise patient that contraception is needed during treatment and for several mo after completion of therapy

Evaluation
Positive therapeutic outcome
• Prevention of rapid division of malignant cells

polymyxin B (℞)
(pol-ee-mix'in)
Aerosporin, polymyxin B Sulfate
Func. class.: Antiinfective
Chem. class: Polymyxin
Pregnancy category B

Action: Interferes with phospholipids, penetrates cell wall; immediately changes bacterial membrane, causing leakage of essential metabolites

Therapeutic Outcome: Bactericidal against *Pseudomonas aeruginosa, Enterobacter aerogenes, Klebsiella pneumoniae, Escherichia coli, Haemophilus influenzae*

Uses: Serious infections or when other antibiotics cannot be used; septicemia, meningitis, UTI, ophth infections (ophth route)

Dosage and routes

P ***Adult and child:*** **IV** inf 15,000-25000 U/kg/day in divided doses q12h, or 25,000 U/kg/day in divided doses q4-8h

P. aeruginosa/H. influenzae

P ***Adult and child >2 yr:*** Intrathecal 50,000 U/day × 3-4 days, then 50,000 U/qod × 2 wks after CSF negative, glucose normal

P ***Child < 2 yr:*** Intrathecal 20,000 U/day × 3-4 days, then 25,000 U/qod × 2 wk after CSF negative

Ocular infections

Adult: Ophth 1-3 gtt qh; may be increased if needed

Available forms: Inj 500,000 U; powder for ophth sol 500,000 U/20-50 ml

Adverse effects

CNS: Dizziness, confusion, weakness, drowsiness, paresthesia, slurred speech, ***coma, seizures,*** headache, stiff neck, fever

EENT (OPHTH): itching, burning, stinging, vision changes

GU: Proteinuria, hematuria, azotemia, leukocyturia

INTEG: Urticaria, pain at inj site, phlebitis, flushing

RESP: Paralysis

SYST: Anaphylaxis, superinfection

Contraindications: Hypersensitivity, severe renal disease

Precaution: Pregnancy **B**

Pharmacokinetics

Absorption	Well absorbed (IM); completely absorbed (IV)
Distribution	Widely distributed
Metabolism	Unknown
Excretion	Kidneys, unchanged (50%-60%)
Half-life	4½-6 hr; increased in renal disease

Pharmacodynamics

	IM	IV	OPHTH
Onset	Rapid	Rapid	Unknown
Peak	1-2 hr	Inf end	Unknown

Interactions

Individual drugs

Tubocurarine: ↑ skeletal muscle relaxation

Succinylcholine: ↑ skeletal muscle relaxation

Gallamine: ↑ skeletal muscle relaxation

Drug classifications

Aminoglycosides: ↑ nephrotoxicity

Anesthetics: ↑ skeletal muscle relaxation

Neuromuscular blockers: ↑ skeletal muscle relaxation

NURSING CONSIDERATIONS

Assessment

- Assess patient for previous sensitivity reaction
- Assess patient for signs and symptoms of infection including characteristics of wounds, sputum, urine, stool, WBC >10,000, fever; obtain baseline information before and during treatment
- Obtain C&S before beginning drug therapy to identify if correct treatment has been initiated
- Assess for allergic reactions: rash, urticaria, pruritus
- Identify urine output; if decreasing, notify prescriber

(may indicate nephrotoxicity); also check for increased BUN, creatinine

• Monitor blood studies: AST (SGOT), ALT (SGPT), CBC, Hct, bilirubin, LDH, alkaline, phosphatase, Coombs' test monthly if patient is on long-term therapy

• Assess bowel pattern daily; if severe diarrhea occurs, drug should be discontinued

• Assess for overgrowth of infection: perineal itching, fever, malaise, redness, pain, swelling, drainage, rash, diarrhea, change in cough, sputum

• Assess for CNS symptoms: insomnia, vertigo, headaches, agitation, confusion

Nursing diagnoses

✓ Infection, risk for (uses)
✓ Diarrhea (adverse reactions)
✓ Injury, risk for (adverse reactions)
✓ Knowledge deficit (teaching)
✓ Noncompliance (teaching)

Implementation

IV **IV route**

• For intermittent inf dilute to 4 mg/ml of D_5W, D_5/0.9% NaCl, 0.9% NaCl, D_5/LR, sodium bicarbonate, sodium lactate, D_5/Plasma-Lyte 56; give over 1 hr or more

• For direct **IV** dissolve 500,000 U of polymyxin B in 10 ml of 0.9% NaCl for a conc of 50,000 U/ml

Y-site compatibility:
Esmolol

Additive compatibilities:
Amikacin, ascorbic acid, diphenhydramine, erythromycin, hydrocortisone, kanamycin, methicillin, penicillin G phenobarbital, potassium, ranitidine, sodium, vit B/C

Additive incompatibilities:
Amphotericin B, cefazolin, cephalothin, chloramphenicol, heparin, magnesium sulfate, prednisolone

Patient/family education

• Teach patient reason for medication and expected results

Evaluation

Positive therapeutic outcome

• Absence of signs/symptoms of infection (WBC <10,000, temp WNL)

• Reported improvement in symptoms of infection

• Absence of red or itching eyes (ophth)

porfirmer (℞)

(pour'fur-meer)

Photofrin

Func. class.: Antineoplastic-misc.

Chem. class.: Photosensitizing agent

Pregnancy category C

Action: Used in photodynamic treatment of tumors (PDT); antitumor and cytotoxic actions are light and O_2 dependent; used with 630 nm laser light

➔ **Therapeutic Outcome:** Prevention of growth of tumor

Uses: Esophageal cancer (completely obstructing)

Dosage and routes

Adult: **IV** 2 mg/kg, then illumination with laser light 40-50 hr after inj; a second laser light application may be given 96-120 hr after inj; may repeat q 30 days × 3

Available forms: Cake/ powder for inj 75 mg

Adverse effects

CNS: Anxiety, confusion, insomnia

CV: Hypotension, hypertension, atrial fibrillation, cardiac failure, tachycardia

GI: Abdominal pain, constipation, diarrhea, dyspepsia, dysphagia, eructation, esophageal edema/bleeding, hematemesis, melena, nausea, vomiting, anorexia

MISC: Dehydration, weight decrease, anemia, photosensitivity reaction, UTI, moniliasis

RESP: ***Pleural effusion,*** pneumonia, dyspnea, resp insufficiency, ***tracheoesophageal fistula***

Contraindications: Porphyria, porphyrin allergy (porfirmer); tracheoesophageal, bronchoesophageal fistula; major blood vessels with eroding tumors (PDT)

G P **Precautions:** Elderly, pregnancy **C,** lactation, children

Pharmacokinetics

Absorption	Unknown
Distribution	Unknown
Metabolism	Unknown
Excretion	Unknown
Half-life	250 hr

Pharmacodynamics

Unknown

Interactions

Drug classifications

Phenothiazines: ↑ photosensitivity

Sulfonamides: ↑ photosensitivity

Sulfonylureas: ↑ photosensitivity

Thiazides: ↑ photosensitivity

NURSING CONSIDERATIONS

Assessment

- Assess for ocular sensitivity; sensitivity to sun, bright lights, car headlights; patients should wear dark sunglasses with an average white light transmittance of <4%
- Assess for chest pain: may be so severe as to necessitate opiate analgesics
- Assess for extravasation at inj site: take care to protect from light

Nursing diagnoses

✓ Infection, risk for (adverse reactions)

✓ Knowledge deficit (teaching)

Implementation

- Give porfirmer as a single slow **IV** inj over 3-5 min at 2mg/kg; reconstitute each vial with 31.8 ml D5 or 0.9% NaCl (2.5 mg/ml), shake well, do not mix with other drugs or sol, protect from light, and use immediately
- Laser light is initiated 630 nm wave length laser light
- Wipe spills with damp cloth, avoid skin/eye contact, use rubber gloves, eye protection; dispose of material in polyethylene bag according to policy

Patient/family education

- Advise patient to report chest pain, eye sensitivity
- Advise patient to wear sunglasses with average white light transmittance of <4%

P

potassium bicarbonate/ potassium acetate/ potassium chloride/ potassium gluconate/ potassium phosphate
Func. class.: Electrolyte
Chem. class.: Potassium
Pregnancy category C

Action: Needed for adequate transmission of nerve impulses and cardiac contraction, renal function, intracellular ion maintenance

→ **Therapeutic Outcome:** Potassium level 3.0-5.0

Uses: Prevention and treatment of hypokalemia

Dosage and routes
Potassium bicarbonate
Adult: PO dissolve 25-50 mEq in water qd-qid

Potassium acetate—hypokalemia
P ***Adult and child:*** PO 40-100 mEq/day in divided doses × 2-4 days

Hypokalemia (prevention)
P ***Adult and child:*** PO 20 mEq/day in 2-4 divided doses

Potassium chloride
Adult: PO 40-100 mEq in divided doses tid-qid; **IV** 20 mEq/hr when diluted as 40 mEq/1000 ml, not to exceed 150 mEq/day

Potassium gluconate
Adult: PO 40-100 mEq in divided doses tid-qid

Potassium phosphate
Adult: **IV** 1 mEq/hr in sol of 60 mEq/L, not to exceed 150 mEq/day; PO 40-100 mEq/day in divided doses

Available forms: Tabs for sol 6.5, 25 mEq; inj for prep of **IV** 2, 4 mEq; ext rel caps 8, 10 mEq; powder for sol 3.3, 5, 6.7, 10, 13.3 mEq/5 ml; tabs 4, 13.4 mEq; ext rel tabs 6.7, 8, 10 mEq; inj for prep of **IV** 1.5, 2, 2.4, 3, 3.2 mEq/ml; elix 6.7 mEq/5 ml; tabs 2, 5 mEq; oral sol 2.375 mEq/5 ml; inj for prep of **IV** 4.4, 4.7 mEq/ml

Adverse effects
CNS: Confusion
CV: Bradycardia, *cardiac depression, dysrhythmias, arrest, peaking T waves, lowered R and depressed RST, prolonged PR interval, widened QRS complex*
GI: Nausea, vomiting, cramps, pain, *diarrhea,* ulceration of small bowel
GU: Oliguria
INTEG: Cold extremities, rash

Contraindications: Renal disease (severe), severe hemolytic disease, Addison's disease, hyperkalemia, acute dehydration, extensive tissue breakdown

Precautions: Cardiac disease, potassium-sparing diuretic therapy, systemic acidosis, pregnancy **C**

Pharmacokinetics and pharmacodynamics unavailable.

Interactions
Drug classifications
Angiotensin converting enzyme inhibitors: ↑ hyperkalemia
Potassium-sparing diuretics: ↑ hyperkalemia

NURSING CONSIDERATIONS
Assessment
- Assess ECG for peaking T waves, lowered R, depressed

RST, prolonged PR interval, widening QRS complex, hyperkalemia; drug should be reduced or discontinued
- Monitor potassium level during treatment (3.5-5.0 mg/dl is normal level)
- Monitor I&O ratio; watch for decreased urinary output; notify prescriber immediately; check urinary pH in patients receiving the drug as a urinary acidifier
- Assess cardiac status: rate, rhythm, CVP, PWP, PAWP if being monitored directly

Nursing diagnoses

✓ Nutrition, altered: less than body requirements (uses)
✓ Knowledge deficit (teaching)

Implementation

IV **IV route**
- Give through large-bore needle to decrease vein inflammation; check for extravasation; administer in P large vein, avoiding scalp vein in child
- After diluting in large volume of **IV** sol give as an **IV** inf slowly to prevent toxicity; never give **IV** bolus or IM

Potassium acetate
Additive compatibility:
Metoclopramide

Y-site compatibility:
Ciprofloxacin

Potassium chloride
Additive compatibilities
Aminophylline, amiodarone, atracurium, bretylium, calcium chloride, cefepime, cephalothin, cephapirin, chloramphenicol, cimetidine, clindamycin, cloxacillin, corticotropin, cytarabine, dimenhydrinate, dopamine, enalaprilat, floxacillin, fluconazole, furosemide, heparin, hydrocortisone, isoproterenol, lidocaine, nafcillin, netilmicin, oxacillin, penicillin G potassium or sodium, piperacillin, verapamil

Potassium chloride
Y-site compatibilities:
Aldesleukin, amifostine, granisetron, lorazepam, midazolam, thiotepa

PO route
- Give with or pc; dissolve effervescent tab, powder in 8 oz cold water or juice; do not give IM, SC
- Store at room temp

Patient/family education
- Teach patient to eat foods rich in potassium after medication is discontinued
- Advise patient to avoid OTC products: antacids, salt substitutes, analgesics, vitamin preparations, unless specifically directed by prescriber
- Advise patient to report hyperkalemia symptoms or continued hypokalemia symptoms
- Tell patient to take cap with full glass of liq; to dissolve powder or tab completely in at least 120 ml water or juice; not to chew time rel or ext rel preparations
- Emphasize importance of regular follow-up

Evaluation

Positive therapeutic outcome
- Absence of fatigue, muscle weakness, and decreased thirst and urinary output, cardiac changes
- Potassium level normal

P

pralidoxime (℞)
(pra-li-dox'eem)
Protopam Chloride
Func. class.: Cholinesterase reactivator
Chem. class.: Quaternary ammonium oxide
Pregnancy category C

Action: Reactivated enzyme metabolizes and inactivates acetylcholine at both muscarinic and nicotinic sites in the periphery

➔ **Therapeutic Outcome:** Prevention of death from organophosphate poisoning

Uses: Cholinergic crisis in myasthenia gravis, organophosphate poisoning antidote, early relief of paralysis of respiratory muscles; used as an adjunct to systemic atropine administration

Dosage and routes
Anticholinesterase overdose
Adult: **IV** 1-2 g, then 250 mg q5 min until desired response
Organophosphate poisoning
Adult: **IV** inf 1-2 g/100 ml 0.9% NaCl over 15-30 min; may repeat in 1 hr; PO 1-3 g q5h
P ***Child:*** **IV** inf 20-40 mg/kg/dose diluted in 100 ml 0.9% NaCl over 15-30 min

Available forms: Inj 600 mg/2 ml; tab 500 mg; emergency kit 1 g/20-ml vial

Adverse effects
CNS: Dizziness, headache, drowsiness, blurred vision, diplopia, impaired accommodation
CV: Tachycardia
GI: Nausea
MS: Weakness, muscle rigidity
RESP: Hyperventilation, ***laryngospasm***

Contraindications: Hypersensitivity, carbamate insecticide poisoning

Precautions: Myasthenia gravis, pregnancy **C,** renal insufficiency, children, lactation P

Pharmacokinetics

Absorption	Variably absorbed (PO), well absorbed (IM), completely absorbed (IV)
Distribution	Widely distributed (extracellular water)
Metabolism	Liver
Excretion	Kidneys, unchanged (90%)
Half-life	1½ hr

Pharmacodynamics

	PO	IV	IM
Onset	Unknown	Unknown	Unknown
Peak	2-3 hr	5-15 min	10-20 min
Duration	Unknown	Unknown	Unknown

Interactions
Individual drugs
Aminophylline: Do not use together
Morphine: Do not use together
Reserpine: Do not use together
Succinylcholine: Do not use together
Theophylline: Do not use together
Drug classifications
Analgesics, narcotic: Do not use together
Barbiturates: Do not use together
Sedative/hypnotics: Do not use together

NURSING CONSIDERATIONS

Assessment

- Monitor liver function studies: AST (SGOT), ALT (SGPT), CPK; liver function enzymes and CPK return to normal levels in 10-14 days
- Assess insecticide that was ingested including amount ingested, time, and if patient used any products to counteract effect; treatment should begin within 24 hr to be completely effective
- Assess for neurologic and muscular effects: weakness, pale skin, hypertension, tachycardia, muscle cramping, twitching; these reactions are the effect of anticholinesterase
- Monitor B/P, VS, I&O ratio; observe for decreased urinary output for 48-72 hr after poisoning to determine atropine toxicity from poisoning effects
- Monitor respiratory status: rate, rhythm, characteristics, tidal volume, vital capacity

Nursing diagnoses

✓ Injury, risk for (uses)
✓ Airway clearance, ineffective (uses)

Implementation

IV IV route

- Give **IV** after diluting 1 g/20 ml sterile water for inj; give directly over 5 min
- Further dilute/100 ml 0.9% NaCl; may be given as an inf over 15-30 min
- Give **IV** slowly after dilution with sterile water; rapid administration may lead to tachycardia, hypertension, rigidity, laryngospasm
- Give concurrent atropine 2-4 mg **IV** or IM if cyanosis is present to block accumulated acetylcholine in respiratory center; repeat q5-10 min until toxicity occurs: dry mouth, flushing, tachycardia, delirium, hallucinations
- Give only with edrophonium (Tensilon) available for myasthenia gravis patient
- Give only with emergency equipment available

Patient/family education

- Explain purpose of drug and expected results

Evaluation

Positive therapeutic outcome

- Decreased effects of organophosphate poisoning
- Decreased effects of anticholesterase overdose

pravastatin (℞)

(pra′va-sta-tin)
Pravachol
Func. class.: Antilipidemic
Pregnancy category **X**

Action: Inhibits biosynthesis of VLDL, LDL, which are responsible for cholesterol development, by inhibiting the enzyme HMG-CoA reductase

➔ **Therapeutic Outcome:** Decreasing cholesterol levels and LDL, increased HDLD

Uses: As an adjunct in primary hypercholesterolemia types IIa, IIb, artherosclerosis

Dosage and routes

Adult: PO 10-20 mg qd at hs (range 10-40 mg qd); elderly may require the lowest dosage

Available forms: Tabs 10, 20, 40 mg

Adverse effects

CNS: Headache, dizziness, psychic disturbances

P

EENT: Lens opacities, common cold, rhinitis, cough
GI: Nausea, constipation, diarrhea, dyspepsia, flatus, abdominal pain, heartburn, ***liver dysfunction,*** pancreatitis, ***hepatitis***
INTEG: Rash, pruritus, photosensitivity
MS: Muscle cramps, myalgia, ***myositis, rhabdomyolysis***

Contraindications: Hypersensitivity, pregnancy **X,** lactation, active liver disease

Precautions: Past liver disease, alcoholism, severe acute infections, trauma, hypotension, uncontrolled seizure disorders, severe metabolic disorders, electrolyte imbalances, renal disease

Pharmacokinetics	
Absorption	Poorly absorbed, erratic
Distribution	Unknown
Metabolism	Liver, extensively
Excretion	Feces (70%-75%); kidneys, unchanged (10%), breast milk (minimal)
Half-life	2 hr

Pharmacodynamics	
Onset	Unknown
Peak	1-1½ hr
Duration	Unknown

Interactions

Individual drugs

Cholestyramine: ↓ action of pravastin
Colestipol: ↓ action of pravastin
Cyclosporine: ↑ risk of myopathy, rhabdomyolysis
Erythromycin: ↑ risk of myopathy, rhabdomyolysis
Gemfibrozil: ↑ risk of myopathy, rhabdomyolysis
Niacin: ↑ risk of myopathy, rhabdomyolysis
Propranolol: ↓ effect of pravastatin
Warfarin: ↑ bleeding

Lab test interferences

↑ CPK, ↑ liver function tests

NURSING CONSIDERATIONS

Assessment

- Assess nutrition: fat, protein, carbohydrates; nutritional analysis should be completed by dietician before treatment
- Monitor triglycerides, cholesterol at baseline and throughout treatment; LDL and VLDL should be watched closely; if increased, drug should be discontinued

Nursing diagnoses

✓ Knowledge deficit (teaching)
✓ Noncompliance (teaching)

Implementation

- Give at hs only; give 1 hr before or 4 hr after bile acid sequestrants
- Store in cool environment in tight, light-resistant container

Patient/family education

- Inform patient that compliance is needed for positive results to occur; not to double doses or skip doses
- Teach patient that risk factors should be decreased: high-fat diet, smoking, alcohol consumption, absence of exercise
- Advise patient to notify prescriber of weakness, tenderness, or limited mobility
- Explain to patient that contraception is necessary, since drug produces teratogenic effects

Evaluation

Positive therapeutic outcome

- Decreased cholesterol serum triglyceride levels and improved ratio with HDL

prazepam (℞)
(praz′e-pam)
Centrax
Func. class.: Sedative/hypnotic; antianxiety agent
Chem. class.: Benzodiazepine
Pregnancy category D
Controlled substance schedule IV

Action: Depresses subcortical levels of CNS, including limbic system, reticular formation; potentiates GABA

Therapeutic Outcome: Decreased anxiety, relaxation, sedation

Uses: Anxiety

Dosage and routes
Adult: PO 10 mg tid; 20-60 mg in divided doses or 20 mg at hs

G ***Elderly:*** PO 10-15 mg/day in divided doses

Available forms: Caps 5, 10, 20 mg; tab 10 mg

Adverse effects
CNS: Dizziness, drowsiness, confusion, headache, anxiety, tremors, stimulation, fatigue, insomnia, weakness
CV: Orthostatic hypotension, ***ECG changes, tachycardia,*** hypotension, palpitations, syncope
EENT: Blurred vision, tinnitus, mydriasis
GI: Constipation, dry mouth, nausea, vomiting, anorexia, diarrhea
INTEG: Rash, dermatitis, itching

Contraindications: Hypersensitivity to benzodiazepines, narrow-angle glaucoma, psychosis, pregnancy **D,** child <18 yr

G **Precautions:** Elderly, debilitated, hepatic disease, renal disease

Pharmacokinetics

Absorption	Slowly absorbed
Distribution	Widely distributed; crosses placenta, blood-brain barrier
Metabolism	Liver, extensively to active metabolites
Excretion	Kidneys, breast milk
Half-life	5-15 hr; active metabolite 30-100 hr

Pharmacodynamics

Onset	Unknown
Peak	6 hr
Duration	Up to 48 hr

Interactions
Individual drugs
Alcohol: ↑ CNS depression
Cimetidine: ↑ action
Disulfiram: ↑ action
Fluoxetine: ↑ action
Isoniazid: ↑ action
Ketoconazole: ↑ action
Levodopa: ↓ action of levodopa
Metoprolol: ↑ action
Propoxyphene: ↑ action
Propranolol: ↑ action
Rifampin: ↓ action of prazepam
Theophylline: ↓ sedative effects
Valproic acid: ↑ action
Drug classifications
Analgesics, opioid: ↑ CNS depression
Antidepressants: ↑ CNS depression
Antihistamines: ↑ CNS depression
Barbiturates: ↓ effect of prazepam
Oral contraceptives: ↑ effect
Lab test interferences
↑ AST (SGOT), ↑ ALT

P

(SGPT), ↑ serum bilirubin
False ↑ 17-OHCS
↓ RAIU

NURSING CONSIDERATIONS

Assessment

- Assess mental status: mood, sensorium, anxiety, affect, sleeping pattern, drowsiness, **G** dizziness, especially elderly; physical dependency, withdrawal symptoms: anxiety, panic attacks, agitation, convulsions, headache, nausea, vomiting, muscle pain, weakness; suicidal tendencies; for indications of increasing tolerance and abuse
- Monitor B/P (with patient lying, standing), pulse; if systolic B/P drops 20 mm Hg, hold drug, notify prescriber
- Monitor hepatic studies: AST (SGOT), ALT (SGPT), bilirubin, creatinine LDH, alkaline phosphatase
- Monitor I&O; indicate renal dysfunction

Nursing diagnoses

- ✓ Anxiety (uses)
- ✓ Depression (uses)
- ✓ Injury, risk for (adverse reactions)
- ✓ Knowledge deficit (teaching)

Implementation

- Give with food or milk for GI symptoms; tab may be crushed if patient is unable to swallow medication whole; provide sugarless gum, hard candy, frequent sips of water for dry mouth

Patient/family education

- Teach patient that drug may be taken with food or fluids, and tab may be crushed or swallowed whole
- Advise patient not to use for everyday stress or longer than 3 mo unless directed by prescriber; not to take more than prescribed amount; may be habit forming; not to double doses or skip doses
- Caution patient to avoid OTC preparations unless approved by prescriber; alcohol and CNS depressants will increase CNS depression
- Advise patient to avoid driving, activities that require alertness, since drowsiness may occur; to avoid alcohol and other psychotropic medications; to rise slowly or fainting may occur, especially **G** elderly; that drowsiness may worsen at beginning of treatment
- ❗ Instruct patient not to discontinue medication abruptly after long-term use; withdrawal symptoms include vomiting, cramping, tremors, seizures

Evaluation

Positive therapeutic outcome

- Decreased anxiety, restlessness, sleeplessness (short-term treatment only)

Treatment of overdose: Lavage, VS, supportive care

prazosin 🔑 (℞)

(pra′zoe-sin)
Minipress, prazosin
Func. class.: Antihypertensive
Chem. class.: α_1-Adrenergic blocker
Pregnancy category C

Action: Peripheral blood vessels dilate, peripheral resistance drops; reduction in blood pressure results from α-adrenergic receptors being blocked

Therapeutic Outcome: Decreased B/P in hypertension; decreased cardiac preload, afterload

Uses: Hypertension

Investigational uses: Benign prostatic hypertrophy to decreased urine outflow obstruction

Dosage and routes

Hypertension

Adult: PO 1 mg bid or tid, increasing to 20 mg qd in divided doses if required, usual range 6-15 mg/day, not to exceed 1 mg initially; max 20-40 mg/day

Benign prostatic hypertrophy

Adult: PO 1-5 mg bid

Available forms: Caps 1, 2, 5 mg

Adverse effects

CNS: Dizziness, headache, drowsiness, anxiety, depression, vertigo, weakness, fatigue

CV: Palpitations, orthostatic hypotension, tachycardia, edema, rebound hypertension

EENT: Blurred vision, epistaxis, tinnitus, dry mouth, red sclera

GI: Nausea, vomiting, diarrhea, constipation, abdominal pain

GU: Urinary frequency, incontinence, impotence, priapism, water and sodium retention

Contraindications: Hypersensitivity

Precautions: Pregnancy **C**, children

Pharmacokinetics	
Absorption	60%
Distribution	Widely distributed
Metabolism	Liver, extensively
Excretion	Kidneys, unchanged (10%), bile (90%)
Half-life	2-3 hr

Pharmacodynamics	
Onset	2 hr
Peak	1-3 hr
Duration	6-12 hr

Interactions

Individual drugs

Alcohol: ↑ hypotension
Indomethacin: ↓ effect
Nitroglycerin: ↑ hypotension

Drug classifications

Antihypertensives: ↑ hypotension
β Blockers: ↑ hypotension
Nitrates: ↑ hypotension

Lab test interferences

↑ Urinary norepinephrine, ↑ VMA

NURSING CONSIDERATIONS

Assessment

- Monitor B/P, orthostatic hypotension, syncope; check for edema in feet, legs daily; monitor I&O, weight daily; notify prescriber of changes
- Assess for allergic reactions: rash, fever, pruritus, urticaria; drug should be discontinued if antihistamines fail to help
- Assess for orthostatic hypotension; tell patient to rise slowly from sitting or lying position

Nursing diagnoses

- ✓ Cardiac output, decreased (uses)
- ✓ Injury, risk for (adverse reactions)
- ✓ Knowledge deficit (teaching)
- ✓ Noncompliance (teaching)

P

Implementation

- Severe hypotension may occur after 1st dose of this medication; decreased hypotension may be prevented by reducing or discontinuing diuretic therapy 3 days before beginning prazosin therapy
- Store in airtight container at 86° F (30° C) or less

Patient/family education

- Instruct patient not to discontinue drug abruptly; stress the importance of complying with dosage schedule, even if feeling better; if dose is missed, take as soon as remembered; take at same time each day
- Advise patient not to use OTC products (cough, cold, allergy) unless directed by prescriber; also to avoid large amounts of caffeine
- Emphasize the need to rise slowly to sitting or standing position to minimize orthostatic hypotension
- Teach patient to notify prescriber of mouth sores, sore throat, fever, swelling of hands or feet, irregular heartbeat, chest pain
- Caution patient to report excessive perspiration, dehydration, vomiting, diarrhea; may lead to fall in B/P
- Caution patient that drug may cause dizziness, fainting, lightheadedness; may occur during 1st few days of therapy; to avoid hazardous activities
- Teach patient how to take B/P and normal readings for age group; instruct to take B/P q7 days

Evaluation

Positive therapeutic outcome

- Decreased B/P in hypertension

Treatment of overdose: Administer volume expanders or vasopressors, discontinue drug, place in supine position

prednisolone (℞)

(pred-niss′oh-lone)

Articulose-50, Delta-Cortef, Prednisolone, Prelone, Key-Pred 25, Key-Pred 50, Predaject-50, Predalone 50, Predcor-25, Predcor-50, Prednisolone Acetate, Hydeltrasol, Key-Pred-SP, Pediapred, Hydeltra-T.B.A., Predalone-T.B.A., Prednisol TBA

Func. class.: Corticosteroid

Chem. class.: Intermediate-acting glucocorticoid

Pregnancy category C

Action: Decreases inflammation by suppressing migration of polymorphonuclear leukocytes, fibroblasts; reversal to increase capillary permeability and lysosomal stabilization, minimal mineralocorticoid

➔ **Therapeutic Outcome:** Decreased inflammation, decreased adrenal insufficiency

Uses: Severe inflammation, immunosuppression, neoplasms

Dosage and routes

Adult: PO 2.5-15 mg bid-qid; IM 2-30 mg (acetate, phosphate) q12h; **IV** 2-30 mg (phosphate) q12h, 2-30 mg in joint or soft tissue (phosphate), 4-40 mg in joint of lesion (tebutate), 0.25-1 ml/wk in joints (acetate-phosphate)

Available forms: Tab 5 mg;

inj 25, 50, 100 mg/ml acetate; inj 20 mg/ml tebutate; inj 20 mg/ml phosphate; inj 80 mg/ml acetate/phosphate

Adverse effects

CNS: Depression, flushing, sweating, headache, mood changes
CV: Hypertension, ***circulatory collapse, thrombophlebitis, embolism,*** tachycardia
EENT: Fungal infections, increased intraocular pressure, blurred vision
GI: Diarrhea, nausea, abdominal distention, ***GI hemorrhage,*** increased appetite, ***pancreatitis***
HEMA: Thrombocytopenia
INTEG: Acne, poor wound healing, ecchymosis, petechiae
MS: Fractures, osteoporosis, weakness

Contraindications: Psychosis, hypersensitivity, idiopathic thrombocytopenia, acute glomerulonephritis, amebiasis, fungal infections, nonasthmatic bronchial disease, child <2 yr

Precautions: Pregnancy **C,** diabetes mellitus, glaucoma, osteoporosis, seizure disorders, ulcerative colitis, CHF, myasthenia gravis

Pharmacokinetics

Absorption	Well absorbed (PO, IM), completely absorbed (IV)
Distribution	Widely distributed; crosses placenta
Metabolism	Liver, extensively
Excretion	Kidney, breast milk
Half-life	2-4 hr

Pharmacodynamics

	PO	IM (phosphate)	IV	IA/IL
Onset	1 hr	Rapid	Rapid	Slow
Peak	2 hr	1 hr	Unknown	Unknown
Duration	1½ days	Unknown	Unknown	Up to 1 mo

Interactions

Individual drugs

Alcohol: ↑ GI effects
Amphotericin B: ↑ hypokalemia
Aspirin: ↑ GI effects
Insulin: ↑ need for insulin
Mezlocillin: ↑ hypokalemia
Phenytoin: ↓ action, ↑ metabolism
Piperacillin: ↑ hypokalemia
Rifampin: ↓ action, ↑ metabolism
Ticarcillin: ↑ hypokalemia

Drug classifications

Barbiturates: ↓ action, ↑ metabolism
Diuretics: ↑ hypokalemia
Hypoglycemic agents: ↑ need for hypoglycemic agents

Lab test interferences

↑ Cholesterol, ↑ sodium, ↑ blood glucose, ↑ uric acid, ↑ calcium, ↑ urine glucose
↓ Calcium, ↓ potassium, ↓ T_4, ↓ T_3, ↓ thyroid ^{131}I uptake test, ↓ urine 17-OHCS, ↓ 17-KS, ↓ PBI
False negative: Skin allergy tests

NURSING CONSIDERATIONS

Assessment

- Monitor potassium, blood sugar, urine glucose while patient is on long-term therapy; hypokalemia and hyperglycemia may occur
- Monitor weight daily; notify prescriber of weekly gain >5 lb; monitor I&O ratio; be alert for

decreasing urinary output and increasing edema
- Monitor B/P q4h, pulse; notify prescriber if chest pain occurs
- Monitor plasma cortisol levels during long-term therapy (normal level; 138-635 nmol/L SI units when drawn at 8 AM)
- Assess adrenal function periodically for HPA axis suppression
- Assess infection: increased temp, WBC even after withdrawal of medication; drug masks infection symptoms
- Assess for potassium depletion: paresthesias, fatigue, nausea, vomiting, depression, polyuria, dysrhythmias, weakness, edema, hypertension, cardiac symptoms
- Assess mental status: affect, mood, behavioral changes, aggression
- Monitor temp; if fever develops, drug should be discontinued
- Assess for systemic absorption: increased temp, inflammation, irritation (top)

Nursing diagnoses

✓ Infection, risk for (adverse reactions)
✓ Knowledge deficit (teaching)
✓ Noncompliance (teaching)

Implementation

IV route

- Give by direct **IV** only sodium phosphate product; give over >1 min; may be given by **IV** inf in D_5W, 0.9% NaCl
- Give after shaking susp (parenteral)
- Give titrated dose; use lowest effective dosage

Y-site compatibilities: Potassium chloride, vitamin B with C

Additive compatibilities: Ascorbic acid, cephalothin, cytarabine, erythromycin, fluorouracil, heparin, methicillin, penicillin G potassium, penicillin G sodium, vitamin B with C

Additive incompatibilities: Calcium gluceptate, methotrexate, polymyxin B sulfate

IM route

- Give IM inj deep in large muscle mass; rotate sites; avoid deltoid; use 21 G needle
- Give in one dose in AM to prevent adrenal suppression; avoid SC administration; may damage tissue

PO route

- Give with food or milk to decrease GI symptoms

Patient/family education

- Advise patient that ID as steroid user should be carried
- Advise patient to notify prescriber if therapeutic response decreases; dosage adjustment may be needed
- Caution patient not to discontinue abruptly; adrenal crisis can result
- Caution patient to avoid OTC products: salicylates, alcohol in cough products, cold preparations unless directed by prescriber
- Teach patient all aspects of drug usage including cushingoid symptoms
- Teach patient symptoms of adrenal insufficiency: nausea, anorexia, fatigue, dizziness, dyspnea, weakness, joint pain
- Advise patient that long-term therapy may be needed to clear infection (1-2 mo depending on type of infection)

Evaluation

Positive therapeutic outcome

- Decreased inflammation

prednisone (℞)
(pred'ni-sone)
Apo-Prednisone, Deltasone, Liquid Pred, Meticorten, Orasone, Panasol-S, Prednicen-M, Prednisone, Sterapred, Winpred
Func. class.: Corticosteroid
Chem. class.: Intermediate-acting glucocorticoid
Pregnancy category C

Action: Decreases inflammation by suppressing migration of polymorphonuclear leukocytes, fibroblasts; reversal to increase capillary permeability and lysosomal stabilization

Therapeutic Outcome: Decreased inflammation, decreased adrenal insufficiency

Uses: Severe inflammation, immunosuppression, neoplasms, multiple sclerosis, collagen disorders, dermatologic disorders

Dosage and routes

Adult: PO 1.5-2.5 mg bid-qid, then qd or qod; maintenance up to 250 mg/day

Nephrosis

P ***Child 18 mo-4 yr:*** 7.5-10 mg qid initially

P ***Child 4-10 yr:*** 15 mg qid initially

P ***Child >10 yr:*** 20 mg qid initially

Multiple sclerosis

Adult: PO 200 mg/day × 1 wk, then 80 mg qod × 1 mo

Available forms: Tabs 1, 2.5, 5, 10, 20, 25, 50 mg; oral sol 5 mg/5 ml; syr 5 mg/5 ml

Adverse effects

CNS: Depression, flushing, sweating, headache, mood changes
CV: Hypertension, ***circulatory collapse, thrombophlebitis, embolism,*** tachycardia
EENT: Fungal infections, increased intraocular pressure, blurred vision
GI: Diarrhea, nausea, abdominal distention, ***GI hemorrhage,*** increased appetite, ***pancreatitis***
HEMA: ***Thrombocytopenia***
INTEG: Acne, poor wound healing, ecchymosis, petechiae
MS: Fractures, osteoporosis, weakness

Contraindications: Psychosis, hypersensitivity, idiopathic thrombocytopenia, acute glomerulonephritis, amebiasis, fungal infections, nonasthmatic P bronchial disease, child <2 yr, AIDS, TB

Precautions: Pregnancy **C,** diabetes mellitus, glaucoma, osteoporosis, seizure disorders, ulcerative colitis, CHF, myasthenia gravis, renal disease, esophagitis, peptic ulcer

Pharmacokinetics	
Absorption	Well absorbed
Distribution	Widely distributed; crosses placenta
Metabolism	Liver, extensively
Excretion	Kidney, breast milk
Half-life	3-4 hr

Pharmacodynamics	
Onset	Unknown
Peak	1-2 hr
Duration	1½ days

Interactions

Individual drugs

Alcohol: ↑ GI effects
Amphotericin B: ↑ hypokalemia
Aspirin: ↑ GI effects

Insulin: ↑ need for insulin
Mezlocillin: ↑ hypokalemia
Ticarcillin: ↑ hypokalemia

Drug classifications

Diuretics: ↑ hypokalemia
Hypoglycemic agents: ↑ need for hypoglycemic agents

Lab test interferences

↑ Cholesterol, ↑ sodium, ↑ blood glucose, ↑ uric acid, ↑ calcium, ↑ urine glucose
↓ Calcium, ↓ potassium, ↓ T_4, ↓ T_3, ↓ thyroid ^{131}I uptake test, ↓ urine 17-OHCS, ↓ 17-KS, ↓ PBI
False negative: Skin allergy tests

NURSING CONSIDERATIONS

Assessment

- Monitor potassium, blood sugar, urine glucose while on long-term therapy; hypokalemia and hyperglycemia may occur
- Monitor weight daily; notify prescriber of weekly gain >5 lb; monitor I&O ratio; be alert for decreasing urinary output and increasing edema
- Monitor B/P q4h, pulse; notify prescriber if chest pain occurs
- Monitor plasma cortisol levels during long-term therapy (normal level 138-635 nmol/L when drawn at 8 AM)
- Assess adrenal function periodically for HPA axis suppression
- Assess infection: increased temp, WBC even after withdrawal of medication; drug masks infection symptoms
- Assess for potassium depletion: paresthesias, fatigue, nausea, vomiting, depression, polyuria, dysrhythmias, weakness, edema, hypertension, cardiac symptoms
- Assess mental status: affect, mood, behavioral changes, aggression
- Monitor temp; if fever develops, drug should be discontinued
- Assess for systemic absorption: increased temp, inflammation, irritation (top)

Nursing diagnoses

- ✓ Infection, risk for (adverse reactions)
- ✓ Knowledge deficit (teaching)
- ✓ Noncompliance (teaching)

Implementation

- Give with food or milk to decrease GI symptoms; use measuring device for liq route

Patient/family education

- Advise patient that ID as steroid user should be carried
- Advise patient to notify prescriber if therapeutic response decreases; dosage adjustment may be needed
- Caution patient not to discontinue abruptly; adrenal crisis can result
- Caution patient to avoid OTC products: salicylates, alcohol in cough products, cold preparations unless directed by prescriber
- Teach patient all aspects of drug usage including cushingoid symptoms
- Teach patient symptoms of adrenal insufficiency: nausea, anorexia, fatigue, dizziness, dyspnea, weakness, joint pain
- Advise patient that long-term therapy may be needed to clear infection (1-2 mo depending on type of infection)

Evaluation

Positive therapeutic outcome

- Decreased inflammation

primidone (℞)

(pri′mi-done)

Apo-Primidone ♣, Myidone, Mysoline, primidone, Sertan ♣

Func. class.: Anticonvulsant

Chem. class.: Barbiturate derivative

Pregnancy category D

Action: Raises seizure threshold by conversion of drug to phenobarbital; decreases neuron firing

➔ **Therapeutic Outcome:** Reduction in seizure activity

Uses: Generalized tonic-clonic (grand mal), complex-partial, psychomotor seizures

Dosage and routes

P ***Adult and child >8 yr:*** PO 250 mg/day; may increase by 250 mg/wk, not to exceed 2 g/day in divided doses qid

P ***Child <8 yr:*** PO 125 mg/day; may increase by 125 mg/wk, not to exceed 1 g/day in divided doses qid

Available forms: Tabs 50, 250 mg; susp 250 mg/5 ml; chew tab 125 mg ♣

Adverse effects

CNS: Stimulation, drowsiness, dizziness, confusion, sedation, headache, flushing, hallucinations, coma, psychosis, ataxia, *vertigo*

EENT: Diplopia, nystagmus, edema of eyelids

GI: Nausea, vomiting, anorexia, hepatitis

GU: Impotence

HEMA: Thrombocytopenia, leukopenia, neutropenia, eosinophilia, megaloblastic anemia, decreased serum folate level, lymphadenopathy

INTEG: Rash, edema, alopecia, lupuslike syndrome

Contraindications: Hypersensitivity, porphyria, pregnancy **D**

Precautions: COPD, hepatic disease, renal disease, P hyperactive children

Pharmacokinetics

Absorption	60%-80%
Distribution	Widely distributed; crosses placenta
Metabolism	Liver, converted to phenobarbital + PEMA
Excretion	Kidneys, breast milk
Half-life	3-24 hr

Pharmacodynamics

Onset	Unknown
Peak	4 hr
Duration	Unknown

Interactions

Individual drugs

Acebutolol: ↓ effectiveness

Acetazolamide: ↓ primidone levels

Alcohol: ↑ CNS depression

Carbamazepine: ↓ primidone

Chloramphenicol: ↓ effectiveness

Doxycycline: ↑ half-life

Griseofulvin: ↓ effectiveness

Isoniazide: ↑ primidone levels

Metoprolol: ↓ effectiveness

Nicotinamide: ↑ primidone levels

Phenobarbital: ↑ toxicity

Propranolol: ↓ effectiveness

Quinidine: ↓ effectiveness

Timolol: ↓ effectiveness

Drug classifications

Antidepressants, tricyclic: ↑ CNS depression

Antihistamines: ↑ CNS depression

Glucocorticoids: ↓ effectiveness

P

Hydantoins: ↑ primidone levels
Narcotics: ↑ CNS depression
Oral contraceptives: ↓ effectiveness
Phenothiazines: ↓ CNS depression
Sedative/hypnotics: ↑ CNS depression
Succinimides: ↓ primidone levels

Lab test interferences

False ↑ Sulfobromophthalein

NURSING CONSIDERATIONS

Assessment

- Assess mental status: mood, sensorium, affect, memory (long, short), especially elderly
- Assess for blood dyscrasias: fever, sore throat, bruising, rash, jaundice, epistaxis (long-term treatment only)
- Assess seizure activity including type, location, duration, and character; provide seizure precaution
- Assess renal studies: urinalysis, BUN, urine creatinine
- Monitor blood studies: RBC, Hct, Hgb, reticulocyte counts weekly for 4 wk then monthly
- Monitor hepatic studies: ALT (SGPT), AST (SGOT), bilirubin, creatinine
- Monitor drug levels during initial treatment
- Assess for signs of physical withdrawal if medication suddenly discontinued
- Assess eye problems: need for ophthalmic examinations before, during, after treatment (slit lamp, fundoscopy, tonometry)
- Assess allergic reaction: red raised rash; if this occurs, drug should be discontinued
- Monitor for toxicity: bone marrow depression, nausea, vomiting, ataxia, diplopia, cardiovascular collapse

Nursing diagnoses

✓ Injury, risk for (side effects)
✓ Knowledge deficit (teaching)

Implementation

- May give with food to decrease gastric irritation
- May crush tab and mix with food or fluid

Patient/family education

- Teach patient to carry ID card or Medic Alert bracelet stating name, drugs taken, condition, prescriber's name, phone number
- Advise patient to avoid driving and other activities that require alertness
- Caution patient to avoid alcohol and CNS depressants; increased sedation may occur
- Teach patient not to discontinue medication quickly after long-term use; taper off over several wk

Evaluation

Positive therapeutic outcome

- Decreased seizure activity

probenecid (℞)

(proe-ben′e-sid)

Benemid, Benuryl ♣, Probalan, probenecid

Func. class.: Uricosuric; antigout

Chem. class.: Sulfonamide derivative

Pregnancy category B

Action: Inhibits tubular reabsorption of urates, with increased excretion of uric acids

➔ Therapeutic Outcome: Decreased uric acid levels

Uses: Hyperuricemia in gout, gouty arthritis; adjunct to cephalosporin or penicillin treatment (gonorrhea)

Dosage and routes

Gonorrhea

Adult: PO 1 g with 3.5 g ampicillin or 1 g 30 min before 4.8 million U of aqueous penicillin G procaine injected into 2 sites IM

Gout/gouty arthritis

Adult: PO 250 mg bid for 1 wk, then 500 mg bid, not to exceed 2 g/day; maintenance 500 mg/day × 6 mo

Adjunct in penicillin/cephalosporin treatment

P ***Adult and child >50 kg:*** PO 500 mg qid

P ***Child <50 kg:*** PO 25 mg/kg, then 40 mg/kg in divided doses qid

Available forms: Tab 0.5 g

Adverse effects

CNS: Drowsiness, headache
CV: Bradycardia
GU: Glycosuria, thirst, frequency, ***nephrotic syndrome***
GI: Gastric irritation, nausea, vomiting, anorexia, ***hepatic necrosis***
INTEG: Rash, dermatitis, pruritus, fever
META: Acidosis, hypokalemia, hyperchloremia, hyperglycemia
RESP: ***Apnea***, irregular respirations

Contraindications: Hypersensitivity, severe hepatic disease, severe renal disease, CrCl <50 mg/min, history of uric acid calculus

Precautions: Pregnancy **B**,
P child <2 yr

Pharmacokinetics	
Absorption	Well absorbed
Distribution	Crosses placenta
Metabolism	Liver
Excretion	Kidneys
Half-life	5-8 hr

Pharmacodynamics	
Onset	½ hr
Peak	2-4 hr
Duration	8 hr

Interactions

Individual drugs

Acyclovir: ↑ toxicity
Allopurinol: ↑ effect
Aspirin: ↑ uricosuric effect
Clofibrate: ↑ effect
Dapsone: ↑ effect
Dyphylline: ↑ effect
Heparin: ↑ effect
Methotrexate: ↑ toxicity
Nitrofurantoin: ↑ toxicity
Penicillamine: ↑ effect
Zidovudine: ↑ effect

Drug classifications

Barbiturates: ↑ effect
Benzodiazepine: ↑ effect
Cephalosporins: ↑ levels
Fluoroquinolones: ↑ levels
NSAIDs: ↑ toxicity
Penicillins: ↑ levels

Lab test interferences

↑ BSP/urinary PSP, ↑ theophylline levels
False positive: Urine glucose with copper sulfate test

NURSING CONSIDERATIONS

Assessment

- Monitor I&O ratio; observe for decrease in urinary output; increase fluids to 2-3 L/day; urine may be alkalized with sodium bicarbonate acetazolamide
- Assess mobility, joint pain, and swelling in the joints
- Monitor CBC, urine pH, uric acid and BUN, creatinine

P

before and periodically during treatment

Nursing diagnoses

- ✓ Pain, chronic (uses)
- ✓ Mobility, impaired (uses)
- ✓ Knowledge deficit (teaching)

Implementation

- Give with food or antacid to decrease GI upset
- Reduce dosage gradually if uric acid levels are normal after 6 mo

Patient/family education

- Advise patient to increase fluids to 2-3 L/day
- Caution patient to avoid salicylates; probenecid levels will be decreased
- Advise patient to report any pain, redness, or hard area, usually in legs
- Instruct patient in importance of complying with medical regimen including weight loss program, diet restrictions, and alcohol intake

Evaluation

Positive therapeutic outcome

- Decreased pain in joints
- Normal serum uric acid levels
- Increased duration of antiinfectives

procainamide (Key Drug) (℞)

(proe'kane-ah-mide)

Procan SR, Promine, procainamide, Procanbid, Pronestyl, Pronestyl-SR

Func. class.: Antidysrhythmic (Class IA)

Chem. class.: Procaine HCl amide analog

Pregnancy category C

Action: Prolongs action potential duration and effective refractory period; reduces disparity in refractory between normal and infarcted myocardium; prevents increased myocardial excitability and conduction contractility

➔ **Therapeutic Outcome:** Prevention of dysrhythmias

Uses: PVCs, atrial fibrillation, PAT, ventricular tachycardia, atrial dysrhythmias, ventricular tachycardia

Dosage and routes

Atrial fibrillation/PAT

Adult: PO 1-1.25 g; may give another 750 mg if needed; if no response, 500 mg-1g q2h until desired response; maintenance 50 mg/kg in divided doses q6h

Ventricular tachycardia

Adult: PO 1 g; maintenance 50 mg/kg/day given in 3-hr intervals; sus rel tab 500 mg-1.25 g q6h

Other dysrhythmias

Adult: **IV** bol 100 mg q5 min, given 25-50 mg/min, not to exceed 500 mg; or 17 mg/kg total, then **IV** inf 2-6 mg/min

Available forms: Caps 250, 375, 500 mg; tabs 250, 375, 500 mg; sus rel tabs 250, 500,

750, 1000 mg; inj **IV** 100, 500 mg/ml

Adverse effects

CNS: Headache, dizziness, confusion, psychosis, restlessness, irritability, weakness

CV: Hypotension, ***heart block, cardiovascular collapse, arrest***

GI: Nausea, vomiting, anorexia, diarrhea, hepatomegaly

HEMA: SLE syndrome, ***agranulocytosis, thrombocytopenia, neutropenia, hemolytic anemia***

INTEG: Rash, urticaria, edema, swelling (rare), pruritus

Contraindications: Hypersensitivity, myasthenia gravis, severe heart block

Precautions: Pregnancy **C**, P lactation, children, renal disease, liver disease, CHF, respiratory depression

Pharmacokinetics

Absorption	Well absorbed
Distribution	Rapidly distributed
Metabolism	Liver
Excretion	Kidneys, unchanged (50%-70%)
Half-life	2½-4½ hr; increased in renal disease

Pharmacodynamics

	PO	PO–ext rel	IV
Onset	½ hr	Unknown	Rapid
Peak	1-1½ hr	Unknown	½-1 hr
Duration	3 hr	Up to 8 hr	3-4 hr

Interactions

Individual drugs

Atropine: ↑ anticholinergic effect

Digoxin: ↑ blood levels, toxicity

Disopyramide: ↑ levels, toxicity

Flecainide: ↑ levels, toxicity

Lidocaine: Bradycardia, arrest

Haloperidol: ↑ anticholinergic effect

Mexiletine: ↑ levels, toxicity

Phenytoin: ↑ blood levels

Quinidine: ↑ levels, toxicity

Warfarin: ↑ level, bleeding

Drug classifications

β-Blockers: ↑ dysrhythmias, arrest

Calcium channel blockers: ↑ dysrhythmias, arrest

Phenothiazines: ↑ anticholinergic effect

Lab test interferences

↑ CPK

NURSING CONSIDERATIONS

Assessment

- Assess for oxygenation or perfusion deficit: decreased B/P, chest pain, dizziness, loss of consciousness
- Assess respiratory status: auscultate lung fields for bibasilar crackles in patients with advanced CHF
- Monitor I&O ratio; electrolytes: potassium, sodium, chloride; watch for decreasing urinary output, possible retention
- Monitor liver function studies: AST (SGOT), ALT (SGPT), bilirubin, alkaline phosphatase
- Monitor ECG continuously to determine drug effectiveness; measure PR, QRS, QT intervals; check for PVCs, other dysrhythmias; check B/P continuously for hypotension, hypertension; for rebound hypertension after 1-2 hr; prolonged PR/QT intervals, QRS complex; if QT or QRS increases by 50% or more, withhold next dose, notify prescriber

- Monitor for dehydration or hypovolemia
- Monitor for CNS symptoms: confusion, psychosis, numbness, depression, involuntary movements; if these occur, drug should be discontinued
- Monitor blood levels (therapeutic level 3-10 μg/ml), ANA titer or NAPA levels; notify prescriber of abnormal results
- Assess cardiac rate, respiration: rate, rhythm, character, chest pain, ventricular tachycardia, supraventricular tachycardia or fibrillation

Nursing diagnoses

✓ Cardiac output, decreased (uses)
✓ Impaired gas exchange (adverse reactions)
✓ Knowledge deficit (teaching)

Implementation

PO route

- Give on an empty stomach with a full glass of water
- May be given with meals if GI irritation occurs; absorption will be decreased
- Tab may be crushed and mixed with fluid or foods for patients with swallowing difficulties; do not break, chew, or crush sus-rel tab

IV **IV route**

- Give by direct **IV** after diluting 100 mg/10 ml of D_5W or sterile water for inj; give 50 mg/min or less
- Give by intermittent inf after diluting to a conc of 2-4 mg/ml 200 mg up to 1 g/50-500 ml D_5W; give over 30 min (2-6 mg/min maintenance); use inf pump for correct dosage
- Do not use dark sol or if precipitate is present

Solution compatibilities: D_5W, D_5/0.9% NaCl, 0.45% NaCl, 0.9% NaCl, water for inj

Y-site compatibilities: Amiodarone, famotidine, heparin, hydrocortisone, potassium chloride, ranitidine, vitamin B with C

Y-site incompatibility: Milrinone

Additive compatibilities: Amiodarone, dobutamine, flumazenil, lidocaine, netilmicin, verapamil

Additive incompatibilities: Esmolol, ethacrynate, milrinone

Patient/family education

- Advise patient to report side effects immediately to prescriber; to take exactly as prescribed; if dose is missed take when remembered if within 3-4 hr of next dose, do not double doses
- Caution patient that dark glasses may be needed for photophobia; to use sunscreen or stay out of sun to prevent burns; avoid temp extremes; impairment of heat-regulating mechanism can occur
- Advise patient to complete follow-up appointment with prescriber including pulmonary function studies, chest x-ray
- Instruct patient that dry mouth may be relieved by frequent sips of water, hard candy, sugarless gum
- Caution patient to make position changes from lying to standing slowly to prevent orthostatic hypotension

Evaluation

Positive therapeutic outcome

- Decreased PVCs, ventricular tachycardia

Treatment of overdose: O_2, artificial ventilation, ECG, administer dopamine for circulatory depression, administer diazepam or thiopental for convulsions, isoproterenol

procarbazine (℞)

(proe-kar'ba-zeen)

Matulane, Natulan ✦

Func. class.: Antineoplastic, alkylating agent

Chem. class.: Hydrazine derivative

Pregnancy category D

Action: Inhibits DNA, RNA, protein synthesis, cell cycle S phase specific; has multiple sites of action; a nonvesicant

➔ **Therapeutic Outcome:** Prevention of rapidly growing malignant cells

Uses: Lymphoma, Hodgkin's disease, cancers resistant to other therapy

Investigational uses: Brain, lung malignancies, other lymphomas, multiple myeloma, malignant melanoma, polycythemia vera

Dosage and routes

Adult: PO 2-4 mg/kg/day for first wk; maintain dosage of 4-6 mg/kg/day until platelets and WBC fall; after recovery, 1-2 mg/kg/day

P ***Child:*** PO 50 mg/day for 7 days, then 100 mg/m^2 until desired response, leukopenia, or thrombocytopenia occurs; 50 mg/day is maintenance after bone marrow recovery

Available forms: Cap 50 mg

Adverse effects

CNS: Headache, dizziness, insomnia, hallucinations, confusion, coma, pain, chills, fever, sweating, paresthesias

EENT: Retinal hemorrhage, nystagmus, photophobia, diplopia

GI: Nausea, vomiting, anorexia, diarrhea, constipation, dry mouth, stomatitis

GU: Azoospermia, cessation of menses

HEMA: ***Thrombocytopenia, anemia, leukopenia, myelosuppression, bleeding tendencies,*** purpura, petechiae, epistaxis

INTEG: Rash, pruritus, dermatitis, alopecia, herpes, hyperpigmentation

MS: Arthralgias, myalgias

RESP: Cough, pneumonitis

Contraindications: Hypersensitivity, thrombocytopenia, bone marrow depression, pregnancy **D**

Precautions: Renal disease, hepatic disease, radiation therapy

Pharmacokinetics

Absorption	Well absorbed
Distribution	Widely distributed; crosses blood-brain barrier
Metabolism	Liver
Excretion	Kidneys
Half-life	1 hr

Pharmacodynamics

Unknown

Interactions

Individual drugs

Alcohol: ↑ CNS depressant, disulfiram reaction

P

Guanadrel: ↑ hypertensive crisis
Guanethidine: ↑ hypertensive crisis
Levodopa: ↑ hypertensive crisis
Meperidine: Avoid use; paradoxic reactions
Radiation: ↑ toxicity, bone marrow suppression
Reserpine: ↑ hypertensive crisis

Drug classifications
Antidepressants: ↑ hypertensive crisis
Antihistamines: ↑ CNS depression
Antineoplastics: ↑ toxicity bone marrow suppression
CNS depressants: ↑ CNS depression
Local anesthetics: ↑ hypertensive crisis
MAOIs: ↑ seizures, temperature
Narcotic analgesics: ↑ CNS depression
Sedative/hypnotics: ↑ CNS depression
Sympathomimetic amines: ↑ hypertensive crisis
Vasoconstrictors: ↑ hypertensive crisis

NURSING CONSIDERATIONS

Assessment

- Monitor CBC, differential, platelet count weekly; withhold drug if WBC is <4000 or platelet count is <75,000; notify prescriber of results if WBC <20,000/mm^3, platelets <150,000/mm^3
- Monitor pulmonary function tests, chest x-ray films before, during therapy; chest film should be obtained q2 wk during treatment; check for dyspnea, rales, unproductive cough, chest pain, tachypnea
- Monitor renal function studies: BUN, serum uric acid, urine CrCl before, during therapy; I&O ratio; report fall in urine output of 30 ml/hr; for decreased hyperuricemia
- Monitor for cold, fever, sore throat (may indicate beginning infection); identify edema in feet, joint and stomach pain, shaking; prescriber should be notified
- Assess for bleeding: hematuria, guaiac, bruising or petechiae, mucosa or orifices q8h, no rectal temp

Nursing diagnoses

✓ Injury, risk for (adverse reactions)
✓ Body image disturbance (adverse reactions)
✓ Infection, risk for (adverse reactions)
✓ Knowledge deficit (teaching)

Implementation

- Give with foods, fluids for GI upset; open cap and give with food/fluids for swallowing difficulty; administer as directed

Patient/family education

- Teach patient to avoid use of products containing aspirin or ibuprofen, razors, commercial mouthwash, since bleeding may occur; to report symptoms of bleeding (hematuria, tarry stools)
- Caution patient to report signs of anemia (fatigue, headache, irritability, faintness, shortness of breath)
- Advise patient to report any changes in breathing or coughing even several mo after treatment; to avoid crowds and persons with respiratory tract or other infections
- Inform patient hair loss is common; discuss the use of wigs or hair pieces

• Caution patient not to have any vaccinations without the advice of the prescriber; serious reactions can occur
• Advise patient that contraception is needed during treatment and for several mo after the completion of therapy

Evaluation

Positive therapeutic outcome
• Absence of swelling at night
• Increased appetite, increased weight

prochlorperazine (℞)

(proe-klor-pair′a-zeen)

Chlorpazine, Compa-Z, Compazine, Contranzine, Provazin ✤, Stemetil ✤, Ultrazine

Func. class.: Antiemetic/antipsychotic

Chem. class.: Phenothiazine, piperazine derivative

Pregnancy category C

Action: Depresses cerebral cortex, hypothalamus, limbic system, which control activity aggression; blocks neurotransmission produced by dopamine at synapse; exhibits a strong α-adrenergic, anticholinergic blocking action; mechanism for antipsychotic effects is unclear; acts centrally by blocking chemoreceptor trigger zone, which in turn acts on vomiting center

➔ **Therapeutic Outcome:** Decreased nausea, vomiting, decreased signs and symptoms of psychosis

Uses: Nausea, vomiting, psychosis

Dosage and routes

Postoperative nausea/vomiting

Adult: IM 5-10 mg 1-2 hr before anesthesia; may repeat in 30 min; **IV** 5-10 mg 15-30 min before anesthesia; **IV** inf 20 mg/L D_5W or NS 15-30 min before anesthesia, not to exceed 40 mg/day

Severe nausea/vomiting

Adult: PO 5-10 mg tid-qid; sus rel 15 mg qd in AM or 10 mg q12h; rec 25 mg/bid; IM 5-10 mg; may repeat q4h, not to exceed 40 mg/day

P ***Child 18-39 kg:*** PO 2.5 mg tid or 5 mg bid; do not exceed 15 mg/day; IM 0.132 mg/kg

P ***Child 14-17 kg:*** PO/rec 2.5 mg bid-tid, not to exceed 10 mg/day; IM 0.132 mg/kg

P ***Child 9-13 kg:*** PO/rec 2.5 mg qd-bid, not to exceed 7.5 mg/day; IM 0.132 mg/kg

Available forms: Syr 5 mg/ml; inj 5 mg/ml; tabs 5, 10, 25 mg; sus rel caps 10, 15, 30 mg; supp 2.5, 5, 25 mg

Adverse effects

CNS: Euphoria, ***depression, EPS,*** restlessness, tremor, dizziness, ***neuroleptic malignant syndrome***

CV: ***Circulatory failure, tachycardia***

GI: Nausea, vomiting, anorexia, dry mouth, diarrhea, constipation, weight loss, metallic taste, cramps, hepatitis

RESP: ***Respiratory depression***

Contraindications: Hypersensitivity to phenothiazines, coma, seizure, encephalopathy, bone marrow depression

P **Precautions:** Children <2 yr, G pregnancy **C**, elderly

P

Pharmacokinetics

Absorption	Variably absorbed (PO); well absorbed (IM)
Distribution	Widely distributed; high concentration in CNS; crosses placenta
Metabolism	Liver, extensively; GI mucosa
Excretion	Kidneys, breast milk
Half-life	Unknown

Pharmacodynamics

	PO	PO–EXT REL	REC	IM	IV
Onset	½ hr	½ hr	1 hr	10-20 min	4-5 min
Peak	Unkn	Unkn	Unkn	Unkn	Unkn
Duration	3-4 hr	10-12 hr	3-4 hr	3-4 hr	3-4 hr

Interactions

Individual drugs

Alcohol: ↑ effects of both drugs, oversedation
Aluminum hydroxide: ↓ absorption
Bromocriptine: ↓ antiparkinsonian activity
Disopyramide: ↑ anticholinergic effects
Epinephrine: ↑ toxicity
Guanethidine: ↓ antihypertensive response
Levodopa: ↓ antiparkinsonian activity
Lithium: ↓ prochlorperizine levels, ↑ extrapyramidal symptoms, masking of lithium toxicity
Magnesium hydroxide: ↓ absorption
Norepinephrine: ↓ vasoresponse, ↑ toxicity
Phenobarbital: ↓ effectiveness, ↑ metabolism

Drug classifications

Antacids: ↓ absorption
Anticholinergics: ↑ anticholinergic effects
Antidepressants: ↑ CNS depression
Antidiarrheals, adsorbent: ↓ absorption
Antihistamines: ↑ CNS depression
Antihypertensives: ↑ hypotension
Antithyroid agents: ↑ agranulocytosis
Barbiturate anesthetics: ↑ CNS depression
β-Adrenergics: ↑ effects of both drugs
General anesthetics: ↑ CNS depression
MAOIs: ↑ CNS depression
Narcotics: ↑ CNS depression
Sedative/hypnotics: ↑ CNS depression

Lab test interferences

↑ Liver function tests, ↑ cardiac enzymes, ↑ cholesterol, ↑ blood glucose, ↑ prolactin, ↑ bilirubin, ↑ PBI, ↑ cholinesterase, ↑ ^{131}I, ↑ alkaline phosphatase, ↑ leukocytes, ↑ granulocytes, ↑ platelets
↓ Hormones (blood and urine)
False positive: Pregnancy tests, PKU, urine bilirubin
False negative: Urinary steroids, 17-OHCS, pregnancy tests

NURSING CONSIDERATIONS

Assessment

- Assess mental status: orientation, mood, behavior, presence and type of hallucinations before initial administration and monthly; this drug should significantly reduce psychotic behavior
- Check for swallowing of PO medication; check for hoarding or giving of medication to other patients
- Monitor I&O ratio; palpate bladder if low urinary output **G** occurs, especially in elderly; urinalysis recommended before, during prolonged therapy

• Monitor bilirubin, CBC, liver function studies monthly
• Assess affect, orientation, LOC, reflexes, gait, coordination, sleep pattern disturbances
• Monitor B/P with patient sitting, standing, and lying; take pulse and respirations q4h during initial treatment; establish baseline before starting treatment; report drops of 30 mm Hg; obtain baseline ECG, Q wave and T wave changes
• Check for dizziness, faintness, palpitations, tachycardia on rising; severe orthostatic hypotension is common
• Identify neuroleptic malignant syndrome: hyperpyrexia, muscle rigidity, increased CPK, altered mental status; drug should be discontinued
• Assess for EPS including akathisia (inability to sit still, no pattern to movements), tardive dyskinesia (bizarre movements of the jaw, mouth, tongue, extremities), pseudoparkinsonism (ragged tremors, pill rolling, shuffling gate); an antiparkinsonism drug should be prescribed
• Assess for constipation, urinary retention daily; if these occur, increase bulk, water in diet

Nursing diagnoses

✓ Thought processes, altered (uses)
✓ Coping, ineffective individual (uses)
✓ Knowledge deficit (teaching)
✓ Noncompliance (teaching)

Implementation

PO route

• Give drug in liq form mixed in glass of juice or cola if hoarding is suspected; do not mix in caffeine drinks, tannics, pectins
• Give decreased dosage in G elderly since metabolism is slowed
• Give PO with full glass of water, milk; or give with food to decrease GI upset
• Store in airtight, light-resistant container; oral sol in amber bottle
• Do not crush or chew sus rel cap

IM route

• Inject slowly in deep muscle mass; do not give SC; aspirate to avoid **IV** administration; do not administer sol with a precipitate; have patient lie down afterward for at least 30 min

IV route

• Give by direct **IV** after diluting **IV** using 0.9% NaCl to 1 mg/1 ml; administer at 1 mg/min or less
• Administer by intermittent inf after diluting 20 mg/L or less LR, Ringer's, dextrose, saline, or any combination

Syringe incompatibilities: Dimenhydrinate, midazolam, pentobarbital, thiopental

Syringe compatibilities: Atropine, butorphanol, chlorpromazine, cimetidine, diamorphine, diphenhydramine, droperidol, fentanyl, glycopyrrolate, hydroxyzine, meperidine, metoclopramide, nalbuphine, pentazocine, perphenazine, promazine, promethazine, ranitidine, scopolamine

Y-site incompatibility: Foscarnet

Y-site compatibilities: Amsacrine, cisplatin, cyclophosphamide, cytarabine, doxorubicin, fluconazole, heparin, hydrocortisone,

P

ondansetron, paclitaxel, potassium chloride, sargramostim, thiotepa, vinorelbine, vitamin B with C

Additive incompatibilities: Aminophylline, amphotericin B, ampicillin, calcium gluceptate, cefoperazone, cephalothin, chloramphenicol, chlorothiazide, floxacillin, furosemide, hydrocortisone sodium succinate, methohexital sodium, penicillin G sodium, phenobarbital, thiopental

Additive compatibilities: Amikacin, ascorbic acid, dexamethasone, dimenhydrinate, erythromycin, ethacrynate, lidocaine, nafcillin, netilmicin, sodium bicarbonate, vitamin B with C

Patient/family education

- Teach patient to use good oral hygiene; frequent rinsing of mouth, sugarless gum for dry mouth
- Caution patient to avoid hazardous activities until drug response is determined; dizziness, blurred vision may occur
- Inform patient that orthostatic hypotension occurs often and to rise from sitting or lying position gradually; to remain lying down after IM inj for at least 30 min; tell patient to avoid hot tubs, hot showers, tub baths, since hypotension may occur; tell patient that in hot weather heat stroke may occur; take extra precautions to stay cool
- Advise patient to avoid abrupt withdrawal of this drug, or EPS may result; drug should be withdrawn slowly
- Teach patient to avoid OTC preparations (cough, hay fever, cold) unless approved by prescriber, since serious drug interactions may occur; avoid use with alcohol, CNS depressants; increased drowsiness may occur; avoid activities requiring mental alertness
- Instruct patient to use a sunscreen and sunglasses to prevent burns
- Teach patient about EPS and necessity of meticulous oral hygiene, since oral candidiasis may occur
- Advise patient to take antacids 2 hr before or after taking this drug
- Advise patient to report sore throat, malaise, fever, bleeding, mouth sores; if these occur, CBC should be drawn and drug discontinued
- Teach patient not to double or skip doses
- Teach patient urine may turn pink to reddish brown
- Instruct patient to report dark urine, clay-colored stools, bleeding, bruising, rash, blurred vision

Evaluation

Positive therapeutic outcome

- Relief of nausea and vomiting
- Decrease in emotional excitement, hallucinations, delusions, paranoia
- Reorganization of patterns of thought, speech

Treatment of overdose: Lavage if orally ingested; provide airway; *do not induce vomiting or use epinephrine*

progesterone (℞)
(proe-jess'ter-one)
Crinone, Progestacert, progesterone, Progesterone in Oil
Func. class.: Progestogen
Chem. class.: Progesterone derivative
Pregnancy category X

Action: Inhibits secretion of pituitary gonadotropins, which prevents follicular maturation, ovulation; stimulates growth of mammary tissue; antineoplastic action against endometrial cancer

Therapeutic Outcome: Decreased abnormal uterine bleeding, absence of amenorrhea

Uses: Contraception, amenorrhea, premenstrual syndrome, abnormal uterine bleeding

Dosage and routes
Infertility
Adult: Vag 90 mg qd
Amenorrhea/uterine bleeding
Adult: IM 5-10 mg qd × 6-8 doses
Contraception
Adult: Insert 1 supp in uterine cavity; active for 1 yr
PMS
Adult: Rec supp/vag supp 200-400 mg

Available forms: Inj 50 mg/ml; powder micronized, vag gel 8%, intrauterine system

Adverse effects
CNS: Dizziness, headache, migraines, depression, fatigue
CV: Hypotension, thrombophlebitis, edema, ***thromboembolism, stroke, pulmonary embolism, MI***
EENT: Diplopia
GI: Nausea, vomiting, anorexia, cramps, increased weight, ***cholestatic jaundice***
GU: Amenorrhea, cervical erosion, breakthrough bleeding, dysmenorrhea, vaginal candidiasis, breast changes, *gynecomastia, testicular atrophy, impotence,* endometriosis, ***spontaneous abortion***
INTEG: Rash, urticaria, acne, hirsutism, alopecia, oily skin, seborrhea, purpura, melasma
META: Hyperglycemia

Contraindications: Breast cancer, hypersensitivity, thromboembolic disorders, reproductive cancer, genital bleeding (abnormal, undiagnosed), cerebral hemorrhage, pregnancy **X**

Precautions: Lactation, hypertension, asthma, blood dyscrasias, gallbladder disease, CHF, diabetes mellitus, bone disease, depression, migraine headache, convulsive disorders, hepatic disease, renal disease, family history of breast or reproductive tract cancer

Pharmacokinetics

Absorption	Unknown
Distribution	Unknown
Metabolism	Unknown
Excretion	Breast milk
Half-life	Unknown

Pharmacodynamics

	IM	REC	VAG
Onset	Unknown	Unknown	Unknown
Peak	Unknown	Unknown	Unknown
Duration	24 hr	24 hr	24 hr

P

Interactions
Individual drugs
Bromocriptine: ↓ effectiveness of bromocriptine
Lab test interferences
↑ Alkaline phosphatase, ↑ nitrogen (urine), ↑ pregnanediol, ↑ amino acids, ↑ factors VII, VIII, IX, X
↓ GTT, ↓ HDL

NURSING CONSIDERATIONS
Assessment
- Monitor B/P at beginning of treatment and periodically; check weight daily; notify prescriber of weekly weight gain >5 lb
- Monitor I&O ratio: be alert for decreasing urinary output, increasing edema, hypertension
- Assess liver function studies: ALT (SGPT), AST (SGOT), bilirubin periodically during long-term therapy
- Assess edema, hypertension, cardiac symptoms, jaundice
- Assess mental status: affect, mood, behavioral changes, depression
- Assess hypercalcemia

Nursing diagnoses
✓ Sexual dysfunction (uses)
✓ Tissue perfusion, altered (adverse reactions)
✓ Injury, risk for (adverse reactions)
✓ Knowledge deficit (teaching)

Implementation
IM route
- Store in dark area
- Give titrated dose; use lowest effective dosage; give oil sol deep in large muscle mass; rotate sites; use after warming to dissolve crystals

Patient/family education
- Teach patient to report breast lumps, vaginal bleeding, edema, jaundice, dark urine, clay-colored stools, dyspnea, headache, blurred vision, abdominal pain, numbness or stiffness in legs, chest pain
- Teach patient to report suspected pregnancy

Evaluation
Positive therapeutic outcome
- Decreased abnormal uterine bleeding
- Absence of amenorrhea
- Prevented pregnancy

promazine (℞)
(proe'ma-zeen)
Promanyl ✤, promazine, Prozine, Sparine
Func. class.: Antipsychotic/neuroleptic
Chem. class.: Phenothiazine, aliphatic
Pregnancy category C

Action: Depresses cerebral cortex, hypothalamus, limbic system, which control activity, aggression; blocks neurotransmission produced by dopamine at synapse; exhibits a strong α-adrenergic, anticholinergic blocking action; as antiemetic, inhibits medullary chemoreceptor trigger zone; mechanism for antipsychotic effects is unclear

Therapeutic Outcome: Decreased signs and symptoms of psychosis, absence of nausea, vomiting

Uses: Psychotic disorders, schizophrenia, nausea, vomiting, alcohol withdrawal

Dosage and routes
Psychosis
Adult: PO 10-200 mg q4-6h; max dose 1000 mg/day; IM

50-150 mg, followed in 30 min with additional dose up to a total dose of 300 mg

P ***Child* >*12 yr:*** PO 10-25 mg q4-6h

Nausea/vomiting

Adult: PO 25-50 mg q4-6h; IM 50 mg; **IV** not recommended, but may use in conc of <25 mg/ml

Available forms: Tabs 25, 50, 100 mg; inj 25, 50 mg/ml

Adverse effects

CNS: Extrapyramidal symptoms: pseudoparkinsonism, akathisia, dystonia, tardive dyskinesia, drowsiness, headache, ***seizures, neuroleptic malignant syndrome***

CV: Orthostatic hypotension, ***cardiac arrest,*** ECG changes, ***tachycardia***

EENT: Blurred vision, glaucoma, dry eyes

GI: Dry mouth, nausea, vomiting, anorexia, constipation, diarrhea, jaundice, weight gain

GU: Urinary retention, urinary frequency, enuresis, impotence, amenorrhea, gynecomastia

HEMA: Anemia, ***leukopenia, leukocytosis, agranulocytosis***

INTEG: Rash, photosensitivity, dermatitis

RESP: ***Laryngospasm,*** dyspnea, ***respiratory depression***

Contraindications: Hypersensitivity, blood dyscrasias, coma, P child <12 yr, brain damage, bone marrow depression, glaucoma

Precautions: Pregnancy **C**, lactation, seizure disorders, hypertension, hepatic disease, cardiac disease

Pharmacokinetics

Absorption	Variably absorbed (PO); well absorbed (IM); completely absorbed (IV)
Distribution	Widely distributed; high concentrations in CNS; crosses placenta
Metabolism	Liver, extensively
Excretion	Kidneys, breast milk
Half-life	Unknown

Pharmacodynamics

	PO	IM
Onset	½ hr	Up to ½ hr
Peak	2-4 hr	Unknown
Duration	4-6 hr	4-6 hr

Interactions

Individual drugs

Alcohol: ↑ effects of both drugs, oversedation

Aluminum hydroxide: ↓ absorption

Bromocriptine: ↓ antiparkinsonian activity

Disopyramide: ↑ anticholinergic effects

Epinephrine: ↑ toxicity

Guanethidine: ↓ antihypertensive response

Levodopa: ↓ antiparkinsonian activity

Lithium: ↓ promazine levels, ↑ EPS, masking of lithium toxicity

Magnesium hydroxide: ↓ absorption

Norepinephrine: ↓ vasoresponse, ↑ toxicity

Phenobarbital: ↓ effectiveness, ↑ metabolism

Drug classifications

Antacids: ↓ absorption

Anticholinergics: ↑ anticholinergic effects

Antidepressants: ↑ CNS depression

Antidiarrheals, adsorbent: ↓ absorption

Antihistamines: ↑ CNS depression

P

Antihypertensives: ↑ hypotension
Antithyroid agents: ↑ agranulocytosis
Barbiturate anesthetics: ↑ CNS depression
β-Adrenergics: ↑ effects of both drugs
General anesthetics: ↑ CNS depression
MAOIs: ↑ CNS depression
Narcotics: ↑ CNS depression
Sedative/hypnotics: ↑ CNS depression

Lab test interferences
↑ Liver function tests, ↑ cardiac enzymes, ↑ cholesterol, ↑ blood glucose, ↑ prolactin, ↑ bilirubin, ↑ PBI, ↑ cholinesterase, ↑ iodine, ↑ alkaline phosphatase, ↑ leukocytes, ↑ granulocytes, ↑ platelets
↓ Hormones (blood and urine)
False positive: Pregnancy tests, PKU, urine bilirubin
False negative: Urinary steroids, 17-OHCS

NURSING CONSIDERATIONS

Assessment

- Assess mental status: orientation, mood, behavior, presence and type of hallucinations before initial administration and monthly; this drug should significantly reduce psychotic behavior
- Check for swallowing of PO medication; check for hoarding or giving of medication to other patients
- Monitor I&O ratio; palpate bladder if low urinary output **G** occurs, especially in elderly; urinalysis recommended before, during prolonged therapy
- Monitor bilirubin, CBC, liver function studies monthly
- Assess affect, orientation, LOC, reflexes, gait, coordination, sleep pattern disturbances
- Monitor B/P with patient sitting, standing and lying, take pulse and respirations q4h during initial treatment; establish baseline before starting treatment; report drops of 30 mm Hg; obtain baseline ECG, Q wave and T wave changes
- Check for dizziness, faintness, palpitations, tachycardia on rising; severe orthostatic hypotension is common
- ! Identify for neuroleptic malignant syndrome: hyperpyrexia, muscle rigidity, increased CPK, altered mental status; drug should be discontinued
- Assess for EPS including akathisia (inability to sit still, no pattern to movements), tardive dyskinesia (bizarre movements of the jaw, mouth, tongue, extremities), pseudoparkinsonism (ragged tremors, pill rolling, shuffling gate); an antiparkinsonian drug should be prescribed
- Assess for constipation, urinary retention daily; if these occur, increase bulk, water in diet

Nursing diagnoses

- ✓ Thought processes, altered (uses)
- ✓ Coping, ineffective individual (uses)
- ✓ Knowledge deficit (teaching)
- ✓ Noncompliance (teaching)

Implementation

PO route

- Give decreased dosage in **G** elderly since metabolism is slowed
- Give PO with full glass of water, milk; or give with food to decrease GI upset
- Store in airtight, light-resistant container

IM route

- Inject in deep muscle mass;

do not give SC; do not administer sol with a precipitate; patient should remain recumbent for at least 30 min to prevent severe hypotension

Patient/family education

• Teach patient to use good oral hygiene; frequent rinsing of mouth, sugarless gum for dry mouth

• Advise patient to avoid hazardous activities until drug response is determined; dizziness, blurred vision may occur

• Inform patient that orthostatic hypotension occurs often and to rise from sitting or lying position gradually; to remain lying down after IM injection for at least 30 min; tell patient to avoid hot tubs, hot showers, tub baths, since hypotension may occur; tell patient that in hot weather heat stroke may occur; take extra precautions to stay cool

• Caution patient to avoid abrupt withdrawal of this drug, or EPS may result; drug should be withdrawn slowly

• Teach patient to avoid OTC preparations (cough, hay fever, cold) unless approved by prescriber, since serous drug interactions may occur; avoid use with alcohol, CNS depressants; increased drowsiness may occur

• Caution patient to use a sunscreen and sunglasses to prevent burns

• Teach patient about EPS and necessity of meticulous oral hygiene, since oral candidiasis may occur

• Instruct patient to take antacids 2 hr before or after taking this drug

• Teach patient to report sore throat, malaise, fever, bleeding, mouth sores; if these occur, CBC should be drawn and drug discontinued

• Teach patient that urine may turn pink or red

Evaluation

Positive therapeutic outcome

• Decrease in emotional excitement, hallucinations, delusions, paranoia

• Reorganization of patterns of thought, speech

Treatment of overdose: Lavage if orally ingested; provide airway; *do not induce vomiting or use epinephrine*

promethazine (℞)

(proe-meth'a-zeen)

Anergan 50, Phenergan, Phenergan Fortis, Phenergan Plain, promethazine HCl

Func. class.: Antihistamine, H_1-receptor antagonist; antiemetic; sedative/hypnotic

Chem. class.: Phenothiazine derivative

Pregnancy category C

Action: Acts on blood vessels, GI, respiratory system by competing with histamine for H_1-receptor site; decreases allergic response by blocking histamine; also acts on chemoreceptor trigger zone to decrease vomiting; increases CNS stimulation, has anticholinergic response

➡ Therapeutic Outcome: Absence of allergy symptoms and rhinitis, absence of nausea/vomiting, sedation

Uses: Motion sickness, rhinitis, allergy symptoms, sedation,

P

nausea, preoperative and postoperative sedation

Dosage and routes
Nausea
Adult: PO/IM/**IV**/rec 10-25 mg; may repeat 12.5-25 mg q4-6h
P ***Child >2 yr:*** PO/IM/**IV**/rec 0.25-0.5 mg/kg q4-6h

Motion sickness
Adult: PO 25 mg bid; give 30-60 min before departure
P ***Child >2 yr:*** PO/IM/rec 12.5-25 mg bid; give 30-60 min before departure

Allergy/rhinitis
Adult: PO 12.5 mg qid, or 25 mg hs
P ***Child >2 yr:*** PO 6.25-12.5 mg tid or 25 mg hs

Sedation
Adult: PO/IM/**IV**/rec 25-50 mg hs
P ***Child >2 yr:*** PO/IM/rec/**IV** 12.5-25 mg hs

Sedation (preoperative/ postoperative)
Adult: PO/IM/**IV** 25-50 mg
P ***Child >2 yr:*** PO/IM/**IV** 12.5-25 mg

Available forms: Tabs 12.5, 25, 50 mg; supp 12.5, 25, 50 mg; inj 25, 50 mg/ml

Adverse effects
CNS: Dizziness, drowsiness, poor coordination, fatigue, anxiety, euphoria, confusion, paresthesia, neuritis
CV: Hypotension, palpitations, tachycardia
EENT: Blurred vision, dilated pupils, tinnitus, nasal stuffiness, dry nose, throat, mouth, photosensitivity
GI: Constipation, dry mouth, nausea, vomiting, anorexia, diarrhea
GU: Retention, dysuria, frequency
HEMA: Thrombocytopenia, agranulocytosis, hemolytic anemia
INTEG: Rash, urticaria, photosensitivity
RESP: Increased thick secretions, wheezing, chest tightness

Contraindications: Hypersensitivity to H_1-receptor antagonist, acute asthma attack, lower respiratory tract disease

Precautions: Increased intraocular pressure, renal disease, cardiac disease, hypertension, bronchial asthma, seizure disorder, stenosed peptic ulcers, hyperthyroidism, prostatic hypertrophy, bladder neck obstruction, pregnancy **C**

Pharmacokinetics

Absorption	Well absorbed (PO, IM); erratically absorbed (rec)
Distribution	Widely distributed; crosses the blood-brain barrier, placenta
Metabolism	Liver
Excretion	Kidneys, breast milk
Half-life	Unknown

Pharmacodynamics

	PO/IM/REC	IV
Onset	20 min	3-5 min
Peak	Unknown	Unknown
Duration	4-6 hr	4-6 hr

Interactions
Individual drugs
Alcohol: ↑ CNS depression
Atropine: ↑ anticholinergic reactions
Disopyramide: ↑ anticholinergic reactions
Haloperidol: ↑ anticholinergic reactions
Quinidine: ↑ anticholinergic reactions

Drug classifications
Antidepressants: ↑ anticholinergic reactions
Antihistamines: ↑ anticholinergic reactions
CNS depressants: ↑ CNS depression
MAOIs: ↑ anticholinergic effect
Narcotics: ↑ CNS depression
Phenothiazines: ↑ anticholinergic reactions
Sedative/hypnotics: ↑ CNS depression

Lab test interferences
False negative: Skin allergy tests (discontinue antihistamines 3 days before testing)
↑ Serum glucose

NURSING CONSIDERATIONS

Assessment

- Assess respiratory status: rate, rhythm, increase in bronchial secretions, wheezing, chest tightness; provide fluids to 2 L/day to decrease secretion thickness
- Monitor I&O ratio: be alert for urinary retention, frequency, dysuria, especially G elderly; drug should be discontinued if these occur
- Monitor CBC during long-term therapy; blood dyscrasias may occur but are rare

Nursing diagnoses

✓ Airway clearance, ineffective (uses)
✓ Injury, risk for (adverse reactions)
✓ Knowledge deficit (teaching)
✓ Noncompliance (teaching, overuse)

Implementation

PO route

- Give with meals to decrease GI upset
- Store in tight, light-resistant container

IM route

- Give IM inj in large muscle mass; aspirate to avoid **IV** administration; do not give SC; necrosis may occur

IV **IV route**

- Give IV directly; give 25 mg or less over 1 min; rapid drop in B/P may occur with rapid administration

Syringe incompatibilities: Dimenhydrinate, heparin, pentobarbital, thiopental

Syringe compatibilities: Atropine, butorphanol, chlorpromazine, cimetidine, diphenhydramine, droperidol, fentanyl, glycopyrrolate, hydromorphone, hydroxyzine, meperidine, metoclopramide, midazolam, pentazocine, perphenazine, prochlorperazine, promazine, ranitidine, scopolamine

Y-site incompatibilities: Cefoperazone, foscarnet, heparin

Y-site compatibilities: Amifostine, amsacrine, aztreonam, ciprofloxacin, cisplatin, cyclophosphamide, cytarabine, doxorubicin, filgrastim, fluconazole, fludarabine, melphalan, ondansetron, sargramostim, thiotepa, vinorelbine

Additive compatibilities: Amikacin, ascorbic acid, netilmicin, vitamin B with C

Additive incompatibilities: Aminophylline, carbenicillin, chloramphenicol, chlorothiazide, floxacillin, furosemide, heparin, hydrocortisone sodium succinate, methicillin, methohexital, penicillin G, pentobarbital, phenobarbital, thiopental

Patient/family education

- Inform patient that a false negative result may occur with skin testing; these procedures should not be scheduled until 3 days after discontinuing use
- Advise patient to take 30 min before departure to prevent motion sickness
- Caution patient to avoid hazardous activities, activities requiring alertness, since dizziness may occur; instruct patient to request assistance with ambulation
- Advise patient to avoid alcohol, other depressants; serious CNS depression may occur
- Teach all aspects of drug use; to notify prescriber if confusion, sedation, hypotension occur; to avoid driving and other hazardous activity if drowsiness occurs; to avoid alcohol and other CNS depressants that may potentiate effect
- Advise patient to take 1 hr ac or 2 hr pc to facilitate absorption
- Caution patient not to exceed recommended dosage; dysrhythmias may occur
- Inform patient hard candy, gum, frequent rinsing of mouth may be used for dryness

Evaluation

Positive therapeutic outcome

- Absence of motion sickness
- Absence of nausea, vomiting

Treatment of overdose: Administer ipecac syrup or lavage, diazepam, vasopressors, barbiturates (short-acting)

propantheline (℞)

(proe-pan′the-leen)
Norpanth, Pro-Banthine, Propanthel ✦, propantheline bromide

Func. class.: GI anticholinergic; antimuscarinic

Chem. class.: Synthetic quaternary ammonium compound

Pregnancy category C

Action: Inhibits muscarinic actions of acetylcholine at postganglionic parasympathetic neuroeffector sites

➔ **Therapeutic Outcome:** Absence of peptic ulcer disease symptoms

Uses: Treatment of peptic ulcer disease, irritable bowel syndrome, duodenography, urinary incontinence

Investigational uses: Antispasmodic uses

Dosage and routes

Adult: PO 15 mg tid ac, 30 mg hs

G ***Elderly:*** PO 7.5 mg tid ac

Antispasmodic

P ***Child:*** PO 2-3 mg/kg/day

Antisecretory

P ***Child:*** PO 1.5 mg/kg/day in 3-4 divided doses

Available forms: Tabs 7.5, 15 mg

Adverse effects

CNS: Confusion, stimulation in G *elderly,* headache, insomnia, dizziness, drowsiness, anxiety, weakness, hallucinations

CV: Palpitations, tachycardia

EENT: Blurred vision, photo-

phobia, mydriasis, cycloplegia, increased ocular tension
GI: Dry mouth, constipation, ***paralytic ileus,*** heartburn, nausea, vomiting, dysphagia, absence of taste
GU: Hesitancy, retention, impotence
INTEG: Urticaria, rash, pruritus, anhidrosis, fever, allergic reactions

Contraindications: Hypersensitivity to anticholinergics, narrow-angle glaucoma, GI obstruction, myasthenia gravis, paralytic ileus, GI atony, toxic megacolon

Precautions: Hyperthyroidism, CAD, dysrhythmias, CHF, ulcerative colitis, hypertension, hiatal hernia, hepatic disease, renal disease, pregnancy **C,** urinary retention, prostatic hypertrophy

Pharmacokinetics	
Absorption	Moderately absorbed
Distribution	Unknown
Metabolism	Unknown
Excretion	Unknown
Half-life	Unknown

Pharmacodynamics	
Onset	½ hr
Peak	2-6 hr
Duration	4-6 hr

Interactions

Individual drugs

Amantadine: ↑ anticholinergic effect
Atropine: ↑ anticholinergic effect
Disopyramide: ↑ anticholinergic effect
Haloperidol: ↑ anticholinergic effect
Potassium chloride, oral: ↑ GI lesions
Quinidine: ↑ anticholinergic effect

Drug classifications

Antacids: ↓ absorption of propantheline
Anticholinergics: ↑ anticholinergic effect
Antidepressants, tricyclic: ↑ anticholinergic effect
Antihistamines: ↑ anticholinergic effect
Phenothiazines: ↑ anticholinergic effect

NURSING CONSIDERATIONS

Assessment

- Assess for the pain of peptic ulcer disease before, during, and after treatment

Nursing diagnoses

- ✓ Pain (uses)
- ✓ Constipation (adverse reactions)
- ✓ Thought processes, impaired (adverse reactions)
- ✓ Knowledge deficit (teaching)

Implementation

- Give 30 min ac and at hs; do not give with antacids; separate by at least 1 hr

Patient/family education

- Teach patient to report blurred vision, chest pain, allergic reactions
- Advise patient not to perform strenuous activity in high temp; heat stroke may result due to decreased perspiration
- Instruct patient to take as prescribed; not to skip doses
- Instruct patient to report change in vision; blurring or loss of sight; drug should be discontinued
- Advise patient not to operate machinery or drive if dizziness occurs
- Caution patient not to take OTC products without approval of prescriber

P

Evaluation
Positive therapeutic outcome
- Decreased pain in peptic ulcer disease

propoxyphene (℞)
(proe-pox'i-feen)
Darvin, Darvon-N, Dolene, Doraphen, Doxaphene, Novapropoxyn ♣, Profene, Pro-Pox, Propoxycon, propoxyphene HCl
Func. class.: Nonnarcotic analgesics
Chem. class.: Synthetic opiate
Pregnancy category C
Controlled substance schedule IV

Action: Depresses pain impulse transmission at the spinal cord level by interacting with opioid receptors

➔ **Therapeutic Outcome:** Decreased pain

Uses: Mild to moderate pain

Dosage and routes
Adult: PO 65 mg q4h prn (HCl)
Adult: PO 100 mg q4h prn (napsylate)

Available forms: Propoxyphene HCl: cap 65 mg, tab 65 mg ♣; Propoxyphene napsylate: tabs 50, 100 mg; cap 100 mg ♣, oral susp 50 mg/5 ml; propoxyphene HCl/acetaminophen: tab 65 mg/650 mg; propoxyphene napsylate/acetaminophen: tabs 50 mg/325 mg, 100 mg/650 mg; propoxyphene/aspirin/caffeine: caps 65 mg/389 mg/32.4 mg

Adverse effects
CNS: Drowsiness, dizziness, confusion, headache, sedation, euphoria, ***convulsions, hyperthermia***
CV: Palpitations, bradycardia, change in B/P, ***dysrhythmias***
EENT: Tinnitus, blurred vision, miosis, diplopia
GI: Nausea, vomiting, anorexia, constipation, cramps
GU: Urinary retention, dysuria
INTEG: Rash, urticaria, bruising, flushing, diaphoresis, pruritus
RESP: ***Respiratory depression***

Contraindications: Hypersensitivity to ASA products (some preparations), addiction (narcotic)

Precautions: Addictive personality, pregnancy **C,** lactation, increased intracranial pressure, MI (acute), severe heart disease, respiratory depression, hepatic disease, renal disease, P child <18 yr

Pharmacokinetics	
Absorption	Well absorbed
Distribution	Widely distributed; crosses placenta
Metabolism	Liver, extensively
Excretion	Kidneys, breast milk
Half-life	6-12 hr

Pharmacodynamics	
Onset	½-1 hr
Peak	2-2½ hr
Duration	4-6 hr

Interactions
Individual drugs
Alcohol: ↑ respiratory depression, hypotension, sedation
Nalbuphine: ↓ analgesia
Pentazocine: ↓ analgesia
Drug classifications
Antihistamines: ↑ respiratory depression, hypotension

CNS depressants: ↑ respiratory depression, hypotension
MAOIs: Use ↓ dosage; reaction is unpredictable
Sedative/hypnotics: ↑ respiratory depression, hypotension
Smoking
↓ analgesic effect
Lab test interferences
↑ Amylase

NURSING CONSIDERATIONS
Assessment
- Assess pain: location, duration, intensity before and 1 hr after administration
- Monitor CNS changes: dizziness, drowsiness, euphoria, LOC, pupil reaction
- Monitor allergic reactions: rash, urticaria

Nursing diagnoses
- ✓ Pain (uses)
- ✓ Sensory-perceptual alteration: visual, auditory (adverse reactions)
- ✓ Breathing pattern, ineffective (adverse reactions)
- ✓ Injury, risk for (adverse reactions)
- ✓ Knowledge deficit (teaching)

Implementation
- Give with antiemetic if nausea, vomiting occur
- Give when pain is beginning to return; determine dosage interval by patient response; continuous dosing of medication is more effective than when given prn
- Withdraw medication slowly after long-term use to prevent withdrawal symptoms
- Store in light-resistant container at room temp
- May be given with food or milk to lessen GI upset

Patient/family education
- Teach patient to avoid CNS depressants: alcohol, sedative/hypnotics for at least 24 hr after taking this drug
- Discuss with patient that dizziness, drowsiness, and confusion are common; to avoid getting up without assistance
- Discuss in detail all aspects of the drug, including purpose and what to expect after anesthesia
- Advise patient to make position changes slowly to lessen orthostatic hypotension

Evaluation
Positive therapeutic outcome
- Decreased pain

Treatment of overdose: Narcan 0.2-0.8 **IV**, O_2, **IV** fluids, vasopressors

propranolol (℞)
(proe-pran'oh-lole)
Apo-Propranolol ✱, Detensol ✱, Inderal, Inderal LA, Inderal 10, Inderal 20, Inderal 40, Inderal 60, Inderal 80, propranolol HCl, Propranolol Intensol, Novopranol ✱
Func. class.: Antihypertensive, antianginal
Chem. class.: β-Adrenergic blocker
Pregnancy category C

Action: Competitively blocks stimulation of β-adrenergic receptor within vascular smooth muscle; produces chronotropic, inotropic activity (decreases rate of SA node discharge, increases recovery time), slows conduction of AV node, decreased heart rate, which decreases O_2 consump-

P

tion in myocardium; also decreases renin-aldosterone-angiotensin system at high doses, inhibits β_2-receptors in bronchial system (high doses)

➡ **Therapeutic Outcome:** Decreased B/P, heart rate

Uses: Chronic stable angina pectoris, hypertension, supraventricular dysrhythmias, migraine, prophylaxis, MI, pheochromocytoma, essential tremor, tetralogy of Fallot, cyanotic spells

Investigational uses: Mitral valve prolapse, anxiety, dysrhythmias associated with thyrotoxicosis

Dosage and routes

Dysrhythmias

Adult: PO 10-30 mg tid-qid; **IV** bol 0.5-3 mg over 1 mg/min; may repeat in 2 min; may repeat q4h thereafter

Hypertension

Adult: PO 40 mg bid or 80 mg qd (ext rel) initially; usual dosage 120-240 mg/day bid-tid or 120-160 mg qd (ext rel)

Angina

Adult: PO 80-320 mg in divided doses bid-qid or 80 mg qd (ext rel); usual dosage 160 mg qd (ext rel)

MI prophylaxis

Adult: PO 180-240 mg/day tid-qid starting 5 days to 3 wk after MI

Pheochromocytoma

Adult: PO 60 mg/day × 3 days preoperatively in divided doses or 30 mg/day in divided doses (inoperable tumor)

Migraine

Adult: PO 80 mg/day (ext rel) or in divided doses; may increase to 160-240 mg/day in divided doses

Essential tremor

Adult: PO 40 mg bid; usual dosage 120 mg/day

Available forms: Ext rel caps 60, 80, 120, 160 mg; tabs 10, 20, 40, 60, 90 mg; inj 1 mg/ml; oral sol 4 mg, 8 mg/ml; conc oral sol 80 mg/ml

Adverse effects

CNS: Depression, hallucinations, dizziness, fatigue, lethargy, paresthesia, bizarre dreams, disorientation
CV: Bradycardia, hypotension, CHF, palpitations, AV block, peripheral vascular insufficiency, vasodilatation
EENT: Sore throat, ***laryngospasm,*** blurred vision, dry eyes
GI: Nausea, vomiting, diarrhea, colitis, constipation, cramps, dry mouth, hepatomegaly, gastric pain, acute pancreatitis
GU: Impotence, decreased libido, UTIs
HEMA: Agranulocytosis, thrombocytopenia
INTEG: Rash, pruritus, fever
META: Hyperglycemia, hypoglycemia
MISC: Facial swelling, weight change, Raynaud's phenomenon
MS: Joint pain, arthralgia, muscle cramps, pain
RESP: Dyspnea, respiratory dysfunction, *bronchospasm*

Contraindications: Hypersensitivity to this drug, cardiac failure, cardiogenic shock, 2nd- or 3rd-degree heart block, bronchospastic disease, sinus bradycardia, CHF

Precautions: Diabetes mellitus, pregnancy **C,** renal disease, lactation, hyperthyroidism, COPD, hepatic disease,

P children, myasthenia gravis, peripheral vascular disease, hypotension, CHF

Pharmacokinetics

Absorption	Well absorbed (PO); slowly absorbed (ext rel); completely absorbed (IV)
Distribution	Widely distributed; crosses blood-brain barrier
Metabolism	Liver, extensively
Excretion	Kidneys
Half-life	3-5 hr; ext rel 8-11 hr

Pharmacodynamics

	PO	PO–Ext Rel	IV
Onset	½ hr	Unknown	Rapid
Peak	1-1½ hr	6 hr	1 min
Duration	6-12 hr	24 hr	4-6 hr

Interactions

Individual drugs

Alcohol: ↑ hypotension (large amounts)
Epinephrine: α-Adrenergic stimulation
Hydralazine: ↑ hypotension, bradycardia
Indomethacin: ↓ antihypertensive effect
Insulin: ↑ hypoglycemia
Methyldopa: ↑ hypotension, bradycardia
Prazosin: ↑ hypotension, bradycardia
Reserpine: ↑ hypotension, bradycardia
Thyroid: ↓ effect of propranolol
Verapamil: ↑ myocardial depression

Drug classifications

Antihypertensive: ↑ hypertension
Cardiac glycosides: ↑ bradycardia
Nitrates: ↑ hypotension
Sulfonylureas: ↓ hypoglycemic effect
Theophyllines: ↓ bronchodilatation

Lab test interferences

False ↑ Urinary catecholamines

NURSING CONSIDERATIONS

Assessment

- Monitor B/P during beginning treatment, periodically thereafter; pulse q4h; note rate, rhythm, quality; check apical/radial pulse before administration; notify prescriber of any significant changes (pulse <50 bpm)
- Check for baselines in renal, liver function tests before therapy begins and periodically thereafter
- Assess for edema in feet, legs daily; monitor I&O, weight daily; check for jugular vein distention, rales bilaterally; dyspnea (CHF)
- Monitor skin turgor, dryness of mucous membranes for hydration status, especially G elderly

Nursing diagnoses

- ✓ Cardiac output, decreased (uses)
- ✓ Injury, potential for (adverse reactions)
- ✓ Knowledge deficit (teaching)
- ✓ Noncompliance (teaching)

Implementation

PO route

- Given ac, hs, tab may be crushed or swallowed whole; do not crush or chew ext rel cap; give with food to prevent GI upset; reduce dosage in renal dysfunction
- Store protected from light, moisture; placed in cool environment

IV **IV route**

- Give by direct **IV** undiluted or diluted 1 mg/10 ml D_5W for inj; administer over 1 min or more

P

• Give by intermittent inf after diluting in 50 ml D_5W, 0.9% NaCl, D_5/0.45% NaCl, D_5/0.9% NaCl, LR; administer over 15 min

Syringe compatibilities: Amrinone, benzquinamide, milrinone

Y-*site incompatibility:* Diazoxide

Y-*site compatibilities:* Amrinone, heparin, hydrocortisone, meperidine, milrinone, morphine, potassium chloride, tacrolimus, vitamin B with C

Additive compatibilities: Dobutamine, verapamil

Solution compatibilities: 0.9% NaCl, 0.45 NaCl, Ringer's, D_5W, D_5/0.9% NaCl, D_5/0.45% NaCl

Patient/family education

• Teach patient not to discontinue drug abruptly, taper over 2 wk; may cause precipitate angina if stopped abruptly
• Teach patient not to use OTC products containing α-adrenergic stimulants (such as nasal decongestants, cold preparations); to avoid alcohol, smoking and to limit sodium intake as prescribed
• Teach patient how to take pulse and B/P at home; advise when to notify prescriber
• Instruct patient to comply with weight control, dietary adjustments, modified exercise program
• Instruct patient to carry/wear Medic Alert ID to identify drug being taken, allergies; tell patient drug controls symptoms but does not cure
• Caution patient to avoid hazardous activities if dizziness, drowsiness is present
• Teach patient to report symptoms of CHF: difficult breathing, especially on exertion or when lying down, night cough, swelling of extremities or bradycardia, dizziness, confusion, depression, fever
• Teach patient to take drug as prescribed, not to double doses, skip doses; take any missed doses as soon as remembered if at least 8 hr until next dose

Evaluation

Positive therapeutic outcome

• Decreased B/P in hypertension (after 1-2 wk)
• Decreased tremors
• Absence of dysrhythmias
• Decreased migraine headaches

Treatment of overdose: Lavage, **IV** atropine for bradycardia, **IV** theophylline for bronchospasm, digitalis, O_2, diuretic for cardiac failure, hemodialysis, **IV** glucose for hyperglycemia, **IV** diazepam (or phenytoin) for seizures

propylthiouracil (℞)

(proe-pill-thye-oh-yoor'a-sill)

propylthiouracil, Propyl-Thyracil ✤, PTU

Func. class.: Thyroid hormone antagonist (antithyroid)

Chem. class.: Thioamide

Pregnancy category D

Action: Blocks synthesis peripherally of T_3, T_4, inhibits organification of iodine

➡ Therapeutic Outcome: Decreased T_3, T_4 levels, hyperthyroid symptoms

Uses: Preparation for thyroidectomy, thyrotoxic crisis, hyperthyroidism, thyroid storm

Dosage and routes

Thyrotoxic crisis

P ***Adult and child:*** PO same as hyperthyroidism with iodine and propranolol

Preparation for thyroidectomy

Adult: PO 600-1200 mg/day

P ***Child:*** PO 10 mg/kg/day in divided doses

Hyperthyroidism

Adult: PO 100 mg tid increasing to 300 mg q8h if condition is severe; continue to euthyroid state, then 100 mg qd-tid

P ***Child >10 yr:*** PO 100 mg tid, continue to euthyroid state, then 25 mg tid to 100 mg bid

P ***Child 6-10 yr:*** PO 50-150 mg in divided doses q8h

P ***Neonates:*** PO 10 mg/kg/day in divided doses

Available forms: Tab 50 mg

Adverse effects

CNS: Drowsiness, headache, vertigo, fever, paresthesias, neuritis

GI: Nausea, diarrhea, vomiting, ***jaundice, hepatitis,*** loss of taste

GU: ***Nephritis***

HEMA: ***Agranulocytosis, leukopenia, thrombocytopenia, hypothrombinemia, lymphadenopathy,*** bleeding, vasculitis, periarteritis

INTEG: Rash, urticaria, pruritus, alopecia, hyperpigmentation, lupuslike syndrome

MS: Myalgia, arthralgia, nocturnal muscle cramps, osteoporosis

Contraindications: Hypersensitivity, pregnancy **D,** lactation

Precautions: Infection, bone marrow depression, hepatic disease

Pharmacokinetics	
Absorption	Rapidly absorbed
Distribution	Crosses placenta; concentration in thyroid gland
Metabolism	Liver
Excretion	Urine, bile, breast milk
Half-life	1-2 hr

Pharmacodynamics	
Onset	30-40 min
Peak	Unknown
Duration	2-4 hr

Interactions

Individual drugs

Heparin: ↑ anticoagulant effect

Lithium: ↑ antithyroid effect

Radiation: ↑ bone marrow depression

Drug classifications

Antineoplastics: ↑ bone marrow depression

Oral anticoagulants: ↑ anticoagulant effect

Phenothiazines: ↑ agranulocytosis

Lab test interferences

↑ Pro-time, ↑ AST (SGOT), ↑ ALT (SGPT), ↑ alkaline phosphatase

NURSING CONSIDERATIONS

Assessment

- Monitor pulse, B/P, temp; I&O ratio; check for edema (puffy hands, feet, periorbits); indicates hypothyroidism
- Check weight daily with same clothing, scale, time of day
- Monitor T_3, T_4, which are increased; check serum TSH, which is decreased; assess free

P

thyroxine index, which is increased if dosage is too low; discontinue drug 3-4 wk before RAIU
- Monitor blood work: CBC for blood dyscrasias (leukopenia, thrombocytopenia, agranulocytosis); liver function tests
- Assess overdose (peripheral edema, heat intolerance, diaphoresis, palpitations, dysrhythmias, severe tachycardia, increased temp, delirium, CNS irritability); drug should be discontinued
- Assess for hypersensitivity (rash, enlarged cervical lymph nodes); drug may have to be discontinued
- Assess for hypoprothrombinemia (bleeding, petechiae, ecchymosis)
- Monitor clinical response: after 3 wk should include increased weight, decreased pulse, decreased T_4
- Assess for bone marrow depression: sore throat, fever, fatigue

Nursing diagnoses

✓ Knowledge deficit (teaching)
✓ Noncompliance (teaching)

Implementation

- Give with meals to decrease GI upset
- Give at same time each day to maintain drug level
- Give lowest dosage that relieves symptoms
- Store in light-resistant container
- Increase fluids to 3-4 L/day, unless contraindicated

Patient/family education

- Advise patient to abstain from breastfeeding after delivery; drug appears in breast milk
- Teach patient to take pulse daily and to keep graph of weight, pulse, mood
- Advise patient to report redness, swelling, sore throat, mouth lesions, which indicate blood dyscrasias
- Caution patient to avoid OTC products that contain iodine; that seafood, other iodine-containing foods may be restricted by prescriber
- Caution patient not to discontinue this medication abruptly; thyroid crisis may occur; stress patient response
- Teach patient that response may take several mo if thyroid is large
- Teach patient symptoms/signs of overdose: periorbital edema, cold intolerance, mental depression; notify prescriber at once
- Teach patient symptoms of inadequate dose: tachycardia, diarrhea, fever, irritability; prescriber should be notified to adjust dosage
- Teach patient to take medication exactly as prescribed, not to skip or double doses; missed doses should be taken when remembered up to 1 hr before next dose
- Instruct patient to carry identification (Medic Alert) indicating medication taken and condition being treated

Evaluation

Positive therapeutic outcome

- Weight gain
- Decreased pulse
- Decreased T_4
- Decreased B/P

protamine (℞)
(proe'ta-meen)
Func. class.: Heparin antagonist
Chem. class.: Low-molecular-weight protein
Pregnancy category C

Action: Binds heparin, making it ineffective

Therapeutic Outcome: Prevention of heparin overdose

Uses: Heparin overdose; neutralizes heparin in procedures

Dosage and routes
P ***Adult and child:*** **IV** 1 mg of protamine/90-115 U heparin given; administer slowly over 1-3 min; give undiluted to 1%, not to exceed 50 mg/10 min

Available forms: Inj 10 mg/ml

Adverse effects
CNS: Lassitude
CV: Hypotension, bradycardia, ***circulatory collapse***
GI: Nausea, vomiting, anorexia
INTEG: *Rash,* dermatitis, urticaria
HEMA: Bleeding, ***anaphylaxis***
RESP: Dyspnea, ***pulmonary edema, severe respiratory distress***

Contraindication: Hypersensitivity

Precautions: Pregnancy **C,** P lactation, children, allergy to fish

Pharmacokinetics

Absorption	Completely absorbed
Distribution	Unknown
Metabolism	Unknown
Excretion	Unknown
Half-life	Unknown

Pharmacodynamics

Onset	5 min
Peak	Unknown
Duration	2 hr

Interactions: None

NURSING CONSIDERATIONS
Assessment
- Monitor blood studies (Hct, platelets, occult blood stools) q3 mo
- Monitor coagulation tests (APTT, ACT) 15 min after dose, then in several hr
- Monitor VS, B/P, pulse q 30 min, plus 3 hr after dose
- Assess for skin rash, urticaria, dermatitis
- Assess for allergy to fish; use with caution in these patients

Nursing diagnoses
✓ Injury, risk for (uses)
✓ Tissue perfusion, altered (uses)
✓ Knowledge deficit (teaching)

Implementation
- Give by direct **IV** after diluting 50 mg/5 ml sterile bacteriostatic water for inj; shake; give 20 mg or less over 1-3 min
- Give by intermittent inf after further diluting with equal volume of NaCl or D_5W and run over 2-3 hr; titrate to APTT, ACT; use inf pump
- Store at 36° to 46° F (2°-8° C)

Additive incompatibilities: Penicillins, cephalosporins

Additive compatibilities: Cimetidine, ranitidine, verapamil

P

Patient/family education
- Explain reason for medication and expected results
- Caution patient to avoid contact activities that may result in bleeding

Evaluation
Positive therapeutic outcome
- Reversal of heparin overdose

pseudoephedrine (OTC)
(soo-doe-e-fed'rin)
Allerid, Children's Sudafed, Decofed Syrup, DeFed-60, Dorcol Children's Decongestant, Drixoral Non-Drowsy Formula, Eltor ✤, Efidac/24, Genaphed, Halofed, Myfedrine, Novafed, Pedia Care Infant's Decongestant, Pseudoephedrine HCl, Pseudogest Decongestant, Pseudo Syrup, Sinustat, Sudafed, Sudafed 12 hour, Sudrin
Func. class.: Adrenergic
Chem. class.: Substituted phenylethylamine
Pregnancy category B

Action: Primary activity through α-adrenergic effects on respiratory mucosal membranes reducing congestion, hyperemia, edema; minimal bronchodilatation secondary to β-adrenergic effects

➔ **Therapeutic Outcome:** Decreased nasal congestion, swelling

Uses: Nasal decongestant, otitis media adjustment, adjunct with antihistamines

Dosage and routes
P ***Adult and child >12 yr:*** PO 60 mg q6h; ext rel 60-120 mg q12h or q24h
P ***Child 6-12 yr:*** PO 30 mg q6h, not to exceed 120 mg/day
P ***Child 2-6 yr:*** PO 15 mg q6h, not to exceed 60 mg/day

Available forms: Ext rel caps 120, 240 mg; oral sol 15 mg, 30 mg/5 ml; drops 7.5 mg/0.8 ml; tabs 30, 60 mg; cap 60 mg; ext rel tabs 120 mg

Adverse effects
CNS: *Tremors, anxiety,* insomnia, headache, dizziness, anxiety, hallucinations, ***seizures***
CV: Palpitations, tachycardia, hypertension, chest pain, ***dysrhythmias***
EENT: Dry nose, irritation of nose and throat
GI: *Anorexia, nausea, vomiting,* dry mouth
GU: Dysuria

Contraindications: Hypersensitivity to sympathomimetics, narrow-angle glaucoma

Precautions: Pregnancy **B,** cardiac disorders, hyperthyroidism, diabetes mellitus, prostatic hypertrophy

Pharmacokinetics

Absorption	Well absorbed
Distribution	Enters CSF, crosses placenta
Metabolism	Liver, partially
Excretion	Kidneys, unchanged (75%); breast milk
Half-life	7 hr

Pharmacodynamics

	PO	PO-EXT REL
Onset	15-30 min	1 hr
Peak	Unknown	Unknown
Duration	4-6 hr	12 hr

Interactions

Individual drugs

Methyldopa: ↓ effect of pseudoephedrine

Rauwolfia: ↓ effect of pseudoephedrine

Drug classifications

β-Blockers: Hypertensive crisis

MAOIs: Hypertensive crisis

Urinary acidifiers: ↓ effect of pseudoephedrine

Urinary alkalizers: ↑ effect of pseudoephedrine

NURSING CONSIDERATIONS

Assessment

- Monitor for nasal congestion; auscultate lung sounds; check for tenacious bronchial secretions; children with otitis media should be assessed for eustachian tube congestion
- Monitor B/P and pulse throughout treatment

Nursing diagnoses

✓ Airway clearance, ineffective (uses)

✓ Knowledge deficit (teaching)

Implementation

- Give ext rel cap and tab whole
- Do not crush, break or chew
- Give several hr before hs if insomnia occurs
- Store at room temp

Patient/family education

- Teach patient reason for drug administration and expected results
- Instruct patient not to use continuously, or more than recommended dose; rebound congestion may occur
- Advise patient to check with prescriber before using other drugs, as drug interactions may occur
- Advise patient to avoid taking near bedtime; stimulation can occur
- Caution patient not to use if stimulation, restlessness, tremors occur

Evaluation

Positive therapeutic outcome

- Decreased nasal congestion

psyllium (OTC)

(sill′i-um)

Cillium, Effer-Syllium, Fiberall, Fiberall Natural Flavor and Orange Flavor, Hydrocil Instant Powder, Karacil ✤, Konsyl-D, Metamucil, Metamucil Instant Mix Lemon Lime, Metamucil Instant Mix Orange, Metamucil Orange Flavor, Metamucil Sugar Free, Metamucil Sugar Free Orange Flavor, Modane Bulk, Natural Vegetable Reguloid, Perdiem, Pro-Lax, Prodiem Plain ✤, Reguloid Natural, Reguloid Orange, Reguloid Sugar Free Orange, Reguloid Sugar Free Regular, Serutan, Siblin, Syllact, V-Lax

Func. class.: Laxative, bulk-forming

Chem. class.: Psyllium colloid

Pregnancy category C

Action: Promotes peristalsis by combining with water in the intestine to form a gel-like substance that is easily evacuated

➔ Therapeutic Outcome: Decreased constipation, decreased diarrhea in colitis

Uses: Chronic constipation, ulcerative colitis, irritable bowel syndrome

P

Dosage and routes

Adult: PO 1-2 tsp in 8 oz water bid or tid, then 8 oz water or 1 premeasured packet in 8 oz water bid or tid, then 8 oz water

P ***Child >6 yr:*** 1 tsp in 4 oz water hs

Available forms: Chew pieces 1.7 g/piece; powder 309, 390, 430, 450, 486, 500, 600, 630, 654, 672, 791, 919, 950 mg/g, 1 g/g; granules 2.5 g/dose

Adverse effects

GI: Nausea, vomiting, anorexia, diarrhea, cramps, intestinal/esophageal blockage

Contraindications: Hypersensitivity, intestinal obstruction, abdominal pain, nausea/vomiting, fecal impaction

Precautions: Pregnancy **C**

Pharmacokinetics	
Absorption	None
Distribution	None
Excretion	Feces
Half-life	Unknown

Pharmacodynamics	
Onset	12-24 hr
Peak	2-4 days
Duration	Unknown

Interactions

Drug classifications

Cardiac glycosides: ↓ absorption of cardiac glycosides

Oral anticoagulants: ↓ absorption of oral anticoagulants

Salicylates: ↓ absorption of salicylates

Lab test interferences

↑ Blood glucose

NURSING CONSIDERATIONS

Assessment

- Monitor blood, urine electrolytes if used often by patient; check I&O ratio to identify fluid loss
- Assess for cramping, rec bleeding, nausea, vomiting; if these symptoms occur, drug should be discontinued; identify cause of constipation; identify whether fluids, bulk, or exercise is missing from lifestyle
- Assess stool for color, consistency, amount, presence of flatulence

Nursing diagnoses

✓ Constipation (uses)
✓ Knowledge deficit (teaching)
✓ Noncompliance (teaching)

Implementation

- Give alone for better absorption; give after mixing with water immediately before use; administer with 8 oz water or juice followed by another 8 oz of fluid
- Administer in AM or PM (oral dose)

Patient/family education

- Discuss with patient that adequate fluid consumption is necessary
- Teach patient that normal bowel movements do not always occur daily
- Caution patient not to use in presence of abdominal pain, nausea, vomiting; tell patient to notify prescriber if constipation is unrelieved or if symptoms of electrolyte imbalance occur (muscle cramps, pain, weakness, dizziness, excessive thirst)
- Teach patient not to use laxatives for long-term therapy; bowel tone will be lost and will decrease
- Teach patient to shake susp well as needed
- Teach patient not to take at hs as a laxative; may interfere

with sleep; also problems with lipid pneumonia
• Teach patient not to use with food or vitamin preparations; delays digestion and absorption of fat-soluble vitamins

Evaluation

Positive therapeutic outcome
• Decreased constipation in 12-24 hr

pyrazinamide (℞)

(peer-a-zin′a-mide)

PMS Pyrazinamide ✤, pyrazinamide, Tebrazid ✤

Func. class.: Antitubercular agent

Chem. class.: Pyrazinoic acid amine/nicoturimide analog

Pregnancy category C

Action: Bactericidal interference with lipid; nucleic acid biosynthesis is possible

Therapeutic Outcome: Bactericidal for *Mycobacterium* species

Uses: Tuberculosis, as an adjunct when other drugs are not feasible

Dosage and routes

Adult: PO 20-35 mg/kg/day qd or individed doses, not to exceed 3 g/day

P ***Child:*** PO 15-30 mg/kg/day qd or divided bid; max 1.5 g/day

Available forms: Tab 500 mg

Adverse effects

CNS: Headache

GI: ***Hepatotoxicity,*** abnormal liver function tests, peptic ulcer

GU: Urinary difficulty, increased uric acid

HEMA: ***Hemolytic anemia***

INTEG: Photosensitivity, urticaria

Contraindications: Hypersensitivity

Precautions: Pregnancy **C**, P child <13 yr

Pharmacokinetics

Absorption	Well absorbed
Distribution	Widely distributed
Metabolism	Liver, extensively
Excretion	Kidneys, breast milk
Half-life	9-10 hr

Pharmacodynamics

Onset	Unknown
Peak	2 hr
Duration	9½ hr; metabolites 12 hr

Interactions: None

NURSING CONSIDERATIONS

Assessment

• C&S studies should be taken before treatment begins, and periodically during treatment
• Monitor serum uric acid, which may be elevated and cause gout symptoms
• Monitor liver studies weekly: ALT (SGPT), AST (SGOT), bilirubin; hepatic status: decreased appetite, jaundice, dark urine, fatigue
• Monitor renal status: before treatment and monthly thereafter: BUN, creatinine, output, sp gr, urinalysis
• Monitor mental status often: affect, mood, behavioral changes; psychosis may occur

Nursing diagnoses

✓ Infection, risk for (uses)
✓ Diarrhea (adverse reactions)
✓ Injury, risk for (adverse reactions)
✓ Knowledge deficit (teaching)
✓ Noncompliance (teaching)

P

Implementation
- Give with meals to decrease GI symptoms
- Give antiemetic if vomiting occurs
- May be given with other antituberculars

Patient/family education
- Instruct patient that compliance with dosage schedule, duration is necessary; that scheduled appointments must be kept or relapse may occur
- Advise diabetic patient to use blood glucose monitor to obtain correct result
- Advise patient to report weakness, fatigue, loss of appetite, nausea, vomiting, yellowing of skin or eyes, tingling/numbness of hands/feet

Evaluation
Positive therapeutic outcome
- Decreased symptoms of TB
- Sputum culture negative × 3

pyridostigmine (℞)
(peer-id-oh-stig'meen)
Mestinon, Mestinon SR ✤, Mestinon Timespan, Regonol
Func. class.: Cholinergic, anticholinesterase
Chem. class.: Tertiary amine carbamate
Pregnancy category C

Action: Inhibits destruction of acetylcholine, which increases concentration at sites where acetylcholine is released; this facilitates transmission of impulses across myoneural junction

Therapeutic Outcome: Decreased action of nondepolarizing muscle relaxant; increased muscle strength in myasthenia gravis

Uses: Nondepolarizing muscle relaxant antagonist, myasthenia gravis

Dosage and routes
Myasthenia gravis
Adult: PO 60-180 mg bid-qid, not to exceed 1.5 g/day; IM/**IV** 1/30 of PO dose; sus rel 180-540 mg qd or bid at intervals of at least 6 hr

Nondepolarizing neuromuscular blocker antagonist
Adult: 0.6-1.2 mg **IV** atropine, then 10-30 mg

Available forms: Tab 60 mg; sus rel tab 180 mg; syr 60 mg/5 ml; inj 5 mg/ml

Adverse effects
CNS: Dizziness, headache, sweating, weakness, ***convulsions***, uncoordination, paralysis, drowsiness, LOC
EENT: Miosis, blurred vision, lacrimation, visual changes
CV: Tachycardia, dysrhythmias, bradycardia, AV block, hypotension, ECG changes, ***cardiac arrest***, syncope
GI: Nausea, diarrhea, vomiting, cramps, increased salivary and gastric secretions, peristalsis
GU: Frequency, incontinence, urgency
INTEG: Rash, urticaria, flushing
RESP: ***Respiratory depression, bronchospasm, constriction, laryngospasm, respiratory arrest***

Contraindications: Bradycardia, hypotension, obstruction of intestine, or renal system, bromide sensitivity

Precautions: Seizure disorders, bronchial asthma, coronary occlusion, hyperthyroidism, dysrhythmias, peptic ulcer, megacolon, poor GI motility, pregnancy **C**

Pharmacokinetics

Absorption	Poorly absorbed (PO)
Distribution	Widely distributed; crosses placenta
Metabolism	Liver, plasma cholinesterase
Excretion	Kidneys
Half-life	2 hr (IV); 4 hr (PO)

Pharmacodynamics

	PO	IM/IV	PO–SUS REL
Onset	20-30 min	2-15 min	½-1 hr
Peak	Unknown	Unknown	Unknown
Duration	3-6 hr	2-4 hr	3-6 hr

Interactions

Individual drugs

Digitalis: Bradycardia
Magnesium: ↓ action of pyridostigmine
Mecamylamine: ↓ action of pyridostigmine
Polymyxin: ↓ action of pyridostigmine
Procainamide: ↓ action of pyridostigmine
Quinidine: ↓ action of pyridostigmine

Drug classifications

Antihistamines: ↑ antagonism
Antidepressants: ↑ antagonism
Phenothiazines: ↑ antagonism
Muscle relaxants, depolarizing: ↑ action of muscle relaxants
Cholinesterase inhibitors: ↑ toxicity

NURSING CONSIDERATIONS

Assessment

- Monitor VS, respiration; ↑ B/P during test and at baseline
- Monitor diabetic patient carefully, since this drug lowers blood glucose

Nursing diagnoses

✓ Breathing pattern, ineffective (uses)
✓ Knowledge deficit (teaching)

Implementation

IV **IV route**

- Give **IV** undiluted, give through Y-tube or 3-way stopcock; give 0.5 mg or less/min
- Give only when atropine sulfate available for cholinergic crisis

Syringe compatibility: Glycopyrrolate

Y-site compatibilities: Heparin, hydrocortisone, potassium chloride, vitamin B with C

PO route

- Give only after all other cholinergics have been discontinued
- Give increased doses if tolerance occurs
- Give larger doses after exercise or fatigue
- Give on empty stomach for better absorption
- Store at room temp

Patient/family education

- Advise patient to wear Medic Alert ID specifying myasthenia gravis, drugs taken

Evaluation

Positive therapeutic outcome

- Increased muscle strength, hand grasp
- Improved gait
- Absence of labored breathing (if severe)

P

Treatment of overdose: Discontinue drug, atropine 1-4 mg **IV**

pyridoxine (vitamin B_6)

(PO,OTC; IM/IV, ℞)
(peer-i-dox'een)
Beesix, Nestrex, pyridoxine HCl, Vitamin B_6, Rodex TD, Hexa-Betalin ✤
Func. class.: Vitamin B_6, water soluble
Pregnancy category A

Action: Needed for fat, protein, carbohydrate metabolism; enhances glycogen release from liver and muscle tissue; needed as coenzyme for metabolic transformations of a variety of amino acids

➔ **Therapeutic Outcome:** Absence of vitamin B_6 deficiency

Uses: Vitamin B_6 deficiency associated with the following: inborn errors of metabolism, seizures, cycloserine, hydralazine penicillamine, isoniazid therapy, oral contraceptives, alcoholism, polyneuritis

Dosage and routes

Vitamin B_6 deficiency

Adult: PO/IM/**IV** 2.5-10 mg until corrected, then 2-5 mg qd

P ***Child:*** PO/IM/**IV** 100 mg until desired response, or 2.5-10 mg/day × 3 wk, then 2-5 mg qd

Inborn errors of metabolism

Adult: IM/**IV**/PO 600 mg or less qd, then 50 mg qd for life

P ***Child:*** IM/PO/**IV** 100 mg, then 2-10 mg IM or 10-100 mg PO qd

Deficiency caused by isoniazid, cycloserine, hydralazine, penicillamine

Adult: PO 100 mg qd × 3 wk, then 50 mg qd

P ***Child:*** PO dose titrated to patient response

Prevention of deficiency caused by isoniazid, cycloserine, hydralazine, penicillamine

Adult: PO 10-50 mg qd

P ***Child:*** PO 0.5-1.5 mg qd

P ***Infant:*** PO 0.1-0.5 mg qd

Available forms: Tabs 10, 25, 50, 100, 200, 250, 500 mg; time rel tabs 100, 150, 500 mg; inj 100 mg/ml; time rel caps 100, 150 mg

Adverse effects

CNS: Paresthesia

INTEG: Pain at inj site

Contraindication: Hypersensitivity

Precautions: Pregnancy **A,** P lactation, children, Parkinson's disease

Pharmacokinetics

Absorption	Well absorbed (PO)
Distribution	Stored in liver, muscle, brain; crosses placenta
Metabolism	Unknown
Excretion	Kidneys, unchanged (not used)
Half-life	Unknown

Pharmacodynamics

Unknown

Interactions

Individual drugs

Chloramphenicol: ↓ effects of pyridoxine

Cycloserine: ↓ effects of pyridoxine

Hydralazine: ↓ effects of pyridoxine

Isoniazid: ↓ effects of pyridoxine
Levodopa: ↓ effects of levodopa
Penicillamine: ↓ effects of pyridoxine
Drug classifications
Immunosuppressants: ↓ effects of pyridoxine
Oral contraceptives: ↓ effects of pyridoxine
Lab Test Interferences
False ↑ Urobilinogen

NURSING CONSIDERATIONS

Assessment

- Monitor pyridoxine levels throughout treatment
- Assess nutritional status: yeast, liver, legumes, bananas, green vegetables, whole grains
- Assess for pyridoxine (B_6) deficiency: nausea, vomiting, dermatitis, cheilosis, seizures, irritability, dermatitis before and during treatment

Nursing diagnoses

✓ Nutrition: less then body requirements (uses)
✓ Knowledge deficit (teaching)
✓ Noncompliance (teaching, overuse)

Implementation

IV IV route

- Give **IV** undiluted or added to most **IV** sol; give 50 mg or less/1 min if undiluted

IM route

- Rotate sites; burning or stinging at site may occur; give by Z-track to minimize pain
- Store in tight, light-resistant container

Syringe compatibility: Doxapram

Additive incompatibilities: Erythromycin, iron salts, kanamycin, riboflavin, streptomycin

PO route

- Ext rel cap and tab should be swallowed whole; do not break, crush, or chew

IM/SC route

- Administer in different site each time to avoid pain

Patient/family education

- Teach patient to avoid other vitamin supplements unless directed by prescriber
- Advise patient to increase meat, bananas, potatoes, lima beans, whole grain cereals in diet which are high in vitamin B_6
- Caution patient not to increase dosage, since serious reactions may occur

Evaluation

Positive therapeutic outcome

- Absence of nausea, vomiting, anorexia, skin lesions, glossitis, stomatitis, edema, convulsions, restlessness, paresthesia

pyrimethamine (℞)

(peer-i-meth'a-meen)

Daraprim, Fansidar (with sulfadoxine)

Func. class.: Antimalarial, antiprotozol

Chem. class.: Folic acid antagonist

Pregnancy category C

Action: Inhibits folic acid metabolism in parasite; prevents transmission by stopping growth of fertilized gametes

➔ Therapeutic Outcome: Prevention of malaria

Uses: Malaria prophylaxis, antiprotozoal action against *Plasmodium vivax*

Investigational uses: *Pneumocystis carinii* pneumonia as an adjunct

P

Dosage and routes
Prophylaxis of malaria
Adult: PO 1 tab qwk or 2 tab q2 wk (Fansidar)
P ***Child 9-14 yr:*** PO ¾ tab qwk or 1½ tab q2 wk (Fansidar)
P ***Child >10 yr:*** PO 25 mg qwk
P ***Child 4-10 yr:*** PO 12.5 mg qwk
P ***Child 4-8 yr:*** PO ½ tab qwk or 1 tab q2 wk (Fansidar)
P ***Child <4 yr:*** PO ¼ tab qwk or ½ tab q2 wk (Fansidar)
P ***Child <4 yr:*** PO 6.25 mg qwk
Acute attacks of malaria
Adult: PO 2-3 tab as a single dose (Fansidar) alone or with quinine or primaquine
P ***Child 9-14 yr:*** 2 tab
P ***Child 4-8 yr:*** 1 tab
P ***Child <4 yr:*** ½ tab
Toxoplasmosis
Adult: PO 100 mg, then 25 mg qd × 4-5 wk, with 1 g sulfadiazine q6h
P ***Child:*** PO 1 mg/kg, then 0.25 mg/kg qd × 4-5 wk, with sulfadiazine 100 mg/kg/day in divided doses q6h

Available forms: Tab 25 mg; combo tab 500 mg sulfadoxine/25 mg pyrimethamine

Adverse effects
CNS: Stimulation, irritability, ***convulsions,*** tremors, ataxia, fatigue
GI: Nausea, vomiting, cramps, anorexia, diarrhea, atrophic glossitis, gastritis
HEMA: ***Thrombocytopenia, leukopenia, pancytopenia, megaloblastic anemia,*** decreased folic acid, ***agranulocytosis***
INTEG: Skin eruptions, photosensitivity
RESP: ***Respiratory failure***

Contraindications: Hypersensitivity, chloroquine-resistant malaria, megaloblastic anemia caused by folate deficiency

Precautions: Blood dyscrasias, seizure disorder, pregnancy **C,** lactation, G6PD disease, renal/hepatic disease

Pharmacokinetics	
Absorption	Well absorbed
Distribution	Widely; crosses placenta
Metabolism	Liver, extensively
Excretion	Kidneys, unchanged (30%); breast milk
Half-life	4 days

Pharmacodynamics	
Onset	Unknown
Peak	2 hr
Duration	Unknown

Interactions
Individual drugs
Folic acid: ↑ synergistic action
Drug classifications
Antiinfectives: ↑ bone marrow suppression

NURSING CONSIDERATIONS
Assessment
- C&S studies should be taken before treatment begins and periodically during treatment
- Monitor serum uric acid, which may be elevated and cause gout symptoms
- Monitor liver studies weekly: ALT (SGPT), AST (SGOT), bilirubin; hepatic status: decreased appetite, jaundice, dark urine, fatigue
- Monitor renal status: before therapy and monthly thereafter: BUN, creatinine, output, sp gr, urinalysis

• Monitor mental status often: affect, mood, behavioral changes; psychosis may occur

Nursing diagnoses

✓ Infection, risk for (uses)
✓ Diarrhea (adverse reactions)
✓ Injury, risk for (adverse reactions)
✓ Knowledge deficit (teaching)
✓ Noncompliance (teaching)

Implementation

• Give with meals to decrease GI symptoms
• Give antiemetic if vomiting occurs

Patient/family education

• Instruct patient that compliance with dosage schedule, duration is necessary; that scheduled appointments must be kept or relapse may occur
• Advise diabetic patient to use blood glucose monitor to obtain correct result
• Advise patient to report weakness, fatigue, loss of appetite, nausea, vomiting, yellowing of skin or eyes, sore throat, glossitis

Evaluation

Positive therapeutic outcome

• Decreased symptoms of toxolasmosis
• Decreased symptoms of *Pneumocystis carinii* pneumonia

quazepam (℞)

(kway'ze-pam)

Doral

Func. class.: Sedative-hypnotic

Chem. class.: Benzodiazepine derivative

Pregnancy category X

Controlled substance schedule IV (USA)

Action: Depresses subcortical levels of CNS, including limbic system, reticular formation; potentiates GABA (gamma aminobutryic acid)

Therapeutic Outcome: Decreased insomnia

Uses: Insomnia (short-term)

Dosage and routes

Adult: PO 15 mg hs; then 7.5-15 mg hs

G ***Elderly:*** PO 15 mg hs × 2 days, then 7.5 mg hs

Available forms: Tabs 7.5, 15 mg

Adverse effects

CNS: Lethargy, drowsiness, daytime sedation, dizziness, confusion, lightheadedness, headache, anxiety, irritability, weakness, tremor, depression
CV: Chest pain, pulse changes, palpitations, tachycardia
GI: Nausea, vomiting, diarrhea, heartburn, abdominal pain, constipation, anorexia, taste alteration
HEMA: ***Leukopenia, granulocytopenia*** (rare)
MISC: Joint pain, congestion, dermatitis, sweating

Contraindications: Hypersensitivity to benzodiazepines, pregnancy **X,** lactation

Q

Precautions: Hepatic disease, renal disease, suicidal individuals, drug abuse, elderly, psychosis, child <18 yr, lactation, depression, pulmonary insufficiency

Pharmacokinetics

Absorption	Well absorbed
Distribution	Crosses placenta, >95% bound to plasma proteins
Metabolism	Liver—extensively, to active metabolite
Excretion	Kidneys
Half-life	39 hr, active metabolite 70-75 hr

Pharmacodynamics

Onset	15-45 min
Peak	2 hr
Duration	8 hr

Interactions

Individual drugs

Alcohol: ↑ CNS depression
Cimetidine: ↑ action
Fluoxetine: ↑ action
Levodopa: ↓ action of levodopa
Propoxyphene: ↑ action
Rifampin: ↓ action of quazepam
Valproic acid: ↑ action

Drug classifications

Analgesics, opioid: ↑ CNS depression
Antidepressants: ↑ CNS depression
Antihistamines: ↑ CNS depression
Barbiturates: ↓ effect of quazepam
Oral contraceptives: ↑ effect of quazepam

Lab test interferences

↑ AST (SGOT)/ALT (SGPT), ↑ serum bilirubin
False ↑ 17-OHCS
↓ RAIU

NURSING CONSIDERATIONS

Assessment

- Assess patient's mental status: mood, sensorium, anxiety, affect, sleeping pattern, drowsiness, dizziness, especially elderly; physical dependency, withdrawal symptoms: anxiety, panic attacks, agitation, convulsions, headache, nausea, vomiting, muscle pain, weakness; suicidal tendencies; for indications of increasing tolerance and abuse
- Monitor B/P (lying, standing), pulse; if systolic B/P drops 20 mm Hg, hold drug, notify prescriber
- Monitor blood studies: CBC during long-term therapy; blood dycrasias have occurred rarely; decreased hematocrit, neutropenia may occur
- Monitor hepatic studies: AST (SGOT), ALT (SGPT), bilirubin, creatinine LDH, alk phosphatase
- Monitor I&O; indicate renal dysfunction

Nursing diagnoses

- ✓ Anxiety (uses)
- ✓ Depression (uses)
- ✓ Injury, risk for (adverse reactions)
- ✓ Knowledge deficit (teaching)

Implementation

- Give with food or milk for GI symptoms; tab may be crushed and mixed with foods or fluids if patient is unable to swallow medication whole
- Give sugarless gum, hard candy, frequent sips of water for dry mouth

Patient/family education

- Inform patient that drug may be taken with food or fluids and that tab may be crushed or swallowed whole

• Caution patient not to use for everyday stress or longer than 3 mo unless directed by prescriber; not to take more than prescribed amount; may be habit-forming; not to double doses or skip doses
• Advise patient to avoid OTC preparations unless approved by health care provider; alcohol and CNS depressants will increase CNS depression
• Caution patient to avoid driving, activities that require alertness because drowsiness may occur; to avoid alcohol ingestion or other psychotropic medications; to rise slowly or fainting may occur, especially G elderly; that drowsiness may worsen at beginning of treatment
• Advise patient not to discontinue medication abruptly after long-term use; withdrawal symptoms include vomiting, cramping, tremors, seizures

Evaluation

Positive therapeutic outcome
• Decreased anxiety, restlessness, sleeplessness (short-term treatment only)

Treatment of overdose: Lavage, VS, supportive care

quinapril (℞)

(kwin′a-pril)

Accupril

Func. class.: Antihypertensive

Chem. class.: Angiotensin-converting enzyme (ACE) inhibitor

Pregnancy category D

Action: Selectively suppresses renin-angiotensin-aldosterone system; inhibits ACE, prevents conversion of angiotensin I to angiotensin II; results in dilation of arterial, venous vessels

Therapeutic Outcome: Decreased B/P in hypertension

Uses: Hypertension, alone or in combination with thiazide diuretics

Dosage and routes

Hypertension

Adult: PO 10 mg qd initially, then 20-80 mg/day divided bid or qd

Congestive heart failure

Adult: PO 2.5 mg initially, then 5-40 mg/day maintenance dose given qd or in 2 divided doses

Available forms: Tabs 5, 10, 20, 40 mg

Adverse effects

CNS: Headache, dizziness, fatigue, somnolence, depression, malaise, nervousness, vertigo
CV: Hypotension, postural hypotension, syncope, palpitations, angina pectoris, MI, tachycardia, vasodilation
GI: Nausea, constipation, vomiting, gastritis, GI hemorrhage, dry mouth
GU: Increased BUN, creatinine, decreased libido, impotence, urinary tract infection
HEMA: ***Thrombocytopenia, agranulocytosis***
INTEG: ***Angioedema,*** rash, sweating, photosensitivity, pruritus
META: Hyperkalemia
MISC: Back pain, amblyopia, pharyngitis
MS: Arthralgia, arthritis, myalgia
RESP: Cough, bronchitis

Q

Contraindications: Hypersensitivity to ACE inhibitors, P pregnancy **D,** children

Precautions: Impaired renal and liver function, dialysis patients, hypovolemia, blood dyscrasias, COPD, asthma, G elderly, lactation

Pharmacokinetics	
Absorption	Well absorbed
Distribution	Unknown, crosses placenta
Metabolism	Unknown
Excretion	Unknown
Half-life	2 hr

Pharmacodynamics	
Onset	½-1 hr
Peak	2-6 hr
Duration	12-24 hr

Interactions

Individual drugs

Alcohol: ↑ hypotension (large amounts)
Allopurinol: ↑ hypersensitivity
Hydralazine: ↑ toxicity
Indomethacin: ↓ antihypertensive effect
Lithium: ↑ serum levels
Prazosin: ↑ toxicity

Drug classifications

Adrenergic blockers: ↑ hypotension
Antacids: ↓ absorption
Antihypertensives: ↑ hypotension
Diuretics: ↑ hypotension
Diuretics, potassium-sparing: ↑ toxicity
Ganglionic blockers: ↑ hypotension
Potassium supplements: ↑ toxicity
Sympathomimetics: ↑ toxicity

Lab test interferences

False positive: Urine acetone

NURSING CONSIDERATIONS

Assessment

- Monitor blood studies: neutrophils, decreased platelets
- Monitor B/P, check for orthostatic hypotension, syncope; if changes occur dosage change may be required
- Monitor renal studies: protein, BUN, creatinine; watch for increased levels that may indicate nephrotic syndrome and renal failure; monitor renal symptoms: polyuria, oliguria, frequency, dysuria
- Establish baselines in renal, liver function tests before therapy begins
- Check potassium levels throughout treatment, although hyperkalemia rarely occurs
- Check for edema in feet, legs daily
- Assess for allergic reactions: rash, fever, pruritus, urticaria; drug should be discontinued if antihistamines fail to help

Nursing diagnoses

✓ Cardiac output, decreased (uses)
✓ Injury, risk for physical (adverse reactions)
✓ Knowledge deficit (teaching)
✓ Noncompliance (teaching)

Implementation

- Store in airtight container at 86° F (30° C) or less
- Severe hypotension may occur after 1st dose of this medication; may be prevented by reducing or discontinuing diuretic therapy 3 days before beginning quinapril therapy

Patient/family education

- Advise patient not to discontinue drug abruptly; advise patient to tell all persons associated with care

• Teach patient not to use OTC products (cough, cold, allergy) unless directed by physician; serious side effects can occur
• Inform patient that xanthines such as coffee, tea, chocolate, cola can prevent action of drug
• Caution patient on the importance of complying with dosage schedule, even if feeling better; to continue with medical regimen to decrease B/P: exercise, cessation of smoking, decreasing stress, diet modifications
• Emphasize the need to rise slowly to sitting or standing position to minimize orthostatic hypotension; not to exercise in hot weather or increased hypotension can occur
• Teach patient to notify prescriber of mouth sores, sore throat, fever, swelling of hands or feet, irregular heartbeat, chest pain, coughing, shortness of breath
• Caution patient to report excessive perspiration, dehydration, vomiting, diarrhea; may lead to fall in B/P
• Caution patient that drug may cause dizziness, fainting, lightheadedness; may occur during 1st few days of therapy; to avoid activities that may be hazardous
• Teach patient how to take B/P, and normal readings for age group

Evaluation

Positive therapeutic outcome
• Decreased B/P in hypertension

Treatment of overdose: 0.9% NaCl **IV** inf, hemodialysis

quinidine gluconate/ quinidine polygalacturonase/ quinidine sulfate ⚷ (℞)

(kwin'i-deen)

Apo-Quinidine ✤, Cin-Quin, Duraquin, Novoquinidin ✤, Quinaglute, Quinalan, quinidine gluconate; Cardioquin; Quinidex Extentabs, quinidine sulfate, Quinora

Func. class.: Antidysrhythmic (Class IA)

Chem. class.: Quinine dextro isomer

Pregnancy category C

Action: Prolongs action, potential duration, and effective refractory period, thus decreasing myocardial excitability; anticholinergic properties

➔ **Therapeutic Outcome:** Treatment of dysrhythmias

Uses: PVCs, atrial fibrillation, PAT, ventricular tachycardia, atrial dysrhythmias

Investigational uses: Malaria/**IV** quinidine gluconate

Dosage and routes

Quinidine sulfate

Atrial fibrillation/flutter

Adult: PO 200 mg q2-3h × 5-8 doses; may increase qd until sinus rhythm is restored; max 4 g/day given only after digitalization

Paroxysmal supraventricular tachycardia

Adult: PO 400-600 mg q2-3h, then 200-300 mg q6-8h or 300-600 mg q8-12h (sus rel)

Q

Premature atrial/ventricular contraction
Adult: PO 200-300 mg q6-8h or 300-600 mg (sus rel) q8-12h, not to exceed 4 g/day

P ***Child:*** PO 6mg/kg or 180 mg/m^2 5/day

Quinidine gluconate
Adult: PO 324-660 mg q6-12h (sus rel); IM 600 mg, then 400 mg q2h; **IV** give 16 mg/min

Quinidine polygalacteronate
Adult: PO 275-825 mg q3-4h × 4 doses, then increase by 137.5-275 mg; repeat up to 4 × until dysrhythmia decreases

P ***Child:*** PO 8.25 mg/kg (247.5 mg/m^2) 5/day

Available forms: (Gluconate) tabs sus rel 324, 330 mg; inj gluconate 80 mg/ml; (sulfate) tabs 200, 300 mg; tabs sus rel 300 mg; (polygalacturonase) tab 275 mg

Adverse effects
CNS: *Headache, dizziness,* involuntary movement, confusion, psychosis, restlessness, irritability, syncope, excitement
CV: *Hypotension, bradycardia, PVCs,* ***heart block, cardiovascular collapse, arrest, Torsades de pointes***
EENT: Cinchonism: tinnitus, blurred vision, hearing loss, mydriasis, disturbed color vision
GI: Nausea, vomiting, anorexia, *diarrhea,* ***hepatotoxicity***
HEMA: ***Thrombocytopenia,*** hemolytic anemia, agranulocytosis, hypoprothrombinemia
INTEG: Rash, urticaria, angioedema, swelling, photosensitivity
RESP: Dyspnea, ***respiratory depression***

Contraindications: Hypersensitivity, blood dyscrasias, severe heart block, myasthenia gravis

Precautions: Pregnancy **C**, P lactation, children, renal disease, K imbalance, liver disease, CHF, respiratory depression

Interactions
Individual drugs
Amiodarone: ↑ toxicity
Cimetidine: ↑ effects of quinidine
Coumadin: ↑ levels of coumadin
Digoxin: ↑ blood levels, ↑ toxicity
Nifedipine: ↓ effects of quinidine

Pharmacokinetics

Absorption	Well absorbed (PO, IM), slowly absorbed (sus-rel)
Distribution	Widely distributed, crosses placenta
Metabolism	Liver
Excretion	Kidney unchanged, breast milk
Half-life	6-8 hr

Pharmacodynamics

	PO (SULFATE)	PO-SR	PO (GLUCONATE)	PO (POLYGALACTERONASE)	IM	IV
Onset	½ hr	Unknown	Unknown	Unknown	½ hr	5 min
Peak	1-1½ hr	4 hr	4 hr	6 hr	½-1½ hr	Unknown
Duration	6-8 hr	8-12 hr	6-8 hr	8-12 hr	6-8 hr	6-8 hr

Phenytoin: ↓ effects of quinidine
Propranolol: ↑ effects of quinidine
Rifampin: ↓ effects of quinidine
Verapamil: ↑ effects of quinidine

Drug classifications

Anticoagulants (oral): ↑ levels of anticoagulant
Anticholinergics: ↑ vagolytic effects
Antacids: ↑ effects of quinidine
Barbiturates: ↓ effects of quinidine
Thiazide diuretics: ↑ effects of quinidine
Antidysrhythmics: ↑ cardiac depression
Phenothiazines: ↑ cardiac depression

Lab test interferences

↑ CPK

NURSING CONSIDERATIONS

Assessment

- Monitor ECG continuously to determine drug effectiveness, measure PR, QRS, QT intervals, check for PVCs, other dysrhythmias; monitor B/P continuously for hypotension, hypertension; for rebound hypertension after 1-2 hr; check for dehydration or hypovolemia
- Monitor I&O ratio; electrolytes: [K (potassium), Na (sodium), Cl (Chloride)]; check weight daily; check for signs of CHG or pulmonary toxicity: dyspnea, fatigue, cough, fever, chest pain; if these occur, drug should be discontinued
- Monitor liver function studies: AST (SGOT), ALT (SGPT), bilirubin, alk phosphatase
- Assess for CNS symptoms: confusion, psychosis, numbness, depression, involuntary movements; if these occur, drug should be discontinued
- Monitor cardiac rate, respiration: rate, rhythm, character, chest pain; watch for ventricular tachycardia, supraventricular tachycardia, or fibrillation that indicates toxicity

Nursing diagnoses

✓ Cardiac output, decreased (uses)
✓ Impaired gas exchange (adverse reactions)
✓ Knowledge deficit (teaching)

Implementation

PO route

- Give on an empty stomach with a full glass of water
- May be given with meals if GI irritation occurs, absorption will be decreased
- Tab may be crushed and mixed with fluid or foods for patients with swallowing difficulties; do not break, chew or crush sus rel tab

IV route

- Give by intermittent inf after diluting 800 mg/50 ml D_5W (gluconate) (16 mg/ml) give at 1 ml/min or less using an inf pump for correct dose
- Do not use colored sol or sol with precipitate
- Diluted quinidine is stable for 24 hr at room temp

Y-site compatibilities:
Diazepam, milrinone

Y-site incompatibility:
Furosemide

Additive compatibilities:
Bretylium, cimetidine, milrinone, ranitidine, verapamil

Additive incompatibility:
Amiodarone

Q

Patient/family education

- Instruct patient to report adverse effects immediately to prescriber
- Caution patient that dark glasses may be needed for photophobia; to use sunscreen, protective clothing, or stay out of sun to prevent burns
- Instruct patient to complete follow-up appointments with health care provider including pulmonary function studies, chest x-ray, ophth and otoscopic examinations

Treatment of overdose: O_2, artificial ventilation, ECG, administer dopamine for circulatory depression, administer diazepam or thiopental for convulsions, isoproterenol

ramipril (℞)

(ra-mi′pril)

Altace

Func. class.: Antihypertensive

Chem. class.: Angiotensin-converting enzyme (ACE) inhibitor

Pregnancy category D

Action: Selectively suppresses renin-angiotensin-aldosterone system; inhibits ACE; prevents conversion of angiotensin I to angiotensin II; results in dilation of arterial, venous vessels

Therapeutic Outcome: Decreased B/P in hypertension

Uses: Hypertension, alone or in combination with thiazide diuretics

Dosage and routes

Adult: PO 2.5 mg qd initially, then 2.5-20 mg/day divided bid or qd; renal impairment: 1.25 mg qd with CrCl <40 ml/min/1.73 m^2, increase as needed to max or 5 mg/day

Available forms: Caps 1.25, 2.5, 5, 10 mg

Adverse effects

CNS: ***Headache, dizziness,*** anxiety, insomnia, paresthesia, fatigue, depression, malaise, vertigo, ***convulsions,*** hearing loss

CV: ***Hypotension,*** chest pain, palpitations, angina, syncope, dysrhythmia

GI: Nausea, constipation, vomiting, dyspepsia, dysphagia, anorexia, diarrhea, abdominal pain

GU: ***Proteinuria,*** increased BUN, creatinine, impotence

HEMA: Decreased Hct, Hgb, ***eosinophilia, leukopenia***

INTEG: ***Angioedema,*** rash, sweating, photosensitivity, pruritus

META: Hyperkalemia

MS: Arthralgia, arthritis, myalgia

RESP: Cough, dyspnea

Contraindications: Hypersensitivity to ACE inhibitors, pregnancy **D,** lactation, P children

Precautions: Impaired renal and liver function, dialysis patients, hypovolemia, blood dyscrasias, COPD, asthma, G elderly

Pharmacokinetics	
Absorption	Well absorbed
Distribution	Not known, crosses placenta
Metabolism	Liver, extensively
Excretion	Urine
Half-life	Ramipril (5 hr), ramiprilat (24 hr)

Pharmacodynamics

Onset	½-1 hr
Peak	6-8 hr
Duration	24-72 hr

Interactions

Individual drugs

Alcohol: ↑ hypotension (large amounts)
Allopurinol: ↑ hypersensitivity
Digoxin: ↑ serum levels
Hydralazine: ↑ toxicity
Indomethacin: ↓ antihypertensive effect
Lithium: ↑ serum levels
Prazosin: ↑ toxicity

Drug classifications

Adrenergic blockers: ↑ hypotension
Antacids: ↓ absorption
Antihypertensives: ↑ hypotension
Diuretics: ↑ hypotension
Diuretics, potassium sparing: ↑ toxicity
Ganglionic blockers: ↑ hypotension
Potassium supplements: ↑ toxicity
Sympathomimetics: ↑ toxicity

Lab test interferences

False positive: Urine acetone

NURSING CONSIDERATIONS

Assessment

- Monitor blood studies: neutrophils, decreased platelets
- Monitor B/P, check for orthostatic hypotension, syncope; if changes occur, dosage may need to be changed
- Monitor renal studies: protein, BUN, creatinine; watch for increased levels that may indicate nephrotic syndrome and renal failure; monitor renal symptoms: polyuria, oliguria, frequency, dysuria
- Establish baselines in renal, liver function tests before therapy begins
- Check potassium levels throughout treatment, although hyperkalemia rarely occurs
- Check for edema in feet, legs daily
- Assess for allergic reactions: rash, fever, pruritus, urticaria; drug should be discontinued if antihistamines fail to help

Nursing diagnoses

- ✓ Cardiac output, decreased (uses)
- ✓ Injury, risk for (side effects)
- ✓ Knowledge deficit (teaching)
- ✓ Noncompliance (teaching)

Implementation

- Store in air-tight container at 86° F (30° C) or less
- Severe hypotension may occur after 1st dose of this medication; decreased hypotension may be prevented by reducing or discontinuing diuretic therapy 3 days before beginning benazepril therapy
- Give **IV** inf of 0.9% NaCl (as ordered) to expand fluid volume if severe hypotension occurs

Patient/family education

- Caution patient not to discontinue drug abruptly; advise patient to tell all persons associated with care
- Teach patient not to use OTC products (cough, cold, allergy) unless directed by physician; serious side effects can occur—xanthines such as coffee, tea, chocolate, cola can prevent action of drug
- Instruct patient on the importance of complying with dosage schedule, even if feeling better; to continue with medical regimen to decrease B/P: exercise, cessation of smoking,

R

decreasing stress, diet modifications
- Emphasize the need to rise slowly to sitting or standing position to minimize orthostatic hypotension; not to exercise in hot weather because increased hypotension can occur
- Teach patient to notify prescriber of mouth sores, sore throat, fever, swelling of hands or feet, irregular heartbeat, chest pain, coughing, shortness of breath
- Caution patient to report excessive perspiration, dehydration, vomiting, diarrhea; may lead to fall in B/P
- Caution patient that drug may cause dizziness, fainting, lightheadedness; may occur during 1st few days of therapy; to avoid activities that may be hazardous
- Teach patient how to take B/P, and normal readings for age group

Evaluation

Positive therapeutic outcome
- Decreased B/P in hypertension

Treatment of overdose: 0.9% NaCl **IV** inf, hemodialysis

ranitidine (℞)

(ra-nit′i-deen)

Apo-Ranitidine ♣, Tritec, Zantac, Zantac-C ♣

Func. class.: H_2 histamine receptor antagonist

Pregnancy category B

Action: Inhibits histamine at H_2 receptor site in the gastric parietal cells, which inhibits gastric acid secretion

➔ **Therapeutic Outcome:** Healing of duodenal ulcers or gastric ulcers; prevention of duodenal ulcers; decreases symptoms of GERD or Zollinger-Ellison syndrome

Uses: Short-term treatment of duodenal and gastric ulcers and maintenance; management of gastroesophageal reflux disease (GERD), Zollinger-Ellison syndrome, active duodenal ulcers with *Helicobacter pylori* in combination with clarithromycin

Investigational uses: Prevention of aspiration pneumonitis, stress ulcers, upper GI bleeding

Dosage and routes

Adult: PO 150 mg bid, 300 mg hs; IM 50 mg q6-8h; **IV** bol 50 mg diluted to 20 ml over 5 min q6-8h; **IV** int inf 50 mg/100 ml D_5 over 15-20 min, q6-8h

Available forms: Tabs 150, 300 mg; inj 0.5, 25 mg/ml; caps ♣ 150, 300 mg; syr 15 mg/ml

Adverse effects

CNS: Headache, sleeplessness, dizziness, confusion, agitation, depression, hallucination
CV: Tachycardia, bradycardia, PVCs
EENT: Blurred vision, increased ocular pressure
GI: Constipation, abdominal pain, diarrhea, nausea, vomiting, ***hepatotoxicity***
GU: Impotence, gynecomastia
INTEG: Urticaria, rash, fever

Contraindications: Hypersensitivity

Precautions: Pregnancy **B**, lactation, P child <12 yr, hepatic disease, renal disease

Pharmacokinetics	
Absorption	Well absorbed (PO, IM), completely absorbed (IV)
Distribution	Widely distributed, crosses placenta
Metabolism	Liver (30%)
Excretion	Kidneys unchanged (70%)
Half-life	2-3 hr, ↑ renal disease

Pharmacodynamics	PO	IV/IM
Onset	Unknown	Unknown
Peak	2-3 hr	15 min
Duration	8-12 hr	8-12 hr

Interactions

Individual drugs

Ketoconazole: ↓ absorption of ranitidine

Drug classifications

Antacids: ↓ absorption of ranitidine

Smoking

↓ effectiveness

Lab test interferences

↑ Alk phosphatase, ↑ AST (SGOT), ↑ creatinine

False positive: Gastric bleeding test

NURSING CONSIDERATIONS

Assessment

- Assess patient with ulcers or suspected ulcers: epigastric or abdominal pain, hematemesis, occult blood in stools, blood in gastric aspirate prior to and throughout treatment, monitor gastric pH (5 should be maintained)
- Monitor I&O ratio, BUN, creatinine, CBC with differential monthly

Nursing diagnoses

✓ Pain (uses)
✓ Knowledge deficit (teaching)

Implementation

PO route

- May be given with or without meals
- Give antacids 1 hr before or 1 hr after this drug

IV **IV route**

Direct **IV**

- Give by direct **IV** after diluting 50 mg/20 ml of 0.9% D_5W, NaCl given over 5 min or more

Intermittent inf

- Give by intermittent inf over 15 min after diluting 50 mg/100 ml D_5W, 0.9% NaCl

Continuous inf

- Give by continuous inf for a concentration 150 mg/250 ml, give 6.25 mg/hr
- Give Zollinger-Ellison patients up to a conc of 2.5 mg/ml at 1 mg/kg/hr initially

Syringe compatibilities: Atropine, cyclizine, dexamethasone, dimenhydrinate, diphenhydramine, fentanyl, glycopyrrolate, hydromorphone, meperidine, metoclopramide, morphine, nalbuphine, oxymorphone, pentazocine, perphenazine, prochlorperazine, promethazine, scopolamine

Syringe incompatibilities: Hydroxyzine, methotrimeprazine, midazolam, pentobarbital, phenobarbital

Y-site compatibilities: Acyclovir, aminophylline, atracurium, bretylium, dobutamine, dopamine, enalaprilat, esmolol, filgrastim, fluconazole, fludarabine, foscarnet, heparin, labetalol, meperidine, morphine, nitroglycerin, ondansetron, pancuronium, procainamide, sargramostim, vecuronium, zidovudine

R

Additive compatibilities: Amikacin, aminophylline, chloramphenicol, doxycycline, furosemide, gentamicin, heparin, lidocaine, penicillin G sodium, potassium chloride, ticarcillin, tobramycin, vancomycin

Additive incompatibilities: Amphotericin B, clindamycin

Patient/family education

- Caution patient that gynecomastia, impotence may occur and are reversible after treatment is discontinued
- Advise patient to avoid driving, other hazardous activities until stabilized on this medication; drowsiness or dizziness may occur
- Caution patient to avoid black pepper, caffeine, alcohol, harsh spices, extremes in temp of food; tell patient to avoid OTC preparations: aspirin, cough, cold preparations because condition may worsen
- Inform patient that smoking decreases the effectiveness of the drug; that smoking cessation should be considered
- Instruct patient that drug must be continued for prescribed time to be effectiveand taken exactly as prescribed; doses should not be doubled; a missed dose should be taken when remembered up to 1 hr before next dose
- Advise patient to report bruising, fatigue, malaise; blood dyscrasias may occur
- Inform patient to report diarrhea, black tarry stools, sore throat, rash, dizziness, confusion, rash or delirium to prescriber immediately

Evaluation

Positive therapeutic outcome

- Decreased pain in abdomen
- Healing of ulcers
- Absence of gastroesophageal reflux

remifentanil 

(re-me-fin′ta-nill)

Ultiva

Func. class.: Narcotic agonist analgesic

Chem. class.: Mu-opioid agonist

Pregnancy category C

Action: Inhibits ascending pain pathways in limbic system, thalamus, midbrain, hypothalamus

Therapeutic Outcome: Maintenance of anesthesia

Uses: In combination with other drugs in general anesthesia, as a primary anesthetic in general surgery

Dosage and routes

Adult: Induction **IV** 0.5-1 μg/kg/min with a hypnotic or volative agent

Available forms: Powder for inj—lyophilized

Adverse effects

CNS: Drowsiness, *dizziness,* confusion, *headache,* sedation, euphoria, delirium, agitation, anxiety

CV: Palpitations, *bradycardia,* change in B/P; facial flushing, syncope, ***asystole***

EENT: Tinnitus, blurred vision, miosis, diplopia

GI: Nausea, vomiting, anorexia, constipation, cramps, dry mouth

GU: Urinary retention, dysuria

INTEG: Rash, urticaria, bruising, flushing, diaphoresis, pruritus
MS: Rigidity
RESP: Respiratory depression, apnea

P **Contraindications:** Child <12 yr, hypersensitivity

Precautions: Pregnancy **C**, lactation, increased intracranial pressure, acute MI, severe heart disease; renal disease, hepatic disease, asthma, respiratory conditions, convulsive G disorders, elderly

Pharmacokinetics

Absorption	Complete
Distribution	Unknown
Metabolism	Unknown
Excretion	Unknown
Half-life	Unknown

Pharmacodynamics

Onset	Immediate
Peak	Unknown
Duration	Unknown

Interactions

Individual drugs

Alcohol: ↑ respiratory depression, hypotension, profound sedation

Drug classifications

Antihistamines: ↑ respiratory depression, hypotension, profound sedation
Sedative/hypnotics: ↑ respiratory depression, hypotension, profound sedative
Phenothiazine: ↑ respiratory depression, hypotension, profound sedation

NURSING CONSIDERATIONS

Assessment

- Monitor I&O ratio, check for decreasing output; may indicate urinary retention, G especially in elderly
- Assess CNS changes: dizziness, drowsiness, hallucinations, euphoria, LOC pupil reaction
- Assess allergic reactions: rash, urticaria
- Assess respiratory dysfunction: respiratory depression, character, rate, rhythm; notify prescriber if respirations are <12/min; CV status, bradycardia, syncope
- Use pain scoring to determine pain perception

Nursing diagnoses

✓ Knowledge deficit (teaching)

Implementation

- Give by direct **IV** over 1½-3 min; use tuberculin syringe
- Store in light-resistant area at room temperature

Patient/family education

- Advise to call for assistance when ambulating or smoking; drowsiness, dizziness may occur
- Advise patient to make position changes slowly to prevent orthostatic hypotension

Evaluation

Positive therapeutic outcome

- Maintenance of anesthesia

reserpine (℞)

(re-ser′peen)
Novoreserpine ✦, Reserfia ✦, reserpine
Func. class.: Antihypertensive
Chem. class.: Antiadrenergic agent (peripherally acting)

Pregnancy category D

Action: Inhibits norepinephrine release, depleting norepi-

R

nephrine stores in adrenergic nerve endings

Therapeutic Outcome: Decreased B/P

Uses: Hypertension

Dosage and routes

Hypertension

Adult: PO 0.25-0.5 mg qd × 1-2 wk, then 0.1-0.25 mg qd for maintenance

Psychiatric disorders

Adult: PO 0.5 mg qd, may range from 0.1-1 mg

Available forms: Tabs 0.1, 0.25 mg

Adverse effects

CNS: *Drowsiness, fatigue, lethargy, dizziness,* depression, anxiety, headache, increased dreaming, nightmares, convulsions, parkinsonism, EPS (high doses)

CV: *Bradycardia,* chest pain, dysrhythmias, prolonged bleeding time, ***thrombocytopenia,*** purpura

EENT: Lacrimation, miosis, blurred vision, ptosis, dry mouth, epistaxis

GI: Nausea, vomiting, cramps, peptic ulcer, dry mouth, increased appetite, anorexia

GU: Impotence, dysuria, nocturia, Na and H_2O retention, edema, breast engorgement, galactorrhea, gynecomastia

INTEG: Rash, purpura, alopecia, flushing, warm feeling, pruritus, ecchymosis

RESP: ***Bronchospasm,*** dyspnea, cough, rales

Contraindications: Hypersensitivity, depression, suicidal patients, active peptic ulcer disease, ulcerative colitis, pregnancy **D,** Parkinson's disease

Precautions: Lactation, seizure disorders, renal disease, P children

Pharmacokinetics	
Absorption	40%-50%
Distribution	Widely distributed, crosses placenta
Metabolism	Liver
Excretion	Feces 50% unabsorbed drug, kidneys small amounts
Half-life	11 days

Pharmacodynamics	
Onset	Unknown
Peak	4 hr
Duration	1-6 wk

Interactions

Individual drugs

Alcohol: ↑ CNS depression

Drug classifications

Amphetamines: ↓ hypotensive effects

Anesthetics: ↑ CNS depression

Antidepressants, tricyclic: ↓ hypotensive effects

β-Blockers: ↑ bradycardia

Cardiac glycosides: ↑ bradycardia

Diuretics: ↑ hypotensive effects

Hypnotics: ↑ CNS depression

MAOIs: avoid use

Narcotics: ↑ CNS depression

Nitrates: ↑ hypotensive effects

Sedatives: ↑ CNS depression

Lab test interferences

↑ VMA excretion, ↑ 5-HIAA excretion, ↑ prolactin

Interference: 17-OHCS, 17-KS

NURSING CONSIDERATIONS

Assessment

• Monitor B/P, orthostatic hypotension, syncope; check for edema in feet, legs daily; check I&O; monitor for weight daily; notify prescriber of changes

• Assess for allergic reactions: rash, fever, pruritus, urticaria; drug should be discontinued if antihistamines fail to help
• Assess for orthostatic hypotension, tell patient to rise slowly from sitting or lying position

Nursing diagnoses

✓ Cardiac output, decreased (uses)
✓ Injury, risk for (adverse reactions)
✓ Knowledge deficit (teaching)
✓ Noncompliance (teaching)

Implementation

• Store in tight container at 86° F (30° C) or less
• May be used in combination with other antihypertensives
• May be given with food to prevent GI symptoms

Patient/family education

• Caution patient not to discontinue drug abruptly and about the importance of complying with dosage schedule, even if feeling better; if dose is missed take as soon as remembered; take dose at same time each day
• Teach patient not to use OTC products (cough, cold, allergy) unless directed by prescriber and to avoid large amounts of caffeine
• Emphasize the need to rise slowly to sitting or standing position to minimize orthostatic hypotension
• Teach patient to notify prescriber of swelling of hands or feet, irregular heartbeat, chest pain
• Caution patient to report excessive perspiration, dehydration, vomiting, diarrhea; may lead to fall in B/P
• Caution patient that drug may cause dizziness, fainting, lightheadedness; may occur during 1st few days of therapy; to avoid hazardous activities
• Teach patient how to take B/P, and normal readings for age group; to take B/P q7 days

Evaluation

Positive therapeutic outcome

• Decreased B/P in hypertension, decrease in psychiatric symptoms

Treatment of overdose: Administer volume expanders or vasopressors; discontinue drug; place patient in supine position

respiratory syncytial virus immune globulin (RSV-IGIV) (℞)

RespiGam

Func. class.: Immune serums

Chem. class.: Immuno globulin G (IgG)

Pregnancy category C

Action: High titer of neutralizing antibody against RSV (respiratory syncytial virus)

➔ **Therapeutic Outcome:** Resolution of infection

Uses: Prevention of serious lower respiratory tract infection caused by RSV in children P <2 yr with bronchopulmonary dysplasia, or premature birth

Dosage and routes

P ***Child <2 yr:*** **IV** INF 1.5 ml/kg/hr × 15 min, then 3 ml/kg/hr 15-30 min; then 6 ml/kg/hr from 30 min to end of inf

R

Available forms: Inj 2500 mg RSV immunoglobulin

Adverse effects

CNS: Fever
CV: Hypertension, tachycardia, fluid overload
GI: Diarrhea, gastroenteritis, vomiting
OTHER: Rash, overdose effect, inj-site inflammation
RESP: Respiratory distress, hypoxia, tachypnea, rales, wheezing

Contraindications: Hypersensitivity to this drug or other human immunoglobulin preparations; IgA deficiency

Precautions: Pregnancy **C**, fluid overload

Pharmacokinetics	
Absorption	Unknown
Distribution	Unknown
Metabolism	Unknown
Excretion	Unknown
Half-life	Unknown

Pharmacodynamics

Unknown

Interactions

Individual drugs

DPT: ↓ immune response
Haemophilus: ↓ immune response
Influenzae B: ↓ immune response
MMR: ↓ immune response

NURSING CONSIDERATIONS

Assessment

• Monitor VS for increase in heart rate, respiratory rate, retractions, rales; a loop diuretic may be needed for fluid overload
• Assess for aseptic meningitis syndrome (AMS): severe headache, drowsiness, photophobia, fever, painful eye movements, nausea, vomiting, muscle rigidity; discontinue RSV-IGIV if these occur

Nursing diagnoses

✓ Infection, risk for (uses)
✓ Knowledge deficit (teaching)

Implementation

• Give by infusion: do not admix; begin infusion within 6 hr and complete within 12 hr after the single-use vial is entered
• Store refrigerated, do not freeze, do not shake vial; discard after use

Patient/family education

• Teach patient the reason for **IV** infusion and expected results

Rh_o (d) immune globulin, human (℞)

HypoRho-D, MICRhoGAM, Mini-Gamulin RH, Hypo Rho-D Mini-Dose, Gamulin Rh, Rhesonatin, RhoGAM

Func. class.: IgG, immunizing agent

Pregnancy category C

Action: Suppresses immune response of nonsensitized Rh_o (D or D^u)-negative patients who are exposed to Rh_o (D or D^u)-positive blood

Therapeutic Outcome: Absence of Rh factor and transfusion error

Uses: Prevention of isoimmunization in Rh-negative women exposed to Rh-positive blood given after abortions, miscarriages, amniocentesis

Dosage and routes

After delivery

Adult: IM 1 vial of fetal packed RBCs <15 ml, or 2 vials of fetal packed RBCs >15 ml;

given within 72 hr of delivery or miscarriage

Before delivery

Adult: IM 1 vial (standard dose) at 26-28 wk, 1 vial (standard dose) 72 hr after delivery

Pregnancy termination <13 wk

Adult: IM 1 vial (micro dose) within 72 hr

Pregnancy termination >13 wk

Adult: IM 1 vial (standard dose) within 72 hr

Fetal-maternal hemorrhage

Adult: IM packed RBCs volume of hemorrhage/15 = needed vials (standard dose)

Transfusion error

Adult: IM—give within 72 hr

Available forms: Inj single-dose vial (50 μg/vial-microdose, 300 μg/vial-standard)

Adverse effects

CNS: Lethargy

INTEG: Irritation at inj site, fever

MS: Myalgia

Contraindications: Previous immunization with this drug, Rh_o (O)-positive/D^u-positive patient

Precautions: Pregnancy **C**

Pharmacokinetics	
Absorption	Well absorbed
Distribution	Unknown
Metabolism	Unknown
Excretion	Unknown
Half-life	Unknown

Pharmacodynamics	
Onset	Rapid
Peak	Unknown
Duration	Unknown

Interactions

Drug classifications

Live virus vaccines: ↓ antibody response to vaccine

NURSING CONSIDERATIONS

Assessment

- Assess for allergies, reactions to immunizations; previous immunization with this drug
- Obtain type and cross-match of mother's blood and of neonate's cord blood; neonate must be Rh_o(D)-positive, mother must be Rh_o(D)-negative and (D^u)-negative, medication should be given if there is a doubt

Nursing diagnoses

✓ Knowledge deficit (teaching)

Implementation

- Give after sending newborn's cord blood to lab after delivery for cross, match, type
- Give IM in deltoid; aspirate to prevent **IV** administration
- Give only equal lot numbers of drug, cross match
- Give only MICrhoGAM for abortions or miscarriages <13 wk unless fetus or father is Rh-negative
- Store in refrigerator

Patient/family education

- Teach patient how drug works; that drug must be given after subsequent deliveries if subsequent babies are Rh-positive

Evaluation

Positive therapeutic outcome

- Prevention of Rh_o(D) sensitization in transfusion error
- Prevention of erythroblastosis fetalis in subsequent Rh_o(D)-positive neonates

ribavarin (℞)

(rye-ba-vye'rin)
Virazole
Func. class.: Synthetic antiviral
Chem. class.: Tricyclic amine
Pregnancy category X

Action: Prevents replication of DNA and RNA synthesis

→ **Therapeutic Outcome:** Resolution of severe lower respiratory tract infections

Uses: Severe lower respiratory P tract infections in infants and children

Investigational uses: Influenza A or B (early)

Dosage and routes

P ***Infant/young children:*** Inh 300 ml of 200 mg/ml sol by mist × 12-18 h/day

Available forms: Powder for reconstitution for aerosol: 6 g/vial

Adverse effects

CNS: Dizziness, faintness
CV: Hypotension, cardiac arrest
EENT: Eye irritation, conjunctivitis, blurred vision, photosensitivity
INTEG: Rash

Contraindications: Hyper- P sensitivity, lactation, child <1 yr, pregnancy **X**

Precautions: Epilepsy, hepatic disease, renal disease

Pharmacokinetics

Absorption	Inh (systemic)
Distribution	To respiratory tract
Metabolism	Liver
Excretion	Respiratory tract
Half-life	9½ hr

Pharmacodynamics

Onset	Unknown
Peak	Inh end
Duration	Unknown

Interactions

Individual drugs

Zidovudine: ↓ antiviral action, ↑ toxicity

Drug classification

Cardiac glycosides: ↑ toxicity

NURSING CONSIDERATIONS

Assessment

- Assess allergies before initiation of treatment, reaction of each medication; list allergies on chart in bright red letters
- Monitor respiratory status: rate, character, wheezing, tightness in chest
- Obtain C&S test results before starting treatment

Nursing diagnoses

- ✓ Infection, risk for (uses)
- ✓ Gas exchange, impaired (uses)
- ✓ Knowledge deficit (teaching)

Implementation

- Give by the viratek SPAG (SPAG-2), do not use other inh equipment
- May be given by an oxygen P hood for infants or a face mask may be attached to the SPAG-2
- Reconstitute 6 g sterile water for inj or inh, place sol in the Erlenmeyer flask and dilute further to 20 mg/ml

Patient/family education

- Teach patient and parents aspects of drug therapy

Evaluation

Positive therapeutic outcome
- Absence of RSV (respiratory syncytial virus)

riboflavin (vitamin B_2) (OTC)
(rye'boo-flay-vin)
Func. class.: Vitamin B_2, water soluble
Pregnancy category A

Action: Needed for respiratory reactions (catalyzes proteins) and for normal vision

Therapeutic Outcome: Prevention or treatment of riboflavin deficiency

Uses: Vit B_2 deficiency or polyneuritis; cheilosis adjunct with thiamine

Dosage and routes

P ***Adult and child >12 yr:*** PO 5-50 mg qd in divided doses

P ***Child <12 yr:*** PO 2-10 mg qd, then 0.6 mg/1000 calories ingested

Available forms: Tabs 10, 25, 50, 100 mg

Adverse effects

GU: Yellow discoloration of urine (large doses)

P **Contraindications:** Child <12 yr

Precautions: Pregnancy **A**

Pharmacokinetics

Absorption	Well absorbed (by active transport)
Distribution	60% protein bound, widely distributed, crosses placenta
Metabolism	Unknown
Excretion	Kidneys (unchanged), excess amounts
Half-life	1-1½ hr

Pharmacodynamics

Unknown

Interactions

Individual drugs

Alcohol: ↑ riboflavin need
Probenicid: ↑ riboflavin need
Tetracycline: ↓ action of tetracycline

Drug classifications

Antidepressants, tricyclic: ↑ riboflavin need
Phenothiazines: ↑ riboflavin need

Lab test interferences

False ↑ Urinary catecholamines
False ↑ urobilinogen

NURSING CONSIDERATIONS

Assessment

- Assess patient's nutritional status: liver, eggs, dairy products, yeast, whole grain, green vegetables
- Assess for vitamin B_2 deficiency: photophobia, cheilosis, stomatitis, ocular swelling

Nursing diagnoses

✓ Nutrition: less than body requirements (uses)
✓ Knowledge deficit (teaching)

Implementation

- Give with food for better absorption
- Store in tight, light-resistant container

Patient/family education

- Inform patient that urine may turn bright yellow
- Instruct patient about addition of needed foods that are rich in riboflavin

Evaluation

Positive therapeutic outcome

- Absence of headache, GI problems, cheilosis, skin lesions, depression, burning, itchy eyes, anemia

R

rifabutin (℞)

(riff'a-byoo-tin)

Mycobutin

Func. class.: Antimycobacterial

Chem. class.: Rifamycin S derivative

Pregnancy category B

Action: Inhibits DNA-dependent RNA polymerase in susceptible strains

➡ Therapeutic Outcome: Antimycobacterial death of *E. coli, B. subtilis,* and *M. avium*

Uses: Prevention of *M. avium* complex in patients with advanced HIV infection

Dosage and routes

Adult: PO 300 mg qd (may take as 150 mg bid)

Available forms: Cap 150 mg

Adverse effects

CNS: Headache, fatigue, anxiety, confusion, insomnia

GI: Nausea, vomiting, anorexia, diarrhea, heartburn, hepatitis

GU: Hematuria

HEMA: Hemolytic anemia, eosinophilia, thrombocytopenia, leukopenia

INTEG: Rash

MISC: Flulike syndrome, shortness of breath, chest pressure

MS: Asthenia, arthralgia, myalgia

Contraindications: Hypersensitivity, active TB

Precautions: Pregnancy **B,** lactation, hepatic disease, blood dyscrasias, children [P]

Pharmacokinetics

Absorption	Well absorbed
Distribution	Widely distributed
Metabolism	Liver
Excretion	Kidney
Half-life	45 hr

Pharmacodynamics

Onset	Unknown
Peak	2-3 hr

Interactions

Individual drugs

Alcohol: ↑ toxicity
Carbamazepine: ↑ toxicity
Cycloserine: ↑ toxicity
Ethionamide: ↑ toxicity
Rifampin: ↑ toxicity

Drug classifications

Antacids, aluminum: ↓ absorption

NURSING CONSIDERATIONS

Assessment

- Assess for active tuberculosis: chest x-ray, sputum culture, blood culture, biopsy of lymph nodes, obtain PPD test; drug should be given only for Mycobacterium avium complex (MAC) and never for TB
- Monitor CBC for neutropenia, thrombocytopenia, eosinophilia

Nursing diagnoses

- ✓ Infection, risk for (uses)
- ✓ Diarrhea (adverse reaction)
- ✓ Injury, risk for (adverse reaction)
- ✓ Knowledge deficit (teaching)
- ✓ Noncompliance (teaching)

Implementation

- Give with meals to decrease GI symptoms; better to take on empty stomach 1 hr ac or 2 hr pc; high fat food slows absorption
- Give antiemetic if vomiting occurs

Patient/family education

- Caution patient that compliance with dosage schedule and duration is necessary
- Instruct patient that scheduled appointments must be kept or relapse may occur
- Instruct patient to notify prescriber if hepatitis, neutropenia, or thrombocytopenia occurs: sore throat, fever, bleeding, bruising, yellow sclera, anorexia, nausea, vomiting, fatigue, weakness
- Advise patient that urine, feces, saliva, sputum, sweat, tears, may be colored red-orange; soft contact lens may become permanently stained
- Caution patients using oral contraceptives to use a nonhormonal method of birth control because rifabutin may decrease efficiency of oral contraceptives

Evaluation

Positive therapeutic outcome

- Decreased symptoms of *M. avium* in patients with HIV

rifampin (℞)

(rif'am-pin)

Rifadin, Rifampicin, Rimactane, Rofact ♣

Func. class.: Antitubercular

Chem. class.: Rifamycin B derivative

Pregnancy category C

Action: Inhibits DNA-dependent polymerase, decreases replication

➔ **Therapeutic Outcome:** Bactericidal against the following organisms: mycobacteria, *Staphylococcus aureus, Hemophilus influenzae, Neisseria meningitides, Legionella pneumophilia*

Uses: Pulmonary tuberculosis, meningococcal carriers (prevention)

Dosage and routes

Tuberculosis

Adult: PO/**IV** 600 mg/day as single dose 1 hr ac or 2 hr pc or 10 mg/kg/day

P ***Child >5 yr:*** PO/**IV** 10-20 mg/kg/day as single dose 1 hr ac or 2 hr pc, not to exceed 600 mg/day, with other antituberculars

Meningococcal carriers

Adult: PO/**IV** 600 mg bid × 2 days

P ***Child >5 yr:*** PO/**IV** 10 mg/kg bid × 2 days, not to exceed 600 mg/dose

P ***Infant 3 mo-1 yr:*** PO 5 mg/kg bid for 2 days

Available forms: Caps 150, 300 mg; inj 600 mg/vial

Adverse effects

CNS: Headache, fatigue, anxiety, drowsiness, confusion

EENT: Visual disturbances

GI: Nausea, vomiting, anorexia, diarrhea, ***pseudomembranous colitis,*** *heartburn,* sore mouth and tongue, pancreatitis

GU: ***Hematuria, acute renal failure, hemoglobinuria***

HEMA: ***Hemolytic anemia, eosinophilia, thrombocytopenia, leukopenia***

INTEG: Rash, pruritus, urticaria

MISC: Flulike syndrome, menstrual disturbances, edema, shortness of breath

MS: Ataxia, weakness

Contraindications: Hypersensitivity

R

Precautions: Pregnancy **C**, lactation, hepatic disease, blood dyscrasias

Pharmacokinetics

Absorption	Well absorbed (PO), completely absorbed (IV)
Distribution	Widely distributed, crosses placenta
Metabolism	Liver—extensively
Excretion	Feces
Half-life	3 hr

Pharmacodynamics

	PO	IV
Onset	Rapid	Rapid
Peak	2-3 hr	Inf end

Interactions

Individual drugs

Alcohol: ↑ toxicity
Chloramphenicol: ↓ effect of chloramphenicol
Disopyramide: ↓ effect of disopyramide
Fluconazole: ↓ effect of fluconazole
Isoniazid: ↑ toxicity
Ketoconazole: ↑ toxicity
Miconazole: ↑ toxicity
Phenytoin: ↓ effect of phenytoin
Quinidine: ↓ effect of quinidine
Theophylline: ↓ effect of theophylline
Tocainide: ↓ effect of tocainide
Verapamil: ↓ effect of verapamil

Drug classifications

Analgesics, narcotic: ↓ effect
Glucocorticoids: ↓ effect
Oral contraceptives: ↓ effect

NURSING CONSIDERATIONS

Assessment

- Monitor liver studies qwk: ALT (SGPT), AST (SGOT), bilirubin
- Monitor renal status: before, qmo: BUN, creatinine, output, sp gr, urinalysis
- Monitor mental status often: affect, mood, behavioral changes; psychosis may occur
- Monitor hepatic status: decreased appetite, jaundice, dark urine, fatigue
- Assess for infection: sputum culture, lung sounds
- C&S tests should be performed prior to beginning treatment, during, and after therapy is completed

Nursing diagnoses

- ✓ Infection, risk for (uses)
- ✓ Diarrhea (adverse reactions)
- ✓ Injury, risk for (adverse reactions)
- ✓ Knowledge deficit (teaching)
- ✓ Noncompliance (teaching)

Implementation

PO route

- Administer with meals to decrease GI symptoms; better to take on empty stomach 1 hr ac or 2 hr pc

IV **IV route**

Intermittent **IV**

- Give by intermittent inf after reconstituting 600 mg/10 ml of sterile water for inj, agitate gently; dilute further in 100 or 500 ml 0.9% NaCl or D_5W; give 100 ml/30 min or 500 ml/3 hr
- Do not mix with other drugs or sols

Patient/family education

- Instruct patient that compliance with dosage schedule, duration is necessary
- Instruct patient that scheduled appointments must be kept or relapse may occur
- Instruct patient to notify prescriber if hepatitis, neutropenia, or thrombocytopenia occurs: sore throat, fever, bleeding, bruising, yellow

sclera, anorexia, nausea, vomiting, fatigue, weakness

- Advise patient that urine, feces, saliva, sputum, sweat, tears, may be colored red-orange; soft contact lens may be permanently stained
- Caution patients using oral contraceptives to use a nonhormonal method of birth control because rifabutin may decrease the efficiency of oral contraceptives

Evaluation

Positive therapeutic outcome

- Decreased symptoms of TB

riluzole (℞)

(ri loo'zole)

Rilutek

Func. class.: ALS agent

Chem. class.: Benzathiazole

Pregnancy category C

Action: Unknown; may act by inhibiting glutamate, interfering with binding of amino acid receptors, inactivation of voltage-dependent sodium channels

➔ Therapeutic Outcome: Decreased symptoms of ALS

Uses: Amyotropic lateral sclerosis (ALS)

Dosage and routes

Adult: PO 50 mg q12h, take 1 hr ac or 2 hr pc

Available forms: Tab 50 mg

Adverse effects

CNS: Hypertonia, depression, dizziness, insomnia, somnolence, vertigo

CV: Hypertension, tachycardia, phlebitis, palpitation, postural hypertension

GI: Nausea, vomiting, dyspepsia, anorexia, diarrhea, flatulence, stomatitis, dry mouth

GU: UTI, dysuria

INTEG: Pruritus, eczema, alopecia, ***exfoliative dermatitus***

RESP: Decreased lung function; rhinitis, increased cough

Contraindications: Hypersensitivity

G P **Precautions:** Neutropenia, renal disease, hepatic disease, elderly, pregnancy **C,** lactation, children

Pharmacokinetics	
Absorption	Well
Distribution	Unknown
Metabolism	Extensively-live
Excretion	Urine, feces
Half-life	Unknown

Pharmacodynamics

Unknown

Interactions

Individual drugs

Amitriptyline: ↓ elimination of riluzole

Cigarette smoke: ↑ elimination of riluzole

Caffeine: ↓ elimination of riluzole

Omeprazole: ↑ elimination of riluzole

Rifampin: ↑ elimination of riluzole

Theophylline: ↓ elimination of riluzole

Drug classifications

Quinolones: ↓ elimination of riluzole

Food

Charcoal-broiled foods: ↑ elimination of riluzole

NURSING CONSIDERATIONS

Assessment

- Monitor LFTs: SGPT, SGOT, bilirubin, GGT, base-

R

line and q mo; monitor liver chemistries
• Assess for neutropenia <500/mm^3

Nursing diagnoses
✓ Physical mobility, impaired (uses)
✓ Knowledge deficit (teaching)

Implementation
• Give 1 hr ac or 2 hr pc; a high-fat meal decreases absorption

Patient/family education
• Advise to report febrile illness, may indicate neutropenia
• Teach reason for drug and expected results

rimantadine (℞)
(ri-man'ti-deen)
Flumadine
Func. class.: Synthetic antiviral
Chem. class.: Tricyclic amine
Pregnancy category C

Action: Prevents uncoating of nucleic acid in viral cell, preventing penetration of virus to host; causes release of dopamine from neurons

➔ **Therapeutic Outcome:** Prevention of influenza type A

Uses: Prophylaxis or treatment of influenza type A

Dosage and routes
Influenza type A prophylaxis
Adult: PO 100 mg bid; in renal hepatic disease, lower dose to 100 mg/day
P ***Child: <10 yr:*** PO 5 mg/kg/day, not to exceed 150 mg

Treatment
Adult: PO 100 mg bid; in renal or hepatic disease, lower dose to 100 mg/day; start treatment at onset of symptoms, continue for at least 1 wk

Available forms: Tab 100 mg; syr 50 mg/5 ml

Adverse effects
CNS: Headache, dizziness, fatigue, depression, hallucinations, tremors, ***convulsions,*** insomnia, poor concentration, asthenia, gait abnormalities
CV: Pallor, palpitations, hypertension
EENT: Tinnitus, taste abnormality, eye pain
GI: Nausea, vomiting, constipation, dry mouth, anorexia, abdominal pain, diarrhea, dyspepsia
INTEG: Rash

Contraindications: Hypersensitivity, lactation, P child <1 yr, pregnancy **C**

Precautions: Epilepsy, hepatic disease, renal disease

Pharmacokinetics

Absorption	Minimally absorbed (PO)
Distribution	Widely distributed, crosses placenta, CSF concentration 50% plasma
Metabolism	Liver
Excretion	95% unchanged—kidneys
Half-life	2-3.5 hr, increased in renal disease

Pharmacodynamics

	PO	IV
Onset	Unknown	Rapid
Peak	1½-2½	Inf end

Interactions
Individual drugs
Amphotericin B: ↑ neurotoxicity, nephrotoxicity
Interferon: ↑ neurotoxicity, nephrotoxicity
Methotrexate: ↑ neurotoxicity, nephrotoxicity
Probenecid: ↑ neurotoxicity, nephrotoxicity
Drug classification
Aminoglycosides: ↑ neurotoxicity, nephrotoxicity

NURSING CONSIDERATIONS
Assessment
- Assess allergies before initiation of treatment, patient's reaction to each medication; list allergies on chart in bright red letters
- Monitor respiratory status: rate, character, wheezing, tightness in chest

Nursing diagnoses
✓ Infection, risk for (uses)
✓ Knowledge deficit (teaching)

Implementation
- Give before exposure to influenza; continue for 10 days after contact
- Give at least 4 hr before hs to prevent insomnia
- Administer pc for better absorption, to decrease GI symptoms; cap may be opened and mixed with food for easy swallowing
- Give in divided doses to prevent CNS disturbances: headache, dizziness, fatigue, drowsiness
- Store in tight, dry container

Patient/family education
- Instruct patient about aspects of drug therapy: need to report dyspnea, dizziness, poor concentration, behavioral changes
- Advise patient to avoid hazardous activities if dizziness occurs
- Caution patient to discuss with prescriber before taking OTC medications, or alcohol—serious drug interactions may result

Evaluation
Positive therapeutic outcome
- Absence of fever, malaise, cough, dyspnea

Treatment of overdose: Withdraw drug, maintain airway, administer epinephrine, aminophylline, O_2, **IV** corticosteroids, physostigmine

risperidone (℞)
(res-pare'a-done)
Risperdal
Func. class: Antipsychotic/neuroleptic
Chem. class.: Benzisoxazole derivative
Pregnancy category C

Action: Unknown; may be mediated through both dopamine type 2 (D_2) and serotinin type 2 ($5\text{-}HT_2$) antagonism

➔ **Therapeutic Outcome:** Decreased hallucination and disorganized thought

Uses: Psychotic disorders

Dosage and routes
Adult: PO 1 mg bid, with incremental increases of 1 mg bid on days 2 and 3 to a dose of 3 mg bid by day 3; then do not increase dose for at least 1 wk

Available forms: Tabs 1, 2, 3, 4 mg

Adverse effects
CNS: Extrapyrimidal symp-

R

toms, pseudoparkinsonism, akathisia, dystonia, tardive dyskinesia, drowsiness, insomnia, agitation, anxiety, headache, ***neuroleptic malignant syndrome***
CV: Orthostatic hypotension, ***tachycardia***
EENT: Blurred vision
GI: Nausea, vomiting, *anorexia, constipation,* jaundice, weight gain
RESP: Rhinitis

Contraindications: Hypersensitivity, lactation, seizure disorders

P **Precautions:** Children, renal disease, pregnancy **C,** hepatic
G disease, elderly, breast cancer

Pharmacokinetics	
Absorption	Unknown
Distribution	Unknown
Metabolism	Liver, extensively
Excretion	Unknown
Half-life	Unknown

Pharmacodynamics	
Onset	Unknown
Peak	Unknown
Duration	Up to 12 hr

Interactions
Individual drugs
Alcohol: ↑ effects of both drugs, oversedation
Lithium: ↑ extrapyramidal symptoms, masking of lithium toxicity
Tegretol: ↑ excretion of risperidone
Drug classifications
Antidepressants: ↑ CNS depression
Antihistamines: ↑ CNS depression
Barbiturate anesthetics: ↑ CNS depression
General anesthetics: ↑ CNS depression
MAOIs: ↑ CNS depression
Narcotics: ↑ CNS depression
Sedative/hypnotics: ↑ CNS depression
Lab test interferences
↑ Liver function tests, ↑ cardiac enzymes, ↑ cholesterol, ↑ blood glucose, ↑ prolactin, ↑ bilirubin, ↑ PBI, ↑ cholinesterase; ↑ I, ↑ alk phosphatase, ↑ leukocytes, ↑ granulocytes, ↑ platelets
↓ Hormones (blood and urine)
False positive: Pregnancy tests, PKU, urine bilirubin
False negative: Urinary steroids, 17-OCHS

NURSING CONSIDERATIONS
Assessment

- Assess mental status: orientation, mood, behavior, presence and type of hallucinations before initial administration and monthly; this drug should significantly reduce psychotic behavior
- Check that patient swallows all PO medication; check for hoarding or giving of medication to other patients
- Monitor I&O ratio, palpate bladder if low urinary output G occurs, especially in elderly; urinalysis recommended before, during prolonged therapy
- Monitor bilirubin, CBC, liver function studies monthly
- Assess affect, orientation, LOC, reflexes, gait, coordination, sleep pattern disturbances
- Monitor B/P with patient in sitting, standing, and lying positions; take pulse and respirations q4h during initial treatment; establish baseline before starting treatment; report drops of 30 mm Hg, obtain baseline ECG; and Q-wave and T-wave changes
- Check for dizziness, faintness, palpitations, tachycardia

on rising; severe orthostatic hypotension is common
- Identify for neuroleptic malignant syndrome: hyperpyrexia, muscle rigidity, increased CPK, altered mental status; drug should be discontinued
- Assess for extrapyramidal symptoms including akathisia (inability to sit still, no pattern to movements), tardive dyskinesia (bizarre movements of the jaw, mouth, tongue, extremities) pseudoparkinsonism (rigidity, tremors, pill rolling, shufling gait); an antiparkinsonian drug should be prescribed
- Assess for constipation, urinary retention daily; if these occur, increase bulk, water in diet

Nursing diagnoses

- ✓ Thought processes, altered (uses)
- ✓ Coping, ineffective individual (uses)
- ✓ Knowledge deficit (teaching)
- ✓ Noncompliance (teaching)

Implementation

- PO with full glass of water, milk; or give with food to decrease GI upset
- Store in airtight, light-resistant container

Patient/family education

- Teach patient to use good oral hygiene; frequent rinsing of mouth, sugarless gum for dry mouth
- Caution patient to avoid hazardous activities until drug response is determined—dizziness, blurred vision may occur
- Inform patient that orthostatic hypotension occurs often—patient should rise from sitting or lying position gradually and remain lying down for at least 30 min after IM inj
- Instruct patient to avoid hot tubs, hot showers, tub baths—hypotension may occur
- Inform patient that heat stroke may occur in hot weather, and to take extra precautions to stay cool
- Advise patient to avoid abrupt withdrawal of this drug, or extrapyramidal symptoms may result; drug should be withdrawn slowly
- Teach patient to avoid OTC preparations (cough, hay fever, cold) unless approved by prescriber—serious drug interactions may occur; avoid use with alcohol, CNS depressants because increased drowsiness may occur

Evaluation

Positive therapeutic outcome

- Decrease in emotional excitement, hallucinations, delusions, paranoia
- Reorganization of patterns of thought, speech

Treatment of overdose: Lavage, provide airway

ritonavir (℞)

(ri-toe′na-veer)

Norvir

Func. class.: Antiviral

Chem. class.: Petidomimetic inhibitor

Pregnancy category B

Action: Inhibits human immunodeficiency virus (HIV) protease and prevents maturation of the infectious virus

Therapeutic Outcome: Improvement of HIV infection

Uses: HIV in combination with AZT, ddc, or alone

R

Dosage and routes
Adult: PO 600 mg bid; if nausea occurs, begin dose at ½ and gradually increase

Available forms: Caps 100 mg; oral sol 80 mg/ml

Adverse effects
CNS: paresthesia, headache
GI: Diarrhea, buccal mucosa ulceration, abdominal pain, nausea, taste perversion, dry mouth
INTEG: Rash
MS: Pain
OTHER: Asthenia

Contraindications: Hypersensitivity

Precautions: Liver disease, P pregnancy **B,** lactation, children

Pharmacokinetics

Absorption	Unknown
Distribution	Unknown
Metabolism	Unknown
Excretion	Unknown
Half-life	Unknown

Pharmacodynamics

Unknown

Interactions
Individual drugs
Clarithromycin: ↑ level of both drugs
ddc: ↑ level of both drugs
Desipramine: ↑ level
Disulfiram: ↑ level
Fluconazole: ↑ levels
Metronidazole: ↑ level
Sulfamethoxazole: ↓ level
Theophylline: ↓ level
Zidovudine: ↓ levels
Lab test interferences
↑ ALT, ↑ GGT, ↑ PT, triglycerides
↓ HCT, ↓ RBC

NURSING CONSIDERATIONS
Assessment
- Assess for signs of infection, anemia
- Assess for liver studies: ALT, AST
- Assess for C&S before drug therapy; drug may be taken as soon as culture is taken; repeat C&S after treatment; determine the presence of other sexually transmitted disease
- Assess for bowel pattern before, during treatment; if severe abdominal pain with bleeding occurs, drug should be discontinued; monitor hydration
- Assess for skin eruptions, rash
- Assess for allergies before treatment, reaction to each medication; place allergies on chart

Nursing diagnoses
✓ Infection, risk for (uses)
✓ Knowledge deficit (teaching)

Patient/family education
- Teach patient to take as prescribed; if dose is missed, take as soon as remembered up to 1 hr before next dose; do not double dose
- Teach patient that drug must be taken in equal intervals around the clock to maintain blood levels for duration of therapy

ropivacaine (℞)
(roe-pi'va-kane)
Naropin
Func. class.: Local anesthetic
Chem. class.: Amide
Pregnancy category B

Action: Competes with calcium for sites in nerve membrane that control sodium transport across cell membrane; decreases rise of depolarization phase of action potential

Therapeutic Outcome: Maintenance of local anesthesia

Uses: Peripheral nerve block, caudal anesthesia, central neural block, vaginal block

Dosage and routes
Varies with route of anesthesia

Available forms: Inj 2, 5, 7.5 mg/ml

Adverse effects
CNS: Anxiety, restlessness, ***convulsions, loss of consciousness,*** drowsiness, disorientation, tremors, shivering
CV: Myocardial depression, cardiac arrest, dysrhythmias, bradycardia, hypotension, hypertension, *fetal bradycardia*
EENT: Blurred vision, tinnitus, pupil constriction
GI: Nausea, vomiting
INTEG: Rash, urticaria, allergic reactions, edema, burning, skin discoloration at injection site, tissue necrosis
RESP: *Status asthmaticus, respiratory arrest, anaphylaxis*

Contraindications: Hypersensitivity, child <12 yr, elderly, severe liver disease

Precautions: Severe drug allergies, pregnancy **B**

Pharmacokinetics	
Absorption	Complete
Distribution	Unknown
Metabolism	Liver
Excretion	Kidneys
Half-life	Unknown

Pharmacodynamics	
Onset	2-8 min
Peak	Unknown
Duration	3-6 hr

Interactions
Individual drugs
Chloroprocaine: ↓ action of ropivacaine
Epinephrine: ↑ dysrhythmias
Enflurane: ↑ dysrhythmias
Halothane: ↑ dysrhythmias
Drug classifications
MAOIs: ↑ hypertension
Antidepressants, tricyclic: ↑ hypertension
Phenothiazines: ↑ hypertension

NURSING CONSIDERATIONS
Assessment
- Assess B/P, pulse, respiration during treatment
- Assess fetal heart tones during labor
- Assess allergic reactions: rash, urticaria, itching
- Assess cardiac status: ECG for dysrhythmias, pulse, B/P during anesthesia

Nursing diagnoses
✓ Knowledge deficit (teaching)

Implementation
- Give only with crash cart, resuscitative equipment nearby
- Give only drugs without preservatives for epidural or caudal anesthesia
- Use new sol; discard unused portions

Evaluation
Positive therapeutic outcome
- Anesthesia necessary for procedure

Treatment of overdose: Airway, O_2, vasopressor, **IV** fluids, anticonvulsants for seizures

R

salmeterol (℞)
(sal-met′er-ole)
Serevent
Func. class.: Adrenergic β_2 agonist
Pregnancy category C

Action: Causes bronchodilatation by action on β_2 (pulmonary) receptors by increasing levels of cAMP, which relaxes smooth muscle; with very little effect on heart rate, maintains improvement in FEV from 3 to 12 hr; prevents nocturnal asthma symptoms

Therapeutic Outcome: Ease of breathing

Uses: Prevention of exercise-induced asthma, bronchospasm

Dosage and routes
Adult: Inh 2 puffs bid (AM and PM)

Available forms: Aerosol

Adverse effects
CNS: Tremors, anxiety, insomnia, headache, dizziness, stimulation, restlessness, hallucinations, flushing, irritability
CV: Palpitations, tachycardia, hypertension, angina, hypotension, dysrhythmias
EENT: Dry nose, irritation of nose and throat
GI: Heartburn, nausea, vomiting
MS: Muscle cramps
RESP: ***Bronchospasm***

Contraindications: Hypersensitivity to sympathomimetics, tachydysrhythmias, severe cardiac disease

Precautions: Lactation, pregnancy **C,** cardiac disorders, hyperthyroidism, diabetes mellitus, hypertension, prostatic hypertrophy, narrow-angle glaucoma, seizures

Pharmacokinetics

Absorption	Unknown
Distribution	Unknown
Metabolism	Unknown
Excretion	Unknown
Half-life	Unknown

Pharmacodynamics

Onset	5-15 min
Peak	4 hr
Duration	12 hr

Interactions
Drug classifications
β-Adrenergic blockers: Block therapeutic effect
Bronchodilators, aerosol: ↑ action of bronchodilator
MAOIs: ↑ chance of hypertensive crisis
Sympathomimetics: ↑ adrenergic side effects

NURSING CONSIDERATIONS
Assessment
- Monitor respiratory function: vital capacity, forced expiratory volume, ABGs, lung sounds, heart rate, rhythm (baseline)

Nursing diagnoses
✓ Airway clearance, ineffective (uses)
✓ Impaired gas exchange (uses)
✓ Knowledge deficit (teaching)

Implementation
- Shake aerosol container, ask patient to exhale, then place mouthpiece in mouth, inhale slowly, hold breath, remove, exhale slowly; allow at least 1 min between inh
- Store in light-resistant container, do not expose to temp over 86° F (30° C)

Patient/family education
- Caution patient not to use OTC medications because

extra stimulation may occur
• Instruct patient to use this medication before other medications and to allow at least 1 min between each, to prevent overstimulation
• Teach patient how to use inhaler; review package insert with patient; to avoid getting aerosol in eyes; blurring may result; to wash inhaler in warm water qd and dry; to avoid smoking, smoke-filled rooms, and persons with respiratory infections
• Instruct patient on administration of dose, not to use more than prescribed; serious side effects may occur

Evaluation

Positive therapeutic outcome
• Absence of dyspnea, wheezing
• Improved airway exchange
• Improved ABGs

Treatment of overdose: Administer a β_2-adrenergic blocker

salsalate (℞)

(sal-sa′late)

Amigesic, Argesic-SA, Arthra-G, Disalcid, Mono-Gesic, Salflex, Salsalate, Salsitab

Func. class.: Nonnarcotic analgesic; nonsteroidal antiinflammatory agent

Chem. class.: Salicylate

Pregnancy category C

Action: Blocks formation of peripheral prostaglandins, which cause pain and inflammation; antipyretic action results from inhibition of hypothalamic heat-regulating center; does not inhibit platelet aggregation

➔ Therapeutic Outcome: Decreased pain, inflammation

Uses: Mild to moderate pain or fever, including arthritis, juvenile rheumatoid arthritis

Dosage and routes

Adult: PO 3 g/day in divided doses

Available forms: Cap 500 mg; tabs 500, 750 mg

Adverse effects

CNS: Stimulation, drowsiness, dizziness, confusion, ***convulsions,*** headache, flushing, hallucinations, coma

CV: Rapid pulse, ***pulmonary edema***

EENT: Tinnitus, hearing loss

ENDO: Hypoglycemia, hyponatremia, hypokalemia, alteration in acid-base balance

GI: Nausea, vomiting, GI bleeding, diarrhea, heartburn, anorexia, ***hepatotoxicity***

HEMA: ***Thrombocytopenia, agranulocytosis, leukopenia, neutropenia, hemolytic anemia,*** increased pro-time

INTEG: Rash, urticaria, bruising

RESP: Wheezing, hyperpnea

Contraindications: Hypersensitivity to salicylates, NSAIDs, GI bleeding, bleeding disorders, **P** children <3 yr, vitamin K deficiency

Precautions: Anemia, hepatic disease, renal disease, Hodgkin's disease, pregnancy **C**, lactation

S

Pharmacokinetics

Absorption	Absorbed in small intestine
Distribution	Rapidly and widely distributed, crosses placenta
Metabolism	Not metabolized
Excretion	Unchanged—kidneys
Half-life	2-3 hr (low doses), 15-30 hr (high doses)

Pharmacodynamics

Onset	30 min
Peak	1-3 hr
Duration	3-6 hr

Interactions

Individual drugs

Alcohol: ↑ bleeding
Cefamandole: ↑ bleeding
Furosemide: ↑ toxic effects
Heparin: ↑ bleeding
Insulin: ↑ effects
Methotrexate: ↑ effects
PABA: ↑ toxic effects
Phenytoin: ↑ effects
Plicamycin: ↑ bleeding
Probenecid: ↓ effects
Spironolactone: ↓ effects
Sulfinpyrazone: ↓ effects
Valproic acid: ↑ effects, ↑ bleeding
Vancomycin: ↑ ototoxicity

Drug classifications

Antacids: ↓ effects of aspirin
Anticoagulants: ↑ effects
Carbonic anhydrase inhibitors: ↑ toxic effects
Nonsteroidal antiinflammatories: ↑ gastric ulcers
Penicillins: ↑ effects
Salicylates: ↓ blood sugar levels
Steroids: ↓ effects of aspirin, ↑ gastric ulcers
Sulfonylamides: ↓ effects
Urinary acidifiers: ↑ salicylate levels
Urinary alkalizers: ↓ effects of aspirin

Lab test interferences

↑ Coagulation studies, ↑ liver function studies, ↑ serum uric acid, ↑ amylase, ↑ CO_2, ↑ urinary protein
↓ Serum potassium, ↓ PBI, ↓ cholesterol, ↓ blood glucose
Interference: Urine catecholamines, pregnancy test

NURSING CONSIDERATIONS

Assessment

- Monitor liver function studies: AST (SGOT), ALT (SGPT), bilirubin, creatinine if patient is on long-term therapy
- Monitor renal function studies: BUN, urine creatinine if patient is on long-term therapy
- Monitor blood studies: CBC, Hct, Hgb, pro-time if patient is on long-term therapy
- Check I&O ratio; decreasing output may indicate renal failure if patient is on long-term therapy
- Assess hepatotoxicity: dark urine, clay-colored stools, yellowing of the skin and sclera, itching, abdominal pain, fever, diarrhea if patient is on long-term therapy
- Assess for allergic reactions: rash, urticaria; if these occur, drug may have to be discontinued
- Assess for ototoxicity: tinnitus, ringing, roaring in ears; audiometric testing needed before, after long-term therapy
- Assess for visual changes: blurring, halos; corneal, retinal damage
- Check edema in feet, ankles, legs
- Identify prior drug history; many drug interactions are possible
- Monitor pain: location,

duration, type, intensity, prior to dose and 1 hr after
• Monitor musculoskeletal status: ROM prior to dose
• Identify fever, length of time, and related symptoms

Nursing diagnoses
✓ Pain (uses)
✓ Mobility, impaired physical mobility (uses)
✓ Knowledge deficit (teaching)
✓ Injury, risk for (side effects)

Implementation
• Administer to patient crushed or whole; chewable tab may be chewed
• Give with food or milk to decrease gastric symptoms; give 30 min ac or 2 hr pc; absorption may be slowed
• Give antacids 1-2 hr after enteric products

Patient/family education
• Advise patient to report any symptoms of hepatotoxicity, renal toxicity, visual changes, ototoxicity, allergic reactions, bleeding (long-term therapy)
• Instruct patient to take with 8 oz of water and sit upright for ½ hr after dose
• Caution patient not to exceed recommended dosage; acute poisoning may result
• Advise patient to read label on other OTC drugs; many contain aspirin
• Inform patient that the therapeutic response takes 2 wk (arthritis)
• Teach patient to report tinnitus, confusion, diarrhea, sweating, hyperventilation
• Caution patient to avoid alcohol ingestion; GI bleeding may occur
• Inform patient that patients who have allergies may develop allergic reactions

Evaluation
Positive therapeutic outcome
• Decreased pain
• Decreased inflammation

Treatment of overdose: Lavage, activated charcoal, monitor electrolytes, VS

saquinavir (℞)
(sa-quen′a-ver)
Invirase
Func. class.: Antiviral
Chem. class.: Synthetic peptide like substrate analog
Pregnancy category B

Action: Inhibits human immunodeficiency virus (HIV) protease

Therapeutic Outcome: Prevents maturation of the infectious virus

Uses: HIV in combination with AZT, zalcitabine, ddc

Dosage and routes
Adult: PO 600 mg tid within 2 hr after a full meal; given with either zalcitabine 0.75 mg tid or AZT 200 mg tid

Available forms: Cap 200 mg

Adverse effects
CNS: Paresthesia, headache
GI: Diarrhea, buccal mucosa ulceration, abdominal pain, nausea
INTEG: Rash
MS: Pain
OTHER: Asthenia

Contraindications: Hypersensitivity

Precautions: Liver disease, pregnancy **B,** lactation, children

S

Pharmacokinetics

Absorption	Unknown
Distribution	Unknown
Metabolism	Unknown
Excretion	Unknown
Half-life	Unknown

Pharmacodynamics

Unknown

Interactions

Individual drugs

Astemizole: ↑ astemizole levels when given with saquinavir
Carbamazepine: ↓ saquinavir levels
Dexamethasone: ↓ saquinavir levels
Phenobarbital: ↓ saquinavir levels
Rifamycin: ↓ saquinavir levels

Lab test interferences

Interference: CPK, glucose (low)

NURSING CONSIDERATIONS

Assessment

- Assess signs of infection, anemia
- Monitor liver studies: ALT, AST
- Monitor C&S before drug therapy; drug may be taken as soon as culture is taken; repeat C&S after treatment; determine the presence of other sexually transmitted diseases
- Assess bowel pattern before, during treatment; if severe abdominal pain with bleeding occurs, drug should be discontinued; monitor hydration
- Assess skin eruptions, rash, urticaria, itching
- Assess allergies before treatment, reaction of each medication; place allergies on chart

Nursing diagnoses

✓ Infection, risk for (uses)
✓ Knowledge deficit (teaching)

Patient/family education

- Advise patient to take as prescribed within 2 hr of a full meal; if dose is missed, take as soon as remembered up to 1 hr before next dose; do not double dose
- Advise patient that drug must be taken in equal intervals around the clock to maintain blood levels for duration of therapy

sargramostim (℞)

(sar-gram'oh-stim)

Leukine, Prokine, rhu GM-CSF, recombinant human

Func. class.: Biologic modifier: cytokine

Chem. class.: Granulocyte/macrophage colony stimulating factor

Pregnancy category C

Action: Stimulates proliferation and differentiation of hematopoietic progenitor cells (granulocyte, macrophage)

Uses: Acceleration of myeloid recovery in patients with non-Hodgkin's lymphoma, acute lymphoblastic leukemia, autologous bone marrow transplantation in Hodgkin's disease; bone marrow transplantation failure or engraftment delay

Dosage and routes

Myeloid reconstitution after autologous bone marrow transplantation

Adult: **IV** 250 μg/m²/day × 3 wk; give over 2 hr, 2-4 hr after autologous bone marrow inf, and not less than 24 hr after last dose of antineoplastics and 12 hr after last dose of radiotherapy, bone marrow transplantation failure, or engraftment delay

Acceleration of myeloid recovery

Adult: **IV** 250 μg/m²/day × 14 days; give over 2 hr; may repeat in 7 days, may repeat 500 μg/m²/day × 14 days after another 7 days if no improvement

Available forms: Powder for inj lyophilized 250, 500 μg

Adverse effects

CNS: Fever, malaise, CNS disorder, weakness, chills

CV: Supraventricular tachycardia, peripheral edema, pericardial effusion

GI: Nausea, vomiting, diarrhea, anorexia, ***GI hemorrhage,*** stomatitis, ***liver damage***

GU: Urinary tract disorder, abnormal kidney function

HEMA: Blood dyscrasias, hemorrhage

INTEG: Alopecia, rash, peripheral edema

MS: Bone pain

RESP: Dyspnea

Contraindications: Hypersensitivity to GM-CSF, yeast products; excessive leukemic myeloid blast in the bone marrow or peripheral blood

Precautions: Pregnancy **C**, P lactation, children; renal, hepatic, lung disease; cardiac disease; pleural, pericardial effusions

Pharmacokinetics	
Absorption	Completely absorbed
Distribution	Unknown
Metabolism	Unknown
Excretion	Unknown
Half-life	2 hr

Pharmacodynamics	
Onset	Rapid
Peak	2 hr
Duration	Unknown

Interactions

Individual drugs

Lithium: ↑ myeloproliferation

Drug classifications

Antineoplastics: Do not use together

Corticosteroids: ↑ myeloproliferation

NURSING CONSIDERATIONS

Assessement

- Monitor blood studies: CBC, differential count before treatment and twice weekly; leukocytosis may occur (WBC >50,000 cells/mm³, ANC >20,000 cells/mm³)
- Monitor renal and hepatic studies before treatment: BUN, creatinine, urinalysis; AST (SGOT), ALT (SGPT), alk phosphatase; monitoring is needed twice a week in renal, hepatic disease
- Assess for hypersensitive reactions/rashes, and local inj site reactions; usually transient
- Assess for increased fluid retention in cardiac disease

Nursing diagnoses

✓ Infection, risk for (uses)
✓ Knowledge deficit (teaching)

Implementation

- Reconstitute with 1 ml sterile water for inj without preservative; do not reenter vial; discard unused portion; direct reconstitution sol at side of vial; rotate contents; do not shake
- Give by intermittent inf after diluting in 0.9% NaCl inj to prepare **IV** inf; if final conc is <10 μg/ml, add human albumin to make a final conc of

S

0.1% to the NaCl before adding sargramostim to prevent absorption; for a final conc of 0.1% albumin, add 1 mg human albumin/1 ml 0.9% NaCl inj; run over 2 hr; give within 6 hr after reconstitution
• Store in refrigerator; do not freeze

Y-site compatibilities: Amikacin, aminophylline, aztreonam, bleomycin, butorphanol, calcium gluconate, carboplatin, carmustine, cefazolin, ceforanide, cefotaxime, cefotetan, ceftizoxime, ceftriaxone, cefuroxime, cimetidine, cisplatin, clindamycin, cyclophosphamide, cytarabine, dacarbazine, dactinomycin, dexamethasone, diphenhydramine, doxorubicin, doxycycline, droperidol, etoposide, famotidine, floxuridine, fluconazole, fluorouracil, furosemide, gentamicin, heparin, ifosfamide, magnesium sulfate, mannitol, mechlorethamine, meperidine, mesna, methotrexate, metoclopramide, metronidazole, mezlocillin, miconazole, minocycline, mitoxantrone, netilmicin, pentostatin, potassium chloride, prochlorperazine, promethazine, ranitidine, teniposide, ticarcillin, ticarcillin/clavulanate, trimethoprim/sulfamethoxazole, vinblastine, vincristine, zidovudine

Y-site incompatibilities: Acyclovir, ampicillin, ampicillin/sulbactam, cefonicid, cefoperazine, ceftazidime, chlorpromazine, ganciclovir, haloperidol, hydrocortisone, hydromorphone, hydroxyzine, idarubicin, imipenem/cilastatin, lorazepam, methylprednisolone sodium succinate, mitomycin, morphine, nalbuphine, ondansetron, piperacillin, sodium bicarbonate, tobramycin

Patient/family education
• Teach patient reason for medication and expected results
• Advise patient to notify nurse or prescriber of side effects

Evaluation

Positive therapeutic outcome
• WBC and differential recovery
• Absence of infection

scopolamine (℞)
(skoe-pol'a-meen)

Transderm-Scop, Isopoto-Hyoscine, Transderm-V ✦, Triptol

Func. class.: Antiemetic, anticholinergic, mydriatic

Chem. class.: Belladonna alkaloid

Pregnancy category C

Action: Inhibits acetylcholine at receptor sites in autonomic nervous system, which controls secretions, free acids in stomach; blocks central muscarinic receptors, which decreases involuntary movements; blocks response of iris sphincter muscle, muscle of accommodation of ciliary body to cholinergic stimulation, resulting in dilation, paralysis of accommodation

➡ Therapeutic Outcome: Absence of vomiting, secretions (preop), involuntary movements

Uses: Reduction of secretions before surgery, calm delirium, motion sickness, uveitis, iritis, cycloplegia, mydriasis; prevention of motion sickness, parkinson symptoms

Dosage and routes

Ophth

Adult: Instill 1-2 gtt before refraction or 1-2 gtt qd-tid for iritis or uveitis

P ***Child:*** Instill 1 gtt bid × 2 days before refraction

Prevention of motion sickness

Adult: Patch 1 placed behind ear 4-5 hr before travel

P Not recommended for children

Parkinson symptoms

Adult: IM/SC/**IV** 0.3-0.6 mg tid-qid diluted using dilution provided

P ***Child:*** SC 0.006 mg/kg tid-qid or 0.2 mg/m^2

Preoperatively

Adult: SC 0.4-0.6 mg

Available forms: Sol 0.25%; patch 0.5 mg delivered in 72 hr; inj 0.3, 0.4, 0.86, 1 mg/ml

Adverse effects

CNS: Confusion, anxiety, restlessness, irritability, delusions, hallucinations, headache, sedation, depression, incoherence, dizziness, excitement, delirium, flushing, weakness

CV: Palpitations, tachycardia, postural hypotension, paradoxical bradycardia

EENT: Blurred vision, photophobia, dilated pupils, difficulty swallowing, mydriasis, cycloplegia

GI: Dryness of mouth, constipation, nausea, vomiting, abdominal distress, ***paralytic ileus***

GU: Hesitancy, retention

INTEG: Urticaria

MISC: Suppression of lactation, nasal congestion, decreased sweating

Contraindications: Hypersensitivity, narrow-angle glaucoma, myasthenia gravis, GI/GU obstruction, hypersensitivity to belladonna, barbiturates

Precautions: Pregnancy **C**,
G elderly, lactation, prostatic hypertrophy, CHF,
P hypertension, dysrhythmia, children, gastric ulcer

Pharmacokinetics

Absorption	Well absorbed (IM, SC, Trans)
Distribution	Crosses placenta, blood-brain barrier
Metabolism	Liver
Excretion	Unknown
Half-life	8 hr

Pharmacodynamics

	SC/IM	IV	TRANS	OPHTH
Onset	30-45 min	10-15 min	4-5 hr	Unknown
Peak	1 hr	1 hr	Unknown	20-30 min
Duration	6 hr	4 hr	72 hr	3-7 days

Interactions

Individual drugs

Alcohol: ↑ CNS depression

Quinidine: ↑ anticholinergic effect

Drug classifications

Antidepressants: ↑ anticholinergic effect

Antihistamines: ↑ anticholinergic effect

Narcotics: ↑ anticholinergic effect

Phenothiazines: ↑ anticholinergic effect

Tricyclics: ↑ anticholinergic effect

S

NURSING CONSIDERATIONS

Assessment

- Assess for eye pain; discontinue use (opticue)
- Monitor I&O ratio; retention commonly causes decreased urinary output
- Assess for Parkinsonism, extrapyramidal symptoms: shuffling gait, muscle rigidity, involuntary movements
- Assess for urinary hesitancy, retention; palpate bladder if retention occurs
- Assess for constipation; increase fluids, bulk, exercise if this occurs
- Assess for tolerance over long-term therapy; dose may have to be increased or changed
- Assess mental status: affect, mood, CNS depression, worsening of mental symptoms during early therapy

Nursing diagnoses

✓ Fluid volume deficit (uses)
✓ Knowledge deficit (teaching)

Implementation

IV SC/IM/IV route

- Administer parenteral dose with patient recumbent to prevent postural hypotension

IV IV route

- Give by direct **IV** after diluting with sterile water; give slowly

Syringe compatibilities: Atropine, benzquinamide, butorphanol, chlorpromazine, cimetidine, dimenhydrinate, diphenhydramine, droperidol, fentanyl, glycopyrrolate, hydromorphone, hydroxyzine, meperidine, metoclopramide, midazolam, morphine, nalbuphine, pentazocine, pentobarbital, perphenazine, prochlorperazine, promazine, promethazine, ranitidine, thiopental

Y-site compatibilities: Heparin, hydrocortisone, potassium chloride, vitamin B with C

Patient/family education

- Tell patient to avoid hazardous activities, activities requiring alertness; dizziness may occur

Trans route

- Instruct patient to wash, dry hands before and after applying to surface behind ear; to change patch q72h; to apply at least 4 hr before traveling
- Advise patient to discontinue use if blurred vision, severe dizziness, drowsiness occurs—another type of antiemetic may be used
- Instruct patient to read labels of all OTC medications; if any scopolamine is found in product, avoid use
- Advise patient to keep medication out of children's reach
- Caution patient to report change in vision; blurring or loss of sight; trouble breathing; inhibition of sweating; flushing

Ophth route

- Teach patient method of instill: pressure on lacrimal sac for 1 min; do not touch dropper to eye
- Inform patient that blurred vision will decrease with repeated use of drug
- Advise patient to wait 5 min to use other drops; blink more than usual
- Caution patient not to discontinue this drug abruptly; to taper off over 1 wk

Evaluation

Positive therapeutic outcome

- Decrease in inflammation, cycloplegic refraction

- Decreased secretions
- Absence of motion sickness

secobarbital (℞)

(see-koe-bar'bi-tal)

secobarbital sodium, Secogen Sodium ✤, Seconal Sodium, Seconal Sodium Pulvules, Seral ✤, Secretin-Ferring

Func. class.: Sedative/hypnotic-barbiturate

Chem. class.: Barbitone (short-acting)

Pregnancy category D

Controlled substance schedule II (USA), schedule G (Canada)

Action: Depresses activity in brain cells primarily in reticular activating system in brainstem; selectively depresses neurons in posterior hypothalamus, limbic structures; decreases seizure activity by inhibition of epileptic activity in CNS

➔ **Therapeutic Outcome:** Sedation, anticonvulsant, improved energy

Uses: Insomnia, sedation, preoperative medication, status epilepticus, acute tetanus convulsions

Dosage and routes

Insomnia

Adult: PO/IM 100-200 mg hs

P ***Child:*** IM 3-5 mg/kg, not to exceed 100 mg, not to inject >5 ml in one site; rec 4-5 mg/kg

Sedation/preoperatively

Adult: PO 200-300 mg 1-2 hr preoperatively

P ***Child:*** PO 50-100 mg 1-2 hr preoperatively; rec 4-5 mg/kg 1-2 hr preoperatively

Status epilepticus

P ***Adult and child:*** IM/**IV** 250-350 mg

Acute psychotic agitation

P ***Adult and child:*** IM/**IV** 5.5 mg/kg q3-4h

Available forms: Caps 50, 100 mg; tab 100 mg; inj 50 mg/ml; powder, rec supp 200 mg

Adverse effects

CNS: Lethargy, drowsiness, hangover, dizziness, paradoxical G stimulation in the elderly and P children, lightheadedness, dependency, CNS depression, mental depression, slurred speech

CV: Hypotension, bradycardia

GI: Nausea, vomiting, diarrhea, constipation

HEMA: ***Agranulocytosis, thrombocytopenia, megaloblastic anemia*** (long-term treatment)

INTEG: Rash, urticaria, pain, abscesses at inj site, angioedema, thrombophlebitis, ***Stevens-Johnson syndrome***

RESP: Depression, ***apnea, laryngospasm, bronchospasm***

Contraindications: Hypersensitivity to barbiturates, respiratory depression, addiction to barbiturates, severe liver impairment, porphyria, uncontrolled severe pain

Precautions: Anemia, pregnancy **D,** lactation, hepatic disease, renal disease, hyper- G tension, elderly, acute/chronic pain

Pharmacokinetics

Absorption	Slow (70%-90%) (PO), IV complete
Distribution	Not known, crosses placenta
Metabolism	Liver (75%)
Excretion	Kidneys (25% unchanged)
Half-life	2-6 days

Pharmacodynamics

	PO	IM	IV
Onset	30-60 min	10-30 min	5 min
Peak	Unknown	Unknown	30 min
Duration	6-8 hr	4-6 hr	4-6 hr

Interactions

Individual drugs

Alcohol: ↑ CNS depression
Chloramphenicol: ↓ effectiveness
Cyclosporine: ↓ effectiveness
Cyclophosphamide: ↑ hematologic toxicity
Dacarbazine: ↓ effectiveness
Quinidine: ↓ effectiveness
Valproic acid: ↑ sedation

Drug classifications

Anticoagulants: ↓ effectiveness
Antidepressants: ↑ CNS depression
Antihistamines: ↑ CNS depression
Glucocorticoids: ↓ effectiveness
MAOIs: ↑ CNS depression
Narcotics: ↑ CNS depression
Oral contraceptives: ↓ effectiveness
Sedatives/hypnotics: ↑ CNS depression
Tricyclics: ↓ effectiveness

NURSING CONSIDERATIONS

Assessment

• Assess patient's mental status: mood, sensorium, affect, memory (long, short), [G] especially in elderly patients; if using as a hypnotic, assess sleep patterns during therapy; drug suppresses REM sleep with dreaming; withdrawal insomnia may occur after short-term use; do not start using drug again—insomnia will improve in 1-3 nights; patient may experience increased dreaming

• Monitor patient for respiratory dysfunction: respiratory depression, character, rate, [IV] rhythm (when using **IV**); hold drug if resp are <10/min or if pupils are dilated. Also check VS q30 min after parenteral route for 2 hr

[!] • Assess patient for barbiturate toxicity: hypotension; pulmonary constriction; cold, clammy skin; cyanosis of lips; CNS depression; nausea; vomiting; hallucinations; delirium; weakness; coma; pupillary constriction, mild symptoms may occur in 8-12 hr without drug

• Assess patient for blood dyscrasias: fever, sore throat, bruising, rash, jaundice, epistaxis (long-term treatment only)

• Assess for pain in postoperative patients; pain threshold is lowered when patients are taking this medication

Nursing diagnoses

✓ Sleep pattern disturbance (uses)
✓ Injury, risk for (adverse reactions)
✓ Knowledge deficit (teaching)

Implementation

• Administer after removal of cigarettes, to prevent fires

• Administer after trying conservative measures for insomnia

PO route

• Tab may be crushed and mixed with food if swallowing

is difficult. Also may be mixed with other fluids ½-1 hr before hs for expected sleeplessness; on empty stomach for best absorption

IM route

• Give in deep muscle mass (gluteal) to minimize irritation to tissues

• Split inj of >5 ml into two because irritation to tissues may occur

IV Direct IV route

• Use large vein to prevent extravasation; if extravasation occurs, use moist heat to the area and procaine sol 5% inj into area

• Give at rate of 65 mg or less/min; titrate to patient response

Syringe incompatibilities: Benzquinamide, dimenhydrinate, diphenhydramine, erythromycin gluceptate, hydroxyzine, kanamycin, oxytetracycline, phenytoin, prochlorperazine, promazine, promethazine, ranitidine, tetracycline

Solution compatibilities: D_5W, $D_{10}W$, 0.45% NaCl, 0.9% NaCl, Ringer's sol, dextrose/saline combinations, dextrose/Ringer's or dextrose/lactated Ringer's combinations

Additive compatibilities: Amikacin, aminophylline

Additive incompatibilities: Cephalothin, chlorpromazine, codeine, ephedrine, hydralazine, hydrocortisone sodium succinate, hydroxyzine, insulin, levorphanol, meperidine, methadone, morphine, norepinephrine, pentazocine, procaine, prochlorazine mesylate, promazine, promethazine, streptomycin, vancomycin

Patient/family education

• Teach patient that hangover is common

• Instruct patient that drug is indicated only for short-term treatment of insomnia and is probably ineffective after 2 wk

• Inform patient that physical dependency may result when used for extended time (45-90 days depending on dose)

• Caution patient to avoid driving or other activities requiring alertness

• Caution patient to avoid alcohol ingestion or CNS depressants; serious CNS depression may result

• Instruct patient not to discontinue medication quickly after long-term use; drug should be tapered over 1 wk

• Emphasize the need to tell all prescribers that a barbiturate is being taken

• Inform patient that withdrawal insomnia may occur after short term use; patient should not start using drug again—insomnia will improve in 1-3 nights; patient may experience increased dreaming

• Inform patient that effects may take 2 nights for benefits to be noticed; teach patient alternate measures to improve sleep: reading, exercise several hours before hs, warm bath, warm milk, TV, self-hypnosis, deep breathing

• Teach patient to make position changes slowly; orthostatic hypotension may occur

• Instruct patient to notify prescriber immediately if bruising or bleeding occur, which may indicate blood dycrasias

Evaluation

Positive therapeutic outcome
- Improved sleeping patterns
- Decreased seizure activity
- Improved energy

Treatment of overdose: Lavage, activated charcoal, warming blanket, vital signs, hemodialysis, alkalinize urine; give **IV** volume expanders, **IV** fluids

selegiline (℞)
(se-le'ji-leen)
Eldepryl, SD-Deprenyl
Func. class.: Antiparkinson agent
Chem. class.: Levorotatory acetylenic derivative of phenethylamine
Pregnancy category C

Action: Increased dopaminergic activity by inhibition of MAO type B activity; not fully understood

Therapeutic Outcome: Decreased symptoms of Parkinson's disease

Uses: Adjunct management of Parkinson's disease in patients being treated with levodopa/carbidopa who have responded poorly to therapy

Dosage and routes

Adult: PO 10 mg/day in divided doses 5 mg at breakfast and lunch; after 2-3 days begin to reduce the dose of levodopa/carbidopa 10%-30%

Available forms: Tab 5 mg

Adverse effects

CNS: Increased tremors, chorea, restlessness, blepharospasm, increased bradykinesia, grimacing, tardive dyskinesia, dystonic symptoms, involuntary movements, increased apraxia, hallucinations, dizziness, mood changes, nightmares, delusions, lethargy, apathy, overstimulation, sleep disturbances, headache, migraine, numbness, muscle cramps, confusion, anxiety, tiredness, vertigo, personality change, back/leg pain
CV: Orthostatic hypotension, hypertension, dysrhythmia, palpitations; angina pectoris, hypotension, tachycardia, edema, sinus bradycardia, syncope
EENT: Diplopia, dry mouth, blurred vision, tinnitus
GI: Nausea, vomiting, constipation, weight loss, anorexia, diarrhea, heartburn, rectal bleeding, poor appetite, dysphagia
GU: Slow urination, nocturia, prostatic hypertrophy, hesitation, retention, frequency, sexual dysfunction
INTEG: Increased sweating, alopecia, hematoma, rash, photosensitivity, facial hair
RESP: Asthma, shortness of breath

Contraindications: Hypersensitivity

Precautions: Pregnancy **C,** P lactation, children

Pharmacokinetics	
Absorption	Well absorbed
Distribution	Widely distributed
Metabolism	Rapidly, liver
Excretion	Metabolites-N-desmethyldeprenyl, amphetamine, methamphetamine
Half-life	Unknown

Pharmacodynamics

Onset	Unknown
Peak	½-2 hr
Duration	Unknown

Interactions

Individual drugs

Meperidine: Do not use—fatal reaction

Levodopa/carbidopa: ↑ side effects

Fluoxetine: ↑ seratonin syndrome (confusion, seizures, fever, hypertension, agitation) discontinue 5 wk prior to selegiline

Drug classifications

Narcotics: Do not use—fatal reaction

Food

Tyramine foods: ↑ hypertension

Lab test interferences

False positive: Urine ketones, urine glucose

False negative: Urine glucose (glucose oxidase)

False ↑ Uric acid, false ↑ urine protein

↓ VMA

NURSING CONSIDERATIONS

Assessment

- Monitor B/P, respiration throughout treatment
- Assess mental status: affect, mood, behavioral changes, depression; perform suicide assessment
- Assess for decreased Parkinson's symptoms: rigidity, unsteady gait, weakness, tremors; these should decrease in severity

Nursing diagnoses

✓ Physical mobility, impaired (uses)

✓ Knowledge deficit (teaching)

Implementation

- Adjust dosage to patient response
- Give with meals; limit protein taken with drug
- Give at doses <10 mg/day because of risks associated with nonselective inhibition of MAO

Patient/family education

- Caution patient to change positions slowly to prevent orthostatic hypotension
- Advise patient to report side effects: twitching, eye spasms —may indicate overdose
- Caution patient to use drug exactly as prescribed; if drug is discontinued abruptly, parkinsonian crisis may occur
- Instruct patient to avoid foods high in tyramine: cheese, pickled products, wine, beer, large amounts of caffeine
- Instruct patient not to exceed recommended dose of 10 ml—might precipitate a hypertensive crisis, report severe headache or other unusual symptoms

Evaluation

Positive therapeutic outcome

- Decreased symptoms of Parkinson's disease

Treatment of overdose: **IV** fluids for hypertension, **IV** dilute pressure agent for B/P titration

S

senna (OTC)

(sin'na)

Black Draught, Dr. Caldwell Senna Laxative, Fletcher's Castoria, Gentlax, Senexon, Senna-Gen, Senokot, Senokotxtra, Senolax

Func. class.: Laxative-stimulant

Chem. class.: Anthraquinone

Pregnancy category C

Action: Stimulates peristalsis by action on Auerbach's plexus; softens feces by increasing water and electrolytes in large intestine

➔ **Therapeutic Outcome:** Decreased constipation

Uses: Acute constipation; bowel preparation for surgery or examination

Dosage and routes

Adult: PO 1-8 tab (Senokot)/day or 1/2 to 4 tsp of granules added to water or juice; rec supp 1-2 hs; syr 1-4 tsp hs (1 tsp = 4 ml), 7.5-15 ml; (Black Draught) 3/4 oz dissolved in 2.5 oz liq given between 2-4 PM the day before procedure (X-Prep)

P ***Child >27 kg:*** ½ adult dose; do not use Black Draught for children

P ***Child 1 mo-1 yr:*** Syr 1.25-2.5 ml (Senokot) hs

Available forms: Supp 625 mg, 30 mg sennosides; powder 662 mg/g, 6, 15 mg sennosides/3 g; tab 8.6 sennosides, 180 mg

Adverse effects

GI: Nausea, vomiting, anorexia, abdominal cramps, diarrhea, flatulence

GU: Pink-red or brown-black discoloration of urine

META: Hypocalcemia, enteropathy, alkalosis, hypokalemia, ***tetany***

Contraindications: Hypersensitivity, GI bleeding, intestinal obstruction, CHF, lactation, abdominal pain, nausea/vomiting, appendicitis, acute surgical abdomen

Precautions: Pregnancy **C**

Pharmacokinetics	
Absorption	Minimally absorbed (PO)
Distribution	Unknown
Metabolism	Not metabolized
Excretion	Kidneys, feces
Half-life	Unknown

Pharmacodynamics	PO	REC
Onset	6-24 hr	Unknown
Peak	Unknown	Unknown
Duration	3-4 days	Unknown

Interactions

Drug classifications

Oral drugs: ↓ absorption

Individual drugs

Disulfiram: Do not use together

NURSING CONSIDERATIONS

Assessment

- Monitor blood, urine electrolytes if used often by patient; check I&O ratio to identify fluid loss
- Assess cramping, rec bleeding, nausea, vomiting; if these symptoms occur, drug should be discontinued; identify cause of constipation; identify whether fluids, bulk, or exercise is missing from lifestyle
- Assess for Mg toxicity: thirst, confusion, decrease in reflexes

• Monitor blood ammonia level (30-70 mg/100 ml); monitor for clearing of confusion, lethargy, restlessness, irritability (hepatic encephalopathy)
• Monitor blood, urine electrolytes if drug is used often by patient

Nursing diagnoses
✓ Bowel elimination, altered: constipation (uses)
✓ Bowel elimination, altered; diarrhea (side effects)
✓ Knowledge deficit (teaching)
✓ Noncompliance (teaching)

Implementation
PO route
• Administration on empty stomach produces more rapid results
• Give with a full glass of water in AM or PM (oral dose); evacuation occurs 6-12 hr later
• Dissolve granules in water or juice before administration
• Shake oral sol before giving

Patient/family education
• Discuss with the patient that adequate fluid consumption is necessary
• Inform patient that normal bowel movements do not always occur daily
• Teach patient not to use in presence of abdominal pain, nausea, vomiting; tell patient to notify prescriber if constipation is unrelieved or if symptoms of electrolyte imbalance occur: muscle cramps, pain, weakness, dizziness, excessive thirst

Evaluation
Positive therapeutic outcome
• Decreased constipation in 8-10 hr

sertraline (℞)
(ser'tra-leen)
Zoloft
Func. class.: Antidepressant
Chem. class.: SSRI
Pregnancy category B

Action: Inhibits serotonin reuptake in the CNS, thus increasing action of serotonin; does not affect dopamine, norepinephrine

➔ **Therapeutic Outcome:** Relief of depression, OCD

Uses: Major depression, obsessive-compulsive disorder (OCD)

Dosage and routes
Adult: PO 50 mg qd; may increase to a maximum of 200 mg/day, do not change dose at intervals of <1 wk; administer qd in AM or PM

Available forms: Tabs 25, 50, 100 mg

Adverse effects
CNS: Insomnia, agitation, somnolence, dizziness, headache, tremor, fatigue, paresthesia, twitching, confusion, ataxia, fever
CV: Palpitations, chest pain
EENT: Vision abnormalities
GI: Diarrhea, nausea, constipation, anorexia, dry mouth, dyspepsia, *vomiting, flatulence*
GU: Male sexual dysfunction, micturition disorder
INTEG: Increased sweating, rash, hot flashes

Contraindications: Hypersensitivity to this drug or SSRIs

Precautions: Pregnancy **B,** G lactation, elderly, hepatic, renal disease, epilepsy

S

Pharmacokinetics

Absorption	Well absorbed
Distribution	Unknown, steady state 1 wk
Metabolism	Liver, extensively
Excretion	Feces (14%)
Half-life	26-104 hr

Pharmacodynamics

Onset	Unknown
Peak	4.5-8.4 hr
Duration	Unknown

Interactions
Individual drugs
Cimetidine: ↑ sertraline
Warfarin: ↑ effect of warfarin
Drug classifications
Antidepressants, tricyclics: ↑ effect
Benzodiazepines: ↑ effect
MAOIs: Hypertensive crisis, convulsions, do not use together
Lab test interferences
↑ AST, ↑ ALT

NURSING CONSIDERATIONS
Assessment
- Assess mental status: mood, sensorium, affect, suicidal tendencies; increase in psychiatric symptoms: depression, panic
- Identify alcohol consumption; if alcohol is consumed, hold dose until AM

Nursing diagnoses
- ✓ Coping, ineffective individual (uses)
- ✓ Injury, risk for (adverse reactions)
- ✓ Knowledge deficit (teaching)
- ✓ Noncompliance (teaching)

Implementation
- Administer dosage hs if oversedation occurs during day; may take entire dose hs; may crush
- Store at room temp; do not freeze

Patient/family education
- Teach patient that therapeutic effects may take 1 wk
- Instruct patient to use caution in driving or other activities requiring alertness because of drowsiness, dizziness, blurred vision; to avoid rising quickly from sitting to standing, G especially elderly
- Advise patient to avoid alcohol ingestion, other CNS depressants
- ! Teach patient not to discontinue medication quickly after long-term use: may cause nausea, headache, malaise
- Caution patient to wear sunscreen or large hat because photosensitivity can occur
- Teach patient to increase fluids, bulk in diet if constipation, urinary retention occur, G especially elderly
- Instruct patient to take gum, hard sugarless candy, or frequent sips of water for dry mouth

Evaluation
Positive therapeutic outcome
- Decrease in depression, OCS
- Absence of suicidal thoughts

Treatment of overdose:
ECG monitoring, induce emesis, lavage, activated charcoal, administer anticonvulsant

simethicone (OTC)

(si-meth'i-kone)

Extra Strength Gas-X, Flatulex Gas Relief, Gas-X, Major Con, Mylanta Gas, Mylicon, Mylicon 80, Ovol ✤, Phazyme, Phazyme 95, Phazyme 125

Func. class.: Antiflatulent

Pregnancy category C

Action: Disperses, prevents gas pockets in GI system; does not decrease gas production

➔ **Therapeutic Outcome:** Belching or flatus

Uses: Flatulence

Dosage and routes

P *Adult and child >12 yr:* PO 40-100 mg pc, hs

Available forms: Chew tabs 40, 80 mg; tabs 50, 60, 95, 125 mg; drops 40 mg/0.6 ml; cap 125 mg

Adverse effects

GI: Belching, rectal flatus

Contraindications: Hypersensitivity

Precautions: Pregnancy **C**

Pharmacokinetics	
Absorption	None
Distribution	None
Metabolism	None
Excretion	None
Half-life	Unknown

Pharmacodynamics	
Onset	Rapid
Peak	Unknown
Duration	3 hr

Interactions: None

NURSING CONSIDERATIONS

Assessment

- Identify the reason for excess gas production; decreased bowel sounds, recent surgery, other GI conditions

Nursing diagnoses

✓ Pain (uses)
✓ Knowledge deficit (teaching)

Implementation

- Give pc and hs
- Shake suspension well before administration
- Chewable tab should be chewed and not swallowed whole

Patient/family education

- Caution patient that tab must be chewed; to shake suspension well before pouring

Evaluation

Positive therapeutic outcome

- Absence of flatulence

simvastatin (℞)

(sim-va-stat'in)

Zocor

Func. class.: Antihyperlipidemic

Chem. class.: Synthetically derived fermentation product

Pregnancy category X

Action: Inhibits HMG-COA reductase enzyme, which reduces cholesterol synthesis; this enzyme is needed for cholesterol production

➔ **Therapeutic Outcome:** Decreasing cholesterol levels and low-density lipoproteins, increased high-density lipoproteins

Uses: As an adjunct in primary hypercholesterolemia (types IIa, IIb), mixed hyperlipidemia, coronary artery disease

S

Dosage and routes
Adult: PO 5-10 mg qd in PM initially, usual range 5-40 mg/day qd in PM, not to exceed 40 mg/day; dosage adjustments may be made at
G 4-wk intervals or more; reduce dose in elderly

Available forms: Tabs 5, 10, 20, 40 mg

Adverse effects
CNS: Headache, tremor, vertigo, peripheral neuropathy
EENT: Lens opacities
GI: Nausea, constipation, diarrhea, dyspepsia, flatus, abdominal pain, heartburn, ***liver dysfunction***
INTEG: Rash, pruritus, alopecia, photosensitivity
MS: Muscle cramps, myalgia, *myositis, rhabdomyolysis*

Contraindications: Hypersensitivity, pregnancy **X,** lactation, active liver disease

Precautions: Past liver disease, alcoholism, severe acute infections, trauma, hypotension, uncontrolled seizure disorders, severe metabolic disorders,
G electrolyte imbalances, elderly, renal desease

Pharmacokinetics

Absorption	85%
Distribution	Unknown
Metabolism	Liver—extensively
Excretion	70% feces, 20% kidneys
Half-life	3 hr

Pharmacodynamics

Onset	Unknown
Peak	1-2½ hr
Duration	Unknown

Interactions
Individual drugs
Cholestyramine: ↓ action of simvastatin
Colestipol: ↓ action of simvastatin
Cyclosporine: ↑ risk of myopathy, rhabdomyolysis
Erythromycin: ↑ risk of myopathy
Gemfibrozil: ↑ risk of myopathy, rhabdomyolysis
Niacin: ↑ risk of myopathy
Warfarin: ↑ risk of bleeding
Food
↑ levels of lovastatin
Lab test interferences
↑ CPK, ↑ liver function tests

NURSING CONSIDERATIONS

Assessment

- Assess nutrition: fat, protein, carbohydrates; nutritional analysis should be completed by dietician before treatment is initiated
- Monitor bowel pattern daily; diarrhea may be a problem
- Monitor triglycerides, cholesterol baseline and throughout treatment; LDL and VLDL should be watched closely; if it increases, drug should be discontinued

Nursing diagnoses

- ✓ Diarrhea (adverse reactions)
- ✓ Knowledge deficit (teaching)
- ✓ Noncompliance (teaching)

Implementation

- Give 30 min before AM and PM meals

Patient/family education

- Inform patient that compliance is needed for positive results to occur; not to double doses
- Advise patient to lower risk factors: high-fat diet, smoking, alcohol consumption, absence of exercise
- Advise patient to notify health care prescriber if the GI symptoms of diarrhea, abdominal or epigastric pain, nausea,

vomiting occur; or if chills, fever, sore throat occur

Evaluation

Positive therapeutic outcome

- Decreased cholesterol levels, serum triglycerides and improved ratio with high-density lipoproteins (HDLs)

sodium bicarbonate (OTC)

Arm and Hammer Pure Baking Soda, Bell/ans, Citrocarbonate, soda mint

Func. class.: Alkalinizer; antacid

Pregnancy category C

Action: Orally neutralizes gastric acid, which forms water, NaCl, CO_2; increases plasma bicarbonate, which buffers H^+ ion concentration; reverses acidosis **IV**

Therapeutic Outcome: Correction of acidosis, gastric acid neutralization

Uses: Acidosis (metabolic), cardiac arrest, alkalinization (systemic/urinary); antacid (PO)

Dosage and routes

Acidosis, metabolic

P ***Adult and child:*** **IV** inf 2-5 mEq/kg over 4-8 hr depending on CO_2, pH

Cardiac arrest

P ***Adult and child:*** **IV** bol 1 mEq/kg, then 0.5 mEq/kg q10 min, then doses based on ABGs

P ***Infant:*** **IV** inf not to exceed 8 mEq/kg/day based on ABGs (4.2% sol)

Alkalinization of urine

Adult: PO 325 mg 2 g qid or 48 mEq/kg (4 g), then 12-24 mEq q4hr

P ***Child:*** PO 12-120 mg/kg/day (1-10 mEq/kg)

Antacid

Adult: PO 300 mg-2 g chewed, taken with water qd-qid

Available forms: Tabs 300, 325, 600, 650 mg; inj 4%, 4.2%, 5%, 7.5%, 8.4%

Adverse effects

CNS: Irritability, headache, confusion, stimulation, tremors, *twitching, hyperreflexia,* ***tetany,*** weakness, ***convulsions*** caused by alkalosis

CV: Irregular pulse, ***cardiac arrest,*** water retention, edema, weight gain

GI: Flatulence, *belching, distention,* ***paralytic ileus,*** acid rebound

GU: Calculi

META: Alkalosis

RESP: Shallow, slow respirations, cyanosis, ***apnea***

Contraindications: Hypertension, peptic ulcer, renal disease, hypocalcemia

Precautions: CHF, cirrhosis, toxemia, renal disease, pregnancy **C**

Pharmacokinetics

Absorption	Unknown
Distribution	Widely distributed—extracellular fluids
Metabolism	Unknown
Excretion	Kidneys
Half-life	Unknown

Pharmacodynamics

	PO	IV
Onset	2 min	Rapid
Peak	½ hr	Rapid
Duration	1-3 hr	Unknown

S

Interactions

Individual drugs

Flecainide: ↑ effects
Ketoconazole: ↓ absorption of ketoconazole
Methenamine: ↓ effect of methenamine
Mexiletine: ↑ blood level of mexiletine
Quinidine: ↑ effects

Drug classifications

Amphetamines: ↑ effects
Anorexiants: ↑ effects
Barbiturates: ↓ effects of barbiturates
Corticosteroids: ↑ sodium, potassium
Fluoroquinolones: ↑ crystalluria
Salicylates: ↓ effect of salicylates

Lab test interferences

↑ Urinary urobilinogen
False positive: Urinary protein, blood lactate

NURSING CONSIDERATIONS

Assessment

- Assess respiratory and pulse rate, rhythm, depth, lung sounds; notify prescriber of abnormalities
- Assess for GI perforation secondary to CO_2 in GI tract; may lead to perforation if ulcer is severe
- Monitor fluid balance (I&O, weight qd, edema); notify prescriber of fluid overload
- Monitor electrolytes: blood pH, PO_2, HCO_3, during beginning treatment; ABGs frequently during emergencies
- Monitor urine pH, urinary output, during beginning treatment
- Monitor extravasation with **IV** administration (tissue sloughing, ulceration, and necrosis)
- Assess for alkalosis: irritability, confusion, twitching, hyperreflexia, stimulation, slow respirations, cyanosis, irregular pulse
- Monitor manifestations of hypokalemia: *Renal:* acidic urine, reduced urine osmolality, nocturia, polyuria, polydipsia; *Cardiac:* hypotension, broad T wave, U wave, ectopy, tachycardia, weak pulse; *Neurologic:* muscle weakness, altered LOC, drowsiness, apathy, lethargy, confusion, depression; *GI:* anorexia, nausea, cramps, constipation, distension, paralytic ileus; *Respiratory:* hypoventilation, respiratory muscle weakness
- Monitor for manifestations of hyponatremia: *CV:* ↑ B/P, cold, clammy skin, hypo or hypervolemia; *GI:* anorexia, nausea, vomiting, diarrhea, abdominal cramps; *Neuro:* lethargy, increased ICP, confusion, headache, seizures, coma, fatigue, tremors, hyperreflexia
- Assess for milk-alkali syndrome: confusion, headache, nausea, vomiting, anorexia, urinary stones, hypercalcemia

Nursing diagnoses

- ✓ Gas exchange, impaired (uses)
- ✓ Fluid volume excess (adverse reactions)
- ✓ Knowledge deficit (teaching)

Implementation

PO route

- Tab must be chewed and taken with 8 oz of water
- Dissolve effervescent tab in water
- May be used to neutralize gastric acid in peptic ulcer disease, given 1 and 3 hr pc and hs

IV **IV route**
- Give **IV** bol in cardiac arrest, may be repeated q10min
- Give by intermittent or continuous inf in prepared sol or diluted in an equal amount of any dextrose/saline combination; administer 2-5mEq/kg over 4-8 hr, not to exceed 50mEq/hr; slower

P rate in children

Syringe compatibilities: Milrinone, pentobarbital

Syringe incompatibilities: Glycopyrrolate, metoclopramide, thiopental

Y-site compatibilities: Acyclovir, famotidine, fludarabine, indomethacin, insulin, melphalan, morphine, paclitaxel, potassium chloride, tolazoline, vitamin B with C

Y-site incompatibilities: Amrinone, calcium chloride, idarubicin, sargramostim, verapamil, vinorelbine

Additive compatibilities: Amikacin, aminophylline, amobarbital, amphotericin B, atropine, bretylium, calcium chloride, calcium gluceptate, cefoxitin, ceftazidime, cephalothin, cephapirin, chloramphenicol, chlorothiazide, cimetidine, clindamycin, cytarabine, droperidol/fentanyl, ergonovine, erythromycin, floxacillin, furosemide, heparin, hyaluronidase, hydrocortisone, kanamycin, lidocaine, metaraminol, methotrexate, methyldopate, multivitamins, nafcillin, netilmicin, nizatidine, oxacillin, oxytocin, phenobarbital, phenylephrine, phenytoin, phytonadione, potassium chloride, prochlorperazine, thiopental, verapamil

Additive incompatibilities: Amoxicillin, ascorbic acid, carboplatin, carmustine, cefotaxime, cisplatin, codeine, dobutamine, epinephrine, hydromorphone, imipenem/cilastatin, insulin, isoproterenol, labetalol, levorphanol, magnesium sulfate, methadone, morphine, norepinephrine, pentazocine, pentobarbital, procaine, secobarbital, streptomycin, succinylcholine, tetracycline, vitamin B with C

Patient/family education
- Instruct patient to chew antacid tab and drink 8 oz water; not to take antacid with milk because milk-alkali syndrome may result; not to use antacid for more than 2 wk
- Advise patient to notify prescriber if indigestion is accompanied by chest pain; dyspnea; diarrhea; dark, tarry stools
- Teach patient about sodium-restricted diet; to avoid use of baking soda for indigestion

Evaluation

Positive therapeutic outcome
- ABGs, electrolytes, blood pH, HCO_3 normal levels
- Decreased gastric pain

sodium biphosphate (OTC)

Fleet Enema, Phospho-Soda

Func. class.: Laxative, saline

Pregnancy category C

Action: Increases water absorption in the small intestine by osmotic action; laxative effect occurs by increased peristalsis and water retention

S

➔ **Therapeutic Outcome:** Absence of constipation

Uses: Constipation, bowel or rectal preparation for surgery, examination

Dosage and routes

Adult: PO 20-30 ml (phospho-soda)

P ***Child:*** PO 5-15 ml (phospho-soda)

P ***Adult and child >12 yr:*** Rec enema (118 ml)

P ***Child 2-12 yr:*** Rec ½ enema (59 ml)

Available forms: Enema 7 g/phosphate and 19 g/biphosphate/118 ml; oral sol 18 g phosphate/48 g biphosphate/100 ml

Adverse effects

GI: Nausea, cramps, diarrhea
META: Electrolyte, fluid imbalances

Contraindications: Hypersensitivity, rectal fissures, abdominal pain, nausea/vomiting, appendicitis, acute surgical abdomen, ulcerated hemorrhoids, Na-restricted diets (Sal-Hepatica, PhosphoSoda)

Precautions: Pregnancy **C**

Pharmacokinetics

Absorption	Up to 20% (Rec)
Distribution	Unknown
Metabolism	Unknown
Excretion	Kidneys
Half-life	Unknown

Pharmacodynamics

	PO	REC
Onset	½-3 hr	5 min
Peak	Unknown	Unknown
Duration	Unknown	Unknown

Interactions: None

NURSING CONSIDERATIONS

Assessment

- Assess stools: color, amount, consistency
- Assess for bowel pattern, bowel sounds (frequency, intensity), flatulence, distention, increased temp, dietary patterns (fluid, bulk), exercise
- Assess for cramping, rec bleeding, nausea, vomiting; if these symptoms occur, drug should be discontinued

Nursing diagnoses

✓ Constipation (uses)
✓ Knowledge deficit (teaching)

Implementation

PO route

- Give on empty stomach
- Mix oral sol in cold water
- Alone for better absorption; do not take within 1 hr of other drugs

Patient/family education

- Advise patient not to use laxatives or enema for long-term therapy; bowel tone will be lost
- Teach patient that normal bowel movements do not always occur daily
- Caution patient not to use in presence of abdominal pain, nausea, vomiting
- Caution patient to notify prescriber if constipation is unrelieved or if symptoms of electrolyte imbalance occur: muscle cramps, pain, weakness, dizziness, excessive thirst
- Instruct patient to maintain adequate fluid consumption to help prevent constipation

Evaluation

Positive therapeutic outcome

- Decrease in constipation

sodium polystyrene sulfonate (℞)

(po-lee-stye'reen)

Kayexalate, SPS Suspension

Func. class.: Potassium-removing resin

Chem. class.: Cation exchange resin

Pregnancy category C

Action: Removes potassium by exchanging sodium for potassium in body; occurs primarily in large intestine

Therapeutic Outcome: Potassium levels within accepted range

Uses: Hyperkalemia in conjunction with other measures

Dosage and routes

Adult: PO 15 g qd-qid; rec enema 30-50 g/100 ml of sorbitol warmed to body temp q6h

P ***Child:*** PO/rec 1 mEq of K exchanged/g of resin, approximate dose 1g/kg q6hr

Available forms: Susp, 15 g polystyrene sulfonate, 21.5 ml sorbitol, 15 g (65 mEq) sodium/60 ml; powder 15 g/4 level tsp

Adverse effects

GI: Constipation, anorexia, nausea, vomiting, diarrhea (sorbitol), ***fecal impaction,*** gastric irritation

META: Hypocalcemia, hypokalemia, hypomagnesemia, sodium retention

Precautions: Pregnancy **C,** renal failure, CHF, severe edema, severe hypertension

Pharmacokinetics

Absorption	None
Distribution	None
Metabolism	None
Excretion	Feces
Half-life	Unknown

Pharmacodynamics

	PO	REC
Onset	2-12 hr	2-12 hr
Peak	Unknown	Unknown
Duration	6-24 hr	4-6 hr

Interactions

Drug classifications

Antacids, calcium or magnesium: ↓ effect of sodium polystyrene

Laxatives: ↓ effect of sodium polystyrene

NURSING CONSIDERATIONS

Assessment

- Assess bowel function daily: amount of stool, color, characteristics
- Assess hypotension: confusion, irritability, muscular pain, weakness
- Monitor for manifestations of hypokalemia: *Renal:* acidic urine, reduced urine osmolality, nocturia, polyuria, polydipsia; *Cardiac:* hypotension, broad T wave, U wave, ectopy, tachycardia, weak pulse; *Neuro:* muscle weakness, altered LOC, drowsiness, apathy, lethargy, confusion, depression; *GI:* anorexia, nausea, cramps, constipation, distension, paralytic ileus; *Respiratory:* hypoventilation, respiratory muscle weakness
- Monitor for manifestations of hypocalcemia: *CNS:* personality changes, anxiety, disturbances, depression, psychosis, nausea, vomiting, *GI:* constipation, abdominal pain from muscle spasm; *CV:* decreased

S

contractility, decreased cardiac output, hypotension, lengthened ST segment, prolonged QT interval; *Integ:* scaling eczema, alopecia, hyperpigmentation; *Neuro:* tetany, muscle twitching, cramping grimacing, seizure, altered deep tendon reflexes, spasm

- Monitor for manifestations of hypomagnesemia; *CNS:* agitation; *Neuro:* muscle twitching, paresthesias, hyperactive reflexes, positive Babinski reflex, dysphagia, nystagmus, seizures, tetany; *GI:* nausea, vomiting, diarrhea, anorexia, abdominal distention; *Cardiac:* ectopy; tachycardia, broad, flat, or inverted T waves; depressed ST segment; prolonged QT; decreased cardiac output; hypotension
- Monitor electrolytes: potassium, sodium, calcium, magnesium

Nursing diagnoses

✓ Constipation (adverse reactions)
✓ Diarrhea (adverse reactions)
✓ Knowledge deficit (teaching)

Implementation

PO route

- Give oral dose as susp mixed with H_2O or syr (20-100 ml)
- Give mild laxative as ordered to prevent constipation and fecal impaction; sorbitol as ordered to prevent constipation

Rec route

- Give by retention enema after mixing with warm water; introduce by gravity, continue stirring, flush with 100 ml of fluid, clamp, and leave in place for at least ½-1 hr
- Complete irrigation of colon after enema with 1-2 qt of nonsodium sol, drain
- Store freshly prepared sol for 24 hr at room temp

Patient/family education

- Explain reason for medication and expected results

Evaluation

Positive therapeutic outcome

- Potassium level normal

somatropin (℞)

(soe-ma-troe'pin)

Genotropin, Humatrope, Norditropin, Nutropin, Nutropin AQ, Saizen, Serostim

Func. class.: Pituitary hormone

Chem. class.: Growth hormone

Pregnancy category C

Action: Stimulates growth; similar to natural growth hormone—both preparations are developed by recombinant DNA technique

➔ **Therapeutic Outcome:** Increase in height as a result of skeletal growth in pituitary growth hormone deficiency

Uses: Pituitary growth hormone deficiency (hypopituitary dwarfism), children with human growth hormone deficiency, AIDs wasting syndrome, cachexia, adults with somatropin deficiency syndrome (SDS)

Dosage and routes

Genotropin: SC 0.16-0.24 mg/kg 1 wk, divided into 6 or 7 inj, give in abdomen, thigh, buttocks

Humatrope: SC/IM 0.18 mg/kg divided into equal doses either on 3 alternate days or 6 x/wk, max wk dose is 0.3 mg/kg

Growth Hormone Deficiency

Nutropin/Nutropin AQ: SC 0.2 mg/kg/wk

Serostim: SC at hs >55 kg 6 mg, 45-55 kg 5 mg, 35-45 kg 4 mg

Norditropin: SC 0.024-0.034 mg/kg 6-7 x/wk

Available forms: Powder for inj (lyophilized) 1.5 mg (4IU/ml), 4 mg (12IU/vial), 5 mg (13IU/vial), 5 mg (15IU/vial), 5 mg (15IU/vial) rDNA origin, 5.8 mg (15IU/ml), 6 mg (18IU ml), 8 mg (24IU/vial), 10 mg (26IU/vial), inj 10 mg (30IU/vial)

Adverse effects

CNS: Headache, **growth of intracranial tumor**

ENDO: Hyperglycemia, ketosis, hypothyroidism

GU: Hypercalciuria

INTEG: Rash, urticaria, pain, inflammation at injection site

MS: Tissue swelling, joint and muscle pain

SYST: Antibodies to growth hormone

Contraindications: Hypersensitivity to benzyl alcohol, closed epiphyses, intracranial lesions

Precautions: Diabetes mellitus, hypothyroidism, pregnancy **C**

Pharmacokinetics

Absorption	Well absorbed (SC/IM)
Distribution	Unknown
Metabolism	Unknown
Half-life	15-60 min

Pharmacodynamics

	IM/SC (GROWTH)
Onset	Unknown
Peak	Unknown
Duration	7 days

Interactions

Drug classifications

Androgens: ↑ epiphyseal closure

Glucocorticosteroids: ↓ growth, ↓ somatotropin response

Thyroid hormones: ↑ epiphyseal closure

NURSING CONSIDERATIONS

Assessment

- Identify growth hormone antibodies if patient fails to respond to therapy
- Monitor thyroid function tests: T_3, T_4, T_7, TSH to identify hypothyroidism
- Assess for allergic reaction: rash, itching, fever, nausea, wheezing
- Assess for hypercalciuria: urinary stones; groin, flank pain; nausea, vomiting, frequency, hematuria, chills
- P Monitor growth rate of child at intervals during treatment

Nursing diagnoses

✓ Body image disturbance (uses)
✓ Knowledge deficit (teaching)

Implementation

- Store in refrigerator for <1 mo; if reconstituted, <1 wk; do not use discolored or cloudy sol

IM route

- Norditropin: After reconstituting 4-8 mg/2 ml diluent
- Humetrope: 5 mg/1.5-5 ml dilute, do not shake
- Nutropin/Nutropin AQ: Reconstitute 5 mg/1-5 ml or 10 mg/1-10 ml bacteriostatic

S

water for inj (benzyl alcohol preserved)

Patient/family education

- Explain reason for medication and expected results
- Advise patient that routine follow-up is needed to monitor growth rate
- Instruct parents on procedure for medication preparation and inj use—request demonstration, return demonstration; provide written instructions

Evaluation

Positive therapeutic outcome

- Growth in children until epiphyseal plates close

sotalol (℞)

(soe-ta′lole)

Betapace, Sotacar ✤

Func. class.: Antidysrhythmic, group II, III

Chem. class.: Nonselective β-blocker

Pregnancy category B

Action: Competitively blocks stimulation of β-adrenergic receptor within vascular smooth muscle; produces chronotropic, inotropic activity (decreases rate of SA node discharge, increases recovery time), slows conduction of AV node, decreases heart rate, which decreases O_2 consumption in myocardium; also decreases renin-aldosterone-angiotensin system at high doses, inhibits β-2 receptors in bronchial system (high doses)

➡ Therapeutic Outcome: Decreased B/P, heart rate, AV conduction

Uses: Life-threatening ventricular dysrhythmias

Dosage and routes

Adult: PO initial 80 mg bid, may increase to total of 240-320 mg/day

Available forms: Tabs 80, 160, 240 mg

Adverse effects

CNS: Dizziness, mental changes, drowsiness, fatigue, headache, catatonia, depression, anxiety, nightmares, paresthesia, lethargy, insomnia, decreased concentration

CV: Orthostatic hypotension, bradycardia, CHF, chest pain, ventricular dysrhythmias, AV block, peripheral vascular insufficiency, palpitations, prodysrhythmia, torsades de pointes

EENT: Tinnitus, visual changes, sore throat, double vision, dry, burning eyes

GI: Nausea, vomiting, diarrhea, dry mouth, flatulence, constipation, anorexia

HEMA: ***Agranulocytosis, thrombocytopenic purpura (rare), thrombocytopenia, leukopenia***

INTEG: Rash, alopecia, urticaria, pruritus, fever

MS: Joint pain, arthralgia, muscle cramps, pain

RESP: ***Bronchospasm,*** dyspnea, wheezing, nasal stuffiness, pharyngitis

OTHER: Facial swelling, decreased exercise tolerance, weight change, Raynaud's disease

Contraindications: Hypersensitivity to β-blockers, cardiogenic shock, heart block (2nd or 3rd degree), sinus bradycardia, CHF, bronchial asthma, congenital or acquired long QT syndrome

Precautions: Major surgery, pregnancy **C,** lactation, diabetes mellitus, renal disease, thyroid disease, COPD, well-compensated heart failure, CAD, nonallergic bronchospasm, electrolyte disturbances, bradycardia, cardiac dysrhythmias, peripheral vascular disease

Pharmacokinetics

Absorption	Variably (30%)
Distribution	Crosses placenta, minimal penetration in CNS
Metabolism	Liver
Excretion	70% unchanged—kidneys
Half-life	10-24 hr, ↑ in renal disease

Pharmacodynamics

Onset	Several hr
Peak	Unknown
Duration	Unknown

Interactions

Individual drugs

Digoxin: ↑ blood levels, ↑ toxicity
Disopyramide: ↑ levels, ↑ toxicity
Flecainide: ↑ levels, ↑ toxicity
Lidocaine: Bradycardia, arrest
Mexiletine: ↑ levels, ↑ toxicity
Phenytoin: ↑ blood levels
Procainamide: ↑ levels, ↑ toxicity
Quinidine: ↑ levels, ↑ toxicity
Warfarin: ↑ level, ↑ bleeding

Drug classifications

Calcium channel blockers: ↑ dysrhythmias, arrest

Lab test interferences

False ↑ Urinary catecholamines

NURSING CONSIDERATIONS

Assessment

- Monitor B/P during beginning treatment, periodically thereafter; pulse q4hr; note rate, rhythm, quality: apical/radial pulse before administration; notify prescriber of any significant changes (pulse <50 bpm)
- Check for baselines in renal, liver function tests before therapy begins
- Assess for edema in feet, legs daily, monitor I&O, daily weight; check for jugular vein distention, rales, bilaterally, dyspnea (CHF)
- Monitor skin turgor, dryness of mucous membranes for hydration status, especially in elderly [G]

Nursing diagnoses

- ✓ Cardiac output, decreased (uses)
- ✓ Injury, risk for (adverse reactions)
- ✓ Knowledge deficit (teaching)
- ✓ Noncompliance (teaching)

Implementation

- Given ac, hs, tab may be crushed or swallowed whole; give with food to prevent GI upset; reduce dosage in renal dysfunction
- Store protected from light, moisture; placed in cool environment

Patient/family education

- Teach patient not to discontinue drug abruptly, taper over 2 wk; may cause precipitate angina if stopped abruptly
- Teach patient not to use OTC products containing α-adrenergic stimulants (such as nasal decongestants, cold preparations); to avoid alcohol and smoking and to limit sodium intake as prescribed
- Teach patient how to take pulse and B/P at home, advise when to notify prescriber

• Instruct patient to comply with weight control, dietary adjustments, modified exercise program
• Caution patient to carry/wear Medic Alert ID to identify drug begin taken, allergies
• Inform patient that drug controls symptoms but does not cure
• Caution patient to avoid hazardous activities if dizziness, drowsiness is present
• Teach patient to report symptoms of CHF: difficulty breathing, especially on exertion or when lying down; night cough; swelling of extremities; bradycardia; dizziness; confusion; depression; fever
• Teach patient to take drug as prescribed, not to double or skip doses; take any missed doses as soon as remembered if at least 4 hr until next dose

Evaluation

Positive therapeutic outcome
• Absence of dysrhythmias

Treatment of overdose: Lavage; **IV** atropine for bradycardia; **IV** theophylline for bronchospasm; digitalis, O_2, diuretic for cardiac failure; hemodialysis; **IV** glucose for hyperglycemia; **IV** diazepam (or phenytoin) for seizures

sparfloxacin (℞)
(spare-floks'a-sin)
Zagram
Func. class.: Antiinfective
Chem. class.: Fluoroquinolone antibacterial
Pregnancy category C

Action: Interferes with conversion of intermediate DNA fragments into high-molecular-weight DNA in bacteria; DNA gyrase inhibitor

Therapeutic Outcome: Bactericidal action against the following organisms: *C. pneumoniae, H. influenzae, H. parainfluenzae, M. catarrhalis*

Uses: Adult infections (including complicated): lower respiratory, community-acquired pneumonia, chronic bronchitis

Dosage and routes
Adult: PO 400 mg loading dose, then 200 mg q24h × 10 days

Available forms: Tabs 200 mg, 500, 750, mg, **IV**

Adverse effects
CNS: Headache, dizziness, insomnia
CV: QT interval prolongation, vasodilation
GI: Nausea, flatulence, abdominal pain, ***pseudomembranous colitis,*** vomiting, diarrhea
INTEG: Pruritus, photosensitivity

Contraindications: Hypersensitivity to quinolones

Precautions: Pregnancy **C,** P lactation, children, renal disease, seizure disorder

Pharmacokinetics	
Absorption	Well absorbed
Distribution	Widely distributed
Metabolism	Liver
Excretion	Kidneys, feces
Half-life	20 hr

Pharmacodynamics
Unknown

Interactions
Individual drugs
Zinc sulfate: ↓ absorption of sparfloxacin

Drug classifications
Antacids: ↓ absorption of sparfloxacin
Lab test interferences
↑ AST (SGOT), ↑ ALT (SGPT)

NURSING CONSIDERATIONS

Assessment

- Assess patient for previous sensitivity reaction
- Assess patient for signs and symptoms of infection including characteristics of wounds, sputum, urine, stool, WBC >10,000, fever; obtain baseline information before and during treatment
- Obtain C&S before beginning drug therapy to identify if correct treatment has been initiated
- Assess for allergic reactions: rash, urticaria, pruritus, chills, fever, joint pain; may occur a few days after therapy begins; epinephrine and resuscitation equipment should be available for anaphylactic reaction
- Identify urine output; if decreasing, notify prescriber (may indicate nephrotoxicity); also check for increased BUN, creatinine
- Monitor blood studies: AST (SGOT), ALT (SGPT), CBC, Hct, bilirubin, LDH, alkaline phosphatase, Coombs' test monthly if patient is on long-term therapy
- Assess bowel pattern qd; if severe diarrhea occurs, drug should be discontinued
- Monitor for bleeding; ecchymosis, bleeding gums, hematuria, stool guaiac daily if on long-term therapy
- Assess for overgrowth of infection: perineal itching, fever, malaise, redness, pain, swelling, drainage, rash, diarrhea, change in cough, sputum

Nursing diagnoses

- ✓ Infection, risk for (uses)
- ✓ Diarrhea (side effects)
- ✓ Injury, risk for (side effects)
- ✓ Knowledge deficit (teaching)
- ✓ Noncompliance (teaching)

Implementation

PO route

- Give around the clock to maintain proper blood levels

IV route

- Check for irritation, extravasation, phlebitis daily
- For intermittent inf, dilute to 1-2 mg/ml of D_5W, 0.9% NaCl; give over 60 min; it will remain stable under refrigeration for 2 wks

Patient/family education

- Advise patient to contact prescriber if vaginal itching, loose foul-smelling stools, furry tongue occur; may indicate superinfection; report itching, rash, pruritus, urticaria
- Instruct patient to take all medication prescribed for the length of time ordered; drug must be taken around the clock to maintain blood levels; do not give medication to others
- Advise patient to notify prescriber of diarrhea with blood or pus

Evaluation

Positive therapeutic outcome

- Absence of signs/symptoms of infection (WBC <10,000, temp WNL)
- Reported improvement in symptoms of infection

spectinomycin (℞)

(spek-ti-noe-mye'sin)
Trobicin
Func. class.: Antibiotic
Chem. class.: Aminocyclitol
Pregnancy category B

Action: Inhibits bacterial synthesis by binding to 30S subunit on ribosome

➔ **Therapeutic Outcome:** Treatment and resolution of gonococcal infection

Uses: Gonorrhea, gonococcal urethritis, cervicitis, proctitis

Dosage and routes

P ***Adult and child >45 kg:*** IM 2-4 g as single dose

P ***Child <45 kg:*** IM 40 mg/kg single dose

Available forms: Powder for inj IM 2, 4 g

Adverse effects

CNS: Dizziness, chills, fever, insomnia, headache, anxiety
GI: Nausea, vomiting, increased BUN
GU: Decreased urine output
HEMA: Anemia
INTEG: Pain at injection site, urticaria, rash, pruritus, fever

Contraindications: Hypersensitivity, syphilis

Precautions: Pregnancy **B**,
P infants, children

Pharmacokinetics

Absorption	Well absorbed
Distribution	Unknown
Metabolism	Liver
Excretion	Kidneys
Half-life	1⅕-2½ hr

Pharmacodynamics

Onset	Rapid
Peak	1 hr

NURSING CONSIDERATIONS

Assessment

- Monitor gonorrhea culture after treatment
- Monitor I&O ratio; report decreased output
- Monitor liver studies: AST (SGOT), ALT (SGPT), serum alk phosphatase following multiple doses
- Monitor blood studies: Hct, Hgb, BUN if multiple diagnoses given
- Monitor serologic test for gonorrhea 3 mo after treatment
- Assess for allergies before treatment, reaction of each medication

Nursing diagnoses

✓ Infection, risk for (uses)
✓ Knowledge deficit (teaching)

Implementation

- Give after shaking vial; IM in deep muscle mass (glutens only); with 20-gauge needle; no more than 5 ml per site
- Store at room temp; reconstituted sol should be discarded after 24 hr

Evaluation

Positive therapeutic outcome

- Negative gonorrhea culture after treatment

spironolactone (℞)
(speer'on-oh-lak'tone)
Aldactone
Func. class: Potassium-sparing diuretic
Chem. class.: Aldosterone antagonist
Pregnancy category D

Action: Competes with aldosterone at receptor sites in the distal tubule in the renal system, resulting in excretion of sodium, chloride, water, bicarbonate, and calcium; potassium, phosphate, and hydrogen are retained

Therapeutic Outcome: Diuretic and antihypertensive effect while retaining potassium; lowered aldosterone levels

Uses: Edema of CHF, hypertension, diuretic induced hypokalemia, primary hyperaldosteronism (diagnosis, short-term treatment, long-term treatment), edema of nephrotic syndrome, cirrhosis of the liver with ascites

Dosage and routes
Edema/Hypertension
Adult: PO 25-200 mg/qd in single or divided doses
Edema
P ***Child:*** PO 3.3 mg/kg/day in single or divided doses
Hypertension
Child: PO 1-2 mg/kg bid
Hypokalemia
Adult: PO 25-100 mg/day; if PO, K supplements are unable to be used
Primary hyperaldosteronism diagnosis
Adult: PO 400 mg/day × 4 days depending on the test, then 100-400 mg/day maintenance

Available forms: Tabs 25, 50, 100 mg

Adverse effects
CNS: Headache, confusion, drowsiness, lethargy, ataxia
ELECT: Hyperchloremic metabolic acidosis, ***hyperkalemia,*** hyponatremia
ENDO: Impotence, gynecomastia, irregular menses, amenorrhea, postmenopausal bleeding, hirsutism, deepening voice
GI: Diarrhea, cramps, bleeding, gastritis, vomiting
HEMA: Agranulocytosis

Contraindications: Hypersensitivity, anuria, severe renal disease, hyperkalemia, pregnancy **D**

Precautions: Dehydration, hepatic disease, lactation, G elderly, renal disease

Pharmacokinetics

PO	
Absorption	GI tract; well absorbed
Distribution	Crosses placenta
Metabolism	Liver to canrenone (active metabolite)
Excretion	Renal; breast milk
Half-life	12-24 hr (canrenone)

Pharmacodynamics

Onset	24-48 hr
Peak	48-72 hr
Duration	Unknown

Interactions
Individual drugs
Aspirin: ↓ action of spironolactone
Lithium: ↑ action, toxicity
Drug classifications
ACE inhibitors: ↑ hyperkalemia

S

Anticoagulants: ↓ effects of anticoagulants
Antihypertensives: ↑ action
Diuretics, potassium-sparing: ↑ hyperkalemia
Potassium products: ↑ hyperkalemia
Salt substitutes: ↑ hyperkalemia

Food

Potassium foods: ↑ hyperkalemia

Lab test interferences

False ↑ Urinary catecholamines
Inteference: Glucose, insulin tolerance tests

NURSING CONSIDERATIONS

Assessment

- Monitor for manifestations of hyperkalemia: *MS:* fatigue, muscle weakness; *Cardiac:* arrhythmias hypotension, *Neuro:* paresthesias, confusion, *Resp:* dyspnea
- Monitor for manifestations of hyponatremia: *CV:* ↑ B/P, cold, clammy skin, hypo or hypervolemia; *GI:* anorexia, nausea, vomiting, diarrhea, abdominal cramps; *Neuro:* lethargy, increased ICP, confusion headache, seizures, coma, fatigue, tremors, hyperreflexia
- Monitor for manifestations of hyperchloremia: *Neuro:* weakness, lethargy, coma; *Resp:* deep rapid breathing
- Assess fluid volume status: I&O ratios and record, count or weigh diapers as appropriate, weight, distended red veins, crackles in lung, color, quality and sp gr of urine, skin turgor, adequacy of pulses, moist mucous membranes, bilateral lung sounds, peripheral pitting edema; dehydration symptoms of decreasing output, thirst, hypotension, dry mouth and mucous membranes should be reported
- Monitor electrolytes: potassium, sodium, calcium, magnesium; also include BUN, ABGs, uric acid, CBC, blood sugar

Associated nursing diagnoses

- ✓ Urinary elmination, altered (adverse reactions)
- ✓ Fluid volume deficit (adverse reactions)
- ✓ Fluid volume excess (uses)
- ✓ Knowledge deficit (teaching)

Implementation

- Give in AM to avoid interference with sleep
- With food, if nausea occurs, absorption may be increased; take at same time each day

Patient/family education

- Teach patient to take the medication early in the day to prevent nocturia
- Instruct patient to take with food or milk if GI symptoms of nausea and anorexia occur
- Teach patient to maintain a record of weight on a weekly basis and notify prescriber of weight loss of >5 lbs
- Caution patient that this drug causes an increase in potassium levels, that foods high in potassium should be avoided; refer to dietician for assistance planning
- Teach patient not to use alcohol, or any over-the-counter medications without prescriber's approval; serious drug reactions may occur
- Emphasize the need to contact prescriber immediately if muscle cramps, weakness, nausea, dizziness, or numbness ocurs

- Teach patient to take own B/P and pulse and record
- Advise patient that dizziness and confusion may occur; avoid driving or other hazardous activities if alertness is decreased
- Teach patient to continue taking medication even if feeling better; this drug controls symptoms but does not cure the condition
- Advise patient with hypertension to continue other treatment (exercise, weight loss, relaxation techniques, cessation of smoking)

Evaluation

Positive therapeutic outcome

- Prevention of hypokalemia (diuretic use)
- Decreased edema
- Decreased B/P
- Decreased aldosterone levels
- Increased diuresis

Treatment of overdose:

- Lavage if taken orally, monitor electrolytes
- Administer sodium bicarbonate for K^2 6.5 mEq/L
- Monitor hydration, CV, renal status

stavudine (℞)

(sta'vu-deen)

Zerit

Func. class.: Antiviral

Chem. class.: Primidone nucleoside

Pregnancy category C

Action: Prevents replication of HIV by the inhibition of the enzyme reverse transcriptase

➔ **Therapeutic Outcome:** Decreasing diarrhea, fatigue, night sweats; increased body weight

Uses: Treatment of advanced HIV infection for patients who have not responded to other antivirals

Dosage and routes

Adult >60 kg: PO 40 mg q12h up to 2 mg/kg/day

Adult <60 kg: 30 mg q12h

Available forms: Caps 15, 20, 30, 40 mg

Adverse effects

CNS: Peripheral neuropathy

GI: Hepatotoxicity

HEMA: Bone marrow suppression, anemia

INTEG: Rash

MS: Myalgia

Contraindications: Hypersensitivity to this drug or zidovudine, didanosine, zalcitabine; severe peripheral neuropathy

Precautions: Advanced HIV infections, pregnancy, lactation, bone marrow suppression, renal disease, liver disease, folic acid or B_{12} deficiency

Pharmacokinetics	
Absorption	Rapidly absorbed, 82% bioavailability
Distribution	Cerebrospinal fluid
Metabolism	Unknown
Excretion	Kidneys, breast milk
Half-life	Elimination: 1-1.6 hr, intracellular: 3-3.5 hr

Pharmacodynamics	
Onset	Unknown
Peak	1 hr
Duration	Unknown

Interactions

Drug classifications

Myelosuppressants: ↑ myelosuppressor

S

NURSING CONSIDERATIONS
Assessment
- Monitor liver studies: AST (SGOT), ALT (SGPT)
- Monitor blood studies: WBC, diff, RBC, Hct, Hgb, platelets
- Monitor renal studies: urinalysis, protein, blood
- Obtain C&S before drug therapy; drug may be taken as soon as culture is taken; C&S may be taken after therapy
- Monitor bowel pattern before, during treatment
- Monitor fluid overload; drug requires large volume to stay in sol
- Assess for weakness, tremors, confusion, dizziness, psychosis; if these occur, drug may have to be decreased or discontinued

Nursing diagnoses
✓ Infection, risk for (uses)
✓ Knowledge deficit (teaching)

Implementation
- Give with or without meals; absorption does not appear to be lowered when taken with food

Patient/family education
- Teach patient signs of peripheral neuropathy: burning, weakness, pain, pricking feeling in the extremities
- Caution patient that this drug should not be given with antineoplastics
- Inform patient that GI complaints and insomnia resolve after 3-4 wk of treatment
- Inform patient that drug is not a cure for AIDS, but will control symptoms
- Advise patient to call prescriber if sore throat, swollen lymph nodes, malaise, fever occur—may indicate presence of other infections
- Caution patient that even with drug administration, patient is still infective and may pass AIDS virus on to others
- Caution patient that follow-up visits must be continued because serious toxicity may occur, blood counts must be done q2wk
- Teach patient that drug must be taken q4hr around clock even during night
- Caution patient that serious drug interactions may occur if OTC products are ingested; check with prescriber first if taking aspirin, acetaminophen, indomethacin
- Inform patient that other drugs may be necessary to prevent other infections
- Inform patient that drug may cause fainting or dizziness

Evaluation
Positive therapeutic outcome
- Decreased symptoms of HIV

streptokinase 🔑 (℞)
(strep-toe-kye'nase)
Kabikinase, Streptase
Func. class.: Thrombolytic enzyme
Chem. class.: β-Hemolytic streptococcus filtrate (purified)
Pregnancy category C

Action: Activates conversion of plasminogen to plasmin (fibrinolysin): plasmin breaks down clots (fibrin), fibrinogen, factors V, VII; occlusion of venous access lines

➔ **Therapeutic Outcome:** Lysis of emboli, or thrombosis in various parts of the body

Uses: Deep vein thrombosis, pulmonary embolism, arterial thrombosis, arterial embolism, arteriovenous cannula occlusion, lysis of coronary artery thrombi after MI, acute evolving transmural MI

Dosage and routes

Lysis of coronary artery thrombi

Adult: CC 20,000 IU, then 2000 IU/min over 1 hr as **IV** inf

Arteriovenous cannula occlusion

Adult: **IV** inf 250,000 IU/2 ml sol into occluded limb of cannula run over ½ hr; clamp for 2 hr; aspirate contents; flush with NaCl sol and reconnect

Thrombosis/embolism /DVT/ pulmonary embolism

Adult: **IV** inf 250,000 IU over ½ hr, then 100,000 IU/hr for 72 hr for deep thrombosis; 100,000 IU/hr over 24-72 hr for pulmonary embolism; 100,000 IU/hr x 24-72 hr for arterial thrombosis or embolism

Acute evolving transmural MI

Adult: **IV** inf 1,500,000 IU diluted to a volume of 45 ml; give within 1 hr; intracoronary inf 20,000 IU by bol, then 2,000 IU/min x 1 hr, total dose 140,000 IU

Available forms: Powder for inj, lyophilized 250,000, 750,000, 1,500,000 IU vial

Adverse effects

CV: Dysrrhythmias, hypotension, non-cardiogenic pulmonary edema, pulmonary embolism

CNS: Headache, fever

EENT: Periorbital edema

GI: Nausea

HEMA: Decreased Hct, ***bleeding***

INTEG: Rash, urticaria, phlebitis at **IV** inf site, itching, flushing

MS: Low back pain

RESP: Altered respirations, SOB, ***bronchospasm***

SYST: ***GI, GU, intracranial retroperitoneal bleeding, surface bleeding, anaphylaxis***

Contraindications: Hypersensitivity, active bleeding, intraspinal surgery, neoplasms of the CNS, ulcerative colitis, enteritis, severe hypertension, severe renal disease, hepatic disease, hypocoagulation, COPD, subacute bacterial endocarditis, rheumatic valvular disease, cerebral embolism/thrombosis/hemorrhage, intraarterial diagnostic procedure or surgery (10 days), recent major surgery

Precautions: Arterial emboli from left side of heart, pregnancy **C**

Pharmacokinetics	
Absorption	Completely absorbed
Distribution	Unknown
Metabolism	>80%—liver, rapidly cleared by reticuloendothelial system
Excretion	Kidneys
Half-life	35 min

Pharmacodynamics	
Onset	Immediate
Peak	Rapid
Duration	<12 hr

S

Interaction

Individual drugs

Aspirin: ↑ bleeding
Dipyridamole: ↑ bleeding
Heparin: ↑ bleeding
Plicamycin: ↑ bleeding
Valproic acid: ↑ bleeding

Drug classifications
Cephalosporins: ↑ bleeding
Anticoagulants, oral: ↑ bleeding
Nonsteroidal antiinflammatories: ↑ bleeding
Lab test interferences
↑ PT, ↑ APTT, ↑ TT
↓ Plasminogen, ↓ fibrinogen

NURSING CONSIDERATIONS
Assessment
- Monitor VS, B/P, pulse, respirations (including peripheral), neurologic signs, temp at least q4h; temp >104° F (40° C) indicates internal bleeding; monitor rhythm closely; ventricular dysrhythmias may occur with hyperfusion; monitor heart, breath sounds, neuro status, peripheral pulses
- Assess for bleeding during first hr of treatment: hematuria, hematemesis, bleeding from mucous membranes, epistaxis, ecchymosis; guaiac, all body fluids, stools; may require transfusion (rare); blood studies (Hct, platelets, PTT, PT, TT, APTT) before starting therapy; PT or APTT must be less than 2 × control before starting therapy TT or PT q3-4h during treatment
- Assess allergy: fever, rash, itching, chills; mild reaction may be treated with antihistamines; report to prescriber
- Monitor ECG on monitor, watch for segment changes, changes in rhythm; sinus bradycardia, ventricular tachycardia, accelerated idioventricular rhythm may occur as a result of reperfusion (coronary thrombosis)
- Monitor ABGs, respiratory rate, (depth, characteristics), pulse, B/P, hemodynamics (pulmonary embolism)
- Monitor peripheral pulses, assess Homan's sign, check for redness, swelling q hr; notify health care prescriber of changes; B/P should not be taken in extremities (deep vein thrombosis)
- Check catheter for ability to aspirate blood from port; patient must exhale and hold breath when inserting and removing syringe to prevent air embolism (catheter/cannula occlusion)
- Assess for Guillain-Barré syndrome that may occur after treatment with this drug
- Assess for respiratory depression

Nursing diagnoses
- ✓ Tissue perfusion, altered (uses)
- ✓ Injury, risk for (adverse reactions)
- ✓ Impaired gas exchange (uses)
- ✓ Knowledge deficit (teaching)

Implementation
- Give after reconstituting with provided diluent; add appropriate amount of sterile water for inj (no preservatives) 20 mg vial/20 ml or 50 mg vial/50 ml to make 1 mg/ml, mix by slow inversion or dilute with NaCl, D_5W to a concentration of 0.5 mg/ml; further dilution, 1.5 to <0.5 mg/ml may result in precipitation of drug; use 18-gauge needle; flush line with NaCl after administration; reconstituted **IV** solution within 8 hr; within 6 hr of coronary occlusion for best results
- Give **IV** loading dose over 30 min to avoid hypotension
- **IV** after dilution with 4-5 g/250 ml NS, D_5W, LR, give over 1 hr; may give by continuous inf after loading dose(s) of 1 g/hr diluted in 50-100 ml of

compatible sol; use inf pump; do not give by direct **IV**

- Give heparin therapy after thrombolytic therapy is discontinued, TT, ACT, or APTT less than 2 × control (about 3-4 hr); **IV** heparin with loading dose is recommended after discontinuing streptokinase to prevent redevelopment of thrombis
- Avoid invasive procedures, injection, taking temp via rec route
- Apply pressure for 30 sec to minor bleeding sites; 30 min to sites of atrial puncture, followed by pressure dressing; inform prescriber if this does not attain hemostasis; apply pressure dressing
- Store powder at room temp or refrigerate; protect from excessive light

Y-site incompatibilities: Dobutamine, dopamine, heparin, nitroglycerine

Y-site compatibilities: Dobutamine, dopamine, heparin, lidocaine, nitroglycerin

Additive incompatibilities: Do not mix with other medications

Patient/family education

- Teach patient reason for medication, signs and symptoms of bleeding, allergic reactions, when to notify prescriber
- Explain that patient is to remain on bed rest to avoid injury

Evaluation

Positive therapeutic outcome

- Lysis of thrombi or emboli

streptomycin (℞)

(strep-toe-mye'sin)

Func. class.: Antiinfective, antitubercular

Chem. class.: Aminoglycoside

Pregnancy category B

Action: Interferes with protein synthesis in bacterial cell by binding to ribosomal subunit, causing inaccurate peptide sequence to form in protein chain, resulting in bacterial death

Therapeutic Outcome: Bactericidal effects for the following organisms: sensitive strains of *M. tuberculosis*, nontuberculous infections caused by sensitive strains of *Y. pestus, Brucella, H. influenzae, K. pneumoniae, E. coli, E. aerogenes, S. viridans, F. tularensis, Proteus*

Uses: Active TB; used in combination for streptococcal and enterococcal infections; endocarditis, tularemia, plague

Dosage and routes

Tuberculosis

Adult: IM 1 g qd × 2-3 mo, then 1 g 2-3 ×/week given with other antitubercular drugs

P ***Child:*** IM 20-40 mg/kg/day in divided doses given with other antitubercular drugs; max 15 mg/kg/day

Streptococcal endocarditis

Adult: IM 1 g q12h × 1 wk with penicillin, then 500 mg bid × 1 wk

Enterococcal endocarditis

Adult: IM 1 g q12h × 2 wk, then 500 mg q12h × 4 wk with penicillin max 15 mg/kg/day

S

Available forms: Inj 1 g: 400 mg/ml

Adverse effects

CNS: Confusion, depression, numbness, tremors, ***convulsions***, muscle twitching, ***neurotoxicity***

CV: Hypotension, myocarditis, palpitations

EENT: ***Ototoxicity***, deafness, visual disturbances

GI: Nausea, vomiting, anorexia, increased ALT (SGPT), AST (SGOT), bilirubin, hepatomegaly, ***hepatic necrosis***, splenomegaly

GU: ***Oliguria, hematuria, renal damage, azotemia, renal failure, nephrotoxicity***

HEMA: ***Agranulocytosis, thrombocytopenia, leukopenia, eosinophilia, anemia***

INTEG: Rash, burning urticaria, dermatitis, alopecia

Contraindications: Severe renal disease, hypersensitivity

Precautions: Neonates, mild renal disease, pregnancy **B**, myasthenia gravis, lactation, G hearing deficits, elderly, Parkinson's disease

Pharmacokinetics

Absorption:	Well absorbed
Distribution	Widely distributed in extracellular fluids, poorly distributed in CSF; crosses placenta
Metabolism	Minimal—liver
Excretion	Mostly unchanged (>90%) kidneys
Half-life	2-2½ hr, increase in renal disease

Pharmacodynamics

Onset	Rapid
Peak	1-2 hr

Interactions

Individual drugs

Amphotericin B: ↑ Ototoxicity, neurotoxicity, nephrotoxicity

Cisplatin: ↑ Ototoxicity, neurotoxicity, nephrotoxicity

Ethacrynic acid: ↑ Ototoxicity, neurotoxicity, nephrotoxicity

Furosemide: ↑ Ototoxicity, neurotoxicity, nephrotoxicity

Mannitol: ↑ Ototoxicity, neurotoxicity, nephrotoxicity

Methoxyflurane:↑ Ototoxicity, neurotoxicity, nephrotoxicity

Polymyxin: ↑ Ototoxicity, neurotoxicity, nephrotoxicity

Succinylcholine: ↑ Neuromuscular blockade, respiratory depression

Vancomycin: ↑ Ototoxicity, neurotoxicity, nephrotoxicity

Drug classifications

Anesthetics: ↑ Neuromuscular blockade, respiratory depression

Aminoglycosides: ↑ Ototoxicity, neurotoxicity, nephrotoxicity

Nondepolarizing neuromuscular blockers:↑ Neuromuscular blockade, respiratory depression

Penicillins: Inactivated in renal disease

NURSING CONSIDERATIONS

Assessment

- Assess patient for previous sensitivity reaction
- Assess patient for signs and symptoms of infection including characteristics of sputum, urine, stool WBC >10,000, temp
- Obtain baseline information before and during treatment
- Complete C&S testing before and beginning drug therapy—this will identify if correct treatment has been initiated

- Assess for allergic reactions: rash, urticaria, pruritus, chills, fever, joint pain; angioedema may occur a few days after therapy begins—epinephrine, resuscitation equipment should be on unit for anaphylactic reaction
- Identify urine output; if decreasing, notify prescriber (may indicate nephrotoxicity); also, increased BUN, creatinine, urine CrCl <80 ml/min
- Monitor blood studies: AST (SGOT), ALT (SGPT), CBC, Hct, bilirubin, LDH, alk phosphatase, Coombs' test monthly if patient is on long-term therapy
- Monitor electrolytes: potassium, sodium, chloride, magnesium monthly if patient is on long-term therapy
- Monitor for bleeding: ecchymosis, bleeding gums, hematuria, stool guaiac daily if on long-term therapy
- Assess for overgrowth of infection: perineal itching, fever, malaise, redness, pain, swelling, drainage, rash, diarrhea, change in cough, sputum
- Obtain weight before treatment; calculation of dosage is usually based on ideal body weight, but may be calculated on actual body weight
- Monitor I&O ratio; urinalysis daily for proteinuria, cells, casts; report sudden change in urine output
- Obtain serum peak 60 min after IM inj, trough level drawn just before next dose; blood level should be 2-4 times bacteriostatic level
- Monitor for deafness by audiometric testing, ringing, roaring in ears, vertigo; assess hearing before, during, after treatment
- Monitor for dehydration: high sp gr, decrease in skin turgor, dry mucous membranes, dark urine
- Monitor for overgrowth of infection including increased temp, malaise, redness, pain, swelling, perineal itching, diarrhea, stomatitis, change in cough, sputum

Nursing diagnoses

- ✓ Infection, risk for (uses)
- ✓ Diarrhea (adverse reactions)
- ✓ Injury, risk for (adverse reactions)
- ✓ Knowledge deficit (teaching)
- ✓ Noncompliance (teaching)

Implementation

- Give deeply in large muscle mass
- Reconstitute with 4.2-4.5 ml sterile water for inj or 0.9% NaCl/1 g (200 mg/ml); 3.2-3.5 ml/1 g (250 mg/ml); 17 ml/5 g (250 mg/ml) (500 mg/ml); give at 500 mg/ml or less

Additive compatibility:
Bleomycin

Y-site compatibility:
Esmolol

Syringe compatibility:
Penicillin G sodium

Syringe incompatibility:
Heparin

Patient/family education

- Teach patient to report sore throat, bruising, bleeding, joint pain, (may indicate blood dyscrasias—rare), ringing, roaring in the ears
- Advise patient to contact prescriber if vaginal itching, loose, foul-smelling stools, furry tongue occur—may indicate superimposed infection

S

Evaluation

Positive therapeutic outcome

- Absence of signs/symptoms of infection
- Reported improvement in symptoms of infection

Treatment of overdose: Withdraw drug, hemodialysis, monitor serum levels of drug, may give ticarcillin or carbenicillin

streptozocin (℞)

(strep-toe-zoe'sin)

Zanosar

Func. class.: Antineoplastic alkylating agent

Chem. class.: Nitrosourea

Pregnancy category C

Action: Alkylates DNA, RNA; inhibits enzymes that allow synthesis of amino acids in proteins; is also responsible for cross-linking DNA strands; activity is not specific to phase of cell cycle

Therapeutic Outcome: Prevention of rapidly growing malignant cells, decreased calcium levels

Uses: Metastatic islet cell carcinoma of pancreas

Investigational uses: Prevention of spread of Hodgkin's disease, metastatic carcinoid tumor, pancreatic adenocarcinoma colon malignancies

Dosage and routes

Adult: **IV** 500 mg/m^2 × 5 days q6 wk until desired response; or 1 g/m^2 qwk × 2 wk, not to exceed 1.5 g/m^2 in 1 dose

Available forms: Powder for inj 1 g

Adverse effects

CNS: Confusion, depression, lethargy

GI: Nausea, vomiting, diarrhea, weight loss, ***hepatotoxicity***

GU: ***Nephrogenic diabetes insipidus***

HEMA: ***Thrombocytopenia, leukopenia, pancytopenia***

Contraindications: Hypersensitivity

Precautions: Radiation therapy, children, lactation, pregnancy **C,** hepatic disease, renal disease

Pharmacokinetics	
Absorption	Complete bioavailability
Distribution	Rapid, crosses placenta
Metabolism	Liver, kidneys—extensively
Excretion	<20% kidneys unchanged
Half-life	35-40 min

Pharmacodynamics	
Onset	Unknown
Peak	Unknown
Duration	Unknown

Interactions

Individual drugs

Doxorubicin: ↑ toxicity

Phenytoin: ↑ toxicity

Radiation: ↑ toxicity, bone marrow suppression

Drug classifications

Aminoglycosides: ↑ risk of nephrotoxicity

Antineoplastics: ↑ toxicity, bone marrow suppression

Live virus vaccines: ↓ antibody response

NURSING CONSIDERATIONS

Assessment

- Assess symptoms indicating severe allergic reaction: rash, pruritus, urticaria, purpuric skin lesions, itching, flushing
- Monitor CBC, differential,

platelet count weekly; withhold drug if WBC count is $<4000/\text{mm}^3$ or platelet count is $<100{,}000/\text{mm}^3$, notify prescriber of results if WBC $<20{,}000/\text{mm}^3$, platelets $<50{,}800/\text{mm}^3$

- Monitor renal function studies: BUN, creatinine, serum uric acid, urine CrCl before and during therapy; I&O ratio; report fall in urine output to <30 ml/hr
- Monitor temp q4hr (may indicate beginning of infection)
- Monitor liver function tests before and during therapy [bilirubin, AST (SGOT), ALT (SGPT), LDH] as needed or monthly; yellowing of skin, sclera, dark urine, clay-colored stools, itchy skin, abdominal pain, fever, diarrhea
- Assess for bleeding: hematuria, stool guaiac, bruising or petechiae, mucosa or orifices q8hr; inflammation of mucosa, breaks in skin
- Identify edema in feet, joint pain, stomach pain, shaking; health care prescriber should be notified
- Identify inflammation of mucosa, breaks in skin

Nursing diagnoses

- ✓ Injury, risk for (adverse reactions)
- ✓ Body image disturbance (adverse reactions)
- ✓ Infection, risk for (adverse reactions)
- ✓ Knowledge deficit (teaching)

Implementation

- Hypoglycemia may occur, have **IV** dextrose available
- Give fluids **IV** or PO before chemotherapy to hydrate patient
- Give antiemetic 30-60 min before giving drug to prevent vomiting, and prn
- Give antibiotics for prophylaxis of infection
- Give topical or systemic analgesics for pain
- Provide liq diet: carbonated beverages; gelatin may be added if patient is not nauseated or vomiting
- Provide rinsing of mouth tid-qid with water, club soda; brushing of teeth bid-qid with soft brush or cotton-tipped applicators for stomatitis; use unwaxed dental floss
- Give **IV** after diluting 1 g/9.5 ml 0.9% NaCl or D_5 (100 mg/ml)
- May be further diluted with 10-200 ml 0.9% NaCl, D_5W give over prescribed rate, usually 15 min

Y-site compatibilities: Filgrastim, melphalan, ondansetron, teniposide, vinorelbine

Patient/family education

- Inform patient that contraceptive measures are recommended during therapy
- Caution patient to avoid use of products containing aspirin or ibuprofen, razors, commercial mouthwash—bleeding may occur; to report symptoms of bleeding (hematuria, tarry stools)
- Instruct patient to report signs of anemia, (fatigue, headache, irritability, faintness, shortness of breath)
- Caution patient not to have any vaccinations without the advice of the prescriber, serious reactions can occur

Evaluation

Positive therapeutic outcome

- Prevention of rapid division of malignant cells

S

succimer (℞)
(sux'i-mer)
Chemet
Func. class: Heavy metal antagonist
Chem. class.: Chelating agent
Pregnancy category C

Action: Binds with ions of lead to form a water-soluble complex that is excreted by kidneys

Therapeutic Outcome: Removal of lead from the body

Uses: Lead poisoning in children with lead levels above 45 µg/dl; may be beneficial in mercury, arsenic poisoning

Dosage and routes

P ***Child:*** PO 10 mg/kg or 350 mg/m^2 q8h × 5 days, then 10 mg/kg or 350 mg/m^2 q12h × 2 wk; another course may be required depending on lead levels; allow 2 wk between courses

Available forms: Cap 100 mg

Adverse effects

CNS: Drowsiness, dizziness, paresthesia, sensorimotor neuropathy
EENT: Otitis media, watery eyes, film in eyes, plugged ears
*GI: **Nausea, vomiting, diarrhea, metallic taste, anorexia***
*GU: **Proteinuria,*** decreased urination, voiding difficulties
HEMA: Increased platelets, intermittent eosinophilia
INTEG: Rash, urticaria, pruritus
META: Increased AST (SGOT), ALT (SGPT), alk phosphatase, cholesterol
RESP: Sore throat, rhinorrhea, nasal congestion, cough
SYST: Back, stomach, head, rib, flank pain; abdominal cramps; chills; fever; flulike symptoms, head cold; headache

Contraindications: Hypersensitivity

Precautions: Pregnancy **C,** P lactation, children <1 yr

Pharmacokinetics

Absorption	Rapidly absorbed
Distribution	Unknown
Metabolism	Liver—extensively
Excretion	Kidneys—unchanged
Half-life	2 days

Pharmacodynamics

Onset	Up to 2 hr
Peak	2-4 hr
Duration	8-12 hr

Interactions

Drug classifications

Heavy metal antagonist, others: Do not use together

NURSING CONSIDERATIONS

Assessment

- Assess VS, B/P, pulse, respirations, weigh daily
- Monitor I&O, kidney function studies, BUN, creatinine, CrCl; watch for decreasing urine output
- Assess neuro status: watch for paresthesias, beginning convulsions
- Monitor urine: pH, albumin, casts, blood, coproporphyrins, calcium
- Assess for febrile reactions that may occur 4-8 hr following drug therapy
- Monitor for cardiac abnormalities: dysrhythmias, hypotension, tachycardia
- Assess for allergic reactions (rash, urticaria); if these occur, drug should be discontinued

Nursing diagnoses

✓ Poisoning, risk for (uses)

✓ Injury, risk for (uses, adverse reactions)
✓ Knowledge deficit (teaching)

Implementation

- Give PO whole or cap contents mixed with food or fluid

Patient/family education

- Explain reason for medication and expected results
- Provide a referral to health department to assess lead levels in home or workplace

Evaluation

Positive therapeutic outcome

- Decreased symptoms of lead intoxication
- Decreased lead level <50 μg/dl

succinylcholine (℞)

(suk-sin-ill-koe'leen)

Anectine, Anectine Flo-Pack, Quelicin, succinylcholine chloride, Sucostrin, Suxamethonium

Func. class.: Neuromuscular blocker (depolarizing—ultra short)

Pregnancy category C

Action: Inhibits transmission of nerve impulses by binding with cholinergic receptor sites, antagonizing action of acetylcholine; causes release of histamine

➔ **Therapeutic Outcome:** Paralysis of skeletal muscles

Uses: Facilitation of endotracheal intubation, skeletal muscle relaxation during orthopedic manipulations

Dosage and routes

Adult: **IV** 25-75 mg, then 2.5 mg/min as needed; IM 2.5 mg/kg, not to exceed 150 mg

P ***Child:*** **IV**/IM 1-2 mg/kg, not to exceed 150 mg IM

Available forms: Inj 20, 50, 100 mg/ml; powder for inj 100/vial; powder for inf 500 mg/vial, 1 g/vial

Adverse effects

CV: Bradycardia, tachycardia; increased, decreased B/P, ***sinus arrest, dysrhythmias***

EENT: Increased secretions, increased IOP

HEMA: ***Myoglobulinemia***

INTEG: Rash, flushing, pruritus, urticaria

MS: Weakness, muscle pain, fasciculation, prolonged relaxation

RESP: ***Prolonged apnea, bronchospasm, cyanosis, respiratory depression***

Contraindications: Hypersensitivity, malignant hyperthermia, decreased plasma pseudocholinesterase, penetrating eye injuries, acute narrow-angle glaucoma

Precautions: Pregnancy **C,** cardiac disease, severe burns, fractures—fasciculation may increase damage—lactation, P children <2 yr, electrolyte imbalances, dehydration, neuromuscular disease, respiratory disease, collagen diseases, glaucoma, eye surgery, penetrating eye wounds, G elderly or debilitated patients

Pharmacokinetics

Absorption	Well absorbed (IM)
Distribution	Widely distributed, crosses placenta
Metabolism	Plasma (90%)
Excretion	Hydrolyzed in urine (active/inactive metabolites)
Half-life	Unknown

Pharmacodynamics

	IV	IM
Onset	1 min	2-3 min
Peak	2-3 min	Unknown
Duration	6-10 min	10-30 min

Interactions

Individual drugs

Clindamycin: ↑ neuromuscular blockade
Enflurane: ↑ neuromuscular blockade
Isofluorophate: ↑ paralysis
Isoflurane: ↑ neuromuscular blockade
Lincomycin: ↑ neuromuscular blockade
Quinidine: ↑ neuromuscular blockade

Drug classifications

Aminoglycosides: ↑ neuromuscular blockade
β-Blockers: ↑ neuromuscular blockade
Local anesthetics: ↑ neuromuscular blockade
Magnesium salts: ↑ neuromuscular blockade
Polymyxin antibiotics: ↑ neuromuscular blockade
Diuretics, potassium-losing: ↑ neuromuscular blockade

NURSING CONSIDERATIONS

Assessment

- Assess for electrolyte imbalances (potassium, magnesium); may lead to increased action of this drug
- Monitor vital signs (B/P, pulse, respirations, airway) until fully recovered; rate, depth, pattern of respirations, strength of hand grip
- Monitor I&O ratio; check for urinary retention, frequency, hesitancy
- Assess for recovery: decreased paralysis of face, diaphragm, leg, arm, rest of body
- Assess for allergic reactions: rash, fever, respiratory distress, pruritus; drug should be discontinued if these occur

Nursing diagnoses

- ✓ Communication, impaired verbal (adverse reactions)
- ✓ Breathing pattern, ineffective (uses)

Implementation

IV route

- Use nerve stimulator by anesthesiologist to determine neuromuscular blockade
- Give anticholinesterase to reverse neuromuscular blockade
- Give by **IV** inf; dilute 1-2 mg/ml in D_5, isotonic saline sol, give 0.5-10 mg/min, titrate to patient response; may be given directly over 1 min

Syringe compatibility:
Heparin

Y-site compatibilities:
Etomidate, potassium chloride, vitamin B with C

Additive compatibilities:
Amikacin, cephapirin, isoproterenol, meperidine, methyldopate, morphine, norepinephrine, scopolamine

Additive incompatibilities:
Barbiturates, nafcillin, sodium bicarbonate

IM route

- Give deep IM, preferably high in deltoid muscle
- Store in refrigerator; store powder at room temp; close container tightly

Patient/family education

- Explain reason for medication and expected results
- Provide reassurance if communication is difficult during

recovery from neuromuscular blockade; postoperative stiffness is normal, soon subsides

Evaluation

Positive therapeutic outcome

• Paralysis of jaw, eyelid, head, neck, rest of body

Treatment of overdose: Edrophonium or neostigmine, atropine, monitor VS; may require mechanical ventilation

sucralfate (℞)

(soo-kral'fate)

Carafate, Sulcrate ✦

Func. class.: Protectant; antiulcer

Chem. class.: Aluminum hydroxide/sulfated sucrose

Pregnancy category B

Action: Forms a complex that adheres to ulcer site, adsorbs pepsin

➔ **Therapeutic Outcome:** Healing of ulcers

Uses: Duodenal ulcer, oral mucositis, stomatitis after radiation of head and neck

Investigational uses: Gastric ulcers, gastroesophageal reflux

Dosage and routes

Adult: PO 1 g qid 1 hr ac, hs

Available forms: Tab 1 g; oral susp 500 mg/5 ml ✦

Adverse effects

CNS: Drowsiness, dizziness

GI: Dry mouth, constipation, nausea, gastric pain, vomiting

INTEG: Urticaria, rash, pruritus

Contraindications: Hypersensitivity

Precautions: Pregnancy **B**,
P lactation, children

Pharmacokinetics

Absorption	Minimally absorbed
Distribution	Unknown
Metabolism	Not metabolized
Excretion	Feces (90%)
Half-life	6-20 hr

Pharmacodynamics

Onset	½ hr
Peak	Unknown
Duration	5 hr

Interactions

Individual drugs

Phenytoin: ↓ absorption

Tetracycline: ↓ absorption

Drug classifications

Fluoroquinolones: ↓ absorption

Fat-soluble vitamins: ↓ absorption

NURSING CONSIDERATIONS

Assessment

• Monitor gastric pH (>5 should be maintained)

Nursing diagnoses

✓ Pain, chronic (uses)
✓ Pain (uses)
✓ Constipation (adverse reactions)
✓ Knowledge deficit (teaching)

Implementation

• Give on empty stomach 1 hr ac and hs

• Storage at room temp

Patient/family education

• Advise patient to avoid black pepper, caffeine, alcohol, harsh spices, extremes in temp of food—may aggravate condition

• Instruct patient to take medication on empty stomach

• Caution patient to take full course of therapy

• Caution patient to avoid

S

antacids within ½ hr of drug or 1 hr after this drug

Evaluation

Positive therapeutic outcome

- Absence of pain or GI complaints

sufentanil (℞)

(soo-fen'ta-nil)

Sufenta

Func. class.: Narcotic analgesic

Chem. class.: Opiate, synthetic

Pregnancy category C

Controlled substance schedule II

Action: Inhibits ascending pain pathways in CNS, increases pain threshold, alters pain perception

Therapeutic Outcome: Anesthesia, decreased pain

Uses: Primary anesthetic, adjunct to general anesthetic

Dosage and routes

Primary anesthetic

***Adult:* IV** 8-30 μg/kg given with 100% O_2, a muscle relaxant

Adjunct

***Adult:* IV** 1-8 μg/kg given with nitrous oxide/O_2

Available forms: Inj 50 μg/ml

Adverse effects

CNS: ***Drowsiness, dizziness, confusion, headache, sedation, euphoria***

CV: Palpitations, bradycardia, change in B/P

EENT: Tinnitus, blurred vision, miosis, diplopia

GI: ***Nausea, vomiting, anorexia, constipation, abdominal cramps***

GU: Increased urinary output, dysuria, urinary retention

INTEG: *Rash*, urticaria, bruising, flushing, diaphoresis, pruritus

RESP: ***Respiratory depression***

Contraindications: Hypersensitivity, addiction (narcotic)

Precautions: Addictive personality, pregnancy **C,** lactation, increased intracranial pressure, MI (acute), severe heart disease, respiratory depression, hepatic disease, renal disease, P child <18 yr

Pharmacokinetics

Absorption	Completely absorbed
Distribution	Crosses placenta
Metabolism	Liver—extensively, small intestines—small amount
Excretion	Kidneys, breast milk
Half-life	2½ hr

Pharmacodynamics

Onset	1½-3 hr
Peak	Unknown
Duration	5 min

Interactions

Individual drugs

Alcohol: ↑ respiratory depression, hypotension, ↑ sedation

Cimetidine: ↑ recovery

Erythromycin: ↑ recovery

Nalbuphine: ↓ analgesia

Pentazocine: ↓ analgesia

Drug classifications

Antihistamines: ↑ respiratory depression, hypotension

CNS depressants: ↑ respiratory depression, hypotension

MAOIs: Do not use 2 wk before alfentanil

Phenothiazines: ↑ respiratory depression, hypotension

Sedative/hypnotics: ↑ respiratory depression, hypotension

Lab test interferences
↑ Amylase

NURSING CONSIDERATIONS
Assessment
- Monitor VS after parenteral route; note muscle rigidity, drug history, liver, kidney function tests
- Monitor respiratory dysfunction: respiratory depression, character, rate, rhythm; notify prescriber if respirations are <10/min
- Monitor for CNS changes: dizziness, drowsiness, hallucinations, euphoria, LOC, pupil reaction
- Monitor allergic reactions: rash, urticaria

Nursing diagnoses
✓ Pain (uses)
✓ Sensory perceptual alteration: visual, auditory (adverse reactions)
✓ Breathing pattern, ineffective (adverse reactions)
✓ Knowledge deficit (teaching)

Implementation
- Give by inj (IM, **IV**), only with resuscitative equipment available; give slowly to prevent rigidity
- Give **IV** undiluted by anesthesiologist or diluted as an inf in 0.9% NaCl
- Store in light-resistant area at room temp

Patient/family education
- Advise patient to report any symptoms of CNS changes, allergic reactions
- Caution patient to avoid CNS depressants: alcohol, sedative/hypnotics for at least 24 hr after this drug
- Discuss with patient that dizziness, drowsiness, and confusion are common, to avoid getting up without assistance
- Discuss in detail all aspects of the drug

Evaluation
Positive therapeutic outcome
- Maintenance of anesthesia

Treatment of overdose:
Narcan 0.2-0.8 **IV**, O_2, **IV** fluids, vasopressors

sulfamethoxazole (℞)
(sul-fa-meth-ox'a-zole)
Apo-Sulfamethoxazole ✱, Gantanol
Func. class.: Antiinfective
Chem. class.: Sulfonamide, intermediate-acting
Pregnancy category C

Action: Interferes with bacterial biosynthesis of proteins by competitive antagonism of PABA

➡ **Therapeutic Outcome:** Bactericidal action against susceptible organisms: Streptococci and staphylococci, *Clostridium perfringens, Clostridium tetani, Nocardia asteroides;* active against gram-negative pathogens, including *Enterobacter, Escherichia coli, Klebsiella, Proteus mirabilis, Proteus vulgaris, Salmonella, Shigella*

Uses: UTIs, chancroid, inclusion conjunctivitis, malaria, meningococcal meningitis, nocardiosis, acute otitis media, toxoplusmosis, trachoma

Dosage and routes
Adult: PO 2 g, then 1 g bid or tid for 7-10 days
P ***Child >2 mo:*** PO 50-60 mg/kg then 25-30 mg/kg

S

bid, not to exceed 75 mg/kg/day

Lymphogranuloma venereum

Adult: PO 1 g bid × 14 days

Available forms: Tab 500 mg

Adverse effects

CNS: Headache, insomnia, hallucinations, depression, vertigo, fatigue, anxiety, convulsions, drug fever, chills, drowsiness

*CV: **Allergic myocarditis***

GI: Nausea, vomiting, abdominal pain, stomatitis, ***hepatitis,*** glossitis, pancreatitis, diarrhea, ***enterocolitis,*** anorexia

*GU: **Renal failure, toxic nephrosis,*** increased BUN, creatinine, crystalluria, hematuria, proteinuria

*HEMA: **Leukopenia, thrombocytopenia, agranulocytosis, hemolytic anemia, aplastic anemia***

INTEG: Rash, dermatitis, urticaria, ***Stevens-Johnson syndrome,*** erythema, photosensitivity, alopecia

*SYST: **Anaphylaxis***

Contraindications: Hypersensitivity to sulfonamides, sulfonylureas, thiazide and loop diuretics, salicylates, sunscreen with PABA, lactation, **P** infants <2 mo (except congenital toxoplasmosis), pregnancy at term

Precautions: Pregnancy **C**, lactation, impaired hepatic function, severe allergy, bronchial asthma

Pharmacokinetics	
Absorption	Well absorbed
Distribution	Widely distributed, crosses placenta
Metabolism	Liver, large amounts
Excretion	Unchanged kidneys (20%), enters breast milk
Half-life	7-12 hr

Pharmacodynamics	
Onset	1 hr
Peak	3-4 hr

Interactions

Individual drugs

Cyclosporine: ↑ nephrotoxicity

Indomethacin: ↑ drug-free concentrations

Methotrexate: ↑ toxicity

Phenytoin: ↑ folic acid deficiency

Probenicid: ↑ drug-free concentrations

Tolbutamide: ↑ effect

Drug classifications

Anticoagulants, oral: ↑ effects of anticoagulant

Barbiturates: ↑ effects

Hypoglycemics, oral: ↑ effects of hypoglycemics

Salicylates: ↑ drug-free concentrations

Thiazide diuretics: ↑ thrombocytopenia

Uricosurics: ↑ effect

Lab test interferences

False positive: Urinary glucose test

NURSING CONSIDERATIONS

Assessment

- Assess patient for previous sensitivity reaction
- Assess patient for signs and symptoms of infection including characteristics of wounds, sputum, urine, stool, WBC >10,000, elevated temp; obtain baseline information before and during treatment

• Complete C & S studies before beginning drug therapy to identify if correct treatment has been initiated
• Assess for allergic reactions: rash, urticaria, pruritus, chills, fever, joint pain; angioedema may occur a few days after therapy begins; epinephrine, resuscitation equipment should be on unit for anaphylactic reaction—AIDS patients are more susceptible
• Monitor blood studies: CBC, Hct, bilirubin, alk phosphatase, monthly if patient is on long-term therapy
• Monitor for bleeding: ecchymosis, bleeding gums, hematuria, stool guaiac daily if patient is on long-term therapy
• Assess for overgrowth of infection: perineal itching, fever, malaise, redness, pain, swelling, drainage, rash, diarrhea, change in cough, sputum

Nursing diagnoses

✓ Infection, risk for (uses)
✓ Diarrhea (adverse reactions)
✓ Injury, risk for (adverse reactions)
✓ Knowledge deficit (teaching)
✓ Noncompliance (teaching)

Implementation

• Give around the clock to maintain proper blood levels; give on empty stomach to increase absorption of drug; do not give within 3 hr of other agents, drug actions may occur
• Give with 8 oz of water to prevent crystalluria

Patient/family education

• Teach patient to report sore throat, bruising, bleeding, joint pain—may indicate blood dyscrasias (rare)
• Advise patient to contact prescriber if vaginal itching, loose, foul-smelling stools, furry tongue occur—may indicate superinfection; report itching, rash, pruritus, urticaria
• Instruct patient to take all medication prescribed for the length of time ordered; drug must be taken around the clock to maintain blood levels; do not give medication to others

Evaluation

Positive therapeutic outcome

• Absence of signs/symptoms of infection (WBC <10,000, temp WNL, absence of urinary pain, hematuria)
• Reported improvement in symptoms of infection
• Negative C&S

sulfasalazine (℞)

(sul-fa-sal′a-zeen)

Azulfidine, Azulfidine EN-Tabs, PMS-Sulfusalazine ♣, S.A.S. ♣, Salazopyrin ♣, sulfasalazine

Func. class.: Antiinflammatory

Chem. class.: Sulfonamide

Pregnancy category C

Action: Prodrug to deliver sulfapyridine and 5-aminosalicylic acid to colon; antinflammatory in connective tissue

➔ **Therapeutic Outcome:** Treatment of ulcerative colitis, rheumatoid arthritis

Uses: Ulcerative colitis, rheumatoid arthritis (delayed rel tab) in patients who inadequately respond to or are intolerant of analgesics/NSAIDs

Investigational uses: Ankylosing spondylitis, collagenous colitis, Crohn's disease, psoriasis

Dosage and routes

Adult: PO 3-4 g/day in divided doses; maintenance 1.5-2 g/day in divided doses q6h

Child >2 yr: PO 40-60 mg/kg/day in 4-6 divided doses, then 20-30 mg/kg/day in 4 doses, max 2 g/day

Rheumatoid Arthritis

Adult: PO 2 g/day in evenly divided doses, initiate treatment with a lower dose of enteric-coated tab

Available forms: Tab 500 mg

Adverse effects

CNS: Headache, confusion, insomnia, hallucinations, depression, vertigo, fatigue, anxiety, ***convulsions***, drug fever, chills

CV: Allergic myocarditis

GI: Nausea, vomiting, abdominal pain, stomatitis, ***hepatitis***, glossitis, pancreatitis, diarrhea, anorexia

GU: Renal failure, toxic nephrosis, increased BUN, creatinine, crystalluria

Contraindications: Hypersensitivity to sulfonamides or salicylates, pregnancy at term, P child <2 yr, intestinal, urinary obstruction

Precautions: Pregnancy **C**, lactation, impaired hepatic function, severe allergy, bronchial asthma, impaired renal function

Pharmacokinetics	
Absorption	Partially absorbed
Distribution	Crosses placenta
Metabolism	Liver
Excretion	Kidneys, breast milk
Half-life	6 hr

Pharmacodynamics	
Onset	1 hr
Peak	1½-6 hr
Duration	6-12 hr

Interactions

Individual drugs

Digoxin: ↓ effectiveness

Methotrexate: ↓ renal excretion

Phenytoin: ↓ hepatic clearance

Drug classifications

Hypoglycemics, oral: ↑ toxicity

Anticoagulants, oral: ↑ toxicity

Food

Iron, folic acid will be poorly absorbed

Lab test interferences

False positive: Urinary glucose test

NURSING CONSIDERATIONS

Assessment

- Monitor I&O ratio; note color, amount, character, pH of urine if drug administered for urinary tract infections; output should be 800 ml less than intake; if urine is highly acidic, alkalization may be needed
- Monitor kidney function studies: BUN, creatinine, urinalysis if on long-term therapy
- Monitor blood dyscrasias: skin rash, fever, sore throat, bruising, bleeding, fatigue, joint pain; monitor CBC before and q3mo
- Assess for allergic reaction: rash, dermatitis, urticaria, pruritus, dyspnea, bronchospasm

Nursing diagnoses

- ✓ Injury, risk for (uses)
- ✓ Knowledge deficit (teaching)

Implementation

- Give with full glass of water to maintain adequate hydration; increase fluids to 2 L/day to decrease crystallization in kidneys; contact lens, urine, skin may be yellow-orange
- Give total daily dose in evenly spaced doses and after meals to help minimize GI intolerance
- Store in tight, light-resistant container at room temp

Patient/family education

- Advise patient to take each oral dose with full glass of H_2O to prevent crystalluria
- Teach patient to avoid sunlight or to use sunscreen to prevent burns
- Teach patient to avoid OTC medication (aspirin, vit C) unless directed by prescriber
- Advise patient to notify prescriber if skin rash, sore throat, fever, mouth sores, unusual bruising, bleeding occur
- Advise patient to use rectal susp at hs and retain all night

Evaluation

Positive therapeutic outcome

- Absence of fever, mucus in stools or pain in joints

sulfinpyrazone (℞)

(sul-fin-peer′a-zone)

Anturane, Sulfinpyrazone

Func. class.: Uricosuric

Chem. class.: Pyrazolone

Pregnancy category C

Action: Inhibits tubular reabsorption of urates, with increased excretion of uric acid; inhibits prostaglandin synthesis, which decreases platelet aggregation

➔ **Therapeutic Outcome:** Decreased uric acid levels, absence of platelet aggregation

Uses: Inhibition of platelet aggregation, gout

Dosage and routes

Inhibition of platelet aggregation

Adult: PO 200 mg qid

Gout/gouty arthritis

Adult: PO 100-200 mg bid × 1 wk, then 200-400 mg bid, not to exceed 800 mg/day

Available forms: Tab 100 mg; cap 200 mg

Adverse effects

CNS: Dizziness, ***convulsions, coma***

EENT: Tinnitus

GI: Gastric irritation, nausea, vomiting, anorexia, ***hepatic necrosis,*** GI bleeding

GU: Renal calculi, hypoglycemia

HEMA: ***Agranulocytosis*** (rare)

INTEG: Rash, dermatitis, pruritus, fever, photosensitivity

RESP: ***Apnea,*** irregular respirations

Contraindications: Hypersensitivity to pyrazolone derivatives, blood dyscrasias, CrCl <50 ml/min, active peptic ulcer, GI inflammation

Precautions: Pregnancy **C**

Pharmacokinetics	
Absorption	Well absorbed
Distribution	Unknown
Metabolism	Liver
Excretion	Feces (metabolites/active drug)
Half-life	4 hr

S

Pharmacodynamics	
Onset	Unknown
Peak	1-2 hr
Duration	4-6 hr

Interactions

Individual drugs:

Acetaminophen: ↑ toxicity
Aspirin: ↑ risk of bleeding
Cefamandole: ↑ risk of bleeding
Cefoperazone: ↑ risk of bleeding
Cefotetan: ↑ risk of bleeding
Niacin: ↓ effect of sulfinpyrazone
Nitrofurantoin: ↑ effect of sulfinpyrazone
Plicamycin: ↑ risk of bleeding
Theophylline: ↓ effect of sulfinpyrazone
Theophylline: ↓ effect of theophylline
Tolbutamide: ↑ effect of tolbutamide
Warfarin: ↑ effect of warfarin
Valproic acid: ↑ risk of bleeding
Verapamil: ↓ effect of sulfinpyrazone

Drug classifications

Antiinflammatories: ↑ risk of bleeding
Anticoagulants: ↑ risk of bleeding
Salicylates: ↓ effect of sulfinpyrazone
Thrombolytics: ↑ risk of bleeding

Lab test interferences

↑ Alk phosphatase, ↑ AST (SGPT) /ALT (SGOT)
False positive: RBC, Hgb

NURSING CONSIDERATIONS

Assessment

- Monitor I&O ratio; observe for decrease in urinary output; increase fluids to 2-3 L/day
- Monitor CBC, platelets, reticulocytes before, during therapy (q3mo)
- Assess mobility, joint pain, and swelling in the joints

Nursing diagnoses

✓ Pain, chronic (uses)
✓ Immobility, impaired physical (uses)
✓ Knowledge deficit (teaching)

Implementation

- Give with food or antacid to decrease GI upset
- Reduce dose gradually if uric acid levels are normal after 6 mo

Patient/family education

- Advise patient to increase fluids to 3-4 L/day
- Caution patient to avoid alcohol, OTC preparationsthat contain alcohol—skin rashes may occur
- Advise patient to report any pain, redness, or hard area, usually in legs
- Instruct patient on importance of complying with medical regimen; bone marrow depression may occur

Evaluation

Positive therapeutic outcome

- Decreased pain in joints
- Normal serum uric acid levels
- Increased duration of antiinfectives

sulfisoxazole (℞)
(sul-fi-sox′a-zole)
Gantrisin, Novosoxazole ✦, sulfisoxazole
Func. class.: Antiinfective
Chem. class.: Sulfonamide, short-acting
Pregnancy category C

Action: Interferes with bacterial biosynthesis of proteinsby competitive antagonism of PABA

Therapeutic Outcome: Bactericidal action against susceptible organisms; gram-positive pathogens, including *Streptococci* and *Staphylococci, Clostridium perfringens, Clostridium tetani, Nocardia asteroides;* active against gram-negative pathogens, including *Enterobacter, Escherichia coli, Klebsiella, Proteus mirabilis, Proteus vulgaris, Salmonella, Shigella*

Uses: Urinary tract; chancroid; trachoma; toxoplasmosis; acute otitis media; malaria, *H. influenzae,* meningitis, meningococcal meningitis, nocardiosis

Dosage and routes
Adult: PO 2-4 g loading dose, then 1-2 g qid × 7-10 days
P ***Child >2 mo:*** PO 75 mg/kg or 2 g/m² loading dose, then 120-150 mg/kg/day or 4 g/m²/day in divided doses q6h, not to exceed 6 g/day

Available forms: Tab 500 mg

Adverse effects
CNS: Headache, insomnia, hallucinations, depression, vertigo, fatigue, anxiety, ***convulsions,*** drug fever, chills, drowsiness
CV: ***Allergic myocarditis***
GI: Nausea, vomiting, abdominal pain, stomatitis, ***hepatitis,*** glossitis, pancreatitis, diarrhea, ***enterocolitis,*** anorexia
GU: ***Renal failure, toxic nephrosis,*** increased BUN, creatinine, crystalluria, hematuria, proteinuria
HEMA: ***Leukopenia, thrombocytopenia, agranulocytosis, hemolytic anemia, aplastic anemia***
INTEG: Rash, dermatitis, urticaria, ***Stevens-Johnson syndrome,*** erythema, photosensitivity, alopecia
SYST: ***Anaphylaxis***

Contraindications: Hypersensitivity to sulfonamides and sulfonylureas, thiazide and loop diuretics, salicylates; sunscreen with PABA,
P lactation, infants <2 mo (except congenital toxoplasmosis); pregnancy at term

Precautions: Pregnancy **C,** lactation, impaired hepatic function, severe allergy, bronchial asthma

Pharmacokinetics

Absorption	Well absorbed
Distribution	Widely distributed, crosses placenta
Metabolism	Liver, mostly
Excretion	Breast milk
Half-life	4-7 hr

Pharmacodynamics

Onset	Unknown
Peak	2-4 hr

Interactions
Individual drugs
Cyclosporine: ↑ nephrotoxicity
Indomethacin: ↑ drug-free concentrations
Methotrexate: ↑ toxicity
Phenytoin: ↑ folic acid deficiency

S

Probenecid: ↑ drug-free concentrations
Tolbutamide: ↑ effects of tolbutamide
Drug classifications
Anticoagulants, oral: ↑ effects of anticoagulant
Barbiturates: ↑ effects of barbiturates
Hypoglycemics, oral: ↑ effects of hypoglycemics
Salicylates: ↑ drug-free concentrations
Thiazide diuretics: ↑ thrombocytopenia
Uricosurics: ↑ effects of uricosurics
Lab test interferences
False positive: Urinary glucose test

NURSING CONSIDERATIONS
Assessment
- Assess patient for previous sensitivity reaction
- Assess patient for signs and symptoms of infection including characteristics of wounds, sputum, urine, stool, WBC >10,000, temp; obtain baseline information before and during treatment
- Complete C&S testing before beginning drug therapy to identify if correct treatment has been initiated
- Assess for allergic reactions: rash, urticaria, pruritus, chills, fever, joint pain; angioedema may occur a few days after therapy begins; epinephrine, resuscitation equipment should be on unit for anaphylactic reaction
- Monitor blood studies: CBC, Hct, bilirubin, alk phosphatase monthly if patient is on long-term therapy
- Monitor for bleeding: ecchymosis, bleeding gums, hematuria, stool guaiac daily if on long-term therapy
- Assess for overgrowth of infection: perineal itching, fever, malaise, redness, pain, swelling, drainage, rash, diarrhea, change in cough, sputum

Nursing diagnoses
- ✓ Infection, risk for (uses)
- ✓ Diarrhea (adverse reactions)
- ✓ Injury, risk for (adverse reactions)
- ✓ Knowledge deficit (teaching)
- ✓ Noncompliance (teaching)

Implementation
- Give around the clock to maintain proper blood levels; give on an empty stomach to increase absorption of drug; do not give within 3 hr of other agents—drug interactions may occur
- Give with 8 oz of water

Patient/family education
- Teach patient to report sore throat, bruising, bleeding, joint pain—may indicate blood dyscrasias (rare)
- Advise patient to contact prescriber if vaginal itching; loose, foul-smelling stools; or furry tongue occur—may indicate superinfection; report itching, rash, pruritus, urticaria
- Instruct patient to take all medication prescribed for the length of time ordered; drug must be taken around the clock to maintain blood levels; medication should not be shared with others

Evaluation
Positive therapeutic outcome
- Absence of signs/symptoms of infection (WBC <10,000, temp WNL, absence of urinary pain, hematuria)

- Reported improvement in symptoms of infection
- Negative C&S

sulindac (℞)

(sul-in'dak)

Apo-Sulin ♣, Clinoril, Novosundac ♣, sulindac

Func. class.: Nonsteroidal antiinflammatory

Chem. class.: Indeneacetic acid derivative

Pregnancy category C

Action: Inhibits prostaglandin synthesis by decreasing an enzyme needed for biosynthesis; analgesic, antiinflammatory, antipyretic

➡ **Therapeutic Outcome:** Decreased pain, inflammation

Uses: Mild to moderate pain, osteoarthritis, rheumatoid, gouty arthritis, ankylosing spondylitis

Dosage and routes

Arthritis

Adult: PO 150 mg bid, may increase to 200 mg bid

Bursitis/acute arthritis

Adult: PO 200 mg bid × 1-2 wk, then reduce dose

Available forms: Tabs 150, 200 mg

Adverse effects

CNS: Dizziness, drowsiness, fatigue, tremors, confusion, insomnia, anxiety, depression

CV: Tachycardia, peripheral edema, palpitations, dysrhythmias

EENT: Tinnitus, hearing loss, blurred vision

GI: Nausea, anorexia, vomiting, diarrhea, jaundice, ***cholestatic hepatitis,*** constipation, flatulence, cramps, dry mouth, peptic ulcer, ***bleeding, ulceration, perforation***

GU: ***Nephrotoxicity: dysuria, hematuria, oliguria, azotemia***

HEMA: ***Blood dyscrasias***

INTEG: Purpura, rash, pruritus, sweating, photosensitivity

Contraindications: Hypersensitivity, asthma, severe renal disease, severe hepatic disease, active ulcers

Precautions: Pregnancy **C,** P lactation, children, bleeding disorders, GI disorders, cardiac disorders, hypersensitivity to other antiinflammatory agents

Pharmacokinetics	
Absorption	Well absorbed
Distribution	Not known
Metabolism	Converted to active drug—liver
Excretion	Minimal unchanged kidneys, breast milk
Half-life	7.8 hr; 16.4-hr active metabolite

Pharmacodynamics	
Onset	Unknown
Peak	2 hr
Duration	Unknown

Interactions

Individual drugs

Acetaminophen (long-term use): ↑ renal reactions

Alcohol: ↑ adverse reactions

Aspirin: ↓ effectiveness, ↑ adverse reactions

Coumadin: ↑ anticoagulant effects

Digoxin: ↑ toxicity, ↑ levels

Insulin: ↓ insulin effect

Lithium: ↑ toxicity

Methotrexate: ↑ toxicity

Phenytoin: ↑ toxicity

Probenecid: ↑ toxicity

Sulfonylurea: ↑ toxicity

Drug classifications
Anticoagulants: ↑ risk of bleeding
Antihypertensives: ↓ effect of antihypertensives
Antineoplastics: ↑ risk of hematologic toxicity
β-Blockers: ↑ antihypertension
Cephalosporins: ↑ risk of bleeding
Diuretics: ↓ effectiveness of diuretics
Glucocorticoids: ↑ adverse reactions
Hypoglycemics: ↓ hypoglycemic effect
Nonsteroidal antiinflammatories: ↑ adverse reactions
Potassium supplements: ↑ adverse reactions
Radiation: ↑ risk of hematologic toxicity
Sulfonamides: ↑ toxicity
Lab test interferences
↑ Liver function studies, ↑ serum potassium, ↑ glucose, ↑ alk phosphatase

NURSING CONSIDERATIONS
Assessment
- Monitor blood counts during therapy; watch for decreasing platelets; if low, therapy may need to be discontinued, restarted after hematologic recovery; and for blood dyscrasia (thrombocytopenia): bruising, fatigue, bleeding, poor healing

Nursing diagnoses
- ✓ Pain (uses)
- ✓ Mobility, impaired physical (uses)
- ✓ Knowledge deficit (teaching)
- ✓ Injury, risk for (adverse reactions)

Implementation
- Administer with food or milk to decrease gastric symptoms—food slows absorption slightly, does not decrease absorption

Patient/family education
- Advise patient that drug must be continued for prescribed time to be effective; to avoid aspirin, alcoholic beverages
- Caution patient to report bleeding, bruising, fatigue, malaise because blood dyscrasias do occur
- Instruct patient to use caution when driving; drowsiness, dizziness may occur
- Teach patient to take with a full glass of water to enhance absorption; do not crush, break or chew

Evaluation
Positive therapeutic outcome
- Decreased pain
- Decreased inflammation
- Increased mobility

sumatriptan (℞)
(soo-ma-trip'tan)
Imitrex
Func. class.: Migraine agent
Chem. class.: 5HT–1-like receptor agonist
Pregnancy category C

Action: Binds selectively to the vascular 5-HT-1 receptor subtype and exerts antimigraine effect; causes vasoconstriction in cranial arteries

➔ **Therapeutic Outcome:** Absence of migraines

Uses: Acute treatment of migraine with or without aura and cluster headache

Dosage and routes

Adult: SC 6 mg or less; may repeat in 1 hr; not to exceed 12 mg/24 hr; PO 25 mg with fluids, max 100 mg

Available forms: Inj 6 mg (12 mg/ml); tabs 25, 50 mg

Adverse effects

CV: Flushing

EENT: Throat, mouth, nasal discomfort, vision changes

GI: Abdominal discomfort

INTEG: Injection site reaction, sweating

MS: Weakness, neck stiffness, myalgia

NEURO: Tingling, hot sensation, burning, feeling of pressure, tightness, numbness, dizziness, sedation, headache, anxiety, fatigue

RESP: Chest tightness, pressure

Contraindications: Angina pectoris, history of MI, documented silent ischemia, Prinzmetal's angina, ischemic heart disease, **IV** use, concurrent ergotamine-containing preparations, uncontrolled hypertension, hypersensitivity, basilar or hemiplegic migraine

Precautions: Postmenopausal women, men >40 yr, risk factors for CAD, hypercholesterolemia, obesity, diabetes, impaired hepatic or renal function, pregnancy **C,** lactation, children, elderly

P G

Pharmacokinetics

Absorption	Well absorbed (SC)
Distribution	10%-20% plasma protein binding
Metabolism	Liver (metabolite)
Excretion	Urine, feces
Half-life	2 hr

Pharmacodynamics

	SC
Onset	10-20 min
Peak	10 min-2 hr
Duration	Up to 24 hr (pain relief)

Interactions

Individual drugs

Ergotamine: ↑ risk of vasospastic reaction

NURSING CONSIDERATIONS

Assessment

- Assess for tingling, hot sensation, burning, feeling of pressure, numbness, flushing, infection site reaction
- Monitor stress level, activity, reaction, coping mechanisms of patient
- Assess neurologic status: LOC, blurring vision, nausea, vomiting, tingling in extremities preceding headache
- Assess for ingestion of tyramine-containing foods (pickled products, beer, wine, aged cheese), food additives, preservatives, colorings, artificial sweeteners, chocolate, caffeine, which may precipitate these types of headaches

Nursing diagnoses

✓ Pain (uses)
✓ Knowledge deficit (teaching)

Implementation

SC route

- Give by SC route only, avoid IM or **IV** administration

Patient/family education

- Teach patient to use the self-dosing system as soon as pain begins, do not use before a migraine is beginning, may repeat dose if migraine returns
- Caution patient not to take more than 2 dose/day or 12 mg/day; allow at least 1 hr between doses

S

• Caution patient to avoid driving or hazardous activities if dizziness or drowsiness occurs
• Teach patient to report chest tightness, heat, flushing, drowsiness, dizziness, fatigue, or any allergic reactions that occur
• Inform patient to report any side effects to prescriber
• Caution patient to use contraception when taking drug, to notify prescriber if pregnancy is suspected or planned

Evaluation

Positive therapeutic outcome
• Decrease in frequency, severity of headache

tacrine (℞)

(tack'rin)

Cognex, Tetrahydroaminoacridine, THA

Func. class.: Reversible cholinesterase

Pregnancy category C

Action: Elevates acetylcholine concentrations (cerebral cortex) by slowing degrading of acetylcholine released in cholinergic neurons; does not alter underlying dementia

➡ **Therapeutic Outcome:** Improvement in symptoms of dementia in Alzheimer's disease

Uses: Treatment of mild to moderate dementia in Alzheimer's disease

Dosage and routes

Adult: PO 10 mg qid × 6 wk, then 20 mg qid × 6 wk, increase at 6-wk intervals if patient tolerating drug well and if transaminase is within normal limits

Available forms: Caps 10, 20, 30, 40 mg

Adverse effects

*CNS: **Dizziness, confusion, insomnia,*** tremor, ***ataxia, somnolence, anxiety, agitation, depression, hallucinations, hostility, abnormal thinking,*** chills, fever

CV: Hypotension or hypertension

*GI: **Nausea, vomiting, anorexia, abdominal pain, constipation,*** dyspepsia, flatulence

*GU: **Frequency, UTI, incontinence***

*INTEG: **Rash,*** flushing

*RESP: **Rhinitis, URI, cough,*** pharyngitis

Contraindications: Hypersensitivity to this drug or acridine derivatives, patients treated with this drug who developed jaundice with a total bilirubin of >3 mg/dL

Precautions: Sick sinus syndrome, history of ulcers, GI bleeding, hepatic disease, bladder obstruction, asthma, pregnancy **C**, lactation, P children

Pharmacokinetics

Absorption	Rapidly absorbed, low
Distribution	55% plasma protein bound
Metabolism	Liver
Excretion	Unknown
Half-life	2-4 hr

Pharmacodynamics

Unknown

Interactions

Individual drugs

Bethanechol: ↑ effect

Cimetidine: ↑ tacrine level
Succinylcholine: ↑ effect
Theophylline: ↑ toxicity

NURSING CONSIDERATIONS
Assessment
- Monitor B/P for hypotension or hypertension
- Assess mental status: affect, mood, behavioral changes, depression, hallucinations, confusion; conduct suicide assessment
- Assess GI status: nausea, vomiting, anorexia, constipation, abdominal pain; add bulk and increase fluids for constipation
- Assess GU status: urinary frequency, incontinence

Nursing diagnoses
✓ Injury, risk for (uses)
✓ Thought processes, altered (uses)
✓ Knowledge deficit (teaching)

Implementation
- Give dosage adjusted to patient's response no more than q6wk
- Provide assistance with ambulation if needed during beginning therapy; dizziness, ataxia may occur
- Give between meals; if GI symptoms occur, may be given with meals

Patient/family education
- Advise patient to report side effects: twitching, eye spasms; may indicate overdose
- Instruct patient to use drug exactly as prescribed at regular intervals, preferably between meals; may be taken with meals for GI upset
- Advise patient to notify prescriber of nausea, vomiting, diarrhea (dose increased or beginning treatment) or rash, very dark or very light stools, jaundice (delayed onset)
- Caution patient not to increase or abruptly decrease dose; serious consequences may result

Evaluation
Positive therapeutic outcome
- Decrease in confusion, improved mood

Treatment of overdose: Withdraw drug, administer tertiary anticholinergics, provide supportive care

tacrolimus (℞)
(tak-roe'li-mus)
Prograf
Func. class.: Immunosuppressant
Chem. clas.: Macrolide
Pregnancy category C

Action: Produces immunosuppression by inhibiting lympho cytes (T)

➡ **Therapeutic Outcome:** Prevention of rejection in organ transplant

Uses: Organ transplants— to prevent rejection

Dosage and routes
P ***Adult and child:*** **IV** 0.15 mg/kg/day × 3 days then PO 0.15 mg/kg bid

Available forms: Inj **IV**

Adverse effects
CNS: Tremors, headache, insomnia, paresthesia, anxiety, hyperesthesia, numbness, dizziness, fatigue
CV: Hypertension
EENT: Blurred vision, photophobia
GI: Nausea, vomiting, diar-

rhea, *oral Candida, gum hyperplasia, hepatotoxicity,* constipation
GU: Urinary tract infections, ***albuminuria, hematuria, proteinuria, renal failure***
HEMA: Anemia, ***leukocytosis, thrombocytopenia purpura***
INTEG: Rash, flushing, itching, alopecia
META: Hirsutism, hyperglycemia, hyperkalemia, hyperuricemia, hypokalemia, hypomagnesemia
RESP: Pleural effusion, atelectasis, dyspnea

Contraindications: Hypersensitivity

Precautions: Severe renal disease, severe hepatic disease, pregnancy **C,** diabetes mellitus, hyperkalemia, hyperuricemia

Pharmacokinetics	
Absorption	Erractically absorbed (PO), completely absorbed (IV)
Distribution	Crosses placenta, 75% protein binding
Metabolism	Liver to metabolite
Excretion	Kidney—minimal, breast milk, bile
Half-life	10 hr

Pharmacodynamics	PO	IV
Onset	Unknown	Unknown
Peak	1-4 hr	Unknown
Duration	12 hr	12 hr

Interactions
Individual drugs
Cyclosporine: ↑ nephrotoxicity, do not use together
Danazol: ↑ toxicity
Erthromycin: ↑ toxicity
Ibuprofen: ↑ oliguria

NURSING CONSIDERATIONS
Assessment
• Monitor blood studies: Hgb, WBC, platelets during treatment monthly; if leukocytes are <3000/mm³, or platelets <100,000/mm³, drug should be discontinued or reduced; decreased hemoglobulin level may indicate bone marrow suppression
• Monitor liver function studies: alk phosphatase, AST (SGOT), ALT (SGPT), amylase, bilirubin, and for hepatotoxicity: dark urine, jaundice, itching, light-colored stools; drug should be discontinued

Nursing diagnoses
✓ Infection, risk for (uses)
✓ Knowledge deficit (teaching)

Implementation
PO route
• Give all medications PO if possible; avoid IM inj because bleeding may occur
• Give with meals to reduce GI upset; nausea is common
• Give for several days before transplant surgery; patients should be placed in protective isolation

IV route
• Give after diluting in 0.9% NaCl or D_5W to a concentration of 0.004 mg/ml to 0.02 mg/ml as a continuous inf

Y-site compatibilities: Acyclovir, aminophylline, amphotericin B, ampicillin, benztropine, calcium gluconate, cefazolin, cefotetan, ceftazidime, chloramphenicol, cimetidine, ciprofloxacin, clindamycin, dexamethasone, digoxin, diphenhydramine, dobutamine, dopamine, doxycycline, erythromycin, esmolol, fluconazole, furosemide, ganciclovir, gentamicin, haloperidol, heparin, hydrocortisone, regular insulin, isoproterenol, leucovorin, lorazepam, methylprednisolone, metoclopramide, metronidazole, mezlocillin, multivitamins, nitroglycerin, oxacillin, penicillin G potassium, perphenazine, phenytoin, piperacillin, potassium chloride, propranolol, ranitidine, sodium bicarbonate

Patient/family education

- Instruct patient to report fever, rash, severe diarrhea, chills, sore throat, fatigue because serious infections may occur; clay-colored stools, cramping may indicate hepatotoxicity
- Caution patient to avoid crowds or persons with known infections to reduce risk of infection

Evaluation

Positive therapeutic outcome

- Absence of graft rejection
- Immunosuppression in autoimmune disorders

tamoxifen (℞)

(ta-mox'i-fen)

Nolvadex, Nolvadex-D ✦, Novo-Tamoxifen ✦, Tamofen ✦, Tamone ✦

Func. class.: Antineoplastic

Chem. class.: Antiestrogen hormone

Pregnancy category D

Action: Inhibits cell division by binding to cytoplasmic estrogen receptors; resembles normal cell complex but inhibits DNA synthesis and estrogen response of target tissue

➔ **Therapeutic Outcome:** Prevention of rapidly growing malignant cells

Uses: Advanced breast carcinoma that has not responded to other therapy in estrogen-receptor-positive patients (usually postmenopausal)

Dosage and routes

Adult: PO 10-20 mg bid

Available forms: Tab 10 mg

Adverse effects

CNS: Hot flashes, headache, lightheadedness, depression

CV: Chest pain

EENT: Ocular lesions, retinopathy, corneal opacity, blurred vision (high doses)

GI: Nausea, vomiting, altered taste (anorexia)

GU: Vaginal bleeding, pruritus vulvae

HEMA: ***Thrombocytopenia, leukopenia***

INTEG: Rash, alopecia

META: Hypercalcemia

Contraindications: Hypersensitivity, pregnancy **D**

Precautions: Leukopenia, thrombocytopenia, lactation, cataracts

Pharmacokinetics	
Absorption	Adequately absorbed
Distribution	Unknown
Metabolism	Liver—extensively
Excretion	Feces—slowly, small amounts (kidneys)
Half-life	1 wk

Pharmacodynamics	
Onset	Unknown
Peak	4-7 hr
Duration	Unknown

Lab test interferences

↑ Serum Ca

NURSING CONSIDERATIONS

Assessment

- Monitor CBC, differential, platelet count weekly; withhold drug if WBC is <4000 or platelet count is <75,000; notify prescriber of results; monitor calcium levels (hypercalcemia is common)

- Assess for tumor flare: increase in bone, tumor pain during beginning treatment; give analgesics as ordered to decrease pain
- Assess for bleeding: hematuria, guaiac, bruising or petechiae, mucosa or orifices q8h, no rec temp

Nursing diagnoses

- ✓ Injury, risk for (adverse reactions)
- ✓ Knowledge deficit (teaching)

Implementation

- Give with food or fluids for GI upset; do not break, crush, or chew enteric products; repeat dose may be needed if vomiting occurs
- Store in light-resistant container at room temp

Patient/family education

- Instruct patient to report any complaints, side effects to health care prescriber; if dose is missed, do not double next dose
- Advise patient that vaginal bleeding, pruritus, hot flashes, can occur, and are reversible after discontinuing treatment
- Instruct patient to report immediately decreased visual acuity, which may be irreversible; stress need for routine eye exams
- Inform patient about who should be told about tamoxifen therapy
- Advise patient to report vaginal bleeding immediately; that tumor flare—increase in size or tumor, increased bone pain—may occur and will subside rapidly; may take analgesics for pain; that premenopausal women must use mechanical birth control method because ovulation may be induced (teratogenic drug)
- Caution patient to use sunscreen and protective clothing to prevent burns because photosensitivity is common
- Teach patient that hair loss may occur during treatment; a wig or hairpiece may make patient feel better; new hair may be different in color, texture
- Inform patient rash or lesions are temporary and may become large during beginning therapy

Evaluation

Positive therapeutic outcome

- Decreased spread of malignant cells in breast cancer

temazepam (℞)

(tem-az'a-pam)

Razepam, Restoril, Temazepam

Func. class.: Sedative/hypnotic

Chem. class.: Benzodiazepine

Pregnancy category X

Controlled substance schedule IV (USA)
schedule F (Canada)

Action: Produces CNS depression at limbic, thalamic, hypothalamic levels of the CNS; may be mediated by neurotransmitter γ-aminobutyric acid (GABA); results are sedation, hypnosis, skeletal muscle relaxation, anticonvulsant activity, anxiolytic action

Therapeutic Outcome: Decreased insomnia

Uses: Insomnia (short-term)

Dosage and routes
Adult: PO 15-30 mg hs

Available forms: Caps 7.5, 15, 30 mg; tabs 15, 30 mg

Adverse effects
CNS: Lethargy, drowsiness, daytime sedation, dizziness, confusion, lightheadedness, headache, anxiety, irritability
CV: Chest pain, pulse changes
GI: Nausea, vomiting, diarrhea, heartburn, abdominal pain, constipation, anorexia
HEMA: ***Leukopenia, granulocytopenia*** (rare)

Contraindications: Hypersensitivity to benzodiazepines, pregnancy **X,** lactation, intermittent porphyria

Precautions: Anemia, hepatic disease, renal disease, suicidal individuals, drug abuse, elderly, psychosis, child <15 yr, acute narrow-angle glaucoma, seizure disorders

G P

Pharmacokinetics

Absorption	Well absorbed
Distribution	Widely distributed, crosses placenta, crosses blood-brain barrier
Metabolism	Liver
Excretion	Kidneys, breast milk
Half-life	10-20 hr

Pharmacodynamics

Onset	½ hr
Peak	2-3 hr
Duration	6-8 hr

Interactions
Individual drugs
Alcohol: ↑ CNS depression
Cimetidine: ↑ action
Disulfiram: ↑ action
Fluoxetine: ↑ action
Isoniazid: ↑ action
Ketoconazole: ↑ action
Levodopa: ↓ action of levodopa
Metoprolol: ↑ action
Propoxyphene: ↑ action
Propranolol: ↑ action
Rifampin: ↓ action of temazepam
Theophylline: ↓ sedative effects
Valproic acid: ↑ action
Drug classifications
Analgesics, opioid: ↑ CNS depression
Antidepressants: ↑ CNS depression
Antihistamines: ↑ CNS depression
Barbiturates: ↓ effect of temazepam
Contraceptives: ↑ effect
Lab test interferences
↑ AST (SGOT)/ALT (SGPT), ↑ serum bilirubin
False ↑ 17 OHCS
↓ RAIU

NURSING CONSIDERATIONS
Assessment

- Assess mental status: mood, sensorium, anxiety, affect, sleeping pattern, drowsiness, dizziness, especially elderly; physical dependency, withdrawal symptoms: anxiety, panic attacks, agitation, convulsions, headache, nausea, vomiting, muscle pain, weakness; suicidal tendencies; for indications of increasing tolerance and abuse
- Monitor B/P (lying, standing), pulse; if systolic B/P drops 20 mm Hg, hold drug, notify prescriber
- Monitor blood studies: CBC during long-term therapy; blood dycrasias have occurred rarely; decreased hematocrit, neutropenia may occur
- Monitor hepatic studies: AST (SGOT), ALT (SGPT), bilirubin, creatinine LDH, alk phosphatase

G

T

• Monitor I&O; indicate renal dysfunction

Nursing diagnoses

✓ Anxiety (uses)
✓ Depression (uses)
✓ Injury, risk for (adverse reactions)
✓ Knowledge deficit (teaching)

Implementation

• Give with food or milk for GI symptoms; if patient is unable to swallow medication whole, tab may be crushed and mixed with foods or fluids
• Give sugarless gum, hard candy, frequent sips of water for dry mouth

Patient/family education

• Inform patient that drug may be taken with food, and that fluids and tab may be crushed or swallowed whole
• Advise patient not to use for everyday stress or longer than 3 mo unless directed by prescriber; not to take more than prescribed amount; may be habit forming; not to double doses or skip doses
• Caution patient to avoid OTC preparations unless approved by health care prescriber; alcohol and CNS depressants will increase CNS depression
• Advise patient to avoid driving, activities that require alertness, because drowsiness may occur; to avoid alcohol ingestion or other psychotropic medications; to rise slowly or fainting may occur, especially G in elderly; that drowsiness may worsen at beginning of treatment
• Caution patient not to discontinue medication abruptly after long-term use; withdrawal symptoms include vomiting, cramping, tremors, seizures

Evaluation

Positive therapeutic outcome

• Decreased anxiety, restlessness, sleeplessness (short-term treatment only)

Treatment of overdose: Lavage, VS, supportive care

teniposide (℞)

(ten-i′poe-side)

Vumon, VM 26

Func. class.: Antineoplastic

Chem. class.: Semisynthetic podophyllotoxin

Pregnancy category D

Action: Inhibits mitotic activity through metaphase to mitosis; inhibits cells from entering mitosis; depresses DNA, RNA synthesis

→ **Therapeutic Outcome:** Prevention of rapid growth of malignant cells

Uses: Childhood acute lymphoblastic leukemia (ALL), refractory childhood acute lymphocytic leukemia

Dosage and routes

P ***Child* IV** inf: Combo teniposide 165 mg/m² and cytarabine 300 mg/m² 2 ×/wk × 8-9 doses or combo teniposide 250 mg/m² and vincristine 1.5 mg/m² qwk × 4-8 wk and prednisone 40 mg/m² PO × 28 days

Available forms: Inj 10 mg/ml

Adverse effects

CNS: Headache, fever
CV: Hypotension
GI: Nausea, vomiting, anorexia, ***hepatotoxicity***, diarrhea, stomatitis
GU: ***Nephrotoxicity***

HEMA: Thrombocytopenia, leukopenia, neutropenia, myelosuppression, anemia
INTEG: Rash, alopecia, phlebitis
RESP: Bronchospasm
SYST: Anaphylaxis

Contraindications: Hypersensitivity, bone marrow depression, severe hepatic disease, severe renal disease, bacterial infection, pregnancy **D**

Precautions: Renal disease, hepatic disease, lactation, P children, gout, depression

Pharmacokinetics

Absorption	Variably absorbed
Distribution	Rapidly distributed, crosses placenta
Metabolism	Liver—some
Excretion	Kidneys, unchanged 45%, breast milk
Half-life	3 hr initial, 15 hr terminal

Pharmacodynamics

Unknown

Interactions

Individual drugs

Radiation: ↑ toxicity, bone marrow suppression

Drug classifications

Antineoplastics: ↑ toxicity, bone marrow suppression

Live virus vaccines: ↑ adverse reactions

NURSING CONSIDERATIONS

Assessment

- Monitor B/P, (baseline and q15 min) during administration
- Monitor CBC, differential, platelet count weekly; withhold drug if WBC is <4000 or platelet count is <75,000; notify prescriber of results and that recovery will take 3 wk
- Assess for dyspnea, rales, unproductive cough, chest pain, tachypnea
- Monitor renal function studies: BUN, serum uric acid, urine CrCl before, during therapy; I&O ratio; report fall in urine output of 30 ml/hr; for decreased hyperuricemia
- Monitor for cold, fever, sore throat (may indicate beginning infection); notify prescriber if these occur
- Assess for bleeding: hematuria, guaiac, bruising or petechiae, mucosa or orifices q8hr, no rec temp; avoid IM inj; use pressure to venipuncture sites
- Identify nutritional status: an antiemetic may need to be prescribed
- Assess for symptoms indicating severe allergic reactions: rash, pruritus, urticaria, itching, flushing, bronchospasm, hypotension; epinephrine and emergency equipment should be nearby

Nursing diagnoses

- ✓ Injury, risk for (adverse reactions)
- ✓ Body image disturbance (adverse reactions)
- ✓ Infection, risk for (adverse reactions)
- ✓ Knowledge deficit (teaching)

Implementation

- Give by intermittent inf; sol should be prepared by qualified personnel only under controlled conditions; gloves, gown, and mask should be worn
- Use Luer-Loc tubing to prevent leakage, do not let sol come in contact with skin; if contact occurs, wash well with soap and water
- Give after diluting 100 mg/250 ml or more D_5W or 0.9% NaCl to a concentration of

T

0.2-0.4 mg/ml, inf over 30-60 min; do not use plastic when preparing this inf
• Use hyaluronidase 150 U/ml to 1 ml NaCl to infiltration area, ice compress for treatment of vesicant activity
• This drug should not be given with or mixed with other drugs

Y-site compatibilities:
Acyclovir, allopurinol, amikacin, aminophylline, amphotericin B, ampicillin, aztreonam, bleomycin, bumetanide, buprenorphine, butorphanol, calcium gluconate, carboplatin, carmustine, cefazolin, cefonicid, cefoperazone, chlorpromazine, cimetidine, ciprofloxacin, cisplatin, clindamycin, cyclophosphamide, cytarabine, dacarbazine, dactinomycin, daunorubicin, dexamethasone, doxorubicin, etoposide, famotidine, floxuridine, fluconazole, fludarabine, fluorouracil, gentamicin, heparin, hydrocortisone, ifosfamide, leucovorin, melphalan, meperidine, mesna, methotrexate, miconazole, mitomycin, mitoxantrone, morphine, nalbuphine, netilmicin, ondansetron, piperacillin, plicamycin, potassium chloride, prochlorperazine, promethazine, ranitidine, sargramostim, sodium bicarbonate, streptozocin, thiotepa, tobramycin, trimethoprim-sulfamethoxazole, vancomycin, vinblastine, vincristine

Patient/family education
• Teach patient to avoid use of products containing aspirin or ibuprofen, razors, commercial mouthwash because bleeding may occur; to report symptoms of bleeding (hematuria, tarry stools)
• Instruct patient to report signs of anemia, (fatigue, headache, irritability, faintness, shortness of breath)
• Instruct patient to report any changes in breathing or coughing even several mo after treatment
• Advise patient that contraception will be necessary during treatment; teratogenesis may occur
• Caution patient that hair may be lost during treatment; a wig or hairpiece may make patient feel better; new hair will be different in color, texture
• Advise patient to avoid vaccinations during treatment; serious reactions may occur
• Teach patient to report signs/symptoms of infection; fever, chills, sore throat; patient should avoid crowds, or persons with known infections

Evaluation
Positive therapeutic outcome
• Decreased spread of malignant, leukemic cells

terazosin (℞)
(ter-ay'zoe-sin)
Hytrin
Func. class.: Antihypertensive
Chem. class.: Adrenergic blocker (peripherally acting)
Pregnancy category C

Action: Peripheral blood vessels are dilated, peripheral resistance lowered; reduction in blood pressure results from α-adrenergic receptors being blocked

Therapeutic Outcome: Decreased B/P in hypertension, decreased symptoms of BPH

Uses: Hypertension, as a single agent or in combination with diuretics or β-blockers, BPH

Dosage and routes

Adult: PO 1 mg hs, may increase doses slowly to desired response; not to exceed 20 mg/day

Available forms: Tabs 1, 2, 5 mg

Adverse effects

CNS: Dizziness, headache, drowsiness, anxiety, depression, vertigo, weakness, fatigue
CV: Palpitations, orthostatic hypotension, tachycardia, edema, rebound hypertension
EENT: Blurred vision, epistaxis, tinnitus, dry mouth, red sclera, nasal congestion, sinusitis
GI: Nausea, vomiting, diarrhea, constipation, abdominal pain
GU: Urinary frequency, incontinence, impotence, priapism
RESP: Dyspnea

Contraindications: Hypersensitivity

Precautions: Pregnancy **C,** P children, lactation

Pharmacokinetics	
Absorption	Well absorbed
Distribution	Not known
Metabolism	Liver—50%
Excretion	Kidneys unchanged—10%, feces unchanged—20%
Half-life	9-12 hr

Pharmacodynamics	
Onset	15 min
Peak	1 hr
Duration	24 hr

Interactions

Individual drugs

Alcohol: ↑ CNS depression

Drug classifications

Antihypertensives: ↑ hypotension
Antiinflamatories, nonsteroidal: ↓ antihypertensive effect
Estrogens: ↓ antihypertensive effect
Nitrates: ↑ hypotensive effects
Sympathomimetics: ↓ antihypertensive effect

Lab test interferences

↑ VMA excretion, ↑ 5-HIAA excretion
Interference: 17-OHCS, 17-KS

NURSING CONSDERATIONS

Assessment

- Monitor B/P, orthostatic hypotension, syncope; check for edema in feet, legs daily; I&O; monitor for weight daily; notify prescriber of changes
- Assess for allergic reactions: rash, fever, pruritus, urticaria; drug should be discontinued if antihistamines fail to help
- Assess for orthostatic hypotension; tell patient to rise slowly from sitting or lying position

Nursing diagnoses

✓ Cardiac output, decreased (uses)
✓ Injury, risk for (adverse reactions)
✓ Knowledge deficit (teaching)
✓ Noncompliance (teaching)

Implementation

- Store in tight container at 86° F (30° C) or less
- May be used in combination with other antihypertensives
- May be given with food to prevent GI symptoms

T

Patient/family education

• Caution patient not to discontinue drug abruptly; the importance of complying with dosage schedule, even if feeling better; if dose is missed take as soon as remembered; take medication at same time each day
• Teach patient not to use OTC products (cough, cold, allergy) unless directed by prescriber; also to avoid large amounts of caffeine
• Emphasize the need to rise slowly to sitting or standing position to minimize orthostatic hypotension
• Teach patient to notify prescriber of mouth sores, sore throat, fever, swelling of hands or feet, irregular heartbeat, chest pain
• Caution patient to report excessive perspiration, dehydration, vomiting, diarrhea; may lead to fall in B/P
• Caution patient that drug may cause dizziness, fainting, lightheadedness; may occur during 1st few days of therapy; to avoid hazardous activities
• Teach patient how to take B/P, and normal readings for age group; to take B/P q7 days

Evaluation

Positive therapeutic outcome
• Decreased B/P in hypertension
• Decreased symptoms of BPH

Treatment of overdose: Administer volume expanders or vasopressors; discontinue drug; place patient in supine position

terbutaline (℞)

(ter-byoo′te-leen)
Brethaire, Brethine, Bricanyl
Func. class.: Selective β_2-agonist; bronchodilator
Chem. class.: Catecholamine
Pregnancy category B

Action: Relaxes bronchial smooth muscle by direct action on β_2-adrenergic receptors through accumulation of cAMP at β-adrenergic receptor sites; results are bronchodilation, diuresis, and CNS and cardiac stimulation; relaxes uterine smooth muscle

➡ **Therapeutic Outcome:** Bronchodilation with ease of breathing

Uses: Bronchospasm

Investigational uses: Premature labor, hyperkalemia

Dosage and routes

Bronchospasm

P ***Adult and child >12 yr:*** Inh 2 puffs q1min, then q4-6h; PO 2.5-5 mg q8h; SC 0.25 mg q8h

Premature labor

Adult: **IV** inf 0.01 mg/min, increased by 0.005 mg q10min, not to exceed 0.025 mg/min; SC 0.25 mg q1h; PO 5 mg q4h × 48 h, then 5 mg q6h as maintenance for above doses

Available forms: Tabs 2.5, 5 mg; aerosol 0.2 mg/actuation; inj 1 mg/ml

Adverse effects

CNS: Tremors, anxiety, insomnia, headache, dizziness, stimulation

CV: Palpitations, tachycardia, hypertension, dysrhythmias, ***cardiac arrest***
GI: Nausea, vomiting

Contraindications: Hypersensitivity to sympathomimetics, narrow-angle glaucoma, tachydysrhythmias

Precautions: Pregnancy **B**, cardiac disorders, hyperthyroidism, diabetes mellitus, prostatic hypertension, lactation, elderly, hypertension, glaucoma

Pharmacokinetics

Absorption	Well absorbed (SC), partially absorbed (PO)
Distribution	Unknown
Metabolism	Liver—partially
Excretion	Unknown
Half-life	Unknown

Pharmacodynamics

	PO	INH	SC	IV
Onset	½ hr	5-15 min	10-15 min	Rapid
Peak	1-2 hr	1-2 hr	½ 1 hr	Unknown
Duration	4-8 hr	4-6 hr	1½-4 hr	Unknown

Interactions

Drug classifications

β-adrenergic blockers: Block therapeutic effect
Bronchodilators, aerosol: ↑ action of bronchodilator
MAOIs: ↑ chance of hypertensive crisis
Sympathomimetics: ↑ adrenergic side effects

NURSING CONSIDERATIONS

Assessment

- Monitor respiratory function: vital capacity, forced expiratory volume, ABGs, lung sounds, heart rate, rhythm (baseline)
- Determine that patient has not received theophylline therapy before giving dose; assess client's ability to self-medicate
- Monitor for evidence of allergic reactions; paradoxical bronchospasm; withhold dose; notify prescriber

Nursing diagnoses

- ✓ Airway clearance, ineffective (uses)
- ✓ Impaired gas exchange (uses)
- ✓ Knowledge deficit (teaching)
- ✓ Noncompliance (teaching)

Implementation

Aerosol route

- Give after shaking; ask patient to exhale, place mouthpiece in mouth, then inhale slowly; hold breath, remove, exhale slowly; allow at least 1 min between inh
- Store in light-resistant container, do not expose to temp over 86° F (30° C)

PO route

- Give PO with meals to decrease gastric irritation; tab may be crushed and mixed with foods and fluids

SC route

- Do not give by IM route

IV route

- Give at 5 μg q 10 min until contractions are stopped, use inf pump for correct dose; after ½-1 hr with no contraction decrease dose by 5 μg; switch to PO dose when possible

Syringe compatibility: Doxapram

Y-site compatibility: Regular insulin

Additive incompatibility: Bleomycin

Additive compatibility: Aminophylline

T

Patient/family education

- Advise patient not to use OTC medications; extra stimulation may occur; to use this medication before other medications and allow at least 5 min between each to prevent overstimulation
- Teach patient how to use inhaler; review package insert with patient; to avoid getting aerosol in eyes because blurring may result; to wash inhaler in warm water qd and dry; to avoid smoking, smoke-filled rooms, persons with respiratory infections
- Teach patient that paradoxical bronchospasm may occur and to stop drug immediately and notify health care prescriber; to limit caffeine products such as chocolate, coffee, tea, and colas
- Instruct patient on administration of dose, not to use more than prescribed; serious side effects may occur; if taking PO regularly and dose is missed, take when remembered; space other doses on new time schedule

Evaluation

Positive therapeutic outcome

- Absence of dyspnea, wheezing after 1 hr
- Improved airway exchange
- Improved ABGs

Treatment of overdose: Administer a β_2-adrenergic blocker

terfenadine (℞)

(ter-fen'i-deen)

Seldane

Func. class.: Antihistamine

Chem. class.: Butyrophenone derivative

Pregnancy category C

Action: Acts on blood vessels, GI, respiratory systems by competing with histamine for H_1-receptor site; decreases allergic response by blocking histamine

Therapeutic Outcome: Absence of allergy symptoms and rhinitis

Uses: Rhinitis, allergy symptoms

Dosage and routes

P ***Adult and child >12 yr:*** PO 60 mg bid

P ***Child <12 yr:*** PO 15-30 mg bid

Available forms: Tab 60 mg, 120 mg ✤; oral susp 6 mg/ml ✤

Adverse effects

CNS: Dizziness, poor coordination

CV: Life-threatening dysrhythmias (rare)

GI: Anorexia, increased liver function tests, dry mouth

GU: Retention

RESP: Increased thick secretions

Contraindications: Hypersensitivity, severe hepatic disease

Precautions: Pregnancy **C**

Pharmacokinetics

Absorption	Completely absorbed
Distribution	Not known
Metabolism	Liver—extensively
Excretion	Feces, biliary
Half-life	Biphasic 3½ hr, 1623 hr

Pharmacodynamics

Onset	1-2 hr
Peak	3-6 hr
Duration	6-12 hr

Interactions
Individual drugs
Alcohol: ↑ CNS depression
Atropine: ↑ anticholinergic reactions
Azithromycin: ↑ dysrhythmias
Clarithromycin: ↑ dysrhythmias
Disopyramide: ↑ anticholin ergic reactions
Erythromycin: ↑ dysrhythmias
Fluconazole: ↑ dysrhythmias
Haloperidol: ↑ anticholinergic reactions
Itraconazole: ↑ dysrhythmias
Ketoconazole: ↑ dysrhythmias
Miconazole: ↑ dysrhythmias
Quinidine: ↑ anticholinergic reactions
Drug classifications
Antidepressants: ↑ anticholinergic reactions
Antihistamines: ↑ anticholinergic reactions
CNS depressants: ↑ CNS depression
MAOIs: ↑ anticholinergic effect
Narcotics: ↑ CNS depression
Phenothiazines: ↑ anticholinergic reactions
Sedative/hypnotics: ↑ CNS depression
Lab test interferences
False negative: Skin allergy tests (discontinue antihistamines 3 days prior to testing)

NURSING CONSIDERATIONS
Assessment
- Assess respiratory status: rate, rhythm, increase in bronchial secretions, wheezing, chest tightness; provide fluids to 2 L/day to decrease secretions thickness
- Monitor I&O ratio: be alert for urinary retention, frequency, dysuria, especially G elderly; drug should be discontinued if these occur
- Monitor CBC during long-term therapy; blood dyscrasias may occur but are rare

Nursing diagnoses
✓ Airway clearance, ineffective (uses)
✓ Injury, risk for (adverse reactions)
✓ Knowledge deficit (teaching)
✓ Noncompliance (teaching—overuse)

Implementation
- Give on an empty stomach 1 hr ac or 2 hr pc to facilitate absorption
- Store in tight, light-resistant container

Patient/family education
- Teach patient all aspects of drug uses; to notify prescriber if dizziness occurs; to avoid driving or other hazardous activity if dizziness occurs; to avoid alcohol or other CNS depressants that may potentiate effect
- Advise patient to take 1 hr ac or 2 hr pc to facilitate absorption
- Caution patient not to exceed recommended dose; dysrhythmias may occur
- Advise patient that hard candy, gum, frequent rinsing of mouth may be used for dryness

T

Evaluation
Positive therapeutic outcome
• Absence of running or congested nose, rashes

Treatment of overdose: Administer ipecac syrup or lavage, diazepam, vasopressors, barbiturates (short-acting)

testosterone cypionate/testosterone enanthate/ testosterone propionate ⚷ (℞)

(tess-toss'te-rone)

Andro L.A. 200, Delatest, Delatestryl, Durathate-200, Everone 100, Everone 200, Testone LA 100, Testone LA 200, testosterone enanthate, Testrin PA, Andro-Cyp 100, Andro-Cyp 200, Andronate 100, Andronate 200, depAndro 100, depAndro 200, Depotest 100, Depotest 200, Depo-Testosterone, Duratest-100, Duratest-200, testosterone cypionate, Testred Cypionate, Testex, testosterone propionate, Testoderm Transdermal

Func. class.: Androgenic anabolic steroid

Chem. class.: Halogenated testosterone derivative

Pregnancy category X

Action: Increases weight by building body tissue; increases potassium, phosphorus, chloride, nitrogen levels; increases bone development; responsible for maintenance of secondary sex characteristics (male)

➡ Therapeutic Outcome: Increased hormone levels in eunuchoidism, decreased tumor growth in female breast cancer, onset of male puberty

Uses: Female breast cancer, eunuchoidism, male climacteric, oligospermia, impotence, osteoporosis, weight loss in AIDS patients, vulvar dystrophies

Dosage and routes

Oligospermia
Adult: IM 100-200 mg q4-6 wk (cypionate or enanthate)

Breast cancer
Adult: IM 50-100 mg 3 ×/wk (propionate) or 200-400 mg q2-4 wk (cypionate or enanthate)

Male climacteric/ eunuchoidism/eunuchism
Adult: IM 10-25 mg 2-4 ×/wk (propionate)

Available forms: Propionate inj 25, 50, 100 mg/ml; enanthate inj 100, 200 mg/ml; cypionate inj 50, 100, 200 mg/ml; patches 4, 6 mg/day

Adverse effects
CNS: Dizziness, headache, fatigue, tremors, paresthesias, flushing, sweating, anxiety, lability, insomnia, carpal tunnel syndrome
CV: Increased B/P
EENT: Conjunctival edema, nasal congestion
ENDO: Abnormal GTT
GI: Nausea, vomiting, constipation, weight gain, ***cholestatic jaundice***
GU: Hematuria, amenorrhea, vaginitis, decreased libido, decreased breast size, clitoral hypertrophy, testicular atrophy
INTEG: Rash, acneiform lesions, oily hair and skin, flushing, sweating, acne vulgaris, alopecia, hirsutism
MS: Cramps, spasms

Contraindications: Severe renal disease, severe cardiac disease, severe hepatic disease, hypersensitivity, pregnancy **X,** lactation, genital bleeding (abnormal)

Precautions: Diabetes mellitus, CV disease, MI

Pharmacokinetics

Absorption	Well but slowly absorbed
Distribution	Crosses placenta
Metabolism	Liver
Excretion	Kidneys, breast milk
Half-life	8 days (cypionate) 10-100 min (Base)

Pharmacodynamics

	IM (base)	IM (cypionate)	IM (enanthate)	IM (propionate)
Onset	Unknown	Unknown	Unknown	Unknown
Peak	Unknown	Unknown	Unknown	Unknown
Duration	1-3 days	2-4 wk	2-4 wk	1-3 days

Interactions

Individual drugs

ACTH: ↑ edema
Insulin: ↓ effects of insulin
Oxyphenbutazone: ↑ effects of oxyphenbutazone

Drug classifications

Adrenal steroids: ↑ edema
Anticoagulants: ↑ pro-time
Oral antidiabetics: ↑ effects of oral antidiabetics

Lab test interferences

↑ Serum cholesterol, ↑ blood glucose, ↑ urine glucose
↓ Serum Ca, ↓ serum K, ↓ T_4, ↓ T_3, ↓ thyroid ^{131}I uptake test, ↓ urine 17-OHCS, ↓ 17-KS, ↓ PBI

NURSING CONSIDERATIONS

Assessment

- Monitor patient's weight daily; notify prescriber if weekly weight gain is >5 lb; assess I&O ratio; be alert for decreasing urinary output, increasing edema
- Monitor B/P q4h
- P Assess growth rate in adolescent because growth rate may be uneven (linear/bone growth) if used for extended periods
- Monitor electrolytes: potassium, sodium, chloride, calcium; cholesterol
- Monitor liver function studies: ALT (SGOT), AST (SGPT), bilirubin
- Assess edema, hypertension, cardiac symptoms, jaundice
- Assess mental status: affect, mood, behavioral changes, aggression
- Assess signs of masculinization in female: increased libido, deepening of voice, decreased breast tissue, enlarged clitoris, menstrual irregularities; male: gynecomastia, impotence, testicular atrophy
- Assess hypercalcemia: lethargy, polyuria, polydipsia, nausea, vomiting, constipation; drug may have to be decreased
- Assess hypoglycemia in diabetics because oral antidiabetic action is increased

Nursing diagnoses

- ✓ Infection, risk for (adverse reactions)
- ✓ Injury, risk for (adverse reactions)
- ✓ Knowledge deficit (teaching)

Implementation

- Administer diet with increased calories, protein; decreased sodium if edema occurs
- Administer supportive drug if anemia occurs
- Give titrated dose; use lowest effective dose
- Give IM deep into upper

outer quadrant of gluteal muscle; route can be painful

Patient/family education

- Inform patient that drug needs to be combined with complete health plan: diet, rest, exercise
- Caution patient to notify prescriber if therapeutic response decreases; not to discontinue this medication abruptly
- Inform women patients to report menstrual irregularities; about changes in sex characteristics
- Discuss that 1-3 mo course is necessary for response in breast cancer

Evaluation

Positive therapeutic outcome

- Decrease size of tumor in breast cancer
- Increased androgen levels

tetracycline (℞)

(tet-ra-sye'kleen)

Achromycin, Achromycin V, Alatel, Apo-Tetra ✦, Nor-Tet, Novotetra ✦, Nu-Tetra ✦, Panmycin, Robitet, Sumycin 250, Sumycin 500, Sumycin Syrup, Teline, Teline 500, Tetracap, tetracycline HCl, tetracycline HCl Syrup, Tetracyn, Tetralan 250, Tetralan 500, Tetralan Syrup, Tetralean ✦, Tetram

Func. class.: Broad-spectrum antiinfective

Chem. class.: Tetracycline

Pregnancy category D

Action: Inhibits protein synthesis and phosphorylation in microorganisms; bacteriostatic

➔ **Therapeutic Outcome:** Bactericidal action against susceptible organisms; gram-positive pathogens: *Bacillus antracis, Clostridium perfringens, Clostridium tetani, Listeria monocytogenes, Nocardia, Propionibacterium acnes, Actinomyces isrealii;* gram-negative pathogens *Haemophilus influenzae, Legionella pneumophilia, Yersenia entercolitica, Yersinia pestis, Neisseria gonorrhoeae, Neisseria meningitidis*

Uses: Syphilis, chlamydia trachomatis, gonorrhea, lymphogranuloma venereum, uncommon gram-positive, gram-negative organisms, rickettsial infections

Dosage and routes

Adult: PO 250-500 mg q6h; IM 250 mg/day or 150 mg q12h; **IV** 250-500 mg q8-12h

P ***Child >8 yr:*** PO 25-50 mg/kg/day in divided doses q6h; IM 15-25 mg/kg/day in divided doses q8-12h; **IV** 10-20 mg/kg/day in divided doses q12h

Gonorrhea

Adult: PO 1.5 g, then 500 mg qid for a total of 9 g over 7 days

Chlamydia trachomatis

Adult: PO 500 mg qid × 7 days

Syphilis

Adult: PO 2-3 g in divided doses × 10-15 days; if syphilis duration >1 yr, must treat 30 days

Brucellosis

Adult: PO 500 mg qid × 3 wk with 1 g streptomycin IM 2 ×/day × 1 wk, and 1 ×/day the second wk

Urethral syndrome in women
Adult: PO 500 mg qid × 7 days

Acne
Adult: 1 g/day in divided doses; maintenance 125-500 mg/day

Available forms: Oral susp 125 mg/5 ml, caps 100, 200, 500 mg; tabs 100, 250, 500 mg; powder for inj

Adverse effects
CNS: Fever, headache, paresthesia
CV: Pericarditis
EENT: Dysphagia, glossitis, decreased calcification (permanent discoloration) of deciduous teeth, oral candidiasis
GI: Nausea, abdominal pain, *vomiting, diarrhea,* anorexia, enterocolitis, ***hepatotoxicity,*** flatulence, abdominal cramps, epigastric burning, stomatitis
GU: Increased BUN
HEMA: Eosinophilia, neutropenia, thrombocytopenia, leukocytosis, hemolytic anemia
INTEG: Rash, urticaria, photosensitivity, increased pigmentation, ***exfoliative dermatitis,*** pruritus, ***angioedema***

Contraindications: Hypersensitivity to tetracyclines,
P children <8 yr, pregnancy **D,** lactation

Precautions: Renal disease, hepatic disease

Pharmacokinetics

Absorption	60%-80% (PO), lower (IM)
Distribution	Widely distributed, some in CSF; crosses placenta
Metabolism	Not metabolized
Excretion	Unchanged—kidneys
Half-life	6-10 hr

Pharmacodynamics

Onset	1-2 hr
Peak	2-3 hr

Interactions
Individual drugs
Calcium: Forms chelates, ↓ absorption
Carbamazepine: ↑ effect of carbamazepine
Colestipol: ↓ absorption of tetracycline
Cholestyramine: ↓ absorption of tetracycline
Iron: Forms chelates, ↓ absorption
Magnesium: Forms chelates, ↓ absorption
Phenytoin: ↓ effect of tetracycline
Sucralfate: Prevents absorption of tetracycline
Drug classifications
Anticoagulants, oral: ↑ effect of anticoagulants
Barbiturates: ↓ effect of tetracycline
Contraceptives, oral: ↓ effect of oral contraception
Food
↓ absorption with dairy products; forms insoluble chelate
Lab test interferences
False ↑ Urinary catecholamines
False negative: Urine glucose with Clinistix, Tes-Tape

T

NURSING CONSIDERATIONS
Assessment
- Assess patient for previous sensitivity reaction
- Assess patient for signs and symptoms of infection including characteristics of wounds, sputum, urine, stool, WBC >10,000, temp; obtain baseline information before and during treatment

• Complete C&S testing before beginning drug therapy to identify if correct treatment has been initiated
• Assess for allergic reactions: rash, urticaria, pruritus, chills, fever, joint pain; angioedema may occur a few days after therapy begins—epinephrine, resuscitation equipment should be on unit for anaphylactic reaction
• Identify urine output; if decreasing, notify prescriber (may indicate nephrotoxicity); also, increased BUN, creatinine
• Monitor blood studies: AST (SGOT), ALT (SGPT), CBC, Hct, bilirubin, LDH, alk phosphatase, monthly if patient is on long-term therapy
• Assess bowel pattern qd; if severe diarrhea occurs, drug should be discontinued
• Monitor for bleeding: ecchymosis, bleeding gums, hematuria, stool guaiac daily if on long-term therapy; blood dyscrasias may occur
• Assess for overgrowth of infection: perineal itching, fever, malaise, redness, pain, swelling, drainage, rash, diarrhea, change in cough, sputum

Nursing diagnoses

✓ Infection, risk for (uses)
✓ Diarrhea (adverse reactions)
✓ Injury, risk for (adverse reactions)
✓ Knowledge deficit (teaching)
✓ Noncompliance (teaching)

Implementation

PO route

• Give around the clock to maintain proper blood levels; give with food to increase absorption of drug; do not give within 3 hr of other agents—drug actions may occur
• Give with 8 oz of water
• Shake liq preparation well before giving; use calibrated device for proper dosing

IM route

• Give IM deep in gluteus only

IV route

• Give after diluting 250 mg or less/5 ml sterile water for inj; may be further diluted with 100 ml or more D_5W or NS; give 100 mg or less over 5 min or more; use sol within 12 hr

Patient/family education

• Teach patient to report sore throat, bruising, bleeding, joint pain—may indicate blood dyscrasias (rare)
• Advise patient to use a sunscreen when outdoors to decrease photosensitivity reaction
• Advise patient to contact prescriber if vaginal itching; loose, foul-smelling stools; furry tongue occur that may indicate superimposed infection; report itching, rash, pruritus, urticaria
• Instruct patient to take all medication prescribed for the length of time ordered; drug must be taken around the clock to maintain blood levels; do not give medication to others

Evaluation

Positive therapeutic outcome

• Absence of signs/symptoms of infection (WBC <10,000, temp WNL, absence of red, draining wounds)
• Reported improvement in symptoms of infection

theophylline (℞)
(thee-off'i-lin)

Accurbron, Aerolate III, Aerolate Jr., Aerolate Slo-Phyllin, Aerolate Sr., Aquaphyllin, Asmalix, Bronkodyl, Constant-T, Elixomin, Elixophyllin, Elixophyllin SR, Lanophyllin, Quibron-T Dividose, Quibron-T/SR Dividose, Respbid, Slo-Bid Gyrocaps, Slo-Phyllin Gyrocaps, Sustaire, Theolair-SR, Theo-24, Theobid Duracaps, Theobid Jr. Duracaps, Theochron, Theoclear-80, Theoclear L.A., Theo-Dur, Theo-Dur Sprinkle, Theolair, Theolair-SR, Theophylline, Theophylline and 5% Dextrose, Theophylline Extended Release, Theophylline Oral, Theophylline S.R., Theo-Sav, Theospan-SR, Theostat 80, Theovent, Theox, T-Phy, Uniphyl

Func. class.: Spasmolytic, bronchodilator

Chem. class.: Xanthine, ethylenediamine

Pregnancy category C

Action: Relaxes smooth muscle of respiratory system by blocking phosphodiesterase, which increases cAMP, which increases bronchodilation, diuresis, circulation, CNS stimulation

Therapeutic Outcome: Ability to breathe without difficulty

Uses: Bronchial asthma, bronchospasm of COPD, chronic bronchitis

Dosage and routes

Bronchospasm, bronchial asthma

Adult: PO 100-200 mg q6h; dosage must be individualized; rec 250-500 mg q9-12h

P ***Child:*** PO 50-100 mg q6h, not to exceed 12 mg/kg/ 24 h

COPD, chronic bronchitis

Adult: PO 30-660 q6-8h pc (sodium glycinate)

P ***Child 1-9 yr:*** PO 5 mg/kg loading dose, then 4 mg/kg q6h

P ***Child 9-16 yr:*** PO 5 mg/kg losding dose, then 3 mg/kg q6h

Available forms: Caps 50, 100, 200, 250 mg; tabs 100, 125, 200, 225, 250, 300 mg; time-release tabs 100, 200, 250, 300, 400, 500 mg; time-release caps 50, 65, 100, 125, 130, 200, 250, 260, 300, 400, 500 mg; elix 80, 11.25 mg/15 mg; sol 80 mg/15 ml; liq 80, 150, 160 mg/15 ml; susp 300 mg/15 ml

Adverse effects

CNS: Anxiety, restlessness, insomnia, dizziness, convulsions, headache, lightheadedness, muscle twitching

CV: Palpitations, sinus tachycardia, hypotension, other dysrhythmias, fluid retention with tachycardia

GI: Nausea, vomiting, anorexia, diarrhea, bitter taste, dyspepsia, gastric distress

INTEG: Flushing, urticaria

RESP: Increased rate

Contraindications: Hypersensitivity to xanthines, tachydysrhythmias

G **Precautions:** Elderly, CHF, cor pulmonale, hepatic disease, active peptic ulcer disease, diabetes mellitus, hyperthyroidism, hypertension, P children, pregnancy **C**

Pharmacokinetics

Absorption	Well absorbed (PO), slowly absorbed (ext rel)
Distribution	Crosses placenta, widely distributed
Metabolism	Liver
Excretion	Kidneys, breast milk
Half-life	3-13, increased in liver disease, CHF, elderly

Pharmacodynamics

	PO	PO-ER	IV
Onset	Rapid	Slow	Immediate
Peak	1 hr	4-8 hr	Inf end
Duration	6 hr	12-24 hr	6-8 hr

Interactions

Individual drugs

Cimetidine: ↑ action of theophylline
Propranolol: ↑ action of theophylline
Erythromycin: ↑ action of theophylline
Lithium: ↓ effect of lithium

Drug classifications

β-Blockers: cardiotoxicity

NURSING CONSIDERATIONS

Assessment

- Monitor theophylline blood levels (therapeutic level is 10-20 μg/ml); toxicity may occur with small increase above 20 μg/ml
- Monitor I&O; diuresis G occurs; dehydration may result P in elderly or children
- Assess for signs of toxicity: irritability, insomnia, restlessness, tremors, nausea, vomiting
- Monitor respiratory rate, rhythm, depth; auscultate lung fields bilaterally; notify prescriber of abnormalities
- Assess for allergic reactions: rash, urticaria; if these occur, drug should be discontinued

Nursing diagnoses

✓ Airway clearance, ineffective (uses)
✓ Knowledge deficit (teaching)

Implementation

PO route

- Give PO pc to decrease GI symptoms; absorption may be affected

IV **IV route**

Additive compatibilities: Cefepime, fluconazole, methylprednisolone, verapamil

Y-site compatibilities: Acyclovir, ampicillin, aztreonam, cefazolin, cefotetan, cimetidine, clindamycin, dexamethasone, diltiazem, dobutamine, dopamine, doxycycline, erythromycin, famotidine, fluconazole, gentamicin, heparin, hydrocortisone, lidocaine, methyldopate, methylprednisolone, metronidazole, nafcillin, nitroglycerin, nitroprusside, penicillin G potassium, piperacillin, potassium chloride, ranitidine, ticarcillin, vancomycin

Patient/family education

- Advise patient to check OTC medications, current prescription medications for ephedrine, which will increase stimulation, and to avoid alcohol, caffeine
- Caution patient to avoid hazardous activities; dizziness may occur
- Inform patient that if GI upset occurs, to take drug with 8 oz water; avoid food; absorption may be decreased
- Teach patient not to crush, dissolve, or chew slow-release products
- Teach patient that contents of bead-filled cap may be

sprinkled over food for children's use

- Advise patient to notify prescriber of toxicity: nausea, vomiting, anxiety, insomnia, convulsions
- Advise patient to notify prescriber of change in smoking habit; dosage may have to be changed

Evaluation

Positive therapeutic outcome

- Ability to breathe more easily

thiamine (vitamin B_1) (PO, OTC; IV, ℞)

Betaxin ✦, Betalin S, Biamine, Revitonus, Thiamilate, thiamine HCl, vitamin B

Func. class.: Vitamin B_1

Chem. class.: Water soluble

Pregnancy category A

Action: Needed for pyruvate metabolism, carbohydrate metabolism

Therapeutic Outcome: Prevention and treatment of thiamine deficiency

Uses: Vitamin B_1 deficiency or polyneuritis, cheilosis adjunct with thiamine beriberi, Wernicke-Korsakoff syndrome, pellagra, metabolic disorders

Dosage and routes

Beriberi

Adult: IM 10-500 mg tid × 2 wk, then 5-10 mg qd × 1 mo

Child: IM 10-50 mg qd × 4-6 wk

Anemia/alcoholism/pregnancy/pellagra

Adult: PO 100 mg qd

Child: PO 10-50 mg qd in divided doses

Beriberi with cardiac failure

Adult and child: **IV** 100-500 mg

Wernicke's encephalopathy

Adult: **IV** 500 mg or less, then 100 mg bid

Available forms: Tab 50, 100, 250, 500 mg; inj 100 mg/ml; enteric-coated tab 20 mg

Adverse effects

CNS: Weakness, restlessness

CV: ***Collapse, pulmonary edema***, hypotension

EENT: Tightness of throat

GI: Hemorrhage, ***nausea, diarrhea***

INTEG: ***Angioneurotic edema***, cyanosis, sweating, warmth

SYST: ***Anaphylaxis***

Contraindications: Hypersensitivity

Precautions: Pregnancy **A**

Pharmacokinetics

Absorption	Well absorbed (PO, IM) completely absorbed (IV)
Distribution	Widely distributed
Metabolism	Liver
Excretion	Kidneys (unchanged— excess amounts)
Half-life	Unknown

Pharmacodynamics

Unknown

Interactions

Drug classifications

Neuromuscular blockers: ↑ effect

NURSING CONSIDERATIONS

Assessment

- Monitor thiamine levels throughout treatment

• Assess nutritional status: yeast, beef, liver, whole or enriched grains, legumes

Nursing diagnoses

✓ Nutrition: less than body requirements (uses)

✓ Knowledge deficit (teaching)

Implementation

IV **IV route**

• **IV** undiluted given over 5 min or diluted with **IV** sol and given as an inf at a rate of 100 mg or less/5 min or more

Syringe compatibility: Doxapram

Y-site compatibility: Famotidine

Additive incompatibilities: Barbiturates; sol with neutral or alkaline pH, such as carbonates, bicarbonates, citrates and acetates; erythromycin, kanamycin, or streptomycin

IM route

• Give by IM inj; rotate sites if pain and inflammation occur; do not mix with alkaline sol; Z-track to minimize pain

• Application of cold may decrease pain

• Store in tight, light-resistant container

Patient/family education

• Teach patient necessary foods to be included in diet: yeast, beef, liver, legumes, whole grains

Evaluation

Positive therapeutic outcome

• Absence of nausea, vomiting, anorexia, insomnia, tachycardia, paresthesias, depression, muscle weakness

thiethylperazine (℞)

(thye-eth-il-per′a-zeen)

Norzine, Torecan

Func. class.: Antiemetic

Chem. class.: Phenothiazine, piperazine derivative

Pregnancy category C

Action: Acts centrally by blocking chemoreceptor trigger zone, which in turn acts on vomiting center

➔ **Therapeutic Outcome:** Control of nausea, vomiting

Uses: Nausea, vomiting

Dosage and routes

Adult: PO/IM/rec 10 mg/qd-tid

Available forms: Tab 10 mg; supp 10 mg; inj 5 mg/ml

Adverse effects

CNS: Euphoria, depression, restlessness, tremor, extrapyramidal symptoms, ***convulsions,*** drowsiness

CV: ***Circulatory failure, tachycardia,*** postural hypotension, ECG changes

GI: Nausea, vomiting, anorexia, dry mouth, diarrhea, constipation, weight loss, metallic taste, cramps

GU: Urinary retention, dark urine

RESP: ***Respiratory depression***

Contraindications: Hypersensitivity to phenothiazines, coma, seizure, encephalopathy, bone marrow depression

P G **Precautions:** Children < 2 yr, pregnancy **C**, elderly

Pharmacokinetics

Absorption	Readily absorbed
Distribution	Crosses placenta
Metabolism	Liver
Excretion	Kidneys, breast milk
Half-life	Unknown

Pharmacodynamics

	PO	REC	IM
Onset	45-60 min	45-60 min	Unknown
Peak	Unknown	Unknown	Unknown
Duration	4 hr	Unknown	Unknown

Interactions

Drug classifications

Antacids: ↓ absorption
Anticholinergics: ↑ anticholinergic effects
Antidepressants: ↑ CNS depression
Antidiarrheals, adsorbent: ↓ absorption
Antihistamines: ↑ CNS depression
Antihypertensives: ↑ hypotension
Antithyroid agents: ↑ agranulocytosis
Barbiturate anesthetics: ↑ CNS depression
β-Adrenergics: ↑ effects of both drugs
General anesthetics: ↑ CNS depression
MAOIs: ↑ CNS depression
Narcotics: ↑ CNS depression
Sedative/hypnotics: ↑ CNS depression

NURSING CONSIDERATIONS

Assessment

- Monitor I&O ratio, palpate bladder if low urinary output occurs, especially in elderly; urinalysis recommended before, during prolonged therapy
- Monitor bilirubin, CBC, liver function studies monthly
- Assess affect, orientation, LOC, reflexes, gait, coordination, sleep pattern disturbances
- Monitor B/P with patient in sitting, standing, and lying positions; take pulse and respirations q4h during initial treatment; establish baseline before starting treatment; report drops of 30 mm Hg
- Check for dizziness, faintness, palpitations, tachycardia on rising; severe orthostatic hypotension is common
- Identify for neuroleptic malignant syndrome: hyperpyrexia, muscle rigidity, increased CPK, altered mental status; drug should be discontinued
- Assess for extrapyramidal symptoms including akathisia (inability to sit still, no pattern to movements), tardive dyskinesia (bizarre movements of the jaw, mouth, tongue, extremities), pseudoparkinsonism (tremors, pill rolling, shuffling gait); antiparkinsonian drug should be prescribed
- Assess for constipation, urinary retention daily; if these occur, increase bulk, water in diet

Nursing diagnoses

- ✓ Thought processes, altered (uses)
- ✓ Coping, ineffective individual (uses)
- ✓ Knowledge deficit (teaching)
- ✓ Noncompliance (teaching)

Implementation

IM route

- Give IM inj in large muscle mass; aspirate to avoid **IV** administration; give slowly; have patient remain supine for 1 hr after administration

Syringe compatibilities: Butorphanol, hydromorphone, midazolam, ranitidine

Patient/family education

- Teach patient to use good oral hygiene; frequent rinsing of mouth, sugarless gum for dry mouth
- Caution patient to avoid hazardous activities until drug response is determined—dizziness, blurred vision may occur
- Inform patient that orthostatic hypotension occurs often and to rise from sitting or lying position gradually
- Instruct patient to remain lying down after IM inj for at least 30 min
- Advise patient to avoid hot tubs, hot showers, tub baths, since hypotension may occur
- Inform patient that heat stroke may occur in hot weather, and to take extra precautions to stay cool
- Teach patient to avoid OTC preparations (cough, hay fever, cold) unless approved by prescriber because serious drug interactions may occur; avoid use with alcohol, CNS depressants because increased drowsiness may occur
- Inform patient to use a sunscreen and sunglasses to prevent burns
- Teach patient about extrapyramidal symptoms
- Instruct patient to report sore throat, malaise, fever, bleeding, mouth sores; if these occur, CBC should be drawn and drug discontinued

Evaluation

Positive therapeutic outcome

- Absence of nausea, vomiting

thioguanine (6-TG) (℞)

(thye-oh-gwah′neen)

thioguanine, Lanvis ✦

Func. class.: Antineoplastic-antimetabolite

Chem. class.: Purine analog

Pregnancy category D

Action: Interferes with synthesis, utilization of purine nucleotides; S phase of cell cycle specific

➡ **Therapeutic Outcome:** Prevention of rapidly growing malignant cells

Uses: Acute leukemias, chronic granulocytic leukemia, lymphomas, multiple myeloma, solid tumors

Dosage and routes

P ***Adult and child:*** PO 2 mg/kg/day, then increase slowly to 3 mg/kg/day after 4 wk

Available forms: Tab 40 mg

Adverse effects

GI: Nausea, vomiting, anorexia, diarrhea, stomatitis, ***hepatotoxicity,*** gastritis, jaundice

GU: ***Renal failure,*** hyperuricemia, oliguria

HEMA: ***Thrombocytopenia, leukopenia, myelosuppression, anemia***

INTEG: Rash, dermatitis, dry skin

Contraindications: Prior drug resistance, leukopenia (2500/mm^3), thrombocytopenia (<100,000/mm^3), anemia, pregnancy **D**

Precautions: Liver disease

Pharmacokinetics

Absorption	Variably absorbed, 30%
Distribution	Crosses placenta
Metabolism	Liver—extensively
Excretion	Kidneys
Half-life	11 hr

Pharmacodynamics

Unknown

Interactions

Individual drugs

Radiation: ↑ toxicity, bone marrow suppression

Drug classifications

Antineoplastics: ↑ toxicity, bone marrow suppression

Lab test interferences

↑ Uric acid (blood, urine)

NURSING CONSIDERATIONS

Assessment

- Assess buccal cavity q8h for dryness, sores or ulceration, white patches, oral pain, bleeding, dysphagia; obtain prescription for viscous lidocaine (Xylocaine)
- Assess symptoms indicating severe allergic reaction: rash, pruritus, urticaria, purpuric skin lesions, itching, flushing
- Monitor CBC, differential, platelet count weekly; withhold drug if WBC count is <4000/mm^3 or platelet count is <100,000/mm^3, notify prescriber of results if WBC <20,000/mm^3, platelets </50,000/mm^3
- Assess for increased uric acid levels, swelling, joint pain (primarily in extremities); patient should be well hydrated to prevent urate deposits
- Monitor renal function studies: BUN, creatinine, serum uric acid, urine CrCl before and during therapy; I&O ratio; report fall in urine output to <30 ml/hr
- Monitor temp q4h (may indicate beginning of infection)
- Monitor liver function tests before and during therapy (bilirubin, AST (SGOT), ALT (SGPT), LDH) as needed or monthly; yellowing of skin, sclera, dark urine, clay-colored stools, itchy skin, abdominal pain, fever, diarrhea
- Assess for bleeding: hematuria, stool guaiac, bruising or petechiae, mucosa or orifices q8h; inflammation of mucosa, breaks in skin
- Identify edema in feet, joint pain, stomach pain, shaking; prescriber should be notified
- Identity inflammation of mucosa, breaks in skin

Nursing diagnoses

- ✓ Injury, risk for (adverse reactions)
- ✓ Body image disturbance (adverse reactions)
- ✓ Infection, risk for (adverse reactions)
- ✓ Knowledge deficit (teaching)

Implementation

- Avoid contact with skin (very irritating), wash completely to remove
- Give fluids **IV** or PO before chemotherapy to hydrate patient
- Give antiemetic 30-60 min before giving drug to prevent vomiting, and prn; antibiotics for prophylaxis of infection
- Give top or syst analgesics for pain
- Provide liq diet: carbonated beverages; gelatin may be added if patient is not nauseated or vomiting
- Provide rinsing of mouth tid-qid with water, club soda;

brushing of teeth bid-qid with soft brush or cotton-tipped applicators for stomatitis; use unwaxed dental floss

- Give 1 hr ac or 2 hr pc to prevent vomiting

Patient/family education

- Inform patient that contraceptive measures are recommended during therapy
- Caution patient to avoid use of products containing aspirin or ibuprofen, razors, commercial mouthwash, bleeding may occur; to report symptoms of bleeding (hematuria, tarry stools)
- Advise patient to report signs of anemia, (fatigue, headache, irritability, faintness, shortness of breath)
- Caution patient not to have any vaccinations without the advice of the prescriber—serious reactions can occur

Evaluation

Positive therapeutic outcome

- Prevention of rapid division of malignant cells

thiopental (℞)

(thye-oh-pen′tal)

Pentothal, thiopental sodium

Func. class.: General anesthetic

Chem. class.: Barbiturate

Pregnancy category C

Controlled substance schedule III

Action: Acts in reticular-activating system to produce anesthesia, raise seizure threshold

Therapeutic Outcome: Sedation, decreased seizure, decreased intracranial pressure

Uses: Short general anesthesia, narcoanalysis, induction anesthesia before other anesthetics

Investigational uses: Increased intracranial pressure

Dosage and routes

Induction

Adult: **IV** 210-280 mg or 3-5 ml/kg

General anesthetic

Adult: **IV** 50-75 mg given at 20-40 sec intervals

Narcoanalysis

Adult: **IV** 100 mg/min, not to exceed 50 ml/min

Sedation or narcosis

Adult: Rec 12-20 mg/lb

Increased intracranial pressure

Adult: 1.5-3.5 mg/kg

Available forms: Powder for inj 2%, 2.5%

Adverse effects

CNS: Retrograde amnesia, prolonged somnolence

CV: Tachycardia, hypotension, ***myocardial depression, dysrhythmias***

EENT: Sneezing, coughing

INTEG: Chills, ***shivering***, necrosis, pain at inj site

MS: Muscle irritability

RESP: Respiratory depression, bronchospasm

Contraindications: Hypersensitivity, status asthmaticus, hepatic/intermittent porphyrias

Precautions: Severe cardiovascular disease, renal disease, hypotension, liver disease, myxedema, myasthenia gravis, asthma, increased intracranial pressure, pregnancy **C**

Pharmacokinetics

Absorption	Rapidly absorbed (rectal)
Distribution	Rapidly—CNS, redistributed to other organs, crosses placenta
Metabolism	Extensively—liver, small amounts converted to phenobarbital
Excretion	Urine
Half-life	11½ hr; ↑ in obese and pregnant patients (term)

Pharmacodynamics

	IV	REC
Onset	½-1 sec	8-10 min
Peak	Unknown	Unknown
Duration	10-30 min	Unknown

Interactions

Individual drugs

Alcohol: ↑ CNS depression
Ketamine: ↑ Hypotension

Drug classifications

Antidepressants: ↑ CNS depression
Antihistamines: ↑ CNS depression
Diuretics: ↑ Hypotension
Narcotics: ↑ CNS depression
Sedative/hypnotics: ↑ CNS depression

Lab test interferences

False ↑ Sulfobromophthalein

NURSING CONSIDERATIONS

Assessment

- Monitor inj site for redness, pain, swelling
- Assess degree of amnesia in G elderly; may be increased
- Assess anterograde amnesia
- Assess vital signs for recovery period in obese patient because half-life may be extended

Nursing diagnoses

✓ Anxiety (uses)
✓ Knowledge deficit (teaching)
✓ Noncompliance (teaching)

Implementation

IV **IV route**

- Dilute with D_5W, 0.9% NaCl, or sterile water for inj; do not use colored sol or sol with a precipitate
- Give test dose before administering 25-75 mg, wait 1-2 sec for response
- Give by continual inf after diluting in compatible sol and give slowly

Syringe compatibilities: Aminophylline, hydrocortisone sodium succinate, neostigmine, pentobarbital, scopolamine, tubocurarine

Syringe incompatibilities: Benzquinamide, chlorpromazine, dimenhydrinate, diphenhydramine, ephedrine, glycopyrrolate, meperidine, morphine, pentazocine, prochlorperazine, promethazine, propiomazine

Additive compatibilities: Chloramphenicol, hydrocortisone sodium succinate, pentobarbital, potassium chloride

Additive incompatibilities: Amikacin, cephapirin, chlorpromazine, codeine, dimenhydrinate, diphenhydramine, hydromorphone, regular insulin, levorphanol, meperidine, methadone, morphine, penicillin G potassium, prochlorperazine, promazine, promethazine, succinylcholine

Solution compatibilities: D_5/0.45% NaCl, D_5W, multiple electrolyte sol, 0.45% NaCl, 0.9% NaCl, 1/6 M sodium lactate

Solution incompatibilities: Dextrose/Ringer's, lactated Ringer's inj combinations, D_{10}/0.9% NaCl, $D_{10}W$, Ringer's, lactated Ringer's inj

T

Patient/family education
- Caution patient to avoid hazardous activities until drowsiness, weakness subside
- Inform patient that amnesia occurs; events may not be remembered

Evaluation
Positive therapeutic outcome
- Induction of sedation, general anesthesia

Treatment of overdose: Discontinue drug; administer vasopressor agents or anticholinergics, artificial ventilation

thioridazine (℞)

(thye-or-rid'a-zeen)
Mellaril, Mellaril Concentrate, Mellaril-5, Novoridazine ✤, thioridazine HCl
Func. class.: Antipsychotic/neuroleptic
Chem. class.: Phenothiazine, piperidine
Pregnancy category C

Action: Depresses cerebral cortex, hypothalamus, limbic system, which control activity, aggression; blocks neurotransmission produced by dopamine at synapse; exhibits strong α-adrenergic, anticholinergic blocking action; mechanism for antipsychotic effects is unclear

➔ **Therapeutic Outcome:** Decreased signs and symptoms of psychosis

Uses: Psychotic disorders, schizophrenia, behavioral problems in children, alcohol withdrawal as adjunct, anxiety, major depressive disorders, organic brain syndrome

Dosage and routes
Psychosis
Adult: PO 25-100 mg tid, max dose 800 mg/day; dose is gradually increased to desired response, then reduced to minimum maintenance

Depression/behavioral problems/organic brain syndrome
Adult: PO 25 tid, range from 10 mg bid-qid to 50 mg tid-qid; decrease dose in elderly [G]

[P] ***Child 2-12 yr:*** PO 0.5-3 mg/kg/day in divided doses

Available forms: Tabs 10, 15, 25, 50, 100, 150, 200, 300 mg; conc 30, 100 mg/ml; susp 25, 100 mg/5 ml; syrup 10 mg/15 ml

Adverse effects
CNS: Extrapyramidal symptoms (rare): pseudoparkinsonism, akathisia, dystonia, tardive dyskinesia, ***seizures, headache,*** confusion
CV: Orthostatic hypotension, ***cardiac arrest,*** ECG changes, ***tachycardia***
EENT: Blurred vision, glaucoma, dry eyes
GI: Dry mouth, nausea, vomiting, anorexia, constipation, diarrhea, jaundice, weight gain
GU: Urinary retention, urinary frequency, enuresis, impotence, amenorrhea, gynecomastia
HEMA: Anemia, ***leukopenia, leukocytosis, agranulocytosis***
INTEG: Rash, photosensitivity, dermatitis
RESP: Laryngospasm, dyspnea, ***respiratory depression***

Contraindications: Hypersensitivity, blood dyscrasias, coma, [P] child <2 yr, brain damage, bone marrow depression

Precautions: Pregnancy **C**, lactation, seizure disorders, hypertension, hepatic disease, cardiac disease

Pharmacokinetics

Absorption	Variably absorbed (tab)
Distribution	Widely distributed, high concentrations in CNS, crosses placenta
Metabolism	Liver, extensively, GI mucosa
Excretion	Kidneys, breast milk
Half-life	26-36 hr

Pharmacodynamics

Onset	Erratic
Peak	2-4 hr
Duration	8-12 hr

Interactions
Individual drugs
Alcohol: ↑ effects of both drugs, oversedation
Aluminum hydroxide: ↓ absorption
Bromocriptine: ↓ antiparkinson activity
Disopyramide: ↑ anticholinergic effects
Epinephrine: ↑ toxicity
Guanethidine: ↓ antihypertensive response
Levodopa: ↓ antiparkinson activity
Lithium: ↓ chlorpromazine levels, ↑ extrapyramidal symptoms, masking of lithium toxicity
Magnesium hydroxide: ↓ absorption
Norepinephrine: ↓ vasoresponse, ↑ toxicity
Phenobarbital: ↓ effectiveness, ↑ metabolism
Drug classifications
Antacids: ↓ absorption
Anticholinergics: ↑ anticholinergic effects
Antidepressants: ↑ CNS depression
Antidiarrheals, adsorbent: ↓ absorption
Antihistamines: ↑ CNS depression
Antihypertensives: ↑ hypotension
Antithyroid agents: ↑ agranulocytosis
Barbiturate anesthetics: ↑ CNS depression
β-adrenergics: ↑ effects of both drugs
General anesthetics: ↑ CNS depression
MAOIs: ↑ CNS depression
Narcotics: ↑ CNS depression
Sedative/hypnotics: ↑ CNS depression
Lab test interferences
↑ Liver function tests, ↑ cardiac enzymes, ↑ cholesterol, ↑ blood glucose, ↑ prolactin, ↑ bilirubin, ↑ PBI, ↑ cholinesterase, ↑ ^{131}I, ↑ alk phosphatase, ↑ leukocytes, ↑ granulocytes, ↑ platelets
↓ Hormones (blood and urine)
False positive: Pregnancy tests, PKU, urine bilirubin
False negative: Urinary steroids, 17-OHCS

NURSING CONSIDERATIONS
Assessment
• Assess mental status: orientation, mood, behavior, presence of hallucinations, and type before initial administration and monthly; this drug should significantly reduce psychotic behavior
• Check for swallowing of PO medication; check for hoarding or giving of medication to other patients
• Monitor I&O ratio, palpate bladder if low urinary output occurs, especially in elderly; urinalysis recommended before, during prolonged therapy
• Monitor bilirubin, CBC, liver function studies monthly
• Assess affect, orientation,

LOC, reflexes, gait, coordination, sleep pattern disturbances

- Monitor B/P sitting, standing and lying, take pulse and respirations q4h during initial treatment; establish baseline before starting treatment; report drops of 30 mm Hg; obtain baseline ECG, Q-wave and T-wave changes
- Check for dizziness, faintness, palpitations, tachycardia on rising; severe orthostatic hypotension is common
- Identify for neuroleptic malignant syndrome: hyperpyrexia, muscle rigidity, increased CPK, altered mental status; drug should be discontinued
- Assess for extrapyramidal symptoms including akathisia (inability to sit still, no pattern to movements), tardive dyskinesia (bizarre movements of the jaw, mouth, tongue, extremities), pseudoparkinsonism (ragged tremors, pill rolling, shuffling gate)—an antiparkinsonian drug should be prescribed
- Assess for constipation, urinary retention daily; if these occur, increase bulk, water in diet

Nursing diagnoses

- ✓ Thought processes, altered (uses)
- ✓ Coping, ineffective individual (uses)
- ✓ Knowledge deficit (teaching)
- ✓ Noncompliance (teaching)

Implementation

- Administer drug in liq form mixed in glass of juice or cola if hoarding is suspected; do not mix in caffeine drinks, tannics, pectins
- G Decrease dose in elderly; metabolism is slowed in the elderly
- Administer PO with full glass of water, milk; or give with food to decrease GI upset
- Store in tight, light-resistant container, oral sol in amber bottle

Patient/family education

- Teach patient to use good oral hygiene; frequent rinsing of mouth, sugarless gum for dry mouth
- Advise patient to avoid hazardous activities until drug response is determined dizziness, blurred vision are common
- Inform patient that orthostatic hypotension occurs often and to rise from sitting or lying position gradually; to avoid hot tubs, hot showers, tub baths because hypotension may occur
- Instruct patient that in hot weather, heat stroke may occur; take extra precautions to stay cool
- Caution patient to avoid abrupt withdrawal of this drug, or extrapyramidal symptoms may result; drug should be withdrawn slowly
- Teach patient to avoid OTC preparations (cough, hay fever, cold) unless approved by prescriber—serious drug interactions may occur; avoid use with alcohol, CNS depressants—increased drowsiness may occur
- Advise patient to use a sunscreen and sunglasses to prevent burns
- Teach patient about extrapyramidal symptoms and necessity for meticulous oral hygiene because oral candidiasis may occur
- Advise patient to take antac-

ids 2 hr before or after this drug

- Instruct patient to report sore throat, malaise, fever, bleeding, mouth sores; if these occur, CBC should be drawn and drug discontinued

Evaluation

Positive therapeutic outcome

- Decrease in emotional excitement, hallucinations, delusions, paranoia
- Reorganization of patterns of thought, speech

Treatment of overdose: Lavage if orally ingested; provide airway; *do not induce vomiting or use epinephrine*

thiotepa (℞)

(thye-oh-tep′a)

Thioplex

Func. class.: Antineoplastic

Chem. class.: Alkylating agent

Pregnancy category D

Action: Responsible for cross-linking DNA strands leading to cell death; activity is not cell–cycle-specific

Therapeutic Outcome: Prevention of rapidly growing malignant cells

Uses: Hodgkin's disease, lymphomas; breast, ovarian, lung, bladder, cancer; neoplastic effusions

Dosage and routes

Adult: **IV** 0.3-0.4 mg/kg at 1-4 wk intervals

Neoplastic effusions

Adult: Intracavity 0.6-0.8 mg/kg

Bladder cancer

Adult: Instill 60 mg/30-60 ml water for inj instilled in bladder for 2 hr once weekly × 4 wk

Available forms: Powder for inj 15 mg

Adverse effects

CNS: Dizziness, headache

GI: Nausea, vomiting, anorexia

GU: Hyperuricemia, ***hematuria, amenorrhea, azoospermia***

HEMA: ***Thrombocytopenia, leukopenia, pancytopenia***

INTEG: Rash, pruritus

Contraindications: Hypersensitivity, pregnancy **D**

Precautions: Radiation therapy, bone marrow suppression, impaired renal or hepatic function

Pharmacokinetics	
Absorption	Variably absorbed
Distribution	Unknown
Metabolism	Liver—extensively
Excretion	Kidneys
Half-life	Unknown

Pharmacodynamics

Unknown

Interactions

Individual drugs

Radiation: ↑ toxicity, bone marrow suppression

Succinylcholine: ↑ apnea

Drug classifications

Antineoplastics: ↑ toxicity, bone marrow suppression

NURSING CONSIDERATIONS

Assessment

- Assess symptoms indicating severe allergic reaction: rash, pruritus, urticaria, itching, flushing
- Monitor CBC, differential, platelet count weekly; withhold drug if WBC count is <4000/

mm^3 or platelet count is <100,000/mm^3; notify prescriber of results if WBC <20,000/mm^3, platelets <150,000/mm^3
• Monitor renal function studies: BUN, creatinine, serum uric acid, urine CrCl before and during therapy; I&O ratio; report fall in urine output to <30 ml/hr
• Monitor temp q4h (may indicate beginning of infection)
• Monitor liver function tests before and during therapy [bilirubin, AST (SGOT), ALT (SGPT), LDH] as needed or monthly; yellowing of skin, sclera, dark urine, clay-colored stools, itchy skin, abdominal pain, fever, diarrhea
• Assess for bleeding: hematuria, stool guaiac, bruising or petechiae, mucosa or orifices q8h; inflammation of mucosa, breaks in skin
• Identify dyspnea, rales, unproductive cough, chest pain, tachypnea
• Identify effects of alopecia on body image; discuss feelings about body changes

Nursing diagnoses

✓ Injury, risk for (adverse reactions)
✓ Body image disturbance (adverse reactions)
✓ Infection, risk for (adverse reactions)
✓ Knowledge deficit (teaching)

Implementation

• Give fluids **IV** or PO before chemotherapy to hydrate patient
• Give antacid before oral agent, give drug after evening meal, before bedtime; antiemetic 30-60 min before giving drug to prevent vomiting, and prn; antibiotics for prophylaxis of infection
• Give top or syst analgesics for pain
• Give liq diet: carbonated beverages; gelatin may be added if patient is not nauseated or vomiting
• Provide rinsing of mouth tid-qid with water, club soda; brushing of teeth bid-qid with soft brush or cotton-tipped applicators for stomatitis; use unwaxed dental floss

IV **IV route**

Direct route

• Give **IV** after diluting 15 mg/1.5 ml of sterile H_2O for inj; give over 1-3 min, use a 0.22 micron filter

Intermittent inf

• May be further diluted in 50-100 ml D_5W, 0.9% NaCl, Ringer's, LR

Syringe compatibilities: Procaine HCl, (2%), epinephrine 1:1000

Y-site compatibilities: Allopurinol, aztreonam, cefepime, melphalan, piperacillin/tazobactam, teniposide

Instill route

• Reconstitute solution, then mix 60 mg/30-60 ml sterile water; instill is by Foley catheter; patient's position may be changed every few min; the patient must retain sol for 2 hr to provide for cell death

Intracavity route

• Reconstitute sol and administer by effusion tube as directed

Patient/family education

• Caution patient to avoid use of products containing aspirin or ibuprofen, razors, commercial mouthwash because bleeding may occur; to report symptoms of bleeding (hematuria, tarry stools)

• Advise patient to report signs of anemia, (fatigue, headache, irritability, faintness, shortness of breath)

• Advise patient to report any changes in breathing or coughing even several mo after treatment; to avoid crowds or persons with respiratory or other infections

• Inform patient that hair may be lost during treatment; a wig or hairpiece may make patient feel better; new hair may be different in color, texture

• Caution patient not to have any vaccinations without the advice of the prescriber because serious reactions can occur

• Advise patient that contraception is needed during treatment and for several mo after the completion of therapy

Evaluation

Positive therapeutic outcome

• Prevention of rapid division of malignant cells

thiothixene (℞)

(thye-oh-thix'een)

Navane, thiothixene

Func. class.: Antipsychotic/neuroleptic

Chem. class.: Thioxanthene

Pregnancy category C

Action: Depresses cerebral cortex, hypothalamus, limbic system, which control activity, aggression; blocks neurotransmission produced by dopamine at synapse; exhibits strong α-adrenergic blocking action; mechanism for antipsychotic effects is unclear

➔ **Therapeutic Outcome:** Decreased signs and symptoms of psychosis

Uses: Psychotic disorders, schizophrenia, acute agitation

Dosage and routes

Adult: PO 2-5 mg bid-qid depending on severity of condition; dose gradually increased to 15-30 mg if needed; IM 4 mg bid-qid; max dose 30 mg qd; administer PO dose as soon as possible

Available forms: Caps 1, 2, 5, 10, 20 mg; conc 5 mg/ml; inj 2 mg/ml; powder for inj 5 mg/ml

Adverse effects

CNS: Extrapyramidal symptoms: pseudoparkinsonism, akathisia, dystonia, tardive dyskinesia, seizures, *headache*

CV: Orthostatic hypotension, hypertension, ***cardiac arrest,*** ECG changes, ***tachycardia***

EENT: Blurred vision, glaucoma

GI: Dry mouth, nausea, vomiting, anorexia, constipation, diarrhea, jaundice, weight gain

GU: Urinary retention, urinary frequency, enuresis, impotence, amenorrhea, gynecomastia

HEMA: Anemia, ***leukopenia, leukocytosis, agranulocytosis***

INTEG: Rash, photosensitivity, dermatitis

RESP: ***Laryngospasm,*** dyspnea, ***respiratory depression***

Contraindications: Hypersensitivity, blood dyscrasias, child <12 yr, bone marrow depression, circulatory collapse, CNS depression, coma, alcoholism, CV disease, hepatic disease, Reye's syndrome, narrow-angle glaucoma

Precautions: Pregnancy **C,** lactation, seizure disorders, hypertension, hepatic disease

Pharmacokinetics

Absorption	Well absorbed (PO, IM)
Distribution	Widely distributed, crosses placenta
Metabolism	Liver
Excretion	Kidneys, breast milk
Half-life	34 hr

Pharmacodynamics

	PO	IM
Onset	Slow	15-30 min
Peak	2-8 hr	1-6 hr
Duration	Up to 12 hr	Up to 12 hr

Interactions

Individual drugs

Alcohol: ↑ effects of both drugs, oversedation
Aluminum hydroxide: ↓ absorption
Bromocriptine: ↓ antiparkinson activity
Disopyramide: ↑ anticholinergic effects
Epinephrine: ↑ toxicity
Guanethidine: ↓ antihypertensive response
Levodopa: ↓ antiparkinson activity
Lithium: ↓ chlorpromazine levels, ↑ extrapyramidal symptoms, masking of lithium toxicity
Magnesium hydroxide: ↓ absorption
Norepinephrine: ↓ vasoresponse, ↑ toxicity
Phenobarbital: ↓ effectiveness, ↑ metabolism

Drug classifications

Antacids: ↓ absorption
Anticholinergics: ↑ anticholinergic effects
Antidepressants: ↑ CNS depression
Antidiarrheals, adsorbent: ↓ absorption
Antihistamines: ↑ CNS depression
Antihypertensives: ↑ hypotension
Antithyroid agents: ↑ agranulocytosis
Barbiturate anesthetics: ↑ CNS depression
β-Adrenergics: ↑ effects of both drugs
General anesthetics: ↑ CNS depression
MAOIs: ↑ CNS depression
Narcotics: ↑ CNS depression
Sedative/hypnotics: ↑ CNS depression

Lab test interferences

↑ Liver function tests, ↑ cardiac enzymes, ↑ cholesterol, ↑ blood glucose, ↑ prolactin, ↑ bilirubin, ↑ PBI, ↑ cholinesterase, ↑ ^{131}I, ↑ alk phosphatase, ↑ leukocytes, ↑ granulocytes, ↑ platelets
↓ Hormones (blood and urine)
False positive: Pregnancy tests, PKU, urine bilirubin
False negative: Urinary steroids, 17-OHCS

NURSING CONSIDERATIONS

Assessment

- Assess mental status: orientation, mood, behavior, presence of hallucinations, and type before initial administration and monthly; this drug should significantly reduce psychotic behavior
- Check for swallowing of PO medication; check for hoarding or giving of medication to other patients
- Monitor I&O ratio, palpate bladder if low urinary output **G** occurs, especially in elderly; urinalysis recommended before, during prolonged therapy
- Monitor bilirubin, CBC, liver function studies monthly
- Assess affect, orientation,

LOC, reflexes, gait, coordination, sleep pattern disturbances
• Monitor B/P sitting, standing and lying, take pulse and respirations q4h during initial treatment; establish baseline before starting treatment; report drops of 30 mm Hg; obtain baseline ECG, Q-wave and T-wave changes
• Check for dizziness, faintness, palpitations, tachycardia on rising; severe orthostatic hypotension is common
• Identify for neuroleptic malignant syndrome: hyperpyrexia, muscle rigidity, increased CPK, altered mental status; drug should be discontinued
• Assess for extrapyramidal symptoms including akathisia (inability to sit still, no pattern to movements), tardive dyskinesia (bizarre movements of the jaw, mouth, tongue, extremities), pseudoparkinsonism (ragged tremors, pill rolling, shuffling gait); an antiparkinson drug should be prescribed
• Assess for constipation, urinary retention daily; if these occur, increase bulk, water in diet

Nursing diagnoses

✓ Thought processes, altered (uses)
✓ Coping, ineffective individual (uses)
✓ Knowledge deficit (teaching)
✓ Noncompliance (teaching)

Implementation

PO route

• Give drug in liq form mixed in glass of juice or cola if hoarding is suspected; do not mix in caffeine drinks, tannics, pectins
• Give decreased dose to elderly because metabolism is slowed in the elderly
• Give PO with full glass of water, milk; or give with food to decrease GI upset
• Store in tight, light-resistant container; store oral sol in amber bottle

IM route

• Dilute 10 mg vial/2.2 ml sterile water for inj to 5 mg/ml
• Inj in deep muscle mass, do not give SC; do not administer sol with a precipitate

Syringe compatibilities: Benztropine, diphenhydramine, hydroxyzine

Patient/family education

• Teach patient to use good oral hygiene; frequent rinsing of mouth, sugarless gum for dry mouth
• Advise patient to avoid hazardous activities until drug response is determined; dizziness, blurred vision is common
• Inform patient that orthostatic hypotension occurs often and to rise from sitting or lying position gradually and to remain lying down after IM inj for at least 30 min; tell patient to avoid hot tubs, hot showers, tub baths because hypotension may occur; tell patient that in hot weather, heat stroke may occur, so to take extra precautions to stay cool
• Caution patient to avoid abrupt withdrawal of this drug, or extrapyramidal symptoms may result; drug should be withdrawn slowly
• Teach patient to avoid OTC preparations (cough, hayfever, cold) unless approved by prescriber, because serious drug interactions may occur; avoid use with alcohol, CNS depressants because increased drowsiness may occur

T

• Caution patient to use a sunscreen and sunglasses to prevent burns
• Teach patient about extrapyramidal symptoms and necessity of meticulous oral hygiene because oral candidiasis may occur
• Tell patient to take antacids 2 hr before or after this drug
• Advise patient to report sore throat, malaise, fever, bleeding, mouth sores; if these occur, CBC should be measured and drug discontinued

Evaluation

Positive therapeutic outcome
• Decrease in emotional excitement, hallucinations, delusions, paranoia
• Reorganization of patterns of thought, speech

Treatment of overdose: Lavage if orally ingested; provide airway; *do not induce vomiting or use epinephrine*

thyroid USP (desiccated) (℞)

(thye'roid)

Armour Thyroid, Cholaxin ✤, S-P-T, Thyrar, Thyroid Strong, thyroid USP

Func. class.: Thyroid hormone

Chem. class.: Active thyroid hormone in natural state and ratio

Pregnancy category A

Action: Increases metabolic rates; controls protein synthesis; increases cardiac output, renal blood blow, O_2 consumption, body temp, blood volume, growth, development at cellular level

➔ **Therapeutic Outcome:** Correction of lack of thyroid hormone

Uses: Hypothyroidism, cretinism (juvenile hypothyroidism), myxedema

Dosage and routes

Hypothyroidism

Adult: PO 65 mg qd, increased by 65 mg q30d until desired response; maintenance dose 65-195 mg qd

G ***Geriatric:*** PO 7.5-15 mg qd, double dose q6-8w until desired response

Cretinism/juvenile hypothyroidism

P ***Child over 1 yr:*** PO up to 180 mg qd titrated to response

P ***Child 4-12 mo:*** PO 30-60 mg qd

P ***Child 1-4 mo:*** PO 15-30 mg qd; may increase q2w; titrated to response; maintenance dose 30-45 mg qd

Myxedema

Adult: PO 16 mg qd, double dose q2w, maintenance 65-195 mg/day

Available forms: Tabs 15, 30, 60, 90, 120 mg; enteric-coated tabs 30, 60, 120 mg; sugar-coated tabs 30, 60, 120, 180 mg; caps pork 60, 90, 120, 180 mg; tabs bovine 30, 60, 120 mg

Adverse effects

CNS: Insomnia, tremors, headache, thyroid storm
CV: Tachycardia, palpitations, angina, dysrhythmias, hypertension, ***cardiac arrest***
GI: Nausea, diarrhea, increased or decreased appetite, cramps
MISC: Menstrual irregularities, weight loss, sweating, heat intolerance, fever

Contraindications: Adrenal insufficiency, MI, thyrotoxicosis

G **Precautions:** Elderly, angina pectoris, hypertension, ischemia, cardiac disease, pregnancy **A**, lactation

Pharmacokinetics

Absorption	Well absorbed
Distribution	Widely distributed, does not cross placenta
Metabolism	Liver, tissues
Excretion	Feces via bile, breast milk
Half-life	T_3—2 days; T_4—1 wk

Pharmacodynamics

Onset	1 hr
Peak	12-48 hr
Duration	Unknown

Interactions

Individual drugs

Cholestyramine: ↓ absorption of thyroid hormone
Colestipol: ↓ absorption of thyroid hormone
Digitalis: ↓ effect of digitalis
Insulin: ↑ requirement for insulin
Phenytoin (IV): ↑ release of thyroid hormone

Drug classifications

Amphetamines: ↑ CNS, cardiac stimulation
β-Adrenergic blockers: ↓ effect of beta blockers
Decongestants: ↑ CNS, cardiac stimulation
Oral anticoagulants: ↑ requirements for anticoagulants
Vasopressors: ↑ CNS, cardiac stimulation

Lab test interferences

↑ CPK, ↑ LDH, ↑ AST (SGOT), ↑ PBI, ↑ blood glucose
↓ TSH, ↓ ^{131}I uptake test, ↓ uric acid, ↓ triglycerides

NURSING CONSIDERATIONS

Assessment

- Identify if the patient is taking anticoagulants, antidiabetic agents; document on chart
- Take B/P, pulse before each dose; monitor I&O ratio and weight every day in same clothing, using same scale, at same time of day
- Monitor height, weight, psychomotor development, and growth rate if given to a P child
- Monitor T_3, T_4, FTIs, which are decreased; radioimmunoassay of TSH, which is increased; radio uptake, which is increased if patient is on too low a dose of medication
- Monitor pro-time—patient may require decreased dosage of anticoagulant; check for bleeding, bruising
- Assess for increased nervousness, excitability, irritability, which may indicate that dose of medication is too high, usually after 1-3 wk of treatment
- Assess cardiac status: angina, palpitation, chest pain, change G in vital signs; the elderly patient may have undetected cardiac problems and baseline ECG should be completed before treatment

Nursing diagnoses

✓ Knowledge deficit (teaching)
✓ Noncompliance (teaching)

Implementation

- Give in AM if possible as a single dose to decrease sleeplessness; at same time each day to maintain drug level
- Give only for hormone imbalances; not to be used for obesity, male infertility, menstrual conditions, lethargy; give

lowest dose that relieves symptoms; lower dose to the elderly and in cardiac diseases
• Store in tight, light-resistant container
• Wean patient off medication 4 wk before RAIU test

Patient/family education
• Teach patient that drug is not a cure but controls symptoms and that treatment is long-term
• Instruct patient to report excitability, irritability, anxiety, sweating, heat intolerance, chest pain, palpitations, which indicate overdose
• Advise patient not to switch brands unless approved by prescriber; bioavailability may differ; do not take with food; absorption will be decreased
• Teach patient that drug may be discontinued after giving birth; thyroid panel will be evaluated after 1-2 mo
• Teach patient that hyperthyroid child will show almost immediate behavior/personality change; that hair loss will occur in child and is temporary
• Caution patient that drug is not to be taken to reduce weight
• Caution patient to avoid OTC preparations containing iodine; read labels; other medications should not be used unless approved by health-care prescriber
• Teach patient to avoid iodine-containing food: iodized salt, soybeans, tofu, turnips, certain kinds of seafood and bread

Evaluation

Positive therapeutic outcome
• Absence of depression
• Weight loss, increased diuresis, pulse, appetite
• Absence of constipation, peripheral edema, cold intolerance, pale, cool dry skin, brittle nails, alopecia, coarse hair, menorrhagia, night blindness, paresthesias, syncope, stupor, coma, rosy cheeks
• Improved levels of T_3, T_4 by laboratory tests
• Child: Age-appropriate weight, height, and psychomotor development

Treatment of overdose: Withhold dose for up to 1 wk, acute overdose—gastric lavage or induce emesis, then activated charcoal; provide supportive treatment to control symptoms

ticarcillin (℞)
(tye-kar-sill′in)
ticar
Func. class.: Broad-spectrum antiinfective
Chem. class.: Extended-spectrum penicillin
Pregnancy category B

Action: Interferes with cell wall replication of susceptible organisms; osmotically unstable cell wall swells, bursts from osmotic pressure

Therapeutic Outcome: Decreased symptoms of infection

Uses: Respiratory, soft tissue, urinary tract infections, bacterial septicemia; effective for gram-positive cocci *(S. aureus, S. faecalis, S. pneumoniae)*, gram-negative cocci *(N. gonorrhoeae)*, gram-positive bacilli *(C. perfringens, C. tetani)*, gram-negative bacilli *(Bacteroides, F. nucleatum, E. coli, P. mirabilis, Salmonella, M. morganii, P. rettgeri, Enterobacter, P. aeruginosa, Serratia, Peptococcus, Peptostreptococcus, Eubacterium)*

Dosage and routes

Adult: IV/IM 12-24 g/day in divided doses q3-6h; infuse over ½-2 hr

P ***Child:*** IV/IM 50-300 mg/kg/day in divided doses q4-8h

Neonate: IV inf 75-100 mg/kg/8-12 hr

Available forms: Inj 1, 3, 6, 20, 30 g

Adverse effects

CNS: Lethargy, hallucinations, anxiety, depression, twitching, ***coma, convulsions***

GI: Nausea, vomiting, diarrhea; increased AST, ALT, abdominal pain, glossitis, colitis

GU: Oliguria, proteinuria, hematuria, *vaginitis, moniliasis,* ***glomerulonephritis***

HEMA: Anemia, increased bleeding time, ***bone marrow depression, granulocytopenia***

META: Hypokalemia

Contraindications: Hypersensitivity to penicillins

Precautions: Hypersensitivity to cephalosporins, pregnancy **B,** lactation

Pharmacokinetics

Absorption	Unknown
Distribution	Widely, breast milk
Metabolism	Liver, small amount
Excretion	Kidneys
Half-life	70 min

Pharmacodynamics

	IM	IV
Onset	Unknown	Unknown
Peak	1 hr	30-45 min
Duration	4-6 hr	4 hr

Interactions

Individual drugs

Aspirin: ↑ ticarcillin concentration

Probenecid: ↑ ticarcillin concentrations

Drug classifications

Aminoglycosides, IV: ↓ effect of ticarcillin

Erythromycins: ↓ effect of ticarcillin

Tetracyclines: ↓ effect of ticarcillin

Lab test interferences

False positive: Urine glucose, urine protein

NURSING CONSIDERATIONS

Assessment

- Monitor I&O ratio; report hematuria, oliguria, since penicillin in high doses is nephrotoxic
- Monitor any patient with compromised renal system, since drug is excreted slowly in poor renal system function; toxicity may occur rapidly
- Monitor liver studies: AST (SGOT), ALT (SGPT)
- Monitor blood studies: WBC, RBC, Hgb, Hct, bleeding time
- Monitor renal studies: urinalysis, protein, blood
- Monitor C&S before drug therapy; drug may be given as soon as culture is taken
- Assess bowel pattern before, during treatment
- Check for skin eruptions after administration of penicillin to 1 wk after discontinuing drug

T

Assess respiratory status: rate, character, wheezing, tightness in chest
Assess allergies before initiation of treatment, reaction of each medication; highlight allergies on chart

Implementation

- Give **IV** after diluting 1 g or less/4 ml sterile H_2O for inj; dilute further with 10-20 ml or more D_5W, NS, or sterile H_2O for inj sol; give 1 g or less/5 min or more or by intermittent inf over ½-2 hr or by continuous inf at prescribed rate

Y-site compatibilities: Acyclovir, allopurinol, aztreonam, cyclophosphamide, diltiazem, famotidine, filgrastim, fludarabine, heparin, IL-2, regular insulin, magnesium sulfate, melphalan, meperidine, morphine, ondansetron, perphenazine, sargramostim, teniposide, theophylline, verapamil, vinorelbine

- Give drug after C&S has been completed
- Have adrenalin, suction, tracheostomy set, endotracheal intubation equipment
- Provide adequate fluid intake (2 L) during diarrhea episodes
- Provide scratch test to assess allergy on order from prescriber; usually done when penicillin is only drug of choice
- Store at room temp, reconstituted sol 72 hr at room temp

Evaluation

Positive therapeutic outcome

- Absence of fever, purulent drainage, redness, inflammation

Patient/family education

- Advise that culture may be taken after completed course of medication
- Teach to report sore throat, fever, fatigue (may indicate superinfection)
- Teach to wear or carry Medic Alert ID if allergic to penicillins
- Advise to notify nurse of diarrhea

Treatment of overdose: Withdraw drug, maintain airway, administer epinephrine, aminophylline, O_2, **IV** corticosteroids for anaphylaxis

ticarcillin/ clavulanate (℞)

(tye-kar-sill'in)

Chem. class: Broad-spectrum antibiotic

Func. class.: Extended-spectrum penicillin

Pregnancy category B

Action: Interferes with cell wall replication of susceptible organisms; osmotically unstable cell wall swells, bursts from osmotic pressure

➔ **Therapeutic Outcome:** Resolution of infection

Uses: Respiratory, soft tissue, urinary tract infections; bacterial septicemia; effective for gram-positive cocci *(S. aureus, S. faecalis, S. pneumoniae),* gram-negative cocci *(N. gonorrhoeae),* gram-positive bacilli *(C. perfringens, C. tetani),* gram-negative bacilli *(Bacteroides, F. nucleatum, E. coli, P. mirabilis, Salmonella, M. morganii, P. rettgeri, Enterobacter, P. aeruginosa, Serratia, Peptococcus, Peptostreptococcus, Eubacterium)*

Dosage and routes

Adult: **IV** inf 1 vial containing ticarcillin 3 g, clavulanate K 0.1 g q4-6h, infuse over 30 min

P ***Child <60 kg:*** **IV** 200-300 mg ticarcillin/kg/day in divided doses q4-6h

Available forms: Inj IM, **IV** 3 g ticarcillin and 0.1 g clavulanate; **IV** inf 3 g ticarcillin and 0.1 g clavulanate

Adverse effects

CNS: Lethargy, hallucinations, anxiety, depression, twitching, ***coma, convulsions***

GI: Nausea, vomiting, diarrhea, increased AST (SGOT), ALT (SGPT), abdominal pain, glossitis, colitis

GU: Oliguria, proteinuria, hematuria, *vaginitis, moniliasis,* ***glomerulonephritis***

HEMA: Anemia, increased bleeding time, ***bone marrow depression, granulocytopenia***

META: Hypokalemia, hypokalemia, alkalosis, hypernatremia

Contraindications: Hypersensitivity to penicillins

Precautions: Hypersensitivity to cephalosporins, pregnancy **B**

Pharmacokinetics

Absorption	Completely absorbed (IV)
Distribution	Widely distributed, crosses blood-brain barrier
Metabolism	Liver
Excretion	Kidneys
Half-life	64-68 min

Pharmacodynamics

	IV
Onset	Unknown
Peak	30-45 min
Duration	4 hr

Interactions

Individual drugs

Cholestyramine: ↓ absorption of thyroid hormone
Colestipol: ↓ absorption of thyroid hormone
Digitalis: ↓ effect of digitalis
Insulin: ↑ requirement for insulin
Phenytoin (IV): ↑ release of thyroid hormone

Drug classifications

Amphetamines: ↑ CNS, cardiac stimulation
β-Adrenergic blockers: ↓ effect of beta blockers
Decongestants: ↑ CNS, cardiac stimulation
Oral anticoagulants: ↑ requirements for anticoagulants
Vasopressors: ↑ CNS, cardiac stimulation

Lab test interferences

False positive: Urine glucose, urine protein Coombs' test

NURSING CONSIDERATIONS

Assessment

- Monitor I&O ratio; report hematuria, oliguria because penicillin in high doses is nephrotoxic
- Monitor any patient with compromised renal system because drug is excreted slowly in poor renal system function; toxicity may occur rapidly
- Monitor liver studies: AST (SGOT), ALT (SGPT)
- Monitor studies: WBC, RBC, H&H, bleeding time
- Monitor renal studies: urinalysis, protein, blood
- Obtain C&S test results before initiating drug therapy; drug may be given as soon as culture is taken
- Assess bowel pattern before, during treatment
- Assess skin eruptions after

T

administration of penicillin to 1 wk after discontinuing drug
• Assess respiratory status: rate, character, wheezing, and tightness in chest
• Assess allergies before initiation of treatment, reaction of each medication; highlight allergies on chart, Kardex

Nursing diagnoses
✓ Infection, risk for (uses)
✓ Knowledge deficit (teaching)

Implementation
IV **IV route**
• Give **IV** after diluting 3.1 g or less/13 ml of sterile H_2O or NaCl (200 mg/ml), shake; may further dilute in 50-100 ml or more normal saline, D_5W, or LR sol and run over ½ hr

Y-site compatibilities: Allopurinol, aztreonam, cefepime, cyclophosphamide, diltiazem, famotidine, filgrastim, fluconazole, fludarabine, foscarnet, heparin, regular insulin, melphalan, meperidine, morphine, ondansetron, perphenazine, sargramostim, teniposide, theophylline, vinorelbine
• Give drug after C&S has been completed
• Have adrenalin, suction, tracheostomy set, endotracheal intubation equipment available
• Give adequate fluid intake (2 L) during diarrhea episodes
• Obtain scratch test results to assess allergy after securing order from prescriber—usually done when penicillin is only drug of choice
• Store at room temp, reconstituted sol for 12-24 hr or 3 7 days refrigerated

Patient/family education
• Advise patient that culture may be taken after completed course of medication
• Instruct patient to report sore throat, fever, fatigue (may indicate super infection)
• Advise patient to wear or carry Medic Alert ID if allergic to penicillins

Evaluation
Positive therapeutic outcome
• Absence of fever, purulent drainage, redness, inflammation

Treatment of overdose: Withdraw drug, maintain airway, administer epinephrine, aminophylline, O_2, **IV** corticosteroids for anaphylaxis

ticlopidine (℞)
(tye-cloe′pi-deen)
Ticlid
Func. class.: Platelet aggregation inhibitor
Pregnancy category B

Action: Inhibits first and second phases of ADP-induced effects in platelet aggregation

➡ **Therapeutic Outcome:** Decreased stroke by decreasing platelet aggregation

Uses: Reducing the risk of stroke in high-risk patients

Dosage and routes
Adult: PO 250 mg bid with food

Available forms: Tab 250 mg

Adverse effects
GI: Nausea, vomiting, diarrhea, GI discomfort, ***cholestatic jaundice, hepatitis,*** increased cholesterol LDL, VLDL
HEMA: Bleeding (epistaxis, hematuria, conjunctival

hemorrhage, GI bleeding), agranulocytosis, neutropenia, thrombocytopenia
INTEG: Rash, pruritus

Contraindications: Hypersensitivity, active liver disease, blood dyscrasias

Precautions: Past liver disease, G renal disease, elderly, preg- P nancy B, lactation, children, increased bleeding risk

Pharmacokinetics

Absorption	Well absorbed
Distribution	Unknown
Metabolism	Liver—extensively
Excretion	Kidneys—unchanged drug
Half-life	Increased with repeat dosing; 4-5 days (multiple doses)

Pharmacodynamics

Onset	Unknown
Peak	1-3 hr
Duration	Unknown

Interactions

Individual drugs

Aspirin: ↑ bleeding tendencies
Cimetidine: ↑ effects of ticlopidine
Digoxin: ↓ plasma levels of ticlopidine
Theophylline: ↑ effects of theophylline

Drug classifications

Antacids: ↓ plasma levels of ticlopidine
Anticoagulants: ↑ bleeding tendencies

NURSING CONSIDERATIONS

Assessment

- Monitor liver function studies: AST (SGOT), ALT (SGPT), bilirubin, creatinine if patient is on long-term therapy (4 mo or more)
- Monitor blood studies: CBC, Hct, Hgb, pro-time if patient is on long-term therapy; thrombocytopenia, neutropenia may occur

Nursing diagnoses

- ✓ Injury, risk for (uses)
- ✓ Knowledge deficit (teaching)

Implementation

- Give with food to decrease gastric symptoms

Patient/family education

- Advise patient that blood work will be necessary during treatment
- Advise patient to report any unusual bleeding to prescriber
- Instruct patient to take with food or just after eating to minimize GI discomfort
- Caution patient to report side effects such as diarrhea, skin rashes, subcutaneous bleeding, signs of cholestasis (yellow skin and sclera, dark urine, light colored stools)

Evaluation

Positive therapeutic outcome

- Absence of stroke

timolol (℞)

(tye'moe-lole)

Apo-Timol ✱, Blocadren, timolol maleate, Timoptic

Func. class.: Antihypertensive; antiglaucoma
Chem. class.: Nonselective β-blocker

Pregnancy category C

Action: Competitively blocks stimulation of β-adrenergic receptor within vascular smooth muscle; produces chronotropic, inotropic activity (decreases rate of SA node discharge, increases recovery time), slows conduction of AV

T

node, decreases heart rate, which decreases O_2 consumption in myocardium; also decreases renin-aldosterone-angiotensin system; at high doses inhibits β-2 receptors in bronchial system

➔ **Therapeutic Outcome:** Decreased B/P, decreased arrhythmias, absence of death from MI, decreased aqueous humor in the eye, absence of migraine headaches

Uses: Mild to moderate hypertension, sinus tachycardia, persistent atrial extrasystoles, tachydysrhythmias, prophylaxis of angina pectoris, reduction of mortality after MI

Investigational uses: Mitral valve prolapse, hypertrophic cardiomyopathy, thyrotoxicosis, tremors, anxiety, pheochromocytoma, tachyarrhythmias, angina pectoris

Dosage and routes

Hypertension

Adult: PO 10 mg bid, or 20 mg qd, may increase by 10 mg q2-3d, not to exceed 60 mg/day

Myocardial infarction

Adult: 10 mg bid beginning 1-4 wk after MI

Glaucoma

Adult: Ophth i gtt qd or bid

P ***Child:*** Ophth i gtt qd or bid (0.25% sol only)

Migraine headache prevention

Adult: PO 10 mg bid, or 20 mg qd, may increase to 30 mg/day, 20 mg in AM, 10 mg in PM

Available forms: Tabs 5, 10, 20 mg; ophth sol 0.25%, 0.5%

Adverse effects

CNS: Insomnia, dizziness, hallucinations, anxiety

CV: Hypotension, bradycardia, ***CHF,*** edema, chest pain, bradycardia, claudication

EENT: Visual changes, sore throat, *double vision,* dry burning eyes

GI: Nausea, vomiting, ***ischemic colitis,*** diarrhea, *abdominal pain,* ***mesenteric arterial thrombosis***

GU: Impotence, urinary frequency

HEMA: Agranulocytosis, thrombocytopenia, purpura

INTEG: Rash, alopecia, pruritus, fever

META: Hypoglycemia

MUSC: Joint pain, muscle pain

RESP: ***Bronchospasm,*** dyspnea, cough, rales

Contraindications: Hypersensitivity to β-blockers, cardiogenic shock, heart block (2nd, 3rd degree), sinus bradycardia, CHF, cardiac failure

Precautions: Major surgery, pregnancy **C**, lactation, diabetes mellitus, renal disease, thyroid disease, COPD, well-compensated heart failure, CAD, nonallergic bronchospasm

Pharmacokinetics	
Absorption	Well absorbed (PO), ophth (minimal)
Distribution	Not known
Metabolism	Liver—extensively
Excretion	Breast milk
Half-life	3-4 hr

Pharmacodynamics	
	PO
Onset	Unknown
Peak	2-4 hr
Duration	12-24 hr

Interactions
Individual drugs
Alcohol: ↑ hypotension (large amounts)
Epinephrine: α-Adrenergic stimulation
Hydralazine: ↑ hypotension, bradycardia
Indomethacin: ↓ antihypertensive effect
Insulin: ↑ hypoglycemia
Methyldopa: ↑ hypotension, bradycardia
Prazosin: ↑ hypotension, bradycardia
Reserpine: ↑ hypotension, bradycardia
Thyroid: ↓ effect of timolol
Verapamil: ↑ myocardial depression
Drug classifications
Antihypertensives: ↑ hypotension
β_2-Agonists: ↓ bronchodilatation
Cardiac glycosides: ↑ bradycardia
Nitrates: ↑ hypotension
Sulfonylureas: ↓ hypoglycemic effect
Theophyllines: ↓ bronchodilation
Lab test interferences
False ↑ Urinary catecholamines

NURSING CONSIDERATIONS
Assessment
- Monitor B/P during beginning treatment, periodically thereafter; pulse q4h; note rate, rhythm, quality: apical/radial pulse before administration; notify prescriber of any significant changes (pulse <50 bpm)
- Check for baselines in renal, liver function tests before therapy begins
- Assess for edema in feet, legs daily, monitor I&O, daily weight; check for jugular vein distention, rales, bilaterally, dyspnea (CHF)
- Monitor skin turgor, dryness of mucous membranes for hydration status, especially G elderly

Nursing diagnoses
- ✓ Cardiac output, decreased (uses)
- ✓ Injury, risk for physical (side effects)
- ✓ Knowledge deficit (teaching)
- ✓ Noncompliance (teaching)

Implementation
PO route
- Given ac, hs, tab may be crushed or swallowed whole; give with food to prevent GI upset; reduced dosage in renal dysfunction
- Store protected from light, moisture; place in cool environment

Patient/family education
- Teach patient not to discontinue drug abruptly; taper over 2 wk; may cause precipitate angina if stopped abruptly
- Advise patient not to use OTC products containing α-adrenergic stimulants (such as nasal decongestants, cold preparations); to avoid alcohol, smoking and to limit sodium intake as prescribed
- Teach patient how to take pulse and B/P at home—advise patient when to notify prescriber
- Instruct patient to comply with weight control, dietary adjustments, modified exercise program
- Advise patient to carry/wear Medic Alert ID to identify drug being taken, any allergies; tell patient drug controls symptoms but does not cure
- Caution patient to avoid

T

hazardous activities if dizziness, drowsiness is present

- Teach patient to report symptoms of CHF; difficult breathing, especially on exertion or when lying down; night cough; swelling of extremities or bradycardia; dizziness; confusion; depression; fever
- Teach patient to take drug as prescribed, not to double doses, skip doses; take any missed doses as soon as remembered if at least 4 hr until next dose

Evaluation

Positive therapeutic outcome

- Decreased B/P in hypertension (after 1-2 wk)
- Absence of dysrhythmias

Treatment of overdose: Lavage, **IV** atropine for bradycardia, **IV** theophylline for bronchospasm, digitalis, O_2, diuretic for cardiac failure, hemodialysis, **IV** glucose for hyperglycemia, **IV** diazepam (or phenytoin) for seizures

tizanidine (℞)

(ti-za′ne-deen)

Zanaflex

Func. class.: α_2-adrenergic agonist

Chem. class.: Imidazoline

Pregnancy category C

Action: Increases presynaptic inhibition of motor neurons and reduces spasticity by α-$_2$-adrenergic agonism

Therapeutic Outcome: Decreased spasticity

Uses: Acute/intermittent management of increased muscle tone associated with spasticity

Dosage and routes

Adult: PO 4 mg, increase gradually by 2-4 mg increments, may repeat dose q6-8h, not to exceed 36 mg/24 hr

Available forms: Tab 4 mg

Adverse effects

CNS: Somnolence, dizziness, speech disorder, dyskinesia, nervousness, hallucination, psychosis

GI: Dry mouth, vomiting, increased ALT (SGPT), abnormal liver function studies, constipation

OTHER: UTI, infection, blurred vision, urinary frequency, flu syndrome, pharyngitis, rhinitis

Contraindications: Hypersensitivity

Precautions: Hypotension, liver disease, pregnancy **C**, P lactation, elderly, children, renal disease

Pharmacokinetics	
Absorption	Complete
Distribution	Widely distributed
Metabolism	Liver
Excretion	Urine, feces
Half-life	2½ hr

Pharmacodynamics	
Onset	Unknown
Peak	1½ hr
Duration	Unknown

Interactions

Individual drugs

Alcohol:↑ CNS depression

Drug classification

Oral contraceptives: ↓ clearance of tizanidine

NURSING CONSIDERATIONS

Assessment

- Assess for hypotension,

gradual dosage increase should lessen hypotensive effects; have patient rise slowly from supine to upright; watch those patients receiving antihypertensives for increased effects

- Assess for increased sedation, dizziness, hallucinations, psychosis; drug may need to be discontinued
- Assess vision by ophthalmic exam, corneal opacities may occur
- Assess liver function studies: 1, 3, 6 mo during treatment and periodically thereafter

Nursing diagnoses

✓ Physical mobility, impaired (uses)
✓ Knowledge deficit (teaching)

Patient/family education

- Teach patient to rise slowly from lying or sitting to upright position
- Teach patient to ask for assistance if dizziness, sedation occur; to avoid drinking alcohol; to avoid operating machinery or driving until effects are known

tobramycin (℞)

(toe-bra-mye'sin)

Nebcin, tobramycin sulfate, Tobrex

Func. class.: Antiinfective

Chem. class.: Aminoglycoside

Pregnancy category D

Action: Interferes with protein synthesis in bacterial cell by binding to ribosomal subunit, causing inaccurate peptide sequence to form in protein chain, causing bacterial death

➡ **Therapeutic Outcome:** Bactericidal effects for the following organisms: *P. aeruginosa, E. coli, Enterobacter, Providencia, Citrobacter, Staphylococcus, Proteus, Klebsiella, Serratia*

Uses: Severe systemic infections of CNS, respiratory, GI, urinary tract, bone, skin, soft tissues, eye

Dosage and routes

Adult: IM/**IV** 3 mg/kg/day in divided doses q8h; may give up to 5 mg/kg/day in divided doses q6-8h

P ***Child:*** IM/**IV** 6-7.5 mg/kg/day in 3-4 equal divided doses

P ***Neonates <1 wk:*** IM up to 4 mg/kg/day in divided doses q12h; **IV** up to 4 mg/kg/day in divided doses q12h diluted in 50-100 mg NS or D_5W; give over 30-60 min

Available forms: Inj 10, 40 mg/ml; powder for inj 1.2 g; inj 20 mg/2 ml; 0.3% ophth

Adverse effects

CNS: Confusion, depression, numbness, tremors, ***convulsions,*** muscle twitching, ***neurotoxicity,*** dizziness, vertigo
CV: Hypotension, hypertension, palpitation
EENT: ***Ototoxicity,*** deafness, visual disturbances, tinnitus
GI: Nausea, vomiting, anorexia, increased ALT (SGOT), AST (SGPT), bilirubin, hepatomegaly, ***hepatic necrosis,*** splenomegaly
GU: ***Oliguria, hematuria, renal damage, azotemia, renal failure, nephrotoxicity***
HEMA: ***Agranulocytosis, thrombocytopenia, leukopenia, eosinophilia,*** anemia
INTEG: Rash, burning, urticaria, dermatitis, alopecia

Contraindications: Severe

T

renal disease, hypersensitivity to aminoglycosides

P Precautions: Neonates, mild renal disease, pregnancy **D,** myasthenia gravis, lactation, hearing deficits, Parkinson's disease

Pharmacokinetics

Absorption	Well absorbed (IM), completely absorbed (IV)
Distribution	Widely distributed in extracellular fluids
Metabolism	Minimal—liver
Excretion	Mostly unchanged (>90%) kidneys
Half-life	2-3 hr, increased in renal disease

Pharmacodynamics

	IM	IV	OPHTH
Onset	Rapid	Rapid	Rapid
Peak	1 hr	Inf end	Unknown

Interactions

Individual drugs

Amphotericin B: ↑ Ototoxicity, neurotoxicity, nephrotoxicity
Cisplatin: ↑ Ototoxicity, neurotoxicity, nephrotoxicity
Ethacrynic acid: ↑ Ototoxicity, neurotoxicity, nephrotoxicity
Furosemide: ↑ Ototoxicity, neurotoxicity, nephrotoxicity
Mannitol: ↑ Ototoxicity, neurotoxicity, nephrotoxicity
Methoxyflurane: ↑ Ototoxicity, neurotoxicity, nephrotoxicity
Polymyxin: ↑ Ototoxicity, neurotoxicity, nephrotoxicity
Succinylcholine: ↑ Neuromuscular blockade, respiratory depression
Vancomycin: ↑ Ototoxicity, neurotoxicity, nephrotoxicity

Drug classifications

Anesthetics: ↑ Neuromuscular blockade, respiratory depression
Aminoglycosides: ↑ Otoxicity, neurotoxicity, neurotoxicity
Nondepolarizing neuromuscular blockers: ↑ Neuromuscular blockade, respiratory depression

NURSING CONSIDERATIONS

Assessment

- Assess patient for previous sensitivity reaction

Syst route

- Assess patient for signs and symptoms of infection including characteristics of wounds, sputum, urine, stool WBC >10,000, temp; obtain baseline information before and during treatment
- Complete C&S testing before beginning drug therapy to identify if correct treatment has been initiated
- Assess for allergic reactions: rash, urticaria, pruritus, chills, fever, joint pain
- Identify urine output; if decreasing, notify prescriber (may indicate nephrotoxicity); also, obtain BUN, creatinine, urine CrCl (<80 ml/min) values
- Monitor blood studies: AST (SGOT), ALT (SGPT), CBC, Hct, bilirubin, LDH, alk phosphatase, Coombs' test monthly if patient is on long-term therapy
- Monitor electrolytes: potassium, sodium, chloride, magnesium monthly if patient is on long-term therapy
- Monitor for bleeding: ecchymosis, bleeding gums, hematuria, stool guaiac daily if patient is on long-term therapy
- Assess for overgrowth of infection: perineal itching, fever, malaise, redness, pain,

swelling, drainage, rash, diarrhea, change in cough, sputum
• Obtain weight before treatment; calculation of dosage is usually based on ideal body weight, but may be calculated on actual body weight
• Monitor I&O ratio; urinalysis daily for proteinuria, cells, casts; report sudden change in urine output
• Monitor VS during inf, watch for hypotension, change in pulse
• Assess **IV** site for thrombophlebitis including pain, redness, swelling q30 min, change site if needed; apply warm compresses to discontinued site
• Obtain serum peak, drawn at 30-60 min after **IV** inf or 60 min after IM inj, trough level drawn just before next dose; blood level should be 2-4 times bacteriostatic level
• Monitor for deafness by audiometric testing, ringing, roaring in ears, vertigo; assess hearing before, during, after treatment
• Monitor for dehydration: high sp gr, decrease in skin turgor, dry mucous membranes, dark urine
• Monitor for overgrowth of infection including increased temp, malaise, redness, pain, swelling, perineal itching, diarrhea, stomatitis, change in cough, sputum

Nursing diagnoses

✓ Infection, risk for (uses)
✓ Diarrhea (adverse reactions)
✓ Injury, risk for (adverse reactions)
✓ Knowledge deficit (teaching)
✓ Noncompliance (teaching)

Implementation

IM route
• Give deeply in large muscle mass

IV **IV route**
• Give **IV** diluted in 50-100 ml NS $D_{10}W$, $D_5/0.9\%$ NaCl, 0.9% NaCl, Ringers, LR, D_5W (adult), infuse over 20-60 min
• Flush after inf with D_5W, 0.9% NaCl
• Separate aminoglycosides and penicillins by ≥1 hr

Syringe incompatibilities: Cefamandole, clindamycin, heparin, sargramostim

Y-site compatibilities: Acyclovir, amsacrine, amiodarone, ciprofloxacin, cyclophosphamide, enalaprilat, esmolol, fluconazole, fludarabine, foscarnet, furosemide, hydromorphone, IL-2, regular insulin, labetalol, magnesium sulfate, meperidine, morphine, perphenazine, tacrolimus, teniposide, theophylline, tolazoline, vinorelbine, zidovudine

Additive incompatibilities: Cefamandole, floxacillin

Additive compatibilities: Aztreonam, bleomycin, calcium gluconate, cefoxitin, ciprofloxacin, clindamycin, furosemide, metronidazole, ranitidine, verapamil

Patient/family education

Syst route
• Teach patient to report sore throat, bruising, bleeding, joint pain—may indicate blood dyscrasias (rare)
• Advise patient to contact prescriber if vaginal itching, loose, foul-smelling stools, furry tongue occur—may indicate superimposed infection

T

• Advise patient to notify prescriber of diarrhea with blood or pus, which may indicate pseudomembranous colitis

Evaluation

Positive therapeutic outcome

• Absence of signs/symptoms of infection (WBC <10,000, temp WNL, absence of red, draining wounds)

• Reported improvement in symptoms of infection

Treatment of overdose: Withdraw drug, hemodialysis, exchange transfusion in the newborn, monitor serum levels of drug, may give ticarcillin or carbenicillin

tocainide (℞)

(toe-kay'nide)

Tonocard

Func. class.: Antidysrhythmic (Class IB)

Chem. class.: Lidocaine analog

Pregnancy category C

Action: Increases electrical stimulation threshold of ventricle, His-Purkinje system, which stabilizes cardiac membrane and decreases automaticity

➔ **Therapeutic Outcome:** Decreased ventricular dysrhythmia

Uses: Life-threatening ventricular dysrhythmias (multifocal/unifocal PVCs), ventricular tachycardia

Dosage and routes

Adult: PO 600 mg loading dose, then 400 mg q8h

Available forms: Tabs 400, 600 mg

Adverse effects

CNS: Headache, dizziness, involuntary movement, confusion, psychosis, restlessness, irritability, paresthesias, tremors, ***seizures***

CV: Hypotension, bradycardia, angina, PVCs, ***heart block, cardiovascular collapse, arrest,*** *CHF,* chest pain, tachycardia, prodysrhythmias

EENT: Tinnitus, blurred vision, hearing loss

GI: Nausea, vomiting, anorexia, diarrhea, hepatitis

HEMA: Blood dyscrasias: leukopenia, agranulocytosis, hypoplastic anemia, thrombocytopenia

INTEG: Rash, urticaria, edema, swelling

RESP: Dyspnea, ***respiratory depression, pulmonary fibrosis***

Contraindications: Hypersensitivity to amides, severe heart block

Precautions: Pregnancy **C,** [P] lactation, children, renal disease, liver disease, CHF, respiratory depression, myasthenia gravis, blood dyscrasias

Pharmacokinetics	
Absorption	Well absorbed
Distribution	Widely distributed, crossed blood-brain barrier
Metabolism	Liver
Excretion	Kidney (up to 50% unchanged)
Half-life	10-17 hr

Pharmacodynamics	
Onset	1 hr
Peak	½-2 hr
Duration	8-12 hr

Interactions

Individual drugs

Cimetidine: ↓ levels of tocainide

Digoxin: ↑ blood levels, ↑ toxicity
Disopyramide: ↑ levels, ↑ toxicity
Flecainide: ↑ levels, ↑ toxicity
Lidocaine: ↑ effect
Mexiletine: ↑ levels, ↑ toxicity
Phenytoin: ↑ blood levels
Procainamide: ↑ levels, ↑ toxicity
Quinidine: ↑ levels, ↑ toxicity
Rifampin: ↓ tocainide levels
Warfarin: ↑ levels, ↑ bleeding

Drug classifications

β-Blockers: ↑ dysrhythmias, arrest
Calcium channel blockers: ↑ dysrhythmias, arrest

Lab test interferences

↑ CPK

NURSING CONSIDERATIONS

Assessment

- Assess for oxygenation or perfusion deficit: decreased B/P, chest pain, dizziness, loss of consciousness
- Assess respiratory status: auscultate lung fields for bibasilar crackles in patients with advanced CHF
- Assess for urinary retention: check for pain, abdominal absorption, palpate bladder; check males with benign prostatic hypertrophy—anticholinergic reaction may cause retention
- Monitor I&O ratio; electrolytes: (potassium, sodium, chloride); watch for decreasing urinary output, possible retention
- Monitor liver function studies: AST (SGOT), ALT (SGPT), bilirubin, alk phosphatase
- Monitor ECG to determine drug effectiveness; measure PR, QRS, QT intervals; check for PVCs, other dysrhythmias; monitor B/P for hypotension, hypertension; for rebound hypertension after 1-2 hr
- Monitor patient for CNS symptoms: confusion, psychosis, numbness, depression, involuntary movements; if these occur, drug should be discontinued
- Assess pulmonary toxicity: dyspnea, fatigue, cough, fever, chest pain; drug should be discontinued if these occur
- Assess cardiac rate, respiration: rate, rhythm, character, chest pain, ventricular tachycardia, supraventricular tachycardia or fibrillation

Nursing diagnoses

- ✓ Cardiac output, decreased (uses)
- ✓ Impaired gas exchange (adverse reactions)
- ✓ Knowledge deficit (teaching)

Implementation

- Give with meals for GI upset occurrences

Patient/family education

- Inform patient or family of reason for use of medication and expected results
- Teach patient method for taking pulse at home and what to report to prescriber
- Advise patient to avoid hazardous activities until drug response is known; dizziness, confusion, sedation may occur
- Advise patient to use a Medic Alert bracelet or other ID indicating medications taken, condition, and prescriber's name and phone number
- Instruct patient to report bleeding, bruising, respiratory symptoms, chills, fever, sore throat to prescriber

T

Evaluation
Positive therapeutic outcome
- Decreased dysrhythmias

Treatment of overdose: Defibrillation, vasopressor for hypotension

tolazamide (℞)
(tole-az'a-mide)
Tolamide, tolazimide, Tolinase
Func. class.: Antidiabetic, oral
Chem. class.: Sulfonylurea (1st generation)
Pregnancy category C

Action: Causes functioning β-cells in pancreas to release insulin, leading to drop in blood glucose levels; may improve binding to insulin receptors or increase the number of insulin receptors with prolonged administration; may also reduce basal hepatic glucose secretion; this drug is not effective if patient lacks functioning β-cells

Therapeutic Outcome: Decreased blood glucose levels in diabetes mellitus

Uses: Type II (NIDDM) diabetes mellitus

Dosage and routes
Adult: PO 100 mg/day for FBS <200 mg/dl or 250 mg/day for FBS >200 mg/dl; dose should be titrated to patient response (1 g or less/day)

Available forms: Tabs 100, 250, 500 mg scored

Adverse effects
CNS: Headache, weakness, fatigue, lethargy, dizziness, vertigo, tinnitus
ENDO: Hypoglycemia
GI: Nausea, vomiting, diarrhea, constipation, gas, ***hepatotoxicity, jaundice,*** heartburn
HEMA: Leukopenia, thrombocytopenia, agranulocytosis, aplastic anemia, pancytopenia, hemolytic anemia
INTEG: Rash(rare), allergic reactions (rare), pruritus, urticaria, eczema, photosensitivity, erythema

Contraindications: Hypersensitivity to sulfonylureas, juvenile or brittle diabetes

Precautions: Pregnancy **C,** elderly, cardiac disease, thyroid disease, severe hypoglycemic reactions, renal disease, hepatic disease

Pharmacokinetics	
Absorption	Well absorbed
Distribution	Bile
Metabolism	Liver to metabolites
Excretion	Kidneys (unchanged)
Half-life	7 hr

Pharmacodynamics	
Onset	1 hr
Peak	4-8 hr
Duration	12-24 hr

Interactions
Individual drugs
Chloramphenicol: ↑ hypoglycemia
Cimetidine: ↑ hypoglycemia
Diazoxide: ↓ effect of both drugs
Guanethidine: ↑ hypoglycemia
Insulin: ↑ hypoglycemia
Methyldopa: ↑ hypoglycemia
Phenobarbital: ↓ action of acetohexamide
Phenytoin: ↓ action of acetohexamide

Rifampin: ↓ action of acetohexamide

Drug classifications

Anticoagulants, oral: ↑ hypoglycemia
Calcium channel blockers: ↓ action of acetohexamide
Corticosteroids: ↓ action of acetohexamide
Diuretics, thiazide: ↓ action of acetohexamide
Estrogens: ↓ action of acetohexamide
MAOIs: ↑ hypoglycemia
Nonsteroidal antiinflammatories: ↑ hypoglycemia
Oral contraceptives: ↓ action of acetohexamide
Phenothiazines: ↓ action of acetohexamide
Salicylates: ↑ hypoglycemia
Sulfonamides: ↑ hypoglycemia
Sympathomimetics: ↓ action of acetohexamide
Thyroid agents: ↓ action of acetohexamide

NURSING CONSIDERATIONS

Assessment

- Assess for hypoglycemic/hyperglycemic reactions that can occur soon pc; hypoglycemic reactions (sweating, weakness, dizziness, anxiety, tremors, hunger); hyperglycemic reactions
- Monitor CBC (baseline, q3mo) during treatment; check liver function tests periodically AST (SGOT), LDH and renal studies: BUN, creatinine during treatment

Nursing diagnoses

✓ Nutrition, altered: more than body requirements (uses)
✓ Nutrition altered: less than body requirements (adverse reactions)
✓ Injury, risk for (adverse reactions)
✓ Knowledge deficit (teaching)
✓ Noncompliance (teaching)

Implementation

- Convert from other oral hypoglycemic agents or insulin dosage of <40 U/day; change may be made without gradual dosage change
- Convert patients taking insulin of >40 U/day gradually by receiving oral hypoglycemic and 50% of previous insulin dosage for 3-5 days
- Monitor serum or urine glucose and ketones 3 times/day during conversion
- Give drug 30 min before breakfast; if large dose is required, may be divided into two; give with meals to decrease GI upset and provide best absorption
- Give tab crushed and mixed with meal or fluids for patients with difficulty swallowing
- Store in tight container in cool environment

Patient/family education

- Teach patient to check for symptoms of cholestatic jaundice: dark urine, pruritus, yellow sclera; if these occur, prescriber should be notified
- Teach patient to use capillary blood glucose test or Chemstrip 3 ×/day
- Teach patient symptoms of hypo/hyperglycemia, what to do about each
- Inform patient that drug must be continued on daily basis; explain consequence of discontinuing drug abruptly
- Teach patient to take drug in morning to prevent hypoglycemic reactions at night
- Caution patient to avoid OTC medications unless approved by a prescriber

T

• Teach patient that diabetes is lifelong illness; that this drug is not a cure
• Instruct patient that all food included in diet plan must be eaten to prevent hypoglycemia
• Advise patient to carry Medic Alert ID for emergency purposes, and to carry a glucagon emergency kit

Evaluation
Positive therapeutic outcome
• Decrease in polyuria, polydipsia, polyphagia, clear sensorium, absence of dizziness, stable gait

Treatment of overdose: Glucose 25 g **IV**, via dextrose 50% sol, 50 cc, or 1 mg glucagon

tolazoline (℞)
(toe-laz'a-leen)
Priscoline
Func. class.: Peripheral vasodilator
Chem. class.: Imidazoline derivative
Pregnancy category C

Action: Peripheral vasodilation occurs by direct relaxation on vascular smooth muscle; also has weak α- and β-adrenergic properties

Therapeutic Outcome: Decreased pulmonary hypertension

Uses: Persistent pulmonary hypertension of newborn; also hypoxic pulmonary hypertension

Dosage and routes
P ***Newborn:*** **IV** 1-2 mg/kg via scalp vein; **IV** inf 1-2 mg/kg/hr

Available forms: Inj 25 mg/ml

Adverse effects
CV: Orthostatic hypotension, ***tachycardia,*** dysrhythmias, hypertension, ***cardiovascular collapse***
GI: Nausea, vomiting, diarrhea, peptic ulcer, ***GI hemorrhage, hepatitis***
GU: Edema, oliguria, hematuria
HEMA: Thrombocytopenia, leukopenia
INTEG: Flushing, tingling, rash, chills, sweating, increased pilomotor activity
RESP: Pulmonary hemorrhage

Contraindications: Hypersensitivity, CVA, CAD

Precautions: Pregnancy **C,** active peptic ulcer, lactation, mitral stenosis

Pharmacokinetics	
Absorption	Complete
Distribution	Unknown
Metabolism	Liver
Excretion	Kidneys
Half-life	3-10 hr

Pharmacodynamics	
Onset	½ hr
Peak	½-1 hr
Duration	3-4 hr

Interactions
Alcohol: ↑ effects
Epinephrine: ↓ B/P, rebound hypertension
Drug classifications
β-Blockers: ↑ effects
Antihypertensives: ↑ effects

NURSING CONSIDERATIONS
Assessment
• Monitor ABGs, electrolytes, P VS in newborn
• Monitor B/P, pulse during treatment until stable; take

B/P with patient in lying and standing position; orthostatic hypotension is common
• Monitor hepatic tests: AST (SGOT), ALT (SGPT), bilirubin; liver enzymes may increase
• Monitor blood studies: CBC, platelets; watch for thrombocytopenia, agranulocytosis
• Monitor hepatic involvement: nausea, vomiting, jaundice; drug should be discontinued if this occurs
• Monitor for bleeding from GI tract: coffee grounds vomitus, increased pulse, pain in upper gastric area
• Assess affected areas for changes in temp, color

Nursing diagnoses

✓ Tissue, perfusion, altered (uses)
✓ Knowledge deficit (teaching)

Implementation

• Give **IV** undiluted; give 10 mg or less over 1 min; in scalp vein may be diluted in D_5, D_5NS, LR, NS, ½NS, Ringer's sol; run over 1 hr
• Give ordered analgesic if headache develops
• Give intraarterially to patient in supine position
• Give to patient who is sitting or lying down during treatment
• Store at room temp, protect from light

Additive compatibility: Verapamil

Y-site compatibilities: Aminophylline, ampicillin, calcium gluconate, cefotaxime, cimetidine, dobutamine, dopamine, furosemide, gentamicin, sodium bicarbonate, tobramycin, vancomycin

Patient/family education

• Advise patient to report jaundice, dark urine, joint pain, fatigue, malaise, bruising, easy bleeding, which may indicate blood dyscrasias
• Instruct patient that it is necessary to quit smoking to prevent excessive vasoconstriction if prescribed for PVD
• Caution to avoid hazardous activities until stabilized on medication; dizziness may occur

Evaluation

Positive therapeutic outcome

• Decrease in pulmonary hypertension or pulse volume, increased temperature in extremities, ability to walk without pain

Treatment of overdose: Administer **IV** fluids, position patient's head in low position

tolbutamide ⚷ (℞)

(tole-byoo'ta-mide)

Mobenol ♣, Novobutamide ♣, Orinase, tolbutamide, Tolbutone ♣

Func. class.: Antidiabetic
Chem. class.: Sulfonylurea (1st generation)

Pregnancy category C

Action: Causes functioning β cells in pancreas to release insulin, leading to drop in blood glucose levels; may improve binding to insulin receptors or increase the number of insulin receptors with prolonged administration; may also reduce basal hepatic secretion; not effective if patient lacks functioning β-cells

T

Therapeutic Outcome: Decreased blood glucose levels in diabetes mellitus

Uses: Type II (NIDDM) diabetes mellitus

Dosage and routes

Adult: PO 1-2 g/day in divided doses, titrated to patient response; **IV** 1 g (Fajan's test)

Available forms: Tabs 250, 500 mg scored; 1 g inj

Adverse effects

CNS: Headache, weakness, paresthesia, tinnitus, dizziness, vertigo

ENDO: Hypoglycemia

GI: Nausea, fullness, heartburn, ***hepatotoxicity, cholestatic jaundice,*** taste alteration, diarrhea

HEMA: Leukopenia, thrombocytopenia, agranulocytosis, aplastic anemia, increased AST (SGOT), ALT (SGPT), alk phosphatase

INTEG: Rash, allergic reactions, pruritus, urticaria, eczema, photosensitivity, erythema

MS: Joint pains

Contraindications: Hypersensitivity to sulfonylureas, juvenile or brittle diabetes

Precautions: Pregnancy **C,** elderly, cardiac disease, thyroid disease, severe hypoglycemic reactions, renal disease, hepatic disease

Pharmacokinetics

Absorption	Well absorbed (PO)
Distribution	Bile
Metabolism	Liver to metabolites
Excretion	Kidneys (unchanged)
Half-life	4-7 hr

Pharmacodynamics

	PO
Onset	1 hr
Peak	3-5 hr
Duration	6-12 hr

Interactions

Individual drugs

Chloramphenicol: ↑ hypoglycemia
Cimetidine: ↑ hypoglycemia
Diazoxide: ↓ effect of both drugs
Guanethidine: ↑ hypoglycemia
Insulin: ↑ hypoglycemia
Methyldopa: ↑ hypoglycemia
Phenobarbital: ↓ action of acetohexamide
Phenytoin: ↓ action of acetohexamide
Rifampin: ↓ action of acetohexamide

Drug classifications

Anticoagulants, oral: ↑ hypoglycemia
Calcium channel blockers: ↓ action of acetohexamide
Corticosteroids: ↓ action of acetohexamide
Diuretics, thiazide: ↓ action of acetohexamide
Estrogens: ↓ action of acetohexamide
MAOIs: ↑ hypoglycemia
Nonsteroidal antiinflammatories: ↑ hypoglycemia
Oral contraceptives: ↓ action of acetohexamide
Phenothiazines: ↓ action of acetohexamide
Salicylates: ↑ hypoglycemia
Sulfonamides: ↑ hypoglycemia
Sympathomimetics: ↓ action of acetohexamide
Thyroid agents: ↓ action of acetohexamide

NURSING CONSIDERATIONS

Assessment

- Assess for hypoglycemic/hyperglycemic reactions that can occur soon pc; hypoglycemic reactions (sweating, weakness, dizziness, anxiety, tremors, hunger); hyperglycemic reactions
- Monitor CBC (baseline, q3mo) during treatment; check liver function tests periodically AST (SGOT), LDH and renal studies: BUN, creatinine during treatment

Nursing diagnoses

✓ Nutrition, altered: more than body requirements (uses)
✓ Nutrition altered: less than body requirements (adverse reactions)
✓ Injury, risk for (adverse reactions)
✓ Knowledge deficit (teaching)
✓ Noncompliance (teaching)

Implementation

- Convert from other oral hypoglycemic agents or insulin dosage of <40 U/day; change may be made without gradual dosage change
- Convert patients taking >40 U/day of insulin gradually by receiving oral hypoglycemic and 50% of previous insulin dosage for 3-5 days
- Monitor serum or urine glucose and ketones 3 times/day during conversion

PO route

- Give drug 30 min before breakfast—if large dose is required, may be divided into two; give with meals to decrease GI upset and provide best absorption
- Give tab crushed and mixed with meal or fluids for patients with difficulty swallowing
- Store in tight container in cool environment

Patient/family education

- Teach patient to check for symptoms of cholestatic jaundice: dark urine, pruritus, yellow sclera; if these occur, prescriber should be notified
- Teach patient to use capillary blood glucose test or Chemstrip 3 ×/day
- Teach patient symptoms of hypo/hyperglycemia, what to do about each
- Instruct patient that drug must be continued on daily basis; explain consequence of discontinuing drug abruptly
- Teach patient to take drug in AM to prevent hypoglycemic reactions at night
- Caution patient to avoid OTC medications unless approved by a prescriber
- Teach patient that diabetes is lifelong illness; that this drug is not a cure
- Instruct patient that all food included in diet plan must be eaten to prevent hypoglycemia
- Advise patient to carry Medic Alert ID and a glucagon emergency kit for emergency purposes

Evaluation

Positive therapeutic outcome

- Decrease in polyuria, polydipsia, polyphagia, clear sensorium, absence of dizziness, stable gait

Treatment of overdose:

Glucose 25 g **IV**, via dextrose 50% sol, 50 cc or 1 mg glucagon

T

tolmetin (℞)
(tole'met-in)
Tolectin DS, Tolectin 200, Tolectin 600, tolmetin sodium
Func. class.: Nonsteroidal antiinflammatory
Chem. class.: Pyrrole acetic acid derivative
Pregnancy category B

Action: Inhibits prostaglandin synthesis by decreasing an enzyme needed for biosynthesis; analgesic, antiinflammatory, antipyretic

➔ **Therapeutic Outcome:** Decreased pain, inflammatory

Uses: Mild to moderate pain, osteoarthritis, rheumatoid arthritis

Dosage and routes
Adult: PO 400 mg tid-qid, not to exceed 2 g/day

P ***Child >2 yr:*** PO 15-30 mg/kg/day in 3 or 4 divided doses

Available forms: Cap 400 mg; tabs 200, 600 mg

Adverse effects
CNS: Dizziness, drowsiness, fatigue, tremors, confusion, insomnia, anxiety, depression
CV: Tachycardia, peripheral edema, palpitations, dysrhythmias, hypertension
EENT: Tinnitus, hearing loss, blurred vision
GI: Nausea, anorexia, vomiting, diarrhea, jaundice, ***cholestatic hepatitis,*** constipation, flatulence, cramps, dry mouth, peptic ulcer, ulceration, bleeding, perforation
GU: ***Nephrotoxicity: dysuria, hematuria, oliguria, azotemia, pseudoproteinuria***
HEMA: ***Blood dyscrasias***
INTEG: Purpura, rash, pruritus, sweating

Contraindications: Hypersensitivity, asthma, severe renal disease, severe hepatic disease, ulcer disease

Precautions: Pregnancy **B,** P lactation, children, bleeding disorders, GI disorders, cardiac disorders, hypersensitivity to other antiinflammatory agents, peptic ulcer disease

Pharmacokinetics

Absorption	Well absorbed
Distribution	Not known
Metabolism	Extensively
Excretion	Unchanged kidneys—20%
Half-life	3-3½ hr

Pharmacodynamics

Onset	Unknown
Peak	2 hr
Duration	Unknown

Interactions
Individual drugs
Acetaminophen (long-term use): ↑ renal reactions
Alcohol: ↑ adverse reactions
Aspirin: ↓ effectiveness, ↑ adverse reactions
Coumadin: ↑ anticoagulant effects
Digoxin: ↑ toxicity, ↑ levels
Insulin: ↓ insulin effect
Lithium: ↑ toxicity
Methotrexate: ↑ toxicity
Phenytoin: ↑ toxicity
Probenecid: ↑ toxicity
Sulfonylurea: ↑ toxicity
Drug classifications
Anticoagulants: ↑ risk of bleeding
Antihypertensives: ↓ effect of antihypertensives
Antineoplastics: ↑ risk of hematologic toxicity

β-Blockers: ↑ antihypertension
Cephalosporins: ↑ risk of bleeding
Glucocorticoids: ↑ adverse reactions
Hypoglycemics: ↓ hypoglycemic effect
Diuretics: ↓ effectiveness of diuretics
Nonsteroidal antiinflammatories: ↑ adverse reactions
Potassium supplements: ↑ adverse reactions
Radiation: ↑ risk of hematologic toxicity
Sulfonamides: ↑ toxicity

Lab test interferences
↑ Serum potassium, ↑ liver function studies, ↑ BUN
False positive: Urine protein

NURSING CONSIDERATIONS

Assessment

- Monitor blood counts during therapy; watch for decreasing platelets; if low, therapy may need to be discontinued, restarted after hematologic recovery; and for blood dyscrasia (thrombocytopenia): bruising, fatigue, bleeding, poor healing

Nursing diagnoses

- ✓ Pain (uses)
- ✓ Mobility, impaired physical (uses)
- ✓ Injury, risk for (adverse reactions)
- ✓ Knowledge deficit (teaching)

Implementation

- Administer with food or milk to decrease gastric symptoms—food will slow absorption slightly, but will not decrease absorption

Patient/family education

- Inform patient that drug must be continued for prescribed time to be effective; to avoid aspirin, alcoholic beverages
- Caution patient to report bleeding, bruising, fatigue, malaise because blood dyscrasias do occur
- Instruct patient to use caution when driving; drowsiness, dizziness may occur
- Teach patient to take with a full glass of water to enhance absorption; do not crush, break or chew

Evaluation

Positive therapeutic outcome

- Decreased pain
- Decreased inflammation
- Increased mobility

topiramate (℞)

(to-pi-ra'mate)
Topamax
Func. class.: Anticonvulsant, misc
Chem. class.: Carbamate derivative
Pregnancy category C

Action: Mechanism of action unknown; may prevent seizure spread as opposed to an elevation of seizure threshold

➔ **Therapeutic Outcome:** Absence of seizures

Uses: Partial seizures, with or without generalization in adults

Dosage and routes

Adjunctive therapy
Adult: PO add 400-800 mg in 2 divided doses

Available forms: Tabs 25, 100, 200 mg

Adverse effects

CNS: Dizziness, fatigue, cogni-

tive disorder, *insomnia,* anxiety, depression, paresthesia
EENT: Diplopia, vision abnormality
ENDO: Weight loss
GI: Diarrhea, anorexia, nausea, dyspepsia, abdominal pain, constipation, dry mouth
GU: Breast pain, dysmenorrhea, menstrual disorder
INTEG: Rash
MISC: Weight loss, leukopenia
RESP: URI, pharyngitis, sinusitis

Contraindications: Hypersensitivity

Precautions: Hepatic disease, renal disease, cardiac disease, G elderly, lactation, children, P pregnancy **C**

Pharmacokinetics	
Absorption	Well absorbed
Distribution	Crosses placenta, plasma protein binding (9%-17%); steady state 4 days
Metabolism	Unknown
Excretion	Kidneys unchanged 55%-97%
Half-life	21 hr

Pharmacodynamics	
Onset	Unknown
Peak	2-4 hr
Duration	Unknown

Interactions

Indivdual drugs

Carbamazepine: ↓ levels of topiramate
Phenytoin: ↓ levels of topiramate
Valproic acid: ↓ levels of topiramate
Digoxin: ↓ levels of digoxin
Alcohol: ↑ levels of alcohol

Drug classifications

CNS depressants: ↑ CNS depression
Carbonic anhydrase inhibitors: ↑ levels of carbonic anhydrase inhibitors
Contraceptives, oral: ↓ level of oral contraceptives
Food: ↓ levels of topiramate

NURSING CONSIDERATIONS

Assessment

- Assess mental status: mood, sensorium, affect, memory (long, short), especially in G elderly
- Assess for blood dyscrasias: fever, sore throat, bruising, rash, jaundice, epistaxis (long-term treatment only)
- Assess seizure actvity including type, location, duration, and character; provide seizure precaution
- Monitor CBC during long-term therapy
- Assess body weight and evidence of cognitive disorder

Nursing diagnoses

✓ Injury, risk for (side effects)
✓ Knowledge deficit (teaching)

Implementation

- May take with food
- ⊘ Do not crush, or break tabs; very bitter

Patient/family education

- Teach patient to carry Medic Alert ID stating name, drugs taken, condition, prescriber's name, phone number
- Advise patient to avoid driving, other activities that require alertness
- Teach patient not to discontinue medication abruptly after long-term use

Evaluation

Positive therapeutic outcome

- Decreased seizure activity

Treatment of overdose:

Lavage, vital signs

topotecan (℞)

(to-poe'ti-kan)

Hycamtin

Func. class: Antineoplastic hormone

Chem. class: Semi-synthetic derivative of camptothecin (topoisomerase inhibitor)

Pregnancy category C

Action: Is an anti-tumor drug with topoisomerase I-inhibitory activity topoisomerase I relieves torsional strain in DNA by causing single-strand breaks; causes double-strand DNA damage

Therapeutic Outcome: Decreased tumor size

Uses: Metastatic carcinoma of the ovary after failure of traditional chemotherapy

Dosage and routes

Adult: **IV** inf 1.5 mg/m^2 over 20 min qd × 5 days starting on day 1 of a 2-day course × 4 courses; may be reduced to 0.25 mg/m^2 for subsequent courses if severe neutropenia occurs

Available forms: Lyophilized powder for inj 4 mg (free base)

Adverse effects

CNS: Arthralgia, asthenia, headache, myalgia, pain

GI: Abdominal pain, constipation, diarrhea, obstruction, nausea, stomatitis, vomiting, increased ALT, AST; anorexia

HEMA: Neutropenia, leukopenia, thrombocytopenia, anemia, sepsis

INTEG: Total alopecia

RESP: Dyspnea

Contraindications: Hypersensitivity, pregnancy **C,** lactation, severe bone marrow depression

Precautions: Children

Pharmacokinetics

Absorption	Rapidly/completely
Distribution	Unknown
Metabolism	Liver
Excretion	Urine, feces to metabolites
Half-life	8 hr

Pharmacodynamics

Unknown

Interactions

Individual drugs

Cisplatin: ↑ myelosuppression

G-CSF: ↑ duration of neutropenia

NURSING CONSIDERATIONS

Assessment

- Monitor liver function studies: AST (SGOT), ALT (SGPT), alk phosphatase, which may be elevated
- Monitor for CNS symptoms: drowsiness, confusion, depression, anxiety
- Monitor CBC, differential, platelet count weekly; withhold drug if WBC is <3500/mm^3 or platelet count is <100,000/mm^3; notify prescriber of these results; drug should be discontinued
- Assess buccal cavity q8h for dryness, sores or ulceration, white patches, oral pain, bleeding, dysphagia
- Assess GI symptoms: frequency of stools, cramping
- Assess signs of dehydration: rapid respiration, poor skin turgor, decreased urine output, dry skin, restlessness, weakness

Nursing diagnoses

- ✓ Infection, risk for (adverse reactions)
- ✓ Knowledge deficit (teaching)

T

Implementation

- Provide increased fluid intake to 2-3 L/day to prevent dehydration, unless contraindicated
- Change **IV** site q48h
- Rinse mouth tid-qid with water, club soda; brushing teeth bid-tid with soft brush or cotton-tipped applicator for stomatitis; use unwaxed dental floss
- Provide nutritious diet with iron, vit K supplements, low fiber, few dairy products

Patient/family education

- Advise to avoid foods with citric acid or hot or rough texture if stomatitis is present; to drink adequate fluids
- Advise to report stomatitis; any bleeding, white spots, ulcerations in mouth; tell patient to examine mouth qd; report symptoms
- Assess to report signs of anemia; fatigue, headache, faintness, shortness of breath, irritability
- Teach to use contraception during therapy

Evaluation

Positive therapeutic outcome

- Decreased tumor size, spread of malignancy

trace elements (chromium, copper, iodide, manganese, selenium, zinc) (℞)

Concentrated Multiple Trace Elements, ConTE-PAK-4, M.T.E.-4 Concentrated, M.T.E.-5, M.T.E.-5 Concentrated, M.T.E.-6, M.T.E.-6 Concentrated, M.T.E.-7, MulTE-PAK-4, MulTE-PAK-5, Multiple Trace Element, Multiple Trace Element Neonatal, Multiple Trace Element Pediatric, Neotrace 4, Ped TE-PAK-4, Pedtrice-4, P.T.E.-4, P.T.E.-5

Func. class.: Mineral supplement

Pregnancy category C

Action: Needed for adequate absorption and synthesis of amino acids

➔ **Therapeutic Outcome:** Replacement for mineral deficiencies

Uses: Prevention of trace element deficiency, a component of TPN

Dosage and routes

Usual dosage may be given in TPN sol

Chromium

Adult: **IV** 10-15 μg qd

P ***Child:*** **IV** 0.14-0.20 μg/kg/day

Copper

Adult: **IV** 0.5-1.5 mg/day

P ***Child:*** **IV** .05-0.2 mg/kg/day

Iodide

Adult: **IV** 1 μg/kg/day

Manganese

Adult: **IV** 1-3 mg/day

Selenium
Adult: 40-120 μg/day
P ***Child:*** 3 μg/kg/day
Zinc
***Adult:* IV** 2-4 mg/day
P ***Child:* IV** 0.05 mg/kg/day

Available forms: Many forms available—see particular elements

Adverse effects
ZINC: Vomiting, oliguria, hypothermia, vision changes, tachycardia, jaundice, coma
SELENIUM: Alopecia, depression, vomiting, GI cramping, nervousness, garlic smell
MANGANESE: Incoordination, headache, irritability, lability, slurred speech, impotence
IODINE: Headache, edema of eyelids, acne, metallic taste, sore mouth, running nose
COPPER: Personality changes, diarrhea, weakness, photophobia, muscle weakness
CHROMIUM: Seizures, coma, nausea, vomiting, ulcers, renal/hepatic toxicity

Precautions: Liver, biliary disease, pregnancy **C,** lactation, severe vomiting or diarrhea

Pharmacokinetics

Absorption	Completely absorbed
Distribution	Widely distributed
Metabolism	Unknown
Excretion	Depends on element
Half-life	Unknown

Pharmacodynamics

Unknown

Interactions: None

NURSING CONSIDERATIONS
Assessment
• Assess trace element levels; notify prescriber if low copper 0.07-0.15 mg/ml, zinc 0.05-0.15 mg/100 ml, manganese 4-20 μg/100 ml, selenium 0.1-0.19 μg/ml
• Assess trace element deficiency if patient is receiving TPN for extended period
• Obtain calorie count to identify nutritional deficiencies
• Assess for toxicity to individual element (see side effects/adverse reactions)

Nursing diagnoses
✓ Nutrition: less than body requirements (uses)
✓ Knowledge deficit (teaching)

Implementation
• Give by **IV** inf, often mixed with TPN sol
• Discard unused portions
• Give by continuous inf diluted in 1 L or more **IV** sol; give at prescribed rate

Patient/family education
• Explain reason for and expected results of medication

Evaluation
Positive therapeutic outcome
• Absence of element deficiency

tramadol (℞)
(trah'mah-dol)
Ultram
Func. class.: Central analgesic
Pregnancy category C

Action: Not completely understood, binds to opioid receptors and inhibits reuptake of norepinephrine, serotonin; does not cause histamine release or affect heart rate

➔ **Therapeutic Outcome:** Relief of pain

T

Uses: Management of moderate to severe pain

Dosage and routes

Adult: PO 50-100 mg prn q4-6h, max 400 mg/day

G ***Elderly >75 yrs:*** PO <300 mg/day in divided dose

Hepatic impairment, adult: PO 50 mg q12h

Available forms: Tab 50 mg

Adverse effects

CNS: Dizziness, CNS stimulation, somnolence, headache, anxiety, confusion, euphoria, seizure, hallucinations

GI: Nausea, constipation, vomiting, dry mouth, diarrhea, abdominal pain, anorexia, flatulence, ***GI bleeding***

CV: Vasodilation, orthostatic hypotension, tachycardia, hypertension, abnormal ECG

INTEG: Pruritus, rash, urticaria, vesicles

GU: Urinary retention/frequency, menopausal symptoms, dysuria, menstrual disorder

Contraindications: Hypersensitivity, acute intoxication with any CNS depressant

Precautions: Seizure disorder, P pregnancy **C,** lactation, children, G elderly, renal, hepatic disease, respiratory depression, head trauma, increased intracranial pressure, acute abdominal condition, drug abuse

Pharmacokinetics

Absorption	Rapidly, almost completely absorbed
Distribution	Steady state 2 days
Metabolism	Extensively in liver, may cross blood-brain barrier
Excretion	Unchanged drug 30% in urine
Half-life	Unknown

Pharmacodynamics

Unknown

Interactions

Individual drugs

Carbamazepine: ↓ of tramadol

Drug classification

MAOIs: Inhibition of norepinephrine and serotonin reuptake; use together with caution

Lab test interferences

↑ Creatinine, ↑ liver enzymes

↓ Hgb

NURSING CONSIDERATIONS

Assessment

- Assess pain: location, type, character; give before pain becomes extreme
- Monitor I&O ratio: check for decreasing output; may indicate urinary retention
- Assess need for drug
- Assess for constipation; increase fluids, bulk in diet
- Monitor CNS changes: dizziness, drowsiness, hallucinations, euphoria, LOC, pupil reaction
- Determine allergic reactions: rash, urticaria

Nursing diagnoses

✓ Pain (uses)

✓ Sensory, perceptual alteration: visual, auditory (adverse reactions)

✓ Injury, risk for (adverse reactions)

✓ Knowledge deficit (teaching)

Implementation

- Give with antiemetic for nausea, vomiting
- Administer when pain is beginning to return; determine dosage interval by patient response
- Store in cool environment, protect from sunlight

Patient/family education
- Teach patient to report any symptoms of CNS changes, allergic reactions
- Teach patient that drowsiness, dizziness, and confusion may occur; to call for assistance
- Instruct patient to make position changes slowly, orthostatic hypotension may occur
- Tell patient to avoid OTC medication and alcohol unless approved by prescriber

Evaluation
Positive therapeutic outcome
- Decreased pain

tranylcypromine (℞)
(tran-ill-sip'roe-meen)
Parnate
Func. class: Antidepressant—MAOI
Chem. class: Nonhydrazine
Pregnancy category C

Action: Increases concentrations of endogenous epinephrine, norepinephrine, serotonin, dopamine in storage sites in CNS by inhibition of MAO; increased concentration reduces depression

➔ **Therapeutic Outcome:** Decreased symptoms of depression after 2-3 wk

Uses: Depression, when uncontrolled by other means

Investigational uses: Bulimia, cocaine addiction, migraines, seasonal affective disorder, panic disorder

Dosages and routes
Adult: PO 10 mg bid; may increase to 30 mg/ day after 2 wk

Available forms: Tab 10 mg

Adverse effects
CNS: Dizziness, drowsiness, confusion, headache, anxiety, tremors, stimulation, weakness, hyperreflexia, mania, insomnia, fatigue, weight gain
CV: Orthostatic hypotension, hypertension, dysrhythmias, ***hypertensive crisis***
EENT: Blurred vision
ENDO: SIADH-like syndrome
GI: Constipation, dry mouth, nausea, vomiting, *anorexia,* diarrhea, weight gain
GU: Change in libido, frequency
HEMA: Anemia
INTEG: Rash, flushing, increased perspiration

Contraindications: Hypersensitivity to MAOIs, G elderly, hypertension, CHF, severe hepatic disease, pheochromocytoma, severe renal disease, severe cardiac disease

Precautions: Suicidal patients, convulsive disorders, severe depression, schizophrenia, hyperactivity, diabetes mellitus, pregnancy **C**

Pharmacokinetics

Absorption	Well absorbed
Distribution	Crosses placenta
Metabolism	Liver, extensively
Excretion	Kidneys, breast milk
Half-life	Unknown

Pharmacodynamics
Unknown

Interactions
Individual drugs
Alcohol: ↑ CNS depression
Dextromethorphan: ↑ hypertensive crisis
Fluoxetine: ↑ serious reactions
Guanethidine: ↓ hypertensive crisis
L-Tryptophan: ↑ effects

Methylphenidate: ↑ hypertensive crisis
Paroxetine: ↑ serious reactions
Sumatriptan: ↑ effects

Drug classifications

Analgesics (opioid): ↑ CNS depression
Antidepressants, tricyclic: ↑ hypertensive crisis
Antihypertensives: ↑ hypotension

Food

Antidiabetics: ↑ effects
β-Blockers: ↑ effects
Diabenzazepine agents: ↑ hypertensive crisis
Diuretics, thiazide: ↑ effects
Rauwolfia alkaloids: ↑ effects
Sulfonamides: ↑ effects
Tyramine: ↑ hypertensive crisis

NURSING CONSIDERATIONS

Assessment

- Monitor B/P (lying, standing), pulse q4h; if systolic B/P drops 20 mm hg hold drug, notify prescriber; take vital signs q4h in patients with cardiovascular disease
- Monitor hepatic studies: AST (SGOT), ALT (SGPT), bilirubin
- Check weight qwk; appetite may increase with drug
- Assess mental status: mood, sensorium, affect, suicidal tendencies; increase in psychiatric symptoms: depression, panic
- Monitor urinary retention, constipation; constipation is P more likely to occur in chil- G dren or elderly
- ! Assess for withdrawal symptoms: headache, nausea, vomiting, muscle pain, weakness; do not usually occur unless drug was discontinued abruptly
- Identify alcohol consumption; if alcohol is consumed, hold dose until morning

Nursing diagnoses

- ✓ Coping, ineffective individual (uses)
- ✓ Injury, risk for (side effects)
- ✓ Knowledge deficit (teaching)
- ✓ Noncompliance (teaching)

Implementation

- Give with food or milk for GI symptoms; crush if patient is unable to swallow medication whole
- Store at room temp; do not freeze

Patient/family education

- Advise patient that therapeutic effects may take 48 hr-3 wk
- Teach patient to use caution in driving or other activities requiring alertness because of drowsiness, dizziness, blurred vision; to avoid rising quickly from sitting to standing, espe- G cially elderly
- Caution patient to avoid alcohol ingestion, other CNS depressants
- Advise patient not to discontinue medication quickly after long-term use: may cause nausea, headache, malaise
- Advise patient to increase fluids, bulk in diet if constipation, urinary retention occur, G especially elderly
- Teach patient to take gum, hard sugarless candy, or frequent sips of water for dry mouth
- Teach patient to avoid high-tyramine foods; cheese (aged), sour cream, beer, wine, pickled products, liver, raisins, bananas, figs, avocados, meat tenderizers, chocolate, yogurt; increased caffeine, ginseng
- Teach patient to report headache, palpitation, neck stiffness

• Instruct patient to wear or carry Medic Alert Bracelet or ID with medications taken, condition treated, and prescriber's name and phone number

Evaluation

Positive therapeutic outcome
- Decrease in depression
- Absence of suicidal thoughts

Treatment of overdose: Lavage, activated charcoal, monitor electrolytes, vital signs, diazepam **IV**, $NaHCO_3$

trazodone (℞)

(tray'zoe-done)

Desyrel, Desyrel Dividose, trazodone HCl

Func. class.: Antidepressant, miscellaneous

Chem. class.: Triazolopyridine

Pregnancy category C

Action: Selectively inhibits serotonin uptake by brain, potentiates behavioral changes

➡ **Therapeutic Outcome:** Decreased symptoms of depression after 2-3 wk

Uses: Depression

Investigational uses: Chronic pain syndromes

Dosage and routes:

Adult: PO 150 mg/day in divided doses; may increase by 50 mg/day q3-4d, not to exceed 600 mg/day

Available forms: Tabs 50, 100, 150, 300 mg

Adverse effects

CNS: Dizziness, drowsiness, confusion, headache, anxiety, tremors, stimulation, weakness, insomnia, nightmares, EPS G (elderly), increase in psychiatric symptoms

CV: Orthostatic hypotension, ECG changes, tachycardia, ***hypertension,*** palpitations

EENT: Blurred vision, tinnitus, mydriasis

GI: Diarrhea, dry mouth, nausea, vomiting, ***paralytic ileus,*** increased appetite, cramps, epigastric distress, jaundice, ***hepatitis,*** stomatitis

GU: Retention, ***acute renal failure, priapism***

HEMA: ***Agranulocytosis, thrombocytopenia, eosinophilia, leukopenia***

INTEG: Rash, urticaria, sweating, pruritus, photosensitivity

Contraindications: Hypersensitivity to tricyclic antidepressants, recovery phase of MI, convulsive disorders, prostatic hypertrophy

Precautions: Suicidal patients, severe depression, increased intraocular pressure, narrow-angle glaucoma, urinary retention, cardiac disease, hepatic disease, hyperthyroidism, electroshock therapy, elective surgery, pregnancy **C**

Pharmacokinetics

Absorption	Well absorbed
Distribution	Widely distributed
Metabolism	Liver, extensively
Excretion	Kidneys—unchanged minimally
Half-life	4½-7½ hr

Pharmacodynamics

Unknown

Interactions

Individual drugs

Alcohol: ↑ CNS depression

Cimetidine: ↑ levels, ↑ toxicity

Clonidine: Severe hypotension, avoid use

T

Disulfiram: Organic brain syndrome
Fluoxetine: ↑ levels, ↑ toxicity
Guanethidine: ↓ effects

Drug classifications

Analgesics:↑ CNS depression
Anticholinergics: ↑ side effects
Antihistamines: ↑ CNS depression
Antihypertensives: may block antihypertensive effect
Barbiturates: ↑ effects
Benzodiazepines: ↑ effects
CNS depressants: ↑ effects
MAOIs: ↑ hypertensive crisis, convulsions
Oral contraceptives: effects, toxicity
Phenothiazines: ↑ toxicity
Sedative/hypnotics: ↑ CNS depression
Sympathomimetics, indirect-acting: ↓ effects

Smoking

↑ metabolism, ↓ effects

Lab test interferences

↑ Serum bilirubin, ↑ blood glucose, ↑ alk phosphatase
↓ VMA, ↓ 5-HIAA, ↓ blood glucose
False increase: Urinary catecholamines

NURSING CONSIDERATIONS

Assessment

- Monitor B/P (lying, standing), pulse q4h; if systolic B/P drops 20 mm hg hold drug, notify prescriber; take vital signs q4h in patients with cardiovascular disease
- Monitor blood studies: CBC, leukocytes, differential, cardiac enzymes if patient is receiving long-term therapy
- Monitor hepatic studies: AST (SGOT), ALT (SGPT), bilirubin
- Check weight qwk; appetite may increase with drug
- Assess ECG for flattening of T wave, bundle branch block, AV block, dysrhythmias in cardiac patients
- Assess for EPS primarily in [G] elderly; rigidity, dystonia, akathisia
- Assess mental status: mood, sensorium, affect, suicidal tendencies; increase in psychiatric symptoms: depression, panic
- Monitor urinary retention, constipation; constipation is [P] more likely to occur in children [G] or elderly
- Assess for withdrawal symptoms: headache, nausea, vomiting, muscle pain, weakness; do not usually occur unless drug was discontinued abruptly
- Identify alcohol consumption; if alcohol is consumed, hold dose until AM

Nursing diagnoses

- ✓ Coping, ineffective individual (uses)
- ✓ Injury, risk for (adverse reactions)
- ✓ Knowledge deficit (teaching)
- ✓ Noncompliance (teaching)

Implementation

- Give with food or milk for GI symptoms; crush if patient is unable to swallow medication whole
- Give dosage hs if oversedation occurs during day; may [G] take entire dose hs; elderly may not tolerate once/day dosing
- Store at room temp; do not freeze

Patient/family education

- Teach patient that therapeutic effects may take 2-3 wk
- Teach patient to use caution in driving or other activities

requiring alertness because of drowsiness, dizziness, blurred vision; to avoid rising quickly from sitting to standing, G especially elderly

- Caution patient to avoid alcohol ingestion, other CNS depressants
- Teach patient not to discontinue medication quickly after long-term use: may cause nausea, headache, malaise
- Advise patient to wear sunscreen or large hat because photosensitivity occurs
- Teach patient to increase fluids, bulk in diet if constipation, urinary retention occur, G especially elderly
- Advise patient to take gum, hard sugarless candy, or frequent sips of water for dry mouth

Evaluation

Positive therapeutic outcome

- Decrease in depression
- Absence of suicidal thoughts

Treatment of overdose: ECG monitoring, induce emesis, lavage, activated charcoal, administer anticonvulsant

tretinoin (vitamin A acid, retinoic acid) (℞)

(tret'i-noyn)

Retin-A, Stievaa ✤, Tretinoin LF IV, Vesanoid

Func. class.: Vitamin A acid/acne product, antineoplastic-misc.

Chem. class.: Tretinoin derivative

Pregnancy category C

Action: Decreases cohesiveness of follicular epithelium, decreases microcomedone formation (top); induces maturation of acute promyelocytic leukemia, exact action is unknown (PO)

➔ **Therapeutic Outcome:** Decreased signs/symptoms of leukemia

Uses: Acne vulgaris (grades 1-3) (top); acute promylocytic leukemia (PO)

Investigational uses: Skin cancer

Dosage and routes

P ***Adult and child:*** Top cleanse area, apply hs; cover lightly

Promyelocytic leukemia

Adult: PO 45 mg/m^2/day given as 2 evenly divided doses until remission, discontinue treatment 30 days after remission or 90 days of treatment, whichever is first

Available forms: Top cream 0.05%, 0.01%; top gel 0.025%, 0.01%; top liq 0.05%; cap 10 mg

Adverse effects

Top

INTEG: Rash, stinging, warmth, redness, erythema, blistering, crusting, peeling, contact dermatitis, hypopigmentation, hyperpigmentation

PO

CNS: Headache, fever, sweating

GI: Nausea, vomiting, ***hemorrhage***, abdominal pain, diarrhea, constipation, dyspepsia, distention, hepatitis

Contraindications: Hypersensitivity to retinoids or sensitive to parabens

Precautions: Pregnancy **D**, lactation, eczema, sunburn

T

Pharmacokinetics

Absorption	Small amounts
Distribution	Unknown
Metabolism	Unknown
Excretion	Kidneys
Half-life	Unknown

Pharmacodynamics

Unknown

Interactions

Individual drugs

Benzoyl peroxide: ↑ peeling
Resorcinol: ↑ peeling
Salicylic acid: ↑ peeling
Sulfur: ↑ peeling

Drug classifications

Abrasive soaps: ↑ peeling
Alcohol astringents: ↑ peeling

NURSING CONSIDERATIONS

Assessment

Top

- Assess part of body involved, including time involved, what helps or aggravates condition, cysts, dryness, itching; lesions may become worse at beginning of treatment

Nursing diagnoses

✓ Skin integrity, impaired (uses)
✓ Body image disturbances (uses)
✓ Knowledge deficit (teaching)

Implementation

Top route

- Apply once daily before hs; cover area lightly using gauze
- Store at room temp
- Wash hands after application

Liq

- Apply with gloves or cotton; apply only to affected areas

Patient/family education

Top

- Instruct patient to avoid application on normal skin, and to avoid getting cream in eyes, nose, other mucous membranes
- Advise patient to avoid sunlight, sunlamps or to use protective clothing or sunscreen to prevent burns
- Advise patient that treatment may cause warmth, stinging; dryness; peeling will occur
- Inform patient that cosmetics may be used over drug; not to use shaving lotions
- Inform patient that rash may occur during first 1-3 wk of therapy
- Caution patient that drug does not cure condition; only relieves symptoms; that therapeutic results may be seen in 2-3 wk but may not be optimal until after 6 wk

Evaluation

Positive therapeutic outcome

- Decrease in size and number of lesions

triamcinolone (℞)
(trye-am-sin'oh-lone)
Amcort, Aristocort, Aristocort Forte, Aristocort Intralesional, Aristospan Intra-Articular, Aristospan Intralesional, Articulose L.A., Atolone, Azmacort, Cenocort A-40, Cenocort Forte, Kenacort, Kenaject-40, Kenalog, Kenalog-10, Kenalog-40, Tac-3, Tac-40, Triam-A, triamcinolone, triamcinolone acetonide, Triam Forte, Triamolone 40, Triamonide 40, Tri-Kort, Trilog, Trilone, Trisoject
Func. class.: Corticosteroid; antiinflammatory
Chem. class.: Glucocorticoid, intermediate-acting
Pregnancy category C

Action: Decreases inflammation by suppression of migration of polymorphonuclear leukocytes, fibroblasts, reversal to increase capillary permeability and lysosomal stabilization

➔ **Therapeutic Outcome:** Decreased inflammation, normal immune response

Uses: Severe inflammation, immunosuppression, neoplasms, asthma (steroid dependent), collagen, respiratory, dermatologic disorders

Dosage and routes
Adult: PO 4-12 mg/day in divided doses qd-qid; IM 40 mg qwk (acetonide, or diacetate), 5-48 mg into neoplasms (diacetate, acetonide), 2-40 mg into joint or soft tissue (diacetate, acetonide), 0.5 mg/sq in of affected intralesional skin (hexacetonide), 2-20 mg into joint or soft tissue (hexacetonide)

P ***Child:*** PO 117 μg/kg/day as a single dose or divided doses

Asthma
Adult: Inh 2 tid-qid, not to exceed 16 Inh/day

P ***Child 6-12 yr:*** Inh 1-2 tid-qid, not to exceed 12 inh/day

Available forms: Tabs 1, 2, 4, 8, 16 mg; syr 2 mg/5 ml, 4.85 mg/5 ml; inj 25, 40 mg/ml diacetate; inj 3, 10, 40 mg/ml acetonide; inj 5, 20 mg/ml hexacetonide; inh 100 μg/spray; intranasal 55 μg/spray

Adverse effects
CNS: Depression, flushing, sweating, headache, mood changes
CV: Hypertension, ***circulatory collapse, thrombophlebitis, embolism,*** tachycardia, edema
EENT: Fungal infections, increased intraocular pressure, blurred vision
GI: Diarrhea, nausea, abdominal distention, ***GI hemorrhage, increased appetite, pancreatitis***
HEMA: ***Thrombocytopenia***
INTEG: Acne, poor wound healing, ecchymosis, petechiae
MS: Fractures, osteoporosis, weakness

Contraindications: Psychosis, hypersensitivity, idiopathic thrombocytopenia, acute glomerulonephritis, amebiasis, fungal infections, nonasthmatic bronchial disease, P child <2 yr, AIDS, TB

Precautions: Pregnancy **C,** diabetes mellitus, glaucoma,

T

osteoporosis, seizure disorders, ulcerative colitis, CHF, myasthenia gravis, renal disease, esophagitis, peptic ulcer

Interactions

Individual drugs

Amphotericin B: ↑ hypokalemia
Azlocillin: ↑ hypokalemia
Insulin: ↑ need for insulin
Mezlocillin: ↑ hypokalemia
Phenytoin: ↓ action, ↑ metabolism
Piperacillin: ↑ hypokalemia
Rifampin: ↓ action, ↑ metabolism
Ticarcillin: ↑ hypokalemia

Drug classifications

Barbiturates: ↓ action, ↑ metabolism
Diuretics: ↑ hypokalemia
Hypoglycemic agents: ↑ need for hypoglycemic agents

Lab test interferences

↑ Cholesterol, ↑ sodium, ↑ blood glucose, ↑ uric acid, ↑ calcium, ↑ urine glucose
↓ Calcium, ↓ potassium, ↓ T_4, ↓ T_3, ↓ thyroid ^{131}I uptake test, ↓ urine 17-OHCS, ↓ 17-KS, ↓ PBI
False negative: Skin allergy tests

Pharmacokinetics

Absorption	Well absorbed (PO, IM)
Distribution	Crosses placenta, widely distributed
Metabolism	Liver—extensively
Excretion	Kidney, breast milk
Half-life	2-5 hr, adrenal suppression 3-4 days

NURSING CONSIDERATIONS

Assessment

- Monitor potassium, blood sugar, urine glucose while on long-term therapy; hypokalemia and hyperglycemia
- Monitor weight daily; notify prescriber of weekly gain >5 lb; I&O ratio; be alert for decreasing urinary output and increasing edema
- Monitor B/P q4h, pulse; notify prescriber if chest pain occurs
- Monitor plasma cortisol levels during long-term therapy (normal level; 138-635 nmol/L SI units when drawn at 8 AM); adrenal function periodically for HPA axis suppression
- Assess for infection: increase temp, WBC even after withdrawal of medication; drug masks infection symptoms
- Assess for potassium depletion: paresthesias, fatigue, nausea, vomiting, depression, polyuria, dysrhythmias, weakness
- Assess mental status: affect, mood, behavioral changes, aggression
- Assess nasal passages during long-term treatment for changes in mucus (nasal)
- Monitor temp; if fever develops, drug should be discontinued
- Assess for systemic absorption: increased temp, inflammation, irritation (top)

Nursing diagnoses

✓ Infection, risk for (adverse reactions)

Pharmacodynamics

	PO	IM	TOP	INH	INTRANASAL
Onset	Unknown	Unknown	Min to hr	1-2 wk	Unknown
Peak	1-2 hr	1-2 hr	Hr to days	Unknown	2-3 wk
Duration	3 days	Unknown	Hr to days	Unknown	Unknown

☑ Knowledge deficit (teaching)
☑ Noncompliance (noncompliance)

Implementation

IM route

• Give IM inj deeply in large muscle mass, rotate sites, avoid deltoid, use 21-gauge needle

• Give in one dose in AM to prevent adrenal suppression; avoid SC administration—may damage tissue

PO route

• Give with food or milk to decrease GI symptoms

Inh route

• Give inh with water to decrease possibility of fungal infections; titrated dose, use lowest effective dose

• Give after cleaning aerosol top daily with warm water, dry thoroughly

• Store in cool environment; do not puncture or incinerate container

Top route

• Apply only to affected areas; do not get in eyes

• Apply medication, then cover with occlusive dressing (only if prescribed), seal to normal skin, change q12h; systemic absorption may occur

• Apply only to dermatoses; do not use on weeping, denuded, or infected areas

• Cleanse skin before applying drug

• Use treatment for a few days after area has cleared

• Store at room temp

Nasal route

• Have patient clear nasal passages before administration; use decongestant if needed; shake inhaler, invert, tilt head backward, insert nozzle into nostril, away from septum; hold other nostril closed and depress activator, inhale through nose, exhale through mouth

Patient/family education

• Advise patient that ID as steroid user should be carried

• Instruct patient to notify patient if therapeutic response decreases; dosage adjustment may be needed; not to discontinue abruptly; adrenal crisis can result

• Caution patient to avoid OTC products: salicylates, alcohol in cough products, cold preparations unless directed by prescriber

• Advise patient on all aspects of drug usage including cushingoid symptoms

• Teach patient symptoms of adrenal insufficiency: nausea, anorexia, fatigue, dizziness, dyspnea, weakness, joint pain

• Teach patient that long-term therapy may be needed to clear infection (1-2 mo depending on type of infection)

Nasal route

• Instruct patient to clear nasal passages if sneezing attack occurs, repeat dose

• Advise patient to continue using product even if mild nasal bleeding occurs; is usually transient

• Teach patient method of instill after providing written instruction from manufacturer

Inh route

• Teach patient proper administration technique; to wash inhaler with warm water and dry after each use

• Teach patient all aspects of drug usage including cushingoid symptoms

Top route

• Instruct patient to avoid

T

sunlight on affected area; burns may occur

Evaluation

Positive therapeutic outcome

- Decrease in runny nose (nasal)
- Decreased dyspnea, wheezing, dry rales on auscultation (inh)
- Ease of respirations, decreased inflammation
- Absence of severe itching, patches on skin, flaking (top)

triamterene (℞)

(try-am′ter-een)

Dyrenium

Func. class.: Potassium-sparing diuretic

Chem. class.: Pteridine derivative

Pregnancy category B

Action: Acts primarily on distal tubule to inhibit reabsorption of sodium, chloride; increase potassium retention and conserve hydrogen ions

➡ **Therapeutic Outcome:** Diuretic and antihypertensive effect while retaining potassium

Uses: Edema, hypertension, diuretic-induced hypokalemia

Dosage and routes

Adult: PO 100 mg bid pc, not to exceed 300 mg/day

Available forms: Caps 50, 100 mg

Adverse effects

CNS: Weakness, headache, dizziness, fatigue

ELECT: Hyperkalemia, hyponatremia, hypochloremia

GI: Nausea, diarrhea, vomiting, dry mouth, jaundice, liver disease

GU: ***Azotemia, interstitial nephritis,*** increased BUN, creatinine, renal stones, bluish discoloration of urine

HEMA: ***Thrombocytopenia, megaloblastic anemia,*** low folic acid levels

INTEG: Photosensitivity, rash

Contraindications: Hypersensitivity, anuria, severe renal, hepatic disease; hyperkalemia

Precautions: Dehydration, hepatic disease, lactation, CHF, renal disease, cirrhosis, pregnancy **B,** lactation

Pharmacokinetics	
Absorption	GI tract; well absorbed
Distribution	Crosses placenta
Metabolism	Liver
Excretion	Renal; breast milk
Half-life	3 hr

Pharmacodynamics	
Onset	2 hr
Peak	6-8 hr
Duration	12-16 hr

Interactions

Individual drugs

Amantadine: ↑ toxicity of amantadine

Cimetidine: ↓ renal clearance of triamterene

Indomethacin: ↑ nephrotoxicity

Drug classifications

ACE inhibitors: ↑ hyperkalemia

Antihypertensives: ↑ action

Diuretics, potassium-sparing: ↑ hyperkalemia

Nonsteroidal antiinflammatories: ↓ nephrotoxicity

Potassium products: ↑ hyperkalemia

Salt substitutes: ↑ hyperkalemia

Food

Potassium foods: ↑ hyperkalemia

Lab test interferences

Interference: Quinidine serum levels, LDH

NURSING CONSIDERATIONS

Assessment

- Monitor for manifestations of hyperkalemia: *Renal:* acidic urine, reduced urine osmolality, nocturia, polyuria, polydipsia; *Cardiac:* hypotension, broad T wave, U wave, ectopy, tachycardia, weak pulse; *Neuro:* muscle weakness, altered LOC, drowsiness, apathy, lethargy, confusion, depression, anorexia, nausea, cramps, constipation, distension, paralytic ileus, hypoventilation, respiratory muscle weakness
- Monitor for manifestations of hyponatremia: *CV:* ↑ B/P, cold, clammy skin, hypo- or hypervolemia; *GI:* anorexia, nausea, vomiting, diarrhea, abdominal cramps; *Neuro:* lethargy, increased ICP, confusion, headache, seizures, coma, fatigue, tremors, hyperreflexia
- Monitor for manifestations of hyperchloremia: *Neuro:* weakness, lethargy, coma; *Resp:* deep rapid breathing
- Assess fluid volume status: I&O ratios and record, weight, distended red veins, crackles in lung, color, quality and sp gr of urine, skin turgor, adequacy of pulses, moist mucous membranes, bilateral lung sounds, peripheral pitting edema; dehydration symptoms of decreasing output, thirst, hypotension, dry mouth and mucous membranes should be reported.
- Monitor electrolytes: potassium, sodium, calcium, magnesium; also include BUN, ABGs, uric acid, CBC, blood sugar

Nursing diagnoses

- ✓ Urinary elmination, altered (adverse reactions)
- ✓ Fluid volume deficit (adverse reactions)
- ✓ Fluid volume excess (uses)
- ✓ Knowledge deficit (teaching)

Implementation

- Give in AM to avoid interference with sleep
- With food, if nausea occurs

Patient/family education

- Teach patient to take medication early in the day to prevent nocturia
- Instruct the patient to take with food or milk if GI symptoms of nausea and anorexia occur
- Teach patient to maintain a record of weight on a weekly basis and notify prescriber of weight loss of 5 lb
- Caution the patient that this drug causes an increase in potassium levels, that foods high in potassium should be avoided; refer to dietician for assistance planning
- Caution the patient not to exercise in hot weather, and stand for prolonged periods of time because orthostatic hypotension will be enhanced
- Advise patient to wear protective clothing and sunscreen in the sun to prevent photosensitivity
- Teach patient not to use alcohol, or any OTC medications without prescriber's approval because serious drug reactions may occur
- Emphasize the need to contact prescriber immediately if

T

muscle cramps, weakness, nausea, dizziness, or numbness occur
- Teach patient to take own B/P and pulse and record
- Advise patient that dizziness and confusion may occur; avoid driving or other hazardous activities if alertness is decreased
- Teach patient to continue taking medication even if feeling better; this drug controls symptoms but does not cure the condition
- Advise the patient with hypertension to continue other medical treatment (exercise, weight loss, relaxation techniques, cessation of smoking)

Evaluation

Positive therapeutic outcome
- Prevention of hypokalemia (diuretic use)
- Decreased edema
- Decreased B/P
- Increased diuresis

Treatment of overdose: Lavage if taken orally; monitor electrolytes; administer sodium bicarbonate for K[2] 6.5 mEq/L; monitor hydration, CV, renal status

triazolam (℞)

(trye-az'oh-lam)

Apo-Triazo ✤, Halcion, Novotriolam ✤, Nu-Triazol ✤

Func. class.: Sedative-hypnotic

Chem. class.: Benzodiazepine

Pregnancy category X

Controlled substance schedule IV (USA), schedule F (Canada)

Action: Produces CNS depression at limbic, thalamic, hypothalamic levels of CNS; may be mediated by neurotransmitter; γ-aminobutyric acid (GABA); results are sedation, hypnosis, skeletal muscle relaxation, anticonvulsant activity, anxiolytic action

Therapeutic Outcome: Decreased anxiety, insomnia

Uses: Insomnia (short-term), sedative/hypnotic

Dosage and routes

Adult: PO 0.125-0.5 mg hs

G ***Elderly:*** PO 0.125-0.25 mg hs

Available forms: Tabs 0.125, 0.25, 0.5 mg

Adverse effects

CNS: Headache, lethargy, drowsiness, daytime sedation, dizziness, confusion, lightheadedness, anxiety, irritability, amnesia, poor coordination

CV: Chest pain, pulse changes

GI: Nausea, vomiting, diarrhea, heartburn, abdominal pain, constipation

HEMA: ***Leukopenia, granulocytopenia*** (rare)

Contraindications: Hypersensitivity to benzodiazepines,

pregnancy **X,** lactation, intermittent porphyria

Precautions: Anemia, hepatic disease, renal disease, suicidal G individuals, drug abuse, elderly, P psychosis, child <15 yr, acute narrow-angle glaucoma, seizure disorders

Pharmacokinetics	
Absorption	Well absorbed
Distribution	Widely distributed, crosses placenta, crosses blood-brain barrier
Metabolism	Liver
Excretion	Kidneys, breast milk
Half-life	2-3 hr

Pharmacodynamics	
Onset	½ hr
Peak	Unknown
Duration	6-8 hr

Interactions

Individual drugs

Alcohol: ↑ CNS depression
Cimetidine: ↑ action
Disulfiram: ↑ action
Fluoxetine: ↑ action
Isoniazid: ↑ action
Ketoconazole: ↑ action
Levodopa: ↓ action of levodopa
Metoprolol: ↑ action
Propoxyphene: ↑ action
Propranolol: ↑ action
Rifampin: ↓ action of triazolam
Theophylline: ↓ sedative effects
Valproic acid: ↑ action

Drug classifications

Analgesics, opioid: ↑ CNS depression
Antidepressants: ↑ CNS depression
Antihistamines: ↑ CNS depression
Barbiturates: ↓ effect of triazolam
Contraceptives: ↑ effect

Lab test interferences

↑ AST (SGOT)/ALT (SGPT), ↑ serum bilirubin
False ↑ 17-OHCS
↓ RAIU

NURSING CONSIDERATIONS

Assessment

- Assess patient's mental status: mood, sensorium, anxiety, affect, sleeping pattern, drowsiness, dizziness, especially G elderly; physical dependency, withdrawal symptoms: anxiety, panic attacks, agitation, convulsions, headache, nausea, vomiting, muscle pain, weakness; suicidal tendencies; for indications of increasing tolerance and abuse
- Monitor patient's B/P (lying, standing), pulse; if systolic B/P drops 20 mm Hg, hold drug, notify prescriber
- Monitor blood studies: CBC during long-term therapy; blood dycrasias have occurred rarely; decreased hematocrit, neutropenia may occur
- Monitor hepatic studies: AST (SGOT), ALT (SGPT), bilirubin, creatinine LDH, alk phosphatase
- Monitor I&O; indicate renal dysfunction

Nursing diagnoses

✓ Anxiety (uses)
✓ Depression (uses)
✓ Injury, risk for (adverse reactions)
✓ Knowledge deficit (teaching)

Implementation

- Give with food or milk for GI symptoms; if patient is unable to swallow medication whole, tab may be crushed and mixed with foods or fluids
- Give sugarless gum, hard candy, frequent sips of water for dry mouth

T

Patient/family education

• Advise patient that drug may be taken with food, or fluids and tab may be crushed or swallowed whole

• Caution patient not to use for everyday stress or longer than 3 mo unless directed by prescriber; not to take more than prescribed amount; may be habit forming; not to double doses or skip doses

• Instruct patient to avoid OTC preparations unless approved by health care prescriber; alcohol and CNS depressants will increase CNS depression

• Caution patient to avoid driving, activities that require alertness because drowsiness may occur; to avoid alcohol ingestion or other psychotropic medications; to rise slowly or fainting may occur, especially G elderly; that drowsiness may worsen at beginning of treatment

• Advise patient not to discontinue medication abruptly after long-term use; withdrawal symptoms include vomiting, cramping, tremors, seizures

Evaluation

Positive therapeutic outcome

• Decreased anxiety, restlessness, sleeplessness (short-term treatment only)

Treatment of overdose: Lavage, VS, supportive care

trifluoperazine (℞)

(trye-floo-oh-per'a-zeen)

Novoflurazine ✦, Solazine ✦, Stelazine, Suprazine, Terfluzine, trifluoperazine HCl, Triflurin

Func. class.: Antipsychotic/neuroleptic

Chem. class.: Phenothiazine, piperazine

Pregnancy category C

Action: Depresses cerebral cortex, hypothalamus, limbic system, which control activity, aggression; blocks neurotransmission produced by dopamine at synapse; exhibits strong α-adrenergic, anticholinergic blocking action; mechanism for antipsychotic effects is unclear

➔ **Therapeutic Outcome:** Decreased signs and symptoms of psychosis

Uses: Psychotic disorders, nonpsychotic anxiety, schizophrenia

Dosage and routes

Adult: PO 2-5 mg bid, usual range 15-20 mg/day, may require 40 mg/day or more; IM 1-2 mg q4-6h

P ***Child >6 yr:*** PO 1 mg qd or bid; IM *not recommended for children,* but 1 mg may be given qd or bid

Nonpsychotic anxiety

Adult: PO 1-2 mg bid, not to exceed 5 mg/day; do not give longer than 12 wk

Available forms: Tabs 1, 2, 5, 10, 20 mg; conc 10 mg/ml; inj 2 mg/ml

Adverse effects

CNS: Extrapyramidal symptoms: pseudoparkinsonism,

akathisia, dystonia, tardive dyskinesia, ***seizures,*** *headache,* ***neuroleptic malignant syndrome***
CV: Orthostatic hypotension, hypertension, ***cardiac arrest,*** ECG changes, ***tachycardia***
EENT: Blurred vision, glaucoma, dry eyes
GI: Dry mouth, nausea, vomiting, anorexia, constipation, diarrhea, jaundice, weight gain
GU: Urinary retention, urinary frequency, enuresis, impotence, amenorrhea, gynecomastia
HEMA: Anemia, ***leukopenia, leukocytosis, agranulocytosis***
INTEG: Rash, photosensitivity, dermatitis
RESP: ***Laryngospasm,*** dyspnea, ***respiratory depression***

Contraindications: Hypersensitivity, cardiovascular disease, coma, blood dyscrasias, severe hepatic disease, child <6 yr, glaucoma

P

Precautions: Breast cancer, seizure disorders, pregnancy **C**, lactation, diabetes mellitus, respiratory conditions, prostatic hypertrophy

Pharmacokinetics

Absorption	Variably absorbed (tab), well absorbed (IM)
Distribution	Widely distributed, high concentrations in CNS, crosses placenta
Metabolism	Liver—extensively
Excretion	Kidneys, breast milk
Half-life	Unknown

Pharmacodynamics

	PO	IM
Onset	Rapid	Immediate
Peak	2-3 hr	1 hr
Duration	12 hr	12 hr

Interactions

Individual drugs

Alcohol: ↑ effects of both drugs, oversedation
Aluminum hydroxide: ↓ absorption
Bromocriptine: ↓ antiparkinson activity
Disopyramide: ↑ anticholinergic effects
Epinephrine: ↑ toxicity
Guanethidine: ↓ antihypertensive response
Levodopa: ↓ antiparkinson activity
Lithium: ↓ chlorpromazine levels, ↑ extrapyramidal symptoms, masking of lithium toxicity
Magnesium hydroxide: ↓ absorption
Norepinephrine: ↓ vasoresponse, ↑ toxicity
Phenobarbital: ↓ effectiveness, ↑ metabolism

Drug classifications

Antacids: ↓ absorption
Anticholinergics: ↑ anticholinergic effects
Antidepressants: ↑ CNS depression
Antidiarrheals, adsorbent: ↓ absorption
Antihistamines: ↑ CNS depression
Antihypertensives: ↑ hypotension
Antithyroid agents: ↑ agranulocytosis
Barbiturate anesthetics: ↑ CNS depression
β-Adrenergics: ↑ effects of both drugs
General anesthetics: ↑ CNS depression
MAOIs: ↑ CNS depression
Narcotics: ↑ CNS depression
Sedative/hypnotics: ↑ CNS depression

Lab test interferences

↑ Liver function tests, ↑ car-

T

diac enzymes, ↑ cholesterol, ↑ blood glucose, ↑ prolactin, ↑ bilirubin, ↑ PBI, ↑ cholinesterase, ↑ alk phosphatase, ↑ leukocytes, ↑ granulocytes, ↑ platelets
↓ Hormones (blood and urine)
False positive: Pregnancy tests, PKU, urine bilirubin
False negative: Urinary steroids, 17-OHCS

NURSING CONSIDERATIONS

Assessment

- Assess mental status: orientation, mood, behavior, presence of hallucinations, and type before initial administration and monthly; drug should significantly reduce psychotic behavior
- Check for swallowing of PO medication; check for hoarding or giving of medication to other patients
- Monitor I&O ratio, palpate bladder if low urinary output G occurs, especially in elderly; urinalysis recommended before, during prolonged therapy
- Monitor bilirubin, CBC, liver function studies monthly
- Assess affect, orientation, LOC, reflexes, gait, coordination, sleep pattern disturbances
- Monitor B/P sitting, standing and lying, take pulse and respirations q4h during initial treatment; establish baseline before starting treatment; report drops of 30 mm Hg; obtain baseline ECG, Q-wave and T-wave changes
- Check for dizziness, faintness, palpitations, tachycardia on rising; severe orthostatic hypotension is common
- ◆ Identify for neuroleptic malignant syndrome: hyperpyrexia, muscle rigidity, increased CPK, altered mental status; drug should be discontinued
- Assess for extrapyramidal symptoms including akathisia (inability to sit still, no pattern to movements), tardive dyskinesia (bizarre movements of the jaw, mouth, tongue, extremities), pseudoparkinsonism (ragged tremors, pill rolling, shuffling gait); an antiparkinson drug should be prescribed
- Assess for constipation, urinary retention daily; if these occur, increase bulk, water in diet
- Assess for hypo/hyper glycemia; appetite patterns

Nursing diagnoses

- ✓ Thought processes, altered (uses)
- ✓ Coping, ineffective individual (uses)
- ✓ Knowledge deficit (teaching)
- ✓ Noncompliance (teaching)

Implementation

PO route

- Drug in liq form mixed in glass of juice or cola if hoarding is suspected; do not mix in caffeine drinks, tannics, pectins
- G • Decreased dose in elderly; metabolism is slowed in the elderly
- PO with full glass of water, milk; or give with food to decrease GI upset
- Storage in tight, light-resistant container, oral sol in amber bottle

IM route

- Inj in deep muscle mass, do not give SC; do not administer sol with a precipitate

IV route

- Give **IV** after diluting 10 mg/9 ml of NS; give 1 mg or less/2 min

Additive compatibilities: Meperidine, netilmicin

Syringe compatibility:
Glycopyrrolate

Patient/family education

- Teach patient to use good oral hygiene; frequent rinsing of mouth, sugarless gum for dry mouth
- Caution patient to avoid hazardous activities until drug response is determined; dizziness, blurred vision is common
- Inform patient that orthostatic hypotension occurs often and to rise from sitting or lying position gradually and to remain lying down after IM inj for at least 30 min
- Caution patient to avoid tubs, hot showers, tub baths because hypotension may occur
- Instruct patient that heat stroke may occur in hot weather, so take extra precautions to stay cool
- Advise patient to avoid abrupt withdrawal of this drug, or extrapyramidal symptoms may result; drug should be withdrawn slowly
- Teach patient to avoid OTC preparations (cough, hay fever, cold) unless approved by prescriber because serious drug interactions may occur; avoid use with alcohol, CNS depressants because increased drowsiness may occur
- Advise patient to use a sunscreen and sunglasses to prevent burns
- Teach patient about extrapyramidal symptoms and necessity of meticulous oral hygiene because oral candidiasis may occur
- Advise patient to take antacids 2 hr before or after this drug
- Instruct patient to report sore throat, malaise, fever, bleeding, mouth sores; if these occur, CBC should be drawn and drug discontinued

Evaluation

Positive therapeutic outcome

- Decrease in emotional excitement, hallucinations, delusions, paranoia
- Reorganization of patterns of thought, speech

Treatment of overdose:
Lavage if orally ingested; provide airway; *do not induce vomiting or use epinephrine*

trihexyphenidyl (℞)

(trye-hex-ee-fen′i-dill)

Artane, Artane Sequels, Novohexidyl ✤, Trihexy-2, Trihexy-5, trihexyphenidyl HCl, Trihexane

Func. class.: Cholinergic blocker; antiparkinson

Chem. class.: Synthetic tertiary amine

Pregnancy category C

Action: Blocks central muscarinic receptors, which decreases involuntary movements, sweating, salivation

➔ **Therapeutic Outcome:** Decreased involuntary movements

Uses: Parkinson symptoms, drug induced extrapyramidal symptoms

Dosage and routes

Parkinson symptoms

Adult: PO 1 mg, increased by 2 mg q3-5d to a total of 6-10 mg/day

T

Drug-induced extrapyramidal symptoms
Adult: PO 1 mg/day; usual dose 5-15 mg/day

Available forms: Tabs 2, 5 mg; caps sus-rel 5 mg; elix 2 mg/5 ml

Adverse effects
CNS: Confusion, anxiety, restlessness, irritability, delusions, hallucinations, headache, sedation, depression, incoherence, dizziness, flushing, weakness
CV: Palpitations, tachycardia, postural hypotension
EENT: Blurred vision, photophobia, dilated pupils, difficulty swallowing, dry eyes, increased intraocular tension, angle-closure glaucoma
GI: Dryness of mouth, constipation, nausea, vomiting, abdominal distress, ***paralytic ileus***
GU: Urinary hesitancy, urinary retention, dysuria
INTEG: Urticaria, rash
MISC: Suppression of lactation, nasal congestion, decreased sweating, increased temp, hyperthermia, heat stroke, numbness of fingers
MS: Weakness, cramping

Contraindications: Hypersensitivity, narrow-angle glaucoma, myasthenia gravis, GI/GU obstruction, tachycardia, myocardial ischemia, unstable CV disease, prostatic hypertrophy

Precautions: Pregnancy **C**, G elderly, lactation, tachycardia, abdominal obstruction, infection, P children, gastric ulcer

Pharmacokinetics

Absorption	Well absorbed
Distribution	Unknown
Metabolism	Unknown
Excretion	Unknown
Half-life	Unknown

Pharmacodynamics

	PO	PO-ER
Onset	1 hr	Unknown
Peak	2-3 hr	Unknown
Duration	6-12 hr	Up to 24 hr

Interactions
Individual drugs
Alcohol: ↑ CNS depression
Disopyramide: ↑ anticholinergic effects
Quinidine: ↑ anticholinergic effects
Drug classifications
Analgesics: ↑ CNS depression
Antacids: ↓ absorption
Antidepressants, tricyclic: ↑ anticholinergic effects
Antihistamines: ↑ anticholinergic effects
Phenothiazines: ↑ anticholinergic effects
Sedatives/hypnotics: ↑ CNS depression

NURSING CONSIDERATIONS
Assessment
- Monitor I&O ratio; retention commonly causes decreased urinary output, distention, frequency, incontinence
- Assess for parkinsonism, extrapyramidal symptoms: shuffling gait, muscle rigidity, involuntary movements, pill rolling, muscle spasms, drooling before and during treatment
- Monitor for urinary hesitancy, retention; palpate bladder if retention occurs
- Monitor for constipation, cramping, pain in abdomen, abdominal distention; increase

fluids, bulk, exercise if this occurs
- Assess for tolerance over long-term therapy; dose may have to be increased or changed
- Assess for mental status: affect, mood, CNS depression, worsening of mental symptoms during early therapy

Nursing diagnoses

✓ Physical mobility, impaired (uses)
✓ Knowledge deficit (teaching)

Implementation
- Give with or pc to prevent GI upset; may give with fluids other than water; offer hard candy, frequent drinks, gum to relieve dry mouth
- Give at hs to avoid daytime drowsiness in patient with parkinsonism
- Store at room temp

Patient/family education
- Teach patient to use caution in hot weather; drug may increase susceptibility to stroke because perspiration is decreased; patient should remain indoors
- Teach patient not to discontinue this drug abruptly; to taper off over 1 wk to prevent withdrawal symptoms (insomnia, involuntary movements, anxiety, tachycardias)
- Caution patient to avoid driving or other hazardous activities; drowsiness, dizziness may occur
- Advise patient to avoid OTC medications: cough, cold preparations with alcohol, antihistamines unless directed by prescriber; increased CNS depression may occur
- Instruct patient to rise from sitting or recumbent position slowly to minimize orthostatic hypotension
- Advise patient to use gum, hard candy, frequent sips of water to decrease dry mouth; if dry mouth continues, saliva substitutes may be prescribed
- Instruct patient that doses should not be doubled, but missed dose may be taken up to 2 hr before next dose

Evaluation

Positive therapeutic outcome
- Absence of involuntary movements (pill rolling, tremors, muscle spasms)

trimethobenzamide (℞)

(trye-meth-oh-ben′za-mide)

Arrestin, Benzacot, Brogan, Stemetic, T-Gen, Tebamide, Ticon, Tigan, Tijet-20, Tribun, Trimazide, trimethobenzamide, trimethobenzamide HCl

Func. class.: Antiemetic, anticholinergic

Chem. class.: Ethanolamine derivative

Pregnancy category C

Action: Acts centrally by blocking chemoreceptor trigger zone, which in turn acts on vomiting center

➔ **Therapeutic Outcome:** Absence of nausea and vomiting

Uses: Nausea, vomiting, prevention of postoperative vomiting

Dosage and routes

Postoperative vomiting

Adult: IM/rec 200 mg before or during surgery; may repeat 3 hr after

Discontinuing anesthesia
P ***Child 13-40 kg:*** PO/rec 100-200 mg tid-qid
P ***Child <13 kg:*** PO/rec 100 mg tid-qid

Nausea/vomiting
Adult: PO 250 mg tid-qid; IM/rec 200 mg tid-qid

Available forms: Caps 100, 250, mg; supp 100, 200 mg; inj 100 mg/ml

Adverse effects
*CNS: **Drowsiness,*** restlessness, headache, dizziness, insomnia, confusion, nervousness, tingling, ***vertigo,*** extrapyramidal symptoms
CV: Hypertension, hypotension, palpitations
EENT: Dry mouth, blurred vision, diplopia, nasal congestion, photosensitivity
GI: Nausea, anorexia, diarrhea, vomiting, constipation
INTEG: Rash, urticaria, fever, chills, flushing

Contraindications: Hypersensitivity to narcotics, shock, **P** children (parenterally)

P **Precautions:** Children, cardiac **G** dysrhythmias, elderly, asthma, pregnancy **C,** prostatic hypertrophy, bladder-neck obstruction, narrow-angle glaucoma, stenosing peptic ulcer, pyloroduodenal obstruction

Pharmacokinetics

Absorption	Unknown
Distribution	Unknown
Metabolism	Liver, extensively
Excretion	Kidneys
Half-life	Unknown

Pharmacodynamics

	PO	IM	REC
Onset	20-40 min	15 min	10-40 min
Peak	Unknown	Unknown	Unknown
Duration	3-4 hr	2-3 hr	3-4 hr

Interactions
Individual drugs
Alcohol: ↑ CNS depression
Drug classifications
Analgesics: ↑ CNS effect
Antidepressants: ↑ CNS effect
Antihistamines: ↑ CNS effect
CNS depressants: ↑ CNS effect
Sedative/hypnotics: ↑ CNS effect

NURSING CONSIDERATIONS

Assessment
- Monitor VS, B/P; check patients with cardiac disease more often
- Assess for signs of toxicity of other drugs or masking of symptoms of disease: brain tumor, intestinal obstructions
- Observe for drowsiness, dizziness
- Assess for nausea, vomiting before and after treatment

Nursing diagnoses
✓ Knowledge deficit (teaching)

Implementation
IM route
- Administer IM inj in large muscle mass; aspirate to avoid **IV** administration

Syringe compatibilities: Glycopyrrolate, hydromorphone, midazolam, nalbuphine

Y-site compatibilities: Heparin, hydrocortisone, potassium chloride, vit B/C

PO route
- Cap may be swallowed whole

or opened and mixed with food or fluids

Patient/family education

• Teach patient to use good oral hygiene; frequent rinsing of mouth, sugarless gum for dry mouth

• Caution patient to avoid hazardous activities until drug response is determined, drowsiness may occur

• Inform patient that orthostatic hypotension occurs often and to rise from sitting or lying position gradually and to remain lying down after IM inj for at least 30 min

• Advise patient to avoid hot tubs, hot showers, tub baths because hypotension may occur

• Inform patient that in hot weather, heat stroke may occur; take extra precautions to stay cool

• Teach patient to avoid OTC preparations (cough, hayfever, cold) unless approved by prescriber because serious drug interactions may occur; avoid use with alcohol, CNS depressants because increased drowsiness may occur

• Teach patient about extrapyramidal symptoms

• Instruct patient to report sore throat, malaise, fever, bleeding, mouth sores; if these occur, CBC should be drawn and drug discontinued

Evaluation

Positive therapeutic outcome

• Decreased nausea, vomiting

trimethoprim/ sulfamethoxazole (co-trimoxazole) (℞)

(trye-meth'oh-prim/sul-fa-meth-ox'a-zole [ko-trye-mox'a-zole])

Apo-Sulfatrim*, Bactrim, Bethaprim, Comoxol, Cotrim, Septra, Sulfatrim

Func. class.: Antibiotic

Chem. class.: Miscellaneous sulfonamide

Pregnancy category C

Action: Sulfamethoxazole (SMZ) interferes with bacterial biosynthesis of proteins by competitive antagonism of PABA when adequate levels are maintained; trimethoprim (TMP) blocks synthesis of tetrahydrofolic acid; combination blocks 2 consecutive steps in bacterial synthesis of essential nucleic acids, protein

Theapeutic Outcome: Absence of infection, based on C&S

Uses: UTI, otitis media, acute and chronic prostatitis, shigellosis, *P. carinii* pneumonitis, chronic bronchitis, chancroid, traveler's diarrhea

Dosage and routes

UTI

Adult: PO 160 mg TMP/800 mg SMZ q12h × 10-14 days

P ***Child:*** PO 8 mg/kg TMP/40 mg/kg SMZ qd in 2 divided doses q12h

Otitis media

P ***Child:*** PO 8 mg/kg TMP/40 mg/kg SMZ qd in 2 divided doses q12h × 10 days

T

Chronic bronchitis
Adult: PO 160 mg TMP/800 mg SMZ q12h × 14 days

Pneumocystis carinii pneumonitis
P ***Adult and child:*** PO 20 mg/kg TMP/100 mg/kg SMZ qd in 4 divided doses q6h × 14 days; IV 15-20 mg/kg/day (based on TMP) in 3-4 divided doses for up to 14 days
• Dosage reduction necessary in moderate to severe renal impairment (CrCl <30 ml/min)

Available forms: Tabs 80 mg trimethoprim/400 mg sulfamethoxazole, 160 mg trimethoprim/800 mg sulfamethoxazole; susp 40 mg/200 mg/5 ml; IV 16 mg/80 mg/ml

Adverse effects

CNS: Headache, insomnia, hallucinations, depression, vertigo, fatigue, anxiety, convulsions, drug fever, chills, aseptic meningitis
CV: Allergic myocarditis
*GI: **Nausea, vomiting, abdominal pain,*** stomatitis, ***hepatitis,*** glossitis, pancreatitis, diarrhea, ***enterocolitis,*** anorexia
GU: ***Renal failure, toxic nephrosis;*** increased BUN, creatinine; crystalluria
HEMA: ***Leukopenia, neutropenia, thrombocytopenia, agranulocytosis, hemolytic anemia, hypoprothrombinemia, Henoch-Schönlein purpura, methemoglobinemia, eosinophilia I***
INTEG: Rash, dermatitis, urticaria, ***Stevens-Johnson syndrome,*** erythema, photosensitivity, pain, inflammation at injection site
RESP: Cough, shortness of breath
SYST: ***Anaphylaxis, SLE***

Contraindications: Hypersensitivity to trimethoprim or sulfonamides, pregnancy at term, megaloblastic anemia, infants <2 mo, CrCl <15 ml/min, lactation

Precautions: Pregnancy **C,** G renal disease, elderly, G6PD deficiency, impaired hepatic function, possible folate deficiency, severe allergy, bronchial asthma

Pharmacokinetics	
Absorption	Rapid
Distribution	Breast milk, crosses placenta, highly protein bound
Metabolism	Liver
Excretion	Kidneys
Half-life	8-13 hr

Pharmacodynamics	
Onset	Unknown
Peak	1-4 hr
Duration	Unknown

Interactions

Individual drugs
Cyclosporine: ↑ nephrotoxicity
Methotrexate: ↑ bone marrow depression
Phenytoin: ↓ hepatic clearance of phenytoin

Drug classifications
Anticoagulants, oral: ↑ anticoagulant effect
Diuretics, thiazide: ↑ thrombocytopenia
Sulfonylureas: ↑ hypoglycemic response

Lab test interferences
↑ Alk phosphatase, ↑ creatinine, ↑ bilirubin
False positive: Urinary glucose test

NURSING CONSIDERATIONS

Assessment

- Assess allergic reactions: rash, fever (AIDS patients more susceptible)
- Monitor I&O ratio; note color, character, pH of urine if drug administered for UTI; output should be 800 ml less than intake; if urine is highly acidic, alkalization may be needed
- Monitor kidney function studies: BUN, creatinine, urinalysis (long-term therapy)
- Assess type of infection, obtain C&S before starting therapy
- Assess blood dyscrasias, skin rash, fever, sore throat, bruising, bleeding, fatigue, joint pain
- Assess allergic reaction: rash, dermatitis, urticaria, pruritus, dyspnea, bronchospasm

Nursing diagnoses

- ✓ Infection, risk for (uses)
- ✓ Knowledge deficit (teaching)
- ✓ Noncompliance (teaching)

Implementation

- Give with full glass of water to maintain adequate hydration; increase fluids to 2 L/day to decrease crystallization in kidneys
- Give medication after C&S; repeat C&S after full course of medication
- Give after diluting 5 ml of drug/125 ml D_5W, run over 1-1½ hr
- Store in tight, light-resistant container at room temp

Patient family education

- Teach patient to take each oral dose with full glass of water to prevent crystalluria; drink 8-10 glasses of water/day
- Teach patient to complete course of full treatment to prevent superinfection
- Teach patient to avoid sunlight or use sunscreen to prevent burns
- Teach patient to avoid OTC medications (aspirin, vit C) unless directed by prescriber
- If diabetic, teach patient to use Clinistix or Tes-Tape
- Teach patient to use alternative contraceptive measures; decreased effectiveness of oral contraceptives may result
- Teach patient to notify prescriber if skin rash, sore throat, fever, mouth sores, unusual bruising, bleeding occur

Evaluation

Positive therapeutic outcome

Absence of pain, fever, C&S negative

triprolidine (℞)

(trye-proe'li-deen)

Actidil, Alleract, Myidil, triprolidine HCl

Func. class.: Antihistamine

Chem. class.: Alkylamine, H_1-receptor antagonist

Pregnancy category C

Action: Acts on blood vessels, GI, respiratory systems by competing with histamine for H_1-receptor site; decreases allergic response by blocking histamine

Therapeutic Outcome: Absence of allergy symptoms and rhinitis

Uses: Rhinitis, allergy symptoms

Dosage and routes

Adult: PO 2.5 mg tid-qid

P ***Child >6 yr:*** PO 1.25 mg tid-qid

P ***Child 4-6 yr:*** PO 0.9 mg tid-qid

P ***Child 2-4 yr:*** PO 0.6 mg tid-qid

P ***Child 4 mo-2 yr:*** PO 0.3 mg tid-qid

Available forms: Tab 2.5 mg; syr 1.25 mg/5 ml

Adverse effects

CNS: Dizziness, drowsiness, poor coordination, fatigue, anxiety, euphoria, confusion, paresthesia, neuritis

CV: Hypotension, palpitations, tachycardia

EENT: Blurred vision, dilated pupils, tinnitus, nasal stuffiness, dry nose, throat, mouth

GI: Constipation, dry mouth, nausea, vomiting, anorexia, diarrhea

GU: Retention, dysuria, frequency

*HEMA: **Thrombocytopenia, agranulocytosis, hemolytic anemia***

INTEG: Rash, urticaria, photosensitivity

RESP: Increased thick secretions, wheezing, chest tightness

Contraindications: Hypersensitivity to H_1-receptor antagonist, acute asthma attack, lower respiratory tract disease

Precautions: Increased IOP, renal disease, cardiac disease, hypertension, bronchial asthma, seizure disorder, stenosed peptic ulcers, hyperthyroidism, prostatic hypertrophy, bladder neck obstruction, pregnancy **C**

Pharmacokinetics	
Absorption	Well absorbed
Distribution	Widely distributed, crosses blood-brain barrier
Metabolism	Liver—extensively
Excretion	Kidneys
Half-life	5 hr

Pharmacodynamics	
Onset	15-60 min
Peak	1-2 hr
Duration	6-8 hr

Interactions

Individual drugs

Alcohol: ↑ CNS depression

Atropine: ↑ anticholinergic reactions

Disopyramide: ↑ anticholinergic reactions

Haloperidol: ↑ anticholinergic reactions

Quinidine: ↑ anticholinergic reactions

Drug classifications

Antidepressants: ↑ anticholinergic reactions

Antihistamines: ↑ anticholinergic reactions

CNS depressants: ↑ CNS depression

MAOIs: ↑ anticholinergic effect

Narcotics: ↑ CNS depression

Phenothiazines: ↑ anticholinergic reactions

Sedative/hypnotics: ↑ CNS depression

Lab test interferences

False negative: Skin allergy tests (discontinue antihistamines 3 days before testing)

NURSING CONSIDERATIONS

Assessment

- Assess respiratory status: rate, rhythm, increase in bronchial secretions, wheezing, chest tightness; provide fluids to 2 L/day to decrease thickness of secretions

• Monitor I&O ratio: be alert for urinary retention, frequency, dysuria, especially in G elderly; drug should be discontinued if these occur
• Monitor CBC during long-term therapy; blood dyscrasias may occur but are rare

Nursing diagnoses
✓ Airway clearance, ineffective (uses)
✓ Injury, risk for (adverse reactions)
✓ Knowledge deficit (teaching)
✓ Noncompliance (teaching—overuse)

Implementation
• Give on an empty stomach, 1 hr ac or 2 hr pc after meals to facilitate absorption
• Store in tight, light-resistant container

Patient/family education
• Teach patient all aspects of drug uses; to notify prescriber if confusion, sedation, hypotension occur; to avoid driving or other hazardous activity if drowsiness occurs; to avoid alcohol or other CNS depressants that may potentiate effect
• Advise patient to take medication 1 hr ac or 2 hr pc to facilitate absorption
• Caution patient not to exceed recommended dose because dysrhythmias may occur
• Inform patient that hard candy, gum, frequent rinsing of mouth may be used for dryness

Evaluation
Positive therapeutic outcome
• Absence of running or congested nose, rashes

Treatment of overdose: Administer ipecac syrup or lavage, diazepam, vasopressors, barbiturates (short-acting)

troglitazone (℞)
(troe-glye'ta-zone)
Rezulin
Func. class.: Antidiabetic, oral
Chem. class.: Thiazolidinedione
Pregnancy category UK

Action: Improves insulin resistance

➔ **Therapeutic Outcome:** Decreased symptoms of diabetes mellitus

Uses: Stable adult-onset diabetes mellitus (type II) NIDDM, nondiabetic obese patients, polycystic ovary syndrome, Werner's syndrome

Dosage and routes
Adult: PO 200 mg bid

Available forms: Tab 200 mg

Adverse effects
CV: Palpitations; increased LDH
GI: Nausea, vomiting, diarrhea, anorexia
GU: Nephrotoxicity
HEMA: Decreased RBC, Hct, Hgb
INTEG: Rash

Contraindications: Hypersensitivity, diabetic ketoacidosis

G **Precautions:** Pregnancy **UK,** elderly, thyroid disease, hepatic, renal disease

Pharmacokinetics	
Absorption	Unknown
Distribution	Unknown
Metabolism	Unknown
Excretion	Unknown
Half-time	Unknown

T

Pharmacodynamics	
Onset	Unknown
Peak	6-12 wk
Duration	Unknown

Interactions: None known

NURSING CONSIDERATIONS
Assessment
- Assess for hypoglycemic reactions (sweating, weakness, dizziness, anxiety, tremors, hunger), hyperglycemic reactions soon after meals
- Assess CBC (baseline, q3mo) during treatment; check liver function tests periodically; AST (SGOT), LDH, FBS, glycosylated Hgb, fasting plasma insulin, plasma lipids, lipoproteins, B/P, body weight during treatment

Nursing diagnoses
✓ Nutrition, altered: more than body requirements (uses)
✓ Knowledge deficit (teaching)

Implementation
- Convert from other oral hypoglycemic agents; change may be made without gradual dosage change; monitor serum or urine glucose and ketones tid during conversion
- Give twice a day; give with meals to decrease GI upset and provide best absorption
- Give tabs crushed and mixed with meal or fluids for patients with difficulty swallowing
- Store in tight container in cool environment

Patient/family education
- Teach patient to use capillary blood glucose test or Chemstrip tid
- Teach patient symptoms of hypo/hyperglycemia, what to do about each
- Advise patient that drug must be continued on daily basis; explain consequence of discontinuing drug abruptly
- Advise patient to avoid OTC medications unless approved by the prescriber
- Advise patient that diabetes is life-long illness; that this drug is not a cure, only controls symptoms
- Advise patient that all food included in diet plan must be eaten to prevent hypoglycemia
- Advise patient to carry Medic Alert ID and glucagon emergency kit for emergencies

Evaluation
Positive therapeutic outcome
- Decrease in polyuria, polydipsia, polyphagia; clear sensorium; absence of dizziness; stable gait; blood glucose at normal level

tubocurarine 🔑 (℞)
(too-boh-cure'a-reen)
Tubarine ✦, Tubocuraine
Func. class.: Neuromuscular blocker
Chem. class.: Synthetic curariform

Pregnancy category C

Action: Inhibits transmission of nerve impulses by binding with cholinergic receptor sites, antagonizing action of acetylcholine; no analgesic response

➔ **Therapeutic Outcome:** Skeletal muscle paralysis during anesthesia

Uses: Facilitation of endotracheal intubation, skeletal muscle relaxation during mechanical ventilation, surgery, or general anesthesia

Dosage and routes

Adult: **IV** bol 0.4-0.5 mg/kg, then 0.08-0.10 mg/kg 20-45 min after 1st dose if needed for prolonged procedures

Available forms: Inj 3 mg/ml, (20 U/ml)

Adverse effects

CV: Bradycardia, tachycardia, increased, decreased B/P

EENT: Increased secretions

INTEG: Rash, flushing, pruritus, urticaria

RESP: Prolonged apnea, bronchospasm, cyanosis, respiratory depression

Contraindications: Hypersensitivity

Precautions: Pregnancy **C**, cardiac disease, lactation, children <2 yr, electrolyte imbalances, dehydration, neuromuscular disease, respiratory disease

Pharmacokinetics

Absorption	Complete bioavailability
Distribution	Extensive, crosses placenta
Metabolism	Liver, small amount
Excretion	Kidneys—unchanged (30%-75%), bile (11%)
Half-life	2 hr

Pharmacodynamics

	IV	IM
Onset	1 min	15-30 min
Peak	5 min	Unknown
Duration	½-1½ hr	Unknown

Interactions

Individual drugs

Clindamycin: ↑ paralysis, length and intensity

Colistin: ↑ paralysis, length and intensity

Lidocaine: ↑ paralysis, length and intensity

Lithium: ↑ paralysis, length and intensity

Magnesium: ↑ paralysis, length and intensity

Polymyxin B: ↑ paralysis, length and intensity

Procainamide: ↑ paralysis, length and intensity

Quinidine: ↑ paralysis, length and intensity

Succinylcholine: ↑ paralysis, length and intensity

Drug classifications

Aminoglycosides: ↑ paralysis, length and intensity

β-Blockers: ↑ paralysis, length and intensity

Diuretics, potassium-losing: ↑ paralysis, length and intensity

General anesthesia: ↑ paralysis, length and intensity

NURSING CONSIDERATIONS

Assessment

- Monitor for electrolyte imbalances (potassium, magnesium), before drug is used; electrolyte imbalances may lead to increased action of this drug
- Monitor vital signs (B/P, pulse, respirations, airway) until fully recovered; rate, depth, pattern of respirations, strength of hand grip; patient should be intubated before use
- Monitor recovery: decreased paralysis of face, diaphragm, leg, arm, rest of body; residual weakness and respiratory problems may occur during recovery period
- Monitor allergic reactions: rash, fever, respiratory distress, pruritus; drug should be discontinued

Nursing diagnoses

- ✓ Breathing pattern, ineffective (uses)
- ✓ Communication, impaired verbal (adverse reactions)
- ✓ Fear (adverse reactions)
- ✓ Knowledge deficit (teaching)

Implementation

- Use peripheral nerve stimulator by anesthesiologist to determine neuromuscular blockade; deep tendon reflexes should be monitored during extended periods
- Give **IV** undiluted by direct **IV** over 1-1½ min, (only by qualified person, usually an anesthesiologist)

Additive incompatibilities: Barbiturates, sodium bicarbonate

Syringe compatibilities: Pentobarbital, thiopental

Solution compatibilities: D_5, $D_{10}W$, 0.9% NaCl, 0.45% NaCl, Ringer's, LR, dextrose/Ringer's or dextrose/LR combinations

Patient/family education

- Provide reassurance if communication is difficult during recovery from neuromuscular blockade
- Provide explanation to patients regarding all procedures or treatments; patient will remain conscious if anesthesia is not given also

Evaluation

Positive therapeutic outcome

- Paralysis of jaw, eyelid, head, neck, rest of body as evaluated by peripheral nerve stimulator

Treatment of overdose: Edrophonium or neostigmine, atropine, monitor VS; patient may require mechanical ventilation

urokinase (℞)

(yoor-oh-kin'ase)

Abbokinase, Abbokinase Open-Cath

Func. class.: Thrombolytic enzyme

Chem. class.: β-hemolytic streptococcus filtrate (purified)

Pregnancy category B

Action: Promotes thrombolysis by directly converting plasminogen to plasmin

Therapeutic Outcome: Lysis of emboli, or thrombosis in various parts of the body

Uses: Venous thrombosis, pulmonary embolism, arterial thrombosis, arterial embolism, arteriovenous cannula occlusion, lysis of coronary artery thrombi after MI

Dosage and routes

Lysis of pulmonary emboli

Adult: **IV** 4400 IU/kg/hr × 12-24 hr, not to exceed 200 ml; then **IV** heparin, then anticoagulants

Coronary artery thrombosis

Adult: Instill 6000 IU/min into occluded artery for 1-2 hr after giving **IV** bol of heparin 2500-10,000 U; may also give as **IV** inf of 2-3 million U over 45-90 min

Venous catheter occlusion

Adult: Instill 5000 IU into line, wait 5 min, then aspirate; repeat aspiration attempts q5min × ½ hr; if occlusion has not been removed, then cap line and wait ½-1 hr, then aspirate; may need 2nd dose if still occluded

Available forms: Powder for

inj, 250,000 IU/vial; powder for catheter clearance

Adverse effects

CNS: Headache, fever
CV: Hypertension, dysrhythmias, hypertension
EENT: Periorbital edema
GI: Nausea, vomiting
HEMA: Decreased Hct, ***bleeding***
INTEG: Rash, urticaria, phlebitis at **IV** inf site, itching, flushing
MS: Low back pain
RESP: Altered respirations, cyanosis, SOB, ***bronchospasm***
SYST: GI, GU, intracranial, retroperitoneal bleeding; surface bleeding; ***anaphylaxis*** (rare)

Contraindications: Hypersensitivity, active bleeding, intraspinal surgery, neoplasms of CNS, ulcerative colitis/enteritis, severe hypertension, renal disease, hepatic disease, hypocoagulation, COPD, subacute bacterial endocarditis, rheumatic valvular disease, cerebral embolism/thrombosis/hemorrhage, intraarterial diagnostic procedure or surgery (10 days), recent major surgery

Precautions: Arterial emboli from left side of heart, pregnancy **B**

Pharmacokinetics	
Absorption	Completely
Distribution	Unknown
Metabolism	Liver
Excretion	Kidneys
Half-life	10-20 min

Pharmacodynamics	
Onset	Rapid
Peak	Rapid
Duration	12 hr

Interactions

Individual drugs

Aspirin: ↑ bleeding
Dipyridamole: ↑ bleeding
Heparin: ↑ bleeding
Plicamycin: ↑ bleeding
Valproic acid: ↑ bleeding

Drug classifications

Cephalosporins: ↑ bleeding
Anticoagulants, oral: ↑ bleeding
Nonsteroidal antiinflammatories: ↑ bleeding

Lab test interferences

↑ PT, ↑ APTT, ↑ TT

NURSING CONSIDERATIONS

Assessment

- Monitor VS, B/P, pulse, respirations (including peripheral), neurologic signs, temp at least q4hr; temp >104° F (40° C) indicates internal bleeding; monitor rhythm closely; ventricular dysrhythmias may occur with hyperfusion; monitor heart, breath sounds, neuro status, peripheral pulses
- Assess for bleeding during first hr of treatment: hematuria, hematemesis, bleeding from mucous membranes, epistaxis, ecchymosis; guaiac all body fluids, stools; blood studies (Hct, platelets, PTT, PT, TT, APTT) before starting therapy; PT or APTT must be less than 2 × control before starting therapy TT or PT q3-4h during treatment
- Assess allergy: fever, rash, itching, chills; mild reaction may be treated with antihistamines; report to health care prescriber
- Monitor ECG on monitor, watch for segment changes, changes in rhythm; sinus bradycardia, ventricular tachycardia, accelerated idioven-

U

tricular rhythm may occur because of reperfusion

Nursing diagnoses

✓ Tissue perfusion, altered (uses)
✓ Injury, high risk for (adverse reactions)
✓ Impaired gas exchange (uses)

Implementation

Int IV

- Give **IV** loading dose over 30 min to avoid hypotension
- **IV** after dilution with 4-5 g/250 ml NS, D_5W, LR, give over 1 hr; may give by continuous inf after loading dose(s) of 1 g/hr diluted in 50-100 ml of compatible sol; use inf pump; do not give by direct **IV**
- Give heparin therapy after thrombolytic therapy is discontinued, TT, ACT, or APTT less than 2 × control (about 3-4 hr)
- Avoid invasive procedures, inj, rec temp
- Apply pressure for 30 sec to minor bleeding sites; 30 min to sites of atrial puncture, followed by pressure dressing; inform prescriber if this does not attain hemostasis; apply pressure dressing
- Store powder at room temp or refrigerate; protect from excessive light

Additive incompatibilities: Do not mix with other medications

Patient/family education

- Teach patient reason for medication, signs and symptoms of bleeding, allergic reactions, when to notify health care prescriber

Evaluation

Positive therapeutic outcome

- Lysis of thrombi or emboli

valproate/valproic acid, divalproex sodium (℞)

(val-proe'ate)

Depakene, Dalpro, Deproic, Epival*, Myproic acid/ Depakote, Depacon

Func. class.: Anticonvulsant

Chem. class.: Carboxylic acid derivative

Pregnancy category D

Action: Increases levels of γ-aminobutyric acid (GABA) in brain, which decreases seizure activity

➡ **Therapeutic Outcome:** Decreased symptoms of epilepsy, bipolar disorder

Uses: Simple (petit mal), complex (petit mal) absence, mixed, manic episode associated with bipolar disorder

Investigational uses: Tonic-clonic (grand mal), myoclonic seizures

Dosage and routes

P ***Adult and child:*** PO 15 mg/kg/day divided in 2-3 doses, may increase by 5-10 mg/kg/day qwk, not to exceed 60 mg/kg/day in 2-3 divided doses

Available forms: Valproic acid caps 250 mg; divalproex delayed rel tabs 125, 250, 500 mg; 125 mg sprinkle cap; valproate sodium syr 250 mg/5 ml

Adverse effects

CNS: Sedation, drowsiness, dizziness, headache, incoordination, paresthesia, depression, hallucinations, behavioral

changes, tremors, aggression, weakness
GI: Nausea, vomiting, constipation, diarrhea, heartburn, anorexia, cramps, ***hepatic failure, pancreatitis, toxic hepatitis,*** stomatitis
GU: Enuresis, irregular menses
HEMA: Thrombocytopenia, leukopenia, lymphocytosis, increased pro-time
INTEG: Rash, alopecia, bruising

Contraindications: Hypersensitivity, pregnancy **D**

Precautions: Lactation

Pharmacokinetics	
Absorption	Unknown
Distribution	Breast milk, crosses placenta, widely distributed
Metabolism	Liver
Excretion	Kidneys
Half-life	9-16 hr

Pharmacodynamics	
Onset	15-30 min
Peak	1-4 hr
Duration	4-6 hr

Interactions
Individual drugs
Cimetidine: ↑ metabolism of valproic acid
Primidone: ↑ CNS depressants
Phenobarbital: ↑ CNS depressants
Phenytoin: ↑ action of phenytoin
Warfarin: ↑ toxicity of warfarin

Drug classifications
Salicylates: ↑ toxicity of valproic acid
Benzodiazepines: ↑ sedation

Lab test interferences
False positive: Ketones

NURSING CONSIDERATIONS
Assessment
- Monitor blood studies: Hct, Hgb, RBC, serum folate, pro-time, vit D if on long-term therapy
- Monitor hepatic studies: AST (SGOT), ALT (SGPT), bilirubin, creatinine, failure
- Monitor blood levels: therapeutic level 50-100 μg/ml
- Assess mental status: mood, sensorium, affect, memory (long, short)
- Assess respiratory dysfunction: respiratory depression, character, rate, rhythm; hold drug if respirations are <12/min or if pupils are dilated

Implementation
- Give tablets or capsules whole
- Give elixir alone; do not dilute with carbonated beverage; do not give syrup to patients on sodium restriction
- Give with food or milk to decrease GI symptoms

Patient family education
- Teach patient that physical dependency may result from extended use
- Instruct patient to avoid driving, other activities that require alertness
- Advise patient not to discontinue medication quickly after long-term use; convulsions may result
- Advise patient to report visual disturbances, rash, diarrhea, light-colored stools, jaundice, protracted vomiting to prescriber

Evaluation
Positive therapeutic outcome
- Decreased seizures

V

valsartan (℞)

(val-zar'tan)

Diovan

Func. class.: Antihypertensive

Chem. class.: Angiotensin II receptor (Type AT_1)

Pregnancy category N/A

Action: Blocks the vasoconstrictor and aldosterone-secreting effects of angiotensin II; selectively blocks the binding of angiotensin II to the AT_1 receptor found in tissues

Therapeutic Outcome: Decreased B/P

Uses: Hypertension, alone or in combination

Dosage and routes

Adult: PO 80-160 mg qd alone or when used in combination

Available forms: Tabs 80, 160 mg

Adverse effects

CNS: Dizziness, insomnia, depression, drowsiness, vertigo

CV: Angina pectoris, 2nd-degree AV block, ***cerebrovascular accident,*** hypotension, *myocardial infarction, dysrhythmias*

EENT: Conjunctivitis

GI: Diarrhea, abdominal pain, nausea, ***hepatotoxicity***

GU: Impotence, nephrotoxicity

HEMA: Anemia, neutropenia

MS: Cramps, myalgia, pain, stiffness

RESP: Cough

Contraindications: Hypersensitivity, pregnancy, severe hepatic disease, bilateral renal artery stenosis

G **Precautions:** Hypersensitivity to ACE inhibitors, congestive heart failure, hypertrophic cardiomyopathy, aortic/mitral valve stenosis, CAD; lactation, P children, G elderly

Pharmacokinetics	
Absorption	Well
Distribution	Bound to plasma proteins
Metabolism	Extensive
Excretion	Feces, urine, breast milk
Half-life	9 hr

Pharmacodynamics	
Onset	Unknown
Peak	2 hr
Duration	24 hr

Interactions: None significant

NURSING CONSIDERATIONS

Assessment

- Assess B/P, pulse q4h; note rate, rhythm, quality
- Monitor electrolytes: potassium, sodium, chloride; total CO_2
- Obtain baselines in renal, liver function tests before therapy begins
- Assess blood studies: BUN, creatinine, LFTs before treatment
- Monitor for edema in feet, legs daily
- Assess for skin turgor, dryness of mucous membranes for hydration status

Nursing diagnoses

- ✓ Fluid volume deficit (side effects)
- ✓ Noncompliance (teaching)
- ✓ Knowledge deficit (teaching)

Implementation

- Administer without regard to meals

Patient/family education

- Teach patient not to take this

drug if breastfeeding or pregnant, or have had an allergic reaction to this drug
• If a dose is missed, instruct patient to take as soon as possible, unless it is within an hour before next dose
• Advise patient to comply with dosage schedule, even if feeling better
• Teach patient to notify prescriber of fever, swelling of hands or feet, irregular heartbeat, chest pain
• Advise patient excessive perspiration, dehydration, diarrhea may lead to fall in blood pressure—consult prescriber if these occur
• Inform patient that drug may cause dizziness, fainting; lightheadedness may occur
• Caution patient to rise slowly to sitting or standing position to minimize orthostatic hypotension

Evaluation
Positive therapeutic outcome
• Decreased B/P

vancomycin
(van-koe-mye'sin)
Vancocin, vancomycin HCl
Func. clas.: Antiinfective, misc.
Chem. class.: Tricyclic glycopeptide
Pregnancy category C

Action: Inhibits bacterial cell wall synthesis

Therapeutic Outcome: Bactericidal for the following organisms: Staphylococci, Streptococci, Corynebacterium, Clostridium

Uses: Resistant staphylococcal infections, pseudomembranous colitis, staphylococcal enterocolitis, group A β-hemolytic streptococci, endocarditis prophylaxis for dental procedures

Dosage and routes
Serious staphylococcal infections
Adult: **IV** 500 mg (7.5 mg/kg) q6h or 1 g (15 mg/kg) q12h max 4 g/day
P ***Child:*** **IV** 40 mg/kg/day divided q6-12h
P ***Neonates:*** **IV** 15 mg/kg initially followed by 10 mg/kg q8-12 h

Pseudomembranous/staphylococcal enterocolitis
Adult: PO 500 mg-2 g/day in 3-4 divided doses for 7-10 days
P ***Child:*** PO 40 mg/kg/day divided q6h, not to exceed 2 g/day
P ***Neonates:*** PO 10 mg/kg/day in divided doses

Endocarditis prophylaxis
Adult: **IV** 1 g over 1 hr, 1 hr before dental procedure
P ***Child:*** 20 mg/kg over 1 hr, 1 hr before procedure

Available forms: Pulvules 125, 250 mg; powder for oral sol 1, 10 g; powder for inj **IV** 500 mg, 1-g, 5-g, 10-g vials

Adverse effects
CV: ***Cardiac arrest, vascular collapse (rare)***
EENT: ***Ototoxicity, permanent deafness,*** tinnitus
GI: Nausea
GU: ***Nephrotoxicity, increased BUN, creatinine, albumin, fatal uremia***
HEMA: ***Leukopenia, eosinophilia, neutropenia***
INTEG: Chills, fever, rash,

V

thrombophlebitis at inj site, urticaria, pruritus, necrosis (Redman's syndrome)
RESP: Wheezing, dyspnea
SYST: ***Anaphylaxis***

Contraindications: Hypersensitivity

Precautions: Renal disease, pregnancy **C**, lactation, G elderly, P neonates

Pharmacokinetics

Absorption	Poorly absorbed (PO), completely absorbed (IV)
Distribution	Widely distributed, crosses placenta
Metabolism	Liver
Excretion	PO—feces, IV—kidneys
Half-life	4-8 hr

Pharmacodynamics

	IV
Onset	Immediate
Peak	Inf end

Interactions

Individual drugs

Amphotericin B: ↑ toxicity
Bacitracin: ↑ toxicity
Cisplatin: ↑ toxicity
Polymyxin B: ↑ toxicity

Drug classifications

Aminoglycosides: ↑ toxicity
Cephalosporins: ↑ toxicity
Nondepolarizing muscle relaxants: ↑ toxicity

NURSING CONSIDERATIONS

Assessment

- Monitor I&O ratio; report hematuria, oliguria because nephrotoxicity may occur
- Monitor any patient with compromised renal system; drug is excreted slowly in poor renal system function; toxicity may occur rapidly
- Monitor blood studies: WBC
- Obtain C&S before drug therapy; drug may be given as soon as culture is taken
- Assess auditory function during, after treatment; hearing loss, ringing, roaring in ears; drug should be discontinued
- Monitor B/P during administration; sudden drop may indicate Red Man's syndrome
- Assess for signs of infection
- Assess respiratory status: rate, character, wheezing, tightness in chest
- Identify allergies before treatment, reaction of each medication; place allergies on chart in bright letters; notify all people giving drugs

Nursing diagnoses

- ✓ Infection, risk for (uses)
- ✓ Knowledge deficit (teaching)

Implementation

IV route

- Give after reconstitution with 10 ml sterile water for inj (500 mg/10 ml); further dilution is needed for **IV**, 500 mg/ 100 ml NS, D_5W given as int inf over 1 hr

Additive compatibilities: Amikacin, atracurium, calcium gluconate, cefepime, cimetidine, corticotropin, dimenhydrinate, hydrocortisone, ofloxacin, potassium chloride, ranitidine, verapamil, vit B/C

Y-site compatibilities: Acyclovir, allopurinol, amiodarone, amsacrine, atracurium, cyclophosphamide, diltiazem, enalaprilat, esmolol, filgrastim, fluconazole, fludarabine, hydromorphone, regular insulin, labetalol, magnesium sulfate, melphalan, meperidine, morphine, ondansetron, paclitaxel, pancuronium, sodium

bicarbonate, tacrolimus, teniposide, theophylline, zidovudine
- Give antihistamine if Red Man's syndrome occurs: decreased B/P, flushing of neck, face
- Give dose based on serum concentration
- Store at room temp for up to 2 wk after reconstitution
- Have adrenalin, suction, tracheostomy set, endotracheal intubation equipment on unit; anaphylaxis may occur
- Provide adequate intake of fluids (2 L) to prevent nephrotoxicity

Patient/family education
- Teach patient aspects of drug therapy: need to complete entire course of medication to ensure organism death (7-10 days); culture may be taken after completed course of medication
- Advise patient to report sore throat, fever, fatigue; could indicate superinfection
- Instruct patient that drug must be taken in equal intervals around clock to maintain blood levels

Evaluation
Positive therapeutic outcome
- Absence of fever, sore throat
- Negative culture after treatment

vasopressin (℞)
(vay-soe-press'in)
Pitressin Synthetic,
Pressyn ✤
Func. class.: Pituitary hormone
Chem. class.: Lysine vasopressin
Pregnancy category C

Action: Promotes reabsorption of water by action on renal tubular epithelium; causes vasoconstriction on muscles in the GI system

➔ **Therapeutic Outcome:** Increased osmolality, decreased urine output in diabetes insipidus

Uses: Diabetes insipidus (nonnephrogenic/ nonpsychogenic), abdominal distention postoperatively, bleeding esophageal varices

Dosage and routes
Diabetes insipidus
Adult: IM/SC 5-10 units bid-qid prn; IM/SC 2.5-5 units q2-3 days (Pitressin Tannate) for chronic therapy
P ***Child:*** IM/SC 2.5-10 units bid-qid prn; IM/SC 1.25-2.5 units q2-3 days (Pitressin Tannate) for chronic therapy

Abdominal distention
Adult: IM 5 units, then q3-4h, increasing to 10 units if needed (aqueous)

Available forms: Inj 20, 5 U/ml (tannate), spray, cotton pledgets

Adverse effects
CNS: Drowsiness, headache, lethargy, flushing
CV: Increased B/P

V

EENT: Nasal irritation, congestion, rhinitis
GI: Nausea, heartburn, cramps
GU: Vulval pain, uterine cramping
MISC: Tremor, sweating, vertigo, urticaria, bronchial constriction

Contraindications: Hypersensitivity, chronic nephritis

Precautions: CAD, pregnancy **C**

Pharmacokinetics

Absorption	Erratically absorbed (IM)
Distribution	Widely distributed extracellular fluid
Metabolism	Liver—rapidly
Excretion	Kidneys, unchanged
Half-life	10-20 min

Pharmacodynamics

	IM	NASAL
Onset	Unknown	1 hr
Peak	Unknown	Unknown
Duration	3-8 hr	3-8 hr

Interactions

Individual drugs

Alcohol: ↓ response
Carbamazepine: ↑ response
Chlorpropamide: ↑ response
Clofibrate: ↑ response
Demeclocycline: ↓ response
Epinephrine (large doses): ↓ response
Heparin: ↓ response
Lithium: ↓ response

Drug classifications

Ganglionic blockers: ↑ vasopressor response

NURSING CONSIDERATIONS

Assessment

- Monitor nasal mucosa for irritation if given by intranasal spray
- Assess intranasal use: nausea, congestion, cramps, headache; usually decreased with decreased dose
- Monitor pulse, B/P when giving drug **IV** or SC
- Monitor I&O ratio, weight daily; check for edema in extremities; if water retention is severe, diuretic may be prescribed; check for water intoxication: lethargy, behavioral changes, disorientation, neuromuscular excitability

Nursing diagnoses

- ✓ Fluid volume excess (side effects)
- ✓ Fluid volume deficit (uses)
- ✓ Knowledge deficit (teaching)

Implementation

IM route

- May be given IM/SC for diagnosis of diabetes insipidus
- Give patient 16 oz water at administration to prevent nausea, vomiting, cramping

Patient/family education

- Teach patient technique for nasal instillation: to insert tube into nasal cavity to instill drug
- Caution patient to avoid OTC products for cough, hay fever products because these preparations may contain epinephrine, decrease drug response; do not use with alcohol
- Advise patient to wear Medic Alert ID specifying therapy, disease process (diabetes insipidus)

Evaluation

Positive therapeutic outcome

- Absence of severe thirst
- Decreased urine output, osmolality

vecuronium (℞)
(ve-kure-oh′nee-yum)
Norcuron
Func. class.: Neuromuscular blocker
Chem. class.: Synthetic curariform
Pregnancy category C

Action: Inhibits transmission of nerve impulses by binding with cholinergic receptor sites, antagonizing action of acetylcholine; no analgesic response

➔ **Therapeutic Outcome:** Skeletal muscle paralysis during anesthesia

Uses: Facilitation of endotracheal intubation; skeletal muscle relaxation during mechanical ventilation, surgery, or general anesthesia

Dosage and routes

P ***Adult and child >9 yr:*** **IV** bol 0.08-0.10 mg/kg, then 0.010-0.015 mg/kg for prolonged procedures

Available forms: 10 mg/5 ml vial

Adverse effects

CNS: Skeletal muscle weakness or paralysis (rarely)
RESP: Prolonged apnea, possible respiratory paralysis

Contraindications: Hypersensitivity

Precautions: Pregnancy **C**, cardiac disease, lactation, P children <2 yr, electrolyte imbalances, dehydration, neuromuscular disease, respiratory, hepatic disease

Pharmacokinetics

Absorption	Completely absorbed
Distribution	Rapid—to extracellular fluids
Metabolism	Liver (20%)
Excretion	Kidneys—unchanged (35%)
Half-life	1½ hr, increased in liver disease

Pharmacodynamics

Onset	1 min
Peak	5 min
Duration	15-25 min

Interactions

Individual drugs

Clindamycin: ↑ paralysis, length and intensity
Colistin: ↑ paralysis, length and intensity
Lidocaine: ↑ paralysis, length and intensity
Lithium: ↑ paralysis, length and intensity
Magnesium: ↑ paralysis, length and intensity
Polymyxin B: ↑ paralysis, length and intensity
Procainamide: ↑ paralysis, length and intensity
Quinidine: ↑ paralysis, length and intensity
Succinylcholine: ↑ paralysis, length and intensity

Drug classifications

Aminoglycosides: ↑ paralysis, length and intensity
β-Blockers: ↑ paralysis, length and intensity
Diuretics, potassium-losing: ↑ paralysis, length and intensity
General anesthesia: ↑ paralysis, length and intensity

V

NURSING CONSIDERATIONS

Assessment

• Monitor for electrolyte imbalances (potassium, magnesium), before drug is used; electrolyte imbalances may lead to increased action of this drug

• Monitor patient's vital signs (B/P, pulse, respirations, airway) until fully recovered; rate, depth, pattern of respirations, strength of hand grip; patient should be intubated before use
• Monitor patient's recovery: decreased paralysis of face, diaphragm, leg, arm, rest of body; residual weakness and respiratory problems may occur during recovery period
• Monitor allergic reactions: rash, fever, respiratory distress, pruritus; drug should be discontinued

Nursing diagnoses
✓ Breathing pattern, ineffective (uses)
✓ Communication, impaired verbal (adverse reactions)
✓ Fear (adverse reactions)
✓ Knowledge deficit (teaching)

Implementation
• Use peripheral nerve stimulator by anesthesiologist to determine neuromuscular blockade; deep tendon reflexes should be monitored during extended periods
• Give by direct **IV** after reconstituting with bacteriostatic water, over 5 min, D_5W, 0.9% NaCl or LR
• Give by direct **IV** after reconstituting dose in 5-10 ml; give by titrating to patient response
• Give by continuous inf after diluting to 10-20 mg/100 ml and by titrating to patient response (only by qualified person, usually an anesthesiologist); do not administer IM
• Store in light-resistant area

Y-site compatibilities: Aminophylline, cefazolin, cefuroxime, cimetidine, dobutamine, dopamine, epinephrine, esmolol, fentanyl, gentamicin, heparin, hydrocortisone, isoproterenol, lorazepam, midazolam, morphine, nitroglycerin, nitroprusside, ranitidine, trimethoprim/sulfamethoxazole, vancomycin

Y-site incompatibility: Barbiturates

Syringe incompatibility: Barbiturates

Patient/family education
• Provide reassurance if communication is difficult during recovery from neuromuscular blockade
• Provide explanation to patients regarding all procedures or treatments; patient will remain conscious if anesthesia is not given also

Evaluation

Positive therapeutic outcome
• Paralysis of jaw, eyelid, head, neck, rest of body as evaluated by peripheral nerve stimulator

Treatment of overdose: Edrophonium or neostigmine, atropine, monitor VS; may require mechanical ventilation

venlafaxine (℞)
(ven-laa-fax'een)
Effexor
Func. class.: Second-generation antidepressant
Pregnancy category C

Action: Potent inhibitor of neuronal serotinin and norepinephrine uptake, weak inhibitor of dopamine; no muscarinic, histaminergic, or α-adrenergic receptors in vitro

➡ Therapeutic Outcome: Relief of depression

Uses: Depression

Dosage and routes
Adult: PO 75 mg/day in 2 or 3 divided doses; taken with food, may be increased to 150 mg/day; if needed may be further increased to 225 mg/day; increments of 75 mg/day should be made at intervals of no less than 4 days; some hospitalized patients may require up to 375 mg/day in 3 divided doses

Available forms: Tabs scored 25, 37.5, 50, 75, 100 mg

Adverse effects
CNS: Emotional lability, vertigo, apathy, ataxia, CNS stimulation, euphoria, hallucinations, hostility, increased libido, hypertonia, hypotonia, psychosis
CV: Migraine, angina pectoris, extrasystoles, postural hypotension, syncope, thrombophlebitis, hypertension
EENT: Abnormal vision, ear pain, cataract, conjunctivitis, corneal lesions, dry eyes, otitis media, photophobia
GI: Dysphagia, eructation, colitis, gastritis, gingivitis, rectal hemorrhage, stomatitis, stomach and mouth ulceration
GU: Anorgasmia, dysuria, hematuria, metrorrhagia, vaginitis, impaired urination, albuminaria, amenorrhea, kidney calculus, cystitis, nocturia, breast and bladder pain, polyuria, uterine hemorrhage, vaginal hemorrhage, moniliasis
INTEG: Ecchymosis, acne, alopecia, brittle nails, dry skin, photosensitivity
META: Peripheral edema, weight gain, diabetes mellitus, edema, glycosuria, hyperlipemia, hypokalemia
MS: Arthritis, bone pain, bursitis, myasthenia tenosynovitis
RESP: Bronchitis, dyspnea, asthma, chest congestion, epistaxis, hyperventilation, laryngitis
SYST: Accidental injury, malaise, neck pain, enlarged abdomen, cyst, facial edema, hangover effect, hernia

Contraindications: Hypersensitivity

Precautions: Mania, pregnancy **C**, lactation, children, elderly

P G

Pharmacokinetics

Absorption	Well absorbed
Distribution	Widely distributed, 27% protein binding
Metabolism	Liver—extensively
Excretion	Kidneys, 87%
Half-life	5-7 hr, 11-13 hr

Pharmacodynamics

Unknown

Interactions
Drug classifications
MAOIs: Hypertensive crisis, convulsions
Lab test interferences
↑ Serum bilirubin, ↑ blood glucose, ↑ alk phosphatase
↓ VMA, ↓ 5-HIAA
False ↑ Urinary catecholamines

NURSING CONSIDERATIONS
Assessment
- Monitor B/P (lying, standing), pulse q4h; if systolic B/P drops 20 mm hg hold drug, notify prescriber; take vital signs q4h in patients with cardiovascular disease
- Monitor blood studies: CBC, leukocytes, differential, cardiac enzymes if patient is receiving long-term therapy
- Monitor hepatic studies: AST (SGOT), ALT (SGPT), bilirubin

V

• Check weight qwk; appetite may increase with drug
• Assess mental status: mood, sensorium, affect, suicidal tendencies; increase in psychiatric symptoms: depression, panic
• Monitor urinary retention, constipation; constipation is
P more likely to occur in children
G or elderly
• Assess for withdrawal symptoms: headache, nausea, vomiting, muscle pain, weakness; do not usually occur unless drug was discontinued abruptly
• Identify alcohol consumption; if alcohol is consumed, hold dose

Nursing diagnoses

✓ Coping, ineffective individual (uses)
✓ Injury, risk for physical (side effects)
✓ Knowledge deficit (teaching)
✓ Noncompliance (teaching)

Implementation

• Give with food or milk for GI symptoms
• Crush if patient is unable to swallow medication whole
• Store at room temp; do not freeze

Patient/family education

• Teach patient that therapeutic effects may take 2-3 wk
• Teach patient to use caution in driving or other activities requiring alertness because of drowsiness, dizziness, blurred vision; to avoid rising quickly from sitting to standing, espe-
G cially elderly
• Teach patient to avoid alcohol ingestion, other CNS depressants

Evaluation

Positive therapeutic outcome

• Decreased depression
• Absence of suicidal thoughts

Treatment of overdose: ECG monitoring, induce emesis, lavage, activated charcoal, administer anticonvulsant

verapamil 🔑 (℞)

(ver-ap'a-mil)

Calan, Calan SR, Isoptin, Isoptin SR, verapamil HCl, verapamil HCl SR, Verelan

Func. class.: Calcium-channel blocker; antihypertensive; antianginal

Chem. class.: Phenylalkylamine

Pregnancy category C

Action: Inhibits calcium ion influx across cell membrane during cardiac depolarization; produces relaxation of coronary vascular smooth muscle; peripheral vascular smooth muscle; dilates coronary vascular arteries; increases myocardial oxygen delivery in patients with vasospastic angina

➔ **Therapeutic Outcome:** Decreased angina pectoris, dysrhythmias, B/P

Uses: Chronic stable angina pectoris, vasospastic angina, dysrhythmias, hypertension

Investigational uses: Prevention of migraine headaches, ventricular outflow obstruction in hypertrophic cardiomyopathy

Dosage and routes

Adult: PO 80 mg tid or qid, increase qwk; **IV** bol 5-10 mg

>2 min, repeat if necessary in 30 min

P ***Child 0-1 yr:* IV** bol 0.1-0.2 mg/kg >2 min with ECG monitoring, repeat if necessary in 30 min

P ***Child 1-15 yr:* IV** bol 0.1-0.3 mg/kg over >2 min, repeat in 30 min, not to exceed 10 mg in a single dose

Available forms: Tabs 40, 80, 120 mg; sus-rel tabs, 120, 180, 240 mg; inj 5 mg/ml; sus-rel caps 120, 180, 240, 360 mg

Adverse effects

CNS: Headache, drowsiness, dizziness, anxiety, depression, weakness, insomnia, confusion, lightheadedness

CV: Edema, CHF, bradycardia, hypotension, palpitations, AV block

GI: Nausea, diarrhea, gastric upset, constipation, increased liver function studies

GU: Nocturia, polyuria

Contraindications: Sick sinus syndrome, 2nd- or 3rd-degree heart block, hypotension less than 90 mm Hg systolic, cardiogenic shock, severe CHF

Precautions: CHF, hypotension, hepatic injury, pregnancy P C, lactation, children, renal disease, concomitant β-blocker therapy

Pharmacokinetics

Absorption	Well absorbed (PO)
Distribution	Not known
Metabolism	Liver—extensively
Excretion	Kidneys
Half-life	Biphasic 4 min, 3-7 hr

Pharmacodynamics

	PO	PO-ER	IV
Onset	1-2 hr	Unknown	1-5 min
Peak	½-1½ hr	5-7 hr	3-5 min
Duration	3-7 hr	24 hr	2 hr

Interactions

Individual drugs

Alcohol: ↑ hypotension
Carbamazepine: ↑ toxicity
Digoxin: ↑ digoxin levels, ↑ bradycardia, CHF
Phenobarbital: ↓ effectiveness
Phenytoin: ↓ effectiveness
Propranolol: ↑ toxicity

Drug classifications

Antihypertensives: ↑ hypotension
β-Adrenergic blockers: ↑ bradycardia, CHF
Nitrates: ↑ nitrates

NURSING CONSIDERATIONS

Assessment

- Assess fluid volume status: I&O ratio and record; weight; distended red veins; crackles in lung; color; quality, and specific gravity of urine; skin turgor; adequacy of pulses; moist mucous membranes; bilateral lung sounds; peripheral pitting edema—dehydration symptoms of decreasing output, thirst, hypotension, dry mouth, and mucous membranes should be reported
- Monitor B/P and pulse, pulmonary capillary wedge pressure (PCWP), central venous pressure, index, often during inf; if B/P drops 30 mm Hg, stop inf and call prescriber
- Monitor ALT (SGPT), AST (SGOT), bilirubin daily; if

V

these are elevated, hepatotoxicity is suspected

- Monitor if platelets are <150,000/mm^3—if so, drug is usually discontinued and another drug started
- Assess for extravasation: change site q48h
- Monitor cardiac status: B/P, pulse, respiration, ECG

Nursing diagnoses

- ✓ Cardiac output, decreased (uses)
- ✓ Knowledge deficit (teaching)

Implementation

PO route

- Give once a day, with food for GI symptoms

IV route

- Give by direct **IV** undiluted (Y-site, 3-way stopcock) over at least 2 min; to prevent serious hypotension, patient should be recumbent for 1 hr or more

Syringe compatibilities: Amrinone, heparin, milrinone

Y-site incompatibilities: Albumin, ampicillin, mezlocillin, nafcillin, oxacillin, sodium bicarbonate

Y-site compatibilities: Amrinone, aprofloxacin, dobutamine, dopamine, famotidine, hydralazine, meperidine, methicillin, milrinone, penicillin G potassium, piperacillin, ticarcillin

Patient/family education

- Caution patient to avoid hazardous activities until stabilized on drug, dizziness is no longer a problem
- Instruct patient to limit caffeine consumption; to avoid alcohol and OTC drugs unless directed by prescriber
- Advise patient to comply with medical regimen: diet, exercise, stress reduction, drug therapy; to notify prescriber of irregular heart beat, shortness of breath, swelling of feet and hands, pronounced dizziness, constipation, nausea, hypotension
- Teach patient to use as directed even if feeling better; may be taken with other cardiovascular drugs (nitrates, β blockers)

Evaluation

Positive therapeutic outcome

- Decreased anginal pain
- Decreased dysrhythmias
- Decreased B/P

Treatment of overdose: Defibrillation, atropine for AV block, vasopressor for hypotension

vinblastine (VLB) (℞)

(vin-blast'een)

Alkaban-AQ, Velban, Velbe ✦, Velsar, vinblastine sulfate

Func. class.: Antineoplastic

Chem. class.: Vinca rosea alkaloid

Pregnancy category D

Action: Inhibits mitotic activity, arrests cell cycle at metaphase; inhibits RNA synthesis, blocks cellular use of glutamic acid needed for purine synthesis; a vesicant

Therapeutic Outcome: Prevention of rapid growth of malignant cells, immunosuppressive

Uses: Breast, testicular cancer; lymphomas; neuroblastoma; Hodgkin's, non-Hodgkin's lymphomas; mycosis fungoides; histiocytosis; Kaposi's sarcoma

Dosage and routes

Adult: **IV** 0.1 mg/kg or 3.7 mg/m^2 q wk or q2 wk, not to exceed 0.5 mg/kg or 18.5 mg/m^2 q wk

P ***Child:*** 2.5 mg/m^2 then dose of 3.75, 5.0, 6.25 and 7.5 at 7-day intervals

Available forms: Inj powder 10 mg for 10 ml **IV** inj

Adverse effects

CNS: Paresthesias, peripheral neuropathy, depression, headache, ***convulsions***

CV: Tachycardia, orthostatic hypotension

GI: Nausea, vomiting, ileus, *anorexia, stomatitis,* constipation, abdominal pain, GI and rectal bleeding, ***hepatotoxicity,*** pharyngitis

GU: Urinary retention, ***renal failure***

HEMA: ***Thrombocytopenia, leukopenia, myelosuppression***

INTEG: Rash, alopecia, photo sensitivity

META: SIADH

RESP: ***Fibrosis, pulmonary infiltrate***

Contraindications: Hypersen-
P sitivity, infants, pregnancy **D**

Precautions: Renal disease, hepatic disease

Pharmacokinetics

Absorption	Complete bioavailability
Distribution	Crosses blood-brain barrier slightly
Metabolism	Liver—active antineoplastic
Excretion	Biliary, kidneys
Half-life	Triphasic—35 min, 53 min, 19 hr

Pharmacodynamics

Unknown

Interactions

Individual drugs

Live virus vaccines: ↑ adverse reactions

Mitomycin: ↑ Bronchospasm

Radiation: ↑ toxicity, bone marrow suppression

Drug classifications

Antineoplastics: ↑ toxicity, bone marrow suppression

NURSING CONSIDERATIONS

Assessment

- Monitor B/P, (baseline and q15 min) during administration
- Monitor CBC, differential, platelet count weekly; withhold drug if WBC is <4000 or platelet count is <75,000; notify prescriber of results, recovery will take 3 wk
- Assess for dyspnea, rales, unproductive cough, chest pain, tachypnea
- Monitor renal function studies: BUN, serum uric acid, urine CrCl before, during therapy; I&O ratio; report fall in urine output of 30 ml/hr; for decreased hyperuricemia
- Monitor for cold, fever, sore throat (may indicate beginning infection); notify health care prescriber if these occur
- Assess for bleeding: hematuria, guaiac, bruising or petechiae, mucosa or orifices q8h, no rectal temp; avoid IM inj; use pressure to venipuncture sites
- Identify nutritional status: an antiemetic may need to be prescribed
- Assess for symptoms indicating severe allergic reactions: rash, pruritus, urticaria, itching, flushing, bronchospasm, hypotension; epinephrine and crash cart should be nearby

V

Nursing diagnoses

- ✓ Injury, risk for (adverse reactions)
- ✓ Body image disturbance (adverse reactions)
- ✓ Infection, risk for (adverse reactions)
- ✓ Knowledge deficit (teaching)

Implementation

- Give by intermittent inf
- Sol should be prepared by qualified personnel only under controlled conditions
- Use Luer-Loc tubing to prevent leakage; do not let sol come in contact with skin; if contact occurs, wash well with soap and water
- Administer **IV** after diluting 10 mg/10 ml NaCl; give through Y-tube or 3-way stopcock or directly over 1 min
- Give hyaluronidase 150 U/ml in 1 ml NaCl, warm compress for extravasation for vesicant activity treatment

Syringe compatibilities: Bleomycin, cisplatin, cyclophosphamide, droperidol, fluorouracil, leucovorin, methotrexate, metoclopramide, mitomycin, vincristine

Y-site compatibilities: Allopurinol, aztreonam, bleomycin, cisplatin, cyclophosphamide, doxorubicin, droperidol, filgrastim, fludarabine, fluorouracil, heparin, leucovorin, melphalan, methotrexate, metoclopramide, mitomycin, ondansetron, sargramostim, teniposide, vincristine

Y-site incompatibility: Furosemide

Patient/family education

- Teach patient to avoid use of products containing aspirin or ibuprofen, razors, commercial mouthwash because bleeding may occur; to report symptoms of bleeding (hematuria, tarry stools)
- Instruct patient to report signs of anemia, (fatigue, headache, irritability, faintness, shortness of breath)
- Caution patient to report any changes in breathing or coughing even several mo after treatment
- Advise patient that contraception will be necessary during treatment; teratogenesis may occur
- Inform patient that hair may be lost during treatment; a wig or hairpiece may make patient feel better; new hair will be different in color, texture
- Advise patient to avoid vaccinations during treatment; serious reactions may occur
- Teach patient to report signs/symptoms of infection: fever, chills, sore throat; patient should avoid crowds and persons with known infections

Evaluation

Positive therapeutic outcome

- Decreased spread of malignant cells

vincristine (VCR)

Key Drug (℞)

(vin-kris'teen)

Oncovin, Vincasar PFS, vincristine sulfate

Func. class.: Antineoplastic

Chem. class.: Vinca alkaloid

Pregnancy category D

Action: Inhibits mitotic activity, arrests cell cycle at metaphase; inhibits RNA synthesis, blocks cellular use of glutamic acid needed for purine synthesis; a vesicant

➔ **Therapeutic Outcome:** Prevention of rapid growth of malignant cells, immunosuppression

Uses: Breast, lung cancer; lymphomas; neuroblastomas; Hodgkin's disease; acute lymphoblastic and other leukemias; rhabdomyosarcoma, Wilms' tumor; osteogenic and other sarcomas

Dosage and routes

Adult: **IV** 1-2 mg/m²/wk, not to exceed 2 mg

P ***Child:*** **IV** 1.5-2 mg/m²/wk, not to exceed 2 mg

Available forms: Inj 1 mg/ml

Adverse effects

CNS: Decreased reflexes, numbness, weakness, motor difficulties, CNS depression, cranial nerve paralysis, ***seizures***

CV: Orthostatic hypotension

GI: Nausea, vomiting, anorexia, stomatitis, constipation, ***paralytic ileus, abdominal pain, hepatotoxicity***

HEMA: ***Thrombocytopenia, leukopenia, myelosuppression, anemia***

INTEG: Alopecia

Contraindications: Hypersensitivity, infants, pregnancy **D**

Precautions: Renal disease, hepatic disease, hypertension, neuromuscular disease

Pharmacokinetics	
Absorption	Complete bioavailability
Distribution	Rapidly, widely distributed; blood-brain barrier
Metabolism	Liver
Excretion	Biliary, in feces, crosses placenta
Half-life	Triphasic 0.85 min, 7.4 min, 1.64 min

Pharmacodynamics	
Onset	Unknown
Peak	Unknown
Duration	1 wk

Interactions

Individual drugs

L-asparaginase: ↓ metabolism of vincristine

Mitomycin: ↑ bronchospasm

Radiation: ↑ toxicity, bone marrow suppression

Drug classifications

Antineoplastics: ↑ toxicity, bone marrow suppression

Live virus vaccines: ↓ antibody response

NURSING CONSIDERATIONS

Assessment

- Monitor CBC, differential, platelet count weekly; withhold drug if WBC is <4000 or platelet count is <75,000; notify prescriber of results; platelets may increase or decrease
- Assess neurologic status: paresthesia, weakness, cranial nerve palsies, orthostatic hypotension, lethargy, agitation, psychosis; notify health care prescriber
- Monitor renal function studies: BUN, serum uric acid, urine CrCl before, during therapy; I&O ratio; report fall in urine output of 30 ml/hr; for decreased hyperuricemia, hyponatremia, and increased fluid retention (SIADH)

V

- Monitor for cold, fever, sore throat (may indicate beginning infection)
- Identify for increased uric acid levels, joint pain in extremities; increase fluid intake to 2-3 L/day unless contraindicated

Nursing diagnoses

- ✓ Injury, risk for (adverse reactions)
- ✓ Body image disturbance (adverse reactions)
- ✓ Infection, risk for (adverse reactions)
- ✓ Knowledge deficit (teaching)

Implementation

- Administer **IV** after diluting with diluent provided or 1 mg/10 ml of sterile H_2O or NaCl; give through Y-tube or 3-way stopcock or directly over 1 min
- Hyaluronidase 150 U/ml in 1 ml NaCl; apply warm compress for extravasation

Syringe compatibilities: Bleomycin, cisplatin, cyclophosphamide, droperidol, fluorouracil, heparin, leucovorin, methotrexate, metoclopramide, mitomycin, ondansetron, vincristine

Syringe incompatibility: Furosemide

Y-site compatibilities: Allopurinol, aztreonam, bleomycin, cisplatin, cyclophosphamide, droperidol, filgrastim, fludarabine, fluorouracil, leucovorin, methotrexate, metoclopramide, mitomycin, ondansetron, sargramostim, vincristine

Y-site incompatibility: Furosemide

Patient/family education

- Teach patient to avoid use of products containing aspirin or ibuprofen, razors, commercial mouthwash because bleeding may occur; to report symptoms of bleeding (hematuria, tarry stools)
- Instruct patient to report signs of anemia, (fatigue, headache, irritability, faintness, shortness of breath)
- Caution patient to report any changes in breathing or coughing, even several mo after treatment
- Advise patient that contraception will be necessary during treatment; teratogenesis may occur
- Inform patient that hair may be lost during treatment; a wig or hairpiece may make patient feel better; new hair will be different in color, texture
- Advise patient to avoid vaccinations during treatment; serious reactions may occur
- Teach patient to report signs/symptoms of infection: fever, chills, sore throat; patient should avoid crowds, or persons with known infections

Evaluation

Positive therapeutic outcome

- Decreased spread of malignancies

vinorelbine (℞)
(vi-nor′el-bine)
Navelbine
Func. class.: Antineoplastic
Chem. class.: Semisynthetic Vinca alkaloid
Pregnancy category D

Action: Inhibits mitotic activity, arrests cell cycle at metaphase; inhibits RNA synthesis, blocks cellular use of glutamic acid needed for purine synthesis; a vesicant

➔ **Therapeutic Outcome:** Decreased spread of malignancy

Uses: Breast cancer; unresectable, advanced non–small-cell lung cancer (NSCLC) stage IV; may be used alone or in combination with cisplatin for stage III or IV NSCLC

Dosage and routes
Adult: **IV** 30 mg/m^2 qwk

Breast cancer
Adult: **IV** 30 mg/m^2 qwk

Available forms: Inj **IV**, powder 10 mg for 10 ml **IV** inj

Adverse effects
CNS: Paresthesias, peripheral neuropathy, depression, headache, ***convulsions,*** weakness, jaw pain
GI: *Nausea, vomiting,* ileus, *anorexia, stomatitis,* constipation, abdominal pain, GI, diarrhea, ***hepatotoxicity***
HEMA: ***Neutropenia, anemia, thrombocytopenia***
INTEG: *Rash,* alopecia, photosensitivity
META: SIADH
MS: Myalgia

Contraindications: Hypersensitivity, infants, pregnancy **D**

Precautions: Renal disease, hepatic disease

Pharmacokinetics	
Absorption	Poor bioavailability (<50%)
Distribution	Unknown
Metabolism	Liver—to metabolite
Excretion	Bile
Half-life	43 hr

Pharmacodynamics	
Onset	Unknown
Peak	1-2 hr
Duration	Unknown

Interactions
Individual drugs
Fluorouracil: ↑ toxicity a possibility

NURSING CONSIDERATIONS
Assessment

- Monitor B/P, (baseline and q15 min) during administration
- Monitor CBC, differential, platelet count weekly; withhold drug if WBC is <4000 or platelet count is <75,000; notify prescriber of results, recovery will take 3 wk
- Assess for dyspnea, rales, unproductive cough, chest pain, tachypnea
- Monitor renal function studies: BUN, serum uric acid, urine CrCl before, during therapy, I&O ratio; report fall in urine output of 30 ml/hr; for decreased hyperuricemia
- Monitor for cold, fever, sore throat (may indicate beginning infection); notify health care prescriber if these occur
- Assess for bleeding: hematuria, guaiac, bruising or petechiae, mucosa or orifices q8h: no rectal temp; avoid IM inj; use pressure to venipuncture sites
- Identify nutritional status: an antiemetic may need to be prescribed
- Assess for symptoms indicating severe allergic reactions: rash, pruritus, urticaria, itching, flushing, bronchospasm, hypotension; epinephrine and crash cart should be nearby

Nursing diagnoses

✓ Injury, risk for (adverse reactions)
✓ Body image disturbance (adverse reactions)

✓ Infection, risk for (adverse reactions)
✓ Knowledge deficit (teaching)

Implementation

Y-site compatibilities: Amikacin, aztreonam, bleomycin, buprenorphine, butorphanol, calcium gluconate, carboplatin, cefotaxime, cisplatin, cimetidine, clindamycin, dexamethasone, enalaprilat, etoposide, famotidine, filgrastim, fluconazole, fludarabine, gentamicin, hydrocortisone, lorazepam, meperidine, morphine, netilmicin, ondansetron, plicamycin, streptozocin, teniposide, ticarcillin, tobramycin, vancomycin, vinblastine, vincristine, zidovudine

- Hyaluronidase 150 U/ml in 1 ml NaCl, warm compress for extravasation for vesicant activity treatment
- Antacid before oral agent; give drug after evening meal before bedtime
- Antiemetic 30-60 min before giving drug and prn to prevent vomiting

Cont inf

- Give 40 mg/m^2 q 3 wk after **IV** bol of 8 mg/m^2; may be given in combination with doxorubicin, fluorouracil, cisplatin

Patient/family education

- Teach patient to use liq diet: cola, Jell-O; dry toast or crackers may be added if patient is not nauseated or vomiting
- Advise patient to rinse mouth 3-4 × day with water and brush teeth 2-3 × day with soft brush or cotton-tipped applicators for stomatitis; use unwaxed dental floss
- Inform patient that a nutritious diet with iron, vitamin supplements is necessary

Evaluation

Positive therapeutic outcome

- Decreased spread of malignant cells

vitamin A (PO, OTC; IM, ℞)

Aquasol A, Del-Vi-A, Vitamin A

Func. class.: Vitamin, fat-soluble

Chem. class.: Retinol

Pregnancy category A

Action: Needed for normal bone and tooth development, visual dark adaptation, skin disease, mucosa tissue repair, assists in production of adrenal steroids, cholesterol, RNA

➔ **Therapeutic Outcome:** Prevention, absence of vitamin A deficiency

Uses: Vitamin A deficiency

Dosage and routes

P ***Adult and child >8 yr:*** PO 100,000-500,000 IU qd 3 days, then 50,000 qd × 2 wk; dose based on severity of deficiency; maintenance 10,000-20,000 IU for 2 mo

P ***Child 1-8 yr:*** IM 5,000-15,000 IU qd × 10 days

P ***Infants <1 yr:*** IM 5,000-15,000 IU × 10 days

Maintenance

P ***Child 4-8 yr:*** IM 15,000 IU qd × 2 mo

P ***Child <4 yr:*** IM 10,000 IU qd × 2 mo

Available forms: Caps 10,000, 25,000, 50,000 IU; drops 5000 IU; inj 50,000 IU/ml; tabs 10,000, 25,000, 50,000 IU

Adverse effects
CNS: Headache, increased intracranial pressure, intracranial hypertension, lethargy, malaise
EENT: Gingivitis, papilledema, exophthalmos, inflammation of tongue and lips
GI: Nausea, vomiting, anorexia, abdominal pain, ***jaundice***
INTEG: Drying of skin, pruritus, increased pigmentation, night sweats, alopecia
MS: Arthralgia, retarded growth, hard areas on bone
META: Hypomenorrhea, hypercalcemia

Contraindications: Hypersensitivity to vit A, malabsorption syndrome (PO)

Precautions: Lactation, impaired renal function, pregnancy **A**

Pharmacokinetics

Absorption	Rapidly absorbed
Distribution	Stored in liver, kidneys, lungs
Metabolism	Liver
Excretion	Breast milk
Half-life	Unknown

Pharmacodynamics

Unknown

Interactions
Individual drugs
Cholestyramine: ↓ absorption of vitamin A
Colestipol: ↓ absorption of vitamin A
Mineral oil: ↓ absorption of vitamin A
Drug classifications
Corticosteroids: ↑ levels of vitamin A
Oral contraceptives: ↑ level of vitamin A

Lab test interferences
False ↑ Bilirubin, ↑ serum cholesterol

NURSING CONSIDERATIONS
Assessment
- Assess nutritional status: increase intake of yellow and dark green vegetables, yellow/orange fruits, vitamin A-fortified foods, liver, egg yolks
- Assess vitamin A deficiency: decreased growth; night blindness; dry, brittle nails; hair loss; urinary stones; increased infection; hyperkeratosis of skin; drying of cornea
- Identify vitamin A deficiency by plasma vitamin A, carotene level
- Assess for chronic vitamin A toxicity: increased calcium, BUN, glucose, cholesterol, triglyceride level

Nursing diagnoses
- ✓ Nutrition: less than body requirements (uses)
- ✓ Knowledge deficit (teaching)

Implementation
PO route
- Give with food (PO) for better absorption; do not give **IV** because anaphylaxis may occur
- Store in tight, light-resistant container

Patient/family education
- Instruct patient that if dose is missed, it should be omitted
- Inform patient that ophth exams may be required periodically throughout therapy
- Instruct patient not to use mineral oil while taking this drug because absorption will be decreased
- Advise patient to notify a prescriber of nausea, vomiting, lip cracking, loss of hair, headache

V

• Caution patient not to take more than the prescribed amount

Evaluation
Positive therapeutic outcome
• Increase in growth rate, weight
• Absence of dry skin and mucous membranes, night blindness

Treatment of overdose: Discontinue drug

(vitamin B_{12}) cyanocobalamin/ (vitamin B_{12}a) hydroxocobalamin

(PO, OTC; IM/SC, ℞)
(sye-an-oh-koe-bal'a-min)
Acti-B_{12} ♣, Alphamine, Anacobin ♣, Bedoz ♣, B_{12}, Resin, Cobex, Crystamine, Crysti-12, Cyanoject, Cyomin, Hydrobexan, Hydro Cobex, Rubesol-1000, Rubion ♣, Rubramin PC, Vitamin B_{12}
Func. class.: Vitamin B_{12}, water-soluble vitamin

Pregnancy category A

Action: Needed for adequate nerve functioning, protein and carbohydrate metabolism, normal growth, RBC development and cell reproduction

Therapeutic Outcome: Prevention, correction of vitamin B_{12} deficiency

Uses: Vitamin B_{12} deficiency; pernicious anemia; Vitamin B_{12} malabsorption syndrome; Schilling test; increased requirements with pregnancy, thyrotoxicosis, hemolytic anemia, hemorrhage, renal and hepatic disease

Dosage and routes
Adult: PO 25 μg qd × 5-10 days, maintenance 100-200 mg IM qmo; IM/SC 30-100 μg qd × 5-10 days, maintenance 100-200 μg IM qmo

P ***Child:*** PO 1 μg qd × 5-10 days, maintenance 60 μg IM qmo or more; IM/SC 1-30 μg qd × 5-10 days, maintenance 60 μg IM qmo or more

Pernicious anemia/ malabsorption syndrome
Adult: IM 100-1000 μg qd × 2 wk, then 100-1000 μg IM qmo

P ***Child:*** IM 100-500 μg over 2 wk or more given in 100-500 μg doses, then 60 μg IM/SC monthly

Schilling test
P ***Adult and child:*** IM 1000 μg in one dose

Available forms: Tabs 25, 50, 100, 250, 500, 1000 μg; inj 100, 120, 1000 μg/ml

Adverse effects
CNS: Flushing, optic nerve atrophy
*CV: **CHF**,* peripheral vascular thrombosis, ***pulmonary edema***
GI: Diarrhea
INTEG: Itching, rash, pain at site
META: Hypokalemia
*SYST: **Anaphylactic shock***

Contraindications: Hypersensitivity, optic nerve atrophy

Precautions: Pregnancy **A,**
P lactation, children, cardiac disease, uremia, iron deficiency, folic acid deficiency

Pharmacokinetics

Absorption	Well absorbed (IM, SC)
Distribution	Crosses placenta
Metabolism	Stored in liver, kidney, stomach
Excretion	50%-90% (urine), breast milk
Half-life	Unknown

Pharmacodynamics

Unknown

Interactions

Individual drugs

Alcohol: ↓ absorption
Aminosalicylic acid: ↓ absorption
Chloramphenicol: ↓ absorption
Cimetidine: ↓ absorption
Colchicine: ↓ absorption

Drug classifications

Aminoglycosides: ↓ absorption
Anticonvulsants: ↓ absorption
Potassium products: ↓ absorption

Lab test interferences

False positive: Intrinsic factor

NURSING CONSIDERATIONS

Assessment

- Assess for deficiency: anorexia, dyspepsia or exertion, palpitations, paresthesias, psychosis, visual disturbances, pallor, red inflamed tongue, neuropathy, edema of legs
- Monitor potassium levels during beginning treatment in patients with megaloblastic anemia
- Monitor CBC for increase in reticulocyte count during 1st wk of therapy, then increase in RBC and hemoglobin; folic acid levels, vitamin B_{12} levels
- Assess nutritional status: egg yolks, fish, organ meats, dairy products, clams, oysters, which are good sources for vit B_{12}
- Monitor for pulmonary edema or worsening of CHF in cardiac patients

Nursing diagnoses

- ✓ Nutrition; less than body requirements (uses)
- ✓ Knowledge deficit (teaching)
- ✓ Noncompliance (teaching) (overuse)

Implementation

PO route

- Give with fruit juice to disguise taste; administer immediately after mixing
- Give with meals if possible for better absorption

IM route

- Give by IM inj for pernicious anemia for life unless contraindicated

IV route

- May be mixed with TPN sol, but **IV** route is not recommended

Y-site compatibilities:

Heparin, hydrocortisone sodium succinate, potassium chloride

Solution compatibilities:

Dextrose/Ringer's or lactated Ringer's combinations, dextrose/saline combinations, D_5W, $D_{10}W$, 0.45% NaCl, Ringer's or lactated Ringer's sol, ascorbic acid

Patient/family education

- Instruct patient that treatment must continue for life if diagnosed as having pernicious anemia
- Advise patient to eat well-balanced diet from the food pyramid and comply with dietary recommendation
- Caution patient not to exceed the RDA of vitamin B_{12} because adverse reactions may occur

V

Evaluation

Positive therapeutic outcome

- Decreased anorexia, dyspnea on exertion, palpitations, paresthesias, psychosis, visual disturbances, edema of legs
- Prevention or correction of vitamin B_{12} deficiency

Treatment of overdose: Discontinue drug

vitamin D (cholecalciferol, vitamin D_3) ergocalciferol, (vitamin D_2) (℞, OTC)

Calciferol, Drisdol, Radiostol ✤, Radiostol Forte ✤, Delta-D, Vitamin D, Vitamin D_3

Func. class.: Vitamin D

Chem. class: Fat soluble

Pregnancy category A (D if >RDA)

Action: Needed for regulation of calcium, phosphate levels; normal bone development; parathyroid activity; neuromuscular functioning

➔ Therapeutic Outcome: Prevention of rickets, osteomalacia, normal calcium/phosphate levels

Uses: Vitamin D deficiency, rickets, renal osteodystrophy, hypoparathyroidism, hypophosphatemia, psoriasis, rheumatoid arthritis

Dosage and routes

Deficiency

Adult: PO/IM 12,000 IU qd, then increased to 500,000 IU/day

P ***Child:*** PO/IM 1500/5000 IU qd × 2-4 wk, may repeat after 2 wk or 600,000 IU as single dose

Hypoparathyroidism

P ***Adult and child:*** PO/IM 200,000 IU given with 4 g calcium tab

Available forms: Tabs 400, 1000, 50,000 IU; caps 25,000, 50,000; oral sol 8000 IU/ml; inj 500,000 IU/ml, 500,000 IU/5 ml

Adverse effects

CNS: Fatigue, weakness, drowsiness, ***convulsions,*** headache, psychosis

CV: Hypertension, dysrhythmias

GI: Nausea, vomiting, anorexia, cramps, diarrhea, constipation, metallic taste, dry mouth, decreased libido

GU: Polyuria, nocturia, ***hematuria, albuminuria, renal failure***

INTEG: Pruritus, photophobia

MS: Decreased bone growth, early joint pain, early muscle pain

Contraindications: Hypersensitivity, hypercalcemia, renal dysfunction, hyperphosphatemia

Precautions: Cardiovascular disease, renal calculi, pregnancy **A**

Pharmacokinetics	
Absorption	Well absorbed
Distribution	Stored in liver
Metabolism	Liver, sun
Excretion	Bile, kidney
Half-life	12-22 hr

Pharmacodynamics	PO	IM
Onset	Unknown	Unknown
Peak	4 hr	Unknown
Duration	15-20 days	Unknown

Interactions
Individual drugs
Cholestyramine: ↓ absorption of vitamin D
Colestipol: ↓ absorption of vitamin D
Mineral oil: ↓ absorption of vitamin D
Drug classifications
Corticosteroids: ↓ effects
Cardiac glycosides: ↑ dysrhythmias
Diuretics, thiazide: ↑ hypercalciuria
Lab test interferences
False ↑ Cholesterol

NURSING CONSIDERATIONS
Assessment
- Monitor BUN, urinary calcium, AST (SGOT), ALT (SGPT), cholesterol, creatinine, uric acid, chloride, magnesium, electrolytes, urine pH, phosphate—may increase; calcium should be kept at 9-10 mg/dl; vitamin D 50-135 IU/dl, phosphate 70 mg/dl; ALK phosphatase—may be decreased
- Monitor for increased blood level—toxic reactions may occur rapidly
- Assess for dry mouth, metallic taste, polyuria, bone pain, muscle weakness, headache, fatigue, tinnitus, change in LOC, irregular pulse, dysrhythmias, increased respirations, anorexia, nausea, vomiting, cramps, diarrhea, constipation—may indicate hypercalcemia
- Assess renal status: decreased urinary output (oliguria, anuria), edema in extremities, weight gain 5 lb, periorbital edema
- Assess nutritional status, diet for sources of vitamin D (milk, cod, halibut, salmon, sardines, egg yolk) calcium (dairy products, dark green vegetables), phosphates (dairy products)

Nursing diagnoses
✓ Nutrition, less than body requirements (uses)
✓ Knowledge deficit (teaching)

Implementation
PO route
- PO may be increased q4wk depending on blood level
- Store in airtight, light-resistant container at room temp

IM route
- Give deeply in large muscle mass, administer slowly, aspirate to avoid **IV** administration, rotate inj site

Patient/family education
- Advise patient to omit dose if missed; to avoid vitamin supplements unless directed by prescriber
- Inform patient of necessary foods to be included in diet
- Advise patient to keep appointments for evaluation because therapeutic and toxic levels are narrow
- Instruct patient to report weakness, lethargy, headache, anorexia, loss of weight; to report nausea, vomiting, abdominal cramps, diarrhea, constipation, excessive thirst, polyuria, muscle and bone pain
- Caution patient to decrease intake of antacids and laxatives containing magnesium

Evaluation
Positive therapeutic outcome
- Calcium levels 9-10 ml/dl
- Decreasing symptoms of bone disease

vitamin E (OTC)

Amino-Opti-E, Aquasol E, Daltose ♣, E-Complex-600, E-Ferol, E Vitamin Succinate, E-200 I.U. Softgels, Gordo-Vite E, Tocopherol, vitamin E, Vita-Plus E Softgells, Vitec

Func. class.: Vitamin E

Chem. class.: Fat soluble

Pregnancy category A

Action: Needed for digestion and metabolism of polyunsaturated fats, decreases platelet aggregation, decreases blood clot formation, promotes normal growth and development of muscle tissue, prostaglandin synthesis

➔ **Therapeutic Outcome:** Prevention and treatment of vitamin E deficiency

Uses: Vitamin E deficiency, impaired fat absorption, hemolytic anemia in premature neonates, prevention of retrolental fibroplasia, sickle cell anemia, supplement in malabsorption syndrome

Dosage and routes

Deficiency

Adult: PO 60-75 IU qd, not to exceed 300 IU/day

P ***Child:*** PO 1 mg/0.6 g of dietary fat

Prevention of deficiency

Adult: PO 30 U/day

Top

P ***Adult and child:*** Top apply to affected areas as needed

Available forms: Caps 100, 200, 400, 500, 600, 800 ♣, 1000 IU; tabs 100, 200, 400 IU; drops 50 mg/ml; chew tab 400 U; ointment, cream, lotion, oil

Adverse effects

CNS: Headache, fatigue

CV: Increased risk thrombophlebitis

EENT: Blurred vision

GI: Nausea, cramps, diarrhea

GU: Gonadal dysfunction

INTEG: Sterile abscess, contact dermatitis

META: Altered metabolism of hormones, thyroid, pituitary, adrenal, altered immunity

MS: Weakness

Contraindications: None significant

Precautions: Pregnancy **A**

Pharmacokinetics

Absorption	20%-80% (PO)
Distribution	Widely distributed, stored in fat
Metabolism	Liver
Excretion	Bile
Half-life	Unknown

Pharmacodynamics

Unknown

Interactions

Individual drugs

Cholestyramine: ↓ absorption

Colestipol: ↓ absorption

Mineral oil: ↓ absorption

Sucralfate: ↓ absorption

Drug classification

Oral anticoagulants: ↑ action of anticoagulants

NURSING CONSIDERATIONS

Assessment

- Monitor vitamin E levels during treatment
- Assess nutritional status: intake of wheat germ, dark green leafy vegetables, nuts, eggs, liver, vegetable oils, dairy products, cereals
- Assess for vitamin E deficiency (usually in neonates): irritability, restlessness, hemolytic anemia

Nursing diagnoses

✓ Nutrition: less than body requirements (uses)
✓ Knowledge deficit (teaching)

Implementation

PO route

- Chewable tab: chew well
- Sol: may be dropped in mouth or mixed with food
- Store in tight, light-resistant container

Top route

- Apply top to moisturize dry skin

Patient/family education

- Inform patient necessary foods to be included in diet high in vitamin E
- Instruct patient to omit if dose missed
- Instruct patient to avoid vitamin supplements unless directed by prescriber because overdose may occur

Evaluation

Positive therapeutic outcome

- Absence of hemolytic anemia
- Adequate vitamin E levels
- Improvement in skin lesions
- Decrease in edema

warfarin (℞)

(war'far-in)

Coumadin, Sofarin, warfarin sodium, Warfilone Sodium ♣

Func. class.: Anticoagulant

Pregnancy category D

Action: Interferes with blood clotting by indirect means; depresses hepatic synthesis of vitamin K-dependent coagulation factors (II, VII, IX, X)

➔ **Therapeutic Outcome:** Prevention of clotting

Uses: Pulmonary emboli, deep vein thrombosis, MI, atrial dysrhythmias, postcardiac valve replacement

Dosage and routes

Adult: PO 10-15 mg/day × 3 days, then titrated to prothrombin time qd

Available forms: Tabs 1, 2, 2.5, 5, 7.5, 10 mg; inj 50 mg/2 ml

Adverse effects

CNS: Fever

GI: Diarrhea, nausea, vomiting, anorexia, stomatitis, cramps, ***hepatitis***

GU: Hematuria

HEMA: Hemorrhage, agranulocytosis, leukopenia, eosinophilia

INTEG: Rash, dermatitis, urticaria, alopecia, pruritus

Contraindications: Hypersensitivity, hemophilia, leukemia with bleeding, peptic ulcer disease, thrombocytopenic purpura, hepatic disease (severe), severe hypertension, subacute bacterial endocarditis, acute nephritis, blood dyscrasias, pregnancy **D,** eclampsia, preeclampsia, lactation

Precautions: Alcoholism, G elderly

Pharmacokinetics	
Absorption	Well absorbed (PO), completely absorbed
Distribution	Crosses placenta, 99% plasma protein binding
Metabolism	Liver
Excretion	Kidney, feces (active, inactive metabolites)
Half-life	½-2½ days

W

Pharmacodynamics

	PO
Onset	12-24 hr
Peak	½-3 days
Duration	3-5 days

Lab test interferences

↑ T_3 uptake
↓ Uric acid

NURSING CONSIDERATIONS

Assessment

- Monitor blood studies (Hct, occult blood in stools) q3mo; partial prothrombin time, which should be 1½-2 × control, PTT; often done qd, APTT, ACT; platelet count q2-3 days; thrombocytopenia may occur
- Monitor B/P, watch for increasing signs of hypertension
- Assess for bleeding: bleeding gums, petechiae, ecchymosis, black tarry stools, hematuria, epistaxis; decreased B/P may indicate bleeding and possible hemorrhage
- Assess for fever, skin rash, urticaria
- Assess for needed dosage change q1-2 wk

Nursing diagnoses

✓ Injury, risk for (uses, adverse reactions)
✓ Tissue perfusion, altered (uses)
✓ Knowledge deficit (teaching)

Implementation

PO route

- Warfarin is usually given with **IV** heparin for 3 or more days, warfarin blood level may take several days

IV IV route

- Protect from light, **IV** form is in short supply

Additive compatibility: Cephapirin

Patient/family education

- Caution patient to avoid OTC preparations unless directed by prescriber—may cause serious drug interactions
- Advise patient that drug may be withheld during active bleeding (menstruation), depending on condition
- Advise patient to use soft-bristle toothbrush to avoid bleeding gums, avoid contact sports, use electric razor, avoid IM inj
- Instruct patient to carry a Medic Alert ID identifying drug taken
- Advise patient to report any signs of bleeding: gums, under skin, urine, stools
- Teach patient to read food labels—limited intake of vitamin K foods is necessary to maintain consistent prothrombin levels

Evaluation

Positive therapeutic outcome

- Decrease of deep vein thrombosis
- Prothrombin time (1.3-2.0 × control)

xylometazoline (OTC)

(xye-loe-met-az'oh-leen)
Otrivin, Otrivin Pediatric Nasal Drops, xylometazoline HCl

Func. class.: Nasal decongestant
Chem. class.: Sympathomimetic amine

Pregnancy category C

Action: Dilates arterioles of nasal membrane, which decreases congestion

➡ **Therapeutic Outcome:** Absence of nasal congestion

Uses: Nasal congestion; adjunct in otitis media

Dosage and routes

P ***Adult and child >12 yr:*** Instill 2-3 gtt or 2 sprays q8-10h (0.1%)

P ***Child <12 yr:*** Instill 2-3 gtt or 1% spray q8-10h (0.05%)

Available forms: Sol 0.05%, 0.1%

Adverse effects

EENT: Irritation, burning, sneezing, stinging, dryness, rebound congestion

INTEG: Contact dermatitis

Contraindications: Hypersensitivity to sympathomimetic amines

Precautions: Pregnancy **C**, glaucoma

Pharmacokinetics	
Absorption	Unknown
Distribution	Unknown
Metabolism	Unknown
Excretion	Unknown
Half-life	Unknown

Pharmacodynamics	
Onset	5-10 min
Peak	Unknown
Duration	5-6 hr

NURSING CONSIDERATIONS

Assessment

- Assess for redness, swelling, pain in nasal passages before and during treatment
- Assess for systemic absorption: hypertension, tachycardia; notify prescriber; systemic absorption occurs at high doses or prolonged use

Nursing diagnoses

✓ Airway clearance, ineffective (uses)
✓ Knowledge deficit (teaching)
✓ Noncompliance (teaching)

Implementation

- Have patient tilt head back, squeeze bulb to create a vacuum and draw correct amount of sol into dropper, insert 2 gtt of sol into nostril, repeat in other nostril
- Store in light-resistant container; do not expose to high temp or let sol come into contact with aluminum
- Give for <4 consecutive days
- Ensure environmental humidification to decrease nasal congestion, dryness

Patient/family education

- Advise patient that stinging may occur for several applications; drying of mucosa may be decreased by environmental humidification
- Caution patient to notify prescriber if irregular pulse, insomnia, dizziness, or tremors occur
- Teach patient proper administration to avoid systemic absorption
- Advise patient to rinse dropper with very hot water to prevent contamination

Evaluation

Positive therapeutic outcome

- Decreased nasal congestion

zafirlukast (℞)

(za-feer'loo-cast)

Accolate

Func. class.: Leukotriene receptor antagonist

Pregnancy category UK

Action: Antagonizes the contractile action of leukotrienes (LTC_4, LTD_4, LTE_4) in airway smooth muscle; inhibits bronchoconstriction caused by antigens

Therapeutic Outcome: Ability to breathe more easily

Uses: Prophylaxis and chronic treatment of asthma in adults/ children >12 yr

Dosage and routes

Adult: PO 20 mg bid, take 1 hr ac or 2 hr pc

Available forms: Tab 20 mg

Adverse effects

CNS: Headache, dizziness
GI: Nausea, diarrhea, abdominal pain, vomiting
OTHER: Infections, pain, asthenia, myalgia, fever, dyspepsia, increased ALT

Contraindications: Hypersensitivity

Precautions: Pregnancy **UK,** elderly, lactation, children, hepatic disease

Pharmacokinetics

Unknown

Pharmacodynamics

Unknown

Interactions

Individual drugs

Aspirin: ↑ plasma levels of zafirlukast
Erythromycin: ↓ plasma levels of zafirlukast
Terfinadine: ↓ plasma levels of zafirlukast
Theophylline: ↓ plasma levels of zafirlukast
Warfarin: ↑ pro-time

Food

↓ Bioavailability of zafirlukast

NURSING CONSIDERATIONS

Assessment

- Assess respiratory rate, rhythm, depth; auscultate lung fields bilaterally; notify prescriber of abnormalities

Nursing diagnoses

- ✓ Breathing pattern, ineffective (uses)
- ✓ Knowledge deficit (teaching)
- ✓ Noncompliance (teaching)

Implementation

- Give after meals for GI symptoms; absorption may be affected

Patient/family education

- Advise patient to check OTC medications, current prescription medications, which will increase stimulation
- Advise patient to avoid hazardous activities; dizziness may occur
- Advise patient that if GI upset occurs, to take drug with 8 oz water; avoid food if possible, absorption may be decreased
- Advise patient to notify prescriber of nausea, vomiting, diarrhea, abdominal pain

Evaluation

Positive therapeutic outcome

- Ability to breathe more easily

zalcitabine (℞)

(zal-sit'a-bin)

HIVID, ddC, Dideoxycitidine

Func. class.: Antiviral
Chem. class.: Synthetic pyrimidine nucleoside analog of 2′-deoxycytidine

Pregnancy category C

Action: Inhibits HIV replication by the conversion of this drug by cellular enzymes to an active antiviral metabolite

Therapeutic Outcome: Improved symptoms of HIV infection

Uses: Advanced HIV infections in adults and children >13 yrs who have been unable to use zidovudine or who have not responded to treatment

Dosage and routes

Adult: PO combined with zidovudine in advanced HIV infection: 0.75 mg administered concomitantly with 200 mg zidovudine q8h; dosage reduction not necessary for patients weighing >30 kg; in presence of peripheral neuropathy initiate dose at 0.375 mg q8h of zalcitabine

Available forms: Tabs 0.375, 0.75 mg

Adverse effects

CNS: Headache, peripheral neuropathy, seizures, confusion, anxiety, hypertonia, abnormal thinking, asthenia, insomnia, CNS depression, pain, dizziness, chills, fever
CV: Hypertension, vasodilation, dysrhythmia, snycope, palpitation, tachycardia
EENT: Ear pain, otitis, photophobia, visual impairment
GI: Pancreatitis, diarrhea, nausea, vomiting, abdominal pain, constipation, stomatitis, dysplasia, liver abnormalities, oral ulcers, flatulence, taste perversion, dry mouth, oral thrush, melena, increased ALT (SGOT), AST (SGPT), alk phosphatase, amylase, increased bilirubin
GU: Uric acid, ***toxic nephropathy,*** polyuria
HEMA: ***Leukopenia, granulocytopenia, thrombocytopenia,*** anemia
INTEG: Rash, pruritus, alopecia, sweating, acne
MS: Myalgia, arthritis, myopathy, muscular atrophy
RESP: Cough, pneumonia, dyspnea, asthma, hypoventilation

Contraindications: Hypersensitivity

Precautions: Renal, hepatic disease, pregnancy **C,** lactation, children (<13 yr), patients with peripheral neuropathy

Pharmacokinetics	
Absorption	Minimally absorbed
Distribution	Unknown
Metabolism	Liver
Excretion	Unknown
Half-life	1.62 hr, increased in renal disease

Pharmacodynamics	
Onset	Unknown
Peak	1½-2½
Duration	Unknown

Interactions

Individual drugs

Amphotericin B: ↑ neurotoxicity, nephrotoxicity
Interferon: ↑ neurotoxicity, nephrotoxicity
Methotrexate: ↑ neurotoxicity, nephrotoxicity
Probenecid: ↑ neurotoxicity, nephrotoxicity

Drug classifications

Aminoglycosides: ↑ neurotoxicity, nephrotoxicity

NURSING CONSIDERATIONS

Assessment

- Assess for peripheral neuropathy: tingling or pain in hands and feet, distal numbness; if these occur during therapy, drug may be decreased or discontinued
- Assess for pancreatitis: abdominal pain, nausea, vomiting, elevated liver enzymes; drug should be discontinued because condition can be fatal
- Assess children by dilated

retinal examination q6mo to rule out retinal depigmentation
- Monitor CBC, differential, platelet count qmo; withhold drug if WBC is <4000 or platelet count is <75,000; notify prescriber of results
- Monitor renal function studies; BUN, serum uric acid, urine CrCl before, during therapy; these may be elevated throughout treatment
- Monitor temp q4h, may indicate beginning infection
- Monitor liver function tests before, during therapy (bilirubin, AST (SGOT), ALT (SGPT), amylase, alk phosphatase as needed or qmo

Nursing diagnoses

- ✓ Infection, risk for (uses)
- ✓ Injury, risk for (adverse reactions)
- ✓ Knowledge deficit (teaching)

Implementation

- Give on empty stomach, q8h around the clock

Patient/family education

- Advise patient to take on empty stomach; not to take dapsone at same time as ddC; to use exactly as prescribed
- Instruct patient to report signs of infection: increased temp, sore throat, flu symptoms; to avoid crowds and those with known infections
- Caution patient to report signs of anemia; fatigue, headache, faintness, shortness of breath, irritability
- Advise patient to report bleeding; avoid use of razors or commercial mouthwash
- Inform patient that hair may be lost during therapy (rare); a wig or hairpiece may make patient feel better
- Caution patient to avoid OTC products or other medications without approval of prescriber
- Caution patient not to have any sexual contact without use of a condom, that needles should not be shared, that blood from infected individual should not come in contact with another's mucus membranes

Evaluation

Positive therapeutic outcome

- Absence of infection; symptoms of HIV

zidovudine 🗝 (℞)
(zye-doe'vue-deen)
Apo-Zidovudine ♣,
Azidothymidine, AZT,
Novo-AZT ♣, Retrovir
Func. class.: Antiviral
Chem. class.: Thymidine analog
Pregnancy category C

Action: Inhibits replication of HIV by incorporating into cellular DNA by viral reverse transcriptase, thereby terminating the cellular DNA chain

➔ **Therapeutic Outcome:** Decreased symptoms of HIV

Uses: Symptomatic HIV infections (AIDS, ARC), confirmed *P. carinii* pneumonia, or absolute CD4 lymphocytes <200/mm^3

Dosage and routes

Adult: PO 200 mg q4h; may have to stop treatment if severe bone marrow depression occurs, and restart after bone marrow recovery; **IV** 1-2 mg/kg q4h, initiate PO as soon as possible

Available forms: Cap 100 mg; inj 200 mg/20 ml; oral syr 50 mg/5 ml

Adverse effects

CNS: Fever, headache, malaise, diaphoresis, dizziness, *insomnia,* paresthesia, somnolence, chills, tremor, twitching, anxiety, confusion, depression, lability, vertigo, loss of mental acuity

EENT: Taste change, hearing loss, photophobia

GI: *Nausea,* vomiting, diarrhea, anorexia, cramps, *dyspepsia,* constipation, dysphagia, *flatulence,* rec bleeding, mouth ulcer

GU: Dysuria, polyuria, frequency, hesitancy

HEMA: ***Granulocytopenia, anemia***

INTEG: Rash, acne, pruritus, urticaria

MS: Myalgia, arthralgia, muscle spasm

RESP: Dyspnea

Contraindications: Hypersensitivity

Precautions: Granulocyte count <1000/mm^3 or Hgb <9.5 g/dl, pregnancy **C,** lactation, P children, severe renal disease, severe hepatic function

Pharmacokinetics

Absorption	Well absorbed (PO), completely absorbed (IV)
Distribution	Widely distributed—crosses placenta, CSF
Metabolism	Liver—mostly
Excretion	Kidneys
Half-life	1 hr

Pharmacodynamics

	PO	IV
Onset	Unknown	Rapid
Peak	½-1½ hr	Inf end
Duration	Unknown	Unknown

Interactions

Individual drugs

Amphotericin B: ↑ neurotoxicity, nephrotoxicity
Interferon: ↑ neurotoxicity, nephrotoxicity
Methotrexate: ↑ neurotoxicity, nephrotoxicity
Probenecid: ↑ neurotoxicity, nephrotoxicity

Drug classifications

Aminoglycosides: ↑ neurotoxicity, nephrotoxicity

NURSING CONSIDERATIONS

Assessment

- Assess for peripheral neuropathy: tingling or pain in hands and feet, distal numbness; if these occur, drug may be decreased or discontinued
- Assess for pancreatitis: abdominal pain, nausea, vomiting, elevated liver enzymes; drug should be discontinued because condition can be fatal
- P Assess children by dilated retinal examination q6mo to rule out retinal depigmentation
- Monitor CBC, differential, platelet count qmo; withhold drug if WBC is <4000 or platelet count is <75,000; notify prescriber of results
- Monitor renal function studies; BUN, serum uric acid, urine CrCl before, during therapy; these may be elevated throughout treatment
- Monitor temp q4h, may indicate beginning infection
- Monitor liver function tests before, during therapy (bilirubin, AST [SGOT], ALT [SGPT]) amylase, alkaline phosphatase prn or qmo

Nursing diagnoses

✓ Infection, risk for (uses)

✓ Injury, risk for physical injury (adverse reactions)
✓ Knowledge deficit (teaching)

Implementation

PO route

- Give on empty stomach, q4h around the clock

IV route

- Give by intermittent inf after diluting with D_5W; give over 1 hr (<4 mg/ml), do not give by direct **IV**

Y-site compatibilities: Acyclovir, allopurinol, amikacin, amphotericin B, aztreonam, ceftazidime, ceftriaxone, cimetidine, clindamycin, dexamethasone, dobutamine, dopamine, erythromycin, fluconazole, fludarabine, gentamicin, heparin, imipenem/cilastatin, lorazepam, metoclopramide, morphine, nafcillin, ondansetron, oxacillin, pentamidine, phenylephrine, piperacillin, potassium chloride, ranitidine, sargramostim, tobramycin, trimethoprim-sulfamethoxazole, vancomycin

Additive incompatibilities: Blood products or protein solutions

Patient/family education

- Caution patient to take on empty stomach; not to take dapsone at same time as ddl; to use exactly as prescribed
- Advise patient to report signs of infection: increased temp, sore throat, flu symptoms; to avoid crowds and those with known infections
- Instruct patient to report signs of anemia: fatigue, headache, faintness, shortness of breath, irritability
- Advise patient to report bleeding; avoid use of razors or commercial mouthwash
- Inform patient that hair may be lost during therapy (rare); a wig or hairpiece may make patient feel better
- Caution patient to avoid OTC products or other medications without approval of prescriber
- Caution patient not to have any sexual contact without use of a condom, needles should not be shared, blood from infected individual should not come in contact with another's mucus membranes

Evaluation

Positive therapeutic outcome

- Decreased infection; symptoms of HIV

zileuton (℞)

(zye-loo'tahn)

Zyflo

Func. class.: Leukotriene pathway inhibitor

Chem. class.: 5-1 poxygenase inhibitor

Pregnancy category C

Action: Inhibits leukotriene (LT) formation; leukotrienes exert their effects by increasing neutrophil, eosinophil migration; aggregation of neutrophils, monocytes; smooth muscle contraction, capillary permeability; these actions further lead to bronchoconstriction, inflammation, edema

Therapeutic Outcome: Ability to breathe more easily

Uses: allergic rhinitis, asthma

Investigational uses: Ulcerative colitis, rheumatoid arthritis

Dosage and routes
Asthma
P ***Adult and child >12 yr:*** PO 600 mg qid, may be given with meal and hs
Ulcerative colitis
Adult: PO 600 mg bid

Available forms: Tab 600 mg

Adverse effects
CNS: Dizziness, insomnia, fatigue, paresthesias, headache
GI: Nausea, abdominal pain, dyspepsia, diarrhea, LFTs abnormalities
INTEG: Hives
MS: Myalgia, asthenia

Contraindications: Hepatic disease, elevations in LFTs 3× upper limits, hypersensitivity

Precautions: Acute attacks of asthma, alcohol consumption, pregnancy **C**

Pharmacokinetics	
Absorption	Rapid
Distribution	Protein-binding 93%
Metabolism	Liver
Excretion	Urine
Half-life	2.1-2.5 hr

Pharmacodynamics	
Onset	Unknown
Peak	1-3 hr
Duration	Unknown

Interactions
Individual drugs
Propranolol: ↑ action of zilenton
Theophylline: ↑ action of zilenton
Drug classifications
Anticoagulants: ↑ effects

NURSING CONSIDERATIONS
Assessment
- Assess CBC, blood chemistry, during treatment
- Assess LFTs before and qmo × 3 mo, their q2-3mo during treatment
- Assess respiratory rate, rhythm, depth; auscultate lung fields bilaterally; notify prescriber of abnormalities
- Assess allergic reactions: rash, urticaria; drug should be discontinued

Nursing diagnoses
- ✓ Breathing pattern, ineffective (uses)
- ✓ Knowledge deficit (teaching)
- ✓ Noncompliance (teaching)

Implementation
- Give PO after meals for GI symptoms; absorption may be affected

Patient/family education
- Advise patient to check OTC medications, current prescription medications for ephedrine, which will increase stimulation; to avoid alcohol
- Advise patient to avoid hazardous activities; dizziness may occur
- Advise patient that if GI upset occurs, to take drug with 8 oz water or food; absorption may be decreased slightly
- Advise patient to notify prescriber of nausea, vomiting, anxiety, insomnia

Evaluation
Positive therapeutic outcome
- Ability to breathe more easily

zinc sulfate

(PO, OTC; IV, ℞)
(zink sul'fate)
Orazinc, PMS Egozine ✤, Verazinc, Zinca-Pak, Zincate, Zinc 15, Zinc-220, zinc sulfate

Func. class.: Trace element; nutritional supplement

Pregnancy category A

Action: Needed for adequate healing, bone and joint development, taste and smell (23% zinc)

Therapeutic Outcome: Replacement of zinc

Uses: Prevention of zinc deficiency, adjunct to vitamin A therapy

Investigational uses: Wound healing

Dosage and routes

Dietary supplement

Adult: PO 25-50 mg/day

Nutritional supplement (**IV**)

Adult: 2.5-4 mg/day, may increase by 2 mg/day if needed

P ***Child to 5 yr:*** **IV** 100 μg/kg/day

P ***Infants: <1500 gm to 3 kg;*** **IV** 300 μg/kg/day

Available forms: Tabs 66, 110 mg; cap 220 mg; inj 1 mg, 5 mg/ml

Adverse effects

GI: Nausea, vomiting, cramps, heartburn, ulcer formation

OVERDOSE: Diarrhea, rash, dehydration, restlessness

Precautions: Pregnancy **A**

Pharmacokinetics

Absorption	Poorly absorbed (PO), completely absorbed (IV)
Distribution	Widely distributed
Metabolism	Liver
Excretion	90%—feces, 10%—kidneys
Half-life	Unknown

Pharmacodynamics

Unknown

Interactions

Individual drugs

Tetracycline: ↓ absorption of tetracycline

NURSING CONSIDERATIONS

Assessment

- Monitor zinc levels during treatment

Nursing diagnoses

- ✓ Nutrition: less than body requirements (uses)
- ✓ Knowledge deficit (teaching)

Implementation

PO route

- Give with meals to decrease gastric upset; restrict dairy products, caffeine, which decrease absorption

IV **IV route**

- Part of total parenteral nutrition (TPN)

Patient/family education

- Inform patient that element must be taken for 2 mo to be effective
- Advise patient to report immediately nausea, diarrhea, rash, severe vomiting, restlessness, abdominal pain, tarry stools

Evaluation

Positive therapeutic outcome

- Absence of zinc deficiency
- Improved wound healing

zolpidem (℞)
(zole-pi'dem)
Ambien
Func. class.: Sedative-hypnotic
Chem. class.: Nonbenzodiazepine of imidazopyridine class
Pregnancy category B

Action: Produces CNS depression at limbic, thalamic, hypothalamic levels of CNS; may be mediated by neurotransmitter γ-aminobutyric acid (GABA); results are sedation, hypnosis, skeletal muscle relaxation, anticonvulsant activity, anxiolytic action

Therapeutic Outcome: Ability to sleep, sedation

Uses: Insomnia, short-term treatment

Dosage and routes
Adult: PO 10 mg hs × 7-10 days only; total dose should not exceed 10 mg

Available forms: Tabs 5, 10 mg

Adverse effects
CNS: Headache, lethargy, drowsiness, daytime sedation, dizziness, confusion, lightheadedness, anxiety, irritability, amnesia, poor coordination
CV: Chest pain, palpitation
GI: Nausea, vomiting, diarrhea, heartburn, abdominal pain, constipation

Contraindications: Hypersensitivity to benzodiazepines

Precautions: Anemia, hepatic disease, renal disease, suicidal individuals, drug abuse, elderly, psychosis, child <18 yr, seizure disorders, pregnancy **B,** lactation

Pharmacokinetics

Absorption	Rapidly absorbed
Distribution	Unknown
Metabolism	Liver—inactive metabolite
Excretion	Kidneys, breast milk
Half-life	2½ hr, increased in elderly

Pharmacodynamics
Unknown

Interactions
Individual drugs
Alcohol: ↑ CNS depression
Fluoxetine: ↑ action
Propoxyphene: ↑ action
Drug classifications
Analgesics, opioid: ↑ CNS depression
Antidepressants: ↑ CNS depression
Antihistamines: ↑ CNS depression
Sedative/hypnotics: ↑ CNS depression
Food
↓ absorption
Lab test interferences
↑ ALT (SGPT), ↑ AST (SGOT), ↑ serum bilirubin
↓ RAI uptake
False ↑ Urinary 17-OHCS

NURSING CONSIDERATIONS
Assessment
• Assess mental status: mood, sensorium, anxiety, affect, sleeping pattern, drowsiness, dizziness, especially elderly; physical dependency, withdrawal symptoms: anxiety, panic attacks, agitation, convulsions, headache, nausea, vomiting, muscle pain, weakness; suicidal tendencies; for indications of increasing tolerance and abuse
• Monitor B/P (lying, stand-

ing), pulse; if systolic B/P drops 20 mm Hg, hold drug, notify prescriber

• Monitor blood studies: CBC during long-term therapy; blood dycrasias have occurred rarely; decreased hematocrit, neutropenia may occur

• Monitor hepatic studies: AST (SGOT), ALT (SGPT), bilirubin, creatinine LDH, alk phosphatase

• Monitor I&O for renal dysfunction

Nursing diagnoses

✓ Anxiety (uses)
✓ Depression (uses)
✓ Injury, risk for (adverse reactions)
✓ Knowledge deficit (teaching)

Implementation

• Give ½-1 hr before hs for sleeplessness; give several hr before patient is to arise (to avoid hangover)

• Store in tight container in cool environment

Patient/family education

• Instruct patient that drug may be taken with food, or fluids and tab may be crushed or swallowed whole

• Caution patient not to use for everyday stress or longer than 3 mo unless directed by prescriber; not to take more than prescribed amount; may be habit forming; not to double or skip doses

• Caution patient to avoid OTC preparations unless approved by health care prescriber; alcohol and CNS depressants will increase CNS depression

• Advise patient to avoid driving, activities that require alertness, because drowsiness may occur; to avoid alcohol ingestion or other psychotropic medications; to rise slowly or fainting may occur, especially **G** elderly; that drowsiness may worsen at beginning of treatment

• Instruct patient not to discontinue medication abruptly after long-term use; withdrawal symptoms include vomiting, cramping, tremors, seizures

Evaluation

Positive therapeutic outcome

• Ability to sleep at night

• Decreased amount of early morning awakening if taking drug for insomnia

Treatment of overdose: Lavage, VS, supportive care

ALPHA-ADRENERGIC BLOCKERS

Action: Binds to α-adrenergic receptors, causing dilatation of peripheral blood vessels; lowers peripheral resistance, resulting in decreased blood pressure.

Uses: Used for pheochromocytoma, prevention of tissue necrosis, and sloughing associated with extravasation of IV vasopressors.

Adverse effects: The most common side effects are hypotension, tachycardia, nasal stuffiness, nausea, vomiting, and diarrhea.

Contraindications: Hypersensitive reactions may occur, and allergies should be identified before these products are given. Patients with myocardial infarction, coronary insufficiency, angina, or other evidence of coronary artery disease should not use these products.

Pharmacokinetics: Onset, peak, and duration vary among products.

Interactions: Vasoconstrictive and hypertensive effects of epinephrine are antagonized by α-adrenergic blockers.

NURSING CONSIDERATIONS

Assessment

- Monitor electrolytes: potassium, sodium chloride, carbon dioxide
- Monitor weight daily, I&O
- Monitor B/P with patient lying, standing before starting treatment, q4h thereafter
- Assess for nausea, vomiting, diarrhea
- Assess for skin turgor, dryness of mucous membranes for hydration status

Nursing diagnoses

- ✓ Altered tissue perfusion (uses)
- ✓ Risk for injury (adverse reactions)
- ✓ Sleep pattern disturbance (adverse reactions)

Implementation

PO Route

- Start with low dose, gradually increasing to prevent side effects
- Give with food or milk for GI symptoms

Evaluation

- Therapeutic response: decreased B/P, increased peripheral pulses

Patient/family education

- Caution patient to avoid alcoholic beverages
- Advise patient to report dizziness, palpitations, fainting
- Instruct patient to change position slowly or fainting may occur

- Teach patient to take drug exactly as prescribed; to avoid all OTC products (cough, cold, allergy) unless directed by prescriber

---

Generic Names

phenoxybenzamine   phentolamine

ANESTHETICS—GENERAL/LOCAL

Action: Anesthetics (general) act on the CNS to produce tranquilization and sleep before invasive procedures. Anesthetics (local) inhibit conduction of nerve impulses from sensory nerves.

Uses: General anesthetics are used to premedicate for surgery, and for induction and maintenance in general anesthesia. For local anesthetics, refer to individual product listing for indications.

Adverse effects: The most common side effects are dystonia, akathisia, flexion of arms, fine tremors, drowsiness, restlessness, and hypotension. Also common are chills, respiratory depression, and laryngospasm.

Contraindications: Persons with CVA, increased intracranial pressure, severe hypertension, cardiac decompensation should not use these products, since severe adverse reactions can occur.

G **Precautions:** Anesthetics (general) should be used with caution in the elderly, cardiovascular disease (hypotension, bradydysrhythmias), P renal disease, liver disease, Parkinson's disease, children <2 yr. The precaution for anesthetics (local) is pregnancy.

Pharmacokinetics: Onset, peak, and duration vary widely among products. Most products are metabolized in the liver and excreted in urine.

Interactions: MAOIs, tricyclics, phenothiazines may cause severe hypotension or hypertension when used with local anesthetics. CNS depressants will potentiate general and local anesthetics.

NURSING CONSIDERATIONS

Assessment

- Monitor VS q10 min during IV administration, q30 min after IM dose

Nursing diagnoses

General

✓ Risk for injury (adverse reactions)
✓ Knowledge deficit (teaching)

Local

✓ Pain (uses)
✓ Knowledge deficit (teaching)

Implementation

- Give anticholinergic preoperatively to decrease secretions
- Administer only with crash cart, resuscitative equipment nearby
- Provide quiet environment for recovery to decrease psychotic symptoms

Evaluation

- Therapeutic response: maintenance of anesthesia, decreased pain

---

Generic Names

General anesthetics:
droperidol
fentanyl citrate
  fentanyl citrate/droperidol
ketamine
methohexital
tetracaine

Local anesthetics:
🔑 lidocaine HCl
midazolam
ropivacaine
thiopental

ANTACIDS

Action: Antacids are basic compounds that neutralize gastric acidity and decrease the rate of gastric emptying. Products are divided into those containing aluminum, magnesium, calcium, or a combination of these.

Uses: Hyperacidity is decreased by antacids in conditions such as peptic ulcer disease, reflux esophagitis, gastritis, or hiatal hernia.

Adverse effects: The most common side effect caused by aluminum-containing antacids is constipation, which may lead to fecal impaction and bowel obstruction. Diarrhea occurs often when magnesium products are given. Alkalosis may occur when systemic products are used. Constipation occurs more frequently than laxation with calcium carbonate. The release of CO_2 from carbonate-containing antacids causes belching, abdominal distention, and flatulence. Sodium bicarbonate may act as a systemic antacid and produce systemic electrolyte disturbances and alkalosis. Calcium carbonate and sodium bicarbonate may cause rebound hyperacidity and milk-alkali syndrome. Alkaluria may occur when products are used on a long-term basis, particularly in persons with abnormal renal function.

Contraindications: Sensitivity to aluminum or magnesium products may cause hypersensitive reactions. Aluminum products should not be used by persons sensitive to aluminum; magnesium products should not be used by persons sensitive to magnesium. Check for sensitivity before administering.

Precautions: Magnesium products should be given cautiously to patients with renal insufficiency and during pregnancy and lactation. Sodium content of antacids may be significant; use with caution for patients with hypertension, CHF, or those on a low-sodium diet.

Pharmacokinetics: Duration is 20-40 min. If ingested 1 hr pc, acidity is reduced for at least 3 hr.

Interactions: Drugs whose effects may be increased by some antacids: quinidine, amphetamines, pseudoephedrine, levodopa, valproic acid, dicumarol. Drugs whose effects may be decreased by some antacids: cimetidine, corticosteroids, ranitidine, iron salts, phenothiazines, phenytoin, digoxin, tetracyclines, ketoconazole, salicylates, isoniazid.

NURSING CONSIDERATIONS

Assessment

- Assess for aggravating and alleviating factors of epigastric pain or hyperacidity; identify the location, duration, and characteristics of epigastric pain
- Assess GI symptoms, including constipation, diarrhea, abdominal pain; if severe abdominal pain with fever occurs, these drugs should not be given
- Assess renal symptoms, including increasing urinary pH, electrolytes

Nursing diagnoses

✓ Pain (uses)
✓ Constipation (adverse reactions)
✓ Diarrhea (adverse reactions)

Implementation

- Give all products with an 8-oz glass of water to ensure absorption in the stomach
- Give another antacid if constipation occurs with aluminum products

Evaluation

- Therapeutic response: absence of epigastric pain, decreased acidity

Patient/family education

- Advise patient not to take other drugs within 1-2 hr of antacid administration, since antacids may impair absorption of other drugs

Generic Names

aluminum hydroxide
bismuth subsalicylate
calcium carbonate
magaldrate
magnesium oxide
sodium bicarbonate

ANTIANGINALS

Action: The antianginals are divided into the nitrates, calcium channel blockers, and β-adrenergic blockers. The nitrates dilate coronary arteries, causing decreased preload, and dilate systemic arteries, causing decreased afterload. Calcium channel blockers dilate coronary arteries, decrease SA/AV node conduction. β-Adrenergic blockers decrease heart rate so that myocardial O_2 use is decreased. Dipyridamole selectively dilates coronary arteries to increase coronary blood flow.

Uses: Antianginals are used in chronic stable angina pectoris, unstable angina, vasospastic angina. Some (i.e., calcium channel blockers and β-blockers) may be used as dysrhythmias and in hypertension.

Adverse effects: The most common side effects are postural hypotension, headache, flushing, dizziness, nausea, edema, and drowsiness. Also common are rash, dysrhythmias, and fatigue.

Contraindications: Persons with known hypersensitivity, increased intracranial pressure, or cerebral hemorrhage should not use some of these products.

Precautions: Antianginals should be used with caution in postural P hypotension, pregnancy, lactation, children, renal disease, and hepatic injury.

Pharmacokinetics: Onset, peak, and duration vary widely among coronary products. Most products are metabolized in the liver and excreted in urine.

Interactions: Please check individual monographs, since interactions vary widely among products.

NURSING CONSIDERATIONS

Assessment

- Orthostatic B/P, pulse
- Assess for pain: duration, time started, activity being performed, character
- Assess for tolerance if taken over long period

- Assess for headache, lightheadedness, decreased B/P; may indicate a need for decreased dosage

Nursing diagnoses

- ✓ Altered tissue perfusion: cardiopulmonary (uses)
- ✓ Pain (uses)
- ✓ Risk for injury (uses)
- ✓ Knowledge deficit (teaching)
- ✓ Decreased cardiac output (adverse reactions)

Implementation

- Store protected from light, moisture; place in cool environment

Evaluation

- Therapeutic response: decreased, prevention of anginal pain

Patient/family education

- Instruct patient to keep tabs in original container
- Instruct patient not to use OTC products unless directed by prescriber
- Advise patient to report bradycardia, dizziness, confusion, depression, fever
- Teach patient to take pulse at home; advise when to notify prescriber
- Advise patient to avoid alcohol, smoking, sodium intake
- Advise patient to comply with weight control, dietary adjustments, modified exercise program
- Teach patient to carry Medic Alert ID to identify drug being taken, allergies
- Caution patient to make position changes slowly to prevent fainting

---

Generic Names

Nitrates:
amyl nitrite
isosorbide
🔑 nitroglycerin

β-adrenergic blockers:
atenolol
dipyridamole
metoprolol

Calcium channel blockers:
amlodipine
bepridil
diltiazem
nadolol
nicardipine
nifedipine
🔑 propranolol
🔑 verapamil

ANTICHOLINERGICS

Action: Anticholinergics inhibit the muscarinic actions of acetylcholine at receptor sites in the autonomic nervous system; anticholinergics are also known as antimuscarinic drugs.

Uses: Anticholinergics are used for a variety of conditions: gastrointestinal anticholinergics are used to decrease motility (smooth muscle tone) in the GI, biliary, and urinary tracts and for their ability to decrease gastric secretions (propantheline, glycopyrrolate); decreasing involuntary movements in parkinsonism (benztropine, trihexyphenidyl); bradydysrhythmias (atropine); nausea and vomiting (scopolamine); and as cycloplegic mydriatics (atropine, hematropine, scopalamine, cyclopentolate, tropicamide).

Adverse effects: The most common side effects are dry mouth, constipation, urinary retention, urinary hesitancy, headache, and dizziness. Also common is paralytic ileus.

Contraindications: Persons with narrow-angle glaucoma, myasthenia gravis, or GI/GU obstruction should not use some of these products.

Precautions: Anticholinergics should be used with caution in patients who are elderly, pregnant, or lactating or in those with prostatic hypertrophy, CHF, or hypertension; use with caution in presence of high environmental temp.

Pharmacokinetics: Onset, peak, and duration vary widely among products. Most products are metabolized in the liver and excreted in urine.

Interactions: Increased anticholinergic effects may occur when used with MAOIs and tricyclic antidepressants and amantadine. Anticholinergics may cause a decreased effect of phenothiazines and levodopa.

NURSING CONSIDERATIONS

Assessment

- Assess I&O ratio; retention commonly causes decreased urinary output
- Assess for urinary hesitancy, retention; palpate bladder if retention occurs
- Assess for constipation; increase fluids, bulk, exercise if this occurs
- Identify tolerance over long-term therapy; dosage may need to be increased or changed
- Assess mental status: affect, mood, CNS depression, worsening of mental symptoms during early therapy

Nursing diagnoses

- ✓ Decreased cardiac output (uses)
- ✓ Constipation (adverse reactions)
- ✓ Knowledge deficit (teaching)

Implementation

IV IM/IV Routes

- Give parenteral dose with patient recumbent to prevent postural hypotension
- Give parenteral dose slowly; keep in bed for at least 1 hr after dose; monitor VS
- Give after checking dose carefully; even slight overdose could lead to toxicity

PO Route

- Give with or after meals to prevent GI upset; may give with fluids other than water
- Store at room temp
- Give hard candy, frequent drinks, sugarless gum to relieve dry mouth

Evaluation

- Therapeutic response: decreased secretions, absence of nausea and vomiting

Patient/family education

- Caution patient to avoid driving and other hazardous activities; drowsiness may occur
- Advise patient to avoid OTC medication: cough, cold preparations with alcohol, antihistamines unless directed by prescriber

---

Generic Names

🔑 atropine	propantheline
🔑 benztropine	scopolamine
biperiden	trihexyphenidyl
glycopyrrolate	

ANTICOAGULANTS

Action: Anticoagulants interfere with blood clotting by preventing clot formation.

Uses: Anticoagulants are used for deep vein thrombosis, pulmonary emboli, myocardial infarction, open heart surgery, disseminated intravascular clotting syndrome, atrial fibrillation with embolization, and in transfusion and dialysis.

Adverse effects: The most serious adverse reactions are hemorrhage, agranulocytosis, leukopenia, eosinophilia, and thrombocytopenia, depending on the specific product. The most common side effects are diarrhea, rash, and fever.

Contraindications: Persons with hemophilia, leukemia with bleeding, peptic ulcer disease, thrombocytopenic purpura, blood dyscrasias, acute nephritis, and subacute bacterial endocarditis should not use these products.

G **Precautions:** Anticoagulants should be used with caution in alcoholism, elderly, and pregnancy.

Pharmacokinetics: Onset, peak, and duration vary widely among products. Most products are metabolized in the liver and excreted in urine.

Interactions: Salicylates, steroids, and nonsteroidal antiinflammatories will potentiate the action of anticoagulants. Anticoagulants may cause serious effects; please check individual monographs.

NURSING CONSIDERATIONS

Assessment

- Monitor blood studies (Hct, platelets, occult blood in stools) q3 mo
- Monitor partial prothrombin time, which should be 1½-2 × control, PPT; often qd, APTT, ACT
- Monitor B/P; watch for increasing signs of hypertension
- Monitor for bleeding gums, petechiae, ecchymosis, black tarry stools, hematuria
- Monitor for fever, skin rash, urticaria
- Monitor for needed dosage change q1-2wk

Nursing diagnoses

✓ Altered tissue perfusion (uses)
✓ Risk for injury (side effects)
✓ Knowledge deficit (teaching)

Implementation

SC Route

- Give at same time each day to maintain steady blood levels
- Do not massage area or aspirate when giving SC inj; give in abdomen between pelvic bones; rotate sites; do not pull back on plunger, leave in for 10 sec; apply gentle pressure for 1 min
- Do not change needles
- Avoid all IM inj that may cause bleeding
- Store in tight container (PO dose)

Evaluation

- Therapeutic response: decrease of deep vein thrombosis

Patient/family education

- Advise patient to avoid OTC preparations that may cause serious drug interactions unless directed by prescriber
- Inform patient that drug may be held during active bleeding (menstruation), depending on condition
- Caution patient to use soft-bristle toothbrush to avoid bleeding gums; avoid contact sports; use electric razor
- Instruct patient to carry a Medic-Alert ID identifying drug taken
- Instruct patient to report any signs of bleeding: gums, under skin, urine, stools

---

Generic Names

ardeparin
danaparoid
enoxaparin
heparin
warfarin

ANTICONVULSANTS

Action: Anticonvulsants are divided into the barbiturates (p. 1321), benzodiazepines (p. 1322), hydantoins, succinimides, and miscellaneous products. Barbiturates and benzodiazepines are discussed in separate sections. Hydantoins act by inhibiting the spread of seizure activity in the motor cortex. Succinimides act by inhibiting spike and wave formation; they also decrease amplitude, frequency, duration, and spread of discharge in seizures.

Uses: Hydantoins are used in generalized tonic-clonic seizures, status epilepticus, and psychomotor seizures. Succinimides are used for absence of (petit mal) seizures. Barbiturates are used in generalized tonic-clonic and cortical focal seizures.

Adverse effects: Bone marrow depression is the most life-threatening adverse reaction associated with hydantoins or succinimides. The most common side effects are GI symptoms. Other common side effects for hydantoins are gingival hyperplasia and CNS effects such as nystagmus, ataxia, slurred speech, and confusion.

Contraindications: Hypersensitive reactions may occur, and allergies should be identified before these products are given.

Precautions: Persons with renal or hepatic disease should be watched closely.

Pharmacokinetics: Onset, peak, and duration vary widely among products. Most products are metabolized in the liver and excreted in urine, bile, and feces.

Interactions: Decreased effects of estrogens, oral contraceptives (hydantoins).

NURSING CONSIDERATIONS

Assessment

- Monitor renal function studies, including BUN, creatinine, serum uric acid, urine creatinine clearance before and during therapy
- Monitor blood studies: RBC, Hct, Hgb, reticulocyte counts weekly for 4 wk then monthly
- Monitor hepatic studies: AST (SGOT), ALT (SGPT), bilirubin, creatinine
- Assess mental status, including mood, sensorium, affect, behavioral changes; if mental status changes, notify prescriber
- Assess for eye problems, including need for ophth examinations before, during, and after treatment (slit lamp, fundoscopy, tonometry)
- Assess for allergic reaction, including red raised rash; if this occurs, drug should be discontinued
- Assess for blood dyscrasias, including fever, sore throat, bruising, rash, jaundice
- Monitor toxicity, including bone marrow depression, nausea, vomiting, ataxia, diplopia, cardiovascular collapse, Stevens-Johnson syndrome

Nursing diagnoses

✓ Risk for injury (uses)
✓ Noncompliance (teaching)
✓ Sleep pattern disturbance (adverse reactions)

Implementation

PO Route

- Give with food, milk to decrease GI symptoms
- Good oral hygiene is important for patients taking hydantoins

Evaluation

- Therapeutic response, including decreased seizure activity; document on patient's chart

Patient/family education

- Advise patient to carry ID card or Medic Alert bracelet stating drugs taken, condition, prescriber's name, phone number
- Advise patient to avoid driving, other activities that require alertness

Generic Names

Hydantoins:
fosphenytoin
phenytoin

Succinimides:
ethosuximide

Miscellaneous:
acetazolamide
carbamazepine
clonazepam
diazepam
felbamate
magnesium sulfate
tiagabine
topiramate

Barbiturates:
amobarbital
phenobarbital
primidone
thiopental

ANTIDEPRESSANTS

Action: Antidepressants are divided into the tricyclics, MAOIs, and miscellaneous antidepressants. The tricyclics work by blocking reuptake of norepinephrine and serotonin into nerve endings and increasing action of norepinephrine and serotonin in nerve cells. MAOIs act by increasing concentrations of endogenous epinephrine, norepinephrine, serotonin, dopamine in storage sites in CNS by inhibition of MAO; increased concentration reduces depression.

Uses: Antidepressants are used for depression and in some cases P enuresis in children.

Adverse effects: The most serious adverse reactions are paralytic ileus, acute renal failure, hypertension, and hypertensive crisis, depending on the specific product. Common side effects are dizziness, drowsiness, diarrhea, dry mouth, urinary retention, and orthostatic hypotension.

Contraindications: The contraindications for antidepressants are convulsive disorders, prostatic hypertrophy, severe renal, hepatic, cardiac disease depending on the type of medication.

Precautions: Antidepressants should be used cautiously in suicidal patients, severe depression, schizophrenia, hyperactivity, diabetes mel- G litus, pregnancy, and the elderly.

Pharmacokinetics: Onset, peak, and duration vary widely among products. Most products are metabolized in the liver and excreted in urine.

Interactions: Please check individual monographs, since interactions vary widely among products.

NURSING CONSIDERATIONS

Assessment

- Monitor B/P (lying, standing), pulse q4h; if systolic B/P drops 20 mm Hg, hold drug, notify prescriber; take VS q4h in patients with cardiovascular disease
- Monitor blood studies: CBC, leukocytes, differential, cardiac enzymes if patient is receiving long-term therapy
- Monitor hepatic studies: AST (SGOT), ALT (SGPT), bilirubin, creatinine
- Monitor weight weekly; appetite may increase with drug
- G Monitor for EPS primarily in elderly: rigidity, dystonia, akathisia
- Assess mental status: mood, sensorium, affect, suicidal tendencies, increase in psychiatric symptoms (depression, panic)
- P G Check for urinary retention, constipation; constipation is more likely to occur in children, elderly
- Assess for withdrawal symptoms: headache, nausea, vomiting, muscle pain, weakness; do not usually occur unless drug was dis continued abruptly
- Identify alcohol consumption; if alcohol is consumed, hold dose until AM

Nursing diagnoses

- ✓ Ineffective individual coping (uses)
- ✓ Risk for injury (uses/adverse reactions)
- ✓ Knowledge deficit (teaching)

Implementation

PO Route

- Give increased fluids, bulk in diet if constipation, urinary retention occur
- Give with food or milk for GI symptoms
- Give gum, hard candy, or frequent sips of water for dry mouth
- Store in tight container at room temp; do not refreeze
- Provide assistance with ambulation during beginning therapy, since drowsiness/dizziness occurs

Evaluation

- Therapeutic response: decreased depression

Patient/family education

- Teach patient that therapeutic effects may take 2-3 wk
- Advise patient to use caution in driving or other activities requiring alertness because of drowsiness, dizziness, blurred vision
- Caution patient to avoid alcohol ingestion, other CNS depressants
- Instruct patient not to discontinue medication quickly after long-term use; may cause nausea, headache, malaise

- Instruct patient to wear sunscreen or large hat, since photosensitivity may occur

---

Generic Names

Tetracyclic:
mirtazapine

Tricyclics:
amitriptyline
amoxapine
clomipramine
doxepin
imipramine
nortriptyline

Miscellaneous:
bupropion
fluoxetine
maprotiline
paroxetine
sertraline
trazodone
venlafaxine

MAOIs:
phenelzine
tranylcypromine

ANTIDIABETICS

Action: Antidiabetics are divided into the insulins that decrease blood sugar, phosphate, and potassium and increase blood pyruvate and lactate; and oral antidiabetics that cause functioning β-cells in the pancreas to release insulin, improves the effect of endogenous and exogenous insulin.

Uses: Insulins are used for ketoacidosis and diabetes mellitus types I (IDDM) and II (NIDDM); oral antidiabetics are used for stable adult-onset diabetes mellitus type II (NIDDM).

Adverse effects: The most common side effect of insulin and oral antidiabetics is hypoglycemia. Other adverse reactions for oral antidiabetics include blood dyscrasias, hepatotoxicity, and, rarely, cholestatic jaundice. Adverse reactions for insulin products include allergic responses and, more rarely, anaphylaxis.

Contraindications: Hypersensitive reactions may occur, and allergies should be identified before these products are given. Oral antidiabetics should not be used in juvenile or brittle diabetes, diabetic ketoacidosis, severe renal disease, or severe hepatic disease.

G **Precautions:** Oral antidiabetics should be used with caution in the elderly, in cardiac disease, pregnancy, lactation, and in the presence of alcohol.

Pharmacokinetics: Onset, peak, and duration vary widely among products. Oral antidiabetics are metabolized in the liver, with metabolites excreted in urine, bile, and feces.
Interactions: Interactions vary widely among products. Check individual monograph for specific information.

NURSING CONSIDERATIONS
Assessment
- Monitor blood, urine glucose levels during treatment to determine diabetes control (oral products)
- Monitor fasting blood glucose, 2 hr PP (60-100 mg/dl normal fasting level) (70-130 mg/dl—normal 2-hr level)
- Assess for hypoglycemic reaction that can occur during peak time

Nursing diagnoses
✓ Altered nutrition: more than body requirements (uses)

Implementation
SC Route
- Give insulin after warming to room temp by rotating in palms to prevent lipodystrophy from injecting cold insulin
- Give human insulin to those allergic to beef or pork
- Rotate inj sites when giving insulin; use abdomen, upper back, thighs, upper arm, buttocks; keep a record of sites

PO Route
- Give oral antidiabetic 30 min ac

Evaluation
- Therapeutic response, including decrease in polyuria, polydipsia, polyphagia, clear sensorium, absence of dizziness, stable gait

Patient/family education
- Advise patient to avoid alcohol and salicylates except on advice of prescriber
- Teach patient symptoms of ketoacidosis: nausea, thirst, polyuria, dry mouth, decreased B/P, dry, flushed skin, acetone breath, drowsiness, Kussmaul respirations
- Teach patient symptoms of hypoglycemia: headache, tremors, fatigue, weakness; and that candy or sugar should be carried to treat hypoglycemia
- Advise patient to test urine for glucose/ketones tid if this drug is replacing insulin
- Advise patient to continue weight control, dietary restrictions, exercise, hygiene

Generic Names

acetohexamide
chlorpropamide
insulin, isophane suspension
insulin lispro
insulin, regular
insulin, regular concentrated
insulin, zinc suspension (extended)
insulin, zinc suspension (Lente)
insulin, zinc suspension (prompt)
miglitol
tolazamide
tolbutamide
troglitazone

ANTIDIARRHEALS

Action: Antidiarrheals work by various actions including direct action on intestinal muscles to decrease GI peristalsis; or by inhibiting prostaglandin synthesis responsible for GI hypermotility; acting on mucosal receptors responsible for peristalsis; or decreasing water content of stools.

Uses: Antidiarrheals are used for diarrhea of undetermined causes.

Adverse effects: The most serious adverse reactions of some products are paralytic ileus, toxic megacolon, and angioneurotic edema. The most common side effects are constipation, nausea, dry mouth, and abdominal pain.

Contraindications: Persons with severe ulcerative colitis, pseudomembranous colitis with some products.

G P **Precautions:** Antidiarrheal should be used with caution in the elderly, pregnancy, lactation, children, dehydration.

Pharmacokinetics: Onset, peak, and duration vary widely among products. Most products are metabolized in the liver and excreted in urine.

Interactions: Please check individual monographs, since interactions vary widely among products.

NURSING CONSIDERATIONS

Assessment

- Monitor electrolytes (potassium, sodium, chloride) if on long-term therapy
- Monitor bowel pattern before; for rebound constipation after termination of medication

- Assess response after 48 hr; if no response, drug should be discontinued
- P • Identify dehydration in children

Nursing diagnoses

- ✓ Diarrhea (uses)
- ✓ Constipation (adverse reactions)
- ✓ Fluid volume deficit (adverse reactions)
- ✓ Knowledge deficit (teaching)

Implementation

PO Route

- Give for 48 hr only

Evaluation

- Therapeutic response: decreased diarrhea

Patient/family education

- Advise patient to avoid OTC products
- Caution patient not to exceed recommended dose

Generic Names

bismuth subsalicylate
diphenoxylate
kaolin/pectin
loperamide

ANTIDYSRHYTHMICS

Action: Antidysrhythmics are divided into four classes and miscellaneous antidysrhythmics:

- Class I increases the action potential duration and the effective refractory period and reduces disparity in the refractory period between a normal and infarcted myocardium; further subclasses include Ia, Ib, Ic
- Class II decreases the rate of SA node discharge, increases recovery time, slows conduction through the AV node, and decreases heart rate, which decreases O_2 consumption in the myocardium
- Class III increases the action potential duration and the effective refractory period
- Class IV inhibits calcium ion influx across the cell membrane during cardiac depolarization; decreases SA node discharge, decreases conduction velocity through the AV node
- Miscellaneous antidysrhythmics include those such as adenosine, which slows conduction through the AV node, and digoxin, which decreases conduction velocity and prolongs the effective refractory period in the AV node

Uses: These products are used for PVCs, tachycardia, hypertension, atrial fibrillation, angina pectoris.
Adverse effects: Side effects and adverse reactions vary widely among products.
Contraindications: Contraindications vary widely among products.
Precautions: Precautions vary widely among products.
Pharmacokinetics: Onset, peak, and duration vary widely among products.
Interactions: Interactions vary widely among products; check individual monograph for specific information.

NURSING CONSIDERATIONS

Assessment

- Monitor ECG continuously to determine drug effectiveness, PVCs, or other dysrhythmias
- Assess for dehydration or hypovolemia
- Monitor B/P continuously for hypotension, hypertension
- Monitor I&O ratio
- Monitor serum potassium
- Assess for edema in feet and legs daily

Nursing diagnoses

✓ Altered tissue perfusion: cardiopulmonary (uses)
✓ Decreased cardiac output (uses)
✓ Diarrhea (adverse reactions)
✓ Impaired gas exchange (adverse reactions)

Evaluation

- Therapeutic response, including decrease in B/P in hypertension, decreased B/P, edema, moist rales in CHF

Patient/family education

- Advise patient to comply with dosage schedule, even if patient is feeling better
- Instruct patient to report bradycardia, dizziness, confusion, depression, fever

---

Generic Names

Class I:
moricizine

Class Ia.
disopyramide
🔑 procainamide
🔑 quinidine

Class II:
acebutolol
esmolol
🔑 propranolol

Class Ib:
lidocaine
mexiletine
phenytoin
tocainide

Class Ic:
flecainide

Class III:
amiodarone
bretylium
ibutilide

Class IV:
verapamil

Miscellaneous:
adenosine
digoxin

ANTIFUNGALS (SYSTEMIC)

Action: Antifungals act by increasing cell membrane permeability in susceptible organisms by binding sterols and decreasing potassium, sodium, and nutrients in the cell.

Uses: Antifungals are used for infections of histoplasmosis, blastomycosis, coccidioidomycosis, cryptococcosis, aspergillosis, phycomycosis, candidiasis, sporotrichosis causing severe meningitis, septicemia, and skin infections.

Adverse effects: The most serious adverse reactions include renal tubular acidosis, permanent renal impairment, anuria, oliguria, hemorrhagic gastroenteritis, acute liver failure, and blood dyscrasias. Some common side effects include hypokalemia, nausea, vomiting, anorexia, headache, fever, and chills.

Contraindications: Persons with severe bone depression or hypersensitivity should not use these products.

Precautions: Antifungals should be used with caution in renal disease, pregnancy, and hepatic disease.

Pharmacokinetics: Onset, peak, and duration vary widely among products. Most products are metabolized in the liver and excreted in urine.

Interactions: Please check individual monographs, since interactions vary widely among products.

NURSING CONSIDERATIONS

Assessment

- Monitor VS q15-30 min during first inf; note changes in pulse, B/P
- Monitor I&O ratio; watch for decreasing urinary output, change in sp gr; discontinue drug to prevent permanent damage to renal tubules

- Monitor blood studies; CBC, potassium, sodium, calcium, magnesium q2 wk
- Monitor weight weekly; if weight increases over 2 lb/wk, edema is present; renal damage should be considered
- Assess for renal toxicity: increasing BUN, is >40 mg/dl or if serum creatinine >3 mg/dl; drug may be discontinued or dosage reduced
- Assess for hepatotoxicity: increasing AST (SGOT), ALT (SGPT), alkaline phosphatase, bilirubin
- Assess for allergic reaction: dermatitis, rash; drug should be discontinued; antihistamines (mild reaction) or epinephrine (severe reaction) administered
- Assess for hypokalemia: anorexia, drowsiness, weakness, decreased reflexes, dizziness, increased urinary output, increased thirst, paresthesias
- Assess for ototoxicity: tinnitus (ringing, roaring in ears), vertigo, loss of hearing (rare)

Nursing diagnoses

✓ Risk for infection (uses)
✓ Risk for injury (adverse reactions)
✓ Knowledge deficit (teaching)

Implementation

IV IV route

- Give by IV using in-line filter (mean pore diameter >1 μm) using distal veins; check for extravasation, necrosis q8h
- Give drug only after C&S confirms organism, drug needed to treat condition; make sure drug is used in life-threatening infections
- Provide protection from light during inf; cover with foil
- Give symptomatic treatment as ordered for adverse reactions: aspirin, antihistamines, antiemetics, antispasmodics
- Store protected from moisture and light; diluted sol is stable for 24 hr

Evaluation

- Therapeutic response: decreased fever, malaise, rash, negative C&S for infecting organism

Patient/family education

- Teach patient that long-term therapy may be needed to clear infection (2 wk-3 mo depending on type of infection)

Generic Names

🔑 amphotericin B
fluconazole
flucytosine
griseofulvin
itraconazole
ketoconazole
🔑 miconazole
nystatin

ANTIHISTAMINES

Action: Antihistamines compete with histamines for H_1 receptor sites. They antagonize in varying degrees most of the pharmacologic effects of histamines.

Uses: Products are used to control the symptoms of allergies, rhinitis, and pruritus.

Adverse effects: Most products cause drowsiness; however, two of the newer products, astemizole and terfenadine, produce little, if any, drowsiness. Other common side effects are headache and thickening of bronchial secretions. Serious blood dyscrasias may occur, but are rare. Urinary retention, GI effects occur with many of these products.

Contraindications: Hypersensitivity to H_1-receptor antagonists occurs rarely. Patients with acute asthma and lower respiratory tract disease should not use these products, since thick secretions may result. Other contraindications include narrow-angle glaucoma, bladder neck obstruction, stenosing peptic ulcer, symptomatic prostatic hypertrophy, newborn, lactation.

Precautions: These products must be used cautiously in conjunction with intraocular pressure, since they increase intraocular pressure. Caution should also be used in patients with renal and cardiac disease, hypertension, and seizure disorders, pregnancy, lactation and in the elderly.

Pharmacokinetics: Onset varies from 20-60 min, with duration lasting 4-12 hr. In general, pharmacokinetics vary widely among products.

Interactions: Barbiturates, narcotics, hypnotics, tricyclic antidepressants, and alcohol can increase CNS depression when taken with antihistamines.

NURSING CONSIDERATIONS

Assessment

- Check I&O ratio; be alert for urinary retention, frequency, dysuria; drug should be discontinued if these occur
- Assess for blood dyscrasias: thrombocytopenia, agranulocytosis (rare)
- Assess for respiratory status, including rate rhythm, increase in bronchial secretions, wheezing, chest tightness
- Assess for cardiac status, including palpitations, increased pulse, hypotension
- Assess CBC during long-term therapy, since hemolytic anemia, although rare, may occur

- Administer with food or milk to decrease GI symptoms; absorption may be decreased slightly
- Administer whole (sustained-release tab)
- Provide hard candy, gum, frequent rinsing of mouth for dryness

Nursing diagnoses

✓ Ineffective airway clearance (uses)

Evaluation

- Therapeutic response: absence of allergy symptoms, itching

Patient/family education

- Advise patient to notify prescriber if confusion, sedation, hypotension occur
- Caution patient to avoid driving and other hazardous activity if drowsiness occurs
- Instruct patient to avoid concurrent use of alcohol and other CNS depressants
- Inform patient to discontinue a few days before skin testing

---

Generic Names

astemizole
azatadine
brompheniramine
cetirizine
chlorpheniramine
clemastine
cyproheptadine
diphenhydramine (key)
fexofenadine
loratadine
promethazine
terfenadine
triprolidine

ANTIHYPERTENSIVES

Action: Antihypertensives are divided into angiotensin converting enzyme (ACE) inhibitors, β-adrenergic blockers, calcium channel blockers, centrally acting adrenergics, diuretics, peripherally acting antiadrenergics, and vasodilators. β-Blockers, calcium channel blockers, and diuretics are discussed in separate sections. ACE inhibitors selectively suppress conversion of renin-angiotensin I to angiotensin II; dilatation of arterial and venous vessels occurs. Centrally acting adrenergics act by inhibiting the sympathetic vasomotor center in the CNS, which reduces impulses in the sympathetic nervous system; blood pressure, pulse rate, and cardiac output decrease. Peripherally acting antiadrenergics inhibit sympathetic vasoconstriction by inhibiting release of norepinephrine and/or depleting norepinephrine stores in adrenergic nerve endings. Vasodilators act on arteriolar smooth muscle by producing direct relaxation or vasodilatation; a reduction in blood pressure, with concomitant increases in heart rate and cardiac output, occurs.

Uses: Used for hypertension and for heart failure not responsive to conventional therapy. Some products are used in hypertensive crisis, angina, and for some cardiac dysrhythmias.

Adverse effects: The most common side effects are marked hypotension, bradycardia, tachycardia, headache, nausea, and vomiting. Side effects and adverse reactions may vary widely between classes and specific products.

Contraindications: Hypersensitive reactions may occur, and allergies should be identified before these products are given. Antihypertensives should not be used in patients with heart block or in children.

Precautions: Antihypertensives should be used with caution in the elderly, in dialysis patients, and in the presence of hypovolemia, leukemia, and electrolyte imbalances.

Pharmacokinetics: Onset, peak, and duration vary widely among products. Most products are metabolized in the liver, with metabolites excreted in urine, bile, and feces.

Interactions: Interactions vary widely among products; check individual monograph for specific information.

NURSING CONSIDERATIONS

Assessment

- Monitor blood studies: neutrophil; decreased platelets occur with many of the products
- Monitor renal studies: protein, BUN, creatinine; watch for increased levels, which may indicate nephrotic syndrome; obtain baselines in renal and liver function studies before beginning treatment
- Assess for edema in feet and legs daily
- Identify allergic reaction, including rash, fever, pruritus, urticaria: drug should be discontinued if antihistamines fail to help
- Identify symptoms of CHF: edema, dyspnea, wet rales, B/P
- Assess for renal symptoms: polyuria, oliguria, frequency

Nursing diagnoses

Altered tissue perfusion (uses)
Decreased cardiac output (uses)
Diarrhea (adverse reactions)
Impaired gas exchange (adverse reactions)

Implementation

- Place patient in supine or Trendelenburg position for severe hypotension

Evaluation

- Therapeutic response: decrease in B/P in hypotension; decreased B/P, edema, moist rales in CHF

Patient/family education

- Instruct patient to comply with dosage schedule, even if feeling better
- Advise patient to rise slowly to sitting or standing position to minimize orthostatic hypotension

---

Generic Names

ACE inhibitors:
enalapril
esoprostenol
fosinopril
quinapril
ramipril

Angiotension II receptors
irbesartan
valsartan

Centrally acting adrenergics:
🔑 clonidine
guanabenz
guanfacine
methyldopa

Peripherally acting antiadrenergics:
guanadrel
benazepril
guanethidine
🔑 prazosin
reserpine
terazosin

Vasodilators:
diazoxide
hydralazine
minoxidil
nitroprusside

Antidrenergic:
combined α-/β-blocker—labetalol

ANTIINFECTIVES

Action: Antiinfectives are divided into several groups, which include but are not limited to penicillins, cephalosporins, aminoglycosides, sulfonamides, tetracyclines, monobactam, erythromycins, and quinolones. These drugs inhibit the growth and replication of susceptible bacterial organisms.

Uses: Used for infections of susceptible organisms. These products are effective against bacterial, rickettsial, and spirochete infections.
Adverse effects: The most common side effects are nausea, vomiting, and diarrhea. Adverse reactions include bone marrow depression and anaphylaxis.
Contraindications: Hypersensitive reactions may occur, and allergies should be identified before these products are given. Cross-sensitivity can occur between products of different classes (penicillins or cephalosporins). Often persons allergic to penicillins are also allergic to cephalosporins.
Precautions: Antiinfectives should be used with caution in persons with renal and liver disease.
Pharmacokinetics: Onset, peak, and duration vary widely among products. Most products are metabolized in the liver, and metabolites are excreted in urine, bile, and feces.
Interactions: Interactions vary widely among products; check individual monograph for specific information.

NURSING CONSIDERATIONS

Assessment

- Assess for nephrotoxicity, including increased BUN, creatinine
- Monitor blood studies: AST (SGOT), ALT (SGPT), CBC, Hct, bilirubin; test monthly if patient is on long-term therapy
- Monitor bowel pattern qd; if severe diarrhea occurs, drug should be discontinued
- Monitor urine output; if decreasing, notify prescriber; may indicate nephrotoxicity
- Assess for allergic reaction, including rash, fever, pruritus, urticaria; drug should be discontinued
- Assess for bleeding: ecchymosis, bleeding gums, hematuria, stool guaiac daily
- Assess for overgrowth of infection: perineal itching, fever, malaise, redness, pain, swelling, drainage, rash, diarrhea, change in cough, sputum

Nursing diagnoses

- Risk for infection (uses)
- Diarrhea (adverse reactions)

Implementation

- Give for 10-14 days to ensure organism death, prevention of superinfection
- Give after C&S completed; drug may be taken as soon as culture is obtained

Evaluation

- Therapeutic response: absence of fever, fatigue, malaise, draining wounds

Patient/family education

- Teach patient to comply with dosage schedule, even if feeling better
- Advise patient to report sore throat, bruising, bleeding, joint pain; may indicate blood dyscrasias (rare)

Generic Names

Aminoglycosides:
amikacin
azithromycin
clarithromycin
gentamicin
kanamycin
neomycin
netilmicin
streptomycin
tobramycin

Cephalosporins:
cefaclor
cefadroxil
cefamandole
cefazolin
cefepime
cefixime
cefmetazole
cefonicid
cefoperazone
ceftibuten
cephalexin
cephalothin
cephapirin
cephradine

Misc
fluoroquinolones
levofloxacin
meropenem
sparfloxacin

Penicillins:
amoxicillin/clavulanate
ampicillin/sulbactam
cloxacillin
dicloxacillin
imipenem/cilastatin
methicillin
mezlocillin
nafcillin
oxacillin
penicillin G benzathine
penicillin G potassium
penicillin G procaine
penicillin G sodium
penicillin V
piperacillin
ticarcillin/clavulanate

Sulfonamides:
sulfasalazine
sulfisoxazole

Tetracyclines:
doxycycline
minocycline
tetracycline

ANTINEOPLASTICS

Action: Antineoplastics are divided into alkylating agents, antimetabolites, antibiotic agents, hormonal agents, and miscellaneous agents. Alkylating agents act by cross-linking strands of DNA. Antimetabolites act by inhibiting DNA synthesis. Antibiotic agents act by inhibiting RNA synthesis and by delaying or inhibiting mitosis. Hormones alter the effect of androgens, luteinizing hormone, follicle-stimulating hormone, or estrogen by changing the hormonal environment.

Uses: Uses vary widely among products and classes of drugs. They are used to treat leukemia, Hodgkin's disease, lymphomas, and other tumors throughout the body.

Adverse effects: Most products cause thrombocytopenia, leukopenia, and anemia, and, if these reactions occur, the drug may need to be stopped until the problem is corrected. Other side effects include nausea, vomiting, glossitis, and hair loss. Some products also cause hepatotoxicity, nephrotoxicity, and cardiotoxicity.

Contraindications: Hypersensitive reactions may occur, and allergies should be identified before these products are given. Also, persons with severe liver and kidney disease should not use these products unless the benefits outweigh the risks.

Precautions: Persons with bleeding, severe bone marrow depression, or renal or hepatic disease should be watched closely.

Pharmacokinetics: Onset, peak, and duration vary widely among products. Most products cross the placenta and are excreted in breast milk and in urine.

Interactions: Toxicity may occur when used with other antineoplastics or radiation.

NURSING CONSIDERATIONS

Assessment

- Monitor CBC, differential, platelet count weekly; withhold drug if WBC is <4000 or platelet count is <75,000; notify prescriber of results
- Monitor renal function studies, including BUN, creatinine, serum uric acid, and urine creatinine clearance before and during therapy
- Monitor I&O ratio; report fall in urine output of 30 ml/hr
- Monitor temp q4h (may indicate beginning infection)
- Monitor liver function tests before and during therapy (bilirubin, AST [SGOT], ALT [SGPT], LDH) prn or monthly

- Assess for bleeding, including hematuria, guaiac, bruising or petechiae, mucosa, or orifices q8h; obtain prescription for viscous lidocaine (Xylocaine)
- Identify yellowing of skin, sclera, dark urine, clay-colored stools, itchy skin, abdominal pain, fever, diarrhea
- Assess for edema in feet, joint pain, stomach pain, shaking
- Assess for inflammation of mucosa, breaks in skin

Nursing diagnoses

✓ Risk for infection (adverse reactions)
✓ Altered nutrition: less than body requirements (adverse reactions)
✓ Altered oral mucous membrane (adverse reactions)

Implementation

- Check IV site for irritation; phlebitis
- Have epinephrine available for hypersensitivity reaction
- Give antibiotics for prophylaxis of infection
- Provide strict medical asepsis, protective isolation if WBC levels are low
- Provide comprehensive oral hygiene, using careful technique and soft-bristle brush

Evaluation

- Therapeutic response: decreased tumor size

Patient/family education

- Advise patient to report signs of infection, including increased temp, sore throat, malaise
- Instruct patient to report signs of anemia, including fatigue, headache, faintness, shortness of breath, irritability
- Instruct patient to report bleeding and to avoid use of razors and commercial mouthwash

---

Generic Names

Alkylating agents:
busulfan
carboplatin
carmustine
chlorambucil
cisplatin
🗝 cyclophosphamide
dacarbazine
lomustine
mechlorethamine
melphalan
streptozocin
thiotepa

Antimetabolites:
cytarabine
🗝 doxorubicin
etoposide
fludarabine
fluorouracil
mercaptopurine
thioguanine (6-TG)

Antibiotic agents:
bleomycin
dactinomycin
daunorubicin
methotrexate
mitomycin
mitoxantrone
plicamycin

Hormonal agents:
aminoglutethimide
estramustine
flutamide
goserelin acetate
leuprolide
megestrol
mitotane
nilutamide
tamoxifen
topotecan

Miscellaneous agents:
altretamine
anastrozole
asparaginase
gemcitabine
interferon alfa-2A, interferon alfa-2B
irinotecan
pentostatin
porfimer
procarbazine
vinblastine
vincristine

ANTIPARKINSONIAN AGENTS

Action: Antiparkinsonian agents are divided into cholinergics and dopamine agonists. Cholinergics work by the blocking or competing at central acetylcholine receptors; dopamine agonists work by decarboxylation to dopamine or by activation of dopamine receptors; monoamine oxidase type B inhibitors increase dopamine activity by inhibiting MAO type B activity.

Uses: These agents are used alone or in combination for patients with Parkinson's disease.

Adverse effects: Side effects and adverse reactions vary widely among products. The most common side effects include involuntary movements, headache, numbness, insomnia, nightmares, nausea, vomiting, dry mouth, and orthostatic hypotension.

Contraindications: Persons with hypersensitivity, narrow-angle glaucoma, and undiagnosed skin lesions should not use these products.

Precautions: Antiparkinsonian agents should be used with caution in P pregnancy, lactation, children, renal, cardiac, hepatic disease, and affective disorder.

Pharmacokinetics: Onset, peak, and duration vary widely among products. Most products are metabolized in the liver and excreted in urine.

Interactions: Please check individual monographs, since interactions vary widely among products.

NURSING CONSIDERATIONS

Assessment

- Monitor B/P, respiration
- Assess mental status: affect, behavioral changes, depression, complete suicide assessment

Nursing diagnoses

✓ Risk for injury (uses)
✓ Risk for impaired mobility (uses)
✓ Knowledge deficit (teaching)

Implementation

- Give drug up until NPO before surgery
- Adjust dosage depending on patient response
- Give with meals; limit protein taken with drug
- Give only after MAOIs have been discontinued for 2 wk
- Assist with ambulation, during beginning therapy if needed
- Test for diabetes mellitus and acromegaly if on long-term therapy

Evaluation

- Therapeutic response: decrease in akathisia, improvement in mood

Patient/family education

- Advise patient to change positions slowly to prevent orthostatic hypotension
- Instruct patient to report side effects: twitching, eye spasm; indicate overdose
- Advise patient to use drug exactly as prescribed; if drug is discontinued abruptly, parkinsonian crisis may occur

---

Generic Names

amantadine
🔑 benztropine
biperiden
bromocriptine
carbidopa-levodopa
🔑 levodopa
selegiline
trihexyphenidyl

ANTIPSYCHOTICS

Action: Antipsychotics/neuroleptics are divided into several subgroups: phenothiazines, thioxanthenes, butyrophenones, dibenzoxazepines, dibenzodiazepines, and indolones and other heterocyclic compounds. Although chemically different, these subgroups share many pharmacologic and clinical properties. All antipsychotics work to block postsynaptic dopamine receptors in the brain that are responsible for psychotic behavior, including hallucinations, delusions, and paranoia.

Uses: Antipsychotic behavior is decreased in conditions such as schizophrenia, paranoia, and mania. These agents are also effective for severe anxiety, intractable hiccups, nausea, vomiting, behavioral problems in children, and before surgery for relaxation.

Adverse effects: The most common side effects include extrapyramidal symptoms such as pseudoparkinsonism, akathisia, dystonia, and tardive dyskinesia, which may be controlled by use of antiparkinsonian agents. Serious adverse reactions such as hypotension, agranulocytosis, cardiac arrest, and laryngospasm have occurred. Other common side effects include dry mouth and photosensitivity.

Contraindications: Persons with liver damage, severe hypertension or coronary disease, cerebral arteriosclerosis, blood dyscrasias, bone marrow depression, parkinsonism, severe depression, or narrow angle glaucoma, children <12 yr, or persons withdrawing from alcohol or barbiturates should not use antipsychotics until these conditions are corrected.

Precautions: Caution must be used when antipsychotics are given to the elderly, since metabolism is slowed and adverse reactions can occur rapidly. Hepatic and renal disease may cause poor metabolism and excretion of the drug. Seizure threshold is decreased with these products; increases in the dose of anticonvulsants may be required. Persons with diabetes mellitus, prostatic hypertrophy, chronic respiratory disease, and peptic ulcer disease should be monitored closely.

Pharmacokinetics: Onset, peak, and duration vary widely with different products and routes. Products are metabolized by the liver, are excreted in urine as metabolites, are highly bound to plasma proteins, cross the placenta, and enter breast milk. Half-life can be extended over 3 days.

Interactions: Because other CNS depressants can cause oversedation, these combinations should be used carefully. Anticholinergics may decrease the therapeutic actions of phenothiazines and also cause increased anticholinergic effects.

NURSING CONSIDERATIONS

Assessment

- Monitor bilirubin, CBC, liver function studies monthly, since these drugs are metabolized in the liver and excreted in urine
- Monitor I&O ratio: palpate bladder if low urinary output occurs, since urinary retention occurs with many of these products
- Assess affect, orientation, LOC, reflexes, gait, coordination, sleep pattern disturbances
- Assess dizziness, faintness, palpitations, tachycardia on rising

- Check B/P with patient lying and standing; wide fluctuations between lying and standing B/P may require dosage or product change, since orthostatic hypotension is occurring
- Assess for EPS, including akathisia, tardive dyskinesia, pseudoparkinsonism

Nursing diagnoses

✓ Altered thought processes (uses)
✓ Sensory-perceptual alterations(uses)

Implementation

- Give antiparkinsonian agent if EPS occur
- Administer liq concentrates mixed in glass of juice or cola, since taste is unpleasant; avoid contact with skin when preparing liq concentrate or parenteral medications
- Supervise ambulation until stabilized on medication; do not involve in strenuous exercise program, since fainting is possible; patient should not stand still for long periods
- Increase fluids to prevent constipation
- Give sips of water, candy, gum for dry mouth

Evaluation

- Therapeutic response: decrease in excitement, hallucinations, delusions, paranoia, reorganization of thought patterns, speech

Patient/family education

- Advise patient to rise from sitting or lying position gradually, since fainting may occur
- Instruct patient to remain lying down for at least 30 min after IM inj
- Caution patient to avoid hot tubs, hot showers, or tub baths, since hypotension may occur
- Advise patient to wear a sunscreen or protective clothing to prevent burns
- Advise patient to take extra precautions during hot weather to stay cool; heat stroke can occur
- Caution patient to avoid driving and other activities requiring alertness until response to medication is known
- Inform patient that drowsiness or impaired mental/motor activity is evident the first 2 wk, but tends to decrease over time

---

Generic Names

Phenothiazines:
🔑 chlorpromazine
fluphenazine
mesoridazine
perphenazine
prochlorperazine
promazine
thioridazine
thiothixene
trifluoperazine

Butyrophenone:
haloperidol

Miscellaneous:
loxapine
molindone
olanzapine
quetiapine
risperidone

ANTITUBERCULARS

Action: Antituberculars act by inhibiting RNA or DNA, or interfering with lipid and protein synthesis, thereby decreasing tubercle bacilli replication.

Uses: Antituberculars are used for pulmonary tuberculosis.

Adverse effects: They vary widely among products. Most products can cause nausea, vomiting, anorexia, and rash. Serious adverse reactions include renal failure, nephrotoxicity, ototoxicity, and hepatic necrosis.

Contraindications: Persons with severe renal disease or hypersensitivity should not use these products.

Precautions: Antituberculars should be used with caution in pregnancy, lactation, and hepatic disease.

Pharmacokinetics: Onset, peak, and duration vary widely among products. Most products are metabolized in the liver and excreted in urine.

Interactions: Please check individual monographs, since interactions vary widely among products.

NURSING CONSIDERATIONS

Assessment

- Assess for signs of anemia: Hct, Hgb, fatigue
- Monitor liver studies weekly: ALT (SGPT), AST (SGOT), bilirubin
- Monitor renal status before treatment and monthly thereafter: BUN, creatinine, output, sp gr, urinalysis
- Monitor hepatic status: decreased appetite, jaundice, dark urine, fatigue

Nursing diagnoses

- ✓ Risk for infection (uses)
- ✓ Risk for injury (adverse reactions)
- ✓ Knowledge deficit (teaching)
- ✓ Noncompliance (teaching)

Implementation

- Give some of these agents on empty stomach, 1 hr ac (only for isoniazid and rifampin) or 2 hr pc
- Give antiemetic if vomiting occurs
- Give after C&S is completed; monthly to detect resistance

Evaluation

- Therapeutic response: decreased symptoms of TB, culture negative

Patient/family education

- Teach patient that compliance with dosage schedule, duration is necessary
- Teach patient that scheduled appointments must be kept; relapse may occur
- Advise patient to avoid alcohol while taking drug
- Advise patient to report flulike symptoms: excessive fatigue, anorexia, vomiting, sore throat; unusual bleeding, yellowish discoloration of skin/eyes

---

Generic Names

ethambutol
isoniazid
pyrazinamide
rifabutin
rifampin
streptomycin

ANTITUSSIVES/EXPECTORANTS

Action: Antitussives suppress the cough reflex by direct action on the cough center in the medulla. Expectorants act by liquefying and reducing the viscosity of thick, tenacious secretions.

Uses: Antitussives/expectorants are used to treat cough occurring in pneumonia, bronchitis, TB, cystic fibrosis, and emphysema; as an adjunct in atelectasis (expectorants); and for nonproductive cough (antitussives).

Adverse effects: The most common side effects are drowsiness, dizziness, and nausea.

Contraindications: Some products are contraindicated in hypothyroidism, iodine sensitivity, pregnancy, and lactation.

G **Precautions:** Some products should be used cautiously in asthma, elderly, and debilitated patients.

Pharmacokinetics: Onset, peak, and duration vary widely among products. Some products are metabolized in the liver and excreted in urine.

Interactions: Please check individual monographs, since interactions vary widely among products.

NURSING CONSIDERATIONS

Assessment

- Assess cough: type, frequency, character including sputum

Nursing diagnoses:

✓ Ineffective breathing pattern (uses)
✓ Ineffective airway clearance (uses)
✓ Knowledge deficit (teaching)

Implementation

- G Give decreased dosage to elderly patients; their metabolism may be slowed
- Increase fluids to liquefy secretions
- Humidify patient's room

Evaluation

- Therapeutic response: absence of cough

Patient/family education

- Advise patient to avoid driving and other hazardous activities until stabilized on this medication
- Caution patient to avoid smoking, smoke-filled rooms, perfumes, dust, environmental pollutants, cleaners that increase cough

---

Generic Names

acetylcysteine
codeine
dextromethorphan
diphenhydramine
guaifenesin
hydrocodone
potassium iodide

ANTIVIRALS

Action: Antivirals act by interfering with DNA synthesis that is needed for viral replication.

Uses: Antivirals are used for mucocutaneous herpes simplex virus, herpes genitalis (HSV_1, HSV_2), advanced HIV infections, herpes simplex virus encephalitis, varicella-zoster encephalomyelitis.

Adverse effects: Serious adverse reactions are fatal metabolic encephalopathy, blood dyscrasias, and acute renal failure. Common side effects are nausea, vomiting, anorexia, diarrhea, headache, vaginitis, and moniliasis.

Contraindications: Persons with hypersensitivity and immunosuppressed individuals with herpes zoster should not use these products.

Precautions: Antivirals should be used with caution in renal disease, liver disease, lactation, pregnancy, and dehydration.

Pharmacokinetics: Onset, peak, and duration vary widely among products. Most products are metabolized in the liver and excreted in urine.

Interactions: Please check individual monographs, since interactions vary widely among products.

NURSING CONSIDERATIONS

Assessment

- Assess for signs of infection, anemia
- Monitor I&O ratio; report hematuria, oliguria, fatigue, weakness; may indicate nephrotoxicity; check for protein in urine during treatment
- Monitor any patient with compromised renal system, since drug is excreted slowly in poor renal system function; toxicity may occur rapidly
- Check liver studies: AST (SGOT), ALT (SGPT)
- Check blood studies: WBC, RBC, Hct, Hgb, bleeding time; blood dyscrasias may occur; drug should be discontinued
- Check renal studies: urinalysis, protein, BUN, creatinine, Cr Cl
- Obtain C&S before drug therapy; drug may be taken as soon as culture is obtained; repeat C&S after treatment
- Assess bowel pattern before, during treatment; if severe abdominal pain with bleeding occurs, drug should be discontinued
- Identify skin eruptions: rash, urticaria, itching
- Assess for allergies before treatment, reaction of each medication; place allergies on chart, Kardex in bright red letters

Nursing diagnoses

✓ Risk for infection (uses)
✓ Risk for injury (adverse reactions)
✓ Knowledge deficit (teaching)

Implementation

- Give increased fluids to 3 L/day to decrease crystalluria when given IB
- Store at room temp for up to 12 hr after reconstitution
- Give adequate intake of fluids (2000 ml) to prevent deposit in kidneys

Evaluation

- Therapeutic response: absence of or control of infection

Patient/family education

- Inform patient that drug does not cure infection, just controls symptoms

- Instruct patient to report sore throat, fever, fatigue; could indicate superinfection
- Advise patient that drug must be taken in equal intervals around the clock to maintain blood levels for duration of therapy
- Advise patient to notify prescriber of side effects of bruising, bleeding, fatigue, malaise; may indicate blood dyscrasias

---

Generic Names

- acyclovir
- amantadine
- cidofovir
- delavirdine
- didanosine
- foscarnet
- ganciclovir
- idoxuridine
- indinavir
- rimantadine
- ritonavir
- saquinavir
- zalcitabine
- zidovudine

BARBITURATES

Action: Barbiturates act by decreasing impulse transmission to the cerebral cortex.

Uses: All forms of epilepsy can be controlled, since the seizure P threshold is increased. Uses also include febrile seizures in children, sedation, insomnia, hyperbilirubinemia, chronic cholestasis with some of these products. Ultra-short acting barbiturates are used as anesthetics.

Adverse effects: The most common side effects are drowsiness and nausea. Serious adverse reactions such as Stevens-Johnson syndrome and blood dyscrasias may occur with high doses and long-term treatment.

Contraindications: Hypersensitivity may occur, and allergies should be identified before administering. Barbiturates are identified as pregnancy category (D) and should not be used in pregnancy. Other contraindications include porphyria and marked impairment of liver function.

Precautions: Caution must be used when these products are given to G the elderly or debilitated; usually smaller doses are needed, since metabolism is slowed. Persons with renal and hepatic disease may show P delayed excretion. Barbiturates may produce excitability in children.

Pharmacokinetics: Onset of action can be slow, up to 1 hr, with a peak of 8 hr and a duration of 3-10 hr. These drugs are metabolized by the liver, excreted by the kidneys, cross the placenta, and enter breast milk.

Interactions: Increased CNS depressant effect may occur with alcohol, MAOIs, sedatives, or narcotics. These products should be used together cautiously. Oral anticoagulants, corticosteroids, griseofulvin, quinidine, oral contraceptives, and theophylline may show a decreased effect when used with barbiturates.

NURSING CONSIDERATIONS

Assessment

- Monitor hepatic and renal studies: AST (SGOT), ALT (SGPT), bilirubin, creatinine, LDH, alkaline phosphatase, BUN if patient is on long-term therapy, since these products are metabolized and excreted by the liver and kidney
- Monitor blood studies: CBC, hematocrit, hemoglobin, and prothrombin time if patient is on long-term therapy, since these products increase the possibility of bleeding and blood dyscrasias
- Identify barbiturate toxicity: hypotension, pulmonary constriction, cold, clammy skin, cyanosis of lips, insomnia, nausea, vomiting, hallucinations, delirium, weakness

Nursing diagnoses

✓ Sleep pattern disturbance (uses)
✓ Risk for injury (adverse reactions)

Evaluation

- Therapeutic response: appropriate sedation or seizure control

Patient/family education

- Inform patient that physical dependency may result when used for extended periods (45-90 days, depending on dosage)
- Advise patient to avoid driving and activities that require alertness, since drowsiness and dizziness may occur
- Caution patient to abstain from alcohol and other psychotropic medications unless prescribed by prescriber
- Instruct patient not to discontinue medication abruptly after long-term use; withdrawal symptoms will occur

---

Generic Names

amobarbital
pentobarbital
phenobarbital (key)
secobarbital
thiopental

BENZODIAZEPINES

Action: Benzodiazepines potentiate the effects of GABA, including any other inhibitory transmitters in the CNS, resulting in decreased anxiety.

Uses: Anxiety is relieved in conditions such as phobic disorders. Benzodiazepines are also used for acute alcohol withdrawal to relieve the possibility of delirium tremens, and some products are used before surgery for relaxation.

Adverse effects: The most common side effects are dizziness, drowsiness, blurred vision, and orthostatic hypotension. Most adverse effects are mediated through the CNS. There is a risk for physical dependence and abuse.

Contraindications: Hypersensitivity, acute narrow-angle glaucoma, children <6 months, liver disease (clonazepam), lactation (diazepam).

Precautions: Caution must be used when these products are given to the elderly or debilitated; usually smaller dosages are needed, since metabolism is slowed. Persons with renal and hepatic disease may show delayed excretion. Clonazepam may increase incidence of seizures.

Pharmacokinetics: Onset of action is ½-1 hr, with a peak of 1-2 hr and a duration of 4-6 hr. These drugs are metabolized by the liver, excreted by the kidneys, cross the placenta, and enter breast milk.

Interactions: Increased CNS depressant effect may occur with other CNS depressants. These products should be used together cautiously. Alcohol should not be used; fatal reactions can occur. The serum concentration and toxicity of digoxin may be increased.

NURSING CONSIDERATIONS

Assessment

- Monitor B/P (with patient lying, standing), pulse; if systolic B/P drops 20 mm Hg, hold drug, notify prescriber; orthostatic hypotension is severe
- Monitor hepatic and renal studies: AST (SGOT), ALT (SGPT), bilirubin, creatinine, LDH, alkaline phosphatase
- Assess for physical dependency, withdrawal symptoms, including headache, nausea, vomiting, muscle pain, weakness after long-term use

Nursing diagnoses

✓ Anxiety (uses)
✓ Risk for injury (adverse reactions)

Implementation

- Give with food or milk for GI symptoms; may give crushed if patient is unable to swallow medication whole

Evaluation

- Therapeutic response: relaxation or decreased anxiety

Patient/family education

- Teach patient that drug should not be used for everyday stress or long term; not to take more than prescribed amount, since drug is habit forming
- Caution patient to avoid driving and activities that require alertness, since drowsiness and dizziness occur
- Caution patient to abstain from alcohol and other psychotropic medications unless prescribed by prescriber
- Advise patient not to discontinue medication abruptly after long-term use; withdrawal symptoms will occur

---

Generic Names

alprazolam
chlordiazepoxide
clonazepam
diazepam
flurazepam
halazepam
lorazepam
midazolam
oxazepam
prazepam
quazepam
temazepam
triazolam

β-ADRENERGIC BLOCKERS

Action: β-Blockers are divided into selective and nonselective blockers. Nonselective blockers produce a fall in blood pressure without reflex tachycardia or reduction in heart rate through a mixture of β-blocking effects; elevated plasma renins are reduced. Selective β-blockers competitively block stimulation of β_1-receptors in cardiac smooth muscle; these drugs produce chronotropic and inotropic effects.

Uses: β-Blockers are used for hypertension, ventricular dysrhythmias, and prophylaxis of angina pectoris.

Adverse effects: The most common side effects are orthostatic hypotension, bradycardia, diarrhea, nausea, vomiting. Serious adverse reactions include blood dyscrasias, bronchospasm, and CHF.

Contraindications: Hypersensitive reactions may occur, and allergies should be identified before these products are given. β-Adrenergic blockers should not be used in heart block, CHF, or cardiogenic shock.

G **Precautions:** β-Blockers should be used with caution in the elderly or in renal and thyroid disease, COPD, CAD, diabetes mellitus, pregnancy, or asthma.

Pharmacokinetics: Onset, peak, and duration vary widely among products. Most products are metabolized in the liver, with metabolites excreted in urine, bile, and feces.
Interactions: Interactions vary widely among products; check individual monograph for specific information.

NURSING CONSIDERATIONS

Assessment

- Monitor renal studies, including protein, BUN, creatinine; watch for increased levels that may indicate nephrotic syndrome; obtain baselines in renal and liver function studies before beginning treatment
- Monitor I&O, weight daily
- Monitor B/P during beginning treatment and periodically thereafter, pulse q4h; note rate, rhythm, quality
- Monitor apical/radial pulse before administration; notify prescriber of significant changes
- Check for edema in feet and legs daily

Nursing diagnoses

✓ Altered tissue perfusion (uses)
✓ Decreased cardiac output (uses)
✓ Diarrhea (adverse reactions)
✓ Impaired gas exchange (adverse reactions)

Implementation

- Give PO ac, hs; tab may be crushed or swallowed whole
- Give reduced dosage in renal dysfunction

Evaluation

- Therapeutic response: decrease in B/P in hypertension; decreased B/P, edema, moist rales in CHF

Patient/family education

- Instruct patient to comply with dosage schedule, even if feeling better
- Caution patient to rise slowly to sitting or standing position to minimize orthostatic hypotension
- Advise patient to report bradycardia, dizziness, confusion, depression, fever
- Teach patient to take pulse at home; advise when to notify prescriber
- Instruct patient to comply with weight control, dietary adjustment, modified exercise program
- Advise patient to wear support hose to minimize effects of orthostatic hypotension

- Advise patient not to discontinue drug abruptly; taper over 2 wk; may precipitate angina

Generic Names

Selective β_1-receptor blockers:
acebutolol
atenolol
esmolol
metoprolol

Nonselective β_1 and β_2-blockers:
carteolol
nadolol
pindolol
propranolol
timolol

Combined α_1, β_1, and β_2-receptor blocker:
labetalol

BRONCHODILATORS

Action: Bronchodilators are divided into anticholinergics, α/β-adrenergics agonists, β-adrenergic agonists, and phosphodiesterase inhibitors. Anticholinergics act by inhibiting interaction of acetylcholine at receptor sites on bronchial smooth muscle; α/β-adrenergic agonists by relaxing bronchial smooth muscle and increasing diameter of nasal passages; β-adrenergic agonists by action on β_2-receptors, which relaxes bronchial smooth muscle; phosphodiesterase inhibitors by blocking phosphodiesterase and increasing cAMP, which mediates smooth muscle relaxation in the respiratory system.

Uses: Bronchodilators are used for bronchial asthma, bronchospasm associated with bronchitis, emphysema, other obstructive pulmonary diseases, and Cheyne-Stokes respirations, as well as prevention of exercise-induced asthma.

Adverse effects: The most common side effects are tremors, anxiety, nausea, vomiting, and irritation in the throat. The most serious adverse reactions include bronchospasm and dyspnea.

Contraindications: Persons with hypersensitivity, narrow-angle glaucoma, tachydysrhythmias, and severe cardiac disease should not use some of these products.

Precautions: Bronchodilators should be used with caution in lactation, pregnancy, hyperthyroidism, hypertension, prostatic hypertrophy, and seizure disorders.

Pharmacokinetics: Onset, peak, and duration vary widely among products. Most products are metabolized in the liver and excreted in urine.

Interactions: Please check individual monographs, since interactions vary widely among products.

NURSING CONSIDERATIONS

Assessment

- Monitor respiratory function: vital capacity, FEV, ABGs, lung sounds, heart rate and rhythm

Nursing diagnoses

✓ Ineffective airway clearance (uses)
✓ Activity intolerance (uses)
✓ Risk for injury (adverse reactions)
✓ Knowledge deficit (teaching)

Implementation

- Give after shaking; exhale, place mouthpiece in mouth, inhale slowly, hold breath, remove, exhale slowly
- Give gum, sips of water for dry mouth
- Give PO with meals to decrease gastric irritation
- Store in light-resistant container; do not expose to temp over 86° F

Evaluation

- Therapeutic response: absence of dyspnea, wheezing

Patient/family education

- Advise patient not to use OTC medications; extra stimulation may occur
- Teach patient use of inhaler; review package insert with patient; to wash inhaler in warm water qd and dry
- Advise patient to avoid getting aerosol in eyes
- Caution patient to avoid smoking, smoke-filled rooms, persons with respiratory tract infections

---

Generic Names

albuterol
aminophylline
atropine
bitolterol
dyphylline
ephedrine
epinephrine
ipratropium
isoproterenol
metaproterenol
oxtriphylline
pirbuterol
terbutaline
theophylline

CALCIUM CHANNEL BLOCKERS

Action: These products inhibit calcium ion influx across the cell membrane in cardiac and vascular smooth muscle. This action produces relaxation of coronary vascular smooth muscle, dilates coronary arteries, slows SA/AV node conduction, and dilates peripheral arteries.

Uses: These products are used for chronic stable angina pectoris, vasospastic angina, dysrhythmias, hypertension, and unstable angina.

Adverse effects: The most common side effects are dysrhythmias and edema. Also common are headache, fatigue, drowsiness, and flushing.

Contraindications: Persons with 2nd- or 3rd-degree heart block, sick sinus syndrome, hypotension of <90 mm Hg systolic, Wolff-Parkinson-White syndrome, or cardiogenic shock should not use these products, since worsening of those conditions may occur.

Precautions: CHF may worsen, since edema may be increased. Hypotension may worsen, since B/P is decreased. Patients with renal and liver disease should use these products cautiously, since they are metabolized in the liver and excreted by the kidneys.

Pharmacokinetics: Onset, peak, and duration vary widely with route of administration. Drugs are metabolized by the liver and excreted in the urine primarily as metabolites.

Interactions: Increased levels of digoxin and theophylline may occur when used with these products. Increased effects of β-blockers and antihypertensives may occur with calcium channel blockers.

NURSING CONSIDERATIONS

Assessment

- Monitor cardiac system, including B/P, pulse, respirations, ECG intervals (PR, QRS, QT)

Nursing diagnoses

✓ Altered tissue perfusion: cardiopulmonary (uses)
✓ Decreased cardiac output (adverse reactions)

Implementation

- Give PO ac and hs

Evaluation

- Therapeutic response: decreased anginal pain, decreased B/P, dysrhythmias

Patient/family education

- Teach patient how to take pulse before taking drug; patient should record or graph pulses to identify changes

- Advise patient to avoid hazardous activities until stabilized on this drug, since dizziness occurs frequently
- Inform patient of need for compliance to all areas of medical regimen, including diet, exercise, stress reduction, drug therapy

---

Generic Names

amlodipine
bepridil
diltiazem
felodipine
isradipine
nicardipine
nifedipine
verapamil

CARDIAC GLYCOSIDES

Action: Products act by inhibiting sodium and potassium ATPase and then making more calcium available to activate contracted proteins. Cardiac contractility and cardiac output are increased.

Uses: These products are used for CHF, atrial fibrillation, atrial flutter, atrial tachycardia, and rapid digitalization in these disorders.

Adverse effects: The most common side effects are cardiac disturbances, headache, hypotension, GI symptoms. Also common are blurred vision and yellow-green halos.

Contraindications: Hypersensitive reactions may occur, and allergies should be identified before these products are given. Also, persons with ventricular tachycardia, ventricular fibrillation, and carotid sinus syndrome should not use these products.

Precautions: Persons with acute MI and those who have or may develop serum potassium, calcium, or magnesium imbalances should use these products cautiously. Also, persons with AV block, severe respiratory disease, hypothyroidism, renal and liver disease, and the elderly should exercise caution when these drugs are prescribed.

Pharmacokinetics: Onset, peak, and duration vary widely with the route of administration. Digitoxin is inactivated by the liver, and inactive metabolites are excreted in urine. Digoxin is excreted in urine mainly as the parent drug and metabolites.

Interactions: Toxicity may occur when used with diuretics, succinylcholine, quinidine, and thioamines. Increased blood levels may occur with propantheline bromide, spironolactone, quinidine, verapamil, aminoglycosides (PO), amiodarone, anticholinergics, and quinine. Diuretics may increase toxicity.

NURSING CONSIDERATIONS

Assessment

- Montior cardiac system, including B/P, pulse, respirations, and increased urine output
- Monitor apical pulse for 1 min before giving drug; if pulse <60, take again in 1 hr; if <60 notify prescriber
- Monitor electrolytes, including potassium, sodium, chloride, calcium, magnesium; renal function studies, including BUN and creatinine; and blood studies, including AST (SGOT), ALT (SGPT), bilirubin
- Monitor I&O ratio, daily weights
- Monitor therapeutic drug levels

Nursing diagnoses

✓ Altered tissue perfusion: cardiopulmonary (uses)
✓ Decreased cardiac output (adverse reactions)

Implementation

- Give potassium supplements if ordered for potassium levels <3

Evaluation

- Therapeutic response: decreased weight, edema, pulse, respiration, and increased urine output

Patient/family education

- Teach patient how to take pulse before taking drug; patient should record or graph pulse to identify changes
- Advise patient to avoid hazardous activities until stabilized on this drug, since dizziness occurs frequently
- Inform patient of need for compliance to all areas of medical regimen, including diet, exercise, stress reduction, drug therapy

---

Generic Names

digitoxin
🔑 digoxin

CHOLINERGICS

Action: Cholinergics act by preventing destruction of acetylcholine, which increases concentration at sites where acetylcholine is released; this exaggerates the effects of acetylcholine and facilitates transmission of impulses across myoneural junction. Cholinergics may also act by stimulating receptors for acetylcholine.

Uses: Cholinergics are used for myasthenia gravis, as antagonists of nondepolarizing neuromuscular blockade, postoperative bladder distention and urinary distention, postoperative ileus.

Adverse effects: The most serious adverse reactions are respiratory depression, bronchospasm, constriction, laryngospasm, respiratory arrest, convulsions, and paralysis. The most common side effects are nausea, diarrhea, and vomiting.

Contraindications: Persons with obstruction of the intestine or renal system should not use these products.

Precautions: Caution should be used in patients with bradycardia, hypotension, seizure disorders, bronchial asthma, coronary occlusion, hyperthyroidism, and in lactation and children.

Pharmacokinetics: Onset, peak, and duration vary widely among products. Most products are metabolized in the liver and excreted in urine.

Interactions: Please check individual monographs since interactions vary widely among products.

NURSING CONSIDERATIONS

Assessment

- Monitor VS, respiration q8h
- Monitor I&O ratio; check for urinary retention or incontinence
- Assess for bradycardia, hypotension, bronchospasm, headache, dizziness, convulsions, respiratory depression; drug should be discontinued if toxicity occurs

Nursing diagnoses

✓ Altered urinary elimination (uses)
✓ Ineffective breathing pattern (uses)
✓ Knowledge deficit (teaching)
✓ Noncompliance (teaching)

Implementation

- Give only with atropine sulfate available for cholinergic crisis
- Give only after all other cholinergics have been discontinued
- Give increased dosages if tolerance occurs
- Give larger doses after exercise or fatigue
- Give on empty stomach for better absorption
- Store at room temp

Evaluation

- Therapeutic response: increased muscle strength, hand grasp, improved muscle gait, absence of labored breathing (if severe)

Patient/family education

- Inform patient that drug is not a cure; it only relieves symptoms (myasthenia gravis)
- Advise patient to wear Medic Alert ID specifying myasthenia gravis, drugs taken

Generic Names

bethanechol
edrophonium
neostigmine
physostigmine
pyridostigmine

CHOLINERGIC BLOCKERS

Action: Cholinergic blockers inhibit or block acetylcholine at receptor sites in the autonomic nervous system.

Uses: Many products are used to decrease secretions before surgery, to reverse neuromuscular blockade, and to decrease motility of GI, biliary, urinary tracts. Other products are used for parkinsonian symptoms, including dystonia associated with neuroleptic drugs.

Adverse effects: The most common side effects are dryness of the mouth and constipation, which can be prevented by frequent rinsing of the mouth and increasing water and bulk in the diet.

Contraindications: Hypersensitivity can occur, and allergies should be identified before administering these products. Persons with GI and GU obstruction should not use these products, since constipation and urinary retention may occur. They are also contraindicated in angle closure glaucoma and myasthenia gravis.

Precautions: Caution must be used when these products are given to G the elderly, since metabolism is slowed. Also, persons with tachycardia or prostatic hypertrophy should use these products with caution.

Pharmacokinetics: Onset, peak, and duration vary with route.

Interactions: Increase in anticholinergic effect occurs when used with narcotics, barbiturates, antihistamines, MAOIs, phenothiazines, amantadine.

NURSING CONSIDERATIONS

Assessment

- Assess I&O ratio; be alert for urinary retention, frequency, dysuria; drug should be discontinued if these occur
- Assess urinary hesitancy, retention; palpate bladder if retention occurs
- Assess constipation; increase fluids, bulk, exercise
- Assess for tolerance over long-term therapy; dosage may need to be changed
- Assess mental status: affect, mood, CNS depression, worsening of mental symptoms during early therapy

Nursing diagnoses

✓ Impaired physical mobility (uses)
✓ Pain (uses)

Implementation

- Give with food or milk to decrease GI symptoms
- Give parenteral dose with patient recumbent to prevent postural hypotension; give dose slowly, monitoring VS
- Give hard candy, gum, frequent rinsing of mouth for dryness

Evaluation

- Therapeutic response: absence of cramps, absence of EPS

Patient/family education

- Caution patient to avoid driving and other hazardous activity if drowsiness occurs
- Advise patient to avoid concurrent use of cough, cold preparations with alcohol, antihistamines unless directed by prescriber
- Caution patient to use with caution in hot weather, since medication may increase susceptibility to heat stroke

---

Generic Names

atropine
benztropine
biperiden
glycopyrrolate
scopolamine
trihexyphenidyl

CORTICOSTEROIDS

Action: Corticosteroids are divided into glucocorticoids and mineralocorticoids. Glucocorticoids decrease inflammation by the suppression of migration of polymorphonuclear leukocytes, fibroblasts, increased capillary permeability, and lysosomal stabilization. They also have varied metabolic effects and modify the body's immune responses to many different stimuli. Mineralocorticoids act by increasing resorption of sodium by increasing hydrogen and potassium excretion in the distal tubule.

Uses: Glucocorticoids are used to decrease inflammation and for immunosuppression. In addition, some products may be given for allergy, adrenal insufficiency, or cerebral edema. Mineralocorticoids are given for adrenal insufficiency or adrenogenital syndrome.

Adverse effects: The most common side effects include change in behavior, including insomnia and euphoria; GI irritation, including peptic ulcer; metabolic reactions; including hypokalemia, hyperglycemia, and carbohydrate intolerance; and sodium and fluid retention. Most adverse reactions are dose dependent.

Contraindications: Hypersensitivity may occur and should be identified before administering. Since these products mask infection, they should not be used in systemic fungal infections or amebiasis. Mothers taking pharmacologic doses of corticosteroids should not nurse.

Precautions: Caution must be used when these products are prescribed for diabetic patients, since hyperglycemia may occur. Also, patients with glaucoma, seizure disorders, peptic ulcer, impaired renal function, CHF, hypertension, ulcerative colitis, or myasthenia gravis
P should be monitored closely if corticosteroids are given. Use with
G caution in children and the elderly and during pregnancy.

Pharmacokinetics: For oral preparations the onset of action occurs between 1-2 hr, and duration can be up to 2 days, with a half-life of 2-4 days. Pharmacokinetics vary widely among products. These products cross the placenta and appear in breast milk.

Interactions: Decreased corticosteroid effect may occur with barbiturates, rifampin, phenytoin; corticosteroid dosage may need to be increased. There is a possibility of GI bleeding when used with salicylates, indomethacin. Steroids may reduce salicylate levels. When using with digitalis glycosides, potassium-depleting diuretics, and amphotericin, serum potassium levels should be monitored.

NURSING CONSIDERATIONS

Assessment

- Monitor potassium, blood sugar, urine glucose while on long-term therapy; hypokalemia and hyperglycemia are common
- Monitor weight daily; notify prescriber if weekly gain of >5 lb, since these products alter fluid and electrolyte balance
- Assess for potassium depletion, including paresthesias, fatigue, nausea, vomiting, depression, polyuria, dysrhythmias, weakness
- Assess for mental status, including affect, mood, behavioral changes, aggression; if severe personality changes occur, including depression, drug may need to be tapered and then discontinued
- Monitor I&O ratio; be alert for decreasing urinary output and increasing edema
- Monitor plasma cortisol levels during long-term therapy (normal level is 138-635 nmol/L when drawn at 8 AM)
- Assess for infection, including increased temp, WBC, even after withdrawal of medication; drug masks symptoms of infection
- Assess for adrenal insufficiency: nausea, anorexia, fatigue, dizziness, dyspnea, weakness, joint pain

Nursing diagnoses

- ✓ Risk for infection (adverse reactions)
- ✓ Body image disturbance (adverse reactions)
- ✓ Risk for violence: self-directed (suicide) (adverse reactions)

Implementation

- Give with food or milk to decrease GI symptoms

Evaluation

- Therapeutic response: decreased inflammation

Patient/family education

- Advise patient that ID as steroid user should be carried
- Advise patient not to discontinue this medication abruptly or adrenal crisis can result
- Teach patient all aspects of drug use, including cushingoid symptoms
- Instruct patient that single daily or alternate-day doses should be taken in the morning before 9 AM (for replacement therapy)
- Instruct patient to take with meals or a snack

Generic Names

Glucocorticoids:
beclomethasone
betamethasone
cortisone
flunisolide
hydrocortisone
methylprednisolone
prednisolone
prednisone (key drug)
triamcinolone

Mineralocorticoid:
fludrocortisone

DIURETICS

Action: Diuretics are divided into subgroups: thiazides and thiazide-like diuretics, loop diuretics, carbonic anhydrase inhibitors, osmotic diuretics, and potassium-sparing diuretics. Each one of these subgroups differs in its mechanism of action. Thiazides and thiazide-like diuretics increase excretion of water and sodium by inhibiting resorption in the early distal tubule. Loop diuretics inhibit resorption of sodium and chloride in the thick ascending limb of the loop of Henle. Carbonic anhydrase inhibitors increase sodium excretion by decreasing sodium-hydrogen ion exchange throughout the renal tubule. Carbonic anhydrase inhibitors also decrease secretion of aqueous humor in the eye and thus decrease intraocular pressure. Osmotic diuretics increase the osmotic pressure of glomerular filtrate, thus decreasing net absorption of sodium. The potassium-sparing diuretics interfere with sodium resorption at the distal tubule, thus decreasing potassium excretion.

Uses: Blood pressure is reduced in hypertension; edema is reduced in CHF; intraocular pressure is decreased in glaucoma.

Adverse effects: Hypokalemia, hyperuricemia, and hyperglycemia occur most frequently with thiazide diuretics. Aplastic anemia, blood dyscrasias, volume depletion, and dehydration may occur when thiazide-like diuretics, loop diuretics, or carbonic anhydrase inhibitors are given. Side effects and adverse reactions vary widely for the miscellaneous products.

Contraindications: Persons with electrolyte imbalances (sodium, chloride, potassium), dehydration, or anuria should not be given these products until the problem is corrected.

G **Precautions:** Caution must be used when diuretics are given to the elderly, since electrolyte disturbances and dehydration can occur rapidly. Hepatic and renal disorders may cause poor metabolism and excretion of the drug.

Pharmacokinetics: Onset, peak, and duration vary widely among the different subgroups of these drugs.

Interactions: Cholestyramine and colestipol decrease the absorption of thiazide diuretics. Concurrent use of thiazides with diazoxide may increase hyperuricemia, hyperglycemia, and antihypertensive effects of thiazides. Ototoxicity may occur when loop diuretics are used with aminoglycosides. Thiazide and loop diuretics may increase therapeutic and toxic effects of lithium.

NURSING CONSIDERATIONS

Assessment

- Monitor weight, I&O daily to determine fluid loss; check skin turgor for dehydration
- Monitor electrolytes: potassium, sodium, chloride: include BUN, blood sugar, CBC, serum creatinine, blood pH, ABGs, uric acid, calcium; electrolyte imbalances may occur quickly
- Monitor B/P with patient lying, standing; postural hypotension may occur, since fluid loss occurs from intravascular spaces first
- Assess for signs of metabolic alkalosis, including drowsiness and restlessness
- Assess for signs of hypokalemia with some products, including postural hypotension, malaise, fatigue, tachycardia, leg cramps, weakness

Nursing diagnoses

- ✓ Fluid volume excess (uses)
- ✓ Decreased cardiac output (adverse reactions)

Implementation

- Give in AM to avoid interference with sleep if using drug as a diuretic
- Give potassium replacement if potassium is less than 3

Evaluation

- Therapeutic reponse: improvement in edema of feet, legs, sacral area daily if medication is being used in CHF; improvement in B/P if medication is being used as a diuretic; improvement in intraocular pressure if medication is being used to decrease aqueous humor in the eye

Patient/family education

- Teach patient to take drug early in the day (diuretic) to prevent nocturia

---

Generic Names

Thiazides:
hydrochlorothiazide

Thiazide-like:
chlorthalidone
indapamide
metolazone

Loop:
bumetanide
furosemide

Carbonic anhydrase inhibitors:
acetazolamide

Potassium-sparing:
amiloride
spironolactone
triamterene

Osmotic:
mannitol

HISTAMINE H_2 ANTAGONISTS

Action: Histamine H_2 antagonists act by inhibiting histamine at H_2 receptor site in parietal cells, which inhibits gastric acid secretion.
Uses: Histamine H_2 antagonists are used for short-term treatment of duodenal and gastric ulcers and maintenance therapy for duodenal ulcer; and for gastroesophageal reflux disease.
Adverse effects: The most serious adverse reactions are agranulocytosis, thrombocytopenia, neutropenia, aplastic anemia, exfoliative dermatitis. The most common side effects are confusion (not with rantidine), headache and diarrhea.

Contraindications: Persons with hypersensitivity should not use these products.

P **Precautions:** Caution should be used in pregnancy, lactation, children <16 yr, organic brain syndrome, hepatic disease, renal disease.

Pharmacokinetics: Onset, peak, and duration vary widely among products. Most products are metabolized in the liver and excreted in urine.

Interactions: Antacids interfere with absorption of histamine H_2 antagonists. Check individual monographs for other interactions.

NURSING CONSIDERATIONS

Assessment

- Monitor gastric pH (>5 should be maintained)
- Monitor I&O ratio, BUN, creatinine

Nursing diagnoses

✓ Pain (uses)
✓ Risk for injury (bleeding)
✓ Knowledge deficit (teaching)

Implementation

- Give with meals for prolonged drug effect
- Give antacids 1 hr before or 1 hr after cimetidine
- Give **IV** slowly; bradycardia may occur; give over 30 min
- Store diluted sol at room temp for up to 48 hr

Evaluation

- Therapeutic response: decreaed pain in abdomen

Patient/family education

- Advise patient that gynecomastia, impotence may occur, but is reversible
- Caution patient to avoid driving and other hazardous activities until patient is stabilized on this medication
- Caution patient to avoid black pepper, caffeine, alcohol, harsh spices, extremes in temp of food
- Caution patient to avoid OTC preparations: aspirin, cough, cold preparations
- Inform patient that drug must be continued for prescribed time to be effective
- Advise patient to report bruising, fatigue, malaise; blood dyscrasias may occur

---

Generic Names

cimetidine
famotidine
ranitidine

IMMUNOSUPPRESSANTS

Action: Immunosuppressants produce immunosuppression by inhibiting T lymphocytes.

Uses: Most products are used for organ transplants to prevent rejection.

Adverse effects: The most serious adverse reactions are albuminuria, hematuria, proteinuria, renal failure, and hepatotoxicity. The most common side effects are oral *Candida* infection, gum hyperplasia, tremors, and headache. The most serious adverse reactions for azathioprine are hematologic (leukopenia and thrombocytopenia) and GI (nausea and vomiting). There is a risk of secondary infection.

Contraindications: Products are contraindicated in hypersensitivity.

Precautions: Caution should be used in severe renal disease, severe hepatic disease, and pregnancy.

Pharmacokinetics: Onset, peak, and duration vary widely among products. Most products are metabolized in the liver and excreted in urine.

Interactions: Please check individual monographs, since interactions vary widely among products.

NURSING CONSIDERATIONS

Assessment

- Monitor renal studies: BUN, creatinine at least monthly during treatment, 3 mo after treatment
- Monitor liver function studies: alkaline phosphatase, AST (SGOT), ALT (SGPT), bilirubin
- Monitor drug blood levels during treatment
- Assess for hepatotoxicity: dark urine, jaundice, itching, light-colored stools; drug should be discontinued

Nursing diagnoses

- ✓ Risk for infection (adverse reactions)
- ✓ Risk for injury (uses)
- ✓ Knowledge deficit (teaching)

Implementation

- Give for several days before transplant surgery
- Give with meals for GI upset or place drug in chocolate milk
- Give with oral antifungal for *Candida* infections

Evaluation

- Therapeutic response: absence of rejection

Patient/family education

- Advise patient to report fever, chills, sore throat, fatigue, since serious infections may occur
- Caution patient to use contraceptive measures during treatment and for 12 wk after ending therapy

---

Generic Names

azathioprine
cyclophosphamide
cyclosporine
methotrexate
muromonab-CD3

LAXATIVES

Action: Laxatives are divided into bulk products, lubricants, osmotics, saline laxative stimulants, and stool softeners. Bulks work by absorbing water and expanding to increase moisture content and bulk in the stool. Lubricants increase water retention in the stool, causing reabsorption of water in the bowel. Stimulants act by increasing peristalsis by direct effect on the intestine. Saline draws water into the intestinal lumen. Osmotics increase distention and promote peristalsis. Stool softeners reduce surface tension of liq in the bowel.
Uses: Laxatives are used as a preparation for bowel, rectal examination, constipation, or as stool softeners.
Adverse effects: The most common side effects are nausea, abdominal cramps, and diarrhea.
Contraindications: Persons with GI obstruction, perforation, gastric retention, toxic colitis, megacolon, abdominal pain, nausea, vomiting, and fecal impaction should not use these products.
Precautions: Caution should be used in rectal bleeding, large hemorrhoids, and anal excoriation.
Pharmacokinetics: Onset, peak, and duration vary among products.
Interactions: Please check individual monographs, since interactions vary widely among products.

NURSING CONSIDERATIONS

Assessment

- Monitor blood, urine electrolytes if drug is used often by patient
- Monitor I&O ratio: to identify fluid loss
- Determine cause of constipation; identify whether fluids, bulk, or exercise is missing from lifestyle
- Assess for cramping, rectal bleeding, nausea, vomiting; if these symptoms occur, drug should be discontinued

Nursing diagnoses

- ✓ Constipation (uses)
- ✓ Diarrhea (adverse reactions)
- ✓ Knowledge deficit (teaching)

Implementation

- Give alone only with water for better absorption; do not take within 1 hr of antacids, milk, or cimetidine

Evaluation

- Therapeutic response: decrease in constipation

Patient/family education

- Teach patient to swallow tab whole; do not chew
- Caution patient not to use laxatives for long-term therapy; bowel tone will be lost; that normal bowel movements do not always occur daily
- Caution patient not to use in presence of abdominal pain, nausea, vomiting
- Advise patient to notify prescriber of abdominal pain, nausea, vomiting
- Advise patient to notify prescriber if constipation is unrelieved or if symptoms of electrolyte imbalance occur: muscle cramps, pain, weakness, dizziness

---

Generic Names

Bulk laxative:
psyllium

Osmotic agents:
glycerin
lactulose

Saline:
magnesium salts
sodium phosphate/biphosphate

Stimulants:
bisacodyl
cascara
phenolphthalein
senna

Stool softeners:
docusate

OPIOID ANALGESICS

Action: These agents depress pain impulse transmission at the spinal cord level by interacting with opioid receptors. Products are divided into opiates and nonopiates.

Uses: Most products are used to control moderate to severe pain and are used before and after surgery.

Adverse effects: GI symptoms, including nausea, vomiting, anorexia, constipation, and cramps are the most common side effects. Other common side effects include lightheadedness, dizziness, sedation. Serious adverse reactions such as respiratory depression, respiratory arrest, circulatory depression, and increased intracranial pressure may result, but are less common and usually dose dependent.
Contraindications: Hypersensitive reactions occur frequently. Check for sensitivity before administering. These drugs should not be used if narcotic addiction is suspected, and they are also contraindicated in acute bronchial asthma and upper airway obstruction.
Precautions: Caution must be used when these products are given to persons with an addictive personality, since the possibility of addiction is so great. Also, persons with increased intracranial pressure may experience an even greater increase in intracranial pressure. Persons with severe heart disease, hepatic or renal disease, respiratory conditions, and seizure disorders should be monitored closely for worsening condition.
Pharmacokinetics: Onset of action is immediate by **IV** route and rapid by IM and PO routes. Peak occurs from 1-2 hr, depending on route, with a duration of 2-8 hr. These agents cross the placenta and appear in breast milk.
Interactions: Barbiturates, other narcotics, hypnotics, antipsychotics, or alcohol can increase CNS depression when taken with narcotics.

NURSING CONSIDERATIONS

Assessment

- Monitor I&O ratio; be alert for urinary retention, frequency, dysuria; drug should be discontinued if these occur
- Assess for respiratory dysfunction, including respiratory depression, rate, rhythm, character; notify prescriber if respirations are <12/min
- Assess for CNS changes: dizziness, drowsiness, hallucinations, euphoria, LOC, pupil reaction
- Assess for allergic reactions: rash, urticaria
- Assess for need for pain medication, use pain scoring

Nursing diagnoses

✓ Pain (uses)
✓ Impaired gas exchange (adverse reactions)

Implementation

- Give with antiemetic if nausea or vomiting occurs
- Give when pain is beginning to return; determine dosage interval by patient response

- Provide assistance with ambulation; patient should not be ambulating during drug peak

Evaluation

- Therapeutic response: decrease in pain

Patient/family education

- Advise patient to report any symptoms of CNS changes, allergic reactions, or shortness of breath
- Caution patient that physical dependency may result when used for extended periods
- Teach patient that withdrawal symptoms may occur, including nausea, vomiting, cramps, fever, faintness, anorexia
- Advise patient to avoid alcohol and other CNS depressants

Generic Names

alfentanil
buprenorphine
butorphanol
codeine
fentanyl
fentanyl transdermal
hydromorphone
levorphanol tartrate
meperidine
methadone HCl
morphine
oxycodone
oxymorphone
pentazocine
propoxyphene
remifentanil
sufentanil

NEUROMUSCULAR BLOCKING AGENTS

Action: Neuromuscular blocking agents are divided into depolarizing and nondepolarizing blockers. They act by inhibiting transmission of nerve impulses by binding with cholinergic receptor sites.

Uses: Neuromuscular blocking agents are used to facilitate endotracheal intubation and skeletal muscle relaxation during mechanical ventilation, surgery, or general anesthesia.

Adverse effects: The most serious adverse reactions are prolonged apnea, bronchospasm, cyanosis, respiratory depression, and malignant hyperthermia. The most common side effects are bradycardia and decreased motility.

Contraindications: Persons that are hypersensitive should not be given this product.

Precautions: Caution should be used in pregnancy, thyroid disease, collagen disease, cardiac disease, lactation, children <2 yr, electrolyte imbalances, dehydration, neuromuscular disease (myasthenia gravis), and respiratory disease.

Pharmacokinetics: Onset, peak, and duration vary widely among products. Most products are metabolized in the liver and excreted in urine.

Interactions: Aminoglycosides potentiate neuromuscular blockade. See individual monographs.

NURSING CONSIDERATIONS

Assessment

- Monitor for electrolyte imbalances (potassium, magnesium); may lead to increased action of this drug
- Monitor VS (B/P, pulse, respirations, airway) q15 min until fully recovered; rate, depth, pattern of respirations, strength of hand grip
- Monitor I&O ratio; check for urinary retention, frequency, hesitancy
- Assess for recovery: decreased paralysis of face, diaphragm, leg, arm, rest of body
- Assess for allergic reactions: rash, fever, respiratory distress, pruritus; drug should be discontinued

Nursing diagnoses

- ✓ Ineffective breathing pattern (uses)
- ✓ Risk for injury (adverse reactions)
- ✓ Knowledge deficit (teaching)

Implementation

- Administer using nerve stimulator by anesthesiologist to determine neuromuscular blockade
- Administer anticholinesterase to reverse neuromuscular blockade
- Administer **IV** undiluted over 1-2 min (only by qualified person, usually an anesthesiologist)
- Store in light-resistant, cool area
- Reassure if communication is difficult during recovery from neuromuscular blockade

Evaluation

- Therapeutic response: paralysis of jaw, eyelid, head, neck, rest of body

---

Generic Names

atracurium
cisatracurium
doxacurium
gallamine
metocurine
mivacurium
pancuronium
pipecuronium
succinylcholine
🔑 tubocurarine
vecuronium

NONSTEROIDAL ANTIINFLAMMATORIES

Action: Nonsteroidals decrease prostaglandin synthesis by inhibiting an enzyme needed for biosynthesis.

Uses: Nonsteroidal antiinflammatories are used to treat mild to moderate pain, osteoarthritis, rheumatoid arthritis, and dysmenorrhea.

Adverse effects: The most serious adverse reactions are nephrotoxicity (dysuria, hematuria, oliguria, azotemia), blood dyscrasias, and cholestatic hepatitis. The most common side effects are nausea, abdominal pain, anorexia, dizziness, and drowsiness.

Contraindications: Persons with hypersensitivity, asthma, severe renal disease, and severe hepatic disease should not use these products.

P **Precautions:** Caution should be used in pregnancy, lactation, children, bleeding disorders, GI disorders, cardiac disorders, hypersensitivity to other antiinflammatory agents, and the elderly. G

Pharmacokinetics: Onset, peak, and duration vary widely among products. Most products are metabolized in the liver and excreted in urine.

Interactions: Please check individual monographs, since interactions vary widely among products.

NURSING CONSIDERATIONS

Assessment

- Monitor renal, liver, blood studies: BUN, creatinine, AST (SGOT), ALT (SGPT), Hgb, before treatment, periodically thereafter
- Monitor audiometric, ophth examination before, during, and after treatment.
- Check for eye, ear problems: blurred vision, tinnitus, may indicate toxicity

Nursing diagnoses

✓ Chronic pain (uses)
✓ Impaired physical mobility (uses)
✓ Knowledge deficit (teaching)
✓ Noncompliance (teaching)

Implementation

- Give with food to decrease GI symptoms; however, best to take on empty stomach to facilitate absorption
- Store at room temp

Evaluation

- Therapeutic response: decreased pain, stiffness in joints, decreased swelling in joints, ability to move more easily

Patient/family education

- Advise patient to report blurred vision, ringing, roaring in ears; may indicate toxicity
- Caution patient to avoid driving, other hazardous activities if G dizziness, drowsiness occurs, especially elderly
- Advise patient to report change in urine pattern, increased weight, edema, increased pain in joints, fever, blood in urine; indicate nephrotoxicity
- Inform patient that therapeutic effects may take up to 1 mo

---

Generic Names

diclofenac	ketorolac
etodolic acid	meclofenamate
fenoprofen	nabumetone
flurbiprofen	naproxen
ibuprofen	piroxicam
indomethacin	sulindac
ketoprofen	tolmetin

SALICYLATES

Action: Salicylates have analgesic, antipyretic, and antiinflammatory effects. The antiinflammatory and analgesic activities may be mediated through the inhibition of prostaglandin synthesis. Antipyretic action results from inhibition of the hypothalamic heat-regulating center.

Uses: The primary uses of salicylates are relief of mild to moderate pain and fever and in inflammatory conditions such as arthritis, thromboembolic disorders, and rheumatic fever.

Adverse effects: The most common side effects are GI symptoms and rash. Serious blood dyscrasias and hepatotoxicity may result when used for long periods at high doses. Tinnitus or impaired hearing may indicate that blood salicylate levels are reaching or exceeding the upper limit of the therapeutic range.

Contraindications: Hypersensitivity to salicylates is common. Check for sensitivity before administering. Persons with bleeding disorders, GI bleeding, and vitamin K deficiency should not use these products, P since salicylates increase prothrombin time. Children should not use these products, since salicylates have been associated with Reye's syndrome.

Precautions: Caution is needed when salicylates are given to patients with anemia, hepatic or renal disease, or Hodgkin's disease. Caution should also be exercised in pregnancy and lactation.

Pharmacokinetics: Onset of action occurs in 15-30 min, with a peak of 1-2 hr and a duration up to 6 hr. These drugs are metabolized by the liver and excreted by the kidneys.

Interactions: Increased effects of anticoagulants, insulin, methotrexate, heparin, valproic acid, and oral sulfonylureas may occur when used with salicylates. Aspirin may decrease serum concentrations of nonsteroidal antiinflammatory agents.

NURSING CONSIDERATIONS

Assessment

- Monitor hepatic and renal studies: AST (SGOT), ALT (SGPT), bilirubin, creatinine, LDH, alkaline phosphatase, BUN if patient is on long-term therapy, since these products are metabolized and excreted by the liver and kidney
- Monitor blood studies: CBC, Hct, Hgb, and prothrombin time if patient is on long-term therapy, since these products increase the possibility of bleeding and blood dyscrasias
- Assess for hepatotoxicity; dark urine, clay-colored stools, yellowing skin and sclera, itching, abdominal pain, fever, diarrhea, which may occur with long-term use
- Assess for ototoxicity: tinnitus, ringing, roaring in ears; audiometric testing is needed before and after long-term therapy

Nursing diagnoses

✓ Pain (uses)
✓ Impaired physical mobility (uses)
✓ Activity intolerance (uses)
✓ Sensory-perceptual alteration: auditory (adverse reactions)
✓ Thermoregulation (uses)

Implementation

- Give with food or milk to decrease gastric irritation; give 30 min ac or 1 hr pc with a full glass of water

Evaluation

- Therapeutic response: decreased pain, fever

Patient/family education

- Advise patient that blood sugar levels should be monitored closely, if patient is diabetic
- Caution patient not to exceed recommended dosage; acute poisoning may result
- Inform patient that therapeutic response takes 2 wk in arthritis
- Caution patient to avoid use of alcohol, since GI bleeding may result

- Advise patient to notify prescriber if ringing in the ears or persistent GI pain occurs
- Advise patient to take with full glass of water to reduce risk of lodging in esophagus

---

Generic Names

aspirin	magnesium salicylate
choline salicylate	salsalate

THROMBOLYTICS

Action: Thrombolytics activate conversion of plasminogen to plasmin (fibrinolysin): plasmin is able to break down clots (fibrin).

Uses: Thrombolytics are used to treat deep vein thrombosis, pulmonary embolism, arterial thrombosis, arterial embolism, arteriovenous cannula occlusion, lysis of coronary artery thrombi after MI, acute evolving transmural MI.

Adverse effects: Serious adverse reactions include GI, GU, intracranial, and retroperitoneal bleeding, and anaphylaxis. The most common side effects are decreased Hct, urticaria, headache, and nausea.

Contraindications: Persons with hypersensitivity, active bleeding, intraspinal surgery, neoplasms of the CNS, ulcerative colitis/enteritis, severe hypertension, renal disease, hepatic disease, hypocoagulation, COPD, subacute bacterial endocarditis, rheumatic valvular disease, cerebral embolism/thrombosis/hemorrhage, intraarterial diagnostic procedure or surgery (10 days), and recent major surgery should not use these products.

Precautions: Caution should be used in arterial emboli from left side of heart and pregnancy.

Pharmacokinetics: Onset, peak, and duration vary widely among products. Most products are metabolized in the liver and excreted in urine.

Interactions: Please check individual monographs, since interactions vary widely among products.

NURSING CONSIDERATIONS

Assessment

- Monitor VS, B/P, pulse, respirations, neurologic signs, temp at least q4h, temp is an indicator of internal bleeding, cardiac rhythm following intracoronary administration; systolic pressure increase of >25 mm Hg should be reported to prescriber
- Assess for neurologic changes that may indicate intracranial bleeding

- Assess retroperitoneal bleeding: back pain, leg weakness, diminished pulses
- Assess for allergy: fever, rash, itching, chill; mild reaction may be treated with antihistamines
- Assess for bleeding during 1st hr of treatment: hematuria, hematemesis, bleeding from mucous membranes, epistaxis, ecchymosis
- Monitor blood studies (Hct, platelets, PTT, PT, TT, APTT) before starting therapy; PT or APTT must be less than 2 times control before starting therapy TT or PT q3-4h during treatment

Nursing diagnoses

✓ Risk for injury (uses)

Implementation

- Administer as soon as thrombi identified; not useful for thrombi over 1 wk old
- Administer cryoprecipitate or fresh, frozen plasma if bleeding occurs
- Administer loading dose at beginning of therapy; may require increased loading doses
- Give heparin after fibrinogen level is over 100 mg/dl; heparin inf to increase PTT to 1.5-2 times baseline for 3-7 days
- About 10% of patients have high streptococcal antibody titers requiring increased loading doses
- Give **IV** therapy using 0.8-μm filter
- Store reconstituted sol in refrigerator; discard after 24 hr
- Provide bed rest during entire course of treatment
- Avoid venous or arterial puncture, injection, rec temp
- Provide treatment of fever with acetaminophen or aspirin
- Apply pressure for 30 sec to minor bleeding sites; inform prescriber if this does not attain hemostasis; apply pressure dressing

Evaluation

- Therapeutic response: resolution of thrombosis, embolism

Generic Names

alteplase
anistreplase
streptokinase (key drug)
urokinase

THYROID HORMONES

Action: Increase metabolic rates, resulting in increased cardiac output, O_2 consumption, body temp, blood volume, growth, development at cellular level, respiratory rate, enzyme system activity

Uses: Products are used for thyroid replacement.

Adverse effects: The most common side effects include insomnia, tremors, tachycardia, palpitations, angina, dysrhythmias, weight loss, and changes in appetite. Serious adverse reactions include thyroid storm.

Contraindications: Persons with adrenal insufficiency, myocardial infarction, or thyrotoxicosis should not use these products.

G **Precautions:** The elderly and patients with angina pectoris, hypertension, ischemia, cardiac disease, or diabetes mellitus or insipidus should be watched closely when using these products. Caution should be used in pregnancy and lactation.

Pharmacokinetics: Pharmacokinetics vary widely among products; check specific monographs.

Interactions

- Impaired absorption of thyroid products may occur when administered with cholestyramine (separate by 4-5 hr)
- Increased effects of anticoagulants, sympathomimetics, tricyclic antidepressants, catecholamines may occur
- Decreased effects of digitalis, glycosides, insulin, hypoglycemics may occur
- Decreased effects of thyroid products may occur with estrogens

NURSING CONSIDERATIONS

Assessment

- Monitor B/P, pulse before each dose
- Monitor I&O ratio
- Monitor weight qd in same clothing, using same scale, at same time of day
- P Monitor height, growth rate if given to a child
- Monitor T_3, T_4, which are decreased; radioimmunoassay of TSH, which is increased; ratio uptake, which is decreased if patient is on too low a dosage of medication
- Assess for increased nervousness, excitability, irritability; may indicate too high doses of medication usually after 1-3 wk of treatment
- Assess for cardiac status: angina, palpitation, chest pain, change in VS

Nursing diagnoses

✓ Knowledge deficit (teaching)
✓ Noncompliance (teaching)
✓ Body image disturbance (adverse reactions)

Implementation

- Give at same time each day to maintain drug level
- Give only for hormone imbalances; not to be used for obesity, male infertility, menstrual conditions, lethargy
- Remove medication 4 wk before RAIU test

Evaluation

- Therapeutic response: absence of depression; increased weight loss, diuresis, pulse, appetite; absence of constipation, peripheral edema, cold intolerance, pale, cool, dry skin, brittle nails, alopecia, coarse hair, menorrhagia, night blindness, paresthesias, syncope, stupor, coma, rosy cheeks

Patient/family education

- P • Advise patient that hair loss will occur in child and is temporary
- Advise patient to report excitability, irritability, anxiety; indicates overdose
- Caution patient not to switch brands unless directed by prescriber
- P • Caution patient that hypothyroid child will show almost immediate behavior/personality change
- Advise patient that treatment drug is not to be taken to reduce weight
- Advise patient to avoid OTC preparations with iodine; read labels; to avoid iodine-containing food, iodinized salt, soybeans, tofu, turnips, some seafood, some bread

---

Generic Names

levothyroxine (T_4)	liotrix
liothyronine (T_3)	thyroid USP

VASODILATORS

Action: Vasodilators act in various ways. Please check individual monograph for specific action.

Uses: Vasodilators are used to treat intermittent claudication, arteriosclerosis obliterans, vasospasm and muscular ischemia, ischemic cerebral vascular disease, hypertension, and angina.

Adverse effects: The most common side effects are headache, nausea, hypotension or hypertension, and ECG changes.

Contraindications: Some drugs are contraindicated in acute MI, paroxysmal tachycardia, and thyrotoxicosis.

Precautions: Caution should be used in uncompensated heart disease or peptic ulcer disease.

Pharmacokinetics: Onset, peak, and duration vary widely among products. Most products are metabolized in the liver and excreted in urine.

Interactions: Please check individual monographs, since interactions vary widely among products.

NURSING CONSIDERATIONS

Assessment

- Assess bleeding time in individuals with bleeding disorders
- Assess cardiac status: B/P, pulse, rate, rhythm, character; watch for increasing pulse

Nursing diagnoses

✓ Decreased cardiac output (uses)
✓ Altered tissue perfusion: cardiovascular/pulmonary (uses)
✓ Knowledge deficit (teaching)

Implementation

- Give with meals to reduce GI symptoms
- Store in tight container at room temp

Evaluation

- Therapeutic response: ability to walk without pain, increased temp in extremities, increased pulse volume

Patient/family education

- Inform patient that medication is not cure, may need to be taken continuously
- Advise patient that it is necessary to quit smoking to prevent excessive vasoconstriction
- Advise patient that improvement may be sudden, but usually occurs gradually over several wk
- Instruct patient to report headache, weakness, increased pulse, since drug may need to be decreased or discontinued
- Instruct patient to avoid hazardous activities until stabilized on medication; dizziness may occur

---

Generic Names

amyl nitrite	minoxidil
dipyridamole	papaverine
hydralazine	tolazoline

VITAMINS

Action: Action varies widely among products and classes; check specific monographs.

Uses: Vitamins are used to correct and prevent vitamin deficiencies.

Adverse effects: There is an absence of side effects or adverse reactions with the water-soluble vitamins (C, B). However, fat-soluble vitamins (A, D, E, K) may accumulate in the body and cause adverse reactions (refer to specific monographs).

Contraindications: Hypersensitive reactions may occur, and allergies should be identified before these products are given.
Pharmacokinetics: Onset, peak, and duration vary widely among products; check individual monograph for specific information.

NURSING CONSIDERATIONS

Nursing diagnoses

✓ Altered nutrition, less than body requirements (uses)

Implementation

- Give PO with food for better absorption
- Store in tight, light-resistant container

Evaluation

- Therapeutic response: absence of vitamin deficiency

Patient/family education

- Advise patient not to take more than prescribed amount

Generic Names

Fat-soluble:
phytonadione
vitamin A
vitamin D
vitamin E

Water-soluble:
ascorbic acid (C)
pyridoxine (B_6)
riboflavin (B_2)
thiamine (B_1)

Miscellaneous:
multivitamins

Appendix A

Selected New Drugs

anagrelide (℞)
(a-na′gre-lide)
Agrylin
Func. class.: Antiplatelet
Chem. class.: Imidazo-quinazolinone
Pregnancy category C

Action: Reduces platelet count (mechanism not clear) and prevents early platelet shape changes in response to aggregating agents thus inhibiting platelet aggregation

Therapeutic Outcome: Inhibition of platelet aggregation

Uses: Essential thrombocythemia

Dosage and routes

Adult: PO 0.5 mg qid or 1 mg bid, may be adjusted after 1 wk, max 10 mg/day or 2.5 mg single dose

Available forms: Caps 0.5, 1.0 mg

Adverse effects

CNS: Headache, dizziness, seizures

CV: Postural hypotension, tachycardia, palpitations, ***CHF, MI,*** cardiomyopathy, cardiomegaly, ***complete heart block, atrial fibrillation,*** arrhythmia

HEMA: Anemia, ***thrombocytopenia,*** ecchymosis, lymphadenoma

INTEG: Rash

Contraindications: Hypersensitivity, hypotension

Precautions: Pregnancy **C**

Pharmacokinetics

Absorption	Unknown
Distribution	Unknown
Metabolism	Liver, extensively
Excretion	Feces/urine
Half-life	1.3 hr

Pharmacodynamics

Onset	Unknown
Peak	1 hr
Duration	>24 hr

NURSING CONSIDERATIONS

Assessment

- Monitor B/P, pulse baseline and during treatment until stable; take B/P with patient lying, standing; orthostatic hypotension is common
- Assess cardiac status: chest pain, what aggravates or ameliorates condition

Nursing diagnoses

✓ Cardiac output, decreased (uses)

✓ Knowledge deficit (teaching)

Implementation

- Give with 8 oz of water; to improve absorption give on an empty stomach
- Store at room temp

Patient/family education

- Teach patient that this medication is not a cure; that drug may have to be taken continuously in evenly spaced doses only as directed; if a dose is missed, take one when remembered up to 4 hr; do not double doses

- Inform patient that it is necessary to quit smoking to prevent excessive vasoconstriction
- Advise patient to rise slowly from sitting or lying down to prevent orthostatic hypotension
- Caution patient not to use alcohol or OTC medication unless approved by prescriber
- Caution patient to avoid hazardous activities until stabilized on medication; dizziness may occur

Evaluation

Positive therapeutic outcome

- Absence of thrombocythemia

ardeparin (℞)

(are-de-pear'in)

Normiflo

Func. class.: Anticoagulant

Chem. class.: Low molecular weight heparin

Pregnancy category C

Action: Prevents conversion of fibrinogen to fibrin and prothrombin to thrombin by enhancing inhibitory effects of antithrombin III

Therapeutic Outcome:

- Absence of deep vein thrombosis

Uses: Prevention of deep vein thrombosis after knee replacement surgery

Dosage and routes

Adult: SC 50 antifactor XaU/kg q12 h the evening of the day of knee replacement surgery or the following AM, continued until patient is fully ambulatory or 2 wk, whichever is first

- To be used SC only

Available forms: Inj 5000, 10,000 anti-XaU/0.5 ml

Adverse effects

CNS: ***Intracranial bleeding,*** fever

GI: Nausea, constipation, ***hepatoxicity***

HEMA: ***Thrombocytopenia,*** anemia

INTEG: Pruritus, superficial wound infection, ecchymosis, rash

SYST: Hypersensitivity, ***hemorrhage, anaphylaxis*** possible

Contraindications: Hypersensitivity to this drug, pork products, heparin, or other anticoagulants; hemophilia, leukemia with bleeding, thrombocytopenic purpura, cerebrovascular hemorrhage, cerebral aneurysm, severe hypertension, other severe cardiac disease

G **Precautions:** Elderly, pregnancy **C,** hepatic disease, severe renal disease, blood dyscrasias, subacute bacterial endocarditis, acute nephritis,
P lactation, child, recent childbirth, peptic ulcer disease, pericarditis, pericardial effusion, recent lumbar puncture, vasculitis, other diseases where bleeding is possible

Pharmacokinetics	
Absorption	Well
Distribution	Widely
Metabolism	Unknown
Half-life	Unknown

Pharmacodynamics
Unknown

Interactions
Drug Classifications

Anticoagulants, oral: ↑ risk of bleeding
Platelet inhibitors: ↑ risk of bleeding
Salicylates: ↑ risk of bleeding

NURSING CONSIDERATIONS
Assessment

- Assess for blood studies (Hct, occult blood in stools) during treatment since bleeding can occur
- Assess for bleeding gums, petechiae, ecchymosis, black tarry stools, hematuria, epistaxis, decrease in Hct, B/P; may indicate bleeding, possible hemorrhage; notify prescriber immediately, drug should be discontinued
- Monitor for hypersensitivity: fever, skin rash, urticaria; notify prescriber immediately

Implementation

- Do not give IM or IV drug route; approved is SC only
- Give by SC only; have patient sit or lie down; SC inj may be around the navel in a U-shape, upper outer side of thigh or upper outer quadrangle of the buttocks; rotate inj sites
- Changing needles is not recommended

Evaluation

- Therapeutic response: absence of deep vein thrombosis

Patient/family education

- Teach patient to avoid OTC preparations that may cause serious drug interactions unless directed by prescriber; may contain aspirin; other anticoagulants
- Teach patient to use soft-bristle toothbrush to avoid bleeding gums, avoid contact sports, use electric razor, avoid IM injection
- Advise patient to report any signs of bleeding: gums, under skin, urine, stools; unusual bruising

Treatment of overdose: Protamine sulfate 1% given IV

azelastine (℞)
(ay'ze-lass-teen)
Astelin
Func. class.: Leukotriene synthesis inhibitor
Chem. class.: Phthalazinone derivative
Pregnancy category C

Action: Inhibits the synthesis and release of leukotrienes; antagonizes action of acetylcholine, histamine, serotonin

➔ Therapeutic Outcome: Decreased nasal stuffiness, itching, swollen eyes

Uses: Seasonal allergic rhinitis

Dosage and routes
Adult and child ≥12 yr: Nasal 2 sprays/nostril bid

Available forms: Spray 137 μg/actuation

Adverse effects
CNS: Sedation (more common with increased dosages), drowsiness
MISC: Weight increase, myalgia

Contraindications: Hypersensitivity

Precautions: Pregnancy **C**

Pharmacokinetics	
Absorption	Unknown
Distribution	Unknown
Metabolism	Liver, extensively
Excretion	Feces
Half-life	25-42 hr

Pharmacodynamics

Onset	Unknown
Peak	4-5 hr
Duration	Unknown

Interactions
Individual drugs
Alcohol: ↑ CNS depression
Drug classifications
CNS depressants: ↑ CNS depression
Narcotics: ↑ CNS depression
Sedative/hypnotics: ↑ CNS depression

NURSING CONSIDERATIONS
Assessment
• Assess respiratory status: rate, rhythm, increase in bronchial secretions, wheezing, chest tightness; provide fluids to 2 L/day to decrease secretion thickness
Nursing diagnoses
✓ Airway clearance, ineffective (uses)
✓ Knowledge deficit (teaching)
✓ Noncompliance (teaching, overuse)
Implementation
• Remove cap/safety clip from spray pump
• Prime pump if using for first time, push 4 times quickly, away from face, blow your nose, then place tip of pump into one nostril, while holding other nostril closed, tilt head forward, and spray into nostril
• Put cover/safety clip back on
Patient/family education
• Teach patient all aspects of drug uses; to notify prescriber if confusion, sedation occur; to avoid driving and other hazardous activity if drowsiness occurs; to avoid alcohol and other CNS depressants that may potentiate effect
• Caution patient not to exceed recommended dosage; dysrhythmias may occur
Evaluation
Positive therapeutic outcome
• Absence of running or congested nose

bromfenac (℞)
(broem'fe-nak)
Duract
Func. class.: Nonsteroidal antiinflammatory
Chem. class.: Phenylacetic acid
Pregnancy category B

Action: Inhibits prostaglandin synthesis by decreasing enzyme needed for biosynthesis; analgesic, antiinflammatory, antipyretic properties

➔ **Therapeutic Outcome:** Decreased pain, inflammation

Uses: Acute, chronic rheumatoid arthritis, osteoarthritis, ankylosing spondylitis, analgesia, primary dysmenorrhea

Dosage and routes
Adult: 25 mg q6-8 h; if taken with high fat meal, then 50 mg may be needed; max daily dose 150 mg

Available forms: Caps 25 mg

Adverse effects
CNS: Dizziness, headache, lightheadedness
CV: **CHF**, tachycardia, peripheral edema, palpitations, dysrhythmias, hypotension, hypertension, fluid retention
EENT: Tinnitus, hearing loss, blurred vision
GI: Nausea, anorexia, vomiting, diarrhea, constipation, flatulence, cramps

GU: Nephrotoxicity: ***dysuria, hematuria, oliguria, azotemia,*** *cystitis, UTI*
HEMA: ***Blood dyscrasias,*** epistaxis, bruising
INTEG: Purpura, rash, pruritus, sweating, erythema, petechiae, photosensitivity, alopecia
RESP: Dyspnea, hemoptysis, pharyngitis, ***bronchospasm, laryngeal edema,*** rhinitis, shortness of breath

Contraindications: Hypersensitivity to aspirin, iodides, other NSAIDs

Precautions: Pregnancy **B**
P lactation, children, bleeding disorders, GI disorders, cardiac disorders, hypersensitivity to other antiinflammatory agents

Pharmacokinetics

Absorption	Unknown
Distribution	Unknown
Metabolism	Liver, kidneys
Excretion	Unknown
Half-life	½-1 hr

Pharmacodynamics

Onset	Unknown
Peak	2-3 hr
Duration	Unknown

Interactions
Individual drugs
Acetaminophen (long-term use): ↑ renal reactions
Alcohol: ↑ adverse reactions
Aspirin: ↓ effectiveness, ↑ adverse reactions to NSAIDs
Coumadin: ↑ anticoagulant effects
Digoxin: ↑ toxicity, ↑ levels
Lithium: ↑ toxicity
Methotrexate: ↑ toxicity
Phenytoin: ↑ toxicity
Probenecid: ↑ toxicity
Sulfonylurea: ↑ toxicity

Drug classifications
Anticoagulants: ↑ risk of bleeding
Antihypertensives: ↓ effect of antihypertensives
Antineoplastics: ↑ risk of hematologic toxicity
β-Blockers: ↑ antihypertension
Cephalosporins: ↑ risk of bleeding
Glucocorticoids: ↑ adverse reactions
NSAIDs: ↑ adverse reactions
Potassium supplements: ↑ adverse reactions
Radiation: ↑ risk of hematologic toxicity
Sulfonamides: ↑ toxicity

NURSING CONSIDERATIONS
Assessment
- Assess for pain of rheumatoid arthritis, osteoarthritis, ankylosing spondylitis; check ROM, inflammation of joints, characteristics of pain
- Monitor blood counts during therapy; watch for decreasing platelets; if low, therapy may need to be discontinued, restarted after hematologic recovery; and for blood dyscrasias (thrombocytopenia): bruising, fatigue, bleeding, poor healing

Nursing diagnoses
- ✓ Pain (uses)
- ✓ Mobility, impaired physical (uses)
- ✓ Injury, risk for (side effects)
- ✓ Knowledge deficit (teaching)

Implementation
- Administer with food or milk to decrease gastric symptoms
- ⊘ Do not crush, dissolve, or chew caps

Patient/family education
- Teach patient that drug must be continued for prescribed time to be effective; to avoid aspirin, alcoholic beverages

- Caution patient to report bleeding, bruising, fatigue, malaise, since blood dyscrasia do occur
- Instruct patient to use caution when driving; drowsiness, dizziness may occur
- Teach patient to take with a full glass of water to enhance absorption
- Instruct patient not to crush, break, or chew caps

Evaluation
Positive therapeutic outcome
- Decreased pain in arthritic conditions

cabergoline (℞)
(ka-bear'joe-leen)
Dostinex
Func. class.: Dopamine receptor/agonist
Chem. class.: Ergot alkaloid derivative
Pregnancy category B

Action: Inhibits prolactin release by activating postsynaptic dopamine receptors

Therapeutic Outcome: Reduced prolactin/secretion

Uses: Prevention of postpartum lactation

Investigational uses: Parkinson's disease, normalization of androgen levels, and improved menstrual cycles in polycystic ovarian syndrome

Dosage and routes
Adult: 0.25 mg 2x/wk, may increase by 0.25 mg 2x/wk at 4 wk intervals, max 1 mg 2x/wk; maintenance therapy may be needed for 6 mo

Available forms: Tabs 0.5 mg

Adverse effects
CNS: Headache, depression, weakness, somnolence, vertigo, paresthesia, nervousness, *dizziness,* fatigue,
CV: ***Orthostatic hypotension,*** decreased B/P,
EENT: Blurred vision
GI: Nausea, vomiting, anorexia, constipation, abdominal pain, dyspepsia
GU: Breast pain, dysmenorrhea
INTEG: Acne, flushing
MISC: Asthenia, malaise, flu-like symptoms

Contraindications: Hypersensitivity to ergot, alkaloids, uncontrolled hypertension

Precautions: Hepatic disease, renal disease, pregnancy **B,** eclampsia, pre-eclampsia, PIH, CV disease

Pharmacokinetics	
Absorption	Unknown
Distribution	Unknown
Metabolism	Liver, completely
Excretion	Urine, feces
Half-life	2.7-14 days

Pharmacodynamics	
Onset	Unknown
Peak	2-3 hr
Duration	24 hr

Interactions
Individual drugs
Droperidol: Do not use together
Haloperidol: Do not use together
Metoclopramide: Do not use together
Drug classifications
Antihypertensives: ↑ hypotension
Butyrophenones: Do not use together
Thioxanthines: Do not use together

Dopamine antagonists: Do not use together

NURSING CONSIDERATIONS

Assessment

- Assess for symptoms of suppression of lactation: decreasing breast tenderness and discomfort, decreasing milk production
- Monitor B/P; establish baseline, compare with other readings; this drug decreases B/P; heart rate, liver function studies, CBC, chest x-ray during prolonged treatment

Nursing diagnoses

✓ Knowledge deficit (teaching)

Implementation

- Give hs so dizziness, orthostatic hypotension do not occur
- Store at room temp in airtight container

Patient/family education

- Advise patient to change position slowly to prevent orthostatic hypotension
- Caution patient to avoid hazardous activity if dizziness, drowsiness occurs during treatment start-up
- Teach patients using drug for lactation suppression that treatment will last up to 3 wk and breast engorgement with milk production may occur after treatment is discontinued

Evaluation

Positive therapeutic outcome

- Decreased breast engorgement with accompanied pain, tenderness

cerivistatin (℞)

(ser-iv'i-sta-tin)
Baycol
Func. class.: Cholesterol-lowering agent
Chem. class.: HMG-CoA reductase inhibitor
Pregnancy category X

Action: Inhibits biosynthesis of VLDL and LDL, which are responsible for cholesterol development

➔ Therapeutic Outcome: Decreased cholesterol levels and LDLs, increased HDLs

Uses: As an adjunct in primary hypercholesterolemia (types IIa, IIb), mixed hyperlipidemia

Dosage and routes

(Patient should first be placed on a cholesterol-lowering diet)

Adult: 0.3 mg qd PM, may be given with a bile-acid–binding resin

Available forms: Tabs 0.2, 0.3 mg

Adverse effects

CNS: Dizziness, headache
EENT: Blurred vision, dysgeusia, lens opacities
GI: Nausea, constipation, diarrhea, dyspepsia, flatus, abdominal pain, heartburn, ***liver dysfunction***
INTEG: Rash, pruritus
MS: Muscle cramps, myalgia, ***myositis, rhabdomyolysis***

Contraindications: Hypersensitivity, pregnancy **X,** lactation, active liver disease

Precautions: Past liver disease, alcoholism, severe acute infections, trauma, hypotension, uncontrolled seizure disorders, severe metabolic disorders, electrolyte imbalances, visual condition, children

P

Pharmacokinetics

Absorption	Unknown
Distribution	Unknown
Metabolism	Unknown
Excretion	Unknown
Half-life	Unknown

Pharmacodynamics

Unknown

Interactions

Individual drugs

Cholestyramine: ↑ action
Colestipol: ↑ action
Cyclosporine: ↑ risk of myopathy
Erythromycin: ↑ risk of myopathy
Gemfibrozil: ↑ risk of myopathy
Itraconazole: ↑ cerivistatin effect
Niacin: ↑ risk of myopathy
Propranolol: ↑ antihyperlipidemic activity
Warfarin: ↑ anticoagulant effect

Lab test interferences

↑ CPK, ↑ liver function tests

NURSING CONSIDERATIONS

Assessment

- Assess nutrition: fat, protein, carbohydrates; nutritional analysis should be completed by dietician before treatment
- Monitor bowel pattern daily; diarrhea may be a problem
- Monitor triglycerides, cholesterol at baseline and throughout treatment; LDL and VLDL should be watched closely; if increased, drug should be discontinued

Nursing diagnoses

✓ Diarrhea (adverse reactions)
✓ Knowledge deficit (teaching)
✓ Noncompliance (teaching)

Implementation

- Give with evening meal; if dosage is increased, take with breakfast and evening meal
- Store in cool environment in airtight, light-resistant container

Patient/family education

- Inform patient that compliance is needed for positive results to occur; not to double doses
- Teach patient that risk factors should be decreased: high-fat diet, smoking, alcohol consumption, absence of exercise
- Advise patient to notify prescriber if the GI symptoms of diarrhea, abdominal or epigastric pain, nausea, vomiting occur; or if chills, fever, sore throat occur

Evaluation

Positive therapeutic outcome

- Decreased cholesterol levels, serum triglyceride
- Improved ratio of HDLs

clopidogrel (℞)

(klo-pid'da-grel)

Plavix

Func. class.: Platelet aggregation inhibitor
Chem. class.: Thienopyridine derivative

Pregnancy category B

Action: Inhibits first and second phases of ADP-induced effects in platelet aggregation

Therapeutic Outcome: Decreased stroke by decreasing platelet aggregation

Uses: Reducing the risk of stroke in high-risk patients

Dosage and routes
Adult: PO 75 mg qd with or without food

Available forms: Tabs 75 mg

Adverse effects
CV: Edema, hypertension
CNS: Headache, dizziness
GI: Nausea, vomiting, diarrhea, GI discomfort,
HEMA: ***Epistaxis,*** purpura,
INTEG: Rash, pruritus
MISC: UTI, depression, hypercholesterolemia, chest pain, fatigue, ***intracranial hemorrhage***
MS: Arthralgia, back pain
RESP: Upper respiratory tract infection, dyspnea, rhinitis, bronchitis, cough

Contraindications: Hypersensitivity, active bleeding

Precautions: Past liver
P disease, pregnancy **B,** lactation, children, increased bleeding risk, neutropenia, agranulocytosis

Pharmacokinetics

Absorption	Well absorbed
Distribution	Unknown
Metabolism	Liver, extensively
Excretion	Kidneys, unchanged drug
Half-life	of platelets 11 days

Pharmacodynamics

Onset	Unknown
Peak	1-3 hr
Duration	Unknown

Interactions
Individual drugs
Aspirin: ↑ bleeding tendencies
Drug classifications
Anticoagulants: ↑ bleeding tendencies
NSAIDs: ↑ bleeding tendencies

NURSING CONSIDERATIONS
Asessment
- Monitor liver function studies: AST (SGOT), ALT (SGPT), bilirubin, creatinine if patient is on long-term therapy (4 mo or more)
- Monitor blood studies: CBC, Hct, Hgb, pro-time if patient is on long-term therapy; thrombocytopenia, neutropenia may occur

Nursing diagnoses
✓ Injury, risk for (uses)
✓ Knowledge deficit (teaching)

Implementation
- Give with food to decrease gastric symptoms

Patient/family education
- Advise patient that blood work will be necessary during treatment
- Advise patient to report any unusual bleeding to prescriber
- Instruct patient to take with food or just after eating to minimize GI discomfort
- Caution patient to report side effects such as diarrhea, skin rashes, subcutaneous bleeding

Evaluation
Positive therapeutic outcome
- Absence of stroke

delavirdine (℞)
(de-la-veer'din)
Rescriptor
Func. class.: Non-nucleoside reverse transcriptase inhibitor (NNRII)
Pregnancy category C

Action: Binds directly to reverse transcriptase and blocks

RNA, DNA causing a disruption of the enzyme's site

Therapeutic Outcome: Improvement of HIV-1 infection

Uses: HIV-1 in combination with zidovudine or didanosine

Dosage and routes

Adult and child ≥16 yr: 400 mg tid

Available forms: Tabs 100 mg

Adverse effects

CNS: Headache, fatigue
GI: Diarrhea, abdominal pain, nausea, vomiting, dyspepsia, ***hepatotoxicity***
GU: Nephrotoxicity
HEMA: Neutropenia, leukopenia, thrombocytopenia, anemia, granulocytopenia
INTEG: Rash
MS: Pain myalgia

Contraindications: Hypersensitivity to this drug or atevirdine

Precautions: Liver disease, pregnancy **C**, lactation, children, renal disease, myleosuppression

Pharmacokinetics	
Absorption	Well
Distribution	Highly protein bound
Metabolism	Liver
Excretion	Kidneys, feces
Half-life	6 hr

Pharmacodynamics

Unknown

Interactions

Drug classifications

Alprazolam: ↑ level of alprazolam
Antacids: ↓ delavirdine levels
Anticonvulsants: ↓ delavirdine levels
Astemizole: ↑ level of astemizole
Cisapride: ↑ level of cisapride
Clarithromycin: ↑ level of clarithromycin or ↑ level of delavirdine
Dapsone: ↑ level of dapsone
Ergots: ↑ ergotism
Felodipine: ↑ level of felodipine
Fluoxetine: ↑ levels of delavirdine
Indinavir: ↑ level of indinavir
Ketoconazole: ↑ level of delavirdine
Midazolam: ↑ level of midazolam
Nifidepine: ↑ level of nifidepine
Oral contraceptives: ↓ action
Protease inhibitors: ↓ action of protease inhibitors
Quinidine and warfarin: ↑ level of both quinidine and warfarin
Rifamycins: ↓ delaviradine levels

NURSING CONSIDERATIONS

Assessment

- Assess signs of infection, anemia
- Assess liver studies: ALT, AST; renal studies
- Assess C&S before drug therapy; drug may be taken as soon as culture is taken; repeat C&S after treatment; determine the presence of other sexually transmitted disease
- Assess bowel pattern before, during treatment; if severe abdominal pain with bleeding occurs, drug should be discontinued; monitor hydration
- Assess skin eruptions; rash, urticaria, itching
- Assess allergies before treatment, reaction to each

medication; place allergies on chart
• Assess plasma delavirdine concentrations (trough 10 micromolar)
• Assess CBC, blood chemistry, plasma HIV RNA, absolute CD4+/CD8+/cell counts/%, serum β-2 microglobulin, serum ICD+24 antigen levels
• Assess for signs of delavirdine toxicity: severe nausea/vomiting, maculopapular rash

Nursing diagnoses

✓ Infection, risk for uses)
✓ Diarrhea (side effects)
✓ Knowledge deficit (teaching)

Patient/family education

• Advise patient to take as prescribed; if dose is missed, take as soon as remembered up to 1 hr before next dose; do not double dose
• Advise patient that drug must be taken in equal intervals around the clock to maintain blood levels for duration of therapy
• Advise patient that tabs may be dissolved in ½ cup of water, stir, when dissolved, drink right away, rinse cup with water, and drink that to get all medication
• Instruct patient to make sure health care provider knows of all the medications being taken
• Advise patient that if severe rash, mouth sores, swelling, aching muscles/joints, or eye redness occur, stop taking and notify health care provider
• Advise patient not to breastfeed if taking this drug

dolasetron (℞)

(do-la'se-tron)
Anzemet
Func. class.: Antiemetic
Chem. class.: 5-HT receptor antagonist
Pregnancy category C

Action: Prevents nausea, vomiting by blocking serotonin peripherally, centrally, and in the small intestine

➔ **Therapeutic Outcome:** Control of nausea, vomiting

Uses: Prevention of nausea, vomiting associated with cancer chemotherapy and prevention of postoperative nausea, vomiting

Investigational uses: Radiotherapy-induced nausea/vomiting

Dosage and routes

Prevention of nausea/vomiting associated with cancer chemotherapy

Adult: **IV** 1.8 mg/kg as a single dose ½ hr prior to chemotherapy

Child 2-16 yr: PO 100 mg 1 hr prior to chemotherapy

Child 2-16 yr: PO 1.8 mg/kg 1 hr prior to chemotherapy

Prevention of postoperative nausea/vomiting

Adult: **IV** 12.5 mg as a single dose 15 min before cessation of anesthesia; PO 100 mg 2 hr before surgery (prevention only)

Child 2-16 yr: **IV** 0.35 mg/kg as a single dose 15 min before cessation of anesthesia; PO 1.2 mg/kg within 2 hr before surgery (prevention only)

Available forms: Tabs 50, 100 mg; inj 20 mg/ml

Adverse effects
CNS: Headache
GI: Diarrhea, constipation, increased AST (SGOT), ALT (SGPT)
MISC: Rash, **bronchospasm**

Contraindication: Hypersensitivity

P G **Precautions:** Pregnancy **B,** lactation, children, elderly

Pharmacokinetics

Absorption	Completely absorbed IV
Distribution	Unknown
Metabolism	Liver, extensively
Excretion	Kidneys
Half-life	Unknown

Pharmacodynamics

Unknown

Interactions Unknown

NURSING CONSIDERATIONS

Assessment
- Assess for absence of nausea, vomiting during chemotherapy
- Assess for hypersensitivity reaction: rash, bronchospasm

Nursing diagnoses
✓ Knowledge deficit (teaching)
✓ Noncompliance (teaching)

Implementation
IV **IV route**
- Store at room temp for 24 hr after dilution

Patient/family education
- Instruct patient to report diarrhea, constipation, rash, or changes in respirations
- Teach patient reason for medication and expected results

Evaluation
Positive therapeutic outcome
- Absence of nausea, vomiting during cancer chemotherapy

follitropin alfa/ follitropin beta (℞)
(fol′ee-tro-pin)
Gonal-F/Follistim
Func. class.: Ovulation stimulant
Chem. class.: Gonadotropin

Pregnancy category X

Action: Stimulates ovarian follicular growth in primary ovarian failure

➔ **Therapeutic Outcome:** Pregnancy

Uses: Induction of ovulation, assisted reproductive technologies (in vitro fertilization)

Dosage and routes
Adult:
Ovulation induction
SC 75 IU, may increase by 37.5 IU after 2 wks, may increase again after 1 wk by 37.5 IU; treatment should not exceed 35 days unless a serum estradiol rise indicates imminent follicular development

Follicle stimulation
SC 150 IU/day on day 2 or 3 of the follicular phase, should not exceed 10 days

Available forms: Gonal-F powder for injection 75 IU, 150 IU; Follistim powder for inj 75 IU

Adverse effects
CNS: Malaise
GI: Nausea, vomiting, constipation, increased appetite, abdominal pain
GU: Polyuria, frequency, birth defects, spontaneous abortions, multiple ovulation, breast pain
INTEG: Rash, dermatitis, urticaria, alopecia

Contraindications: Hypersensitivity, pregnancy **X,** undiagnosed vaginal bleeding, intracranial lesion, ovarian cyst not caused by polycystic ovarian disease

Precautions: Lactation, arterial thromboembolism

Pharmacokinetics	
Absorption	Unknown
Distribution	Unknown
Metabolism	Unknown
Excretion	Feces
Half-life	Unknown

NURSING CONSIDERATIONS

Implementation

- Give immediately after dissolving contents of ampule in 1-2 ml of sterile saline, discard unused portion
- Administer drug at same time qd to maintain drug level

Patient/family education

- Teach patient that multiple births are common after taking this drug
- Teach patient to notify prescriber of low abdominal pain; may indicate ovarian cyst, cyst rupture
- Teach patient method of taking, recording basal body temp to determine whether ovulation has occurred
- Teach patient that if ovulation can be determined (there is a slight decrease, then a sharp increase for ovulation), to attempt coitus 3 days before and qod until after ovulation
- Teach patient to notify prescriber immediately if pregnancy is suspected

Evaluation

Positive therapeutic outcome

- Ovulation, pregnancy

grepafloxacin (℞)

(gre-pa-floks'a-sin)

Raxar

Func. class.: Antiinfective

Chem. class.: Fluoroquinolone

Pregnancy category C

Action: Interferes with conversion of intermediate DNA fragments into high-molecular-weight DNA in bacteria; DNA gyrase inhibitor

Uses: Acute sinusitis, acute chronic bronchitis, community acquired pneumonia, nongonococcal urethritis, cervicitis, uncomplicated gonorrhea by *S. pneumoniae, H. influenzae, H. parainfluenzae, M. catarrhalis*

Dosage and routes

Adult: PO 400-600 mg qd for 7-10 days uncomplicated gonorrhea; PO 400 mg as a single dose

Available forms: Tabs 200 mg

Adverse effects

CNS: Headache, dizziness, insomnia, anxiety

GI: Nausea, flatulence, vomiting, diarrhea, abdominal pain, ***pseudomembranous colitis***

GU: Vaginitis, crystalluria

INTEG: Rash, pruritus, photosensitivity

Contraindications: Hypersensitivity to quinolones, photosensitivity

Precautions: Pregnancy **C,** P lactation, children

Pharmacokinetics	
Absorption	Unknown
Distribution	Unknown
Metabolism	Liver
Excretion	Urine (unchanged)
Half-life	Unknown

Lab test interferences
↓ Glucose, ↓ lymphocytes

NURSING CONSIDERATIONS

Assessment

- Assess for previous sensitivity reaction
- Assess for signs and symptoms of infection: characteristics of sputum, WBC >10,000, fever; obtain baseline information before and during treatment
- Obtain C&S before beginning drug therapy to identify if correct treatment has been initiated
- Assess for allergic reactions: rash, urticaria, pruritus, chills, fever, joint pain; may occur a few days after therapy begins; epinephrine and resuscitation equipment should be available for anaphylactic reaction
- Monitor bowel pattern qd; if severe diarrhea occurs, drug should be discontinued
- Assess for overgrowth of infection: perineal itching, fever, malaise, redness, pain, swelling, drainage, rash, diarrhea, change in cough, sputum

Patient/family education

- Teach patient to contact prescriber if vaginal itching, loose, foul-smelling stools, furry tongue occur; may indicate superinfection; report itching, rash, pruritus, urticaria
- Teach patient to notify prescriber of diarrhea with blood or pus

Evaluation

Positive therapeutic outcome

- Absence of signs/symptoms of infection (WBC <10,000/mm^3, temp WNL)

interferon alfacon-1 (℞)

(in-ter-feer'on al'fa-kon)
Infergen
Func. class.: Recombinant type I interferon

Action: Induces biologic responses and has antiviral, antiproliferative, and immunomodulatory effects

Therapeutic Outcome: Decreased signs/symptoms of Hepatitis C

Uses: Chronic hepatitis C infections

Investigational uses: Hairy cell leukemia when used with G-CSF

Dosage and routes
Adult: SC 9 micrograms as a single inj 3×/wk × 24 wk

Available forms: Inj 9, 15 mg

Adverse effects
CNS: Headache, fatigue, fever, rigors, insomnia, dizziness
CV: Hypertension, palpitation
EENT: Tinnitus, earache, conjunctivitis, eye pain
GI: Abdominal pain, nausea, diarrhea, anorexia, dyspepsia, vomiting, constipation, flatulence, hemorrhoids, decreased salivation
GU: Dysmenorrhea, vaginitis, menstrual disorders
HEMA: ***Granulocytopenia, thrombocytopenia, leukopenia,*** ecchymosis
INTEG: Alopecia, pruritus, rash, erythema, dry skin
MS: Back, limb, neck, skeletal pain
PSYCH: Nervousness, depression, anxiety, lability, abnormal thinking
RESP: Pharyngitis, upper

respiratory infection, cough sinusitis, rhinitis, respiratory tract congestion, epistaxis, dyspnea, bronchitis

Contraindications: Hypersensitivity to alpha interferons, or products from *E.coli*

Precautions: Thyroid disorders, myelosuppression, hepatic, cardiac disease, lactation, children <18 yrs

Pharmacokinetics	
Absorption	Unknown
Distribution	Unknown
Metabolism	Unknown
Excretion	Unknown
Half-life	Unknown

Pharmacodynamics	
Onset	Unknown
Peak	24-36 hr
Duration	Unknown

Interactions: None known

NURSING CONSIDERATIONS

Assessment

- Assess platelet counts, heme concentration, ANC, serum creatinine concentration, albumin, bilirubin, TSH, T4
- Assess for myelosuppression, low dose is neutrophil count is <500 × 10 6/1 or if platelets are < 50 × 10 9/L
- Assess for hypersensitivity; discontinue immediately if hypersensitivity occurs

Nursing diagnoses

✓ Infection, risk for (uses)
✓ Knowledge deficit (teaching)

Patient/family education

- Provide patient or family member with written, detailed instructions about the drug
- Caution patient to use contraception during treatment

Evaluation

Positive therapeutic outcome

- Decreased hepatitis C signs/symptoms

irbesartan (℞)

(er-be-sar′tan)

Avapro

Func. class.: Antihypertensive

Chem. class.: Angiotensin II receptor (Type AT_1)

Pregnancy category
C (1st trimester);
D (2nd/3rd trimester)

Action: Blocks the vasoconstrictor and aldosterone-secreting effects of angiotensin II; selectively blocks the binding of angiotensin II to the AT_1 receptor found in tissues

➔ **Therapeutic Outcome:** Decreased B/P

Uses: Hypertension, alone or in combination

Investigational uses: Heart failure, hypertensive patients with diabetic nephropathy caused by type II diabetes

Dosage and routes

Adult: PO 150 mg qd; may be increased to 300 mg qd

Available forms: Tabs 75, 150, 300 mg

Adverse effects

CNS: Dizziness, anxiety, headache, fatigue

GI: Diarrhea, dyspepsia

RESP: Cough, upper respiratory infection,

Contraindications: Hypersensitivity

Precautions: Hypersensitivity to ACE inhibitors; Pregnancy category **C** 1st trimester, **D** 2nd, 3rd trimester; lactation, children, elderly, renal disease

Pharmacokinetics

Absorption	Well
Distribution	Bound to plasma proteins (90%)
Metabolism	Liver (minimal)
Excretion	Feces, urine
Half-life	11-15 hr

Pharmacodynamics

Unknown

Interactions: None significant

NURSING CONSIDERATIONS
Assessment

- Assess B/P, pulse q4h; note rate, rhythm, quality
- Monitor electrolytes: potassium, sodium, chloride
- Obtain baselines in renal, liver function tests before therapy begins
- Monitor for edema in feet, legs daily
- Assess for skin turgor, dryness of mucous membranes for hydration status

Nursing diagnoses

✓ Fluid volume deficit (side effects)
✓ Noncompliance (teaching)
✓ Knowledge deficit (teaching)

Implementation

- Administer without regard to meals

Patient/family education

- Advise patient to comply with dosage schedule, even if feeling better
- Inform patient that drug may cause dizziness, fainting; lightheadedness may occur
- Caution patient to rise slowly to sitting or standing position to minimize orthostatic hypotension

Evaluation
Positive therapeutic outcome

- Decreased B/P

letrozole (℞)

(let'tro-zohl)

Femara

Func. class.: Antineoplastic, nonsteroidal aromatase inhibitor

Pregnancy category D

Action: Binds to the heme group of aromatase; inhibits conversion of androgens to estrogens to reduce plasma estrogen levels; 30% of breast cancers decrease in size when deprived of estrogen

➔ Therapeutic Outcome: Decreased spread of malignancy

Uses: Metastatic breast cancer in postmenopausal women

Dosage and routes
Adult: PO 2.5 mg qd

Available forms: Tab 2.5 mg

Adverse effects
CNS: Somnolence, dizziness, depression, anxiety, ***headache, lethargy***
CV: Hypertension
GI: Nausea, vomiting, anorexia, ***hepatotoxicity,*** constipation, heartburn, diarrhea
INTEG: Rash, pruritus, alopecia, sweating, hot flashes
RESP: Dyspnea, cough

Contraindications: Hypersensitivity, pregnancy **D**

Precautions: Hepatic disease, respiratory disease

Pharmacokinetics

Absorption	Well absorbed
Distribution	Widely
Metabolism	Liver
Excretion	Kidneys
Half-life	Unknown

Pharmacodynamics

Unknown

NURSING CONSIDERATIONS

Assessment

• Monitor renal function studies: BUN, serum uric acid, urine CrCl, electrolytes before, during therapy; I&O ratio; report fall in urine output of 30 ml/hr

• Monitor temperature q4h; may indicate beginning infection

• Monitor liver function tests before, during therapy (bilirubin, AST, ALT, LDH) as needed or monthly; RBC, Hct, Hgb, since these may be decreased; lymphocyte count, thyroid function tests

• Monitor inflammation of mucosa, breaks in skin, yellowing of skin and sclera, dark urine, clay-colored stools, itchy skin, abdominal pain, fever, diarrhea

Nursing diagnoses

✓ Injury, risk for (adverse reactions)

✓ Body image disturbance (adverse reactions)

✓ Infection, risk for (adverse reactions)

✓ Knowledge deficit (teaching)

Implementation

• Give with food or fluids for GI upset

• Give in equal intervals q6h

Patient/family education

• Instruct patient to report side effects

• Advise patient to avoid use of alcohol, which potentiates this drug

Evaluation

Positive therapeutic outcome

• Prevention of rapid division of malignant cells, postmenopausal cancer, prostate cancer

Treatment of overdose: Induce vomiting, provide supportive care

mibefradil (℞)

(mi-be-fray'dill)

Posicor

Func. class.: Calcium channel blocker; antihypertensive; antianginal

Chem. class.: Benzimidazoyle-substituted tetraline derivative

Pregnancy category C

Action: Inhibits calcium ion influx across cell membrane during cardiac depolarization; produces relaxation of coronary vascular smooth muscle; peripheral vascular smooth muscle; dilates coronary vascular arteries; increases myocardial oxygen delivery in patients with vasospastic angina; only calcium channel blocker that blocks both T-type and L-type

➔ Therapeutic Outcome: Decreased angina pectoris

Uses: Chronic stable angina pectoris

Dosage and routes

Adult: PO 50-100 mg qd

Available forms: Tabs 50, 100 mg

Adverse effects

CNS: Headache, dizziness

CV: Bradycardia, hypotension, palpitation, AV block, Wenckebach episodes
GI: Gastric upset, heartburn
HEMA: Intravascular hemolysis

Contraindications: Sick sinus syndrome, 2nd- or 3rd-degree heart block, hypotension less than 90 mm Hg systolic, cardiogenic shock, severe CHF

Precautions: CHF, hypotension, hepatic injury, pregnancy **C**, lactation, children, renal disease, concomitant β-blocker therapy, elderly

P G

Pharmacokinetics

Absorption	Unknown
Distribution	Unknown
Metabolism	Liver
Excretion	Kidneys
Half-life	27 hr

Pharmacodynamics

Onset	Unknown
Peak	2 hr
Duration	24 hr

Interactions

Drug classifications

β-Adrenergic blockers: ↑ depressant effects on myocardial contractility

NURSING CONSIDERATIONS

Assessment

- Assess fluid volume status: I&O ratio and record; weight; distended red veins; crackles in lung; color; quality, and sp gr of urine; skin turgor; adequacy of pulses; moist mucous membranes; bilateral lung sounds; peripheral pitting edema—dehydration symptoms of decreasing output, thirst, hypotension, dry mouth, and mucous membranes should be reported
- Monitor if platelets are <150,000/mm^3—if so, drug is usually discontinued and another drug started
- Assess for extravasation: change site q48h
- Monitor cardiac status: B/P, pulse, respiration, ECG

Nursing diagnoses

✓ Cardiac output, decreased (uses)
✓ Knowledge deficit (teaching)

Implementation

- Give once a day, with food for GI symptoms

Patient/family education

- Caution patient to avoid hazardous activities until stabilized on drug, dizziness is no longer a problem
- Instruct patient to limit caffeine consumption; to avoid alcohol and OTC drugs unless directed by prescriber
- Advise patient to comply with medical regimen: diet, exercise, stress reduction, drug therapy; to notify prescriber of irregular heart beat, shortness of breath, swelling of feet and hands, pronounced dizziness, constipation, nausea, hypotension
- Teach patient to use as directed even if feeling better; may be taken with other cardiovascular drugs (nitrates, β-blockers)

Evaluation

Positive therapeutic outcome

- Decreased anginal pain

Treatment of overdose:

Defibrillation, atropine for AV block, vasopressor for hypotension

nelfinavir (℞)

(nell-fin′a-ver)

Viracept

Func. class.: Antiviral

Chem. class.: HIV protease inhibitor

Pregnancy category B

Action: Inhibits human immunodeficiency virus (HIV) protease

Therapeutic Outcome: Prevents maturation of the infectious virus

Uses: HIV alone or in combination

Dosage and routes

Adult: PO 750 mg tid

Child: PO 20-30 mg/kg tid

Available forms: Tabs 250 mg; oral powder 50 mg/g

Adverse effects

CNS: Headache, poor concentration, fatigue, anxiety, depression

CV: Bleeding

ENDO: Hypoglycemia, hyperlipidemia

GI: Diarrhea, nausea, anorexia, dyspepsia

HEMA: Anemia, leukopenia, thrombocytopenia, Hgb abnormalities

INTEG: Rash, dermatitis

OTHER: Asthenia

Contraindications: Hypersensitivity to protease inhibitors

Precautions: Liver disease, pregnancy **B,** lactation, hemophilia, PKU, renal disease

Pharmacokinetics

Absorption	Unknown
Distribution	98% protein binding
Metabolism	Liver, (minimal)
Excretion	Feces
Half-life	3½-5 hr

Pharmacodynamics

Onset	Unknown
Peak	2-4 hr
Duration	Unknown

Interactions

Individual drugs

Astemizole: ↑ astemizole levels when given with nelfinavir

Carbamazepine: ↓ nelfinavir levels

Dexamethasone: ↓ nelfinavir levels

Lamivudine: ↓ effect of lamivudine

Oral contraceptives: ↓ effect of contraceptive

Rifamycin: ↓ nelfinavir levels

Zidovudine: ↓ effect of zidovudine

NURSING CONSIDERATIONS

Assessment

- Assess signs of infection, anemia
- Monitor liver studies: ALT, AST
- Monitor C&S before drug therapy; drug may be taken as soon as culture is taken; repeat C&S after treatment; determine the presence of other sexually transmitted diseases
- Assess bowel pattern before, during treatment; if severe abdominal pain with bleeding occurs, drug should be discontinued; monitor hydration
- Assess skin eruptions, rash, urticaria, itching
- Assess allergies before treatment, reaction of each medication; place allergies on chart

Nursing diagnoses

- ✓ Infection, risk for (uses)
- ✓ Knowledge deficit (teaching)

Patient/family education
• Advise patient to take with meal or snack; if dose is missed, take as soon as remembered up to 1 hr before next dose; do not double dose

pramipexole (℞)
(pra-mi-pex'ol)
Mirapex
Func. class.: Antiparkinsonian agent
Chem. class.: Dopamine-receptor agonist, nonergot
Pregnancy category C

Action: Selective agonist for D_2 receptors (presynaptic/postsynaptic sites); binding at D_3 receptor contributes to antiparkinson effects

➔ Therapeutic Outcome: Decreased symptoms of Parkinson's disease (involuntary movements)

Uses: Parkinsonism

Dosage and routes
Maintenance treatment
Adult: PO 1.5-4.5 mg qd in 3 divided doses

Initial treatment
Adult: PO from a starting dose of 0.375 mg/day given in 3 divided doses; increase gradually at 5-7 day intervals until total daily dose of 4.5 mg is reached

Available forms: Tabs 0.125, 0.25, 1.0, 1.5 mg

Adverse effects
CNS: Agitation, insomnia, psychosis, hallucinations, depression, dizziness
CV: Orthostatic hypotension
EENT: Blurred vision
GI: Nausea, anorexia, constipation
GU: Impotence

Contraindications: Hypersensitivity

Precautions: Renal disease, cardiac disease, MI with dysrhythmias, affective disorders, psychosis

Pharmacokinetics

Absorption	Well absorbed
Distribution	Widely distributed
Metabolism	Liver, minimally
Excretion	Kidneys, unchanged
Half-life	8-14 hr

Pharmacodynamics

Unknown

Interactions
Individual drugs
Cimetidine: ↑ pramipexole levels
Diltiazem: ↑ pramipexole levels
Levodopa: ↑ pramipexole levels
Quinidine: ↑ pramipexole levels
Ranitidine: ↑ pramipexole levels
Triamterene: ↑ pramipexole levels

Drug classifications **Dopamine antagonists:** ↓ pramipexole levels

NURSING CONSIDERATIONS
Assessment
• Monitor B/P, respiration during initial treatment; hypotension or hypertension should be reported
• Assess mental status: affect, mood, behavioral changes, depression; complete suicide assessment
• Monitor renal function studies
• Assess for involuntary move-

ments in parkinsonism: akinesia, tremors, staggering gait, muscle rigidity, drooling; these symptoms should improve with therapy

Nursing diagnoses

- ✓ Mobility, impaired (uses)
- ✓ Injury, risk for (uses)
- ✓ Knowledge deficit (teaching)
- ✓ Noncompliance (teaching)

Implementation

PO route

- Give drug until NPO before surgery
- Adjust dosage to patient response
- Give with meals to decrease GI upset

Patient/family education

- Advise patient that therapeutic effects may take several wk to a few mo
- Caution patient to change positions slowly to prevent orthostatic hypotension
- Instruct patient to use drug exactly as prescribed; if drug is discontinued abruptly, parkinsonian crisis may occur; if treatment is to be discontinued, taper over 1 wk

Evaluation

Positive therapeutic outcome

- Decreased akathisia, other involuntary movements
- Increased mood

quetiapine (℞)

(kwe-tie'a-peen)

Seroquel

Func. class.: Antipsychotic/neuroleptic

Pregnancy category C

Action: Functions as an antagonist at multiple neurotransmitter receptors in the brain including $5HT_{1A}$, $5HT_2$, dopamine D_1, D_2, H_1, adrenergic α-$_1$, α-$_2$ receptors

➔ **Therapeutic Outcome:** Decreased hallucination and disorganized thought

Uses: Psychotic disorders

Dosage and routes

Adult: PO 25 mg bid, with incremental increases of 25-50 mg bid-tid on days 2 and 3 to a dose of 300-400 mg qd given bid-tid

Available forms: Tabs 25, 100, 200 mg

Adverse effects

CNS: Extrapyrimidal symptoms, pseudoparkinsonism, akathisia, dystonia, tardive dyskinesia, drowsiness, insomnia, agitation, anxiety, *headache,* ***neuroleptic malignant syndrome,*** dizziness

CV: Orthostatic hypotension, *tachycardia*

GI: Nausea, anorexia, constipation, abdominal pain, dry mouth

INTEG: Rash

MISC: Asthenia, back pain, fever, ear pain

RESP: Rhinitis

Contraindications: Hypersensitivity

P **Precautions:** Children, lactation, long-term use, seizures, dementia, pregnancy **C,** hepatic disease, elderly, breast cancer G

Pharmacokinetics	
Absorption	Rapidly
Distribution	Widely
Metabolism	Liver, extensively
Excretion	Urine, feces
Half-life	≥6 hr

Pharmacodynamics

Onset	Unknown
Peak	1.5 hr
Duration	Up to 12 hr

Interactions
Individual drugs
Cimetidine: ↓ clearance of quetiapine
Levodopa: ↓ effect of levodopa
Lorazepam: ↓ clearance of lorazepam
Phenytoin: ↑ clearance of quetiapine
Thioridazine: ↑ clearance of quetiapine

Drug classifications
Barbiturates: ↑ clearance of quetiapine
Dopamine agonists: ↓ effects of dopamine agonists
Glucocorticoids: ↑ clearance of quetiapine

NURSING CONSIDERATIONS
Assessment
- Assess mental status: orientation, mood, behavior, presence and type of hallucinations before initial administration and monthly; this drug should significantly reduce psychotic behavior
- Check that patient swallows all PO medication; check for hoarding or giving of medication to other patients
- Monitor I&O ratio, palpate bladder if low urinary output occurs, especially in elderly; P urinalysis recommended before, during prolonged therapy
- Monitor bilirubin, CBC, liver function studies monthly
- Assess affect, orientation, LOC, reflexes, gait, coordination, sleep pattern disturbances
- Monitor B/P with patient in sitting, standing, and lying positions; take pulse and respirations q4h during initial treatment; establish baseline before starting treatment; report drops of 30 mm Hg; obtain baseline ECG; and Q-wave and T-wave changes
- Check for dizziness, faintness, palpitations, tachycardia on rising; severe orthostatic hypotension is common
- Identify for neuroleptic malignant syndrome: hyperpyrexia, muscle rigidity, increased CPK, altered mental status; drug should be discontinued
- Assess for extrapyramidal symptoms including akathisia (inability to sit still, no pattern to movements), tardive dyskinesia (bizarre movements of the jaw, mouth, tongue, extremities) pseudoparkinsonism (rigidity, tremors, pill rolling, shuffling gait); an antiparkinson drug should be prescribed
- Assess for constipation, urinary retention daily; if these occur, increase bulk, water in diet

Nursing diagnoses
- ✓ Thought processes, altered (uses)
- ✓ Coping, ineffective individual (uses)
- ✓ Knowledge deficit (teaching)
- ✓ Noncompliance (teaching)

Implementation
- PO with full glass of water, milk; or give with food to decrease GI upset
- Store in airtight, light-resistant container

Patient/family education
- Teach patient to use good oral hygiene; frequent rinsing of mouth, sugarless gum for dry mouth
- Caution patient to avoid hazardous activities until drug

response is determined—dizziness, blurred vision may occur
- Inform patient that orthostatic hypotension occurs often—patient should rise from sitting or lying position gradually
- Instruct patient to avoid hot tubs, hot showers, tub baths—hypotension may occur
- Inform patient that heat stroke may occur in hot weather, and to take extra precautions to stay cool
- Advise patient to avoid abrupt withdrawal of this drug, or extrapyramidal symptoms may result; drug should be withdrawn slowly
- Teach patient to avoid OTC preparations (cough, hayfever, cold) unless approved by prescriber—serious drug interactions may occur; avoid use with alcohol, CNS depressants because increased drowsiness may occur

Evaluation
Positive therapeutic outcome
- Decrease in emotional excitement, hallucinations, delusions, paranoia
- Reorganization of patterns of thought, speech

Treatment of overdose: Lavage, provide airway

ropinirole (℞)
(roe-pin′e-role)
Requip
Func. class.: Antiparkinsonian agent
Chem. class.: Dopamine-receptor agonist, nonergot
Pregnancy category C

Action: Selective agonist for D_2 receptors (presynaptic/postsynaptic sites); binding at D_3receptor contributes to antiparkinson effects

➔ Therapeutic Outcome: Decreased symptoms of Parkinson's disease (involuntary movements)

Uses: Parkinsonism

Dosage and routes
Adult: PO 0.25 mg tid, titrate weekly to a max of 24 mg/day

Available forms: Tabs 0.25, 0.5, 1, 2, 5 mg

Adverse effects
CNS: Dystonia, *agitation, insomnia,* dizziness, psychosis, hallucinations, depression
CV: Orthostatic hypotension, hypotension, syncope, palpitations, tachycardia, hypertension
EENT: Blurred vision
GI: Nausea, vomiting, anorexia, dry mouth, constipation, dyspepsia, flatulence
GU: Impotence, urinary frequency
INTEG: Rash, sweating
RESP: Pharyngitis, rhinitis, sinusitis, bronchitis, dyspnea

Contraindications: Hypersensitivity

Precautions: Renal disease, cardiac disease, dysrhythmias, affective disorders, psychosis

Pharmacokinetics

Absorption	Well absorbed
Distribution	Widely distributed
Metabolism	Liver, extensively
Excretion	Kidneys
Half-life	6 hr

Pharmacodynamics

Unknown

Interactions
Individual drugs
Cimetidine: ↑ effect of ropinirole
Ciprofloxacin: ↑ ropinirole effect
Diltiazem: ↑ ropinirole effect
Enoxacin: ↑ ropinirole effect
Erythromycin: ↑ ropinirole effect
Estrogen: ↓ oral clearance of ropinirole
Fluvoxamine: ↑ ropinirole effect
Levodopa: ↑ effect of levodopa
Mexiletine: ↑ ropinirole effect
Norfloxacin: ↑ ropinirole effect
Tacrine: ↑ ropinirole effect

NURSING CONSIDERATIONS
Assessment
- Monitor B/P, respiration during initial treatment; hypotension or hypertension should be reported
- Assess mental status: affect, mood, behavioral changes, depression; complete suicide assessment
- Assess for involuntary movements in parkinsonism: akinesia, tremors, staggering gait, muscle rigidity, drooling; these symptoms should improve with therapy

Nursing diagnoses
✓ Mobility, impaired (uses)
✓ Injury, risk for (uses)
✓ Knowledge deficit (teaching)
✓ Noncompliance (teaching)

Implementation
- Give drug until NPO before surgery
- Adjust dosage to patient response
- Give with meals to decrease GI upset

Patient/family education
- Advise patient that therapeutic effects may take several wk to a few mo
- Caution patient to change positions slowly to prevent orthostatic hypotension
- Instruct patient to use drug exactly as prescribed; if drug is discontinued abruptly, parkinsonian crisis may occur

Evaluation
Positive therapeutic outcome
- Decreased akathisia, other involuntary movements
- Increased mood

sildenafil (℞)
(sil-den′a-fill)
Viagra
Func. class.: Erectile agent
Chem. class.: Selective inhibitor of cGMP-PDE5
Pregnancy category B

Action: Enhances the effect of nitric oxide (NO) by inhibiting phosphodiesterase type 5 (PDE5), which is necessary for degrading cGMP in the carpus cavernosum

➔ Therapeutic Outcome: Ability to achieve and maintain erection

Uses: Treatment of erectile dysfunction

Dosage and routes
Adult: PO 50 mg 1 hr before sexual activity; may be increased to 100 mg or decreased to 25 mg; max qd

Available forms: Tabs 25, 50, 100 mg

Adverse effects
CNS: Headache, flushing, dizziness

OTHER: Dyspepsia, nasal congestion, UTI, abnormal vision, diarrhea, rash

Contraindications: Hypersensitivity

Precautions: Anatomical penile deformities, sickle cell anemia, leukemia, multiple myeloma, pregnancy **B**

Pharmacokinetics

Absorption	Rapidly, bioavailability (40%)
Distribution	Unknown
Metabolism	Liver (active metabolities)
Excretion	Feces, urine
Half-life	4 hr

Pharmacodynamics

Onset	Unknown
Peak	½-1½ hr
Duration	Unknown

Interactions
Individual drugs

Cimetidine: ↑ sildenafil levels
Erythromycin: ↑ sildenafil levels
Ketoconazole: ↑ sildenafil levels
Itraconazole: ↑ sildenafil levels
Rifampin: ↓ sildenafil levels

NURSING CONSIDERATIONS
Assessment
- Identify organic nitrates that should not be used with this drug

Nursing diagnoses
✓ Noncompliance (teaching)
✓ Knowledge deficit (teaching)

Implementation
- Give approximately 1 hr before sexual activity, do not use more than once a day

Patient/family education
- Teach patient that drug does not protect against sexually transmitted diseases, including HIV
- Teach patient that drug absorption is reduced with a high fat meal

Evaluation
Positive therapeutic outcome
- Ability to achieve and maintain an erection

sodium hyaluronate (℞)
(so'dee-um hy-al-yur'o-nate)
Hyalgan, Synvisc
Func. class.: Joint agent

Action: Improves elasticity and viscosity of synovial fluid

➔ Therapeutic Outcome: Decreased pain in joint

Uses: Osteoarthritis of the knee

Dosage and routes
Adult: Intra-articular inj 2 ml injected qwk into affected knee, for a total treatment cycle of 3-5 inj/treatment cycle

Available forms: Tabs 0.4 mg

Adverse effects
LOCAL: Pain at inj site, pruritus

SYST: Headache

Contraindications: Hypersensitivity to hyaluronan, infections in area to be injected

P **Precautions:** Pregnancy, lactation, children

NURSING CONSIDERATIONS
Assessment
- Check site for bruising, swelling, pain

tamsulosin (℞)
(tam-sue-lo'sen)

Flumax

Func. class.: Selective α-adrenergic blocker

Chem. class.: Sulfamoyl phenethylamine derivative

Pregnancy category B

Therapeutic Outcome: Decreased symptoms of BPH

Uses: Symptoms of benign prostatic hyperplasia

Dosage and routes

Adult: PO 0.4 mg qd, increasing up to 0.8 mg qd if required after 2 wk

Available forms: Tabs 1, 2, 4, 8 mg

Adverse effects

CNS: Dizziness, headache, asthenia

CV: Chest pain

EENT: Amblyopia

GI: Nausea, diarrhea

GU: Decreased libido, abnormal ejaculation

MS: Back pain

RESP: Rhinitis, pharyngitis, cough

Contraindications: Hypersensitivity

P **Precautions:** Pregnancy **B**, children, lactation, hepatic disease, coronary artery disease, severe renal disease

Pharmacokinetics

Absorption	Well absorbed
Distribution	Not known; 98% plasma protein bound
Metabolism	Liver, extensively
Excretion	Kidneys
Half-life	9-15 hr

Pharmacodynamics

Unknown

Interactions

Drug classifications

α_1-Adrenergic blockers: Do not use together

NURSING CONSIDERATIONS
Assessment
- Monitor CBC with diff and liver function studies; B/P and heart rate
- Monitor urodynamic studies/urinary flow rates, residual volume

Nursing diagnoses
- ✓ Cardiac output, decreased (uses)
- ✓ Injury, potential for physical (side effects)
- ✓ Knowledge deficit (teaching)
- ✓ Noncompliance (teaching)

Implementation
- Store in tight container at 86° F (30° C) or less
- May be given with food to prevent GI symptoms

Patient/family education
- Teach patient not to discontinue drug abruptly; emphasize the importance of complying with dosage schedule, even if feeling better; if dose is missed take as soon as remembered; take at same time each day
- Teach patient not to use OTC products (cough, cold,

allergy) unless directed by prescriber; also to avoid large amounts of caffeine

• Caution patient that drug may cause dizziness, may occur during 1st few days of therapy; to avoid hazardous activities

Evaluation

Positive therapeutic outcome

• Decreased symptoms of benign prostatic hyperplasia

tiagabine (℞)

(tie-ah-ga'been)

Gabatril

Func. class.: Anticonvulsant

Pregnancy category C

Action: Mechanism unknown; may increase seizure threshold

Uses: Adjunct treatment of partial seizures

Dosage and routes

Adult: PO 4 mg qd, may increase by 4-8 mg qwk until desired response, max 56 mg/day

P ***Child 12-18 yr:*** PO 4 mg qd, may increase by 4 mg at beginning of wk 2, may increase by 4-8 mg of wk until desired response, max 32 mg/day

Available forms: Tabs 4, 12, 16, 20 mg

Adverse effects

CNS: Dizziness, anxiety, somnolence, ataxia, amnesia, unsteady gait, depression

CV: Vasodilation

GI: Nausea, diarrhea, vomiting

INTEG: Pruritus, rash

RESP: Pharyngitis, coughing

Contraindications: Hypersensitivity to this drug

Precautions: Hepatic disease, P renal disease, pregnancy **C**, G lactation, child <12 yr, elderly

Pharmacokinetics

Absorption	>95%
Distribution	Unknown
Metabolism	Liver
Excretion	Kidneys
Half-life	7-9 hr

Pharmacodynamics

Unknown

Interactions: Unknown

NURSING CONSIDERATIONS

Assessment

• Monitor renal studies: urinalysis, BUN, urine creatinine q3mo

• Monitor hepatic studies: ALT (SGPT), AST (SGOT), bilirubin

• Assess description of seizures

• Assess mental status: mood, sensorium, affect, behavioral changes; if mental status changes, notify prescriber

• Assess eye problems, need for ophthalmic examinations before, during, after treatment (slit lamp, funduscopy, tonometry)

• Assess allergic reaction: purpura, red raised rash; if these occur, drug should be discontinued

Implementation

• Store at room temp away from heat and light

• Provide hard candy, frequent rinsing of mouth, gum for dry mouth

• Provide assistance with ambulation during early part of treatment; dizziness occurs

• Provide seizure precautions: padded side rails; move objects that may harm patient

• Provide increased fluids, bulk in diet for constipation

Patient/family education

- Advise patient to carry Medic Alert ID stating patient's name, drugs taken, condition, prescriber's name and phone number
- Advise patient to avoid driving, other activities that require alertness
- Teach patient not to discontinue medication quickly after long-term use

Evaluation

Positive therapeutic outcome

- Decreased seizure activity; document on patient's chart

Treatment of overdose: Lavage, VS

tiludronate (℞)

(till-oo'droe-nate)

Skelid

Func. class.: Parathyroid agent (calcium regulator)

Chem. class.: Bisphosphonate

Pregnancy category C

Action: Decreases bone reabsorption and new bone development

Therapeutic Outcome: Decreased bone reabsorption and reduced calcium levels WNL

Uses: Paget's disease

Dosage and routes

Adult: PO 400 mg qd, with 8 oz water × 3 mo

Available forms: Tab 240 mg

Adverse effects

CNS: Headache, somnolence, dizziness, anxiety, vertigo, nervousness, involuntary movements

ENDO: Hyperparathyroidism

GI: *Nausea, diarrhea,* dry mouth, gastritis, vomiting, flatulence, gastric ulcers

GU: *Nephrotoxicity,* UTI

INTEG: Rash, epidermal necrosis, pruritus, sweating

MS: *Bone pain,* decreased mineralization of nonaffected bones, pathologic fractures

RESP: Rhinitis, rales, sinusitis, URI

Contraindications: Hypersensitivity to bisphosphonates, pathologic fractures, **P** children, colitis, severe renal disease with creatinine >5 mg/dl

Precautions: Pregnancy **C,** renal disease, lactation, restricted vit D/Ca, GI disease

Pharmacokinetics	
Absorption	Rapid
Distribution	Unknown, steady state 10 days
Metabolism	None
Excretion	Feces (unabsorbed), kidney (unchanged)
Half-life	150 hrs

Pharmacodynamics	
Onset	Unknown
Peak	Unknown
Duration	6 mo

Interactions

Drug classifications

Antacids: ↓ absorption of tiludronate

Mineral supplements with magnesium, calcium, or aluminum: ↓ absorption of tiludronate

Individual drugs

Aspirin: ↓ effect of tiludronate

Indomethacin: ↑ effect of tiludronate

NURSING CONSIDERATIONS

Assessment

- Assess for GI symptoms, polyuria, flushing, head swell-

ing, tingling, headache—may indicate hypercalcemia; nervousness, irritability, twitching, seizures, spasm, paresthesia indicates hypocalcemia at start of treatment
• Identify nutritional status; evaluate diet for sources of vitamin D (milk, some seafood), calcium (dairy products, dark green vegetables), phosphates
• Monitor BUN, creatinine, uric acid, chloride, electrolytes, urine pH, urinary calcium, magnesium, phosphate, urinalysis (calcium should be kept at 9-10 mg/dl), albumin, alk phosphatase baseline and q3-6 mo; check urine sediment for casts throughout treatment
• Assess for increased drug level—toxic reactions occur rapidly; have calcium chloride or gluconate on hand if calcium level drops too low; check for tetany

Nursing diagnoses
✓ Injury, risk for (adverse reactions)
✓ Pain, chronic (uses)
✓ Knowledge deficit (teaching)

Implementation
• Administer on empty stomach to improve absorption (2 hr ac), with 6-8 oz water

Patient/family education
• Caution patient to notify prescriber of hypercalcemic relapse: renal calculi, nausea, vomiting, thirst, lethargy, deep bone or flank pain
• Teach patient to follow a low-calcium diet as prescribed (Paget's disease, hypercalcemia)
• Advise patient to notify prescriber of diarrhea, nausea; dose may be divided to lessen these symptoms

Evaluation
Positive therapeutic outcome
• Calcium levels 9-10 mg/dl
• Decreasing symptoms of Paget's disease including pain

tizanidine (℞)
(tye-za'na-deen)
Zanaflex
Func. class.: Skeletal muscle relaxant, central acting
Chem. class.: Imidazole
Pregnancy category C

Action: Unknown; possesses central α_2-adrenergic agonist properties; reduces excitation of spinal cord interneurons; also acts on the basal ganglia, producing muscle relaxation

➔ **Therapeutic Outcome:** Decreased spasticity of muscles

Uses: Spinal cord injury, spasticity in multiple sclerosis, tension headache

Dosage and routes
Adult: Reduce dose in renal failure; 4-36 mg qd in 3 divided doses

Spasticity:
Adult: PO 4 mg as a single dose; may increase in 2-4 mg steps until desired response, may repeat q6-8 hr up to 3 doses/24 hr, max 36 mg/day

Tension headache:
Adult: PO 2 mg tid, may increase by 4-6 mg tid after 2 wk interval

Available forms: Tabs 4 mg

Adverse effects
CNS: Dizziness, asthenia, somnolence, *fatigue, insomnia,* severe sedation

CV: Hypotension
GI: Nausea, constipation, vomiting, diarrhea, ***hepatotoxicity,*** *dry mouth,* anorexia
GU: Urinary frequency, UTI
INTEG: Rash, pruritus, sweating, skin ulcer

Contraindications: Hypersensitivity

Precautions: Renal disease, hepatic disease, stroke, cardiac disease, pregnancy **C,** G elderly

Pharmacokinetics

Absorption	Complete
Distribution	Widely
Metabolism	Liver, extensively
Excretion	Kidneys, feces
Half-life	2½ hr

Pharmacodynamics

Onset	Unknown
Peak	1-2 hr
Duration	3-6 hr

Interactions

Individual drugs

Alcohol: CNS depression

Drug classifications

Antidepressants, tricyclic: ↑ CNS depression
Barbiturates: ↑ CNS depression
Diuretics: ↑ hypotensive effects
Narcotics: ↑ CNS depression
Oral contraceptives: ↑ adverse reactions of tizanidine
Sedative/hypnotics: ↑ CNS depression

Lab test interferences

↑ AST (SGOT), ↑ alkaline phosphatase

NURSING CONSIDERATIONS

Assessment

- Monitor B/P, heart rate
- Perform neuroexam in spasticity: deep tendon reflexes, muscle tone, clonus, sensory function
- Monitor Liver, renal function tests, electrolytes, CBC with diff during long-term treatment
- Assess for allergic reactions: rash, fever, respiratory distress; severe weakness, numbness in extremities
- Assess CNS depression: dizziness, drowsiness, psychiatric symptoms
- Check dosage, as individual titration is required

Nursing diagnoses

✓ Mobility, impaired uses
✓ Injury, risk for (adverse reactions)
✓ Knowledge deficit (teaching)

Implementation

- Give with meals for GI symptoms; gum, frequent sips of water for dry mouth
- Store in airtight container at room temperature

Patient/family education

- Advise patient not to discontinue medication quickly; spasticity, will occur; drug should be tapered off over 1-2 wk
- Advise patient not to take with alcohol, other CNS depressants, take as directed, if dose is missed, take as soon as remembered, unless it is almost time for next dose
- Caution patient to avoid altering activities while taking this drug; to avoid hazardous activities if drowsiness or dizziness occurs; to rise from sitting or lying slowly to prevent fainting
- Advise patient to avoid using OTC medication: cough preparations, antihistamines unless directed by prescriber
- Notify prescriber if fainting, hallucinations, dark urine, stomach pain, yellowing of skin/eyes occur

Evaluation
Positive therapeutic outcome
- Decreased pain, spasticity

toremifene (℞)
(tore′me-feen)
Fareston
Func. class.: Antineoplastic
Chem. class.: Antiestrogen hormone
Pregnancy category D

Action: Inhibits cell division by binding to cytoplasmic estrogen receptors; resembles normal cell complex but inhibits DNA synthesis and estrogen response of target tissue

Therapeutic Outcome: Prevention of rapidly growing malignant cells

Uses: Advanced breast carcinoma that has not responded to other therapy in estrogen-receptor-positive patients (usually postmenopausal)

Dosage and routes
Adult: PO 60 mg qd

Available forms: Tabs 60 mg

Adverse effects
CNS: Hot flashes, headache, lightheadedness, depression
CV: Chest pain
EENT: Ocular lesions, retinopathy, corneal opacity, blurred vision (high doses)
GI: Nausea, vomiting, altered taste (anorexia)
GU: Vaginal bleeding, pruritus vulvae
HEMA: Thrombocytopenia, leukopenia
INTEG: Rash, alopecia
META: Hypercalcemia

Contraindications: Hypersensitivity, pregnancy **D**

Precautions: Leukopenia, thrombocytopenia, lactation, cataracts

Pharmacokinetics

Absorption	Adequately absorbed
Distribution	Unknown
Metabolism	Liver, extensively
Excretion	Feces, slowly, small amounts (kidneys)
Half-life	Unknown

Pharmacodynamics

Onset	Unknown
Peak	3 hr
Duration	Unknown

Interactions
Lab test interferences
↑ Serum Ca

NURSING CONSIDERATIONS
Assessment
- Monitor CBC, differential, platelet count weekly; withhold drug if WBC is <4000 or platelet count is <75,000; notify prescriber of results; monitor calcium levels (hypercalcemia is common)
- Assess for tumor flare: increase in bone, tumor pain during beginning treatment; give analgesics as ordered to decrease pain
- Assess for bleeding: hematuria, guaiac, bruising or petechiae, mucosa or orifices q8h, no rec temp

Nursing diagnoses
- ✓ Injury, risk for (adverse reactions)
- ✓ Knowledge deficit (teaching)

Implementation
- Give with food or fluids for GI upset; do not break, crush, or chew enteric products; repeat dose may be needed if vomiting occurs
- Store in light-resistant container at room temp

Patient/family education

- Instruct patient to report any complaints, side effects to health care prescriber; if dose is missed, do not double next dose
- Advise patient that vaginal bleeding, pruritus, hot flashes, can occur, and are reversible after discontinuing treatment
- Instruct patient to report immediately decreased visual acuity, which may be irreversible; stress need for routine eye exams
- Inform patient about who should be told about toremifene therapy
- Advise patient to report vaginal bleeding immediately; that tumor flare—increase in size or tumor, increased bone pain—may occur and will subside rapidly; may take analgesics for pain; that premenopausal women must use mechanical birth control method because ovulation may be induced (teratogenic drug)
- Caution patient to use sunscreen and protective clothing to prevent burns because photosensitivity is common
- Teach patient that hair loss may occur during treatment; a wig or hairpiece may make patient feel better; new hair may be different in color, texture
- Inform patient rash or lesions are temporary and may become large during beginning therapy

Evaluation

Positive therapeutic outcome

- Decreased spread of malignant cells in breast cancer

trandolapril (℞)
(tran-doe'la-prill)
Mavik
Func. class.: Antihypertensive
Chem. class.: Angiotensin-converting enzyme inhibitor
Pregnancy category
D (2nd/3rd trimester);
C (1st trimester)

Action: Selectively suppresses renin-angiotensin-aldosterone system; inhibits ACE; prevents conversion of angiotensin I to angiotensin II, resulting in dilatation of arterial and venous vessels and lowered B/P

➔ **Therapeutic Outcome:** Decreased B/P in hypertension

Uses: Hypertension alone or in combination

Dosage and routes
Adult: PO 1 mg/day, 2 mg/day in African Americans, make dosage adjustment ≥wk

Available forms: Tabs 1, 2, 4 mg

Adverse effects
CNS: Dizziness, paresthesias, headache, fatigue, drowsiness, depression, sleep disturbances
CV: Hypotension, MI, palpitations, angina, TIAs, stroke, bradycardia, dysrhythmias
GI: Nausea, vomiting, cramps, diarrhea, constipation, ileus, pancreatitis, hepatitis
GU: ***Proteinuria, renal failure***
HEMA: Agranulocytosis, ***neutropenia,*** leukopenia, anemia
INTEG: Rash, purpura

MISC: Hyperkalemia, hyponatremia, impotence
RESP: Dyspnea, cough

Contraindications: Hypersensitivity, history of angioedema, pregnancy **D** (2nd/3rd trimester)

Precautions: Renal disease, hyperkalemia, hepatic disease, bilateral renal stenosis, post kidney transplant, aortal/mitral valve stenosis, cirrhosis, severe renal disease, untreated CHF, autoimmune diseases, severe hypertension

Pharmacokinetics

Absorption	40-60%
Distribution	Unknown
Metabolism	Liver
Excretion	Kidneys, feces
Half-life	0.6-1.1 hr, 16-24 hr

Pharmacodynamics

Onset	½ hr
Peak	4-10 hr
Duration	>8 days

Interactions

Individual drugs

Alcohol: ↑ hypotension (large amounts)
Allopurinol: ↑ hypersensitivity
Capsaicin: ↑ coughing
Digoxin: ↑ serum levels of digoxin
Hydralazine: ↑ toxicity
Indomethacin: ↓ antihypertensive effect
Lithium: ↑ serum levels of lithium
Prazosin: ↑ toxicity

Drug classifications

Adrenergic blockers: ↑ hypotension
Antacids: ↓ absorption
Antihypertensives: ↑ hypotension
Diuretics: ↑ hypotension
Diuretics, potassium-sparing: ↑ toxicity
Ganglionic blockers: ↑ hypotension
Phenothiazines: ↑ antihypertensive effects
Potassium supplements: ↑ toxicity of potassium
Sympathomimetics: ↑ toxicity

NURSING CONSIDERATIONS

Assessment

- Monitor blood studies: neutrophils, decreased platelets
- Monitor B/P, orthostatic hypotension, syncope; if changes occur dosage change may be required
- Monitor renal studies: protein, BUN, creatinine; increased levels may indicate nephrotic syndrome and renal failure
- Monitor renal symptoms: polyuria, oliguria, frequency, dysuria
- Establish baselines in renal, liver function tests before therapy begins
- Check potassium levels throughout treatment, although hyperkalemia rarely occurs
- Check for edema in feet, legs daily
- Assess for allergic reactions: rash, fever, pruritus, urticaria; drug should be discontinued if antihistamines fail to help

Nursing diagnoses

✓ Cardiac output, decreased (uses)
✓ Injury, potential for (adverse reactions)
✓ Knowledge deficit (teaching)
✓ Noncompliance (teaching)

Implementation

- Store in air-tight container at 86° F (36° C) or less

Patient/family education

- Advise patient not to discontinue drug abruptly; advise

patient to tell all persons associated with health care

- Teach patient not to use OTC products (cough, cold, allergy medications) unless directed by physician; serious side effects can occur; xanthines, such as coffee, tea, chocolate, cola can prevent action of drug
- Instruct patient on the importance of complying with dosage schedule, even if feeling better; to continue with medical regimen to decrease B/P: exercise, cessation of smoking, decreasing stress, diet modifications
- Emphasize the need to rise slowly to sitting or standing position to minimize orthostatic hypotension; not to exercise in hot weather, which can cause increased hypotension
- Advise patient to notify prescriber of mouth sores, sore throat, fever, swelling of hands or feet, irregular heartbeat, chest pain, coughing, shortness of breath
- Caution patient to report excessive perspiration, dehydration, vomiting, diarrhea; may lead to fall in B/P
- Caution patient that drug may cause dizziness, fainting, lightheadedness; may occur during 1st few days of therapy; to avoid activities that may be hazardous
- Teach patient how to take B/P, and normal readings for age group

Evaluation

Positive therapeutic outcome

- Decreased B/P in hypertension

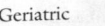

Treatment of overdose: Lavage, **IV** atropine for bradycardia, **IV** theophylline for bronchospasm, digitalis, O_2, diuretic for cardiac failure, hemodialysis

Appendix B

Recent FDA Drug Approvals

GENERIC NAME	TRADE NAME	USE
alatrofloxacin	Trovan*	Bacterial infections
arbutamine	GenESA	Diagnosis of coronary artery disease
beclapermin	Regranex	Diabetic neuropathic ulcers
cefdinir	Omnicef	Bacterial infections
daclizumab	Zenapax	Immunosuppressive
emedastine	Emadine	Allergic conjunctivitis
eprosartan	Teveten	Essential hypertension
fenoldopam	Corlopam	Severe hypertension
fomepizole	Antizol	Antifreeze poisoning
montelukast	Singulair	Chronic asthma
naratriptan	Amerge	Migraine headaches
oprevelkin	Neumega	Prevention of severe thrombocytopenia
raloxifene	Evista	Estrogen receptor modulator
repaglinide	Prandin	Non–insulin-dependent diabetes
sibutramine	Meridia	Weight loss
tolcapone	Tasmar	Parkinson's disease
trovafloxacin	Trovan*	Bacterial infections
ursodiol	URSO	Biliary cirrhosis
zolmitriptan	Zomig	Migraine headaches

* *Note:* Trovafloxacin, which is administered PO, and alatrofloxacin (a trovafloxacin prodrug, preservative free), which is administered IV, are both being marketed under the trade name Trovan.

Appendix C

Combination Products

A-200 Shampoo: 33% pyrethrins/4% piperonyl
Aceta with Codeine: acetaminophen 300 mg/codeine 30 mg
Actifed: pseudoephedrine 60 mg/tripolidine 2.5 mg
Actifed Allergy Nighttime: pseudoephedrine 30 mg/ acetaminophen 500 mg
Actifed Sinus Daytime: pseudoephedrine 30 mg/acetaminophen 500 mg
Actifed Sinus Nighttime: pseudoephedrine 30 mg/ diphenhydramine 25 mg/acetaminophen 500 mg
Adderall 10 mg: dextroamphetamine sulfate 5 mg/ dextroamphetamine saccharate 2.5 mg/amphetamine sulfate 2.5 mg/amphetamine aspartate 2.5 mg
Adderall 20 mg: dextroamphetamine sulfate 5 mg/ dextroamphetamine saccharate 5 mg/amphetamine sulfate 5 mg/ amphetamine aspartate 5 mg
Advil Cold & Sinus: pseudoephedrine 30 mg/ibuprofen 20 mg
AK-Cide Ophthalmic Suspension (ointment): 10% sulfacetamide/0.5% prednisolone
Aldactazide 25/25: spironolactone 25 mg/hydrochlorothiazide 25 mg
Aldactazide 50/50: spironolactone 50 mg/hydrochlorothiazide 50 mg
Aldoclor-150: methyldopa 250 mg/chlorothiazide 150 mg
Aldoclor-250: methyldopa 250 mg/chlorothiazide 250 mg
Aldoril-15: methyldopa 250 mg/hydrochlorothiazide 15 mg
Aldoril-25: methyldopa 250 mg/hydrochlorothiazide 25 mg
Aldoril D30: methyldopa 500 mg/hydrochlorothiazide 30 mg
Aldoril D50: methyldopa 500 mg/hydrochlorothiazide 50 mg
Alka-Seltzer Effervescent, Original: sodium bicarbonate 1916 mg/citric acid 1000 mg/aspirin 325 mg
Alka-Seltzer Plus Night-Time Cold Liqui-Gels: doxylamine 6.25 mg/dextromethorphan 10 mg/pseudoephedrine 30 mg/ acetaminophen 250 mg
Alka-Seltzer Plus Cold & Cough Liqui-Gels: dextromethorphan 10 mg/pseudoephedrine 30 mg/chlorpheniramine 2 mg/ acetaminophen 250 mg
Alka-Seltzer Plus Cold & Cough: phenylpropanolamine 20 mg/ chlorpheniramine 2 mg/dextromethorphan 10 mg/aspirin 325 mg
Alka-Seltzer Plus Cold Medicine: chlorpheniramine 2 mg/ phenylpropanolamine 20 mg/aspirin 325 mg
Alka-Seltzer Plus Night-Time Cold: phenylpropanolamine 20 mg/doxylamine 6.25 mg/dextromethorphan 15 mg/ aspirin 500 mg

Allerest Maximum Strength: pseudoephedrine 30 mg/chlorpheniramine 2 mg

All-Nite Cold Formula Liquid: pseudoephedrine 10 mg/doxylamine 1.25 mg/dextromethorphan 5 mg/acetaminophen 167 mg/5 ml

Amaphen: acetaminophen 325 mg/butalbital 50 mg/caffeine 40 mg

Ambenyl: diphenhydramine 12.5 mg/codeine 10 mg/5 ml

Anacin: aspirin 400 mg/caffeine 32 mg

Anacin Maximum Strength: aspirin 500 mg/caffeine 32 mg

AnacinPM (Aspirin Free): diphenhydramine 25 mg/acetaminophen 500 mg

Anaplex HD Syrup: hydrocodone 1.7 mg/phenylephrine 5 mg/chlorpheniramine 2 mg

Anaplex Liquid: chlorpheniramine 2 mg/pseudoephedrine 30 mg

Anatuss: guaifenesin 100 mg/dextromethorphan 15 mg/phenylpropanolamine 25 mg/acetaminophen 325 mg

Anatuss Syrup: guaifenesin 100 mg/dextromethorphan 15 mg/phenylpropanolamine 25 mg

Anexsia 5/500: hydrocodone 5 mg/acetaminophen 500 mg

Anexsia 7.5/650: hydrocodone 7.5 mg/acetaminophen 650 mg

Anexsia 10/650: hydrocodone 10 mg/acetaminophen 650 mg

Antrocol Elixir: atropine 0.195 mg/phenobarbital 16 mg

Apresazide 25/25: hydralazine 25 mg/hydrochlorothiazide 25 mg

Aprodine Syrup: pseudoephedrine 30 mg/tripolidine 1.25 mg

Aralen Phosphate with Primaquine Phosphate: chloroquine 300 mg/primaquine 45 mg

Arthritis Foundation Nighttime: acetaminophen 500 mg/diphenhydramine 25 mg

Arthritis Pain Formula: aspirin 500 mg/aluminum hydroxide 25 mg/magnesium hydroxide 100 mg

Ascriptin A/D: aspirin 325 mg/aluminum hydroxide 75 mg/magnesium hydroxide 75 mg/calcium carbonate 75 mg

Aspirin-Free Bayer Select Allergy Sinus: pseudoephedrine 30 mg/chlorpheniramine 2 mg/acetaminophen 500 mg

Aspirin-Free Bayer Select Head & Chest Cold: pseudoephedrine 30 mg/guaifenesin 100 mg/dextromethorphan 10 mg/acetaminophen 500 mg

Aspirin Free Excedrin: acetaminophen 500 mg/caffeine 65 mg

Aspirin Free Excedrin Dual: acetaminophen 500 mg/calcium carbonate 111 mg/magnesium carbonate 64 mg/magnesium oxide 30 mg

Atropine/Meperidine Injection: meperidine 50 mg/atropine 0.4 mg/ml

Atropine/Meperidine Injection: meperidine 75 mg/atropine 0.4 mg/ml

Augmentin/Clavulin: amoxicillin 250 mg/clavulanate 125 mg; amoxicillin 500 mg/clavulanate 125 mg; amoxicillin 125 mg/clavulanate 31.5 mg/5 ml; amoxicillin 250 mg/clavulanate 31.5 mg/5 ml

Axotal: aspirin 650 mg/butalbital 50 mg

Azo-Gantanol: sulfisoxazole 500 mg/phenazopyridine 100 mg
Azo-Gantrisin: sulfisoxazole 500 mg/phenazopyridine 50 mg
B&O Supprettes: belladonna extract 16.2 mg/opium 60 mg
B-A-C: aspirin 650 mg/butalbital 50 mg/caffeine 40 mg/buffers
Bactrim: trimethoprim 80 mg/sulfamethoxazole 400 mg
Bactrim DS: trimethoprim 160 mg/sulfamethoxazole 800 mg
Bancap: acetaminophen 325 mg/butalbital 50 mg
Bancap HC: acetaminophen 500 mg/hydrocodone 5 mg
Barbidonna: belladonna alkaloids/atropine 0.025 mg/hyoscyamine 0.1286 mg/phenobarbital 16 mg/scopolamine 0.0074 mg
Barbidonna #2: belladonna alkaloids, atropine 0.025 mg/hyoscyamine 0.1286 mg/phenobarbital 32 mg/scopolamine 0.0074 mg
Bayer Plus, Extra Strength: aspirin 500 mg/calcium carbonate/magnesium carbonate/magnesium oxide
Bayer Select Chest Cold: dextromethorphan 15 mg/acetaminophen 500 mg
Bayer Select Flu Relief: acetaminophen 500 mg/pseudoephedrine 30 mg/dextromethorphan 15 mg/chlorpheniramine 2 mg
Bayer Select Head Cold: pseudoephedrine 30 mg/acetaminophen 500 mg
Bayer Select Maximum Strength Headache: acetaminophen 500 mg/caffeine 65 mg
Bayer Select Maximum Strength Menstrual: acetaminophen 500 mg/pamabrom 25 mg
Bayer Select Maximum Strength Night-Time Pain Relief: acetaminophen 500 mg/diphenhydramine 25 mg
Bayer Select Maximum Strength Sinus Pain Relief: acetaminophen 500 mg/diphenhydramine 25 mg
Bayer Select Maximum Strength Sinus Pain Relief: acetaminophen 500 mg/pseudoephedrine 30 mg
Bayer Select Night Time Cold: acetaminophen 500 mg/pseudoephedrine 30 mg/dextromethorphan 15 mg/tripolidine 1.25 mg
BC Powder: aspirin 650 mg/caffeine 32 mg/salicylamide 195 mg
Bellatal: phenobarbital 16.2 mg/hyoscyamine 0.1027 mg/atropine 0.0194 mg/scopolamine 0.0065 mg
Bellergal-S: ergotamine 0.6 mg/belladonna alkaloids 0.2 mg
Bel-Phen-Ergot-S: phenobarbital 40 mg/ergotamine 0.6 mg/belladonna alkaloids 0.2 mg
Benadryl Allergy Decongestant Liquid: diphenhydramine 12.5 mg/pseudoephedrine 30 mg/5 ml
Benylin Expectorant Liquid: dextromethorphan 5 mg/guaifenesin 100 mg/5 ml
Benylin Multi-Symptom: dextromethorphan 5 mg/pseudoephedrine 15 mg/guaifenesin 100 mg
Benzamycin: erythromycin 30 mg/benzoyl peroxide 50 mg/gm
Bicillin C-R: 150,000 U penicillin G procaine/150,000 U penicillin G benzathine/ml
Bion Tears: 0.1% dextran 70/0.3% hydroxypropyl methylcellulose

Blephamide Suspension/Ointment: 0.2% prednisolone/10% sulfacetamide
Bromfed Capsules: brompheniramine 12 mg/pseudoephedrine 120 mg
Bromo-Seltzer: sodium bicarb 2.781 mg/acetaminophen 325 mg/citric acid 2.224 mg
Bromophen T.D.: brompheniramine 12 mg/phenylephrine 15 mg/phenylpropanolamine 15 mg
Bronchial Capsules: theophylline 150 mg/guaifenesin 90 mg
Bronkaid Dual Action: ephedrine 25 mg/guaifenesin 400 mg
Brontex: codeine 10 mg/guaifenesin 300 mg
Buff-A-Comp No. 3: aspirin 325 mg/codeine 30 mg/caffeine 40 mg/butalbital 50 mg
Bufferin: aspirin 325 mg/calcium carbonate 158 mg/magnesium oxide 63 mg/magnesium carbonate 34 mg
Bufferin AF Nite-Time: acetaminophen 500 mg/diphenhydramine 38 mg
Butibel: belladonna extract 15 mg/butabarbital 15 mg
Cafatine PB: ergotamine 1 mg/caffeine 100 mg/belladonna alkaloids 0.125 mg/pentobarbital 30 mg
Cafatine Suppositories: ergotamine 2 mg/caffeine 100 mg
Cafergot: ergotamine 1 mg/caffeine 100 mg
Cafergot Suppositories: ergotamine 2 mg/caffeine 100 mg
Caladryl Lotion: 8% calamine and camphor/2.2% alcohol/pramoxine/diazolidinyl urea
Calcet: calcium 152.8 mg/vitamin D 100 IU
Calcidrine Syrup: codeine 8.4 mg/calcium iodide 152 mg/5 ml
Cama Arthritis Pain Reliever: aspirin 500 mg/magnesium oxide 150 mg/aluminum hydroxide 125 mg
Capital with Codeine: acetaminophen 120 mg/codeine 12 mg/5 ml
Capozide 25/25: captopril 25 mg/hydrochlorothiazide 25 mg
Capozide 50/15: captopril 50 mg/hydrochlorothiazide 15 mg
Cardec DM Syrup: pseudoephedrine 60 mg/carbinoxamine 4 mg/dextromethorphan 15 mg/5 ml
Cetacaine Topical: 14% benzocaine/2% tetracaine/0.5% benzalkonium/0.005% cetyl dimethyl ethyl ammonium
Ceta Plus: hydrocodone 5 mg/acetaminophen 500 mg
Cetapred Ophthalmic Ointment: 0.25% prednisolone/10% sodium sulfacetamide
Cheracol Syrup: codeine 10 mg/guaifenesin 100 mg/5ml
Chlor-Trimeton Allergy Decongestant: chlorpheniramine 4 mg/pseudoephedrine 60 mg
Chlor-Trimeton 12 Hour Relief: pseudoephedrine 120 mg/chlorpheniramine 8 mg
Claritin-D: loratidine 5 mg/pseudoephedrine 120 mg
Clindex: chlordiazepoxide 5 mg/clidinium 2.5 mg
Clinoxide: chlordiazepoxide 5 mg/clidinium 2.5 mg
Clipoxide: chlordiazepoxide 5 mg/clidinium 2.5 mg
Clomycin Ointment: bacitracin 500 U/neomycin 3.5 gm/polymyxin B 500 U/lidocaine 40 mg

Co-Apap: pseudoephedrine 30 mg/chlorpheniramine 2 mg/ dextromethorphan 15 mg/acetaminophen 325 mg
Co-Gesic: acetaminophen 500 mg/hydrocodone 5 mg
Codamine Syrup: hydrocodone 5 mg/phenylpropanolamine 25 mg
Codehist DH Elixir: pseudoephedrine 30 mg/chlorpheniramine 2 mg/codeine 10 mg/5ml
Codiclear DH Syrup: hydrocodone 5 mg/guaifenesin 100 mg/ 5ml
Codimal DH Syrup: hydrocodone 1.66 mg/phenylephrine 5 mg/ pyrilamine 8.33 mg/5ml
Codimal LA: chlorpheniramine 8 mg/pseudoephedrine 120 mg
Codimal PH Syrup: codeine 10 mg/phenylephrine 5 mg/ pyrilamine 8.33 mg/5ml
Col-Probenecid: probenecid 500 mg/colchicine 0.5 mg
ColBenemid: probenecid 500 mg/colchicine 0.5 mg
Coldrine: pseudoephedrine 30 mg/acetaminophen 500 mg
Coly-Mycin S Otic: 1% hydrocortisone/neomycin 3.3 mg/colistin 3 mg/0.5% thonzonium/ml
Combipres 0.1: chlorthalidone 15 mg/clonidine 0.1 mg
Comhist: phenylephrine 10 mg/chlorpheniramine 2 mg/ phenyltoloxamine 25 mg
Comtrex Liquid: chlorpheniramine 0.67 mg/acetaminophen 108.3 mg/dextromethorphan 3.3 mg/pseudoephedrine 10 mg/5ml
Comtrex Allergy-Sinus: chlorpheniramine 2 mg/acetaminophen 500 mg/pseudoephedrine 30 mg
Comtrex Liqui-Gels: acetaminophen 325 mg/ phenylpropanolamine 12.5 mg/chlorpheniramine 2 mg/ dextromethorphan 10 mg
Comtrex Maximum Strength Multi-Symptoms Cold and Flu Relief: pseudoephedrine 30 mg/dextromethorphan 15 mg/ chlorpheniramine 2 mg/acetaminophen 500 mg
Congespirin: phenylephrine 1.25 mg/acetaminophen 81 mg
Congess SR: guaifenesin 250 mg/pseudoephedrine 120 mg
Congestac: guaifenesin 400 mg/pseudoephedrine 60 mg
Contac Cough & Sore Throat Liquid: dextromethorphan 5 mg/ acetaminophen 125 mg/5ml
Contac Day Cold and Flu: pseudoephedrine 60 mg/ dextromethorphan 30 mg/acetaminophen 650 mg/5ml
Contac 12 Hour Capsules: phenylpropanolamine 75 mg/ chlorpheniramine 8 mg
Contac Night Cold and Flu Caplets: pseudoephedrine 60 mg/ diphenhydramine 50 mg/acetaminophen 650 mg
Contuss Liquid: phenylpropanolamine 20 mg/phenylephrine 5 mg/guaifenesin 100 mg/5ml
Cope: aspirin 421 mg/caffeine 32 mg/magnesium hydroxide 50 mg/aluminum hydroxide 25 mg
Coricidin: chlorpheniramine 2 mg/acetaminophen 325 mg
Coricidin 'D': phenylpropanolamine 12.5 mg/chlorpheniramine 2 mg/acetaminophen 325 mg
Correctol: docusate 100 mg/phenolphthalein 65 mg

Cortic Ear Drops: hydrocortisone 10 mg/pramoxine 10 mg/ chloroxylenol 1 mg/ml
Cortisporin Ophthalmic/Otic Suspension: 0.35% neomycin/ polymyxin B 10,000 U/1% hydrocortisone/ml
Cortisporin topical: 0.5% neomycin/polymyxin B 10,000 U/0.5% hydrocortisone
Corzide 40/5: nadolol 40 mg/bendroflumethiazide 5 mg
Cough-X: dextromethorphan 5 mg/benzocaine 2 mg
Creon: lipase 8,000 U/amylase 30,000 U/protease 13,000 U/pancreatin 300 mg
Cyclomydril Ophthalmic Solution: 0.2% cyclopentolate/1% phenylephrine
D-S-S Plus: docusate sodium 100 mg/casanthranol 30 mg
Dallergy: chlorpheniramine 4 mg/phenylephrine 10 mg/ methscopolamine 1.25 mg
Dallergy-D Syrup: phenylephrine 5 mg/chlorpheniramine 2 mg/5 ml
Damason-P: hydrocodone 5 mg/aspirin 500 mg
Darvocet-N 50: acetaminophen 325 mg/propoxyphene 50 mg
Darvocet-N 100: propoxyphene 100mg/acetaminophen 650 mg
Darvon Compound-65: propoxyphene 65 mg/aspirin 389 mg/ caffeine 32.4 mg
Deconsal II: pseudoephedrine 60 mg/guaifenesin 600 mg
Deconamine SR: pseudoephedrine 120 mg/chlorpheniramine 8 mg
Demazin: phenylpropanolamine 25 mg/chlorpheniramine 4 mg
Demi-Regroton: chlorthalidone 25 mg/reserpine 0.125 mg
Demulen 1/50: ethinyl estradiol 50 mcg/ethynodiol diacetate 1 mg
Deprol: meprobamate 400 mg/benactyzine 1 mg
Dermoplast Spray 20% : 0.5% menthol/methylparaben/aloe/ lanolin
Dexacidin Ophthalmic Ointment: 0.1% dexamethasone/0.35% neomycin/polymyxin B 10,000 U/gm
Dexasporin Ophthalmic Ointment: 0.1% dexamethasone/0.35% neomycin/polymyxin B 10,000 U/gm
DHC Plus: dihydrocodeine 16 mg/acetaminophen 356.4 mg/ caffeine 30 mg
Dialose Plus: docusate 100 mg/phenolphthalein 60 mg
Di-Gel Liquid: aluminum hydroxide 200 mg/magnesium hydroxide 200 mg/simethicone 20 mg/5ml
Di-Gel Advanced Formula: magnesium hydroxide 128 mg/ calcium carbonate 280 mg/simethicone 20 mg
Dilaudid Cough Syrup: guaifenesin 100 mg/hydromorphone 1 mg
Dilor-G: dyphylline 200 mg/guaifenesin 200 mg
Dimetane Decongestant: brompheniramine 4 mg/phenylephrine 10 mg
Dimetapp: brompheniramine 4 mg/phenylpropanolamine 25 mg

Dimetapp Cold & Flu: phenylpropanolamine 12.5 mg/brompheniramine 2mg/acetaminophen 500 mg
Dimetapp Extentabs: brompheniramine 12 mg/phenylpropanolamine 75 mg
Dimetapp Sinus: pseudoephedrine 30 mg/ibuprofen 200 mg
Diupres-250: chlorothiazide 250 mg/reserpine 0.125 mg
Diupres-500: chlorothiazide 500 mg/reserpine 0.125 mg
Diutensin-R: methychlorthiazide 2.5 mg/reserpine 0.1 mg
Doan's PM Extra Strength: magnesium salicylate 500 mg/diphenhydramine 25 mg
Dolacet: hydrocodone 5 mg/acetaminophen 500 mg
Dolene-AP-65: acetaminophen 650 mg/propoxyphene 65 mg
Donnatal: phenobarbital 16.2 mg/hyoscyamine 0.1037 mg/atropine 0.194 mg/scopolamine 0.0065 mg
Donnatal Elixir: atropine 0.0194 mg/5 ml, scopolamine 0.0065 mg/5 ml, ethanol 23%, hyoscyamine 0.1037 mg/5 ml, phenobarbital 16 mg/5 ml
Donnatal Extentabs: atropine 0.0582 mg/scopolamine 0.0195 mg/ hyoscyamine 0.3111 mg/phenobarbital 48.6 mg
Donnatal No. 2 Tablets: atropine 0.0194 mg/scopolamine 0.0065 mg/hyoscyamine 0.1037 mg/phenobarbital 32.4 mg
Donnazyme: pancreatin 500 mg/lipase 1000 U/protease 12,500 U/amylase 12,500 U
Doxapap-N: propoxyphene 100 mg/acetaminophen 650 mg
Doxidan: docusate 60 mg/phenolphthalein 65 mg
Dristan Cold Multi-Symptom Formula: acetaminophen 325 mg/phenylephrine 5 mg/chlorpheniramine 2 mg
Drixoral Allergy Sinus: pseudoephedrine 60 mg/dexbrompheniramine 3 mg/acetaminophen 500 mg
Drixoral Cough & Congestion Liquid Caps: pseudoephedrine 60 mg/dextromethorphan 30 mg
Drixoral Cough & Sore Throat Liquid Caps: dextromethorphan 15 mg/acetaminophen 325 mg
Drize: phenylpropanolamine 75 mg/chlorpheniramine 12 mg
DT: diphtheria toxoid 2 Lf U/tetanus toxoid 5 Lf U/0.5 ml dose
DTP: diphtheria toxoid 6.5 Lf U/tetanus toxoid 5 Lf U/pertussis 4 Lf U/0.5 ml dose
Duocet: hydrocodone 5 mg/acetaminophen 500 mg
Duo-Medihaler: phenylephrine 0.24 mg/isoproterenol 0.16 mg
Dura-Vent: phenylpropanolamine 75 mg/guaifenesin 600 mg
Dura-Vent/A: phenylpropanolamine 75 mg/chlorpheniramine 10 mg
Dura-Vent/DA: phenylephrine 20 mg/chlorpheniramine 8 mg/methscopolamine 25 mg
Dyazide: hydrochlorothiazide 25 mg/triamterene 37.5 mg
Dynafed Asthma Relief: ephedrine 25 mg/guaifenesin 200 mg
Dyflex-G: dyphylline 200 mg/guaifenesin 200 mg
Dyphylline GG Elixir: dyphylline 100 mg/guaifenesin 100 mg/5 ml
E-L: acetaminophen 650 mg/propoxyphene 65 mg

E-Pilo-2 Ophthalmic Solution: 1% epinephrine bitartrate/2% pilocarpine
E-Pilo-4 Ophthalmic Solution: 1% epinephrine bitartrate/4% pilocarpine
Elase Ointment: fibrinolysin 1 U/desoxyribonuclease 666.6 U/gm
Elase-Chloromycetin Ointment: fibrinolysin 1 U/desoxyribonuclease 666.6 U/chloramphenicol 10 mg
Elixophyllin KI Elixir: theophylline 80 mg/potassium iodide 130 mg
Elixophyllin-GG Liquid: guaifenesin 100 mg/theophylline 100 mg/5 ml
EMLA Cream: lidocaine 2.5 mg/prilocaine 2.5 mg
Empirin #3: aspirin 325 mg/codeine 30 mg
Empirin #4: aspirin 325 mg/codeine 60 mg
Enovid 5 mg: mestranol 75 mcg/norethynodrel 5 mg
Enovid 10 mg: mestranol 150 mcg/norethynodrel 9.85 mg
Entex: phenylephrine 5 mg/phenylpropanolamine 45 mg/guaifenesin 200 mg
Entex LA: phenylpropanolamine 75 mg/guaifenesin 400 mg
Epifoam Aerosol Foam: 1% hydrocortisone/1% pramoxine
Equagesic: aspirin 325 mg/meprobamate 20 mg
Ercaf: ergotamine 1 mg/caffeine 100 mg
Esgic-Plus: butalbital 50 mg/acetaminophen 500 mg/caffeine 40 mg
Esimil: guanethidine 10 mg/hydrochlorothiazide 25 mg
Etrafon: perphenazine 2 mg/amitriptyline 25 mg
Etrafon Forte: perphenazine 4 mg/amitriptyline 25 mg
Ex-Lax, Extra Gentle: docusate sodium 75 mg/phenolphthalein 65 mg
Excedrin Extra Strength: aspirin 250 mg/acetaminophen 250 mg/caffeine 65 mg
Excedrin P.M.: acetaminophen 500 mg/diphenhydramine 38 mg
Excedrin Sinus Extra Strength: pseudoephedrine 30 mg/acetaminophen 500 mg
Fedahist: pseudoephedrine 60 mg/chlorpheniramine 4 mg
Fedahist Expectorant Syrup: guaifenesin 200 mg/pseudoephedrine 20 mg/5 ml
Feen-A-Mint Pills: docusate sodium 100 mg/phenolphthalein 65 mg
Fergon Plus: ferrous gluconate 58 mg/ascorbic acid 75 mg/vitamin B_{12} 7.5 mcg/intrinsic factor 150 mg
Ferro-Sequels: docusate sodium 100 mg/ferrous fumarate 150 mg
Fioricet: acetaminophen 325 mg/caffeine 40 mg/butalbital 50 mg
Fiorinal: aspirin 325 mg/caffeine 40 mg/butalbital 50 mg
Fiorinal with Codeine: aspirin 325 mg/caffeine 40 mg/butalbital 50 mg/codeine 30 mg
FML-S Ophthalmic Suspension: 0.1% flurometholone/10% sulfacetamide
Gaviscon Liquid: aluminum hydroxide 31.7 mg/magnesium carbonate 119.3 mg/5ml
Gaviscon: magnesium trisilicate 20 mg/aluminum hydroxide 80 mg

Gelprin: acetaminophen 125 mg/aspirin 240 mg/caffeine 32 mg
Gelusil: aluminum hydroxide 200 mg/magnesium hydroxide 200 mg/simethicone 25 mg
Genagesic: acetaminophen 650 mg/propoxyphene 65 mg
Genatuss DM Syrup: guaifenesin 100 mg/dextromethorphan 10 mg/5ml
Glyceryl-T: theophylline 150 mg/guaifenesin 90 mg
Granulex Aerosol: trypsin 0.1 mg/balsam peru 72.5 mg/castor oil 650 mg/0.82 ml
Halotussin-DM Sugar Free Liquid: guaifenesin 100 mg/ dextromethorphan 10 mg/5 ml
HemFe: ferrous fumarate 100 mg/ascorbic acid 125 mg/vitamin B_{12} 5 mcg/desiccated gastric substance 50 mg/docusate sodium 25 mg
Hycodan: hydrocodone 5 mg/homatropine 1.5 mg
Hycomine Compound: chlorpheniramine 2 mg/acetaminophen 250 mg/phenylephrine 10 mg/hydrocodone 5 mg/caffeine 30 mg
Hycomine Syrup: hydrocodone 5 mg/phenylpropanolamine 25 mg
Hycotuss Expectorant: guaifenesin 100 mg/hydrocodone 5 mg/ 10% alcohol
Hydergine: dihydroergocornine 0.167 mg/dihydroergocristine 0.167 mg/dihydroergocryptine 0.167 mg
Hydro-Serp: hydrochlorothiazide 50 mg/reserpine 0.125 mg
Hydrocet: hydrocodone 5 mg/acetaminophen 500 mg
Hydrogesic: hydrocodone 5 mg/acetaminophen 500 mg
Hydropres-25: hydrochlorothiazide 25 mg/reserpine 0.125 mg
Hydropres-50: hydrochlorothiazide 50 mg/reserpine 0.125 mg
Hydroserpin #1: hydrochlorothiazide 25 mg/reserpine 0.125 mg
Hyzaar: losartan 50mg/hydrochlorothiazide 12.5 mg/potassium 4.24 mg
Ibert Filmtab: ferrous sulfate 105 mg/ascorbic acid 150 mg/ B-complex vitamins
Iberet Liquid: ferrous sulfate 78.75 mg/ascorbic acid 112.5 mg/ B-complex vitamins/5ml
Inderide 40/25: propranolol 40 mg/hydrochlorothiazide 25 mg
Iophen-C Liquid: iodinated glycerol 30 mg/codeine 10 mg/5 ml
Isollyl Improved: aspirin 325 mg/caffeine 40 mg/butalbital 50 mg
Isophen-DM Liquid: iodinated glycerol 30 mg/dextromethorphan 10 mg/5 ml
Kinesed Tablets: atropine 0.02 mg/scopolamine 0.007 mg/ hyoscyamine 0.1 mg/phenobarbital 16 mg
Kondremul with Phenolphthalein: phenolphthalein 150 mg/ 55% mineral oil/Irish moss/15 ml
Levin with Phenobarbital: 1-hyoscyamine 0.125 mg/ phenobarbital 15 mg
Librax: chlordiazepoxide 5 mg/clidinium 2.5 mg
Lida-Mantel-HC-Cream: 0.5% hydrocortisone/3% lidocaine
Limbitrol DS 10-25: chlordiazepoxide 10 mg/amitriptyline 25 mg

Lobac: salicylamide 200 mg/phenyltoloxamine 20 mg/ acetaminophen 300 mg
Loestrin Fe 1.5/30: norethindrone acetate 1.5 mg/ethinyl estradiol 30 μg
Lo Ovral: ethinyl estradiol 30 μg/norgestrel 0.3 mg
Lopressor HCT 50/25: metoprolol 50 mg/hydrochlorothiazide 25 mg
Lopressor HCT 100/25: metoprolol 100 mg/ hydrochlorothiazide 25 mg
Lorcet: acetaminophen 500 mg/hydrocodone 5 mg
Lorcet-HD: hydrocodone 5 mg/acetaminophen 500 mg
Lorcet Plus: acetaminophen 650 mg/hydrocodone 7.5 mg
Lorcet 10/650: acetaminophen 650 mg/hydrocodone 10 mg
Lortab 2.5/500: hydrocodone 2.5 mg/acetaminophen 500 mg
Lortab 5/500: hydrocodone 5 mg/acetaminophen 500 mg
Lortab ASA: aspirin 500 mg/hydrocodone 5 mg
Lotensin HCT 20/25: benazepril 20 mg/hydrochlorothiazide 25 mg
Lotrel: amlopidine 2.5 mg/benazepril 10 mg
Lotrisone Topical: 0.5% betamethasone/1% clotrimazole
Lufyllin-EPG Elixir: ephedrine 24 mg/dyphylline 150 mg/ guaifenesin 300 mg/phenobarbital 24 mg
Lufyllin-GG: dyphylline 200 mg/guaifenesin 200 mg
M-M-R-II: measles/mumps/rubella
M-R Vax II: measles/rubella
Maalox Plus: aluminum hydroxide 200 mg/magnesium hydroxide 200 mg/simethicone 25 mg
Mapap Cold Formula: acetaminophen 325 mg/chlorpheniramine 2 mg/pseudoephedrine 30 mg/dextromethorphan 15 mg
Mapap with Codeine: acetaminophen 120 mg/codeine 12 mg/ 5 ml
Marax: ephedrine 25 mg/theophylline 130 mg/hydroxyzine 10 mg
Marax DF Syrup: theophylline 80 mg/ephedrine 18.75/ hydroxyzine 7.5 mg
Maxitrol Ophthalmic Suspension: 0.35% neomycin/0.1% dexamethasone/polymyxin B 10,000 U/ml
Maxzide: hydrochlorothiazide 50 mg/triamterene 75 mg
Menrium 5-2: chlordiazepoxide 5 mg/esterified estrogens 0.2 mg
Mepergan Injection: meperidine 25 mg/promethazine 25 mg
Mepergan Fortis: meperidine 50 mg/promethazine 25 mg
Metimyd Ophthalmic Suspension: 0.5% prednisolone/10% sodium sulfacetamide
Midol Maximum Strength Multi-Symptom: acetaminophen 500 mg/pyrilamine 15 mg
Midol PM: acetaminophen 500 mg/diphenhydramine 25 mg
Midol, Teen: acetaminophen 400 mg/pamabrom 25 mg
Midrin: isometheptene 65 mg/acetaminophen 325 mg/ dichloralphenazone 100 mg
Minizide 2: prazosin 2 mg/polythiazide 0.5 mg
Minizide 5: prazosin 5 mg/polythiazide 0.5 mg
Modane Plus: docusate sodium 100 mg/phenolphthalein 65 mg

Moduretic: hydrochlorothiazide 50 mg/amiloride 5 mg
Motrin IB Sinus: pseudoephedrine 30 mg/ibuprofen 200 mg
Mycolog II Topical: 0.1% triamcinolone acetonide/nystatin 100,000 U/gm
Mylanta Gelcaps: calcium carbonate 311 mg/magnesium carbonate 232 mg
Mylanta: aluminum hydroxide 200 mg/magnesium hydroxide 200 mg/simethicone 20 mg
Naldecon: chlorpheniramine 2.5 mg/phenylephrine 5 mg/phenylpropanolamine 20 mg/phenyltoloxamine 7.5 mg/5 ml
Naldecon: phenylephrine 10 mg/phenylpropanolamine 40 mg/phenyltoloxamine 15 mg/chlorpheniramine 5 mg
Naldecon DX: dextromethorphan 15 mg/guaifenesin 200 mg/phenylpropanolamine 18 mg/5 ml
Naldecon DX Children's Syrup: dextromethorphan 7.5 mg/guaifenesin 100 mg/phenylpropanolamine 9 mg/5 ml
Naldecon CX Adult Liquid: guaifenesin 200 mg/phenylpropanolamine 12.5 mg/codeine 10 mg/5 ml
Naldecon EX Children's Syrup: guaifenesin 100 mg/phenylpropanolamine 6.25 mg
Naldegesic: acetaminophen 325 mg/pseudoephedrine 15 mg
Nasatab LA: guaifenesin 500 mg/pseudoephedrine 120 mg
Naquival: trichlormethiazide 4 mg/reserpine 0.1 mg
Neo-Cortef Ointment: neomycin 0.5%/hydrocortisone 1%
Neo Decadron Cream: neomycin 0.5%/dexamethasone 0.1%
Neosporin Ointment: polymyxin B 5000 U/bacitracin zinc 400 U/neomycin 5 mg/g
Neosporin Ophthalmic: neomycin 1.75 mg/polymyxin B 10,000 U/gramicidin 0.025 mg/ml
Neosporin Ophthalmic: neomycin 3.5 mg/polymyxin B 10,000 U/bacitracin zinc 400 U/g
Neosporin Plus Cream: polymyxin B 10,000 U/neomycin 3.5 mg/lidocaine 40 mg
Neotal: neomycin 5 mg/polymyxin B 5000 U/bacitracin zinc 400 U
Neothylline-GG Tablets: dyphylline 200 mg/guaifenesin 200 mg
Neotrace-4: zinc sulfate 1.5 mg/copper sulfate 0.1 mg/manganese sulfate 0.025 mg/chromium chloride 0.85 mcg/ml
Neutra-Phos: phosphorus 25 mg/sodium 164 mg/potassium 278 mg
Nitrotym-Plus: nitroglycerin 2.5 mg/butabarbital 48 mg
Nolamine: chlorpheniramine 4 mg/phenindamine 24 mg/phenylpropanolamine 50 mg
Norgesic: orphenadrine 25 mg/aspirin 385 mg/caffeine 30 mg
Norgesic Forte: orphenadrine 50 mg/aspirin 770 mg/caffeine 60 mg
Normozide 100/25: labetalol 100 mg/hydrochlorothiazide 25 mg
Normozide 200/25: labetalol 200 mg/hydrochlorothiazide 25 mg
Normozide 300/25: labetalol 300 mg/hydrochlorothiazide 25 mg
Novacet Lotion: sulfacetamine 10%/sulfur 5%

Novafed A: pseudoephedrine 120 mg/chlorpheniramine 8 mg
Novahistine DH Liquid: chlorpheniramine 2 mg/ pseudoephedrine 30 mg/codeine 10 mg/5 ml
Novahistine DMX Liquid: guaifenesin 100 mg/dextromethorphan 10 mg/pseudoephedrine 30 mg/5 ml
Novahistine Elixir: phenylephrine 5 mg/chlorpheniramine 2 mg/ alcohol 5%/5 ml
Novahistine Expectorant: guaifenesin 100 mg/pseudoephedrine 30 mg/codeine 10 mg/5 ml
Novolin 70/30: isophane insulin suspension, human 70%/regular insulin injection, human 30%/100 U/ml
NuLytely: PEG 3350 420 g/sodium bicarbonate 5.72 g/sodium chloride 11.2 g/potassium chloride 1.48 g
NyQuil Hot Therapy: acetaminophen 1000 mg/pseudoephedrine 60 mg/dextromethorphan 30 mg/doxylamine 12.5 mg/packet
NyQuil Nightime Cold/Flu Medicine Liquid: pseudoephedrine 10 mg/doxylamine 1.25 mg/dextromethorphan 5 mg/ acetaminophen 167 mg/25% alcohol/5 ml
Octicair Otic: hydrocortisone 1%/neomycin 5 mg/polymyxin B 10,000 U/ml
Ophthocort: chloramphenicol 1%/polymyxin B 10,000 U/hydrocortisone 1%
Ophthocort: chloramphenicol 1%/polymyxin B 10,000 U/hydrocortisone 0.5%
Optimyd: prednisolone 0.5%/sulfacetamide 10%
Ornada Spansules: phenylpropanolamine 75 mg/chlorpheniramine 12 mg
Ornex No Drowsiness Caplets: acetaminophen 325 mg/ pseudoephedrine 30 mg
Ortho-Novum 1/35: 35 μg ethinyl estradiol/1 mg norethindrone
Ortho-Novum 1/50: 50 μg mestranol/1 mg norethindrone
Ortho-Novum 7/7/7: Phase I: 0.5 mg norethindrone/35 μg ethinyl estradiol; Phase II: 0.75 mg norethindrone, 35 μg ethinyl estradiol
Ortho-Novum 10/11: Phase I: 0.5 mg norethindrone/35 μg ethinyl estradiol; Phase II: 1 mg norethindrone/35 μg ethinyl estradiol
Otocort: hydrocortisone 1%/neomycin 5 mg/polymyxin B 10,000 U/ml
P-A-C Tablets: aspirin 400 mg/caffeine 32 mg
Pamprin, Maximum Pain Relief: acetaminophen 250 mg/ pamabrom 25 mg/magnesium salicylate 250 mg
Panacet 5/500: hydrocodone 5 mg/acetaminophen 500 mg
Panasal 5/500: hydrocodone 5 mg/aspirin 500 mg
Pancrease Capsules: amylase 20,000 U/protease 25,000 U/lipase 4,000 U (microspheres)
Pedia Care Cough-Cold Liquid: pseudoephedrine 15 mg/ chlorpheniramine 1 mg/dextromethorphan 5 mg
Pedia Care NightRest Cough-Cold Liquid: pseudoephedrine 15 mg/chlorpheniramine 1 mg/dextromethorphan 7.5 mg

Pediacof Syrup: codeine 5 mg/phenylephrine 2.5 mg/ chlorpheniramine 0.75 mg/potassium iodide 75 mg/ 5% alcohol/5 ml
Pediacon EX Drops: phenylpropanolamine 6.25 mg/guaifenesin 50 mg
Pediatric Multiple Trace Element: zinc sulfate 0.5 mg/copper sulfate 0.1 mg/manganese sulfate 0.03 mg/chromium chloride 1 mcg/ml
Pediazole Suspension: erythromycin 200 mg/sulfisoxazole 600 mg/ml
Pedtrace-4: zinc sulfate 0.5 mg/copper sulfate 0.1 mg/manganese sulfate 0.025 mg/chromium chloride 0.85 mcg/ml
Percocet: oxycodone 5 mg/acetaminophen 325 mg
Percodan: oxycodone 4.88 mg/aspirin 325 mg
Percodan-Demi: aspirin 325 mg/oxycodone 2.25 mg/oxycodone terephthalate 0.19 mg
Percodan-Roxiprin: aspirin 325 mg/oxycodone 4.5 mg/ oxycodone terephthalate 0.38 mg
Peri-Colace-Capsules: docusate 100 mg/casanthranol 30 mg
Peri-Colace Syrup: docusate 60 mg/casanthranol 30 mg/15 ml
Phenaphen-650 with Codeine: acetaminophen 650 mg/codeine 30 mg
Phenerbel-S: ergotamine 0.6 mg/belladonna alkaloids 0.2 mg/ phenobarbital 40 mg
Phenergan VC Syrup: phenylephrine 5 mg/promethazine 6.25 mg/5 ml
Pherazine DM Syrup: dextromethorphan 15 mg/promethazine 6.25 mg/7% alcohol/5 ml
Phillips' Laxative Gelcaps: docusate 83 mg/phenolphthalein 90 mg
Phrenilin: acetaminophen 325 mg/butalbital 50 mg
Phrenilin Forte: acetaminophen 650 mg/butalbital 50 mg
PMB-200: conjugated estrogens 0.45 mg/meprobamate 200 mg
PMB-400: conjugated estrogens 0.45 mg/meprobamate 400 mg
Polaramine Expectorant Liquid: guaifenesin 100 mg/ dexchlorpheniramine 2 mg/pseudoephedrine 20 mg
Polycitra Syrup: potassium citrate 550 mg/sodium citrate 550 mg/citric acid 334 mg
Poly-Histine Elixir: pheniramine 4 mg/pyrilamine 4 mg/ phenyltoloxamine 4 mg/4% alcohol
Poly-Histine DM Syrup: brompheniramine 2 mg/ phenylpropanolamine 12.5 mg/dextromethorphan 10 mg/5 ml
Poly-Histine CS Syrup: phenylpropanolamine 12.5 mg/ brompheniramine 2 mg/codeine 10 mg
Poly-Pred Ophthalmic Suspension: 0.5% prednisolone/0.35% neomycin/polymyxin B 10,000 U
Polysporin Ointment: polymyxin B 10,000 U/bacitracin zinc 500 U/g
Polysporin Ophthalmic Ointment: polymyxin B 10,000 U/bacitracin zinc 500 U

Polytrim Ophthalmic: trimethoprim 1 mg/polymyxin B 10,000 U/ml
Pred-G S.O.P.: prednisolone 0.6%/gentamicin base 0.3%/ chlorobutanol 0.5%,
Prednisolone Acetate and Prednisolone Sodium Phosphate: prednisolone acetate 80 mg/prednisolone sodium phosphate 20 mg/ml
Prefrin-A: phenylephrine 0.12%/pyrilamine 0.1%/antipyrine 0.1%
Premarin with Methyltestosterone: conjugated estrogens 0.625 mg/methyltestosterone 5 mg
Premarin with Methyltestosterone: conjugated estrogens 1.25 mg/methyltestosterone 10 mg
Prinzide 10-12.5: lisinopril 10 mg/hydrochlorothiazide 12.5 mg
Prinzide 20-12.5: lisinopril 20 mg/hydrochlorothiazide 12.5 mg
Prinzide 20-25: lisinopril 20 mg/hydrochlorothiazide 25 mg
Probenecid with Colchicine: probenecid 500 mg/cholchicine 0.5 mg
Pro Pox with APAP: acetaminophen 650 mg/propoxyphene 65 mg
Prosed/DS: methenamine 81.65 mg/phenylsalicylate 36.2 mg/ methylene blue 10.8 mg/benzoic acid 9 mg/atropine 0.06 mg/ hyoscyamine 0.06 mg
P.T.E.-4: zinc sulfate 1 mg/copper sulfate 0.1 mg/manganese sulfate 0.025 mg/chromium chloride 1 µg/ml
P.T.E.-5: zinc sulfate 1 mg/copper sulfate 0.1 mg/manganese sulfate 0.025 mg/chromium chloride 1 µg/selenious acid 15 µg/ml
P-V-Tussin Syrup: chlorpheniramine 2 mg/phenindamine 5 mg/ phenylephrine 5 mg/pyrilamine 6 mg/5 ml
Quibron Capsules: theophylline 150 mg/guaifenesin 90 mg
Rauzide: bendroflumethiazide 4 mg/powdered rauwolfia serpentina 50 mg
Regroton: chlorthalidone 50 mg/reserpine 0.25 mg
Renese-R: polythiazide 2 mg/reserpine 0.25 mg
Repan: acetaminophen 325 mg/caffeine 40 mg/butalbital 50 mg
Rezide: hydrochlorothiazide 15 mg/hydralazine 25 mg/reserpine 0.1 mg
R-HCTZ-H: hydrochlorothiazide 15 mg/hydralazine 25 mg/ reserpine 0.1 mg
Riopan Plus Chewable Tablets: magaldrate 540 mg/simethicone 20 mg
Riopan Plus Suspension: magaldrate 5409 mg/simethicone 20 mg/5 ml
Robaxisal: methocarbamol 400 mg/aspirin 325 mg
Rounox and Codeine 15: acetaminophen 325 mg/codeine 15 mg
Rounox and Codeine 30: acetaminophen 325 mg/codeine 30 mg
Rounox and Codeine 60: acetaminophen 325 mg/codeine 60 mg
Roxicet Oral Solution: acetaminophen 325 mg/oxycodone 5 mg/5 ml
Salutensin: hydroflumethiazide 50 mg/reserpine 0.125 mg
Salutensin Demi: hydroflumethiazide 25 mg/reserpine 0.125 mg

Semprex-D: acrivastine 8 mg/pseudoephedrine 60 mg
Senokot-S: docusate 50 mg/senna concentrate 187 mg
Septra: sulfamethoxazole 400 mg/trimethoprim 80 mg
Septra DS: sulfamethoxazole 800 mg/trimethoprim 160 mg
Ser-A-Gen: hydrochlorothiazide 15 mg/hydralazine 25 mg/ reserpine 0.1 mg
Seralazide: hydrochlorothiazide 15 mg/hydralazine 25 mg/ reserpine 0.1 mg
Ser-Ap-Es: hydrochlorothiazide 15 mg/reserpine 0.1 mg/ hydralazine 25 mg
Serpasil-Apresoline #1: reserpine 0.1 mg/hydralazine 25 mg
Serpasil-Apresoline #2: reserpine 0.2 mg/hydralazine 50 mg
Serpasil-Esidrix #1: hydrochlorothiazide 25 mg/reserpine 0.1 mg
Serpasil-Esidrix #2: hydrochlorothiazide 50 mg/reserpine 0.1 mg
Serpazide: hydrochlorothiazide 15 mg/hydralazine 25 mg/ reserpine 0.1 mg
Sinemet 25-100: carbidopa 10 mg/levodopa 100 mg
Sinemet 25-250: carbidopa 25 mg/levodopa 250 mg
Sinemet CR: carbidopa 50 mg/levodopa 200 mg
Sinus Excedrin Extra Strength: acetaminophen 500 mg/ pseudoephedrine 30 mg
Sinus Relief Tablets: acetaminophen 325 mg/pseudoephedrine 30 mg
Sinutab: acetaminophen 325 mg/chlorpheniramine 2 mg/ pseudoephedrine 30 mg
Sinutab Maximum Strength: acetaminophen 500 mg, pseudoephedrine 30 mg/chlorpheniramine 2 mg
Sinutab Without Drowsiness: acetaminophen 325 mg/ pseudoephedrine 30 mg
Slophyllin GG Syrup: theophylline 150 mg/guaifenesin 90 mg
Soma Compound: carisprodol 200 mg/aspirin 325 mg
Soma Compound with Codeine: carisprodol 200 mg/aspirin 325 mg/codeine 16 mg
Spirozid: spironolactone 25 mg/hydrochlorothiazide 25 mg
Statrol: neomycin 3.5 mg/polymyxin B 10,000 U
Sudafed Plus: pseudoephedrine 60 mg/chlorpheniramine 4 mg
Synophylate-GG Syrup: theophylline 100 mg/guaifenesin 33.3 mg/5 ml
Talacen: acetaminophen 650 mg/pentazocine 25 mg
Talwin Compound: aspirin 325 mg/pentazocine 12.5 mg
Tavist-D: clemastine 1.34 mg/phenylpropanolamine 75 mg
Tecnal: aspirin 330 mg/caffeine 40 mg/butalbital 50 mg
Tenoretic 50: atenolol 50 mg/chlorthalidone 25 mg
Tenoretic 100: atenolol 100 mg/chlorthalidone 25 mg
Tetramune: Purified Haemophilus B saccharide 10 μg/CRM protein 25 μg/12.5 Lf U inactivated diphtheria/5 Lf U inactivated tetanus/protective pertussis 4 U/0.5 ml
Thalfed: theophylline 120 mg/ephedrine 25 mg/phenobarbital 8 mg
Timolide 10/25: timolol 10 mg/hydrochlorothiazide 25 mg

Titralac Plus Suspension: calcium carbonate 500 mg/simethicone 20 mg
Titralac Tablets: calcium carbonate 420 mg/glycine 150 mg
Tobra Dex: tobramycin 0.3%/dexamethasone 0.1%/ chlorobutanol 0.5%
Trace Metals Additive: zinc chloride 0.8 mg/copper chloride 0.2 mg/manganese chloride 0.16 mg/chromium chloride 2 μg/ml
Trac-Tabs 2X: methenamine 120 μg/methylene blue 6 mg/ phenylsalicylate 30 mg/hyoscyamine 0.03 mg/benzoic acid 7.5 mg
Tri-Ad: acetaminophen 325 mg/butalbital 50 mg/caffeine 40 mg
Triaminic-12: phenylpropanolamine 75 mg/chlorpheniramine 12 mg
Triavil 2-10: perphenazine 2 mg/amitriptyline 10 mg
Triavil 4-10: perphenazine 4 mg/amitriptyline 10 mg
Triavil 2-25: perphenazine 2 mg/amitriptyline 25 mg
Triavil 4-25: perphenazine 4 mg/amitriptyline 25 mg
Triavil 4-50: perphenazine 4 mg/amitriptyline 50 mg
Tri-Hydroserpine: hydrochlorothiazide 15 mg/hydralazine 25 mg/reserpine 0.1 mg
Trinalin Repetabs: azatadine 1 mg/pseudoephedrine 120 mg
Twin-K: 20 mEq of potassium gluconate/potassium citrate
Two-Dyne: acetaminophen 325 mg/butalbital 50 mg/caffeine 40 mg
Tylenol with Codeine Elixir: acetaminophen 120 mg/codeine 12 mg/5 ml
Tylenol with Codeine No. 1: acetaminophen 300 mg/codeine 7.5 mg
Tylenol with Codeine No. 2: acetaminophen 300 mg/codeine 15 mg
Tylenol with Codeine No. 3: acetaminophen 300 mg/codeine 30 mg
Tylenol with Codeine No. 4: acetaminophen 300 mg/codeine 60 mg
Ty-Pap with Codeine Elixir: acetaminophen 120 mg/codeine 12 mg/15 ml
UAA: methenamine 40.8 mg/phenylsalicylate 18.1 mg/atropine 0.03 mg/hyoscyamine 0.03 mg/benzoic acid 4.5 mg/methylene blue 5.4 mg
Unilax Softgel: docusate 230 mg/yellow phenolphthalein 30 mg
Unipress: hydrochlorothiazide 15 mg/reserpine 0.1 mg/ hydralazine 25 mg
Uridon Modified: methenamine 40.8 mg/phenylsalicylate 18.1 mg/atropine 0.03 mg/hyoscyamine 0.03 mg/benzoic acid 4.5 mg/methylene blue 5.4 mg
Urimar-T: methenamine 81.6 mg/sodium biphosphate 40.8 mg/ phenylsalicylate 36.2 mg/methylene blue 10.8 mg/hyoscyamine 0.12 mg
Urinary Aseptic No. 2: methenamine 40.8 mg/phenylsalicylate

18.1 mg/atropine 0.03 mg/hyoscyamine 0.03 mg/benzoic acid 4.5 mg/methylene blue 5.4 mg

Urised: methenamine 40.8 mg/phenylsalicylate 18.1 mg/atropine 0.03 mg/hyoscyamine 0.03 mg/benzoic acid 4.5 mg/methylene bluc 5.4 mg

Urisedamine: methenamine 500 mg/hyoscyamine 0.15 mg

Uritin: methenamine 40.8 mg/phenylsalicylate 18.1 mg/atropine 0.03 mg/hyoscyamine 0.03 mg/benzoic acid 4.5 mg/methylene blue 5.4 mg

Urogesic Blue: methenamine 81.6 mg/sodium biphosphate 40.8 mg/phenylsalicylate 36.2 mg/methylene blue 10.8 mg/ hyoscyamine 0.12 mg

Uro Phosphate: methenamine 300 mg/sodium acid phosphate 434.78 mg

Uroquid-Acid No. 2: methenamine 500 mg/sodium acid phosphate 500 mg

Vanquish: aspirin 227 mg/acetaminophen 194 mg/caffeine 33 mg/aluminum hydroxide 25 mg/magnesium hydroxide 50 mg

Vaseretic: enalapril 10 mg/hydrochlorothiazide 25 mg

Vasocidin Ophthalmic Ointment: sulfacetamide 10%/ prednisolone 0.5%

Vasocidin Ophthalmic Ointment: sulfacetamide 10%/ prednisolone 0.5%/phenylephrine 0.125%

Vasocidin Ophthalmic Solution: sulfacetamide 10%/prednisolone 0.5%

Vasocidin Ophthalmic Solution: sulfacetamide 10%/prednisolone 0.25%/phenylephrine 0.125

Vasocon-A Ophthalmic Solution: naphazoline 0.05%/antazoline 0.5%

Vasosulf: sulfacetamide 15%/phenylephrine 0.125

Vicodin: acetaminophen 500 mg/hydrocodone 5 mg

Vicodin ES: acetaminophen 750 mg/hydrocodone 7.5 mg

Vioform-Hydrocortisone Mild Cream: iodochlorhydroxyquin 3%/hydrocortisone 0.5%

Wigraine: ergotamine 1 mg/caffeine 100 mg

Wigraine Suppositories: ergotamine 2 mg/caffeine 100 mg

WinGel: aluminum hydroxide 180 mg/magnesium hydroxide 160 mg

Wygesic: acetaminophen 650 mg/propoxyphene 65 mg

Zestoretic 20-12.5: lisinopril 20 mg/hydrochlorothiazide 12.5 mg

Zestoretic 20-25: lisinopril 20 mg/hydrochlorothiazide 25 mg

Ziac 2.5: bisoprolol 2.5 mg/hydrochlorothiazide 6.2 mg

Ziac 5: bisoprolol 5 mg/hydrochlorothiazide 6.2 mg

Ziac 10: bisoprolol 10 mg/hydrochlorothiazide 6.2 mg

Zincfrin: phenylephrine 0.12%/zinc sulfate 0.25

Appendix D

Rarely Used Drugs

clioquinol (OTC)

Functional class: Local antiinfective

Dosage and routes: Top apply to affected area bid or tid × 7 days only

Uses: Cutaneous infections: athlete's foot, eczema, and other fungal infections

Contraindications: Hypersensitivity to iodine, chloroxine

clobetasol (℞)

Functional class: Topical corticosteroid

Dosage and routes:
Adult and child: Top apply to affected area bid

Uses: Psoriasis, eczema, contact dermatitis, pruritus; usually reserved for severe dermatoses that have not responded to less potent formulation

Contraindications: Hypersensitivity to corticosteroids, fungal infections

clocortolone (℞)

Functional class: Topical corticosteroid

Dosage and routes:
Adult and child: Top apply to affected area tid or qid

Uses: Psoriasis, eczema, contact dermatitis, pruritus

Contraindications: Hypersensitivity to corticosteroids, fungal infections

clotrimazole (℞) (OTC)

Functional class: Local antiinfective

Dosage and routes:
Adult and child: Top rub into affected area bid × 1-4 wk; loz dissolve in mouth 5 times/day × 2 wk; intravag 1 applicator/1 tab × 1-2 wk hs; oral troches 10 mg 5 times/day × 14 days

Uses: Tinea pedis, tinea cruris, tinea corporis, tinea versicolor, *C. albicans* infection of the vagina, vulva, throat, mouth

Contraindications: Hypersensitivity

flunisolide (℞)

Functional class: Steroid, intranasal

Dosage and routes:
Adult: Instill 2 sprays in each nostril bid, then increase to tid if needed, not to exceed 8 sprays/day in each nostril
Child 6-14 yr: Instill 1 spray in each nostril tid or 2 sprays bid, not to exceed 4 sprays/day in each nostril

Adult and child >6 yr: Spray 2 puffs bid, not to exceed 4 puffs bid

Uses: Rhinitis (seasonal or perennial), nasal polyps; chronic steroid-dependent asthma (inh)

Contraindications: Hypersensitivity, child <12 yr; fungal, bacterial infection of nose

hydroxychloroquine (℞)

Functional class: Antimalarial, antiarthritic

Dosage and routes:
Malaria:
Adult and child: PO 5 mg/kg/wk on same day of week, not to exceed 400 mg; treatment should begin 2 wk before entering endemic area; continue 8 wk after leaving; if treatment begins after exposure, 800 mg for adult, 10 mg/kg for children in 2 divided doses 6 hr apart
Lupus erythematosus
Adult: PO 400 mg qd-bid; length depends on patient response; maintenance 200-400 mg qd
Rheumatoid arthritis
Adult: PO 400-600 mg qd, then 200-300 mg qd after good response

Uses: Malaria caused by *Plasmodium vivax, P. malariae, P. ovale, P. falciparum* (some strains); SLE, rheumatoid arthritis

Contraindications: Hypersensitivity, retinal field changes, porphyria, children (long-term)

hydroxyprogesterone (℞)

Functional class: Progestin, hormone

Dosage and routes:
Menstrual disorders
Adult: IM 125-375 mg q4wk; discontinue after 4 cycles
Uterine cancer:
Adult: IM 1 g 5-7 times/wk

Uses: Uterine carcinoma, menstrual disorders (abnormal uterine bleeding, amenorrhea)

Contraindications: Breast cancer, hypersensitivity, thromboembolic disorders, reproductive cancer, genital bleeding (abnormal, undiagnosed), pregnancy

isotretinoin (℞)

Functional class: Dermatologic antiacne agent

Dosage and routes:
Adult: PO 0.5-2 mg/kg/day in 2 divided doses × 15-20 wk; if relapse occurs, repeat after 8 wk off drug

Uses: Severe recalcitrant cystic acne

Contraindications: Hypersensitivity, inflamed skin, pregnancy **X**

papaverine (℞)

Functional class: Peripheral vasodilator

Dosage and routes:
Adult: PO 100-300 mg 3-5 times day; sus rel cap 150-300 mg q8-12h; IM/**IV** 30-120 mg q3h prn; Intracavernosal

(IC) 30 mg/0.5-1 mg phentolamine or 60 mg alone

Uses: Arterial spasm resulting in cerebral and peripheral ischemia, myocardial ischemia associated with vascular spasm or dysrhythmias, angina pectoris, peripheral pulmonary embolism, visceral spasm as in ureteral, biliary, GI colic, peripheral vascular disease

Contraindications: Hypersensitivity, complete AV heart block

phenoxybenzamine (℞)

Functional class: Antihypertensive

Dosage and routes:

Adult: PO 10 mg qd; increase by 10 mg qod; usual range 20-40 mg bid-tid

Child: PO 0.2 mg/kg or 6 mg/m^2/day, max 10 mg, may increase at 4-day intervals; maintenance dosage 0.4-1.2 mg/kg/day or 12-36 mg/m^2/day given in divided doses tid or qid

Uses: Pheochromocytoma

Contraindications: Hypersensitivity, CHF, angina, cerebral vascular insufficiency, coronary arteriosclerosis

Appendix E

Controlled Substance Chart

DRUGS	UNITED STATES	CANADA
Heroin, LSD, peyote, marijuana, mescaline	Schedule I	Schedule H
Opium (morphine), meperidine, amphetamines, cocaine, short-acting barbiturates (secobarbital)	Schedule II	Schedule G
Glutethimide, paregoric, phendimetrazine	Schedule III	Schedule F
Chloral hydrate, chlordiazepoxide, diazepam, mazindol, meprobamate, phenobarbital (Canada-G)	Schedule IV	Schedule F
Antidiarrheals with opium (Canada-G), antitussives	Schedule V	Schedule F

Appendix F

FDA Pregnancy Categories

A No risk demonstrated to the fetus in any trimester

B No adverse effects in animals, no human studies available

C Only given after risks to the fetus are considered; animal studies have shown adverse reactions, no human studies available

D Definite fetal risks, may be given in spite of risks if needed in life-threatening conditions

X Absolute fetal abnormalities; not to be used anytime during pregnancy

Appendix G

Nomogram for Calculation of Body Surface Area

Place a straight edge from the patient's height in the left column to his or her weight in the right column. The point of intersection on the body surface area column indicates the body surface area (BSA). Reproduced from Behrman RE, and Vaughn VC (editors): Nelson's textbook of pediatrics, ed 12, Philadelphia, 1983. WB Saunders.

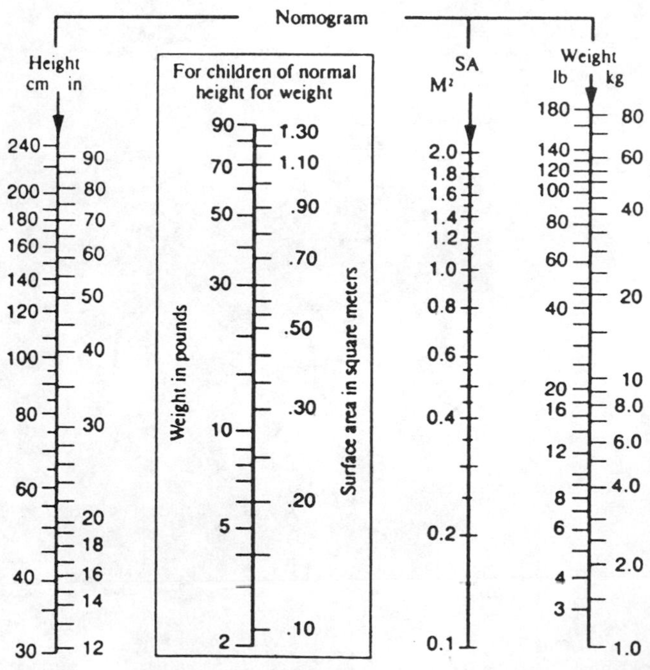

Appendix H

Commonly Used Abbreviations

abd abdomen
ABG arterial blood gas
ac before meals
ACE angiotensin-converting enzyme
ADA American Diabetes Association
ADH antidiuretic hormone
ALT alanine aminotransferase
ANA antinuclear antibody
AP anteroposterior
APTT activated partial thromboplastin time
ASA acetylsalicylic acid, aspirin
ASHD arteriosclerotic heart disease
AST aspartate aminotransferase (SGOT)
AV atrioventricular
bid twice a day
BM bowel movement
BMR basal metabolic rate
B/P blood pressure
BPH benign prostatic hypertrophy
BPM beats per minute
BS blood sugar
BUN blood urea nitrogen
C Celsius (centigrade)
Ca cancer
CAD coronary artery disease
cap capsule
Cath catheterization or catheterize
CBC complete blood cell count
CC chief complaint
cc cubic centimeter
CHF congestive heart failure
cm centimeter
CNS central nervous system
CO_2 carbon dioxide
CONT continuous
COPD chronic obstructive pulmonary disease
CPAP continuous positive airway pressue
CPK creatinine phosphokinase
CPR cardiopulmonary resuscitation
CrCl creatinine clearance
C&S culture and sensitivity
C sect cesarean section
CSF cerebrospinal fluid
CV cardiovascular
CVA cerebrovascular accident
CVP central venous pressure
D&C dilatation and curettage
DIR INF direct infusion
dr dram
D_5W 5% glucose in distilled water
ECG electrocardiogram (EKG)
EDTA ethylenediamine tetraacetic acid
EEG electroencephalogram
EENT ear, eye, nose, and throat
EPS extrapyramidal symptom
ESR erythrocyte sedimentation rate

EXT REL extended release
EXTRA extra strength
STREN suspension
SUSP
FBS fasting blood sugar
FHT fetal heart tones
FSH follicle-stimulating hormone
g gram
GABA γ-aminobutyric acid
GI gastrointestinal
gr grain
GTT glucose tolerance test
gtt drops
GU genitourinary
H_2 histamine$_2$
HCG human chorionic gonadotropin
Hct hematocrit
HDCV human diploid cell rabies vaccine
Hgb hemoglobin
H & H hematocrit and hemoglobin
5-HIAA 5-hydroxyindoleacetic acid
HIV human immunodeficiency virus (AIDS)
H_2O water
HOB head of bed
HR heart rate
hr hour
hs at bedtime
IgG immunoglobulin G
IM intramuscular
INF infusion
INH inhalation
inj injection
I&O intake and output
IPPB intermittent positive-pressure breathing
ITP idiopathic thrombocytopenic purpura
IUD intrauterine device
IV intravenous
IVP intravenous pyelogram
K potassium
kg kilogram
L liter
lb pound
LDH lactic dehydrogenase
LE lupus erythematosus
LH luteinizing hormone
LLQ left lower quadrant
LMP last menstrual period
LOC level of consciousness
LR lactated Ringer's solution
LUQ left upper quadrant
M meter
m minim
m^2 square meter
MAOI monoamine oxidase inhibitor
mEq milliequivalent
mg milligram
μg microgram
MI myocardial infarction
min minute
ml milliliter
mm millimeter
mo month
Na sodium
neg negative
NPO nothing by mouth (Lat. *nulla per os*)
NS normal saline
O_2 oxygen
OBS organic brain syndrome
OD right eye
OR operating room
os left eye
OTC over-the-counter
OU each eye
oz ounce
$\bar{p}$ after
P56 plasma-lyte 56
$PaCO_2$ arterial carbon dioxide tension (pressure)
PaO_2 arterial oxygen tension (pressure)

PAT paroxysmal atrial tachycardia
PBI protein-bound iodine
PCWP pulmonary capillary wedge pressure
PEEP positive end-expiratory pressure
PERRLA pupils equal, round, react to light and accommodation
pH hydrogen ion concentration
PO by mouth
postop postoperative
PP postprandial
preop preoperative
prn as required
PT prothrombin time
PTT partial thromboplastin time
PVC premature ventricular contraction
q every
qAM every morning
qd every day
qh every hour
q2h every 2 hours
q3h every 3 hours
q4h every 4 hours
q6h every 6 hours
q12h every 12 hours
qid four times daily
qod every other day
qPM every night
qs sufficient quantity
qt quart
R right
RAIU radioactive iodine uptake
RBC red blood count or cell
RLQ right lower quadrant
ROM range of motion
RUQ right upper quadrant
SC subcutaneous
SIMV synchronous intermittent mandatory ventilation
SL sublingual
SLE systemic lupus erythematosus
SOB shortness of breath
sol solution
ss one half
suppos suppository
sus rel sustained release
Syr syrup
T&A tonsillectomy and adenoidectomy
tab tablet
tbsp tablespoon
temp temperature
tid three times daily
tinc tincture
TPN total parenteral nutrition
top topical
TRANS transdermal
TSH thyroid-stimulating hormone
tsp teaspoon
TT thrombin time
U unit
UA urinalysis
UTI urinary tract infection
UV ultraviolet
vag vaginal
VMA vanillylmandelic acid
vol volume
VS vital sign
WBC white blood cell count
wk week
wt weight
yr year
> greater than
< less than
= equal
° degree
% percent
γ gamma
β beta

Appendix I

Bibliography

American Society of Health-System Pharmacists: American hospital formulary service drug information '97, Bethesda, Md, 1997, The Society.

Clark J, Queener S, and Karb V: Pharmacologic basis of nursing practice, ed 5, St. Louis, 1998, Mosby.

Drug information for the health care professional (USP DI), ed 15, United States Pharmaceutical Convention, Rockville, Md, 1997.

Gahart B: Intravenous medications, ed 12, St. Louis, 1998, Mosby.

Goodman A and others: Goodman and Gilman's the pharmacological basis of therapeutics, ed 10, New York, 1998, Pergamon Press.

McKenry LM and Salerno E: Mosby's pharmacology in nursing, ed 18, St. Louis, 1996, Mosby.

Trissel L: Handbook on injectable drugs, ed 9, Bethesda, Md, 1997, American Society of Hospital Pharmacists, Inc.

Appendix J

IV Drug/Solution Compatibility Chart

	D_5	D_{10}	D_5 ½S	D_5 S	NS	R	LR	OTHER
Acetazolamide	C	C	C	C	C	C	C	
Acyclovir	C							
Alpha$_1$-proteinase inhibitor								Sterile water for inj
Alprostadil	C	C			C			
Alteplase								Sterile water for inj
Amdinocillin	C	C	C	C	C	C	C	D_5 in R
Amikacin	C				C			
Aminocaproic acid			C	C	C	C		D in distilled water
Ammonium Cl					C			May add KCl to solution
Amphotericin B	C							
Ampicillin	C				C			
Amrinone lactate					C			0.45% saline
Antithrombin III	C				C			Sterile water for inj
Ascorbic acid	C				C	C	C	Sodium lactate
Azlocillin	C		C		C			
Atenolol	C				C			0.45% saline
Aztreonam	C	C			C	C	C	Normosol-R
Bretylium tosylate	C				C			
Cefamandole	C				C			
Cefazolin	C				C			
Cefotetan	C				C			
Cefoxitin	C	C			C	C	C	Aminosol
Ceftrazidime	C		C	C	C	C	C	M/G Sodium lactate
Ceftriaxone	C				C			
Cefuroxime	C		C	C		C		M/G Sodium lactate
Cephalothin	C				C	C	C	M/G Sodium lactate

This chart is not inclusive and is based on manufacturers' recommendations.

Key

C = Compatible
D_5 = Dextrose 5%
D_{10} = Dextrose 10%
D_5½S = Dextrose 5% in saline 0.45%
D_5S = Dextrose 5% in saline 0.9%
NS = Sodium chloride 0.9% (normal saline)
R = Ringer's solution
LR = Lactated Ringer's solution

			D_5					
	D_5	D_{10}	½S	S	NS	R	LR	OTHER
Cephapirin	C				C			
Ciprofloxacin	C				C			
Cyclosporine	C				C			Use only glass containers
Dobutamine					C			Sodium lactate
Dopamine	C		C	C	C		C	M/G Sodium lactate
Doxycycline	C				C			Invert sugar 10%
Edetate Na	C	C						Isotonic saline
Ganciclovir	C				C	C	C	
Gentamicin	C				C			Normosol-R
Heparin Na	C	C			C	C		
Ifosfamide	C				C		C	Sterile water for inj
Isoproterenol	C			C	C	C		Invert sugar 5% & 10%
Kanamycin	C				C			
Metaraminol	C			C	C	C	C	Normosol-R
Methicillin	C			C				
Metoclopramide	C			C		C	C	
Mezlocillin	C	C	C	C	C	C	C	Fructose 5%
Moxalactam	C	C	C	C	C	C	C	M/G Sodium lactate
Netilmicin	C	C		C	C	C	C	Normosol-R
Norepinephrine	C	C		C			C	
Nitroglycerin	C	C			C			
Piperacillin	C			C	C		C	
Ritodrine	C							
Ticarcillin	C				C		C	
Tobramycin	C				C			
Vidarabine	C	C			C			

Appendix K

Ophthalmic, Nasal, and Topical Products

OPHTHALMIC PRODUCTS

ANESTHETICS
proparacaine
(proe-par'a-kane)
AK-Taine, Alcaine, I-Paracine, Kainair, Ophthaine, Ophthestic
tetracaine
(tet'ra-kane)

α-ADRENERGIC BLOCKER
dapiprazole
(da-pip'ra-zole)
Rev-Eyes

ANTIINFECTIVES
idoxuridine-IDU
(eye-dox-yoor'i-deen)
Herplex, Stoxil
natamycin
(nat-a-mye'sin)
Natacyn
sulfacetamide sodium
(sul-fa-seet'a-mide)
AK-Sulf, Bleph-10 Liquifilm, Bleph-10 S.O.P., Isopto Cetamide, Ophthacet, Sodium Sulamyd, sodium sulfacetamide 10%, sodium sulfacetamide 15%, sodium sulfacetamide 30%, SOSS-10, Sulfair 15
trifluridine
(trye-floor'i-deen)
Viroptic

β-BLOCKERS
levobunolol
(lee-voe-byoo'no-lole)
Betagen
metipranolol
(met-ee-pran'oh-lole)
Optipranolol

CHOLINERGICS
(Direct-acting)
carbachol
(kar'ba-kole)
Iosopto Carbachol, Miostat
pilocarpine
(pye-loe-kar'peen)
Adsorbocarpine, Akarpine, Isopto Carpine, Ocu-Carpine, Ocusert-Pilo, Pilagan, Pilocar, pilocarpine, Pilopine HS, Piloptic-1, Piloptic-2, Pilostat, Pilopto-Carpine

(cholinesterase inhibitors)
demecarium
(dem-e-kare'ee-um)
Humorsol
ecothiophate
(ek-oh-thye'eh-fate)
Ecostigmine Iodide, Phospholine Iodide

isoflurophate
(eye-soe-floor'oh-fate)
Floropryl

CYCLOPLEGIC MYDRIATICS
cyclopentolate
(sye-kloe-pen'toe-late)
AK-Pentolate, Cyclogly, I-Pentolate
homatropine
(home-a'troe-peen)
AK-Homatropine, I-Homatrine, Isopto Homatropine, Minims Homatropine ✤, Spectro-Homatropine
tropicamide
(troe-pik'a-mide)
Mydriacyl, Tropicacyl, I-Piramide

GLUCOCORTICOIDS
fluorometholone
(flure-oh-meth'oh-lone)
Flarex, Fluor-Op, FML, FML Forte, FML Liquifilm
medrysone
(me'dri-sone)
HMS

NONSTEROIDAL ANTIINFLAMMATORIES
suprofen
(soo-proe'fen)
Profenal

SYMPATHOMIMETICS
apraclonidine
(a-pra-klon'i-deen)
Iopidine
dipivefrin
(dye-pi'vef-rin)
Propine

Pregnancy category: demecarium, isoflurophate **X;** apraclonidine, cyclopentolate, ecothipate, glucocorticoids, levobunalol, metipranolol, pilocarpine, proparacaine, suprofen, tetracaine **C;** dapiprazole, dipivefrin **B**

Action

Antiinflammatories: Decreases inflammation, resulting in decreased pain, photophobia, hyperemia, cellular infiltration

Uses: Inflammation of eye, eyelids, conjunctiva, cornea; uveitis, iridocyclitis, allergic conditions, burns, foreign bodies, postoperatively in cataract

Carbonic anhydrase inhibitor: Converted to epinephrine, which decreases aqueous production and increases outflow

Uses: Open-angle glaucoma, ocular hypertension

Direct-acting miotic: Acts directly on cholinergic receptor sites; induces miosis, spasm of accommodation, fall in intraocular pressure, caused by stimulation of ciliary, pupillary sphincter muscles, which leads to pulling away of iris from filtration angle, resulting in increased outflow of aqueous humor

Uses: Primary glaucoma, early stages of wide-angle glaucoma (less useful in advanced stages), chronic open-angle glaucoma, acute narrow-angle glaucoma before emergency surgery; also neutralizes mydriatics used during eye exam; may be used alternately with mydriatics to break adhesions between iris and lens

β-Adrenergic blockers: Reduces production of aqueous humor by unknown mechanism

Uses: Ocular hypertension, chronic open-angle glaucoma

Anesthetics: Decreases ion permeability by stabilizing neuronal membrane

Uses: Cataract extraction, tonometry, gonioscopy, removal of foreign objects, corneal suture removal, glaucoma surgery (ophth); pruritus, sunburn, toothache, sore throat, cold sores, oral pain, rectal pain and irritation, control of gagging (top)

Antiinfectives: Inhibits folic acid synthesis by preventing PABA use, which is necessary for bacterial growth

Uses: Conjunctivitis, superficial eye infections, corneal ulcers, prophylaxis against infection after removal of foreign matter from the eye

Interactions

Antiinfectives

Individual drugs

Gentamicin, ophth: ↑ antagonism

Mild silver nitrate: Incompatible with this drug

Silver nitrate: Incompatible with this drug

Antiinflammatories

Individual drugs

Acetylcholine: ↓ effect

Carbachol: ↓ effect

β-Blockers

Individual drugs

Metoprolol: ↑ effect

Propranolol: ↑ effect

Adverse effects

CNS: Headache

CV: Hypertension, tachycardia, dysrhythmias

EENT: Burning, stinging

GI: Bitter taste

Contraindications: Hypersensitivity

Precautions: Pregnancy, lactation, children, aphakia, hypersensitivity to carbonic anhydrase inhibitors, sulfonamides, thiazide diuretics, ocular inhibitors, hepatic and renal insufficiency

NURSING CONSIDERATIONS

Assessment

- Monitor ophth exams and intraocular pressure readings
- Monitor blood counts, liver, renal function tests and serum electrolytes during long-term treatment

Nursing diagnoses

✓ Sensory-perceptual alteration: visual (uses)

✓ Knowledge deficit (teaching)

Implementation

Ophth route

- Store at room temp away from light

Patient/family education

- Teach patient how to instill drops
- Advise patient that drug may cause burning, itching, blurring, dryness of eye area

Evaluation

Positive therapeutic response

- Absence of increased intraocular pressure

NASAL AGENTS

desoxyephedrine
(des-oxy-e-fed'rin)
Vicks Inhaler
ephedrine
(e-fed'rin)
Kondon's Nasal Jelly, Pretz-D, Vicks Vatronol
epinephrine
(ep-i-neff'rin)
Adrenalin
naphazoline
(naff-a-zoe'leen)
Privine
oxymetazoline
(ox-i-met-az'oh-leen)
Afrin, Afrin Children's Nose Drops, Allerest 12-Hour Nasal, Chlorphed-LA, Coricidin Nasal Mist, Dristan Long Lasting, Duramist Plus, Duration, Genasal, NTZ Long-Acting Nasal, Nafrine ♣, Neo-Synephrine 12 Hour, Nostrilla, oxymetazoline HCl, Sinarest 12-Hour, Sinex Long-Acting, Twice-A-Day Nasal, 4-Way Long Acting Nasal
phenylephrine
(fen-ill-eff'rin)
Alconefrin 12, Children's Nostril, Neo-Synephrine, Sinex
propylhexadrine
(proe-pil-hex'a-dreen)
Benzedrex Inhaler
tetrahydrozoline
(tet-ra-hye-dro'zoe-leen)
Tyzine

xylometazoline
(zye-loe-met-a-zoe'leen)
Func. class.: Nasal decongestant
Chem. class.: Sympathomimetic amine
Pregnancy category C

Action: Produces vasoconstriction (rapid, long acting) of arterioles, thereby decreasing fluid exudation, mucosal engorgement by stimulation of α-adrenergic receptors in vascular smooth muscle

➔ **Therapeutic Outcome:** Absence of nasal congestion

Uses: Nasal congestion

Dosage and routes

Desoxyephedrine

P ***Adults and child >6 yr:*** 1-2 Inh in each nostril q2h or less

Ephedrine
Adult: Fill dropper to level marked, use in each nostril q4h or less

Naphazoline
P ***Adult and child >6 yr:*** 1-2 drops/spray q6h or less

Oxymetazoline
P ***Adult and child >6 yr:*** Instill 2-3 gtt or sprays to each nostril bid

P ***Child 2-6 yr:*** Instill 2-3 gtt or sprays 0.025% sol bid, not to exceed 3 days

Available forms: Nasal sol 0.025%, 0.05%

Epinephrine
P ***Adult and child >6 yr:*** Apply with swab, drops, spray prn

Phenylephrine
P ***Adult and child >12 yr:*** 2-3 drops/spray (0.25-0.5%) in each nostril: q3-4hr or less; or

2-3 drops/spray (1%) in each nostril q4hr or less

P *Child 6-12 yr:* 2-3 drops/spray (0.25%) in each nostril q3-4hr

P *Infants >6 mo:* 1-2 drops (0.16%) in each nostril q3hr

Propylhexadrine

P *Adult and child >6 yr:* 1-2 inh in each nostril q2h or less

Tetrahydrozoline

P *Adult and child >6 yr:* 2-4 drops (0.1%) q3-4h prn or 3-4 sprays in each nostril q4hr prn

P *Child 2-6 yr:* 2-3 drops (0.05%) in each nostril q4-6h prn

Xylometazoline

P *Adult and child >12 yr:* 2-3 drops/spray (0.1%) in each nostril q8-10hr

P *Child 2-12 yr:* 2-3 drops (0.05%) in each nostril q8-10hr

Adverse effects

CNS: Anxiety, restlessness, tremors, weakness, insomnia, dizziness, fever, headache
EENT: Irritation, burning, sneezing, stinging, dryness, rebound congestion
GI: Nausea, vomiting, anorexia
INTEG: Contact dermatitis

Contraindications: Hypersensitivity to sympathomimetic amines

P G **Precautions:** Child <6 yr, elderly, diabetes, cardiovascular disease, hypertension, hyperthyroidism, increased intracranial pressure, prostatic hypertrophy, pregnancy **C**, glaucoma

Interactions

Individual drugs

Mecamylamine: ↑ hypotension
Methyldopa: ↑ hypotension
Reserpine: ↑ hypotension

Drug classifications

β-Adrenergic blockers: ↑ hypertension
MAOIs: ↑ hypertension

NURSING CONSIDERATIONS

Assessment

- Asssess for redness, swelling: pain in nasal passages before and during treatment
- Assess for syst absorption: hypertension, tachycardia; notify prescriber; syst absorption occurs at high doses or after prolonged use

Nursing diagnoses

✓ Airway clearance, ineffective (uses)
✓ Knowledge deficit (teaching)
✓ Noncompliance (teaching)

Implementation

Nasal route

- Have patient tilt head back, squeeze bulb to create a vacuum, and draw correct amount of sol into dropper; insert 2 gtt of sol into nostril; repeat in other nostril
- Store in light-resistant container; do not expose to high temp or let sol come into contact with aluminum
- Give for <4 consecutive days
- Provide environmental humidification to decrease nasal congestion, dryness

Patient/family education

- Advise patient that stinging may occur for several applications; drying of mucosa may be decreased by environmental humidification
- Caution patient to notify prescriber if irregular pulse, insomnia, dizziness, or tremors occur

- Teach patient proper administration to avoid syst absorption
- Advise patient to rinse dropper with very hot water to prevent contamination

Evaluation

Positive therapeutic outcome

- Decreased nasal congestion

TOPICAL GLUCOCORTICOIDS

alclometasone
(al-kloe-met'a-sone)
Adovate

amcinonide
(am-sin'oh-nide)
Cyclocort

betamethasone
(bay-ta-meth'a-sone)
Alphatrex, Beben ✤, Betacort ✤, Betaderm, Betatrex, Beta-Val, Betmethacort, Bethovate ✤, Celestoderm ✤, Dermabet, Diprolene, Diprosone, Ectosonel ✤, Maxivate, Metaderm ✤, Novo-betamet, Psorion, Uticort, Valisone, Valnac

clobetasol
(kloe-bay'ta-sol)
Dermovate ✤, Temovate

clocortolone
(kloe-kore'toe-lone)
Cloderm

desonide
(dess'oh-nide)
Des Owen, Tridesilon

desoximetasone
(dess-ox-i-met'a-sone)
Topicort

dexamethasone
(dex-a-meth'a-sone)
Aeroseb-Dex, Decaderm, Decaspray

diflorasone
(dye-flor'a-sone)
Florone, Maxiflor, Psorcon

fluocinolone
(floo-oh-sin'oh-lone)
Fluocin, Licon, Lidemol ✤, Lidex, Lyderm ✤, Topsyn ✤, Vasoderm

flurandrenolide
(flure-an-dren'oh-lide)
Cordran, Cordran SP, Cordran Tape, Drenison 1/4 ✤, Drenison Tape ✤

fluticasone
(floo-tik'a-sone)
Cutivate

halcinonide
(hal-sin'oh-nide)
Halog, Halog-E

halobetasol
(hal-oh-bay'ta-sol)
Ultravate

hydrocortisone
(hye-droe-kor'ti-sone)
Actiocort, Aeroseb-HC, Ala-Cort, Allercort, Alpha-derm, Anusol HC, Bactine, Barriere-HC ♣, Calde-CORT Anti-Itch, Carmol HC, Cetacort, Cortacet ♣, Cortaid, Cortate ♣, Cort-Dome, Cortef ♣, Corticaine, Corticreme ♣, Cortifair, Cortizone, Cortoderm ♣, Cortril, Delcort, Dermacort, Demi-Cort, Dermtex HC, Emo-Cort, Epifoam, FoilleCort, Gly-Cort, Gynecort, Hi-Cor, Hycort, Hyderm ♣, Hydro-Tex, Hytone, Lacti-Care-HC, Lanacort, Lemoderm, Locoid, My Cort, Novoehydrocort ♣, Nutracort Pharm, Pharmacort, Pentacort, Rederm, Rhulicort S-T Cort, Synacort, Sarna HC ♣, Texa-Cort, Unicort ♣, Westcort
mometasone
(moe-met'a-sone)
Elocon
prednicarbate
(pred-ni-kar'bate)
Dermatop
triamcinolone
(trye-am-sin'oh-lone)
Aristocort, Flutex, Kenac, Kenalog, Kenonel, Triaderm ♣, Trianide ♣, Triderm, Trymex
Func. class.: Corticosteroid, synthetic
Chem. class.: Fluorinated corticosteroid
Pregnancy category C

Action: Antipruritic, antiinflammatory

Therapeutic Outcome: Decreased inflammation

Uses: Psoriasis, eczema, contact dermatitis, pruritus; usually reserved for severe dermatoses that have not responded to less potent formulation

Dosage and routes

Adult and child: Apply to affected area

Adverse effects

INTEG: Acne, atrophy, epidermal thinning, purpura striae

Contraindications: Hypersensitivity, viral infections, fungal infections

Precautions: Pregnancy **C**

Interactions: None

NURSING CONSIDERATIONS

Assessment

- Monitor temp; if fever develops, drug should be discontinued
- Check for systemic absorption; increased temp, inflammation, irritation

Nursing diagnoses

✓ Infection, risk for (adverse reactions)
✓ Knowledge deficit (teaching)
✓ Noncompliance (teaching)

Implementation

Top route

- Apply only to affected areas; do not get in eyes
- Leave site uncovered or lightly covered; occlusive dressing is not recommended—systemic absorption may occur
- Use only on dermatoses; do not use on weeping, denuded, or infected area
- Cleanse before application of drug

• Continue treatment for a few days after area has cleared
• Store at room temp

Patient/family education
• Caution patient to avoid sunlight on affected area; burns may occur
• Advise patient to limit treatment to 14 days

Evaluation
Positive therapeutic outcome
• Absence of severe itching, patches on skin, flaking

TOPICAL ANTIFUNGALS

amphotericin B
(am-foe-ter'i-sin)
Fungizone
ciclopirox
(sye-kloe-peer'ox)
Loprox
clioquinol
(klye-oh-kwin'ole)
Vioforim
clotrimazole
(kloe-trye'ma-zole)
Canestew ♣, Clotrimaderm ♣, Lotrimin, Lotrimin AF, Mycelex, Mycelex OTC, Myclo ♣, Neozol ♣
econazole
(ee-kon'a-zole)
Spectazole
haloprogin
(hal-oh-proe'jin)
Halotex
ketoconazole
(kee-toe-kon'a-zole)
Nizoral
miconazole
(mye-kon'a-zole)
Micatin, Monistat-Derm
naftifine
(naff'ti-feen)
Naftin
nystatin
(nye-stat'in)
Mycostatin, Nodostine ♣, Nilstat, Nyoderm ♣, Nystex
oxiconazole
(ox-i-kon'a-zole)
Oxistat
terbinafine
(ter-bin'a-feen)
Lamisil
tolnaftate
(tole-naf'tate)
Absorbine Antifungal, Absorbine Jock Itch, Absorbine Jr. Antifungal, Aftate For Athlete's Foot, Aftate for Jock Itch, Desenex Spray, Genaspor, NP-27, Quinsana Plus, Tinactin, Ting, tolnaftate, Zeasorb-AF
undecylenic acid (topical)
(un-de'sye-len-ik)
Caldesene, Cruex, Decylenes, Desenex, Desenex Maximum Strength, Protectol

Action: Interferes with fungal cell membrane permeability

Therapeutic Outcome: Absence of itching and white patches of the skin

Uses: Tinea cruris, tinea pedis, diaper rash, minor skin irritations; amphotericin B is used for *Candida* infections

Dosage and routes
Massage into affected area, surrounding area qd or bid, continue for 7-14 days, not to exceed 4 wk

Adverse effects
INTEG: Burning, stinging, dryness, itching, local irritation

Contraindications: Hypersensitivity

Precautions: Pregnancy B,
P lactation, children

Interactions: None

NURSING CONSIDERATIONS
Assessment
• Assess skin for fungal infections: peeling, dryness, itching before and throughout treatment
• Assess for continuing infection: increased size, number of lesions

Nursing diagnoses
✓ Skin integrity, impaired (uses)
✓ Infection, risk for (uses)
✓ Knowledge deficit (teaching)

Implementation
Top route
• Apply to affected area, surrounding area; do not cover with occlusive dressings
• Store below 30° C (86° F)

Patient/family education
• Instruct patient to apply with glove to prevent further infection; not to cover with occlusive dressings
• Teach patient that long-term therapy may be needed to clear infection (2 wk-6 mo depending on organism); compliance is needed even after feeling better
• Teach patient proper hygiene; hand-washing technique, nail care, use of concomitant top agents if prescribed
• Caution patient to avoid use of OTC creams, ointments, lotions unless directed by prescriber
• Instruct patient to use medical asepsis (hand washing) before, after each application; to change socks and shoes on a day during treatment of tinea pedis
• Advise patient to report to health care prescriber if infection persists or recurs; if blisters, burning, oozing, swelling
• Caution patient to avoid alcohol because nausea, vomiting, hypertension may occur
• Caution patient to use sunscreen or avoid direct sunlight to prevent photosensitivity
• Advise patient to notify health care prescriber of sore throat, fever, skin rash, which may indicate overgrowth of organisms

Evaluation
Positive therapeutic outcome
• Decrease in size, number of lesions

TOPICAL ANESTHETICS

benzocaine
(ben'zoe-kane)
Anbesol Maximum Strength, Baby Anbesol, Children's Chloraseptic, Medamint, Orabase Baby, Oracin, Ora-Jel, Oratect, Spec-T Anesthetic, T-Caine, Tyrobenz
dibucaine
(dye'byoo-kane)
dibucaine, Nupercainal
pramoxine
(pra-mox'een)
Fleet Relief, Prax, ProctoFoam, Tronolane, Tronothane
Func. class.: Topical anesthetic
Pregnancy category C

Action: Inhibits conduction of nerve impulses from sensory nerves

Therapeutic Outcome: Decreasing inflammation, itching, pain

Uses: Oral irritation, sore throat, toothache, cold sore, canker sore, sunburn, minor cuts, insect bites, pain, itching

Dosage and routes
P ***Adult and child:*** Top apply qid as needed; rec insert tid and after each BM

Adverse effects
INTEG: Rash, irritation, sensitization

Contraindications: Hypersensitivity, P infants <1 yr, application to large areas

P **Precautions:** Child <6 yr, sepsis, pregnancy **C,** denuded skin

Interactions: None

NURSING CONSIDERATIONS
Assessment
- Assess pain: location, duration, characteristics before and after administration
- Assess for infection: redness, drainage, inflammation; this drug should not be used until infection is treated

Nursing diagnoses
✓ Pain (uses)
✓ Knowledge deficit (teaching)

Implementation
- Store in tight, light-resistant container; do not freeze, puncture, or incinerate aerosol container

Patient/family education
- Teach patient to avoid contact with eyes
- Instruct patient not to use for prolonged periods: use for <1 wk; if condition remains, prescriber should be contacted

Evaluation
Positive therapeutic outcome
- Decreased redness, swelling, pain

VAGINAL ANTIFUNGALS

butoconazole
(byoo'toe-kon-a-zole)
Femstat
clotrimazole
(kloe-trye'ma-zole)
Canesten ♣, Gyne-Lotrimin, Mycelex G, Mycelex Twin Pak, Myclo ♣
miconazole
(mye-kon'a-zole)
Monistat, Monistat 3, Monistat 7, Monistat Dual Pak
nystatin
(nye-stat'in)
mycostatin, Nilstat, Nadostine ♣, Nyoderm ♣, O-V Statin
terconazole
(ter-kon'a-zole)
Terazol
tioconazole
(tye-oh-kon'a-zole)
Gyne-Trosyd ♣, Vagistat

Pregnancy category A: nystatin; **B:** clotrimazole; **C:** butoconazole, terconazole, tioconazole

Action: Interferes with fungal DNA replication; binds sterols in fungal cell membranes, which increases permeability, leaking of nutrients

Therapeutic Outcome: Fungistatic/fungicidal against susceptible organisms: *Candida* only

Uses: Vaginal, vulval, vulvovaginal candidiasis (moniliasis)

Dosage and routes

Butoconazole
Adult: Vag 5 g (1 applicator) hs × 3-6 days

Clotrimazole
Adult: 100 mg (1 vag tab, 100 mg) hs × 1 wk, or 200 mg (2 vag tab, 100 mg) hs × 3 nights, or 500 mg (1 vag tab, 500 mg); or 5 g (1 applicator) hs × 1-2 wks

Miconazole
Adult: 200 mg supp hs × 3 day or 100 mg supp × 1 wk

Nystatin
Adult: 100,000 U gd × 2 wk

Terconazole
Adult: Vag 5 g (1 applicator) hs × 7 days

Tioconazole
Adult: 1 applicator hs × 1

Adverse effects
GU: Vulvovaginal burning, itching, pelvic cramps
INTEG: Rash, urticaria, stinging, burning
MISC: Headache, body pain

Contraindications: Hypersensitivity

Precautions: Children <2 yrs, pregnancy, lactation

Interactions: None

NURSING CONSIDERATIONS

Assessment
• Assess for allergic reaction; burning, stinging, itching, discharge, soreness

Nursing diagnoses
✓ Skin integrity, impaired (uses)
✓ Infection, risk for (uses)
✓ Knowledge deficit (teaching)

Implementation
Top route
• Administer 1 applicatorful every night high into the vagina
• Store at room temp in dry place

Patient/family education

- Instruct patient in asepsis (hand washing) before, after each application
- Teach patient to apply with applicator only; to avoid use of any other vaginal product unless directed by prescriber; sanitary napkin may prevent soiling of undergarments
- Instruct patient to abstain from sexual intercourse until treatment is completed; reinfection and irritation may occur
- Advise patient to notify prescriber if symptoms persist

Evaluation

Positive therapeutic outcome

- Decrease in itching or white discharge (vaginal)

Disorders Index

Index

Entries can be identified as follows: generic name, Trade Name, DRUG CATEGORY, *Combination Product.*

B

Entries can be identified as follows: generic name, Trade Name, DRUG CATEGORY, *Combination Product.*

Entries can be identified as follows: generic name, Trade Name, DRUG CATEGORY, *Combination Product.*

Entries can be identified as follows: generic name, Trade Name, DRUG CATEGORY, *Combination Product.*

Entries can be identified as follows: generic name, Trade Name, DRUG CATEGORY, *Combination Product.*

Entries can be identified as follows: generic name, Trade Name, DRUG CATEGORY, *Combination Product*.

G

Entries can be identified as follows: generic name, Trade Name, DRUG CATEGORY, *Combination Product.*

H

Entries can be identified as follows: generic name, Trade Name, DRUG CATEGORY, *Combination Product.*

Entries can be identified as follows: generic name, Trade Name, DRUG CATEGORY, *Combination Product.*

L

Entries can be identified as follows: generic name, Trade Name, DRUG CATEGORY, *Combination Product.*

Entries can be identified as follows: generic name, Trade Name, DRUG CATEGORY, *Combination Product.*

O

P

Entries can be identified as follows: generic name, Trade Name, DRUG CATEGORY, ***Combination Product.***

Entries can be identified as follows: generic name, Trade Name, DRUG CATEGORY, *Combination Product.*

Q

R

Entries can be identified as follows: generic name, Trade Name, DRUG CATEGORY, *Combination Product.*

Entries can be identified as follows: generic name, Trade Name, DRUG CATEGORY, *Combination Product.*

W

Entries can be identified as follows: generic name, Trade Name, DRUG CATEGORY, *Combination Product.*

X

Z

Standard Precautions

In 1996, the Centers for Disease Control and Prevention published a set of recommendations to protect health care workers, patients, and others from the spread of infection. These recommendations are called *Standard Precautions.* The precautions are used in the care of all patients regardless of their diagnosis or disease. The precautions will not work if they are not used correctly. It is the health care worker's responsibility to select the correct personal protective equipment for the procedure being performed. The principles of standard precautions are also applied when handling or cleaning equipment or supplies that are potentially contaminated.

1. Wear gloves any time that you may contact blood, any moist body fluid (except sweat), secretions, excretions, nonintact skin, or mucous membranes.
2. Remove your gloves, wash your hands, and reapply clean gloves if your gloves become soiled with infective material.
3. Even if you are wearing gloves, remove them, wash your hands, and apply clean gloves *immediately before* contact with mucous membranes or nonintact skin.
4. Wear a protective cover gown of waterproof material if your clothing is likely to have substantial contact with infective material or if splashing of body fluids is likely
5. Wear a face shield or goggles to protect your eyes if splashing of secretions is likely.
6. Any time a face shield or goggles is worn, wear a surgical mask to protect the mucous membranes of your nose and mouth. A surgical mask may be worn in certain sterile procedures without protective eyewear. However, protective eyewear is *never* worn without a surgical mask.
7. Handle needles, razors, broken glass, and other sharp objects with care. Needles should never be recapped. All sharps should be disposed of in a puncture-resistant sharps container.
8. Wash your hands before and after each patient contact.
9. Wash your hands before you apply and after you remove gloves. Do not assume that handwashing is unnecessary because gloves were worn. Do not wash your hands with gloves on them.
10. Gloves are used for the care of one patient only, then discarded.
11. Follow your facility policy for disposal of gloves and other contaminated items. These items are generally not disposed of in open trash containers. Facilities have designated disposal sites for these biohazardous waste materials.
12. Use resuscitation barrier devices as an alternative to mouth-to-mouth resuscitation.

13. Linen should be handled in a manner that prevents contamination of the outside of the container. Linen from isolation rooms was previously doubled bagged. Double bagging is no longer recommended, since all linen is handled as potentially infectious. Double bag linen only if the outside of the bag becomes contaminated during the bagging process.

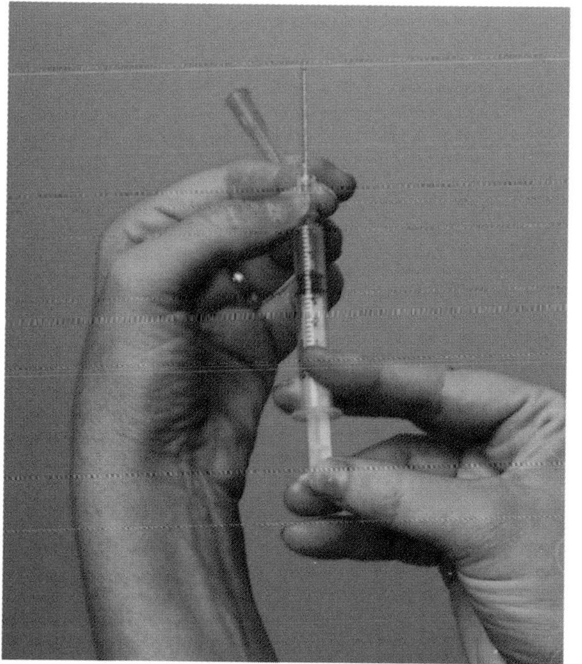

A

Plate 1 Preparing an injection from a vial. **A,** Take syringe and remove needle cap. Pull back on plunger to draw amount of air into syringe equivalent to volume of medication to be aspirated from vial.

Continued.

B

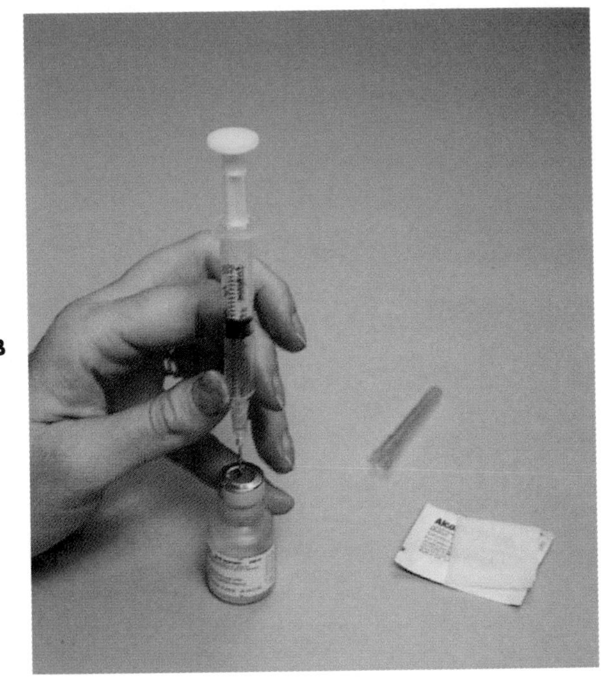

Plate 1, cont'd B, Insert tip of needle, with bevel pointing up, through center of rubber seal. Apply pressure on tip of needle during insertion.

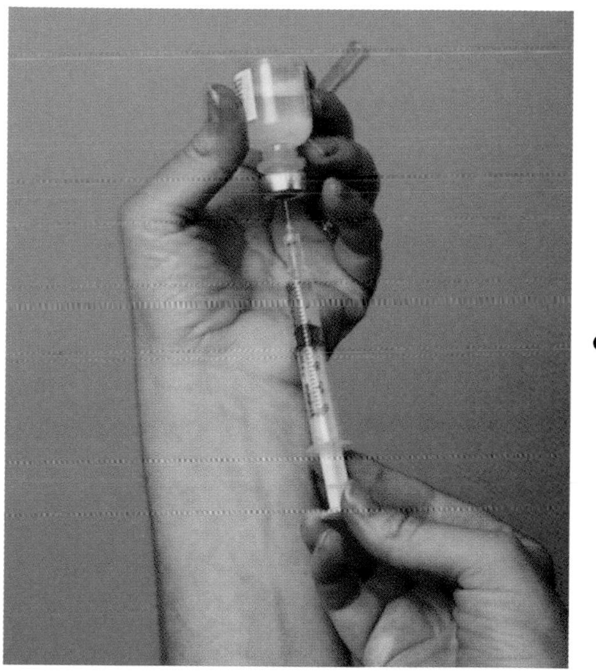

C

Plate 1, cont'd C, Allow air pressure to fill syringe gradually with medication. Pull back slightly on plunger if necessary.

Continued.

D

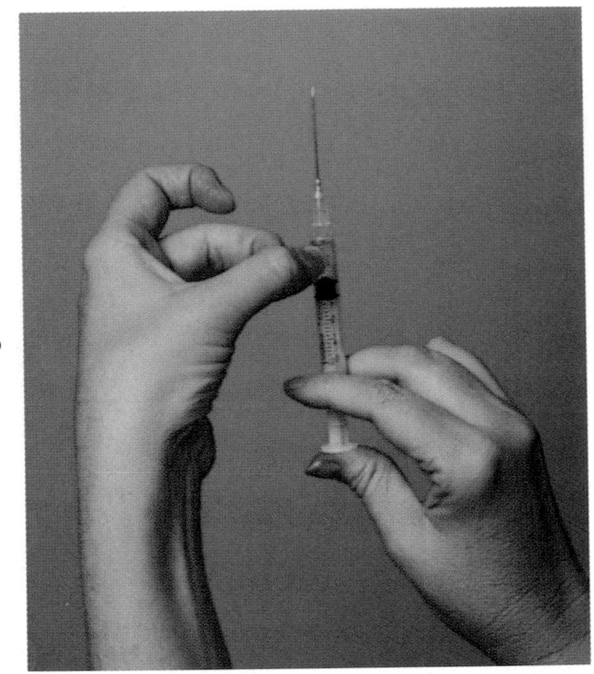

Plate 1, cont'd D, Remove remaining air from syringe by holding it and needle upright. Tap barrel to dislodge air bubbles. Draw back slightly on plunger and then push plunger upward to eject air.

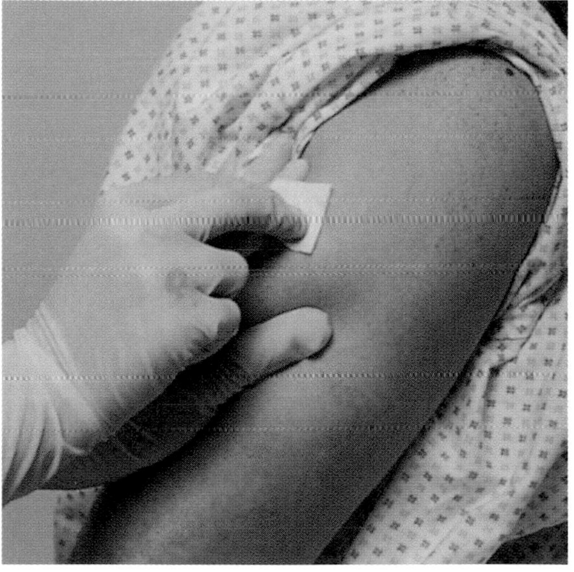

Plate 2 Administering an injection. Cleanse site with antiseptic swab. Apply swab at center of site and rotate outward in circular direction for about 5 cm (2 inches).

A

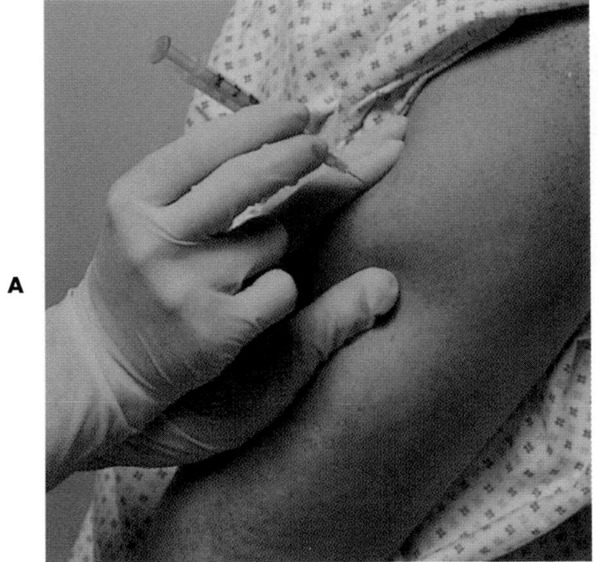

Plate 3 **A,** Hold syringe correctly between thumb and forefinger of dominant hand.

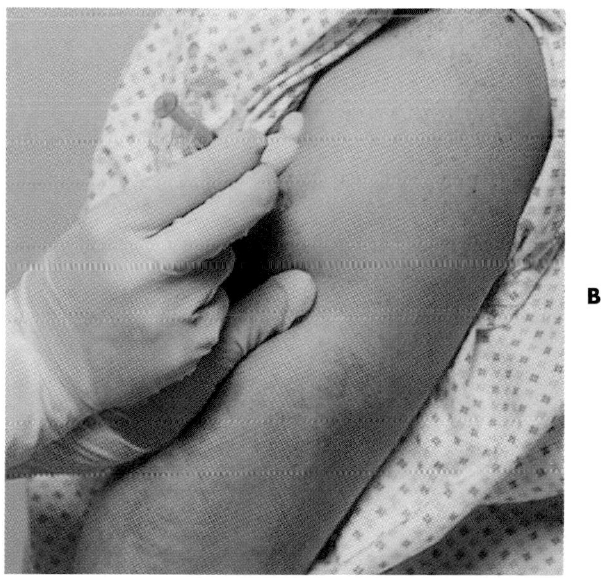

B

Plate 3, cont'd B, Position nondominant hand at proper anatomical landmarks and spread skin tightly. Inject needle quickly at a 90° angle (IM).

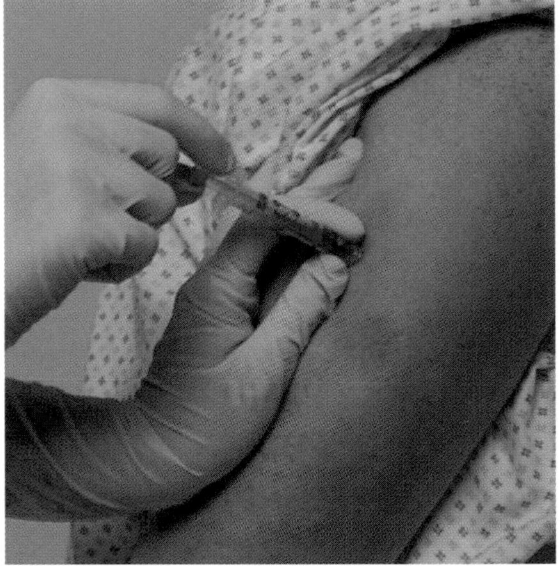

Plate 4 Move dominant hand to end of plunger. Avoid moving syringe while pulling back on plunger (IM).

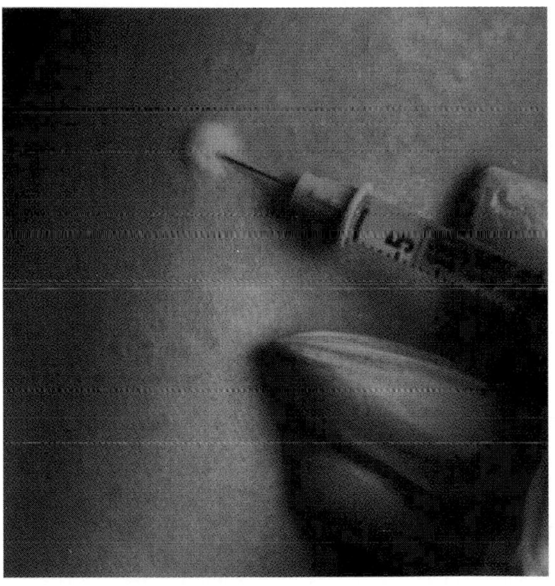

Plate 5 During intradermal injection, note formation of small bleb on the skin's surface.

A

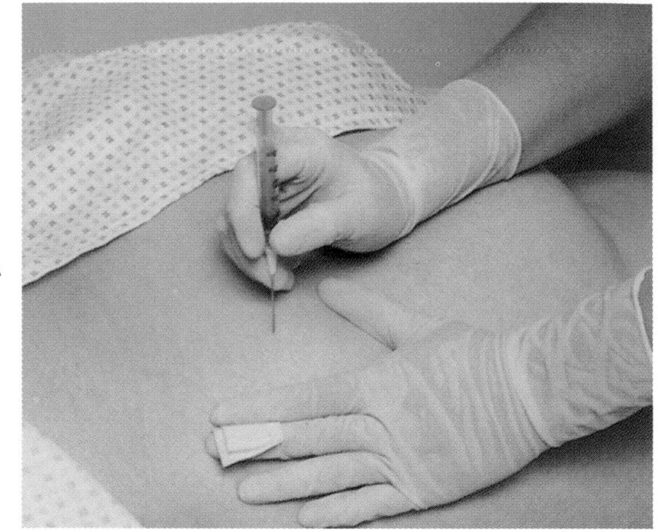

B

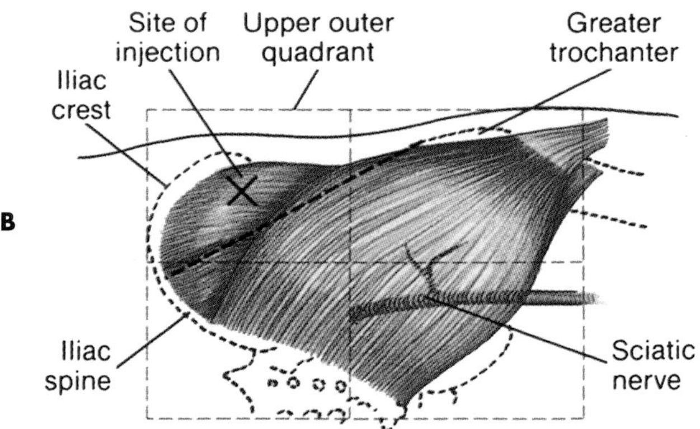

Plate 6 **A,** Site of IM injection into the left dorsogluteal muscle. **B,** Imaginary diagonal line extending from the posterior iliac spine to the greater trochanter is the landmark for selecting the dorsogluteal injection site.

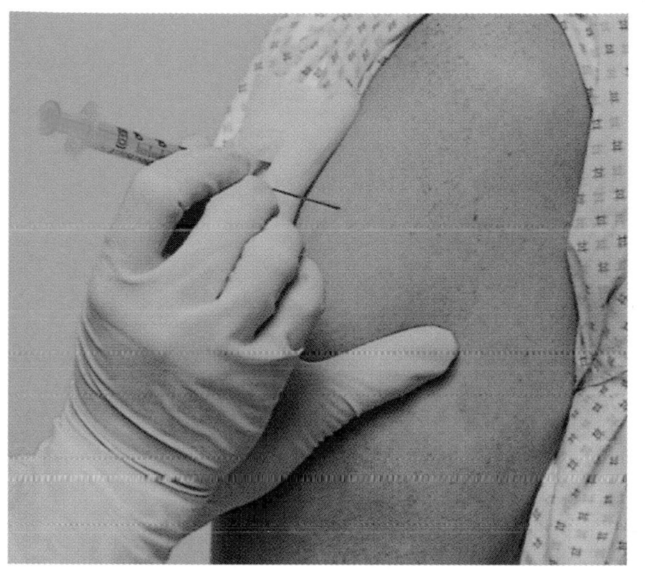

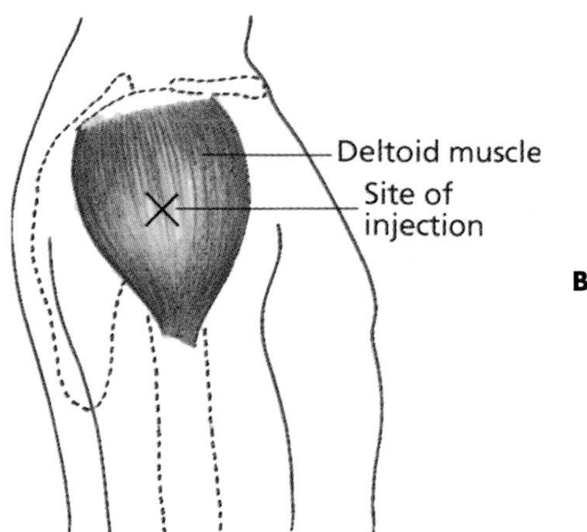

Plate 7 **A,** Site of IM injection into the deltoid muscle. **B,** Site of deltoid muscle injection below acromion process.

A

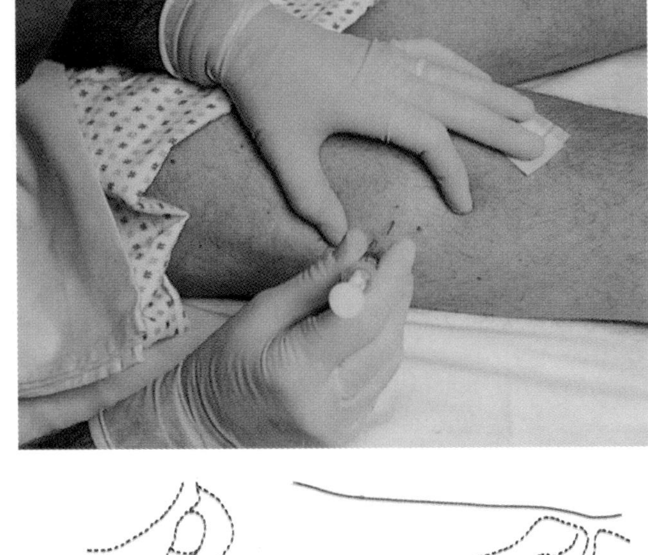

B

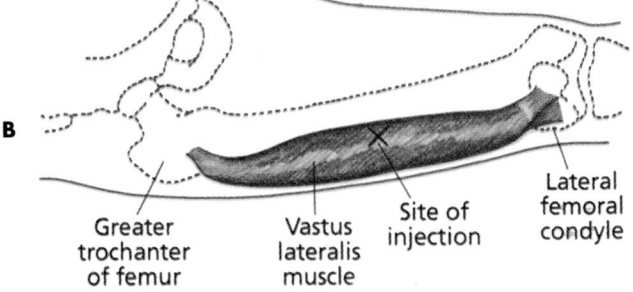

Plate 8 **A,** Injection site into the vastus lateralis muscle. **B,** Anatomical view of the site for IM injection into the vastus lateralis muscle.

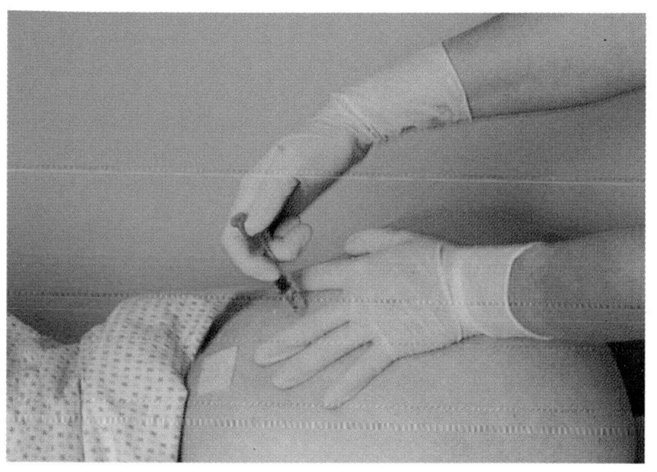

A

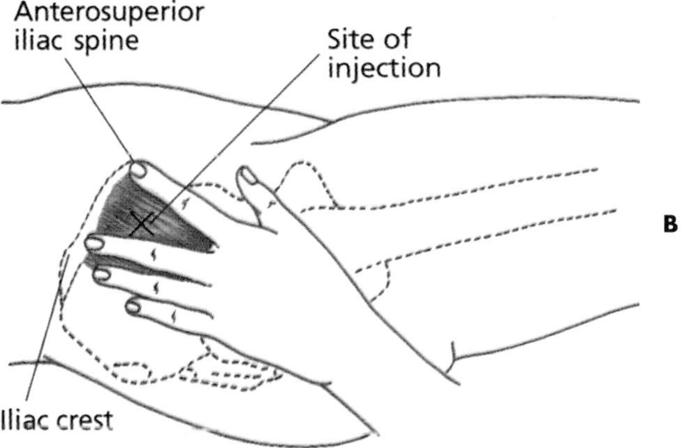

B

Plate 9 **A,** Injection site into ventrogluteal muscle avoids major nerves and blood vessels. **B,** Anatomical view of ventrogluteal muscle injection site.

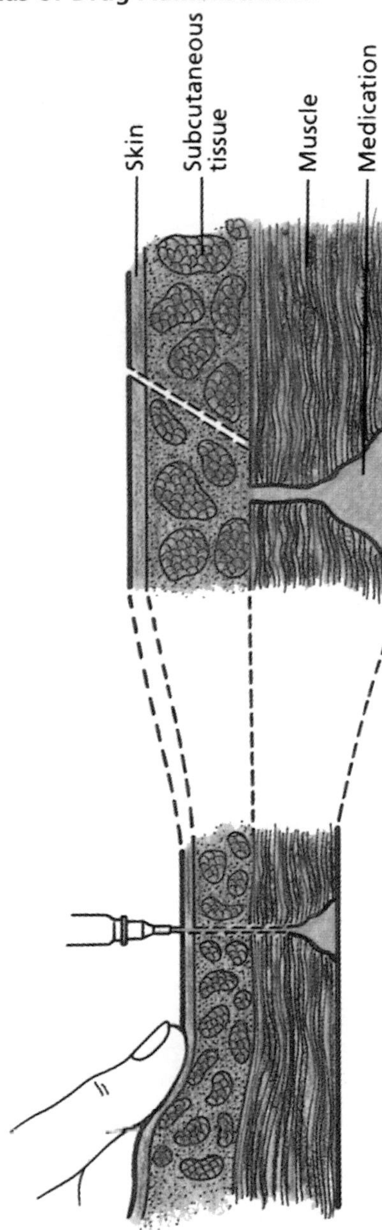

Plate 10 The Z-track method of injection prevents the deposit of medication through sensitive tissues.

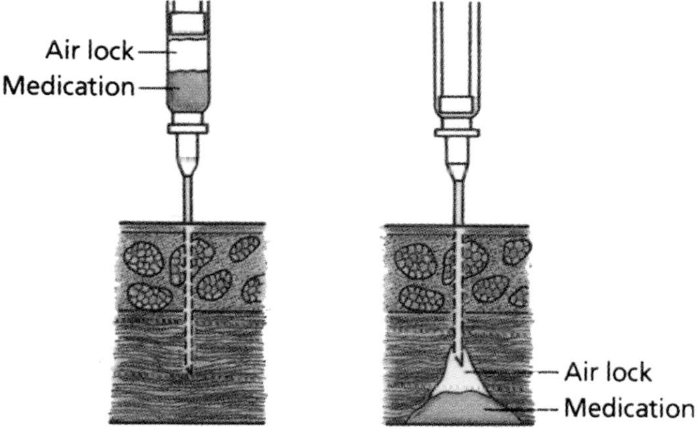

Plate 11 Administering IM injection by the air-lock technique prevents tracking of medication through SQ tissues.

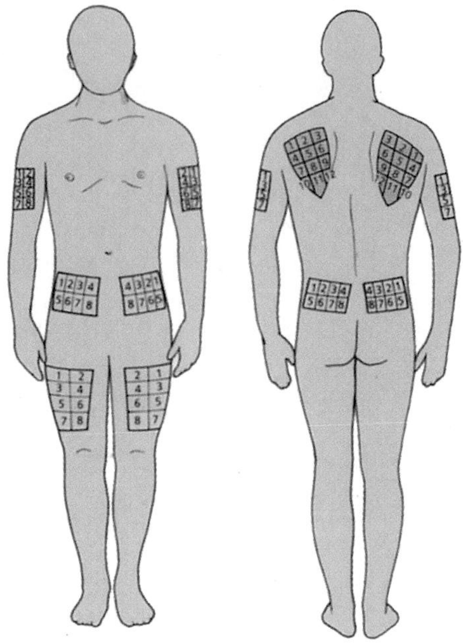

Plate 12 Common sites for SQ injections. Note how sites might be rotated.

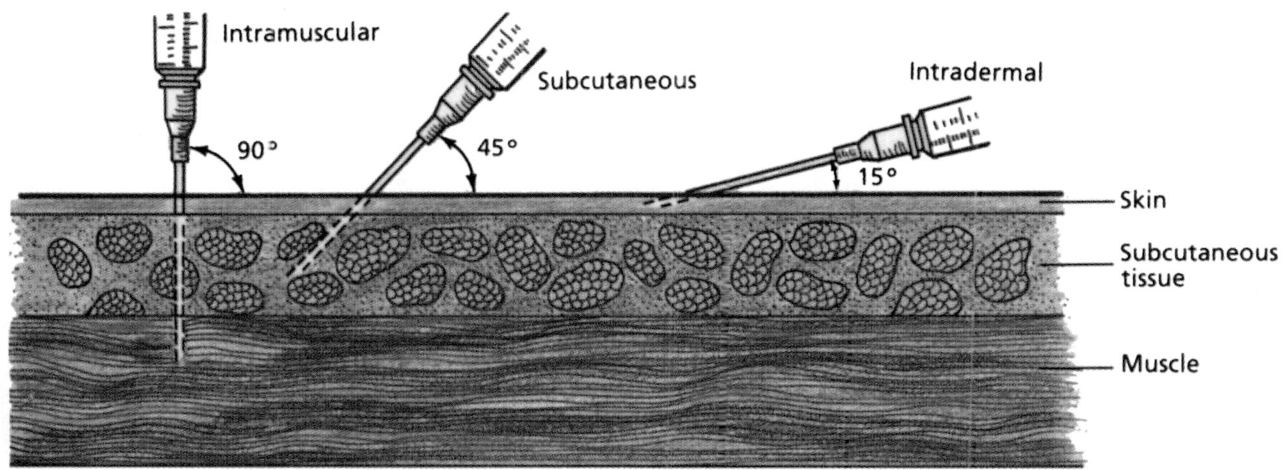

Plate 13 Comparison of the angles of insertion for IM (90°), SQ (45°), and intradermal (15°) injections.

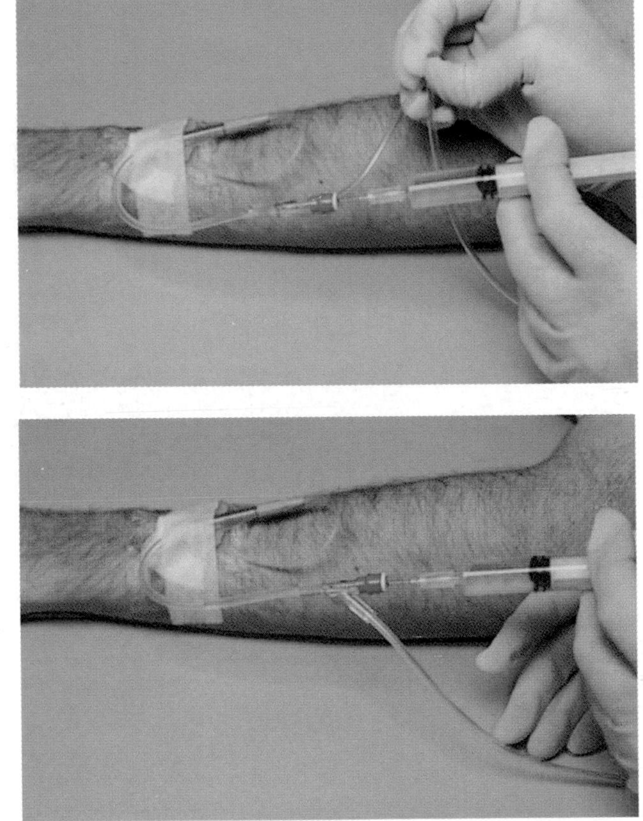

Plate 14 For legend, see opposite page.

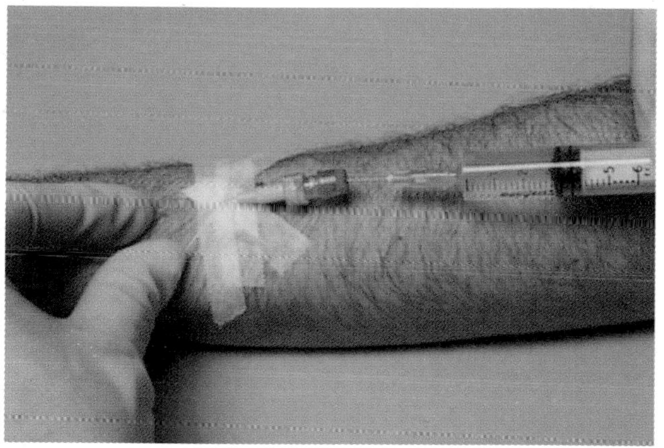

C

Plate 14 cont'd **A,** Occlude IV line by pinching tubing just above injection port. **B,** Inject medication slowly after aspirating with blood return. **C,** Administering medications by IV push. Insert needle of syringe containing prepared drug through center of diaphragm.

A

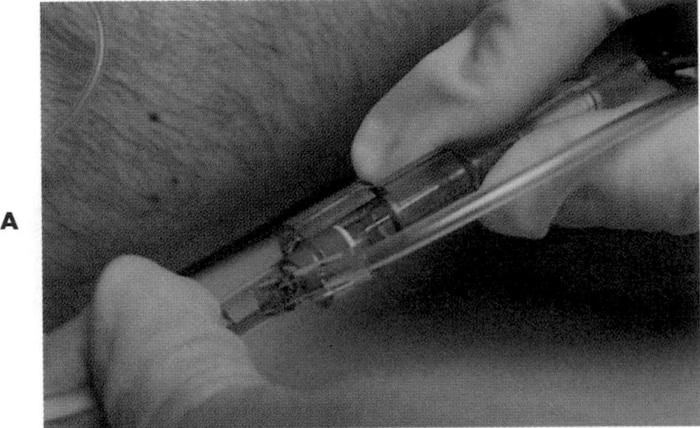

B

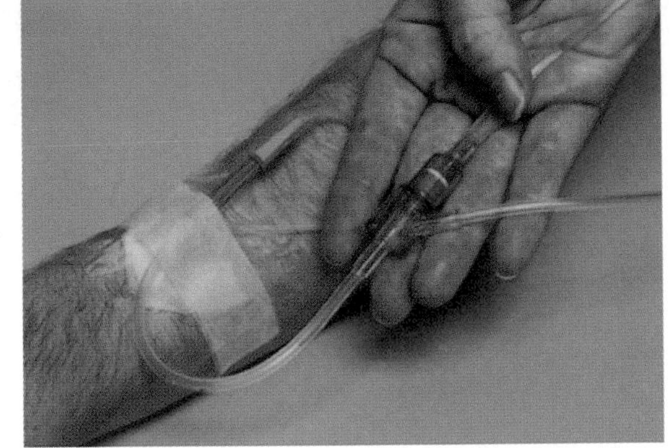

Plate 15 Administering IV medication by piggyback or volume administration sets. **A,** Connect covered sterile needle to end of infusion tubing after removing cover. **B,** Use needle-lock device to secure needle of secondary piggyback through injection port of main line.

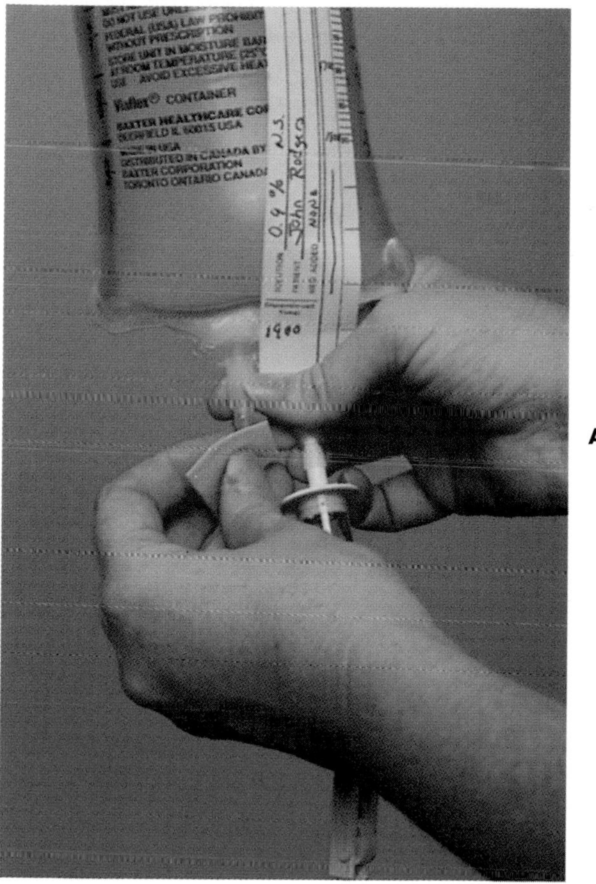

Plate 16 **A,** Wipe medication port with alcohol or antiseptic swab before adding medication to new container.

Continued.

B

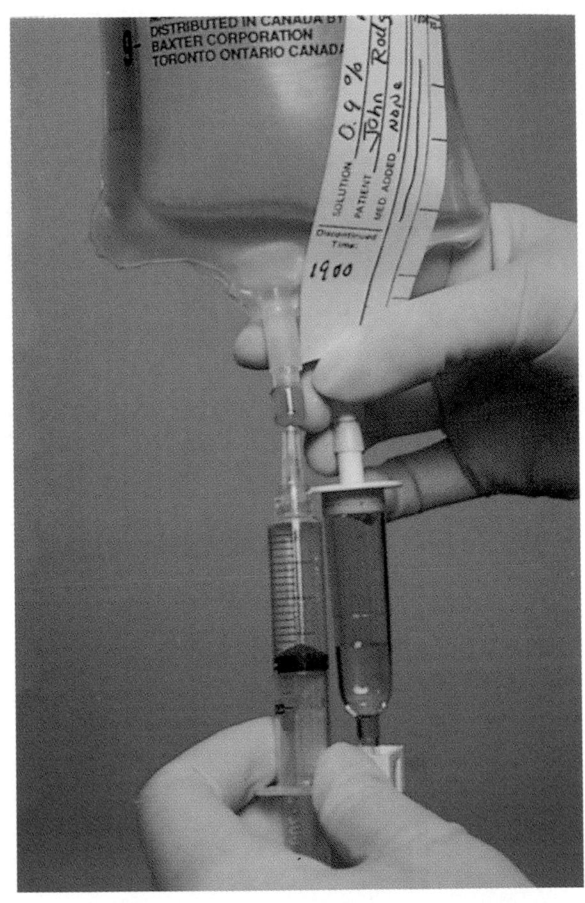

Plate 16, cont'd B, Adding medication to IV fluid containers. Remove needle cap from syringe through center of injection port or site and then inject medication.

Mosby's Pharmacology Patient Teaching Disk version 2.0*

[illegible]

2000 Update to Mosby's Drug Guide for Nurses
Third Edition

Following are monographs for 35 drugs that have received FDA approval since the publication of *Mosby's Drug Guide for Nurses,* 3rd edition. These monographs follow the same format as those in the book. They are arranged in alphabetical order by generic name, and trade names are given for all medications in common use. Each monograph contains the same subsections as those listed and described on pages v through vii of the preface to this book.

Drug Monographs in This Insert

GENERIC	TRADE	GENERIC	TRADE
alatrofloxacin/ trovafloxacin	Trovan	montelukast	Singulair
		naratriptan	Amerge
basiliximab	Simulect	palivizumab	Synagis
calfactant	Infasurf	paricalcitol	Zemplar
candesartan	Atacand	raloxifene	Evista
capecitabine	Xeloda	repaglinide	Prandin
cefdinir	Omnicef	rifapentine	Priftin
celecoxib	Celebrex	risedronate	Actonel
citalopram	Celexa	rituximab	Rituxan
daclizumab	Zenapax	rizatriptan	Maxalt
efavirenz	Sustiva	sibutramine	Meridia
eptifibatide	Integrilin	telmisartan	Micardis
etanercept	Enbrel	tirofiban	Aggrastat
fenoldopam	Corlopam	tolcapone	Tasmar
halofantrine	Halfan	tolterodine	Detrol
infliximab	Remicade	trastuzumab	Herceptin
leflunomide	Arava	valrubicin	Valstar
lepirudin	Refludan	zolmitriptan	Zomig

alatrofloxacin/ trovafloxacin (℞)

(ah-lat-troh-floks'ah-sin/ troh-vah-floks'a-sin)

Trovan

Func. class.: Antiinfective

Chem. class.: Fluoroquinolone

Pregnancy category C

Action: Interferes with conversion of intermediate DNA fragments into high-molecular-weight DNA in bacteria; DNA gyrase inhibitor

➔ **Therapeutic Outcome:** Bacterial action against the following: Nosocomial pneumonia: *E. coli, P. aeruginosa, H. influenzae, S. aureus*; community-acquired pneumonia: *S. pneumoniae, H. influenzae, S. aureus, K. pneumoniae, M. pneumoniae, M. catarrhalis, L. pneumophilia, C. pneumoniae*

Uses: Nosocomial pneumonia, community-acquired pneumonia, chronic bronchitis, acute sinusitis, complicated intraabdominal infections, gyn/pelvic infection, skin/skin structure infections, UTIs, chronic bacterial prostatitis, urethral gonorrhea in males, PID, cervicitis caused by susceptible organisms

Dosage and routes

Adult: **IV**/PO 200-300 mg qd for 7-14 days, depending on infection

Available forms: Sol for inj 5 mg/ml (alatrofloxacin); tabs 100, 200 mg (trovafloxacin)

Adverse effects

CNS: Headache, dizziness, insomnia, anxiety

GI: Nausea, flatulence, vomiting, diarrhea, abdominal pain, ***pseudomembranous colitis***

GU: Vaginitis, crystalluria

INTEG: Rash, pruritus, photosensitivity

Contraindications: Hypersensitivity to quinolones, seizure disorders, cerebral atherosclerosis, photosensitivity

Precautions: Pregnancy (C), lactation, children

Pharmacokinetics	
Absorption	Unknown
Distribution	Unknown
Metabolism	Liver
Excretion	Kidneys, unchanged
Half-life	Unknown

Pharmacodynamics	
Onset	Unknown
Peak	Unknown
Duration	Unknown

Interactions

None significant

Lab test interferences

↓ glucose, ↓ lymphocytes

NURSING CONSIDERATIONS

Assessment

- Assess for previous sensitivity reaction to fluoroquinolones
- Monitor for signs and symptoms of infection: characteristics of sputum, WBC >10,000, fever; obtain baseline information before and during treatment
- Obtain C&S before beginning drug therapy to identify if correct treatment has been initiated
- Assess for allergic reactions: rash, urticaria, pruritus, chills,

fever, joint pain; may occur a few days after therapy begins; epinephrine and resuscitation equipment should be available for anaphylactic reaction
- Assess bowel pattern qd; if severe diarrhea occurs, drug should be discontinued
- Assess for overgrowth of infection, perineal itching, fever, malaise, redness, pain, swelling, drainage, rash, diarrhea, change in cough, sputum
- Identify urine output; if decreasing, notify prescriber (may indicate nephrotoxicity); also check for increased BUN, creatinine
- Monitor blood studies: AST (SGOT), ALT (SGPT), CBC, Hct, bilirubin, LDH, alkaline phosphatase, Coombs' test monthly if patient is on long-term therapy
- Monitor electrolytes: potassium, sodium, chloride monthly if patient is on long-term therapy

Nursing diagnoses

- ✓ Infection, risk for (uses)
- ✓ Diarrhea (side effects)
- ✓ Injury, risk for (side effects)
- ✓ Knowledge deficit (teaching)
- ✓ Noncompliance (teaching)

Implementation

IV route

- Check for irritation, extravasation, phlebitis daily

Incompatibilities:

Do not use with magnesium in the same IV line

Solution compatibilities:

D_5, ½% NaCl, D_5/0.2% NaCl, LR

Patient/family education

- Teach patient to report sore throat, bruising, bleeding, joint pain; may indicate blood dyscrasias (rare)
- Advise patient to contact prescriber if vaginal itching, loose, foul-smelling stools, furry tongue occur, may indicate superinfection; report itching, rash, pruritus, urticaria
- Instruct patient to take all medication prescribed for the length of time ordered; drug must be taken around the clock to maintain blood levels; do not give medication to others
- Advise patient to notify prescriber of diarrhea with blood or pus

Evaluation

Positive therapeutic outcome

- Absence of signs/symptoms of infection (WBC <10,000, temp WNL)
- Reported improvement in symptoms of infection

basiliximab (℞)

(bas-ih-liks'ih-mab)

Simulect

Func. class.: Immunosuppressive

Chem. class.: Murine/human monoclonal antibody (Interleukin-2) receptor antagonist

Pregnancy category B

Action: Binds to and blocks the IL-2 receptor, which is selectively expressed on the surface of activated T-lymphocytes; impairs the immune system to antigenic challenges

➡ **Therapeutic Outcome:** Prevention of graft rejection

Uses: Acute allograft rejection

in renal transplant patients when used with cyclosporine and corticosteroids

Dosage and routes

Adult: **IV** 20 mg × 2 doses; 1st dose within 2 hr before transplant surgery; 2nd dose given 4 days after transplantation

Child 2-15 yr: 12 mg/m^2 × 2 doses; 1st dose within 2 hr before transplant surgery; 2nd dose given 4 days after transplantation

Available forms: Powder for inj 20 mg

Adverse effects

CNS: Pyrexia, chills, tremors, headache, insomnia

CV: Chest pain, angina, ***cardiac failure,*** hypotension

GI: Vomiting, nausea, diarrhea, constipation, abdominal pain

MISC: Infection, moniliasis

MS: Arthralgia, myalgia

RESP: Dyspnea, wheezing, ***pulmonary edema***

Contraindications: Hypersensitivity

Precautions: Pregnancy (B), infections, elderly, lactation, children

Pharmacokinetics	
Absorption	Unknown
Distribution	Unknown
Metabolism	Unknown
Excretion	Unknown
Half-life	Unknown

Pharmacodynamics	
Onset	Unknown
Peak	Unknown
Duration	Unknown

Interactions

Unknown

NURSING CONSIDERATIONS

Assessment

- Monitor blood studies: Hgb, WBC, platelets during treatment qmo; if leukocytes are <3000/mm^3, drug should be discontinued
- Monitor liver function studies: alk phosphatase, AST (SGOT), ALT (SGPT), bilirubin
- Assess hepatotoxicity: dark urine, jaundice, itching, light-colored stools; drug should be discontinued

Nursing diagnoses

- ✓ Infection, risk for (adverse reactions)
- ✓ Knowledge deficit (teaching)

Implementation

- Administer all medications PO if possible; avoid IM injection, since infection may occur

IV route

- After adding 5 ml sterile water for inj, shake gently to dissolve, reconstitute to a vol of 50 ml with 0.9% NaCl or D_5, gently invert bag, do not shake

Patient/family education

- Instruct patient to report fever, chills, sore throat, fatigue, since serious infection may occur

Evaluation

Positive therapeutic outcome

- Absence of graft rejection

calfactant (℞)

(cal-fak'tant)

Infasurf

Func. class.: Natural lung surfactant extract

Pregnancy category N/A

Action: Replenishes surfactant and restores surface activity to the lungs in premature infants

Therapeutic Outcome: Ability of neonate to breathe without assistance

Uses: Prevention and treatment (rescue) of respiratory distress syndrome in premature infants

Dosage and routes

INTRATRACHEAL INSTILL:
3 ml/kg of birth wt, given as 2 doses of 1.5 ml/kg, repeat doses of 3 ml/kg of birth wt, until up to 3 doses 12 hr apart have been given

Available forms: Susp 35 mg phospholipids/ml in 0.9% NaCl with 0.65 mg proteins in single-use vials containing 6 ml susp

Adverse effects

RESP: Pulmonary air leaks, pulmonary interstitial emphysema, apnea, pulmonary hemorrhage

SYST: Patent ductus arteriosus, intracranial hemorrhage, severe intracranial hemorrhage, necrotizing enterocolitis, posttreatment sepsis, posttreatment infection, bradycardia, oxygen desaturation, pallor, vasoconstriction, hypotension, hypertension

Precautions: Bradycardia, rales, infections

Pharmacokinetics

Absorption	Unknown
Distribution	Lung
Metabolism	Recycled
Excretion	Unknown
Half-life	Unknown

Pharmacodynamics

Onset	Few min
Peak	Unknown
Duration	Becomes lung associated within hours of administration

Interactions

None

NURSING CONSIDERATIONS

Assessment

- Assess respiratory rate, rhythm, character, chest expansion, color, transcutaneous saturation, ABGs; monitor ECG
- Check endotracheal tube placement before dosing; monitor for apnea after endotracheal administration
- Check for reflux of drug into the endotracheal tube during administration; stop drug administration if this occurs, and if needed increase peak inspiratory pressure on the ventilator by 4-5 cm H_2O until tube is cleared
- Assess infant for repeat dosing using radiographic confirmation of respiratory distress syndrome; repeat doses should be given as noted above; ventilator settings for repeat doses F_{IO_2} are decreased by 0.2 or amount to prevent cyanosis; ventilator rate of 30/min; inspiratory time <1 sec; if infant's pretreatment rate was >30, leave unchanged during dosing; resume usual ventilator management after dosing

Nursing diagnoses

- ✓ Gas exchange, impaired (uses)
- ✓ Knowledge deficit (teaching)

Implementation

- Administer after suctioning; give by endotracheal administration only by persons trained in neonatal intubation and ventilation
- Use a no. 5 Fr end-hole catheter inserted into the endotracheal tube with the tip protruding just beyond the end of the endotracheal tube; shorten the catheter before insertion; do not insert the drug into the mainstream bronchus
- Divide each dose into quarters and administer with infant in different positions
- Determine the dosing by weight of infant; slowly withdraw the contents into the plastic syringe through a 20-G needle; do not filter or shake; attach the premeasured no. 5 Fr catheter to syringe; fill with drug and discard excess through the catheter so only dose to be given remains in syringe
- For prevention dosing, stabilize, weigh, and intubate the infant; give drug within 15 min of birth if possible; position infant and inj first quarter dose through catheter over 2-3 sec; remove catheter and manually ventilate with O_2 to prevent cyanosis (60 bpm) and sufficient positive pressure to promote adequate air exchange and chest wall excursion
- For **rescue dosing,** give drug as soon as infant is placed on ventilator after birth; immediately before administering dose, change ventilator settings to 60/min, inspiratory time 0.5 sec, FIO_2 1; position infant and inj first quarter through catheter over 2-3 sec; remove catheter; return to mechanical ventilator
- Ventilate infant for >30 sec or until stable after prevention or rescue strategy; reposition for next dose; same procedure for subsequent dosing; do not suction for at least 1 hr after dosing unless airway obstruction is evident; resume ventilator therapy after dosing
- Reduce peak ventilator inspiratory pressures immediately if chest expansion improves substantially after dose
- Suction all infants before administration to prevent mucus plugging; if endotracheal tube obstruction is suspected, remove the obstruction and replace tube immediately
- Store in refrigerator; protect from light; warm to room temp for >20 min or warm in hand 8 min before giving; do not use artificial warming methods; enter a vial only once; unopened, unused vials that have been warmed to room temp may be rerefrigerated within 8 hr of warming; do not warm and return to refrigerator more than once

Patient/family education

- Explain disease process and purpose of medication to parents; communicate neonate's progress

Evaluation

Positive therapeutic outcome

- Significant improvement in respiratory status (oxygenation, arterial blood gases WNL)

candesartan (℞)

(can-deh-sar'tan)

Atacand

Func. class.: Antihypertensive

Chem. class.: Angiotensin II receptor (Type AT_1)

Pregnancy category C, 1st trimester; D, 2nd/3rd trimester

Action: Blocks the vasoconstrictor and aldosterone-secreting effects of angiotensin II; selectively blocks the binding of angiotensin II to the AT_1 receptor found in tissues

Therapeutic Outcome: Decreased B/P

Uses: Hypertension, alone or in combination

Dosage and routes

Adult: PO 16 mg qd initially in patients who are not volume depleted, range 8-32 mg/day; may be given with a diuretic

Available forms: Tabs 4, 8, 16, 32

Adverse effects

CNS: Dizziness, fatigue, headache

GI: Diarrhea, nausea

MS: Arthralgia, pain

RESP: Cough, upper respiratory infection

SYST: Angioedema

Contraindications: Hypersensitivity

Precautions: Hypersensitivity to ACE inhibitors; pregnancy (C) 1st trimester, (D) 2nd and 3rd trimesters; lactation; children; elderly

Pharmacokinetics

Absorption	Well
Distribution	Bound to plasma proteins
Metabolism	Extensive
Excretion	Feces, urine, breast milk
Half-life	9 hr

Pharmacodynamics

Onset	Unknown
Peak	2 hr
Duration	24 hr

Interactions

None significant

NURSING CONSIDERATIONS

Assessment

- Assess B/P, pulse q4h; note rate, rhythm, quality
- Monitor electrolytes: potassium, sodium, chloride; total CO_2
- Obtain baselines in renal, liver function tests before therapy begins
- Assess blood studies: BUN, creatinine, LFTs before treatment
- Monitor for edema in feet, legs daily
- Assess for skin turgor, dryness of mucous membranes for hydration status

Nursing diagnoses

- ✓ Fluid volume deficit (side effects)
- ✓ Noncompliance (teaching)
- ✓ Knowledge deficit (teaching)

Implementation

PO route

- Administer without regard to meals

Patient/family education

- Teach patient not to take the drug if breastfeeding or pregnant, or have had an allergic reaction to this drug

• If a dose is missed, instruct patient to take as soon as possible, unless it is within an hour before next dose
• Advise patient to comply with dosage schedule, even if feeling better
• Teach patient to notify prescriber of fever, swelling of hands or feet, irregular heartbeat, chest pain
• Advise patient excessive perspiration, dehydration, diarrhea may lead to fall in blood pressure—consult prescriber if these occur
• Inform patient that drug may cause dizziness, fainting; lightheadedness may occur
• Caution patient to rise slowly to sitting or standing position to minimize orthostatic hypotension

Evaluation

Positive therapeutic outcome
• Decreased B/P

capecitabine (℞)

(cap-eh-sit'ah-bean)

Xeloda

Func. class.: Antineoplastic, antimetabolite

Chem class.: Fluoropyrimidine carbamate

Pregnancy category D

Action: Competes with physiologic substrate of DNA synthesis, thus interfering with cell replication in the S phase of cell cycle (before mitosis)

➔ **Therapeutic Outcome:** Decreasing symptoms of breast cancer

Uses: Metastatic breast cancer

Dosage and routes

Adult: PO 2500 mg/m^2/day in 2 divided doses q12h at end of meal × 2 wk, then 1 wk rest period; given in 3 wk cycles

Available forms: Tabs 150, 500 mg

Adverse effects

CNS: Dizziness, headache, paresthesia, fatigue, insomnia
GI: Nausea, vomiting, anorexia, diarrhea, stomatitis, abdominal pain
HEMA: Neutropenia, lymphopenia, thrombocytopenia, myelosuppression, anemia
INTEG: Hand and foot syndrome, dermatitis, nail disorder
OTHER: Hyperbilirubinemia, eye irritation, pyrexia, edema, myalgia, limb pain

Contraindications: Hypersensitivity to 5-fluorouracil, infants, pregnancy (D)

Precautions: Renal disease, hepatic disease, lactation, children, elderly

Pharmacokinetics

Absorption	Readily, food ↓
Distribution	Unknown
Metabolism	Liver, extensively
Excretion	Kidneys
Half-life	45 min

Pharmacodynamics

Onset	Unknown
Peak	1½ hr
Duration	Unknown

Interactions

Individual drugs

Leucovorin: ↑ toxicity

Drug classifications

Antacids: ↑ capecitabine

NURSING CONSIDERATIONS

Assessment

• Assess buccal cavity q8h for dryness, sores or ulceration, white patches, pain, bleeding, dysphagia; obtain prescription for viscous lidocaine (Xylocaine)

• Assess symptoms indicating severe allergic reation: rash, pruritus, urticaria, purpuric skin lesions, itching, flushing; drug should be discontinued

• Monitor CBC, differential, platelet count weekly; withhold drug if WBC count is $<4000/mm^3$ or platelet count is $<100,000/mm^3$; notify prescriber of results if WBC $<20,000/mm^3$, platelets $<150,000/mm^3$

• Monitor temp q4h (may indicate beginning of infection)

• Monitor liver function tests before and during therapy (bilirubin, AST [SGOT], ALT [SGPT], LDH) as needed or monthly; note yellowing of skin or sclera, dark urine, clay-colored stools, itchy skin, abdominal pain, fever, diarrhea

• Assess for bleeding: hematuria, stool guaiac, bruising or petechiae, mucosa or orifices q8h; inflammation of mucosa, breaks in skin

Nursing diagnoses

- ✓ Injury, risk for (adverse reactions)
- ✓ Body image disturbance (adverse reactions)
- ✓ Infection, risk for (adverse reactions)
- ✓ Knowledge deficit (teaching)

Implementation

PO route

• Give antiemetic 30-60 min before giving drug to prevent vomiting and prn; give antibiotics for prophylaxis of infection

• Provide liq diet: carbonated beverages; gelatin may be added if patient is not nauseated or vomiting

• Help patient to rinse mouth tid-qid with water or club soda, brush teeth bid-qid with soft brush or cotton-tipped applicators for stomatitis, use unwaxed dental floss

Patient/family education

• Measures are recommended during therapy; drug is teratogenic to fetus

• Advise patient to avoid use of products containing aspirin or ibuprofen, razors, commercial mouthwash, since bleeding may occur; to report symptoms of bleeding (hematuria, tarry stools)

• Instruct patient to report signs of anemia (fatigue, headache, irritability, faintness, shortness of breath)

Evaluation

Positive therapeutic outcome

• Prevention of rapid division of malignant cells

cefdinir (℞)

(sef′dih-ner)

Omnicef

Func. class.: Antibiotic, broad-spectrum

Chem class.: Cephalosporin (3rd generation)

Pregnancy category B

Action: Inhibits bacterial cell synthesis, which renders cell wall osmotically unstable, leading to cell death

Therapeutic Outcome: Bactericidal effects for the following: gram-negative organisms *Haemophilus influenzae*, gram-positive organisms *Streptococcus pneumoniae*, *S. pyogenes*, *Staphylococcus aureus*

Uses: Uncomplicated skin and skin structure infections, community-acquired pneumonia, acute exacerbations of chronic bronchitis, acute maxillary sinusitis, pharyngitis, tonsillitis

Dosage and routes

Uncomplicated skin and skin structure infections/community-acquired pneumonia

Adult and child ≥13 yr: PO 300 mg q12h × 10 days

Acute exacerbations of chronic bronchitis/acute maxillary sinusitis

Adult and child ≥13 yr: PO 300 mg q12h or 600 mg q24h × 10 days

Pharyngitis/tonsillitis

Adult and child ≥13 yr: PO 300 mg q12h or 600 mg q24h × 10 days

Available forms: Caps 300 mg, oral susp 125 mg/ml

Adverse effects

CNS: Headache, dizziness, weakness, paresthesia, fever, chills

GI: Nausea, vomiting, diarrhea, anorexia, pain, glossitis, bleeding; increased AST (SGOT), ALT (SGPT), bilirubin, LDH, alk phosphatase; abdominal pain

GU: Proteinuria, vaginitis, pruritus, candidiasis, increased BUN, ***nephrotoxicity, renal failure***

HEMA: ***Leukopenia, thrombocytopenia, agranulocytosis,*** anemia, ***neutropenia, lymphocytosis, eosinophilia, pancytopenia, hemolytic anemia (rare)***

INTEG: Rash, urticaria, dermatitis, thrombophlebitis

SYST: ***Anaphylaxis***

Contraindications: Hypersensitivity to cephalosporins; infants <1 mo

Precautions: Hypersensitivity to penicillins, pregnancy (B), lactation, renal disease

Pharmacokinetics	
Absorption	Well absorbed
Distribution	Widely distributed; crosses placenta
Metabolism	Not metabolized
Excretion	Kidneys, unchanged; enters breast milk
Half-life	Unknown

Pharmacodynamics	
	PO
Onset	Unknown
Peak	Unknown

Interactions

Individual drugs

Probenecid: ↓ excretion of drug and ↑ blood levels

Vancomycin: ↑ toxicity

Drug classifications

Aminoglycosides: ↑ toxicity

Anticoagulants: ↑ bleeding

Erythromycins: ↓ effects

Tetracyclines: ↓ effects

Thrombolytics: ↑ bleeding

Lab test interferences

False: ↑ Creatinine (serum urine), false ↑ urinary 17-KS

False positive: Urinary protein, direct Coombs' test, urine glucose

Interference: Cross-matching

NURSING CONSIDERATIONS

Assessment

- Assess patient for previous sensitivity reaction to penicillins or other cephalosporins; cross-sensitivity between penicillins and cephalosporins is common
- Assess patient for signs and symptoms of infection, including characteristics of wounds, sputum, urine, stool, WBC >10,000, earache, fever; obtain baseline information and during treatment
- Obtain C&S before beginning drug therapy to identify if correct treatment has been initiated
- Assess for allergic reactions: rash, urticaria, pruritus, chills, fever, joint pain; angioedema may occur a few days after therapy begins; epinephrine and resuscitation equipment should be available for anaphylactic reaction
- Identify urine ouput; if decreasing, notify prescriber (may indicate nephrotoxicity); also check for increased BUN, creatinine
- Monitor blood studies: AST (SGOT), ALT (SGPT), CBC, Hct, bilirubin, LDH, alkaline phosphatase, Coombs' test monthly if patient is on long-term therapy
- Monitor electrolytes: potassium, sodium, chloride monthly if patient is on long-term therapy
- Assess bowel pattern qd; if severe diarrhea occurs, drug should be discontinued; may indicate pseudomembranous colitis
- Monitor for bleeding: ecchymosis, bleeding gums, hematuria, stool guaiac daily if on long-term therapy
- Assess for overgrowth of infection: perineal itching, fever, malaise, redness, pain, swelling, drainage, rash, diarrhea, change in cough, sputum

Nursing diagnoses

- ✓ Infection, risk for (uses)
- ✓ Diarrhea (side effects)
- ✓ Injury, risk for (side effects)
- ✓ Knowledge deficit (teaching)
- ✓ Noncompliance (teaching)

Implementation

PO route

- Give oral suspension after adding 39 ml water to the 60 ml bottle; 65 ml water to the 12.0 ml bottle; discard unused portion after 10 days

Patient/family education

- Teach patient to report sore throat, bruising, bleeding, joint pain; may indicate blood dyscrasias (rare)
- Advise patient to contact physician if vaginal itching, loose, foul-smelling stools, furry tongue occur; may indicate superinfection
- Advise patient to notify prescriber of diarrhea with blood or pus, which may indicate pseudomembranous colitis

Evaluation

Positive therapeutic outcome

- Absence of signs/symptoms of infection (WBC <10,000, temp WNL, absence of red, draining wounds, earache)
- Reported improvement in symptoms of infection
- Negative C&S

Treatment of anaphylaxis:

Epinephrine, antihistamines, resuscitate if needed

celecoxib (℞)
(cel-eh-cox'ib)
Celebrex
Func. class.: Nonsteroidal antiinflammatory
Pregnancy category C

Action: Inhibits prostaglandin synthesis by decreasing enzyme needed for biosynthesis; analgesic, antiinflammatory, antipyretic properties

➔ **Therapeutic Outcome:** Decreased pain, inflammation

Uses: Acute, chronic rheumatoid arthritis, osteoarthritis

Dosage and routes
Osteoarthritis
Adult: PO 200 mg/day as a single dose
Rheumatoid arthritis
Adult: PO 100-200 mg bid

Available forms: Caps 100, 200 mg

Adverse effects
CNS: Fatigue, anxiety, depression, nervousness, paresthesia
*CV: **Tachycardia**,* angina, ***MI**, palpitations, dysrhythmias, hypertension, fluid retention*
EENT: Tinnitus, hearing loss, blurred vision, glaucoma, cataract, conjunctivitis, eye pain
*GI: Nausea, anorexia, vomiting, constipation, dry mouth, diverticulitis, gastritis, gastroenteritis, hemorrhoids, hiatal hernia, stomatitis, **GI bleeding***
GU: Nephrotoxicity: dysuria, hematuria, oliguria, azotemia, cystitis, UTI
HEMA: Blood dyscrasias, *epistaxis, bruising, anemia*
INTEG: Purpura, *rash, pruritus, sweating, erythema, petechiae, photosensitivity, alopecia*
RESP: Pharyngitis, shortness of breath, pneumonia, coughing

Contraindications: Hypersensitivity to aspirin, iodides, other NSAIDs, asthma

Precautions: Pregnancy C, P lactation, children, bleeding disorders, GI disorders, cardiac disorders, hypersensitivity to other antiinflammatory agents

Pharmacokinetics	
Absorption	Well absorbed (PO)
Distribution	Crosses placenta, bound to plasma proteins
Metabolism	Liver
Excretion	Kidneys
Half-life	Unknown

Pharmacodynamics	
Onset	Unknown
Peak	3 hr
Duration	Unknown

Interactions
Individual drugs
Aspirin: ↓ effectiveness, ↑ adverse reactions
Coumadin: ↑ anticoagulant effects
Lithium: ↑ toxicity
Drug classifications
ACE inhibitors: may ↓ effects of ACE inhibitors
Anticoagulants: ↑ risk of bleeding
Antineoplastics: ↑ risk of hematologic toxicity
Glucocorticoids: ↑ adverse reactions
Diuretics: ↓ effectiveness of diuretics
NSAIDs: ↑ adverse reactions

NURSING CONSIDERATIONS
Assessment
• Assess for pain of rheumatoid arthritis, osteoarthritis;

check ROM, inflammation of joints, characteristics of pain

- Monitor blood counts during therapy; watch for decreasing platelets; if low, therapy may need to be discontinued, restarted after hematologic recovery; and for blood dyscrasias (thrombocytopenia): bruising, fatigue, bleeding, poor healing

Nursing diagnoses

- Pain (uses)
- Mobility, impaired physical (uses)
- Injury, risk for (side effects)
- Knowledge deficit (teaching)

Implementation

PO route

- Administer with food or milk to decrease gastric symptoms
- Do not crush, dissolve, or chew caps

Patient/family education

- Teach patient that drug must be continued for prescribed time to be effective; to avoid other NSAIDs
- Caution patient to report bleeding, bruising, fatigue, malaise, since blood dyscrasia do occur
- Teach patient to take with a full glass of water to enhance absorption; do not crush, break, or chew

Evaluation

Positive therapeutic outcome

- Decreased pain in arthritic conditions
- Decreased inflammation in arthritic conditions

citalopram (℞)

(sigh-tal'oh-pram)
Celexa
Func. class.: Antidepressant
Chem class.: Selective serotonin reuptake inhibitor (SSRI)
Pregnancy category B

Action: Inhibits CNS neuron uptake of serotonin but not of norepinephrine

Therapeutic Outcome: Decreased symptoms of depression after 2-3 wk

Uses: Major depressive disorder

Dosage and routes

Adult: PO 20 mg qd AM or PM, may increase if needed to 40 mg/day after 1 wk; maintenance: after 6-8 wk of initial treatment, continue for 24 wk (32 wk total), reevaluate long-term usefulness

Available forms: Tabs 20, 40 mg

Adverse effects

CNS: Headache, nervousness, insomnia, drowsiness, anxiety, tremor, dizziness, fatigue, sedation, poor concentration, abnormal dreams, agitation, ***convulsions***
CV: Hot flashes, palpitations, angina pectoris, ***hemorrhage***, hypertension, first-degree tachycardia
EENT: Visual changes, ear/eye pain, photophobia, tinnitus
GI: Nausea, diarrhea, dry mouth, anorexia, dyspepsia, constipation, cramps, vomiting, taste changes, flatulence, decreased appetite

GU: Dysmenorrhea, decreased libido, urinary frequency, urinary tract infection, amenorrhea, cystitis, impotence
INTEG: Sweating, rash, pruritus, acne, alopecia, urticaria
MS: Pain, arthritis, twitching
RESP: Infection, pharyngitis, nasal congestion, sinus headache, sinusitis, cough, dyspnea, bronchitis, asthma, hyperventilation, pneumonia
SYST: Asthenia, viral infection, fever, allergy, chills

Contraindications: Hypersensitivity

P G **Precautions:** Pregnancy (B), lactation, children, elderly

Pharmacokinetics	
Absorption	Well absorbed
Distribution	Unknown
Metabolism	Liver
Excretion	Kidneys, steady state 28-35 days
Half-life	Unknown

Pharmacodynamics	
Onset	Unknown
Peak	Unknown
Duration	Unknown

Interactions
Individual drugs
Alcohol: ↑ CNS depression
Carbamazepine: ↑ toxicity
Lithium: ↑ toxicity
Drug classifications
Antifungals, azole: ↑ citalopram levels
Barbiturates: ↑ CNS depression
Benzodiazepines: ↑ CNS depression
β-blockers: ↑ plasma levels of β-blockers
CNS depressants: ↑ CNS depression
Macrolides: ↑ citalopram levels
MAOI: Hypertensive crisis, convulsions
Sedative/hypnotics: ↑ CNS depression
- Do not use with MAOIs

Lab test interferences:
↑ Serum bilirubin, ↑ blood glucose, ↑ alk phosphatase, ↓ VMA, ↓ 5-HIAA, ↓ blood glucose
False: ↑ Urinary catecholamines

NURSING CONSIDERATIONS
Assessment
- Monitor B/P (lying, standing), pulse q4h; if systolic B/P drops 20mm hg, hold drug and notify prescriber; take vital signs q4h in patients with cardiovascular disease
- Monitor blood studies: CBC, leukocytes, differential, cardiac enzymes if patient is receiving long-term therapy; check platelets, bleeding can occur
- Monitor hepatic studies: AST (SGOT), ALT (SGPT), bilirubin
- Check weight qwk; appetite may increase with drug
- Assess ECG for flattening of T wave, bundle branch block, AV block, dysrhythmias in cardiac patients
- Assess EPS primarily in elderly: rigidity, dystonia, akathisia
- Assess mental status: mood, sensorium, affect, suicidal tendencies; increase in psychiatric symptoms: depression, panic
- Monitor urinary retention, constipation; constipation is P G more likely to occur in children or elderly

• Assess for withdrawal symptoms: headache, nausea, vomiting, muscle pain, weakness; do not usually occur unless drug is discontinued abruptly

• Identify patient's alcohol consumption; if alcohol is consumed, hold dose until AM

Nursing diagnoses

- Coping, ineffective individual (uses)
- Injury, risk for (side effects)
- Knowledge deficit (teaching)
- Noncompliance (teaching)

Implementation

• Give with food or milk for GI symptoms

• Give dosage hs if oversedation occurs during day

• Store at room temp; do not freeze

Patient/family education

• Teach patient that therapeutic effects may take 2-3 wk

• Instruct patient to use caution in driving or other activities requiring alertness because of drowsiness, dizziness, blurred vision; to avoid rising quickly from sitting to standing, especially elderly

• Caution patient to avoid alcohol ingestion, other CNS depressants

• Advise patient not to discontinue medication quickly after long-term use: may cause nausea, headache, malaise

• Instruct patient to increase fluids, bulk in diet if constipation, urinary retention occur, especially elderly

• Advise patient to take gum, hard sugarless candy, or frequent sips of water for dry mouth

Evaluation

Positive therapeutic outcome

• Decrease in depression

• Absence of suicidal thoughts

daclizumab (℞)

(dah-kliz'uh-mab)

Zenapax

Func. class.: Immunosuppressive

Chem class.: Humanized IgG1 monoclonal antibody

Pregnancy category C

Action: Binds to the IL-2 (Interleukin-2) receptor antagonist

Therapeutic Outcome: Prevention of graft rejection

Uses: Acute allograft rejection in renal transplant patients

Dosage and routes

Adult: **IV** 1 mg/kg as part of a regimen that includes cyclosporine and corticosteroids, mix calculated vol with 50 ml of 0.9% NaCl and give via peripheral/central vein over 15 min

Available forms: Inj conc 25 mg/ml

Adverse effects

CNS: Chills, tremors, headache, prickly sensation

CV: Hypertension, tachycardia, thrombosis, bleeding

GI: Vomiting, nausea, diarrhea, constipation, abdominal pain, pyrosis

GU: Oliguria, dysuria, renal tubular necrosis, renal damage, hydronephrosis

INTEG: Impaired wound healing

RESP: Dyspnea, wheezing, ***pulmonary edema,*** coughing, atelectasis, congestion

Contraindications: Hypersensitivity

Precautions: Pregnancy (C), child <2 yr, lactation, elderly

Pharmacokinetics

Unknown

Pharmacodynamics

Unknown

Interactions
Unknown

NURSING CONSIDERATIONS

Assessment

- Monitor blood studies: Hgb, WBC, platelets during treatment qmo; if leukocytes are <3000/mm^3, drug should be discontinued
- Monitor liver function studies: alk phosphatase, AST (SGOT), ALT (SGPT), bilirubin
- Assess for hepatotoxicity: dark urine, jaundice, itching, light-colored stools; drug should be discontinued

Nursing diagnoses

- ✓ Injury, risk for (uses)
- ✓ Knowledge deficit (teaching)

Implementation

- Give all other medications PO if possible; avoid IM injection, since infection may occur

IV route

- Solution compatibilities 0.9% NaCl

Patient/family education

- Teach patient to report fever, chills, sore throat, fatigue, since serious infection may occur

Evaluation

Positive therapeutic outcome

- Absence of graft rejection

efavirenz (℞)

(ef-ah-veer'enz)
Sustiva
Func. class.: Antiviral
Chem class.: Nonnucleoside reverse transcriptase inhibitor (NNRII)
Pregnancy category C

Action: Binds directly to reverse transcriptase and blocks RNA, DNA causing a disruption of the enzyme's site

➡ **Therapeutic Outcome:** Improvement of HIV-1 infection

Uses: HIV-1 in combination with other antiretrovirals

Dosage and routes

Adult: PO 600 mg qd hs in combination with protease inhibitor or nucleoside analog reverse transcriptase inhibitors (NRTIs)

Child:
10-<15 kg: PO 200 mg qd hs
15-<20 kg: PO 250 mg qd hs
20-<25 kg: PO 300 mg qd hs
25-<32.5 kg: PO 350 mg qd hs
32.5-<40 kg: PO 400 mg qd hs
≥40 kg: Adult dose

Available forms: Caps 50, 100, 200 mg

Adverse effects

CNS: Headache
GI: Diarrhea, abdominal pain, *nausea*

INTEG: Rash, dizziness, fatigue, impaired concentration, insomnia, abnormal dreams, depression

Contraindications: Hypersensitivity

Precautions: Liver disease, pregnancy (C), lactation, children <3 yr, renal disease, myelosuppression

Pharmacokinetics

Absorption	Well
Distribution	Highly protein bound
Metabolism	Liver
Excretion	Kidneys, feces
Half-life	Terminal 52-76 hr

Pharmacodynamics

Unknown

Interactions

Individual drugs

Astemizole: ↑ level of astemizole
Cisapride: ↑ level of cisapride
Indinavir: ↑ level of indinavir
Ritonavir: ↑ levels of both drugs
Saquinavir: ↓ level of saquinavir
Warfarin: ↑ level of warfarin

Drug classifications

Benzodiazepines: Do not give together
Ergots: ↑ ergotism

NURSING CONSIDERATIONS

Assessment

- Assess signs of infection, anemia
- Assess liver studies: ALT, AST; renal studies
- Assess C&S before drug therapy; drug may be taken as soon as culture is taken; repeat C&S after treatment; determine the prescence of other sexually transmitted disease
- Assess bowel pattern before, during treatment; if severe abdominal pain with bleeding occurs, drug should be discontinued; monitor hydration
- Assess skin eruptions; rash, urticaria, itching
- Assess allergies before treatment, reaction to each medication; place allergies on chart
- Assess CBC, blood chemistry, plasma HIV RNA, absolute CD4+/CD8+/cell counts/%, serum β-2 microglobulin, serum ICD+24 antigen levels, cholesterol, hepatic enzymes
- Assess for signs of toxicity: severe nausea/vomiting, maculopapular rash

Nursing diagnoses

- ☑ Infection, risk for (uses)
- ☑ Diarrhea (side effects)
- ☑ Knowledge deficit (teaching)

Patient/family education

- Advise patient to take as prescribed; if dose is missed, take as soon as remembered; do not double dose
- Instruct patient to make sure health care provider knows of all the medications being taken
- Advise patient that if severe rash occurs, stop taking and notify health care provider
- Advise patient not to breastfeed if taking this drug

Evaluation

Positive therapeutic outcome

- Improvement in symptoms of HIV-1 infection

eptifibatide (℞)
(ep-tih-fib'ah-tide)
Integrilin
Func. class.: Antiplatelet agent
Chem class.: Glycoprotein IIb/IIIa inhibitor
Pregnancy category B

Action: Platelet glycoprotein antagonist. This agent reversibly prevents fibrinogen, von Willebrand's factor from binding to the glycoprotein IIb/IIIa receptor, inhibiting platelet aggregation

Therapeutic Outcome: Decreased platelets

Uses: Acute coronary syndrome including those with PCI (percutaneous coronary intervention)

Dosage and routes
Acute coronary syndrome
Adult: **IV BOL** 180 μg/kg as soon as diagnosed, then **IV CONT** 2 μg/kg/min until discharge or CABG up to 72 hr; may decrease inf rate to 0.5 μg/kg/min if undergoing PCI; continue inf for 20-24 hr postprocedure, allowing up to 96 hr of treatment
PCI in patients without acute coronary syndrome
Adult: **IV BOL** 135 μg/kg given immediately before PCI; then 0.5 μg/kg/min × 20-24 hr

Adverse effects
CV: ***Stroke,*** hypotension
SYST: ***Bleeding***

Contraindications: Hypersensitivity, active internal bleeding; history of bleeding, stroke within 1 mo; major surgery with severe trauma, severe hypotension, history of intracranial bleeding, intracranial neoplasm, arteriovenous malformation/aneurysm, aortic dissection, dependence on renal dialysis

Precautions: Bleeding, pregnancy (B), lactation, children, elderly, renal function impairment

Pharmacokinetics	
Absorption	Unknown
Distribution	Unknown
Metabolism	Limited
Excretion	Kidneys
Half-life	2.5 hr

Pharmacodynamics	
Onset	Unknown
Peak	Unknown
Duration	Unknown

Interactions
Individual drugs
Aspirin: ↑ bleeding
Heparin: ↑ bleeding

NURSING CONSIDERATIONS
Assessment
- Monitor platelets, Hgb, Hct, creatinine, PT/APTT baseline, within 6 hr of loading dose and qd thereafter; patients undergoing PCI should have ACT monitored; maintain APTT 50-70 sec unless PCI is to be performed; during PCI, ACT should be 300-350 sec; if platelets drop <100,000/mm^3, obtain additional platelet counts; if thrombocytopenia is confirmed, discontinue drug
- Monitor ECG continuously

Nursing diagnoses
- ✓ Tissue perfusion, altered (uses)
- ✓ Knowledge deficit (teaching)

Implementation
IV route

- After withdrawing the bolus dosc from 10 ml vial, give IV push over 1-2 min; follow bolus dose with continuous inf using inf pump, give drug undiluted directly from the 100 ml vial, spike the 100 ml vial with a vented infusion set, use caution when centering the spike on the circle of the stopper top
- Discontinuing drug prior to CABG

Evaluation
Positive therapeutic outcome

- Decreased platelets

etanercept (℞)
(eh-tan'er-sept)
Enbrel
Func. class.: Biological
Pregnancy category B

Action: Binds to tumor necrosis factor (TNF), which decreases inflammation and immune response.

Therapeutic Outcome: Decreased pain, inflammation

Uses: Acute, chronic rheumatoid arthritis that has not responded to other treatments

Dosage and routes
Osteoarthritis
Adult: SC 25 mg 2×/wk, may be given with other drugs for rheumatoid arthritis

Child 4-17 yr: SC 0.4 mg/kg, max 25 mg, 2×/wk

Available forms: Powder for inj: 25 mg

Adverse effects
CNS: Headache, asthenia, dizziness
GI: Abdominal pain, dyspepsia
INTEG: Rash, inj site reaction
RESP: Pharyngitis, rhinitis, cough, URI, non-URI, sinusitis

Contraindications: Hypersensitivity, sepsis

Precautions: Pregnancy (B), P lactation, children <4 yr

Pharmacokinetics	
Absorption	Rapidly
Distribution	Unknown
Metabolism	Unknown
Excretion	Unknown
Half-life	115 hr

Pharmacodynamics	
Onset	Unknown
Peak	Unknown
Duration	Unknown

Interactions
Drug classifications
Immunizations: Do not give concurrently
Vaccines: Do not give concurrently

NURSING CONSIDERATIONS
Assessment
- Assess for pain of rheumatoid arthritis; check ROM, inflammation of joints, characteristics of pain

Nursing diagnoses
- ✓ Pain (uses)
- ✓ Mobility, impaired physical (uses)
- ✓ Injury, risk for (side effects)
- ✓ Knowledge deficit (teaching)

Implementation
SC route

- Administer after reconstituting 1 ml of supplied diluent, slowly inject diluent into vial, swirl contents, do not shake, sol should be clear/colorless, do not use if cloudy or discolored

• Do not admix with other sol or medications; do not use filter

Patient/family education

• Teach patient that drug must be continued for prescribed time to be effective; to avoid aspirin, alcoholic beverages

• Instruct patient to use caution when driving; dizziness may occur

• Teach patient about self-administration, if appropriate: inj should be made in thigh, abdomen, upper arm; rotate sites at least 1 in from old site

Evaluation

Positive therapeutic outcome

• Decreased pain in arthritic conditions

• Decreased inflammation in arthritic conditions

fenoldopam (℞)
(feh-nahl'doh-pam)
Corlopam
Func. class.: Antihypertensive
Chem class.: Vasodilator
Pregnancy category B

Action: Antagonizes D_1-like dopamine receptors; binds to α_2-adrenoreceptors; increases renal blood flow

➡ **Therapeutic Outcome:** B/P, decreased

Uses: Hypertensive crisis when urgent decrease of pressure required; including malignant hypertension

Dosage and routes

Adult: CONT IV titrate initial dose upward or downward no more frequently than q15 min; increments should range between 0.05-0.1 μg/kg/min; initial doses of 0.03-0.1 μg/kg/min titrated slowly result in less reflex tachycardia

Available forms: Inj conc 10 mg/ml

Adverse effects

CNS: Headache, anxiety, dizziness

CV: ***Hypotension,*** ST-T-wave changes, angina pectoris, palpitations, ***MI, ischemic heart disease***

GI: Nausea, vomiting, constipation, diarrhea

HEMA: ***Leukocytosis,*** bleeding

META: Increased BUN, glucose, LDH, creatinine, hypokalemia

Contraindications: Hypersensitivity, sulfite sensitivity

Precautions: Tachycardia, pregnancy (B), lactation, children, intraocular pressure, hypokalemia

Pharmacokinetics	
Absorption	Unknown
Distribution	Steady state 20 min
Metabolism	Unknown
Excretion	Unknown
Half-life	5 min (elimination)

Pharmacodynamics	
Onset	Unknown
Peak	Unknown
Duration	Unknown

Interactions

Drug classifications

β-Blockers: Avoid use

NURSING CONSIDERATIONS
Assessment
- Monitor B/P q5min until stabilized, then q1h × 2 hr, then q4h
- Monitor pulse, jugular venous distension q4h
- Monitor electrolytes, blood studies: K, Na, Cl, CO_2, CBC, serum glucose
- Monitor weight daily, I&O
- Assess edema in feet, legs daily
- Assess skin turgor, dryness of mucous membranes for hydration status
- Assess rales, dyspnea, orthopnea
- Assess IV site for extravasation, rate
- Assess postural hypotension, take B/P sitting, standing

Nursing diagnoses
- ☑ Tissue perfusion, altered (uses)
- ☑ Knowledge deficit (teaching)
- ☑ Noncompliance (teaching)

Implementation
IV route
- Administer after diluting contents of ampules in 0.9% NaCl, or 5% dextrose inj (40 µg/ml); then add 4 ml of conc. (40 mg of drug/1000 ml); 2 ml of conc. (20 mg of drug/500 ml); 1 ml of conc. (10 mg of drug/250 ml)
- Give to patient in recumbent position; keep in that position for 1 hr after administration
- Diluted sol is stable in normal light/temp for 24 hr

Evaluation
Positive therapeutic outcome
- Decreased B/P

halofantrine (℞)
(hay-loh-fan'trin)
Halfan
Func. class.: Antimalarial
Chem class.: Phenanthrenemethanol
Pregnancy category X

Action: Inhibits parasite replications, transcription of DNA to RNA by forming complexes with DNA of parasite

Therapeutic Outcome: Absence of malaria after treatment

Uses: Mild to moderate malaria

Dosage and routes
Adult: PO 500 mg q6h × 3 doses; may need to repeat after 1 wk

Available forms: Tabs 250 mg

Adverse effects
CV: Dysrhythmias
GI: Nausea, vomiting, anorexia, diarrhea

Contraindications: Hypersensitivity

Precautions: Severe GI disease, severe hepatic disease, cardiac dysrhythmias

Pharmacokinetics	
Absorption	Unknown
Distribution	Unknown
Metabolism	Liver
Excretion	Kidneys
Half-life	Unknown

Pharmacodynamics	
Onset	Unknown
Peak	Unknown
Duration	Unknown

Interactions
Unknown

NURSING CONSIDERATIONS

Assessment

- Monitor B/P, pulse, watch for tachycardia
- Monitor liver studies qwk: ALT (SGPT), AST (SGOT), bilirubin

Nursing diagnoses

- ✓ Infection, risk for (uses)
- ✓ Diarrhea (side effects)
- ✓ Knowledge deficit (teaching)

Implementation

PO route

- Give 1 hr before or 2 hr after meals at same time each day to maintain level
- Store in tight, light-resistant container

Patient/family education

- Advise patient to take exactly as prescribed, to take full course that is prescribed

Evaluation

Positive therapeutic outcome

- C&S—negative
- Decreased symptoms of malaria

infliximab (℞)

(in-fliks'ih-mab)
Remicade
Func. class.: Monoclonal antibody
Pregnancy category C

Action: Monoclonal antibody that neutralizes the activity of tumor necrosis factor alpha (TNFα) that has been found in Crohn's disease; decreased infilitration of inflammatory cells

➔ **Therapeutic Outcome:** Decreased cramping and blood in stools

Uses: Crohn's disease; fistulizing, moderate-severe

Dosage and routes

Crohn's disease (moderate-severe)
***Adult:* IV** inf 5 mg/kg
Crohn's disease (fistulizing)
***Adult:* IV** inf 5 mg/kg initially, then repeat dose 2 wk, 6 wk after 1st dose

Available forms: Powder for inj 100 mg

Adverse effects

CNS: Headache, dizziness, *depression, vertigo, fatigue, anxiety, fever*
CV: Chest pain, hypertension and hypotension, tachycardia
GI: Nausea, vomiting, abdominal pain, stomatitis, constipation, dyspepsia, flatulence
GU: Dysuria, frequency
HEMA: ***Anemia***
INTEG: Rash, dermatitis, urticaria, dry skin, sweating, flushing, hematoma, pruritus
MS: Myalgia, back pain, arthralgia
RESP: URI, pharyngitis, bronchitis, cough, dyspnea, sinusitis
SYST: ***Anaphylaxis***

Contraindications: Hypersensitivity to murines

P G **Precautions:** Pregnancy (C), lactation, children, elderly

Pharmacokinetics	
Absorption	Unknown
Distribution	Vascular compartment
Metabolism	Unknown
Excretion	Unknown
Half-life	9½ days

Pharmacodynamics	
Onset	Unknown
Peak	Unknown
Duration	Unknown

Interactions
Unknown

NURSING CONSIDERATIONS
Assessment
- Assess GI symptoms: nausea, vomiting, abdominal pain
- Take periodic blood counts (CBC)
- Assess CV status: B/P, pulse, chest pain
- Assess for allergic reaction: rash, dermatitis, urticaria, dyspnea, hypotension; discontinue if severe

Nursing diagnoses
✓ Injury, risk for (uses)
✓ Diarrhea (uses)
✓ Knowledge deficit (teaching)

Implementation
IV inf route
- Administer immediately after reconstitution; reconstitute with 10 ml of sterile water for inj, further dilute total dose/ 250 ml 0.9% NaCl inj to a total conc of between 0.4 and 4 mg/ml; use 21G or smaller needle for reconstitution, direct sterile water at glass wall of vial, gently swirl
- Give over ≥2 hr, use polyethylene-lined infusion with in-line, sterile, low-protein-bind filter
- Provide refrigerated storage, do not freeze

Evaluation
Positive therapeutic outcome
- Absence of blood in stool
- Reported improvement in comfort
- Weight gain

leflunomide (℞)
(leh-floo'noh-mide)
Arava
Chem. class.: Pyrimidine synthesis inhibitor
Pregnancy category X

Action: Inhibits an enzyme involved in pyrimidine synthesis and has antiproliferative effect

➔ **Therapeutic Outcome:** Decreased pain, joint swelling, increased mobility

Uses: Rheumatoid arthritis

Dosage and routes
Adult: **PO** loading dose 100 mg/day × 3 days maintenance 20 mg/day, may be decreased to 10 mg/day if not well tolerated

Available forms: Tabs 10, 20, 100 mg

Adverse effects
CNS: Dizziness, insomnia, depression, paresthesia
CV: Palpitations, hypertension, chest pain, angina pectoris, migraine
GI: Nausea, anorexia, vomiting, constipation, flatulence
INTEG: Rash, pruritus
RESP: Pharyngitis, rhinitis, bronchitis, cough, respiratory infection, pneumonia, sinusitis

Contraindications: Hypersensitivity, pregnancy (X), lactation

Precautions: Hepatic, renal disorders

Pharmacokinetics

Absorption	Unknown
Distribution	Unknown
Metabolism	Liver
Excretion	Kidneys
Half-life	Unknown

Pharmacodynamics

Onset	Unknown
Peak	Unknown
Duration	Unknown

Interactions
Individual drugs
Activated charcoal: ↓ effect of leflunomide
Cholestyramine: ↓ effect of leflunomide
Drug classifications
NSAIDs: ↑ NSAID effect
Hepatotoxic agents: ↑ side effects of leflunomide

NURSING CONSIDERATIONS
Assessment
• Monitor liver function studies: if ALT elevations are > twofold ULN, reduce dose to 10 mg/day

Nursing diagnoses
✓ Mobility, impaired (uses)
✓ Pain (uses)
✓ Knowledge deficit (teaching)

Implementation
PO route
• Give PO with food for GI upset

Patient/family education
• Teach patient that drug must be continued for prescribed time to be effective
• Instruct patient to take with food, milk, or antacids to avoid GI upset
• Advise patient to use caution when driving; drowsiness, dizziness may occur
• Advise patient to take with a full glass of water to enhance absorption
• Advise patient to avoid pregnancy while taking this drug

Evaluation
Positive therapeutic outcome
• Increased joint mobility without pain
• Decreased joint swelling

lepirudin (℞)
(lep-ih-roo'din)
Refludan
Func. class.: Anticoagulant
Chem. class.: Hirudin
Pregnancy category B

Action: Direct inhibitor of thrombin that is highly specific

Therapeutic Outcome: Absence of thrombocytopenia, stroke, MI, or other thromboembolic conditions

Uses: Heparin-induced thrombocytopenia and other thromboembolic conditions

Dosage and routes
Adult: IV 0.4 mg/kg (≤110 kg) over 15-20 sec; then 0.15 mg/kg (≤110 kg/hr) as a cont inf for 2-10 days or longer

Available forms: Powder for inj 50 mg

Adverse effects
CNS: Fever
CV: ***Heart failure, pericardial effusion, ventricular fibrillation***
GI: GI bleeding, abnormal LFTs
GU: ***Hematuria,*** abnormal kidney function
HEMA: ***Hemorrhage, thrombocytopenia***
INTEG: Allergic skin reactions

RESP: Pneumonia
SYST: Multiorgan failure, sepsis

Contraindications: Hypersensitivity to hirudins

Precautions: Intracranial bleeding, renal function impairment, lactation, children, hepatic disease, pregnancy (B)

Pharmacokinetics

Absorption	Unknown
Distribution	Unknown
Metabolism	Possibly by the release of amino acids during catabolism
Excretion	50% unchanged in urine
Half-life	Unknown

Pharmacodynamics

Onset	Unknown
Peak	Unknown
Duration	Unknown

Interactions

Drug classifications

Coumadin derivatives: ↑ risk of bleeding

Thrombolytics: ↑ action of lepirudin

NURSING CONSIDERATIONS

Assessment

- Obtain baseline in APTT before treatment; do not start treatment if APTT ratio is ≥2.5, then APTT 4 hr after initiation of treatment and at least qd thereafter; if APTT is above target, stop infusion for 2 hr, then restart at 50%, take APTT in 4 hr; if below target, increase inf rate by 20%, take APTT in 4 hr, do not exceed inf rate of 0.21 mg/kg/hr without checking for coagulation abnormalities
- Monitor APTT, which should be 1.5-2.5 × control
- Assess bleeding gums, petechiae, ecchymosis, black tarry stools, hematuria/epistaxis, B/P, vaginal bleeding, puncture sites; indicate bleeding and possible hemorrhage
- Assess fever, skin rash, urticaria

Nursing diagnoses

- ✓ Tissue perfusion, altered (uses)
- ✓ Injury, risk for (side effects)
- ✓ Knowledge deficit (teaching)

Implementation

- Administer after reconstitution and further dilution under sterile conditions; use water for Inj or 0.9% NaCl; for further dilution 0.9% NaCl or D_5; for rapid and complete reconstitution, inject 1 ml of diluent into vial and shake gently, use immediately, warm to room temp before use
- Avoid all IM injections that may cause bleeding

IV route

- Administer IV bol: Use sol with conc. of 5 mg/ml, reconstitute 5 mg (1 vial)/1 ml of water for inj or 0.9% NaCl, use body wt for correct calculation as to weight
- Administer IV inf: Use sol with a conc. of 0.2 or 0.4 mg/ml; reconstitute 100 mg (2 vials) with 1 ml each (2 ml) water for inj or 0.9% NaCl, transfer to inf. bag with either 500 or 250 ml of 0.9% NaCl or D_5

Patient/family education

- Teach patient to use soft-bristle toothbrush to avoid bleeding gums, avoid contact sports, use electric razor, avoid IM injection
- Teach patient to report any

signs of bleeding: gums, under skin, urine, stools

Evaluation

Positive therapeutic outcome

- Absence of thrombocytopenia without significant bleeding

montelukast (℞)

(mon-teh-loo'kast)

Singulair

Func. class.: Leukotriene receptor

Chem class.: Cysteinyl

Pregnancy category B

Action: Inhibits leukotriene (LTD_4) formation; leukotrienes exert their effects by increasing neutrophil, eosinophil migration; aggregation of neutrophils, monocytes; smooth muscle contraction, capillary permeability; these actions further lead to bronchoconstriction, inflammation, edema

Therapeutic Outcome: Ability to breathe with ease

Uses: Chronic asthma

Dosage and routes

Asthma

Adult and child ≥ 15 yr: PO 10 mg qd PM

Child 6-14 yr: PO 5 mg chew tab qd PM

Available forms: Tabs 10 mg; tabs, chew 5 mg

Adverse effects

CNS: Dizziness, fatigue, headache

GI: Abdominal pain, dyspepsia, LFT abnormalities

INTEG: Rash

MS: Asthenia

RESP: Influenza, cough, nasal congestion

Contraindications: Hypersensitivity

Precautions: Acute attacks of asthma, alcohol consumption, pregnancy (B), lactation, child <6 yr, aspirin sensitivity

Pharmacokinetics	
Absorption	Rapidly
Distribution	Protein binding 99%
Metabolism	Liver
Excretion	Bile
Half-life	2.7-5.5 hr

Pharmacodynamics	
Onset	Unknown
Peak	3-4 hr
Duration	Unknown

Interactions

Individual drugs

Phenobarbitol: ↑ montelukast levels

Rifampin: ↑ montelukast levels

NURSING CONSIDERATIONS

Assessment

- Assess adult patients carefully for symptoms of Churg-Strauss syndrome (rare), including eosinophilia, vasculitic rash, worsening pulmonary symptoms, cardiac complications, and/or neuropathy
- Monitor CBC, blood chemistry during treatment
- Monitor LFTs before and qmo × 3 mo, then q2-3 mo during treatment (ALT; AST)
- Assess respiratory rate, rhythm, depth; auscultate lung fields bilaterally; notify prescriber of abnormalities
- Assess allergic reactions: rash, urticaria; drug should be discontinued

Nursing diagnoses
- ✓ Airway clearance, ineffective (uses)
- ✓ Activity intolerance (uses)
- ✓ Knowledge deficit (teaching)

Implementation
PO route
- Give PO in PM qd

Patient/family education
- Instruct patient to check OTC and current prescription medications for ephedrine, which will increase stimulation; to avoid alcohol
- Advise patient to avoid hazardous activities; dizziness may occur
- Teach patient that drug is not to be used for acute asthma attacks

Evaluation
Positive therapeutic outcome
- Increased ease of breathing
- Decreased bronchospasm

naratriptan (℞)
(nair'ah-trip-tan)
Amerge
Func. class.: Migraine agent
Chem class.: 5-HT_1-like receptor agonist
Pregnancy category C

Action: Binds selectively to the vascular 5-HT_1 receptor subtype, exerts antimigraine effect; causes vasoconstriction in cranial arteries

➡ **Therapeutic Outcome:** Decreased intensity and incidence of migraines

Uses: Acute treatment of migraine with or without aura

Dosage and routes
Adult: PO 1 or 2.5 mg with fluids, if headache returns, repeat once after 4 hr, max 5 mg/24 hr

Available forms: Tab 1, 2.5 mg

Adverse effects
GI: Nausea
MS: Weakness, neck stiffness, myalgia
NEURO: Dizziness, sedation, fatigue

Contraindications: Angina pectoris, history of MI, documented silent ischemia, ischemic heart disease, concurrent ergotamine-containing preparations, uncontrolled hypertension, hypersensitivity, severe renal disease (CrCl <15 ml/min); severe hepatic disease (child-Pugh grade C)

Precautions: Postmenopausal women, men >40 yr, risk factors for CAD, hypercholesterolemia, obesity, diabetes, impaired hepatic or renal function, pregnancy (C), lactation, children, elderly, peripheral vascular disease

Pharmacokinetics	
Absorption	Unknown
Distribution	28%-31% protein binding
Metabolism	Liver (metabolite)
Excretion	Urine/feces
Half-life	6 hr

Pharmacodynamics	
Onset	Unknown
Peak	30 min
Duration	Unknown

Interactions
Drug classifications
Ergot derivatives: ↑ vasospastics effects
SSRIs: ↑ weakness, hyperreflexia, incoordination
Drugs/smoking: ↑ the clearance of naratriptan

NURSING CONSIDERATIONS

Assessment

- Assess for stress level, activity, recreation, coping mechanisms
- Assess neurologic status: LOC blurred vision, nausea, vomiting, tingling in extremities preceding headache

Nursing diagnoses

- ✓ Pain (uses)
- ✓ Knowledge deficit (teaching)
- ✓ Noncompliance (teaching)

Implementation

- Give with fluids
- Provide a quiet, calm environment with decreased stimulation for noise, bright light, excessive talking

Patient/family education

- Teach patient to report any side effects to prescriber
- Teach patient to use contraception while taking drug
- Advise patient not to use if another 5-HT agonist or an ergot preparation has been used in the past 24 hrs

Evaluation

Positive therapeutic outcome

- Absence of migraine headaches

palivizumab (℞)

(pal-ih-viz'uh-mab)
Synagis
Func. class.: Monoclonal antibody
Pregnancy category N/A

Action: A humanized monoclonal antibody that exhibits neutralizing and fusion-inhibitory activity against respiratory syncytial virus (RSV)

Therapeutic Outcome: Absence of RSV

Uses: Prevention of serious lower respiratory tract disease caused by RSV in pediatric patients

Dosage and routes
Child: IM 15 mg/kg, those patients who develop RSV should receive monthly doses during RSV season

Available forms: Lyophilized inj 100 mg

Adverse effects
EENT: Otitis media, rhinitis, pharyngitis
GI: Nausea, vomiting, diarrhea, increased AST
INTEG: Rash, inj site reaction
RESP: URI

Contraindications: Hypersensitivity, adults, cyanotic congenital heart disease

Precautions: Thrombocytopenia, coagulation disorders, established RSV, congenital heart disease, chronic lung disease, systemic allergic reactions

Pharmacokinetics

Absorption	Unknown
Distribution	Unknown
Metabolism	Unknown
Excretion	Unknown
Half-life	20 days

Pharmacodynamics

Onset	Unknown
Peak	Unknown
Duration	Unknown

Interactions
Unknown

NURSING CONSIDERATIONS
Assessment
• Assess for presence of RSV infection, drug is given to prevent infection
• Assess for side effects and report if allergic reaction is evident

Nursing diagnoses
✓ Infection, risk for (uses)
✓ Knowledge deficit (teaching)

Implementation
• Give IM only
• Give after adding 1 ml of sterile water for inj per 100 mg vial, gently swirl, let stand at room temp for 20 min until sol clarifies; given within 6 hr of reconstitution

Patient/family education
• Teach patient to report upper respiratory infections, earaches, rash, sore throat

Evaluation
Positive therapeutic outcome
• Absence of RSV

paricalcitol (℞)
(par-ih-cal'sih-tol)
Zemplar
Func. class.: Vit D analog
Chem class.: Fat-soluble vitamin
Pregnancy category C

Action: Reduces parathyroid hormone (PTH) levels; suppresses PTH levels in patients with chronic renal failure with absence of hypercalcemia/hyperphosphatemia. Serum PO_4, Ca, CaXP may increase

Therapeutic Outcome: Decreased symptoms of hypoparathyroidism

Uses: Hypoparathyroidism

Dosage and routes
Adult: **IV** BOL 0.04-0.1 μg/kg (2.8-7 μg) no more than qod during dialysis; may increase by 2-4 μg q2-4wk

Available forms: Inj 5 μg/ml

Adverse effects
CNS: Lightheadedness
CV: Palpitations
GI: Nausea, vomiting, anorexia, dry mouth
OTHER: Pneumonia, edema, chills, fever, flu, sepsis

Contraindications: Hypersensitivity, hypercalcemia

Precautions: Cardiovascular disease, renal calculi, pregnancy (C), elderly, lactation, children

Pharmacokinetics

Absorption	Unknown
Distribution	Unknown
Metabolism	Unknown
Excretion	Unknown
Half-life	Unknown

Pharmacodynamics	
Onset	Unknown
Peak	Unknown
Duration	Unknown

Interactions
Individual drugs
Digitalis: ↑ toxicity

NURSING CONSIDERATIONS
Assessment
- Monitor Ca, PO_4, 2×/wk qwk during initial therapy; after dose is established take calcium and phosphorus qmo

Nursing diagnoses
✓ Knowledge deficit (teaching)

Implementation
IV route
- Give by IV bolus only

Patient/family education
- Advise patient to report weakness, lethargy, headache, anorexia, loss of weight
- Teach patient to report nausea, vomiting, palpitations

Evaluation
Positive therapeutic outcome
- Decreased hypoparathyroidism in chronic renal disease

raloxifene (℞)
(ral-ox'ih-feen)
Evista
Func. class.: Selective estrogen receptor modulator (SERM)
Chem class.: Benzthiophene
Pregnancy category X

Action: Reduces resorption of bone and decreases bone turnover; mediated through estrogen receptor binding

➔ **Therapeutic Outcome:** Absence of osteoporosis in postmenopausal women

Uses: Prevention of osteoporosis in postmenopausal women

Dosage and routes
Hormone replacement
Adult: PO 60 mg qd

Available forms: Tabs 60 mg

Adverse effects
CNS: Insomnia, migraines, depression
CV: Hot flashes
GI: Nausea, vomiting, diarrhea, anorexia, cramps
GU: Vaginitis, UTI, leukorrhea, endometrial disorder, breast pain
INTEG: Rash, sweating
META: Weight gain, peripheral edema
MS: Arthralgia, myalgia, leg cramps, arthritis
RESP: Sinusitis, pharyngitis, increased cough, pneumonia, laryngitis

Contraindications: Hypersensitivity, pregnancy (X), lactation

Precautions: Lactation, venous thromboembolic events, hepatic disease

Pharmacokinetics	
Absorption	Unknown
Distribution	Highly protein bound
Metabolism	Unknown
Excretion	Feces, breast milk
Half-life	28 hr (elimination)

Pharmacodynamics	
Onset	Unknown
Peak	Unknown
Duration	Unknown

Interactions
Individual drugs
Ampicillin: ↓ action of raloxifene
Cholestyramine: ↓ action of raloxifene
Drug classifications
Anticoagulants: ↓ action of anticoagulants
Highly protein-bound drugs: Administer cautiously
Lab test interferences
↑ Apolipoproteins A_1 and B, ↑ lipoprotein, ↑ fibrinogen, ↑ LDL cholesterol, ↑ total cholesterol, ↑ corticosteroid-binding globulin, ↑ thyroxine-binding globulin (TBG)
↓ calcium, ↓ total protein, ↓ albumin, ↓ platelets

NURSING CONSIDERATIONS
Assessment
- Monitor blood glucose of diabetic patients
- Monitor weight daily, notify prescriber of weekly weight gain >5 lb
- Monitor B/P q4h, watch for increase caused by H_2O and Na retention
- Monitor liver function studies, including AST (SGOT), ALT (SGPT), bilirubin, alk phosphatase
- Monitor I&O ratio; decreasing urinary output, increasing edema

Nursing diagnoses
✓ Immobility, risk for (uses)
✓ Knowledge deficit (teaching)

Implementation
PO route
- Administer without regard to meals

Patient/family education
- Teach patient to weigh weekly, report gain >5 lb
- Teach patient to discontinue drug 72 hr before prolonged bedrest
- Advise patient to avoid maintaining one position for long periods
- Advise patient to take calcium supplements, vit D if intake is inadequate
- Advise patient to increase exercise using weights
- Advise patient to stop smoking and to decrease alcohol consumption
- Inform patient that this drug does not help control hot flashes
- Teach patient to report fever, acute migraine, insomnia, emotional distress; urinary tract infection or vaginal burning/itching; swelling, warmth, or pain in calves

Evaluation
Positive therapeutic outcome
- Prevention of osteoporosis

repaglinide (℞)
(re-pag'lih-nide)
Prandin
Func. class.: Antidiabetic
Chem class.: Meglitinides
Pregnancy category C

Action: Causes functioning β-cells in pancreas to release insulin, leading to drop in blood glucose levels; closes ATP-dependent potassium channels in the β-cell membrane; this leads to opening of calcium channels; increased calcium influx induces insulin secretion

➡ **Therapeutic Outcome:** Blood glucose controlled

Uses: Stable adult-onset diabetes mellitus (type II) NIDDM

Dosage and routes

Adult: PO 0.5-4 mg

Available forms: Tabs 0.5, 1, 2 mg

Adverse effects

CNS: Headache, weakness, paresthesia

ENDO: ***Hypoglycemia***

GI: Nausea, vomiting, diarrhea, constipation, dyspepsia

INTEG: Rash, allergic reactions

MS: Back pains, arthralgia

RESP: URI, sinusitis, rhinitis, bronchitis

Contraindications: Hypersensitivity to meglitinides, diabetic ketoacidosis, type I diabetes

Precautions: Pregnancy (C), elderly, cardiac disease, severe renal disease, severe hepatic disease, thyroid disease, severe hypoglycemic reactions, lactation, children

Pharmacokinetics

Absorption	Complete
Distribution	98% protein binding, crosses placenta
Metabolism	Liver
Excretion	Urine/feces
Half-life	1 hr

Pharmacodynamics

Onset	2-4 hr
Peak	2-8 hr
Duration	24 hr

Interactions

Individual drugs

Carbamazepine: ↑ repaglinide metabolism
Chloramphenicol: ↑ effect of repaglinide
Erythromycin: ↓ repaglinide metabolism
Isoniazid: ↓ action of repaglinide
Phenobarbital: ↓ action of repaglinide
Phenytoin: ↓ action of repaglinide
Probenecid: ↑ effect of repaglinide
Rifampin: ↓ action of repaglinide
Troglitazone: ↑ repaglinide metabolism

Drug classifications

Antifungals: ↓ repaglinide metabolism
Barbiturates: ↑ repaglinide metabolism
β-Blockers: ↑ repaglinide effect
Calcium channel blockers: ↓ repaglinide effect
Corticosteroids: ↓ repaglinide effect
Coumarins: ↑ repaglinide effect
Diuretics, thiazide: ↓ repaglinide effect
Estrogens: ↓ repaglinide effect
NSAIDs: ↑ repaglinide effect
Oral contraceptives: ↓ repaglinide effect
Phenothiazines: ↓ repaglinide effect
Salicylates: ↑ repaglinide effect
Sulfonamides: ↑ repaglinide effect
Sympathomimetics: ↓ repaglinide effect
Thyroid preparations: ↓ repaglinide effect

NURSING CONSIDERATIONS

Assessment

- Assess for hypoglycemic or hyperglycemic reaction, which can occur soon after meals

Nursing diagnoses

✓ Nutrition, altered (more than body requirements) (uses)

☑ Knowledge deficit (teaching)
☑ Noncompliance (teaching)

Implementation

PO route

- 15 min before meals; 2, 3, or 4 ×/day preprandially
- Skip dose if meal is skipped; add dose if meal is added
- Store in tight container in cool environment

Patient/family education

- Advise patient to avoid alcohol; explain disulfiram reaction
- Teach patient to use a capillary blood glucose test while on this drug
- Teach patient the symptoms of hypoglycemia and hyperglycemia; what to do about each
- Teach patient that drug must be continued on daily basis; explain consequence of discontinuing drug abruptly
- Advise patient to avoid OTC medications unless ordered by prescriber
- Advise patient that diabetes is a lifelong illness; drug will not cure disease
- Advise patient to eat all food included in diet plan to prevent hypoglycemia; to have glucagon emergency kit available
- Instruct patient to carry a Medic Alert ID for emergency purposes

Evaluation

Positive therapeutic outcome

- Decrease in polyuria, polydipsia, polyphagia, clear sensorium, absence of dizziness, stable gait

Treatment of overdose

Glucose 25 g IV via dextrose 50% solution, 50 ml or 1 mg glucagon

rifapentine (℞)

(riff'ah-pen-teen)

Priftin

Func. class.: Antitubercular
Chem class.: Rifamycin derivative

Pregnancy category C

Action: Inhibits DNA-dependent polymerase, decreases tubercle bacilli replication

Therapeutic Outcome: Resolution of pulmonary TB

Uses: Pulmonary tuberculosis, must be used with at least one other antitubercular

Dosage and routes

Intensive phase

Adult: **PO** 600 mg (four 150 mg tabs 2×/wk), with an interval of 72 hr between doses × 2 mo; must be given with at least one other antitubercular

Continuation phase

Adult: **PO** continue with 1×/wk × 4 mo in combination with isoniazid or other appropriate antitubercular

Available forms: Tabs 150 mg

Adverse effects

CNS: Headache, fatigue, anxiety, dizziness
EENT: Visual disturbances
GI: Nausea, vomiting, anorexia, diarrhea, bilirubinemia, hepatitis, increased ALT, AST, ***heartburn, pancreatitis***
GU: ***Hematuria,*** pyuria, proteinuria, urinary casts
HEMA: ***Thrombocytopenia, leukopenia, neutropenia, lymphopenia,*** anemia, ***leukocytosis,*** purpura, hematoma

INTEG: Rash, pruritus, urticaria, acne
MISC: Edema, aggressive reaction
MS: Gout, arthrosis

Contraindications: Hypersensitivity to rifamycins

Precautions: Pregnancy (C), lactation, hepatic disease, blood dyscrasias, children <12 yr

Pharmacokinetics

Absorption	Unknown
Distribution	Unknown
Metabolism	Unknown
Excretion	Unknown
Half-life	Unknown

Pharmacodynamics

Onset	Unknown
Peak	Unknown
Duration	Unknown

Interactions

Individual drugs

Amitriptyline: ↓ action of amitriptyline
Chloramphenicol: ↓ action of chloramphenicol
Clarithromycin: ↓ action of clarithromycin
Clofibrate: ↓ action of clofibrate
Cyclosporine: ↓ action of cyclosporine
Dapsone: ↓ action of dapsone
Delaviridine: ↓ action of delaviridine
Diazepam: ↓ action of diazepam
Digoxin: ↓ action of digoxin
Diltiazem: ↓ action of diltiazem
Disopyramide: ↓ action of disopyramide
Doxycycline: ↓ action of doxycycline
Fluconazole: ↓ action of fluconazole
Haloperidol: ↓ action of haloperidol
Indinavir: ↓ action of indinavir
Itraconazole: ↓ action of itraconazole
Ketoconazole: ↓ action of ketoconazole
Methadone: ↓ action of methadone
Mexiletine: ↓ action of mexiletine
Nelfinavir: ↓ action of nelfinavir
Nifedipine: ↓ action of nifedipine
Nortriptyline: ↓ action of nortriptyline
Phenytoin: ↓ action of phenytoin
Quinidine: ↓ action of quinidine
Quinine: ↓ action of quinine
Ritonavir: ↓ action of ritonavir
Saquinavir: ↓ action of saquinavir
Sildenafil: ↓ action of sildenafil
Tacrolimus: ↓ action of tacrolimus
Theophylline: ↓ action of theophylline
Tocainide: ↓ action of tocainide
Verapamil: ↓ action of verapamil
Zidovudine: ↓ action of zidovudine

Drug classifications

Anticoagulants: ↓ action of anticoagulants
Antidiabetics: ↓ action of antidiabetics
Barbiturates: ↓ action of barbiturates
Corticosteroids: ↓ action of corticosteroids

Fluoroquinolones: ↓ action of fluoroquinolones
Oral contraceptives: ↓ action of oral contraceptives
Protease inhibitors: Use extreme caution
Thyroid preparations: ↓ action of thyroid preparations
Food/Drug:
Food: ↑ drug concentration by 44%
Lab test interferences:
Interference: Folate level, vit B_{12}

NURSING CONSIDERATIONS
Assessment
- Monitor baselines in CBC, AST, ALT, bilirubin, platelets
- Assess for infection: sputum culture, lung sounds
- Assess signs of anemia: Hct, Hgb, fatigue
- Monitor liver studies qmo: ALT (SGPT), AST (SGOT), bilirubin
- Monitor renal status qmo: BUN, creatinine, output, specific gravity, urinalysis
- Assess hepatic status: decreased appetite, jaundice, dark urine, fatigue

Nursing diagnoses
- ✓ Infection, risk for (uses)
- ✓ Diarrhea (side effects)
- ✓ Knowledge deficit (teaching)
- ✓ Noncompliance (teaching)

Implementation
PO route
- Give PO, may be given with food for GI upset
- Give antiemetic if vomiting occurs
- Administer after C&S is completed; qmo to detect resistance

Patient/family education
- Advise patient that compliance with dosage schedule, duration is necessary
- Instruct patient that scheduled appointments must be kept; relapse may occur
- Teach patient that urine, feces, saliva, sputum, sweat, tears may be colored red-orange; soft contact lenses may be permanently stained
- Teach patient to use alternate method of contraception, oral contraceptive action may be decreased
- Teach patient to report flulike symptoms: excessive fatigue, anorexia, vomiting, sore throat; unusual bleeding, yellowish discoloration of skin, eyes

Evaluation
Positive therapeutic outcome
- Decreased symptoms of TB
- Culture-negative

risedronate (℞)
(rih-sed'roh-nate)
Actonel
Func. class.: Bone-resorption inhibitor
Chem class.: Biphosphonate
Pregnancy category C

Action: Absorbs calcium phosphate crystal in bone and may directly block dissolution of hydroxyapatite crystals of bone; inhibits bone resorption, apparently without inhibiting bone formation, mineralization

➡ **Therapeutic Outcome:** Increased bone mass, activity without fractures

Uses: Paget's disease

Investigational uses: Osteoporosis in postmenopausal women

Dosage and routes:
Adult: PO 30 mg qd × 2 mo; patients with Paget's disease should receive calcium and vit D if dietary intake is lacking; if relapse occurs, retreatment is advised

Available forms: Tabs 30 mg

Adverse effects
CNS: Dizziness, headache
CV: Chest pain
GI: Abdominal pain, anorexia, diarrhea, *nausea*
MS: Bone pain, arthralgia

Contraindications: Hypersensitivity to biphosphonates

Precautions: Children, lactation, pregnancy (C), renal disease

Pharmacokinetics	
Absorption	Unknown
Distribution	To bones
Metabolism	Unknown
Excretion	Kidneys
Half-life	Unknown

Pharmacodynamics	
Onset	Unknown
Peak	Unknown
Duration	Unknown

Interactions
Drug classifications
Calcium supplement: ↓ absorption of risedronate
Antacids: ↓ absorption of risedronate
Food/Drug:
Food: ↓ bioavailability: take ½ hr before food or drinks

NURSING CONSIDERATIONS
Assessment
- Monitor electrolytes: renal function studies; Ca, P, Mg, K
- Assess for hypercalcemia: paresthesia, twitching, laryngospasm, Chvostek's/ Trousseau's signs

Nursing diagnoses
✓ Immobility, impaired (uses)
✓ Nutrition, altered, less than body requirements (uses)
✓ Knowledge deficit (teaching)

Implementation
- Give PO for 2 months to be effective in Paget's disease
- Give with a full glass of water; patient should be in upright position
- Administer supplemental calcium and vit D in Paget's disease
- Store in cool environment, out of direct sunlight

Evaluation
Positive therapeutic outcome
- Increased bone mass, absence of fractures

rituximab (℞)
(rih-tuks'ih-mab)
Rituxan
Func. class.: Misc. antineoplastic
Chem class.: Murine/ human monoclonal antibody
Pregnancy category C

Action: Directed against the CD20 antigen that is found on malignant B lymphocytes; CD20 regulates a portion of cell-cycle initiation/ differentiation

➔ **Therapeutic Outcome:** Decreased tumor size, prevention of spread of cancer

Uses: Non-Hodgkin's lymphoma (CD20 positive, B-cell)

Dosage and routes

Adult: **IV** inf 375 mg/m^2 qwk × 4 doses; give at 50 mg/hr for 1st inf; if hypersensitivity does not occur, increase rate by 50 mg/hr q½h, max 400 mg/hr; slow/interrupt inf if hypersensitivity occurs; other inf can be given at 100 mg/hr and increased by 100 mg/hr, max 400 mg/hr

Available forms: Inj 10 mg/ml

Adverse effects

GI: Nausea, vomiting, anorexia
HEMA: Leukopenia, neutropenia, thrombocytopenia
INTEG: Irritation at site, rash
OTHER: Fever, chills, asthenia, headache, angioedema, hypotension, myalgia, bronchospasm

Contraindications: Hypersensitivity, murine proteins

Precautions: Lactation, children, elderly, pregnancy (C)

Pharmacokinetics	
Absorption	Unknown
Distribution	Unknown
Metabolism	Unknown
Excretion	Unknown
Half-life	42-79 min

Pharmacodynamics	
Onset	Unknown
Peak	Unknown
Duration	Unknown

Interactions

Unknown

NURSING CONSIDERATIONS

Assessment

- Monitor CBC, differential, platelet count weekly; withhold drug if WBC is <3500/mm^3, or platelet count <100,000/mm^3; notify prescriber of these results; drug should be discontinued
- Assess food preferences: list likes, dislikes
- Assess GI symptoms: frequency of stools
- Assess signs of dehydration: rapid respirations, poor skin turgor, decreased urine output, dry skin, restlessness, weakness

Nursing diagnoses

- ✓ Injury, risk for (side effects)
- ✓ Knowledge deficit (teaching)

Implementation

IV infusion

- Administer after diluting to a final conc. of 1-4 mg/ml; use 0.9% NaCl, D_5W, gently invert bag to mix; do not mix with other drugs
- Increase fluid intake to 2-3 L/day to prevent dehydration, unless contraindicated
- Change IV site q48h
- Provide nutritious diet with iron, vitamin supplement, low fiber, few dairy products
- Store vials at 36°-40° F, protects vials from direct sunlight, inf sol is stable at 36°-46° F × 24 hr and room temp for another 12 hr

Patient/family education

- Teach patient to report adverse reactions

Evaluation

Positive therapeutic outcome

- Decrease in tumor size, decrease in spread of cancer

rizatriptan (℞)

(rye-zah-trip'tan)
Maxalt, Maxalt-MLT
Func. class.: Migraine agent
Chem class.: 5-HT_1-like receptor agonist
Pregnancy category C

Action: Binds selectively to the vascular 5-HT_1 receptor subtype, exerts antimigraine effect; causes vasoconstriction in cranial arteries

Therapeutic Outcome: After treatment, relief of migraine

Uses: Acute treatment of migraine

Dosage and routes
Adult: **PO** 5-10 mg single dose, redosing separate by 2 hr or more; max 30 mg/24 hr

Available forms: Maxalt: Tabs 5, 10 mg; Maxalt-MLT: Tabs, orally disintegrating 5, 10 mg

Adverse effects
CNS: Dizziness, headache, fatigue
GI: Nausea, dry mouth
RESP: Chest tightness, pressure

Contraindications: Angina pectoris, history of MI, documented silent ischemia, Prinzmetal's angina, ischemic heart disease, concurrent ergotamine-containing preparations, uncontrolled hypertension, hypersensitivity, basilar or hemiplegic migraine

Precautions: Postmenopausal women, men >40 yr, risk factors for CAD, hypercholesterolemia, obesity, diabetes, impaired hepatic or renal function, pregnancy (C), lactation, children, elderly

Pharmacokinetics

Absorption	Unknown
Distribution	Unknown
Metabolism	Liver (metabolite)
Excretion	Urine/feces
Half-life	2-3 hr

Pharmacodynamics

Onset	10 min-2 hr
Peak	Unknown
Duration	Unknown

Interactions
Individual drugs
Cimetidine: ↑ action of rizatriptan
Ergot: ↑ vasospastic effects
Propranolol: ↑ action of rizatriptan
Drug classifications
Ergot derivatives: ↑ vasospastic effects
MAOIs: ↑ action of rizatriptan

NURSING CONSIDERATIONS
Assessment
- Assess for tingling, hot sensation, burning, feeling of pressure, numbness, flushing, injection site reaction
- Assess for stress level, activity, recreation, coping mechanisms
- Assess neurologic status: LOC, blurring vision, nausea, vomiting, tingling in extremities preceding headache
- Monitor for ingestion of tyramine foods (pickled products, beer, wine, aged cheese), food additives, preservatives, colorings, artificial sweeteners, chocolate, caffeine, which may precipitate these types of headaches

Nursing diagnoses

- Pain (uses)
- Knowledge deficit (teaching)

Implementation

• Provide quiet, calm environment with decreased stimulation for noise, bright light, excessive talking

Patient/family education

• Teach patient use of orally disintegrating tab: instruct patient not to open blister until use, to peel blister open with dry hands, to place tab on tongue, where it will dissolve, and to swallow with saliva (contains phenylalanine)
• Advise patient to report any side effects to prescriber
• Advise patient to use alternate contraception while taking drug if oral contraceptives are being used

Evaluation

Positive therapeutic outcome
• Decrease in frequency, severity of headache

sibutramine (℞)

(si-byoo'tra-meen)
Meridia
Func. class.: Appetite suppressant
Pregnancy category UK

Action: Inhibits reuptake of serotonin, norepinephrine, dopamine

Therapeutic Outcome: Weight loss with B/P in normal range

Uses: Obesity in conjunction with other treatments

Dosage and routes
Adult: PO 10 mg qd; may be increased to 15 mg qd after 4 wk, or lowered to 5 mg qd depending on response

Available forms: Caps 5, 10, 15 mg

Adverse effects
CNS: Headache, insomnia, seizures, stimulation, drowsiness, dizziness, nervousness, emotional lability
CV: Hypotension, palpitations, vasodilation, tachycardia
EENT: Laryngitis, pharyngitis, rhinitis, sinusitis
GI: Anorexia, constipation, dry mouth, taste aberration, nausea, increased appetite
GU: Dysmenorrhea
INTEG: Rash, sweating

Contraindications: Hypersensitivity, hypothyroidism, anorexia nervosa, severe hepatic/renal disease, uncontrolled hypertension, history of CAD, CHF, dysrhythmias, pregnancy, lactation, CVA

Precautions: History of seizures, elderly, children <16 yr, narrow-angle glaucoma

Pharmacokinetics	
Absorption	Unknown
Distribution	Widely
Metabolism	Liver (extensively)
Excretion	Unknown
Half-life	14 hr (metabolites)

Pharmacodynamics	
Onset	Unknown
Peak	Unknown
Duration	Unknown

Interactions
Individual drugs
Dextromethorphan: Fatal serotonin syndrome, do not use together
Dihydroergotamine: Fatal

serotonin syndrome, do not use together
Fentanyl: Fatal serotonin syndrome, do not use together
Ketoconazole: ↑ levels of sibutramine
Lithium: Fatal serotonin syndrome, do not use together
Meperidine: Fatal serotonin syndrome, do not use together
Naratriptan: Fatal serotonin syndrome, do not use together
Pentazocine: Fatal serotonin syndrome, do not use together
Sumatriptan: Fatal serotonin syndrome, do not use together
Tryptophan: Fatal serotonin syndrome, do not use together
Zolmitriptan: Fatal serotonin syndrome, do not use together

Drug classifications

Appetite suppressants, centrally acting: Fatal serotonin syndrome, do not use together
Decongestants: Hypertension
MAOIs: Fatal serotonin syndrome, do not use together
SSRIs: Fatal serotonin syndrome, do not use together

NURSING CONSIDERATIONS

Assessment

- Monitor B/P, pulse during treatment; if B/P or pulse rises or if palpitations, tachycardia occur, drug may need to be discontinued
- Assess patient's current dosage of antihypertensives, antidiabetics; these may need to be adjusted
- Assess need for medication and results when combined with other weight-loss strategies

Nursing diagnoses

- ✓ Knowledge deficit (teaching)
- ✓ Noncompliance (teaching)

Implementation

- Give PO with or without meals qd

Patient/familiy education

- Instruct patient to discuss all other medications taken (including OTC) with health care provider; serious—even fatal—interactions can occur
- Advise patient to take exactly as prescribed, and not to exceed recommended dose

Evaluation

Positive therapeutic outcome

- Decrease in weight over time

telmisartan (℞)

(tel-mih-sar'tan)

Micardis

Func. class.: Antihypertensive

Chem class.: Angiotensin II receptor (Type AT_1)

Pregnancy category C

Action: Blocks the vasoconstrictor and aldosterone-secreting effects of angiotensin II; selectively blocks the binding of angiotensin II to the AT_1 receptor found in tissues

➡ Therapeutic Outcome: ↓ B/P

Uses: Hypertension, alone or in combination

Investigational uses: Heart failure

Dosage and routes

Adult: PO 40 mg qd; range 20-80 mg

Available forms: Tabs 40, 80 mg

Adverse effects
CNS: Dizziness, insomnia, anxiety
GI: Diarrhea, dyspepsia, *anorexia, vomiting*
MS: Myalgia, pain
RESP: Cough, *upper respiratory infection*

Contraindications: Hypersensitivity

Precautions: Hypersensitivity to ACE inhibitors; Pregnancy (C) 1st trimester, (D) 2nd and 3rd trimesters; lactation, children, elderly

Pharmacokinetics	
Absorption	Unknown
Distribution	Highly protein bound
Metabolism	Liver (extensively)
Excretion	Urine/feces
Half-life	Terminal 24 hr

Pharmacodynamics	
Onset	Unknown
Peak	Unknown
Duration	Unknown

Interactions
Digoxin: ↑ digoxin peak, trough concentrations

NURSING CONSIDERATIONS
Assessment
- Monitor B/P, pulse q4h; note rate, rhythm, quality
- Monitor electrolytes: K, Na, Cl
- Monitor baselines in renal, liver function tests before therapy begins
- Assess edema in feet, legs qd
- Assess skin turgor, dryness of mucous membranes for hydration status

Nursing diagnoses
✓ Tissue perfusion, altered (uses)
✓ Knowledge deficit (teaching)
✓ Noncompliance (teaching)

Implementation
- Give without regard to meals
- Give increased dose to black patients, B/P response may be reduced

Patient/family education
- Instruct patient to comply with dosage schedule, even if feeling better
- Advise patient to notify prescriber of mouth sores, fever, swelling of hands or feet, irregular heartbeat, chest pain
- Teach patient that excessive perspiration, dehydration, vomiting, diarrhea may lead to fall in blood pressure; consult prescriber if these occur
- Teach patient that drug may cause dizziness, fainting; lightheadedness may occur

Evaluation
Positive therapeutic outcome
- Decreased B/P

tirofiban (℞)
(tie-roh-fee'ban)
Aggrastat
Func. class.: Antiplatelet
Chem class.: Nonpeptide antagonist
Pregnancy category B

Action: Activation of platelet glycoprotein (GP) IIb/IIIa receptor that leads to binding of fibrinogen and von Willebrand's factor, which causes platelet aggregation

➔ **Therapeutic Outcome:** Increased platelet count

Uses: Acute coronary syndrome

Dosage and routes
Adult: IV 0.4 μg/kg/min × 30 min, then 0.1 μg/kg/min; give ½ dose in renal disease

Available forms: Inj for sol 250 μg/ml, inj 50 μg/ml

Adverse effects
CV: Bradycardia
CNS: Dizziness
HEMA: Bleeding
INTEG: Rash
OTHER: Dissection, coronary artery edema, pain in legs/pelvis, sweating

Contraindications: Hypersensitivity, active internal bleeding, stroke, major surgery, severe trauma, intracranial neoplasm, aneurysm, hemorrhage

Precautions: Pregnancy (B), lactation, elderly, renal disease, bleeding tendencies

Pharmacokinetics

Absorption	Unknown
Distribution	Plasma clearance 20%-25%
Metabolism	Liver
Excretion	Urine/feces
Half-life	2 hr

Pharmacodynamics

Onset	Unknown
Peak	Unknown
Duration	Unknown

Interactions
Individual drugs
Aspirin: ↑ bleeding
Heparin: ↑ bleeding
Levothyroxine: ↑ clearance of tirofiban
Omeprazole: ↑ clearance of tirofiban

NURSING CONSIDERATIONS

Assessment

- Monitor B/P pulse during treatment until stable; take B/P lying, standing; orthostatic hypotension is common
- Monitor platelet counts, Hct, Hgb, prior to treatment, within 6 hr of loading dose and at least qd thereafter

Nursing diagnoses
✓ Tissue perfusion, altered (uses)

Implementation

- IV: Give ½ dose in renal disease
- Dilute inj: withdraw and discard 100 ml from a 500 ml bag of sterile 0.9% NaCl or D_5W and replace this vol with 50 ml of tirofiban inj from one vial
- Tirofiban inj for sol is premixed in containers of 500 ml 0.9% NaCl (50 mg/ml)
- Minimize other arterial/venous punctures IM inj, catheter use, intubation, to reduce bleeding risks

Patient/family education

- Advise patient that it is necessary to quit smoking to prevent excessive vasoconstriction
- Teach patient to avoid hazardous activities; dizziness may occur

Evaluation
Positive therapeutic outcome

- Increased platelet count

tolcapone (℞)

(toll'cah-pone)

Tasmar

Func. class.: Antiparkinson agent

Chem class.: Catecholamine inhibitor

Pregnancy category C

Action: Selective, reversible inhibitor of catecholamine; used as adjunct to levodopa/carbidopa therapy

Therapeutic Outcome: Increased ability to move and speak

Uses: Parkinsonism

Dosage and routes

Adult: PO 100-200 mg tid, with levodopa/carbidopa therapy; max 600 mg/day

Available forms: Tabs 100, 200 mg

Adverse effects

CNS: Dystonia, dyskinesia, dreaming, ***fatigue, headache, confusion,*** psychosis, hallucination, dizziness

CV: ***Orthostatic hypotension,*** chest pain, hypotension

EENT: Cataract, eye inflammation

GI: ***Nausea, vomiting, anorexia, abdominal distress,*** diarrhea, constipation

GU: UTI, urine discoloration, uterine tumor, micturition disorder

HEMA: Hemolytic anemia, leukopenia, agranulocytosis

INTEG: Sweating, alopecia

Contraindications: Hypersensitivity

Precautions: Renal disease, cardiac disease, hepatic disease, hypertension, pregnancy (C), asthma, lactation

Pharmacokinetics

Absorption	Rapidly
Distribution	Protein binding 99%
Metabolism	Liver (extensively)
Excretion	Urine (60%), feces (40%)
Half-life	2-3 hr

Pharmacodynamics

Onset	Unknown
Peak	Unknown
Duration	Unknown

Interactions

Individual drugs

α-Methyldopa: May influence pharmacokinetics

Apomorphine: May influence pharmacokinetics

Dobutamine: May influence pharmacokinetics

Isoproterenol: May influence pharmacokinetics

Drug classifications

MAOIs: ↓ normal catecholamine metabolism; MAO-B inhibitor may be used

NURSING CONSIDERATIONS

Assessment

- Monitor liver function enzymes: AST (SGOT), ALT (SGPT), alk phosphatase, LDH, bilirubin, CBC
- Assess involuntary movements in parkinsonism: akinesia, tremors, staggering gait, muscle rigidity, drooling
- Monitor B/P, respiration during initial treatment; hypo/hypertension should be reported
- Monitor mental status: affect, mood, behavioral changes

Nursing diagnoses

✓ Physical mobility, impaired (uses)

☑ Injury, risk for (uses)
☑ Knowledge deficit (teaching)

Implementation

PO route

- Administer tid with levodopa/carbidopa therapy
- Provide assistance with ambulation during beginning therapy

Patient/family education

- Advise patient to change positions slowly to prevent orthostatic hypotension
- Advise patient that urine, sweat may change color
- Teach patient that food taken within 1 hr ac or 2 hr pc increases action of drug by 20%
- Teach patient to report nausea, vomiting, anorexia

Evaluation

Positive therapeutic outcome

- Decrease in akathisia, increased mood

tolterodine (℞)

(toll-tehr'oh-deen)

Detrol

Func. class.: Overactive bladder product

Chem class.: Muscarinic receptor antagonist

Pregnancy category C

Action: Relaxes smooth muscles in urinary tract by inhibiting acetylcholine at postganglionic sites

➡ **Therapeutic Outcome:** Decreased symptoms of overactive bladder

Uses: Overactive bladder (frequency, urgency)

Dosage and routes

Adult: PO 2 mg bid, hepatic disease 1 mg bid

Available forms: Tabs 1, 2 mg

Adverse effects

CNS: Anxiety, paresthesia, fatigue, *dizziness,* headache

CV: Chest pain, hypertension

EENT: Vision abnormalities, xerophthalmia

GI: Nausea, vomiting, anorexia, abdominal pain, constipation, dry mouth, dyspepsia

GU: Dysuria, retention, frequency, UTI

INTEG: Rash, pruritus

RESP: Bronchitis, cough, pharyngitis, URI

Contraindications: Hypersensitivity, uncontrolled narrow-angle glaucoma, urinary retention, gastric retention

Precautions: Pregnancy (C), lactation, children, renal/hepatic disease, controlled narrow-angle glaucoma

Pharmacokinetics

Absorption	Rapidly
Distribution	Highly protein bound
Metabolism	Liver (extensively)
Excretion	Urine/feces
Half-life	Unknown

Pharmacodynamics

Onset	Unknown
Peak	Unknown
Duration	Unknown

Interactions

Drug classifications

Antibiotics, macrolide: ↑ action of tolterodine

Antifungals: ↑ action of tolterodine

Food/Drug:

↑ bioavailability of tolterodine

NURSING CONSIDERATIONS
Assessment
• Assess urinary patterns: distention, nocturia, frequency, urgency, incontinence
• Assess allergic reactions: rash; if this occurs, drug should be discontinued

Nursing diagnoses
✓ Urinary elimination, altered (uses)
✓ Incontinence, functional (uses)
✓ Knowledge deficit (teaching)
✓ Activity intolerance (uses)

Patient/family education
• Advise patient to avoid hazardous activities; dizziness may occur

Evaluation
Positive therapeutic outcome
• Decreased urinary frequency, urgency

trastuzumab (℞)
(tras-tuz'uh-mab)
Herceptin
Func. class.: Miscellaneous antineoplastic
Chem class.: Humanized monoclonal antibody
Pregnancy category B

Action: DNA-derived monoclonal antibody selectively binds to extracellular portion of human epidermal growth factor receptor 2; it inhibits proliferation of cancer cells

➔ **Therapeutic Outcome:** Decreasing symptoms of breast cancer

Uses: Breast cancer; metastatic with overexpression of HER2

Dosage and routes
***Adult:* IV** 4 mg/kg given over 90 min, then maintenance 2 mg/kg given over 30 min; do not give as IV push or BOL

Available forms: Lyophilized powder 440 mg

Adverse effects
CNS: ***Dizziness, numbness, paresthesias,*** depression, insomnia, neuropathy, peripheral neuritis
CV: Tachycardia, *CHF*
GI: Nausea, vomiting, anorexia, diarrhea
HEMA: Anemia, leukopenia
INTEG: ***Rash,*** acne, herpes simplex
META: Edema, peripheral edema
MISC: ***Flulike syndrome; fever, headache, chills***
MS: Arthralgia, bone pain
RESP: Cough, dyspnea, pharyngitis, rhinitis, sinusitis

Contraindications: Hypersensitivity to this drug, Chinese hamster ovary cell protein

Precautions: Pregnancy (B), lactation, children, elderly, cardiac disease, anemia, leukopenia

Pharmacokinetics	
Absorption	Unknown
Distribution	Unknown
Metabolism	Unknown
Excretion	Unknown
Half-life	1.7-12 days

Pharmacodynamics	
Onset	Unknown
Peak	Unknown
Duration	Unknown

Interactions
Unknown

NURSING CONSIDERATIONS
Assessment
• Assess for symptoms of

infection; may be masked by drug
- Assess CNS reaction: LOC, mental status, dizziness, confusion

Nursing diagnoses
- ✓ Infection, risk for (side effects)
- ✓ Nutrition, altered, less than body requirements (side effects)
- ✓ Knowledge deficit (teaching)

Implementation
- Give acetaminophen as ordered to alleviate fever and headache
- Increase fluid intake to 2-3 L/day

IV route
- Administer after reconstituting vial with 20 ml bacteriostatic water for inj, 1.1% benzyl alcohol preserved (supplied) to yield 21 mg/ml, mark date on vial 28 days from reconstitution date, if pt is allergic to benzyl alcohol, reconstitute with sterile water for inj—use immediately
- Do not mix or dilute with other drugs or dextrose sol

Patient/family education
- Advise patient to take acetaminophen for fever
- Teach patient to avoid hazardous tasks, since confusion, dizziness may occur
- Teach patient to report signs of infection: sore throat, fever, diarrhea, vomiting
- Inform patient that emotional lability is common; instruct patient to notify prescriber if severe or incapacitating

Evaluation
Positive therapeutic outcome
- Decrease in size of tumors

valrubicin (℞)
(val-roo'bih-sin)
Valstar
Func. class.: Antineoplastic, antibiotic
Chem class.: Anthracycline glycoside
Pregnancy category C

Action: A semisynthetic analog of doxorubicin that inhibits DNA synthesis primarily; replication is decreased by binding to DNA, which causes strand splitting; active throughout entire cell cycle; a vesicant

➡ **Therapeutic Outcome:** Decreasing symptoms of breast cancer

Uses: Bladder cancer

Dosage and routes
Adult: **INTRAVESICALLY** 800 mg qwk × 6 wk, delay administration ≥2 wks after transurethral resection or fulguration

Available forms: Sol for intravesical instillation: 40 mg/ml

Adverse effects
CV: Chest pain
GI: Nausea, vomiting, anorexia, diarrhea
GU: UTI, urinary retention, hematuria
HEMA: Thrombocytopenia, leukopenia, anemia
INTEG: Rash

Contraindications: Hypersensitivity to anthracyclines or Cremophor E1, urinary tract infection, small bladder

Precautions: Pregnancy (C), lactation, children

Pharmacokinetics

Absorption	Unknown
Distribution	Penetrates bladder wall
Metabolism	Not metabolized
Excretion	Unknown
Half-life	Unknown

Pharmacodynamics

Onset	Unknown
Peak	Unknown
Duration	Unknown

Interactions
Unknown

NURSING CONSIDERATIONS

Assessment

- Monitor I&O ratio; report fall in urine output of <30 ml/hr
- Monitor temperature q4h; fever may indicate beginning infection
- Monitor local irritation, pain, burning at injection site

Nursing diagnoses

- ✓ Infection, risk for (side effects)
- ✓ Nutrition, altered, less than body requirements (side effects)
- ✓ Knowledge deficit (teaching)

Implementation

- Administer after urinary catheter is inserted under aseptic conditions, drain bladder and instill the diluted 75 ml valrubicin by gravity for several min, withdraw catheter; drug should be retained for 2 hr, then void
- Use procedure for handling and disposal of cytotoxic agents
- Do not use polyvinyl chloride (PVC) or IV tubing
- Prepare/store valrubicin sol in glass, polypropylene, or polyolefin tubing/containers
- For instillation, 5 ml vials (200 mg valrubicin/5 ml/vial) should be warmed to room temp, withdraw 20 ml from the 4 vials and dilute with 55 ml 0.9% NaCl inj to 75 ml of diluted valrubicin sol
- Valrubicin sol is clear red, at lower temps a waxy precipitate may form, warm in hand until sol is clear
- Perform strict hand-washing technique, gloves, protective clothing
- Provide increased fluid intake to 2-3 L/day to prevent urate, calculi formation
- Store at room temperature for 12 hr after reconstituting

Patient/family education

- Advise patient to report any complaints, side effects to nurse or prescriber
- Teach patient that urine and other body fluids may be red-orange for 48 hr
- Teach patient that contraceptive measures are recommended during therapy

Evaluation

Positive therapeutic outcome

- Decreased tumor size, spread of malignancy

zolmitriptan (℞)

(zole-mih-trip'tan)

Zomig

Func. class.: Migraine agent

Chem class.: 5-HT_1-like receptor agonist

Pregnancy category C

Action: Binds selectively to the vascular 5-HT_1 receptor subtype, exerts antimigraine effect;

causes vasoconstriction in cranial arteries

Therapeutic Outcome: Decreased severity, frequency of headache

Uses: Acute treatment of migraine with or without aura

Dosage and routes
Adult: **PO** ≤2.5 mg (tab may be broken), may repeat after 2 hr, max 10 mg/24 hr

Available forms: Tabs 2.5, 5 mg

Adverse effects
CV: Palpitations
GI: Abdominal discomfort
MS: Weakness, neck stiffness, myalgia
NEURO: Tingling, hot sensation, burning, feeling of pressure, tightness, numbness, dizziness, sedation
RESP: Chest tightness, pressure

Contraindications: Angina pectoris, history of MI, documented silent ischemia, ischemic heart disease, concurrent ergotamine-containing preparations, uncontrolled hypertension, hypersensitivity, basilar or hemiplegic migraine

Precautions: Postmenopausal women, men >40 yr, risk factors for CAD, hypercholesterolemia, obesity, diabetes, impaired hepatic or renal function, pregnancy (C), lactation, children, elderly

Pharmacokinetics

Absorption	Unknown
Distribution	25% protein binding
Metabolism	Liver (metabolite)
Excretion	Urine/feces
Half-life	3-3½ hr

Pharmacodynamics

Onset	Unknown
Peak	Unknown
Duration	2-3½ hr

Interactions
Individual drugs
Cimetidine: ↑ half-life of zolmitriptan
Ergot: ↑ vasospastic effects
Drug classifications
Ergot derivatives: ↑ vasospastic effects
MAOIs: Do not use within 2 wk
SSRIs: ↑ weakness, hyperreflexia, incoordination

NURSING CONSIDERATIONS

Assessment

- Assess tingling, hot sensation, burning, feeling of pressure, numbness, flushing
- Assess for stress level, activity, recreation, coping mechanisms
- Assess neurologic status: LOC, blurring vision, nausea, vomiting, tingling in extremities preceding headache
- Monitor ingestion of tyramine foods (pickled products, beer, wine, aged cheese), food additives, preservatives, colorings, artificial sweeteners, chocolate, caffeine, which may precipitate these types of headaches
- Assess for serotonin syndrome, if also taking an SSRI

Nursing diagnoses

- ✓ Pain (uses)
- ✓ Noncompliance (teaching)
- ✓ Knowledge deficit (teaching)

Implementation

- Give with fluids as soon as symptoms of migraine occur

• Provide quiet, calm environment with decreased stimulation for noise, bright light, excessive talking

Patient/family education

• Teach patient to report any side effects to prescriber

• Advise patient to use contraception while taking drug

Evaluation

Positive therapeutic outcome

• Decrease in frequency, severity of headache

9997635086

Mosby's Pharmacology Patient Teaching Disk version 2.0*

This easy-to-use program allows you to view and print handy PATIENT TEACHING GUIDES for 25 commonly used drugs (see installation instructions below). When you start the program, the initial screen will display a list of generic drug names. Simply click on the name of the drug to bring up the patient teaching guide you want. Click on "Print" to print out a copy.

Each guide provides the drug's generic name and pronunciation, its R_X or OTC status, and the following sections:

- "About This Medication"—Lists the type of drug, trade names (including Canada only), common uses, and other helpful information, such as availability of generic and brand names and various forms of the drug
- "How to Take This Medication"—Tells whether to take the drug with food, foods to avoid, whether or not the drug may be crushed, dosing regimen, and other important information
- "Warnings and Side Effects"—Describes common side effects, lists those that the patient should report immediately, and (where applicable) describes signs of overdose and what to do
- "Special Precautions"—Lists special situations to inform the health care provider about, including known allergies, pregnancy, other drugs being taken, and preexisting medical conditions; also provides a list of "do's and don'ts" to follow while taking the medication

Installation for Windows 3.1

1. Start Microsoft Windows and insert disk.
2. From the Program Manager's File menu, choose RUN.
3. Type A:SETUP and press ENTER.
4. Follow the on-screen prompts for installation.

Installation for Windows 95/Windows NT

1. Start Microsoft Windows 95 and insert disk.
2. From the Taskbar choose START, then RUN.
3. Type A:SETUP and press ENTER.
4. Follow the on-screen prompts for installation.

* Additional pharmacology patient teaching guides are included in *Mosby's Patient Teaching Guides in Pharmacology* by Leda McKenry. For more information or to order, call Mosby toll-free at 1-800-426-4546.